The Biomedical Engineerin
Third Edition

Tissue Engineering and Artificial Organs

The Electrical Engineering Handbook Series

Series Editor
Richard C. Dorf
University of California, Davis

Titles Included in the Series

The Biomedical Engineering Handbook
Third Edition

Edited by
Joseph D. Bronzino

Biomedical Engineering Fundamentals

Medical Devices and Systems

Tissue Engineering and Artificial Organs

The Biomedical Engineering Handbook
Third Edition

Tissue Engineering and Artificial Organs

Edited by
Joseph D. Bronzino

Trinity College
Hartford, Connecticut, U.S.A.

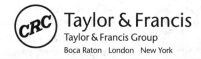

Taylor & Francis
Taylor & Francis Group
Boca Raton   London   New York

A CRC title, part of the Taylor & Francis imprint, a member of the
Taylor & Francis Group, the academic division of T&F Informa plc.

Published in 2006 by
CRC Press
Taylor & Francis Group
6000 Broken Sound Parkway NW, Suite 300
Boca Raton, FL 33487-2742

International Standard Book Number-10: 0-8493-2123-9 (Hardcover)
International Standard Book Number-13: 978-0-8493-2123-8 (Hardcover)
Library of Congress Card Number 2005044776

Library of Congress Cataloging-in-Publication Data

Tissue engineering and artificial organs / edited by Joseph D. Bronzino.
    p. cm. -- (The electrical engineering handbook series)
  Includes bibliographical references and index.
  ISBN 0-8493-2123-9 (alk. paper)
  1. Tissue engineering. 2. Artificial organs. I. Bronzino, Joseph D., 1937- II. Title. III. Series.

R857.T55T547 2006
612.028--dc22
                                                    2005044776

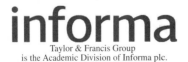
Taylor & Francis Group
is the Academic Division of Informa plc.

Visit the Taylor & Francis Web site at
http://www.taylorandfrancis.com

and the CRC Press Web site at
http://www.crcpress.com

Introduction and Preface

During the past five years since the publication of the Second Edition — a two-volume set — of the *Biomedical Engineering Handbook*, the field of biomedical engineering has continued to evolve and expand. As a result, this Third Edition consists of a three-volume set, which has been significantly modified to reflect the state-of-the-field knowledge and applications in this important discipline. More specifically, this Third Edition contains a number of completely new sections, including:

- Molecular Biology
- Bionanotechnology
- Bioinformatics
- Neuroengineering
- Infrared Imaging

as well as a new section on ethics.

In addition, all of the sections that have appeared in the first and second editions have been significantly revised. Therefore, this Third Edition presents an excellent summary of the status of knowledge and activities of biomedical engineers in the beginning of the 21st century.

As such, it can serve as an excellent reference for individuals interested not only in a review of fundamental physiology, but also in quickly being brought up to speed in certain areas of biomedical engineering research. It can serve as an excellent textbook for students in areas where traditional textbooks have not yet been developed and as an excellent review of the major areas of activity in each biomedical engineering subdiscipline, such as biomechanics, biomaterials, bioinstrumentation, medical imaging, etc. Finally, it can serve as the "bible" for practicing biomedical engineering professionals by covering such topics as a historical perspective of medical technology, the role of professional societies, the ethical issues associated with medical technology, and the FDA process.

Biomedical engineering is now an important vital interdisciplinary field. Biomedical engineers are involved in virtually all aspects of developing new medical technology. They are involved in the design, development, and utilization of materials, devices (such as pacemakers, lithotripsy, etc.) and techniques (such as signal processing, artificial intelligence, etc.) for clinical research and use; and serve as members of the health care delivery team (clinical engineering, medical informatics, rehabilitation engineering, etc.) seeking new solutions for difficult health care problems confronting our society. To meet the needs of this diverse body of biomedical engineers, this handbook provides a central core of knowledge in those fields encompassed by the discipline. However, before presenting this detailed information, it is important to provide a sense of the evolution of the modern health care system and identify the diverse activities biomedical engineers perform to assist in the diagnosis and treatment of patients.

Evolution of the Modern Health Care System

Before 1900, medicine had little to offer the average citizen, since its resources consisted mainly of the physician, his education, and his "little black bag." In general, physicians seemed to be in short supply, but the shortage had rather different causes than the current crisis in the availability of health care professionals. Although the costs of obtaining medical training were relatively low, the demand for doctors' services also was very small, since many of the services provided by the physician also could be obtained from experienced amateurs in the community. The home was typically the site for treatment and recuperation, and relatives and neighbors constituted an able and willing nursing staff. Babies were delivered by midwives, and those illnesses not cured by home remedies were left to run their natural, albeit frequently fatal, course. The contrast with contemporary health care practices, in which specialized physicians and nurses located within the hospital provide critical diagnostic and treatment services, is dramatic.

The changes that have occurred within medical science originated in the rapid developments that took place in the applied sciences (chemistry, physics, engineering, microbiology, physiology, pharmacology, etc.) at the turn of the century. This process of development was characterized by intense interdisciplinary cross-fertilization, which provided an environment in which medical research was able to take giant strides in developing techniques for the diagnosis and treatment of disease. For example, in 1903, Willem Einthoven, a Dutch physiologist, devised the first electrocardiograph to measure the electrical activity of the heart. In applying discoveries in the physical sciences to the analysis of the biologic process, he initiated a new age in both cardiovascular medicine and electrical measurement techniques.

New discoveries in medical sciences followed one another like intermediates in a chain reaction. However, the most significant innovation for clinical medicine was the development of x-rays. These "new kinds of rays," as their discoverer W.K. Roentgen described them in 1895, opened the "inner man" to medical inspection. Initially, x-rays were used to diagnose bone fractures and dislocations, and in the process, x-ray machines became commonplace in most urban hospitals. Separate departments of radiology were established, and their influence spread to other departments throughout the hospital. By the 1930s, x-ray visualization of practically all organ systems of the body had been made possible through the use of barium salts and a wide variety of radiopaque materials.

X-ray technology gave physicians a powerful tool that, for the first time, permitted accurate diagnosis of a wide variety of diseases and injuries. Moreover, since x-ray machines were too cumbersome and expensive for local doctors and clinics, they had to be placed in health care centers or hospitals. Once there, x-ray technology essentially triggered the transformation of the hospital from a passive receptacle for the sick to an active curative institution for all members of society.

For economic reasons, the centralization of health care services became essential because of many other important technological innovations appearing on the medical scene. However, hospitals remained institutions to dread, and it was not until the introduction of sulfanilamide in the mid-1930s and penicillin in the early 1940s that the main danger of hospitalization, that is, cross-infection among patients, was significantly reduced. With these new drugs in their arsenals, surgeons were able to perform their operations without prohibitive morbidity and mortality due to infection. Furthermore, even though the different blood groups and their incompatibility were discovered in 1900 and sodium citrate was used in 1913 to prevent clotting, full development of blood banks was not practical until the 1930s, when technology provided adequate refrigeration. Until that time, "fresh" donors were bled and the blood transfused while it was still warm.

Once these surgical suites were established, the employment of specifically designed pieces of medical technology assisted in further advancing the development of complex surgical procedures. For example, the Drinker respirator was introduced in 1927 and the first heart–lung bypass was done in 1939. By the 1940s, medical procedures heavily dependent on medical technology, such as cardiac catheterization and angiography (the use of a cannula threaded through an arm vein and into the heart with the injection of radiopaque dye) for the x-ray visualization of congenital and acquired heart disease (mainly valve disorders due to rheumatic fever) became possible, and a new era of cardiac and vascular surgery was established.

Following World War II, technological advances were spurred on by efforts to develop superior weapon systems and establish habitats in space and on the ocean floor. As a by-product of these efforts, the development of medical devices accelerated and the medical profession benefited greatly from this rapid surge of technological finds. Consider the following examples:

1. Advances in solid-state electronics made it possible to map the subtle behavior of the fundamental unit of the central nervous system — the neuron — as well as to monitor the various physiological parameters, such as the electrocardiogram, of patients in intensive care units.
2. New prosthetic devices became a goal of engineers involved in providing the disabled with tools to improve their quality of life.
3. Nuclear medicine — an outgrowth of the atomic age — emerged as a powerful and effective approach in detecting and treating specific physiologic abnormalities.
4. Diagnostic ultrasound based on sonar technology became so widely accepted that ultrasonic studies are now part of the routine diagnostic workup in many medical specialties.
5. "Spare parts" surgery also became commonplace. Technologists were encouraged to provide cardiac assist devices, such as artificial heart valves and artificial blood vessels, and the artificial heart program was launched to develop a replacement for a defective or diseased human heart.
6. Advances in materials have made the development of disposable medical devices, such as needles and thermometers, as well as implantable drug delivery systems, a reality.
7. Computers similar to those developed to control the flight plans of the *Apollo* capsule were used to store, process, and cross-check medical records, to monitor patient status in intensive care units, and to provide sophisticated statistical diagnoses of potential diseases correlated with specific sets of patient symptoms.
8. Development of the first computer-based medical instrument, the computerized axial tomography scanner, revolutionized clinical approaches to noninvasive diagnostic imaging procedures, which now include magnetic resonance imaging and positron emission tomography as well.
9. A wide variety of new cardiovascular technologies including implantable defibrillators and chemically treated stents were developed.
10. Neuronal pacing systems were used to detect and prevent epileptic seizures.
11. Artificial organs and tissue have been created.
12. The completion of the genome project has stimulated the search for new biological markers and personalized medicine.

The impact of these discoveries and many others has been profound. The health care system of today consists of technologically sophisticated clinical staff operating primarily in modern hospitals designed to accommodate the new medical technology. This evolutionary process continues, with advances in the physical sciences such as materials and nanotechnology, and in the life sciences such as molecular biology, the genome project and artificial organs. These advances have altered and will continue to alter the very nature of the health care delivery system itself.

Biomedical Engineering: A Definition

Bioengineering is usually defined as a basic research-oriented activity closely related to biotechnology and genetic engineering, that is, the modification of animal or plant cells, or parts of cells, to improve plants or animals or to develop new microorganisms for beneficial ends. In the food industry, for example, this has meant the improvement of strains of yeast for fermentation. In agriculture, bioengineers may be concerned with the improvement of crop yields by treatment of plants with organisms to reduce frost damage. It is clear that bioengineers of the future will have a tremendous impact on the qualities of human life. The potential of this specialty is difficult to imagine. Consider the following activities of bioengineers:

- Development of improved species of plants and animals for food production
- Invention of new medical diagnostic tests for diseases
- Production of synthetic vaccines from clone cells

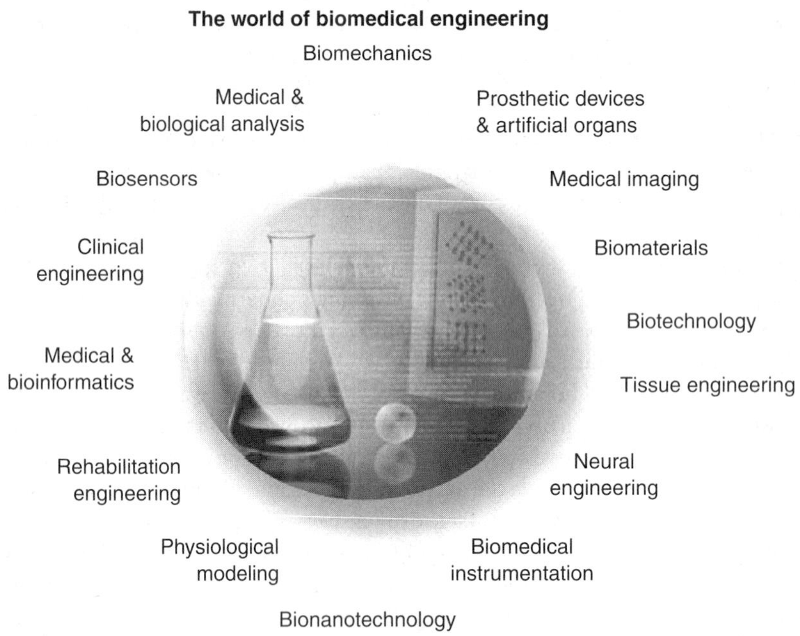

The world of biomedical engineering

Biomechanics

Medical &
biological analysis

Prosthetic devices
& artificial organs

Biosensors

Medical imaging

Clinical
engineering

Biomaterials

Biotechnology

Medical &
bioinformatics

Tissue engineering

Rehabilitation
engineering

Neural
engineering

Physiological
modeling

Biomedical
instrumentation

Bionanotechnology

FIGURE 1 The world of biomedical engineering.

- Bioenvironmental engineering to protect human, animal, and plant life from toxicants and pollutants
- Study of protein–surface interactions
- Modeling of the growth kinetics of yeast and hybridoma cells
- Research in immobilized enzyme technology
- Development of therapeutic proteins and monoclonal antibodies

Biomedical engineers, on the other hand, apply electrical, mechanical, chemical, optical, and other engineering principles to understand, modify, or control biologic (i.e., human and animal) systems, as well as design and manufacture products that can monitor physiologic functions and assist in the diagnosis and treatment of patients. When biomedical engineers work within a hospital or clinic, they are more properly called clinical engineers.

Activities of Biomedical Engineers

The breadth of activity of biomedical engineers is now significant. The field has moved from being concerned primarily with the development of medical instruments in the 1950s and 1960s to include a more wide-ranging set of activities. As illustrated above, the field of biomedical engineering now includes many new career areas (see Figure 1), each of which is presented in this handbook. These areas include:

- Application of engineering system analysis (physiologic modeling, simulation, and control) to biologic problems
- Detection, measurement, and monitoring of physiologic signals (i.e., biosensors and biomedical instrumentation)
- Diagnostic interpretation via signal-processing techniques of bioelectric data
- Therapeutic and rehabilitation procedures and devices (rehabilitation engineering)
- Devices for replacement or augmentation of bodily functions (artificial organs)
- Computer analysis of patient-related data and clinical decision making (i.e., medical informatics and artificial intelligence)

- Medical imaging, that is, the graphic display of anatomic detail or physiologic function
- The creation of new biologic products (i.e., biotechnology and tissue engineering)
- The development of new materials to be used within the body (biomaterials)

Typical pursuits of biomedical engineers, therefore, include:

- Research in new materials for implanted artificial organs
- Development of new diagnostic instruments for blood analysis
- Computer modeling of the function of the human heart
- Writing software for analysis of medical research data
- Analysis of medical device hazards for safety and efficacy
- Development of new diagnostic imaging systems
- Design of telemetry systems for patient monitoring
- Design of biomedical sensors for measurement of human physiologic systems variables
- Development of expert systems for diagnosis of disease
- Design of closed-loop control systems for drug administration
- Modeling of the physiological systems of the human body
- Design of instrumentation for sports medicine
- Development of new dental materials
- Design of communication aids for the handicapped
- Study of pulmonary fluid dynamics
- Study of the biomechanics of the human body
- Development of material to be used as replacement for human skin

Biomedical engineering, then, is an interdisciplinary branch of engineering that ranges from theoretical, nonexperimental undertakings to state-of-the-art applications. It can encompass research, development, implementation, and operation. Accordingly, like medical practice itself, it is unlikely that any single person can acquire expertise that encompasses the entire field. Yet, because of the interdisciplinary nature of this activity, there is considerable interplay and overlapping of interest and effort between them. For example, biomedical engineers engaged in the development of biosensors may interact with those interested in prosthetic devices to develop a means to detect and use the same bioelectric signal to power a prosthetic device. Those engaged in automating the clinical chemistry laboratory may collaborate with those developing expert systems to assist clinicians in making decisions based on specific laboratory data. The possibilities are endless.

Perhaps a greater potential benefit occurring from the use of biomedical engineering is identification of the problems and needs of our present health care system that can be solved using existing engineering technology and systems methodology. Consequently, the field of biomedical engineering offers hope in the continuing battle to provide high-quality care at a reasonable cost. If properly directed toward solving problems related to preventive medical approaches, ambulatory care services, and the like, biomedical engineers can provide the tools and techniques to make our health care system more effective and efficient; and in the process, improve the quality of life for all.

Joseph D. Bronzino
Editor-in-Chief

Editor-in-Chief

Joseph D. Bronzino received the B.S.E.E. degree from Worcester Polytechnic Institute, Worcester, MA, in 1959, the M.S.E.E. degree from the Naval Postgraduate School, Monterey, CA, in 1961, and the Ph.D. degree in electrical engineering from Worcester Polytechnic Institute in 1968. He is presently the Vernon Roosa Professor of Applied Science, an endowed chair at Trinity College, Hartford, CT and President of the Biomedical Engineering Alliance and Consortium (BEACON), which is a nonprofit organization consisting of academic and medical institutions as well as corporations dedicated to the development and commercialization of new medical technologies (for details visit www.beaconalliance.org).

He is the author of over 200 articles and 11 books including the following: *Technology for Patient Care* (C.V. Mosby, 1977), *Computer Applications for Patient Care* (Addison-Wesley, 1982), *Biomedical Engineering: Basic Concepts and Instrumentation* (PWS Publishing Co., 1986), *Expert Systems: Basic Concepts* (Research Foundation of State University of New York, 1989), *Medical Technology and Society: An Interdisciplinary Perspective* (MIT Press and McGraw-Hill, 1990), *Management of Medical Technology* (Butterworth/Heinemann, 1992), *The Biomedical Engineering Handbook* (CRC Press, 1st ed., 1995; 2nd ed., 2000; Taylor & Francis, 3rd ed., 2005), *Introduction to Biomedical Engineering* (Academic Press, 1st ed., 1999; 2nd ed., 2005).

Dr. Bronzino is a fellow of IEEE and the American Institute of Medical and Biological Engineering (AIMBE), an honorary member of the Italian Society of Experimental Biology, past chairman of the Biomedical Engineering Division of the American Society for Engineering Education (ASEE), a charter member and presently vice president of the Connecticut Academy of Science and Engineering (CASE), a charter member of the American College of Clinical Engineering (ACCE) and the Association for the Advancement of Medical Instrumentation (AAMI), past president of the IEEE-Engineering in Medicine and Biology Society (EMBS), past chairman of the IEEE Health Care Engineering Policy Committee (HCEPC), past chairman of the IEEE Technical Policy Council in Washington, DC, and presently editor-in-chief of Elsevier's BME Book Series and Taylor & Francis' *Biomedical Engineering Handbook*.

Dr. Bronzino is also the recipient of the Millennium Award from IEEE/EMBS in 2000 and the Goddard Award from Worcester Polytechnic Institute for Professional Achievement in June 2004.

Contributors

Alptekin Aksan
University of Minnesota
Center for Engineering in
    Medicine/Surgical Services
Massachusetts General Hospital
Harvard Medical School
Shriners Hospital for Children
Boston, Massachusetts

Kyle D. Allen
University of Texas Dental Branch
Department of Oral and
    Maxillofacial Surgery
Houston, Texas

Robert C. Allen
Emory University
Atlanta, Georgia

Jose F. Alvarez-Barreto
School of Chemical Engineering
    and Materials Science
Bioengineering Center
University of Oklahoma
Norman, Oklahoma

James M. Anderson
Department of Pathology
Macromolecular Science and
    Biomedical Engineering
Case Western Reserve University
Cleveland, Ohio

Anthony Atala
Department of Urology
Wake Forest University Baptist
    Medical Center
Winston-Salem, North Carolina

Kyriacos A. Athanasiou
University of Texas Dental Branch
Department of Oral and
    Maxillofacial Surgery
Department of Bioengineering
Rice University
Houston, Texas

John G. Aunins
Merck Research Laboratories
Rahway, New Jersey

James W. Baish
Bucknell University
Lewisburg, Pennsylvania

Scott Banta
Columbia University
New York, New York

Raj Bawa
Bawa Biotechnology
    Consulting LLC
Arlington, Virginia
Rensselaer Polytechnic
    Institute, NVCC
Troy, New York

S.R. Bawa
Bawa Biotechnology
    Consulting LLC
Schenectady, New York

C. Becker
Department of Pharmaceutical
    Technology
University of Regensburg
Regensburg, Germany

B.L. Beckstead
Department of Bioengineering
University of Washington
Seattle, Washington

François Berthiaume
Center for Engineering in
    Medicine/Surgical Services
Massachusetts General Hospital
Harvard Medical School
Shriners Hospital for Children
Boston, Massachusetts

Robert R. Birge
Department of Chemistry
University of Connecticut
Storrs, Connecticut

William Bentley
University of Maryland
    Biotechnology Institute
Baltimore, Maryland

Michael Betenbaugh
Johns Hopkins University
Baltimore, Maryland

Nicole Bleckwenn
University of Maryland
    Biotechnology Institute
Baltimore, Maryland

Steven T. Boyce
Department of Surgery
University of Cincinnati
College of Medicine
Cincinnati, Ohio

Joseph D. Bronzino
Trinity College/Biomedical
    Engineering Alliance and
    Consortium (BEACON)
Hartford, Connecticut

Nenad Bursac
Department of Biomedical
    Engineering
Duke University
Durham, North Carolina

Baohong Cao
Department of Orthopaedic
    Surgery
University of Pittsburgh
Pittsburgh, Pennsylvania

Arnold I. Caplan
Skeletal Research Center
Case Western Reserve University
Cleveland, Ohio

Shawn D. Carrigan
McGill University
Montreal, Quebec, Canada

Ayse B. Celil
Bone Tissue Engineering Center
Department of Biological Sciences
Carnegie Mellon University
Pittsburgh, Pennsylvania

Christina Chan
Center for Engineering in
    Medicine/Surgical Services
Massachusetts General Hospital
Harvard Medical School
Shriners Hospital for Children
Boston, Massachusetts
Michigan State University
Chemical Engineering and
    Materials Science
East Lansing, Michigan

Gang Cheng
Department of Chemical
    Engineering
Institute of Biosciences and
    Bioengineering
Rice University
Houston, Texas

K.S. Chian
School of Mechanical and
    Production Engineering
Nanyang Technological University
Singapore

Clark K. Colton
Massachusetts Institute of
    Technology
Cambridge, Massachusetts

Michael Connolly
Integrated Nano-Technologies
Henrietta, New York

Nathan R. Domagalski
Carnegie Mellon University
Pittsburgh, Pennsylvania

Michael Domach
Carnegie Mellon University
Pittsburgh, Pennsylvania

Kimberly L. Douglas
McGill University
Montreal, Quebec, Canada

Rebekah A. Drezek
Department of Bioengineering
Rice University
Houston, Texas

Rena N. D'Souza
University of Texas Health Science
    Center at Houston
Dental Branch, Department of
    Orthodontics
Houston, Texas

Atul Dubey
Department of Mechanical and
    Industrial Engineering
Northeastern University
Boston, Massachusetts
Department of Mechanical and
    Aerospace Engineering
Rutgers University
Piscataway, New Jersey

Brian Dunham
Department of
    Otolaryngology/Head and Neck
    Surgery
Department of Biomedical
    Engineering
Johns Hopkins School of Medicine
Baltimore, Maryland

Wafa M. Elbjeirami
Department of Biochemistry and
    Cell Biology
Rice University
Houston, Texas

Jennifer H. Elisseeff
Department of Biomedical
    Engineering
Johns Hopkins University
Baltimore, Maryland

Mary C. Farach-Carson
Department of Biological Sciences
University of Delaware
Newark, Delaware

John P. Fisher
University of Maryland
College Park, Maryland

Robert J. Fisher
The SABRE Institute
Massachusetts Institute of
    Technology
Cambridge, Massachusetts

William H. Fissell
Department of Internal Medicine
University of Michigan
Ann Arbor, Michigan

Paul Flint
Department of
    Otolaryngology/Head and Neck
    Surgery
Johns Hopkins School of Medicine
Baltimore, Maryland

Pierre M. Galletti
(deceased)

Andrés J. García
Woodruff School of Mechanical
    Engineering
Petit Institute for Bioengineering
    and Bioscience
Georgia Institute of Technology
Atlanta, Georgia

C.M. Giachelli
Department of Bioengineering
University of Washington
Seattle, Washington

Andrea S. Gobin
Department of Bioengineering
Rice University
Houston, Texas

W.T. Godbey
Laboratory for Gene Therapy and
  Cellular Engineering
Department of Chemical and
  Biomolecular Engineering
Tulane University
New Orleans, Louisiana

Aaron S. Goldstein
Department of Chemical
  Engineering
Virginia Polytechnic Institute and
  State University
Blacksburg, Virginia

A. Göpferich
Department of Pharmaceutical
  Technology
University of Regensburg
Regensburg, Germany

K. Jane Grande-Allen
Department of Bioengineering
Rice University
Houston, Texas

Scott Guelcher
Bone Tissue Engineering Center
Department of Biological Sciences
Carnegie Mellon University
Pittsburgh, Pennsylvania

Naomi J. Halas
Department of Electrical and
  Computer Engineering
Rice University
Houston, Texas

Jie Han
NASA Ames Research Center
Moffett Field, California

Sarina G. Harris
Cornell University
Ithaca, New York

Kiki B. Hellman
The Hellman Group, LLC
Clarksburg, Maryland

Jason R. Hillebrecht
Department of Chemistry
University of Connecticut
Storrs, Connecticut

Theodore R. Holford
Susan Dwight Bliss Professor of
  Public Health (Biostatistics)
Yale University School of Medicine
New Haven, Connecticut

Jeffrey O. Hollinger
Bone Tissue Engineering Center
Department of Biological Sciences
Carnegie Mellon University
Pittsburgh, Pennsylvania

Johnny Huard
Department of Orthopaedic
  Surgery
University of Pittsburgh
Pittsburgh, Pennsylvania

H. David Humes
Departments of Internal Medicine
University of Michigan and
  Ann Arbor Veteran's Affairs
  Medical Center
Ann Arbor, Michigan

Marcos Intaglietta
University of California
La Jolla, California

Chid Iyer
Sughrue Mion PLLC
Washington, D.C.

Esmaiel Jabbari
Department of Orthopedic
  Surgery
Department of Physiology and
  Biomedical Engineering
Mayo Clinic College of Medicine
Rochester, Minnesota

Michel Jaffrin
Université de Technologie de
  Compiègne
Compiègne, France

John A. Jansen
Department of Biomaterials
University Medical Center
  St. Radboud
Nijmegen, The Netherlands

Hugo O. Jauregui
Rhode Island Hospital
Providence, Rhode Island

Cindy Jung
Georgia Institute of Technology
Atlanta, Georgia

Robert Kaiser
University of Washington
Seattle, Washington

Kristi L. Kiick
Department of Materials Science
  and Engineering
University of Delaware
Newark, Delaware

Jeremy F. Koscielecki
Department of Chemistry
University of Connecticut
Storrs, Connecticut

David N. Ku
Georgia Institute of Technology
Atlanta, Georgia

Joseph M. Le Doux
Emory University
Atlanta, Georgia

Catherine Le Visage
Department of Biomedical
  Engineering
Johns Hopkins School of Medicine
Baltimore, Maryland

Ann L. Lee
Merck Research Laboratories
Rahway, New Jersey

Kam Leong
Department of Biomedical
    Engineering
Johns Hopkins School of Medicine
Baltimore, Maryland

Xinran Li
Cornell University
Ithaca, New York

Yong Li
Department of Orthopaedic
    Surgery
University of Pittsburgh
Pittsburgh, Pennysylvania

E.N. Lightfoot
University of Wisconsin
Madison, Wisconsin

Lichun Lu
Department of Orthopedic
    Surgery
Department of Physiology and
    Biomedical Engineering
Mayo Clinic College of Medicine
Rochester, Minneapolis

Michael J. Lysaght
Brown University
Providence, Rhode Island

Stephen B. Maebius
Foley & Lardner
Washington, D.C.

Surya K. Mallapragada
Department of Chemical
    Engineering
Iowa State University
Ames, Iowa

C. Mavroidis
Department of Mechanical and
    Industrial Engineering
Northeastern University
Boston, Massachusetts

Zaki Megeed
Center for Engineering in
    Medicine/Surgical Services
Massachusetts General Hospital
Shriners Burns Hospital for
    Children
Harvard Medical School
Boston, Massachusetts

Antonios G. Mikos
Department of Bioengineering
Rice University
Houston, Texas

Michael Miller
Department of Plastic Surgery
University of Texas
Houston, Texas

Amit S. Mistry
Department of Bioengineering
Rice University
Houston, Texas

David J. Mooney
Departments of Chemical
    Engineering, Biomedical
    Engineering
Biologic and Materials Sciences
University of Michigan
Ann Arbor, Michigan
Division of Engineering and
    Applied Sciences
Harvard University
Cambridge, Massachusetts

Michael J. Moore
Department of Orthopedic
    Surgery
Department of Physiology and
    Biomedical Engineering
Mayo Clinic College of Medicine
Rochester, Minnesota

John Moran
Vasca, Inc.
Tewksbury, Massachusetts

J.M. Munson
Laboratory for Gene Therapy and
    Cellular Engineering
Department of Chemical and
    Biomolecular Engineering
Tulane University
New Orleans, Louisiana

Tatsuo Nakamura
Kyoto University
Kyoto, Japan

Robert M. Nerem
Georgia Institute of Technology
Atlanta, Georgia

Shuming Nie
Emory University
Georgia Institute of Technology
Atlanta, Georgia

Joo L. Ong
Department of Biomedical
    Engineering
University of Tennessee
Memphis, Tennessee

Robert A. Peattie
Oregon State University
Corvallis, Oregon

Hairong Peng
Department of Orthopaedic
    Surgery
University of Pittsburgh
Pittsburgh, Pennsylvania

Yuchen Qui
Cordis Corporation
Miami Lakes, Florida

J. Daniell Rackley
Department of Urology
Wake Forest University Baptist
    Medical Center
Winston-Salem, North Carolina

B.D. Ratner
Department of Bioengineering
University of Washington
Seattle, Washington

Genard Reach
Hôpital Hostel-Dieu Paris
Paris, France

Jennifer B. Recknor
Department of Chemical
    Engineering
Iowa State University
Ames, Iowa

A. Hari Reddi
Center for Tissue Regeneration
    and Repair
Department of Orthopaedic
    Surgery
University of California
Davis School of Medicine
Sacramento, California

David E. Reisner
Inframat Corporation
Willington, Connecticut

A.C. Ritchie
School of Mechanical and
    Production Engineering
Nanyang Technological University
Singapore

Gerson Rosenberg
Pennsylvania State University
Hershey, Pennsylvania

Gualberto Ruaño
Genomas Inc.
Hartford, Connecticut

P. Quinten Ruhé
Department of Biomaterials
University Medical Center
    St. Radboud
Nijmegen, The Netherlands

W. Mark Saltzman
Department of Biomedical
    Engineering
Yale University
New Haven, Connecticut

Tina Sauerwald
Centocor R&D Inc.
Radnor, Pennsylvania

Rachael H. Schmedlen
Department of Bioengineering
Rice University
Houston, Texas

Gaurav Sharma
Department of Mechanical and
    Industrial Engineering
Northeastern University
Boston, Massachusetts

Songtao Shi
National Institutes of Health
National Institute of Dental and
    Craniofacial Research
Craniofacial and Skeletal Diseases
    Branch
Bethesda, Maryland

Xinfeng Shi
Department of Bioengineering
Rice University
Houston, Texas

Yasuhiko Shimizu
Kyoto University
Kyoto, Japan

Yan-Ting Shiu
Department of Bioengineering
University of Utah
Salt Lake City, Utah

Michael L. Shuler
Cornell University
Ithaca, New York

Vassilios I. Sikavitsas
School of Chemical Engineering
    and Materials Science
Bioengineering Center
University of Oklahoma
Norman, Oklahoma

Sunil Singhal
Department of General Surgery
Johns Hopkins School of Medicine
Baltimore, Maryland

Andrew Michael Smith
Emory University
Georgia Institute of Technology
Atlanta, Georgia

David Smith
Teregenics, LLC
Pittsburgh, Pennsylvania

Paul H.M. Spauwen
Department of Plastic and
    Recontructive Surgery
University Medical Center
    St. Radboud
Nijmegen, The Netherlands

Srikanth Sundaram
Harvard Medical School
Boston, Massachusetts
Rutgers University
Piscataway, New Jersey

Dorothy M. Supp
Shriners Hospital for Children
Cincinnati Burns Hospital
Cincinnati, Ohio

Maryam Tabrizian
McGill University
Montreal, Quebec, Canada

Weihong Tan
Department of Chemistry and
    Shands Cancer Center
University of Florida
Gainesville, Florida

John M. Tarbell
The City College of New York
New York, New York

Arno W. Tilles
Center for Engineering in
    Medicine/Surgical Services
Massachusetts General Hospital
Harvard Medical School
Shriners Hospitals for Children
Boston, Massachusetts

Mehmet Toner
Center for Engineering in
    Medicine/Surgical Services
Massachusetts General Hospital
Harvard Medical School
Shriners Hospital for Children
Boston, Massachusetts

Ajay Ummat
Department of Mechanical and
    Industrial Engineering
Northeastern University
Boston, Massachusetts

Robert F. Valentini
Brown University
Providence, Rhode Island

David B. Volkin
Merck Research Laboratories
Rahway, New Jersey

Roger C. Wagner
Department of Biological
    Sciences
University of Delaware
Newark, Delaware

S. Patrick Walton
Michigan State University
East Lansing, Michigan

Lin Wang
Department of Chemistry
  and Shands Cancer
  Center
University of Florida
Gainesville, Florida

Jennifer L. West
Department of Bioengineering
Rice University
Houston, Texas

Andreas Windemuth
Genomas
Hartford, Connecticut

Robert M. Winslow
SANGART Inc.
La Jolla, California

Joop G.C. Wolke
Department of Biomaterials
University Medical Center
  St. Radboud
Nijmegen, The Netherlands

Mark E.K. Wong
University of Texas Dental
  Branch
Department of Oral and
  Maxillofacial Surgery
Department of Bioengineering
Rice University
Houston, Texas

Fan Yang
Department of Biomedical
  Engineering
Johns Hopkins University
Baltimore, Maryland

Yunzhi Yang
Department of Biomedical
  Engineering
University of Tennessee
Memphis, Tennessee

Ioannis V. Yannas
Massachusetts Institute of
  Technology
Cambridge, Massachusetts

David M. Yarmush
Center for Engineering in
  Medicine/Surgical Services
Massachusetts General
  Hospital
Shriners Burns Hospital for
  Children
Harvard Medical School
Boston, Massachusetts

Martin L. Yarmush
Center for Engineering in
  Medicine/Surgical Services
Massachusetts General
  Hospital
Shriners Burns Hospital for
  Children
Harvard Medical School
Boston, Massachusetts

Michael J. Yaszemski
Department of Orthopedic
  Surgery
Department of Physiology and
  Biomedical Engineering
Mayo Clinic College of Medicine
Rochester, Minneapolis

Diana M. Yoon
Department of Chemical
  Engineering
University of Maryland
College Park, Maryland

Yu Ching Yung
Departments of Chemical
  Engineering
University of Michigan
Ann Arbor, Michigan

Zongtao Zhang
Inframat Corporation
Willington, Connecticut

Craig Zupke
Amgen Corporation
Thousand Oaks, California

Andrew L. Zydney
University of Delaware
Newark, Delaware

Kyriacos Zygourakis
Department of Chemical
  Engineering
Institute of Biosciences and
  Bioengineering
Rice University
Houston, Texas

Contents

SECTION III   Biotechnology

Martin L. Yarmush and Mehmet Toner

SECTION IV   Bionanotechnology

David E. Reisner

SECTION V ⟨ Tissue Engineering ⟩

John P. Fisher and Antonios G. Mikos

SECTION VI Prostheses and Artificial Organs

Pierre M. Galletti (deceased) and Robert M. Nerem

SECTION VII   Ethics

David E. Reisner

I

Molecular Biology

Michael Domach
Carnegie Mellon University

W HETHER IT IS DEVELOPING NEW DRUGS, fathoming how a material will behave in the
body or coaxing stem cells to develop into a particular type of tissue, a sometimes bewildering
array of molecular actors produced by cells that dictate outcome have been identified. The
understanding of the deterministic molecular basis for cellular events and responses also continues to
expand and improve. Within the sciences, chemistry and other fields have "fused" their expertise with
"molecular biology," and the same can now be said for some subfields in bioengineering. Accordingly, this
volume of the handbook now includes a section on Molecular Biology.

The subject of Molecular Biology is large and ultimately overlaps with tissue engineering, metabolic
engineering, gene therapy, and other technologies that are covered well in this handbook. Thus, the main
aim of this section is to bring the traditional engineer quickly up to speed on the basics of Molecular Biology
and some key technological applications. This base can then be used to augment the understanding of
some other sections in the handbook.

In Chapter 1, a historical perspective and definitions are provided in order to explain how Molecular
Biology emerged, and to provide facility with the language of the science. Some technological aspects
are also covered such as DNA manipulation. Because this is an engineering as opposed to a science
handbook, an introduction to new technologies and issues inspired by advances in molecular biology are
then provided in Chapters 2 and 3. These two chapters cover bacterial and eukaryotic cells.

1

Historical Perspective and Basics of Molecular Biology

Nathan R. Domagalski
Michael Domach
Carnegie Mellon University

1.1 Introduction

This chapter provides first a historical perspective on the origins of molecular biology. A historical perspective is important because the emergence of molecular biology has radically altered how living systems are viewed by scientists and biomedical engineers. It is thus useful for a biomedical engineer to be acquainted with the evolution of the discipline in order to fully appreciate the technological and social impact of molecular biology. For example, a mechanistic basis for the origin of many diseases can now be established, which paves the way for developing new treatments. It is also now possible to manipulate living systems for technological purposes, such as developing bacteria that can produce the therapeutic, human insulin. Acquiring the capability to manipulate the genetic potential of organisms and ultimately humans also raises new important ethical issues (see Section VII, Ethics). After summarizing the major historical developments, the "Central Dogma of Molecular Biology" will be presented and salient mechanistic details will be provided. This chapter concludes with some largely stable Internet resources that can provide quick definitions of terms, documentaries of prominent molecular biologists and their accomplishments, as well as other useful resources that can be used while reading this section.

1.2   Molecular Biology: A Historical Perspective

Nineteenth-century biologists and their predecessors emphasized the collection and inventorying of life on Earth. The physical or other similarities between organisms led to classification schemes. As new organisms were discovered or new ideas emerged, schemes were often debated and then reorganized. Thus, unlike physics or chemistry, unifying rules and descriptions that had a mechanistic basis and could account for behavior were scant in biology.

Toward the end of the 19th century, scientists began to gaze within cells, and as result, some striking observations were made that began to demystify biological systems. In 1897, Buchner found that cell-free extracts (i.e., the molecules found within yeast cells) executed chemical reactions. His finding was significant because a debate had been underway for decades. The question driving the debate was "What exactly is the role of cells, such as yeast, in practical processes such as wine making?" Hypotheses were abundant. The German chemist Jutus von Liebig, for example, proposed in 1839 that yeast emit certain vibrations that can reorganize molecules, which accounts for the yeast-mediated conversion of sugar to alcohol. In 1876, William Kuhne coined the term enzyme to imply that something contained within yeast is associated with processes, such as converting sugar to alcohol. Bucher's experiments were powerful because the results showed that cells are not required for chemical reactions to occur. Rather, it seemed plausible that the "rules" of chemistry apply to living systems as opposed to "vibrations" or other phenomena unique to living systems being operative. Many now credit the Bucher brothers with launching the modern field of biochemistry. In 1894, Emil Fisher developed a theoretical model for how enzymes function. Later in 1926, *Charles Sumner* provided some useful closure *and* a method for characterizing cells at the molecular level. He and his colleagues showed that enzymes are proteins *and* crystallization is one means that can be used to isolate specific enzymes from cells.

The omnipresence of deoxyribonucleic acid (DNA) within cells piqued curiosity. Miescher discovered the DNA molecule in 1869, which was 3 years after Mendel published his experiments on heredity in plants. Mendle's work incorporated the notion that a "gene" is a conserved and transmittable unit of trait information. However, science had to wait until 1943 for the link to be made between the manifestation of traits and the presence of DNA within a cell. Oswald Theodore Avery (1877–1955) and his coworkers showed that by simply adding the DNA from a virulent form of the bacterium *Pneumococcus* to a suspension of nonvirulent *Pneumococcus*, the nonvirulent bacterium acquired the traits of the virulent form. With this link established, the nature of the DNA molecule became a subject of intense interest. In 1951, Pauling and Corey proposed that the DNA molecule forms an α-helix structure, and experimental evidence was reported by Watson and Crick in 1953.

By the 1950s, knowledge had accumulated to the extent that it was known that (1) enzymes catalyze reactions, (2) cellular reactions are understandable in terms of organic chemistry fundamentals, (3) the DNA molecule possesses the information for traits, and (4) the DNA molecule has an intriguing spatial organization that may "somehow" confer information storage and expression capabilities. Additionally, it had been established that all DNA molecules contain four bases: adenine (A), thymine (T), guanine (G), and cytosine (C). However, how information is actually stored in DNA and used were still mysteries. Interestingly, basic questions on how life "works" were unresolved while at the same time,

Yuri Alexeyevich Gagarin's (1961) and John Glenn's (1962) pioneering orbits of the Earth extended the reach of human life to space.

Molecular biology had now supplanted descriptive biology, and inspired further research. Through the 1950s to the mid1960s, many workers from varied disciplines solved many key problems in molecular biology. In 1958, François Jacob and Jacques Monod predicted the existence of a molecule that is a working copy of the genetic information contained in DNA (messenger RNA), and the information is conveyed from where DNA is stored (the cell's nucleus) to where proteins are produced (the ribosomes). In 1966, Marshall Nirenberg and colleagues cracked the genetic code. They showed that sequences of three of the four bases (e.g., AAT, GCT) that compose DNA specifies each of the 20 different amino acids used by a cell to produce proteins. In 1971, this accumulated knowledge enabled Stanley Cohen and Herbert Boyer to insert into a bacterial cell the DNA that encodes an amphibian protein, and, in turn, compel the bacterium to produce a protein from a vastly different organism. The prospect of using bacteria and simple raw materials (e.g., glucose) to produce human-associated and other proteins with therapeutic or commercial value led to the formation of the company Genentech in 1976. More recently, the DNA from humans and other sources has been successfully sequenced, which should lead to further commercial and medical impacts, as well as ethical challenges.

Section 1.3 and Section 1.4 present the Central Dogma of Molecular Biology/Molecular Genetics and summarizes salient features of how cells function at the molecular level.

1.3   The Central Dogma of Modern Molecular Biology

The Central Dogma of Molecular Biology/Molecular Genetics in its original form proposes that information encoded by DNA is first transcribed to a working copy. The working copy is messenger RNA (mRNA). The information contained by a given mRNA is then translated to produce a particular protein. The collection of proteins/enzymes a cell possesses at any point in time, in turn, has a strong bearing on a cell's behavior and capabilities.

The central dogma has been proven to be largely correct. Salient aspects of how the central dogma is manifested at the molecular level are described below. Thereafter, an important deviant from the Central Dogma and additional refinements are presented.

1.3.1   DNA Base Composition, Connectivity, and Structure

Because DNA contains information, it follows that the composition of DNA must play a role in the information that the molecule encodes. DNA is composed of four different mononucleotide building blocks. As shown in Figure 1.1, a mononucleotide molecule has three "parts" (1) a five-carbon ribose sugar, (2) an organic nitrogen-containing base, and (3) one (i.e., "mono") phosphate group (PO_4). The ribose sugar can possess one or two hydroxyl groups (–OH); the "deoxy" form, which is present in DNA, has one hydroxyl. Five bases are commonly found within cells: adenine (A), guanine (G), cytosine (C), uracil (U), and thymine (T). A, G, C, and T are the four bases that appear in the nucleotides that comprise the DNA molecule, and thus the base present distinguishes one building block from another. A, G, C, and U appear in ribonucleic acid (RNA) molecules. Thus, DNA and RNA molecules differ by the number of hydroxyl constituents possessed by the ribose, and whether thymine (DNA) or uracil (RNA) is the base present.

The number of bound phosphates can vary in a nucleotide. When phosphate is absent, the molecule is referred to as a nucleoside or a deoxynucleoside, depending on the hydroxylation-state of the sugar. Up to three phosphate groups can be present. When one or more phosphates are present, the compound is commonly referred to by the base present, how many phosphates are present, and whether the deoxy-form of the sugar is used. For example, when the base adenine is present and there are two phosphates, the corresponding deoxyribonucleotide and ribonucleotide are typically referred to by the abbreviations, dADP and ADP. The former and latter abbreviations indicate "deoxy-adenine diphosphate" and

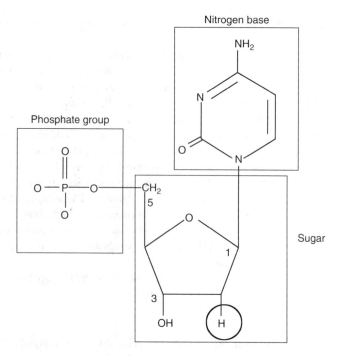

FIGURE 1.1   The mononucleotide, deoxycytidine 5′-phosphoric acid. A less formal, or more likely used name and abbreviation are deoxy cytosine monophosphate and dCMP, respectively. Replacing the circled hydrogen with a hydroxyl group (OH) would produce cytosine monophosphate (CMP). The 3′ and 5′ carbons are marked as well as the 1′ carbon, which is the starting point of the labeling system in the five-carbon sugar (pentose) ring.

"adenine diphosphate," respectively. Overall, the deoxy monophosphates, dAMP, dTMP, dGMP, and dCMP, are the constituents of the DNA molecule.

The mononucleotides in DNA are connected by phosphodiester bonds as shown in Figure 1.2a. This polymeric chain is commonly called single stranded DNA (abbreviated as ssDNA). Based on the numerical labeling of the carbon atoms in ribose, links exist between the third and fifth carbons of successive riboses; hence, "3′–5′ bridges or links" are said to exist. Also, based on this numbering scheme, practitioners note that a strand has either a "free 3′ or 5′ hydroxyl end."

When discussing the nucleotide composition or sequence present in DNA from a particular source, experts often drop naming formalities and simply use the bases' names or abbreviations, because the base distinguishes the building blocks. For example, the "G + C percent content" of the DNA from one organism is often compared to the content in the DNA from another organism in order to highlight a difference between the two organisms. The sequence in which the nucleotide building blocks appear in a section of a DNA molecule is also abbreviated. For example, GCCATCC, refers to the order in which the guanine-, cytosine-, adenine-, and thymine-containing mononucleotides appear in a section of DNA.

Within a cell, the DNA molecule actually consists of two hydrogen-bonded antiparallel strands as depicted in Figure 1.2b. The strands are "antiparallel" because the end of one strand has a free 3′ OH while the adjacent end of the companion strand has a free 5′ OH. Thus, one strand is said to run in 3′ → 5′ direction, while the other has the opposite 5′ → 3′ "polarity." This allows the A, G, C, and T bases on the two strands to interact via hydrogen bonding, as illustrated in Figure 1.2c. An A on one strand can interact with a T residue on the other strand via two hydrogen bonds. Likewise, G and C residues on adjacent strands interact, but the interaction is stronger because three hydrogen bonds can be formed in a G–C association. The interaction between bases on different strands is referred to as base-pairing, and a complex of two strands is known as a duplex or doubled stranded DNA (abbreviated as dsDNA).

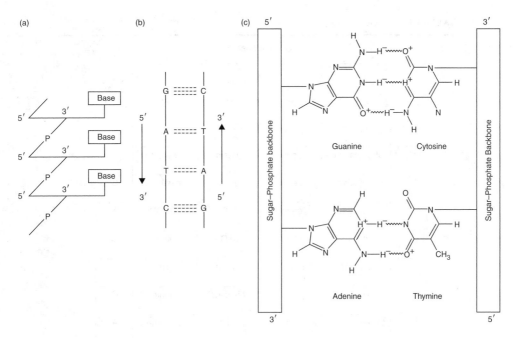

FIGURE 1.2 Connections and pairing of strands in the DNA duplex. (a) A connected strand has a direction where the example shown has a "free" 3′ end. (b) In the cell, two strands run in an "antiparallel direction" allowing the G–C and A–T residues to base pair thereby holding the duplex together. (c) The illustration demonstrates that hydrogen bonding, shown as zig-zag lines, dictates which bases are complimentary to one another. Three hydrogen bonds form between guanine and cytosine. Similarly, two hydrogen bonds form between adenine and thymine (or uracil in RNA).

Although individually rather weak when compared to ionic or covalent bonds, the cumulative effect of numerous hydrogen bonds results in a rather strong and stable molecular interaction. Finally, the two strands of DNA have to be complementary in that every position an A (or G) appears, the other strand must have a T (or C) present. The base-paired, duplex assumes an α-helical structure.

The DNA molecule represents only a small fraction of the total weight of a cell. However, each DNA molecule itself is quite large in terms of molecular weight. The DNA molecule found in the bacterium *Escherichia coli*, for example, contains about 4.2 million base pairs, which represents a molecular weight on the order of 2.8 billion Daltons.

1.3.2 Base Sequence, Information, and Genes

Some details on the molecular species that actually decipher and then use the information in DNA for producing a functional protein will be described after summarizing how information storage is accomplished at the "base sequence information level." A sequence of three bases encodes for an amino acid in a protein. That is, when the information encoded by a strand of DNA is read in a fixed direction, the "word" formed from three letters (e.g., ATT) denotes that a particular amino acid should be added to a lengthening protein chain. There are a total of 20 amino acids; hence, at the minimum 20 code words are required. Words consisting of different three-letter combinations of A, G, C, and T can yield $4^3 = 64$ unique "code words," which exceed the 20 required for all the amino acids; hence, there are 44 extra "words." The extra words result in synonyms for amino acids, which is known as degeneracy. Other extra "words" provide signals for where a protein's code starts and stops. A sequence of three bases that encode for a particular amino acid is called a codon or triplet. Table 1.1 summarizes the genetic code. The set of all codons that encode the amino acid sequence of a protein is called a structural gene.

TABLE 1.1   The Genetic Code

		Second position				
		U	C	A	G	
First position (5′ end)	U	phenylalanine	serine	tyrosine	cysteine	U
		phenylalanine	serine	tyrosine	cysteine	C
		leucine	serine	STOP	STOP	A
		leucine	serine	STOP	tryptophan	G
	C	leucine	proline	histidine	arginine	U
		leucine	proline	histidine	arginine	C
		leucine	proline	glutamine	arginine	A
		leucine	proline	glutamine	arginine	G
	A	isoleucine	threonine	asparagine	serine	U
		isoleucine	threonine	asparagine	serine	C
		isoleucine	threonine	lysine	arginine	A
		methionine[a]	threonine	lysine	arginine	G
	G	valine	alanine	aspartic acid	glycine	U
		valine	alanine	aspartic acid	glycine	C
		valine	alanine	glutamic acid	glycine	A
		valine	alanine	glutamic acid	glycine	G

[a] Also START.

1.3.3 Codon Information to a Protein

As shown in Figure 1.3, the information encoded by a gene on one DNA strand is first translated by the enzyme, RNA polymerase (RNApol). The copy of the gene RNApol has helped to produce what is called messenger RNA (mRNA). The raw materials for mRNA synthesis are ATP, CTP, GTP, and UTP. The analogous mRNA copy is complementary to the original DNA; hence, wherever G, C, A, and T appear in the DNA-encoded gene, C, G, U, and A appear in the mRNA.

Thinking mechanistically, if mRNA synthesis is blocked, then a protein cannot be produced. Therefore, one logical place to exercise control over gene expression is at the level of mRNA synthesis. One example of gene regulation is illustrated in Figure 1.3. As shown, a binding site upstream from the gene, known as an operator region, is often used to control whether mRNA is produced or not. A protein called a repressor normally binds to a repressor region that lies within the operator region. When the repressor is bound,

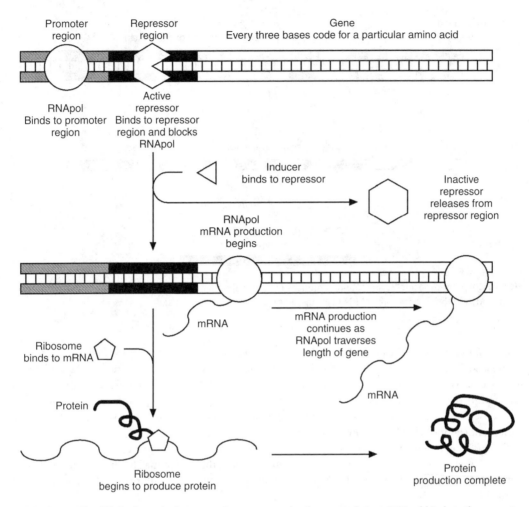

FIGURE 1.3 Simplified schematic demonstrating one example of gene regulation. RNApol binds to the promoter region forward of a gene. However, an active repressor may bind to the repressor region and block the RNApol from translating the gene into a molecule of mRNA. Binding of an inducer molecule to the repressor leads to inactivation and causes the repressor to release from the DNA. RNApol is now free to produce mRNA from the gene. Ribosomes next bind to the mRNA, sequentially adding amino acids in a growing chain that becomes a protein.

RNApol's access to the gene is blocked. The repressor normally possesses another binding site. The second site can bind a ligand that serves as a signal for indicating that the protein the gene codes for is now needed. Such a ligand is termed an inducer. When the inducer binds, the repressor's three-dimensional structure is altered such that its ability to bind to the operator site is significantly reduced. Consequently, the tendency for the repressor to dissociate from the promoter site increases. The result of repressor dissociation is that RNApol can now access the gene and commence mRNA synthesis. It is important to note that there are many variations in how binding is used to regulate gene expression that differ from the scenario in Figure 1.3. For example, in addition to providing RNApol access to a gene, binding between RNApol and other molecular "signals" occur that actually increase the avidity of RNApol–DNA binding.

Ribosomes, which are large protein–nucleic acid complexes, bind to the newly produced mRNA usually before synthesis of the entire strand is even complete. In fact, multiple ribosomes will bind to the same mRNA molecule thereby creating a polyribosome. Ribosomes mediate the sequential addition of amino acids, where each amino acid is prescribed by the complementary codon information now contained in the mRNA. What occurs is that all 20 amino acids have been "prepped" by being enzymatically esterified

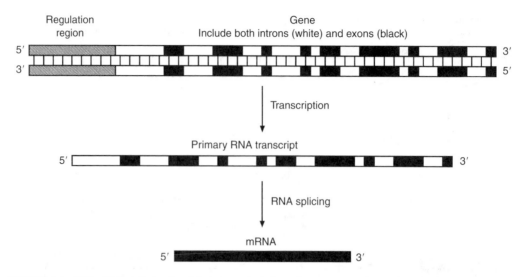

FIGURE 1.4 RNA splicing. Genes found in humans include coding sequences (introns) and noncoding sequences (exons). After both transcription and RNA splicing, an mRNA molecule is created.

to an amino acid-specific transfer RNA (tRNA). Each tRNA possesses a binding site that binds to one amino acid's codon(s) on the mRNA; the binding site on the tRNA is called an anticodon. The enzymes that mediate the attachment of a particular amino acid to its tRNA are very specific for both the amino acid and its tRNA. Any sloppiness could result in a tRNA being "charged" with the wrong amino acid. The consequence of an error is that the wrong amino acid would be added to a protein even though the correct anticodon-codon binding event occurred.

The growing strand of amino acids are joined together by an amide linkage known as a peptide bond. Without knowing structural or functional information, this strand may be simply referred to as a polypeptide. However, when the polypeptide is organized into an active conformation, it is finally called a protein.

Although this description of the Central Dogma is operative in many microorganisms, there are other significant intermediate steps that are required by higher organisms. One such step is RNA splicing. As shown in Figure 1.4, a typical gene in, for example, a human cell is composed of numerous coding (exons) and noncoding (introns) stretches of DNA sequences. While bacterial proteins are predominantly encoded by a continuous, uninterrupted DNA sequence, most higher cells, such as those that compose humans, must have the translated introns removed to produce a molecule of mRNA. After the entire gene is translated into a large RNA molecule known as a primary transcript, a complex of RNA modification enzymes deletes the introns and splices the exons into a true mRNA molecule. The splicing process is known as ligation. Subsequently, the mRNA is processed by the mechanisms described previously.

1.3.4 DNA Replication

While the base composition of DNA explains much, a lingering issue is how DNA replication occurs and results in the faithful transmission of genetic information when a parent cell divides and forms two cells. DNA replication has been proven to be a semiconservative replication process. When a cell undergoes asexual division to form two cells, each daughter cell must obtain identical amounts of DNA, and each copy should contain all the information that the parent possessed. It has been established that each strand in a parental duplex serves as a template for its reproduction. Enzymes called DNA polymerases replicate each strand. The result is that the resulting two duplexes that are derived from the parental duplex each possess one of the original strands from the parental DNA.

1.3.5   mRNA Dynamics

For the Central Dogma to work, the control of gene expression should depend on whether or not mRNA synthesis occurs. Implicit in this requirement is mRNA must have a short lifetime in cells. If the lifetime of mRNA was on the order of cell lifetime or more, then "ON–OFF" controls of mRNA synthesis would have little effect because working copies of mRNA from many genes would be ample and omnipresent. It has been found that in bacterial cells, for example, the lifetime of mRNA is on the order of minutes. From the engineering standpoint, an interesting control system and dynamics is thus manifested by many cells. "ON–OFF" controls dictate whether new mRNA is produced or not, and the transduced output from repressor–promoter binding (mRNA) has a short lifetime, which leads to "sharp" ON–OFF dynamics for the production of specific, gene-encoded proteins.

1.3.6   Variations and Refinements of the Central Dogma

Some viruses do not directly follow the DNA → mRNA → protein path. Retroviruses, for example, are composed of RNA and consequently replicate by a pathway of RNA → DNA → mRNA → protein. After a retrovirus infects a cell, the viral RNA cargo is converted to DNA via the enzyme, reverse transcriptase. The viral DNA then integrates into the host cell's DNA. Expression of the viral genes by the host's transcriptional and translational machinery build the components for new viruses. Self-assembly of the components then occurs. Retroviruses are not biological curiosities; they are the agents of diseases, such as human T-cell leukemia and acquired immune deficiency syndrome (AIDS).

Another variant is found on the border of living vs. self-assembling/propagating systems. We note this case because of its medical importance. Prions are altered proteins that lead to diseases, such as Creutzfeldt–Jakob Disease in humans, Chronic Wasting Disease in deer and elk, and Bovine Spongiforme Encephalopathy in cattle. It is now thought that a prion is a protein that has been altered to be significantly more resistant to natural degradation mechanisms as well as the heat treatment that occurs during sterilization or the preparation of food. When a prion encounters a natural form of its precursor protein, a binding interaction is thought to occur that converts the normal protein into a likewise degradation-resistant form. Subsequent binding events result in a chain reaction that propagates the accumulation of prions. The accumulation of prions can interfere with normal neurological function leading to the aforementioned diseases. Prions are currently under intense investigation. Future research will reveal if the "protein-only hypothesis" is a sufficient explanation, or if an expanded or alternate mechanistic model is required to explain prion formation and propagation.

It is now also known that controls beyond ON–OFF mRNA synthesis also play a role in whether the information in a gene is expressed within cells. These other controls do not necessarily negate the utility of the Central Dogma as a model. Rather, from the control engineering standpoint, these additional mechanisms represent different interesting means of "fine tuning" and adding additional levels of control over gene expression. At the protein level, where enzymes are gene products, some enzymes possess binding sites to which reaction products or other metabolites can bind. When binding occurs, the rate of the enzyme-catalyzed reaction is either accelerated or decreased leading to feedback and feed-forward control of the pace at which some expressed gene products function.

The prior description of mRNA regulation (see Figure 1.3) has many steps. Thus, it is not surprising to find that other processes can also influence the rate and extent to which the information in a gene can be manifested as an active functional protein. Such translational level controls can entail competition for ribosomes by the numerous mRNAs from different genes. Alternately, the base interactions that occur in a duplex DNA molecule that lead to the α-helix can also result in structural organization in mRNA. For example, the bases within an mRNA strand can self-complement thereby leading to the formation of hairpin loops. Such "secondary structures" that result from a primary structure (the base sequence) can influence how fast and successfully the ribosomal-mediated translation process occurs.

Lastly, the control architecture of cellular gene expression is not limited to the previously described case of one promoter-one signal-one structural gene. Different genes can be expressed from a particular set of environmental "signals" when shared control elements and/or molecular components are used. One example entails the "stress response of cells." Here, nutrient deprivation or another "signal" unleashes the expression of various genes that collectively enhance the survival chances for a cell. Sometimes these "circuits" utilize different transcriptional molecular components, which thereby provides for subsystem isolation and specialization. Alternately, even microbes are capable of intercellular communication, a trait more typically attributed to different cells in a complex biosystem, such as a human. Examples of such distributed and specialized control circuits will be provided in the next chapter.

1.4   Molecular Biology Leads to a Refined Classification of Cells

The science of classification is called taxonomy and the organization of life by ancestor-descendent (evolutionary) relationships is called phylogeny. The characterization and comparison of key intracellular molecules has altered prior classification and relationship schemes.

The components of the ribosomes found in cells are the basis for modern taxonomy. A ribosome is composed of different parts that enable mRNA binding and amino acid addition. The parts are called subunits. Different subunits are characterized and distinguished by centrifugation. Based on such physical sorting, the subunits are assigned S-values, where "S" stands for a Svedberg unit. The larger the value of S, the more readily a subunit is driven to the bottom of a centrifuge tube. The sedimentation unit's namesake, Theodor Svedberg (1884–1971), studied the behavior of macromolecules and small particles; for his pioneering work, he received the Noble Prize in 1926.

One key part of a ribosome is the 16S rRNA component, which is found in the 30S subunit along with proteins. Many seemingly different cells are actually similarly based on their constituent 16S rRNA. Not only is the S-value the same, the genes that encode for the 16S RNAs in seemingly different cells exhibit similar base sequences. When the degree of base overlap in a coding sequence is extensive, the DNAs from different sources are said to exhibit high homology. Other cells, however, have been found to possess significantly different components that make up the intact ribosome. The S-value can also vary somewhat. For example, in mammalian cells, the rRNA that fulfills the 16S rRNA function in bacterial cells settles somewhat faster at 18S on the Svedberg scale. More notably, the genes that encode 18S mammalian and 16S bacterial rRNA exhibit low homology. Thus, cells are grouped together based on the homology of their 16S rRNA-encoding genes.

The current classification of cell types and how they are believed to have evolved from one ancestor are shown in Figure 1.5. The three types are Bacteria, Archaea, and Eucarya. *Bacteria* are unicellular organisms capable of reproduction. Bacteria vary in size and shape; a typical length scale is 1 μm (10^{-6} m). *Archaea* resemble bacteria in many ways. They are about the same size and they can metabolize an array of raw materials. One notable difference is that *Archaea* are often found in extreme environments, such as hot springs and acidic waters. Such environments may resemble those present in the early days of the Earth; hence, *Archaea* are believed to be remnants of the early Earth. The ability of *Archaea* to function well

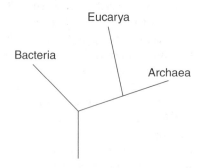

FIGURE 1.5   Family tree of three cell types originating and then diverging from one ancestor.

in extreme environments has also intensified some people's curiosity about the possibility of life beyond the Earth. Others regard *Archaea* proteins and other molecular constituents as potentially useful catalysts and medicinal compounds due to their stability or environmental coping properties (see polymerase chain reaction, which is discussed later). *Eucarya* include the cells that compose the human body. One distinguishing characteristic is that unlike *Bacteria* or *Archaea*, *Eucarya* have compartments within them. The compartments are called organelles. One important organelle is the nucleus, which houses the DNA molecule.

1.5 Mutations

What traits an organism presents is called the phenotype, and the traits are linked to the instructions encoded in the DNA. The raw instructions are, in turn, called the genotype. An alteration in an organism's genetic code is termed a mutation.

Mutations can occur that involve large sections of DNA. Some common examples are described below:

- Translocations involve the interchange of large segments of DNA between two different chromosomes. Gene expression can change when the gene is located at the translocation breakpoint, or if the gene is reattached such that its expression is controlled by a new promoter region that responds to a different inducer.
- Inversions occur when a region of DNA flips its orientation with respect to the rest of the chromosome. An inversion can have the same consequences as a translocation.
- Sometimes large regions of a chromosome are deleted, which can lead to a loss of important genes.
- Sometimes chromosomes can lose track of where they are supposed to go during cell division. One of the daughter cells will end up with more or less than its share of DNA. This is called a chromosome nondisjunction. When a new cell gets less or more than its share of DNA, it may have problems with gene dosage. Fewer or more copies of a gene can affect the amount of gene-encoded protein present in a cell.

More modest alterations occur at the single base level and are called point mutations. Common examples and consequences are summarized below:

- A nonsense mutation creates a stop codon where none previously existed. The resulting protein is thus shortened, which can eliminate functionality.
- A missense mutation changes the amino acid "recipe." If an AGU is changed to an AGA, the protein will have an arginine where a serine was meant to go. This amino acid substitution might alter the shape or properties of the protein. The sickle cell mutation is an example of a missense mutation occurring on a structural gene. Hemoglobin has two subunits. One subunit is normal in people with sickle cell disease. The other subunit has the amino acid valine at position 6 in the protein chain instead of glutamic acid.
- A silent mutation has no effect on protein sequence. Changing one base results in a redundant codon for a particular amino acid.
- Within a gene, small deletions or insertions of a number of bases not divisible by three will result in a frame shift. Consider the coding sequence:

AGA UCG ACG UUA AGC → arginine–serine–threonine–leucine–serine

Inserting a C–G base pair between bases 6 and 7 would generate the following altered code and amino acid errors following the insertion:

AGA UCG CAC GUU AAG C → arginine–serine–histidine–valine–lysine

A frame shift could also introduce a stop codon, which would yield an incomplete protein.

Mutations can also alter gene expression. For example, a mutated promoter region may lose the ability to bind a repressor. Consequently, gene expression always occurs. Such a cell is often called a constitutive mutant and the gene product is constitutively expressed. Alterations in the sequence that encodes for the repressor protein could also result in constitutive expression in that the altered repressor protein can no longer bind to the promoter region and block mRNA synthesis.

1.6 Nucleic Acid Processing Mechanisms and Inspired Technologies with Medical and Other Impacts

The experiment performed by Avery and colleagues revealed the function of DNA via a natural process whereby a bacterium imported raw DNA, and after incorporating the DNA into its genetic material, cellular properties were consequently altered. Today, DNA is routinely inserted into many types of cells for the purpose of altering what cells do or produce. Cell transformation (bacterial) or transfection (mammalian) relies on exploiting the many natural DNA uptake, modification, and repair processes that cells use. This section first reviews the types of enzymes that can alter DNA, and then provides an example of their use in technological processes.

1.6.1 Nucleic Acid Modification Enzymes

To remain viable and sustain reproduction, cells have to replicate DNA, destroy unwanted RNA, repair broken DNA strands, eliminate any foreign DNA inserted by viruses, and execute other maintenance and defense functions. Three important enzymes have been found to enable these functions within cells: nucleases, ligases, and polymerases.

Nucleases are enzymes that cut both DNA and RNA. These enzymes may be further classified as cutting both DNA and RNA, DNA-only (DNases), or RNA-only (RNases). Additionally, enzymes that cut strands of nucleic acids starting at the ends are known as exonucleases. Those enzymes that instead cut only at internal sites are called endonucleases. Exonucleases have a variety of uses, such as removing unwanted DNA or RNA. Although some nucleases will cleave nucleic acids indiscriminately, restriction enzymes are high specificity endonucleases that only cut double-stranded DNA wherever a particular internal base sequence occurs. Sequence specificity is certainly the greatest strength of this type of nuclease. For example, the restriction enzyme *EcoR* I only cuts when the sequence 5′-GAATTC-3′ occurs. When DNA is exposed to this particular restriction enzyme, double-stranded fragments with sticky ends are formed as shown in Figure 1.6. The ends are called "sticky" because each free single strand end has the ability to base pair with any complimentary base sequence. A given organism tends to have only a few restriction enzymes, and those few enzymes are generally unique to the organism. However, the wide diversity of organisms that exist in nature has resulted in the discovery of a large number of different restriction enzymes.

Just as strands of nucleic acids may be cut, they can also be repaired. In fact, the ligase's functionality can simply be thought of as the reverse of that of a restriction enzyme. A critical difference, however, is that the ligase is not site specific. DNA ligase is an enzyme that seals breaks in the sugar–phosphate backbone that can occur within one strand of a duplex. DNA ligase is thus used to repair broken DNA.

Lastly, DNA polymerase catalyzes the synthesis of duplex DNA from a single strand of DNA when a primer is used to initiate the process. The primer is simply a short strand of complimentary nucleic acids. DNA replicates in nature using RNA primers. Once the polymerase has elongated the strand to some extent, organisms possess a special repair mechanism that removes the RNA primer and replaces it with DNA. In contrast, DNA replication in the laboratory is usually accomplished by using oligonucleotides (DNA primers). How the primer-based synthesis of duplex DNA works is shown in Figure 1.7.

Perhaps one of the most important properties of a polymerase is its fidelity. The possibility always exists that a noncomplimentary nucleotide can be inadvertently added to an elongating strand. A polymerase's fidelity is defined as the frequency at which wrong nucleotide addition errors occur. Because

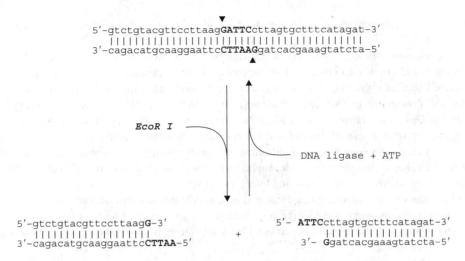

```
           ▼
5'-gtctgtacgttccttaagGATTCcttagtgctttcatagat-3'
   |||||||||||||||||||||||||||||||||||||||||||
3'-cagacatgcaaggaattcCTTAAGgatcacgaaagtatcta-5'
                      ▲
```

EcoR I

DNA ligase + ATP

```
5'-gtctgtacgttccttaagG-3'                5'- ATTCcttagtgctttcatagat-3'
   |||||||||||||||||||          +           |||||||||||||||||||
3'-cagacatgcaaggaattcCTTAA-5'            3'- Ggatcacgaaagtatcta-5'
```

FIGURE 1.6 Cutting and joining DNA. *EcoR* I is an example of a restriction endonuclease that cleaves dsDNA at a specific, internal recognition sequence (shown here as 5'-GAATTC-3'). By contrast, a nonspecific DNA ligase can join the two complimentary DNA molecules by repairing the sugar–phosphate backbone.

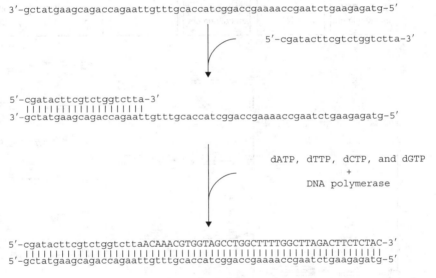

```
3'-gctatgaagcagaccagaattgtttgcaccatcggaccgaaaaccgaatctgaagagatg-5'
```

5'-cgatacttcgtctggtctta-3'

```
5'-cgatacttcgtctggtctta-3'
   ||||||||||||||||||||
3'-gctatgaagcagaccagaattgtttgcaccatcggaccgaaaaccgaatctgaagagatg-5'
```

dATP, dTTP, dCTP, and dGTP
+
DNA polymerase

```
5'-cgatacttcgtctggtcttaACAAACGTGGTAGCCTGGCTTTTGGCTTAGACTTCTCTAC-3'
   ||||||||||||||||||||||||||||||||||||||||||||||||||||||||||||
5'-gctatgaagcagaccagaattgtttgcaccatcggaccgaaaaccgaatctgaagagatg-5'
```

FIGURE 1.7 DNA polymerase. PCR is a routine procedure for amplifying DNA. Primers first anneal to a complimentary sequence on the target ssDNA molecule. Next, DNA polymerase synthesizes the remainder of the complimentary sequence from the four deoxyribonucleotide triphosphates.

of the potentially life-threatening mutations such errors may cause, organisms have an enzymatic proof-reading mechanism. Although the details may differ slightly between organisms, in general if an incorrect nucleotide is added, the proof-reading enzymes pause the polymerase, remove the troubled nucleotide, and then allow the polymerase to continue the elongation process.

1.6.2 Copying DNA in the Laboratory

Many aspects of how cells replicate their DNA can now be reproduced in the laboratory without using intact cells. When a subset of biomolecular components is used in, for example, a beaker to execute a cellular reaction, the reproduced natural process is said to be conducted *in vitro* (e.g., "*in vitro* DNA replication").

Conducting primer-based, DNA polymerase-catalyzed reactions *in vitro* is the basis for both gene amplification and crime scene investigation technologies. One application is the synthesis of a large quantity of a particular protein. Using *in vitro* DNA replication, the sequence that encodes the gene for this desirable protein may be amplified. Obtaining more DNA would enable the insertion of the gene into a bacterium. Given the relative ease with which bacteria can be cultivated and processed on a large scale, the exogenous protein may be then produced in a quantity that far exceeds that of the parent organism. Another use of the technology of gene amplification involves producing both normal and mutated protein products. Such altered proteins can provide insights on the gene's properties and the effect of the mutations of protein's three-dimensional structure and biological activity.

The laboratory process of amplifying DNA is known as polymerase chain reaction (PCR). To demonstrate how this process works, consider the amplification of a gene encoded within a fragment of dsDNA as shown in Figure 1.8. The process begins outside the laboratory by designing a pair of DNA primers.

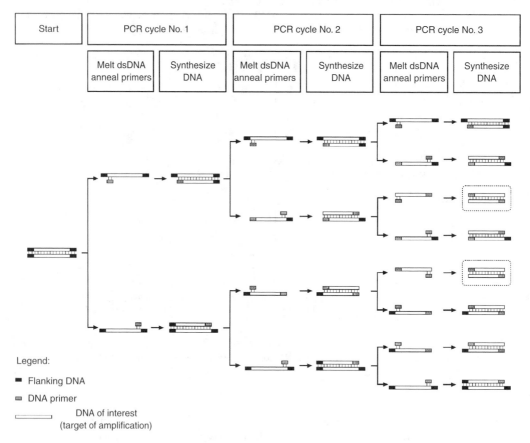

FIGURE 1.8 Amplification of DNA by PCR. A fragment of DNA may be amplified by means of the PCR. The starting fragment of double stranded DNA (dsDNA) consists of the sequence of interest as well as flanking sequences. At the beginning of each cycle, the temperature rises and dsDNA is melted into single stranded DNA (ssDNA). After reducing the temperature, DNA primers anneal to the sequence of interest. The temperature is elevated to the ideal conditions for the DNA polymerase and complimentary strands are synthesized. The cycle is repeated until the sequence of interest has been amplified in great numbers. Any dsDNA, which includes the flanking sequence, will soon become only a very small percentage of the population. After 20 or more cycles, the dsDNA sequence of interest (circled in PCR cycle No. 3) will be the dominant product.

With a design in hand, the primers may then be synthesized using a gene machine, which adds the bases A, T, G, and T in a user-specified order. As a side note, most scientists typically do not synthesize their own primers. Rather, they submit a design over the Internet to a commercial supplier who produces and purifies the primers for a modest fee. Next, a buffered mixture is prepared with the dsDNA fragment (which is often called the template), the primers, the four deoxyribonucleotide triphosphates (dNTPs), and DNA polymerase. The mixture is loaded into a thermal cycler, which is a device that precisely controls temperature according to a specified program. A cycle of PCR starts by heating the mixture so that the individual strands of the dsDNA fragment separate into two single strands of DNA (ssDNA). This "melting" of the dsDNA is the result of the thermal energy exceeding the strength of the G–C and A–T associations. The mixture is cooled and the complimentary primer binds to each ssDNA molecule. The temperature is then elevated to the ideal conditions for the DNA polymerase to function and new DNA is synthesized, starting from the primer and elongating to the end of template. This marks the end of a cycle and each dsDNA molecule has been doubled into two new dsDNA molecules. Since PCR is normally carried out for at least 20 cycles, the product is a million-fold increase over the original starting material.

As mentioned previously, the fidelity of the polymerase determines the frequency at which incorrect nucleotides will be added to the growing strand of DNA. Although *Taq* DNA polymerase is widely used for PCR, it lacks a proof-reading mechanism and will introduce errors after several cycles of amplification. Any application requiring very low error rates, such as molecular cloning, analysis of rare mutations, or amplification of very small quantities of template DNA, should use high fidelity polymerases. The increase in fidelity is due to the presence of proof-reading activity. Several DNA polymerases, including *Pfu* and Deep Vent, are commercially available that will greatly minimize incorrect incorporation of nucleotides. As the name "Deep Vent" suggests, these enzymes are found in *Archaea*, which illustrates one technologically important use of molecules found in the organisms that dwell in extreme environments.

PCR and restriction enzymes have many practical uses outside of life science or biotechnology laboratories. DNA from blood, hair follicle, or other samples from evidence gathered in a murder investigation can be cut with restriction enzymes to produce a fragment profile that has a high probability of belonging only to one person. Such a fingerprint enables victim identification, or whether the accused is linked to the blood trail. If the sample from the crime scene is small, PCR can be first used to increase the amount of DNA prior to treatment with restriction enzymes. Interestingly, the early uses of "DNA" fingerprinting in the criminal justice system were in appeal cases to exonerate some inmates on "Death Row" as opposed to strengthening criminal prosecutions.

1.6.3 Basic Bacterial Transformation Techniques

When bacterial cells are manipulated to internalize and use the instructions encoded by a piece of foreign DNA, the process is known as bacterial transformation. Using bacteria to produce a protein based on human genetic instructions has many advantages. A historical example is provided by the protein insulin. Before gaining the means to produce human proteins in microbes, insulin was obtained from animals that produce a similar protein. Insulin from pigs and cows differ from the human molecule by one and three amino acids, respectively. Although the animal-derived insulin substitute works, the differences between the human and animal insulin molecules can result in immune system activation. One adverse consequence is that a higher dose of the animal-derived insulin is required to offset the effort the immune system exerts on removing the "foreign" molecule from the body. Now that transformation technology is readily available, microbes can be used to express the actual human gene directly rather than searching for a surrogate protein from another species. Additional benefits are bacteria such as *E. coli* reproduce quickly and require only basic, inexpensive raw materials, such as glucose and salts. Hence, the production costs associated with therapeutic production can be managed. Many practitioners use the term "metabolic engineering" to refer to the directed alteration and management of cellular synthetic machinery for the purpose of producing a target molecule.

The first step in any transformation is selection of an appropriate host. That is, one must decide which microorganism will express the exogenous DNA. The choice can play an important role in subsequent steps, including the overall success of transformation, the relative ease of purifying the protein product, and even as basic a concept as whether the microorganism is even capable of producing an active form of the given protein. Sometimes this choice is an obvious one and on other occasions, it can pose a considerable challenge.

For the purpose of our example, let us choose the Gram-negative[1] microorganism *E. coli*, which is a well-known bacteria that is routinely used by many investigators. Although *E. coli* can be toxic to humans due to the lipopolysaccharide constituents of its cell wall, numerous strains have been isolated that cannot propagate in the human body and are generally regarded as safe. Having been studied for many years, *E. coli* also offers a great opportunity to utilize a number of proven technologies.

DNA is generally inserted into a microorganism by one of two methods. The exogenous DNA can be carried on a plasmid or integrated into the host's chromosome. In either case, the key is that the foreign DNA utilizes a means of replication as it is transferred from a parent to progeny during cell division.

A plasmid is a closed-circular piece of dsDNA that persists apart from the cell's chromosome. In nature, plasmids carry only a small amount of information, such as the genes needed for a cell to survive a particular environment. When this environmental pressure is removed, the plasmid is no longer needed and the cells tend to loose the plasmid after several generations. Laboratories often use plasmids that carry a gene-encoding factor that confers resistance to a particular antibiotic. Therefore, if a cell carries the plasmid, it can grow in the presence of the antibiotic. Likewise, the plasmid may be lost from the cells if the antibiotic is removed. Such survivability is an important tool that is routinely exploited when screening for successful transformants.

By contrast, integration means that the foreign DNA is somehow inserted within the cell's chromosome, and thus becomes a permanent part of the genome. The experimental techniques necessary for integration can be quite varied and challenging, but integration offers a significant advantage over using plasmids for inserting DNA into a cell. In particular, the integration is generally permanent and the maintenance of specific environmental conditions is not required for the cell to maintain the foreign DNA. There are exceptions when the foreign DNA integrated within the genome is lost, but such loss is generally a rare event.

Although integration may be accomplished by many different means, it frequently shares methods common to plasmid transformation. Plasmids are a very popular method transformation tool largely because many plasmids have been well characterized and are easy to manipulate. Since the plasmid is a vehicle constructed for the purpose of carrying exogenous genes into a cell, a plasmid in the transformation context is commonly called a vector. As such, our discussion of bacterial transformation will proceed with a closer examination of plasmids and their use.

Using the human insulin gene as an example, the goals are (1) to insert the foreign insulin-encoding DNA into a plasmid, and (2) then insert the altered plasmid into *E. coli*. Let us also presume that the chosen plasmid includes a gene for survival in the presence of the antibiotic ampicillin. Such a survival gene will provide a means for screening for and isolating a successful transformant when manipulated cells are grown in ampicillin-containing growth medium.

As shown in Figure 1.8, the first step is to amplify the source of human insulin DNA. Using PCR and an appropriate primer design, the DNA encoding for insulin is amplified and flanked with restriction sites of our choosing. These restriction sites are a consequence of the primer design. After purifying the PCR product, the amplified DNA is treated with restriction enzymes, which create sticky ends. The plasmid is also exposed to the same restriction enzymes. To foster the binding of the complimentary sequences, the treated insulin-encoding DNA and the plasmid are mixed. Finally, a DNA ligase repairs the sugar–phosphate backbone, yielding a plasmid that now possesses the human insulin gene.

The new plasmid, carrying the genes for human insulin as well as ampicillin resistance can now be inserted into *E. coli*. There are several common insertion techniques, each with their strengths and

---

[1]Gram negative and Gram positive refer to whether a stain is lost or retained by microbes after application and destaining procedures, respectively. The difference in stainability relates to the cell wall structure, which, in turn, provides a means for contrasting different types of bacteria.

weaknesses. These techniques, in order of relative ease, are heat shock, electroporation, and protoplast fusion. Furthermore, a cell that has been treated to optimize a given means of DNA uptake is described as competent.

Although many commercial suppliers offer competent *E. coli* for heat shock, it is fairly easy to create such cells in the laboratory. Under appropriate conditions, the bacteria is cultured, harvested, washed, and finally frozen. In general, bacteria grown in batch cultures will experience a peak ability to uptake foreign DNA. This peak may be correlated to cell concentration or a particular time point during the growth and nutrient exhaustion process. Banks exist that can provide many types of competent cells. In other cases, for a given organism, ample empirical evidence has recorded when such peaks in competence occur. Other investigators that seek to produce their own competent cells exploit the information published on peaks.

Frozen competent cells are first thawed and then mixed with a plasmid. After incubating the mixture on ice for some time, it is quickly exposed to an elevated temperature, which creates small pores in the cell surface. The plasmid enters the cell through these pores. Thereafter, the pores are quickly closed by exposure to cold. The cells are then allowed to relax for about an hour to permanently re-seal the pores. Finally, the cells are spread onto media and incubated overnight. In our example, the plasmid provides resistance to the antibiotic ampicillin. When ampicillin is added to the growth medium, only cells that carry the plasmid can survive, which, in turn, provides a useful first step in screening for successful transformants.

Another method of plasmid insertion into the cell is electroporation. Using competent cells specially prepared for electroporation, a device called an electroporator exposes the cells to a high strength electric field. Much like heat shock, electroporation creates pores in the cells' surface for DNA to enter. From this point, the methodology is just like that used when heat shock is employed; the cells are allowed to relax, grow on antibiotic-containing media overnight, and then screened for surviving transformants.

Electroporation routinely provides more successful transformants than heat shock. This can be very important when working with bacteria that are difficult to transform. Fortunately, *E. coli* is quite easy to transform and electroporation is generally not required. Some Gram-positive bacteria like *Bacillus subtilis*, a cousin of the agent of the disease anthrax, are easier to transform via electroporation.

Protoplast fusion is the last method to be addressed. It is an old technique that is rarely used today because it is quite demanding. However, protoplast fusion can be useful when other methods have failed. Although the details differ from one bacterium to another, the central concept is that the cell wall is chemically and/or enzymatically removed. The resulting protoplasts, which are spherical cells that lack a cell wall, are then mixed with plasmid and a chemical, such as polyethylene glycol (PEG). The PEG causes the protoplasts to fuse with one another, often trapping DNA within the newly formed protoplasts in the process. The transformed protoplasts are carefully cultured under osmotically controlled conditions to both regenerate their cell walls and bear the new plasmid. Antibiotic resistance conferred by the plasmid again facilitates the screening process.

By using antibiotic selection, some of the successfully transformed cells can be isolated. In many cases, this is the end of the process; namely, *E. coli* has acquired the instructions for producing a new protein, such as insulin. In other cases, *E. coli* is simply used to amplify the DNA further via growing a quantity of plasmid-containing cells. After processing the amplified DNA isolated from *E. coli*, the DNA may be used for transforming another type of cell. Chromosomal integration is a possible end point for plasmid-based strategies as well. Such integration, if it does not knock out an essential gene, is advantageous because the new DNA is permanently imbedded in the genome as opposed to be associated with a peripheral plasmid.

The use of recombinant DNA technology has yielded a number of microbial-produced therapeutics. The transformed bacteria are grown in specialized vessels called bioreactors or fermenters. The growth vessel and solution of raw materials and nutrients (growth medium) are first sterilized. Thereafter, a starter culture of transformed cells is added. As the cells grow, they are supplied with oxygen and nutrients to foster their growth and to manage their metabolism such that the recombinant gene product is produced at a high level. A partial listing of products of medical importance is provided in Table 1.2.

TABLE 1.2   Examples of Products Produced from Transformed
Microbes

Product	Medical use
Insulin	Diabetes management
Factor VIII	Treatment for hemophilia A
Factor IX	Treatment for hemophilia B
Human Growth Hormone	Treatment of dwarfism
Erythropoietin	Treatment of anemia
Tissue Plasminogen Activator	Blot clot dissolution
Interferon	Augment immune system function

1.6.4   Transfecting Eucaryotic Cells

It is also possible to transfect eucaryotic cells. The steps and strategies can resemble that used to transform bacterial cells. For example, plasmids can be used to transfect yeast cells. However, additional challenges can arise due to the compartmental nature of eucaryotic cells. In this case, the foreign DNA to be inserted has to cross the cell wall and/or membrane and travel through several physical compartments before the nuclear DNA is encountered. Then, recombination with nuclear DNA must successfully occur before enzymes that destroy DNA have a chance to diminish the outcome.

It is desirable to perfect eucaryotic transfection for a number of reasons. Some proteins with therapeutic value have sugar residues attached to them. Such proteins are known as glycosylated proteins. As is the case for insulin production, it would be beneficial to use cell culture-based processes to produce specific glycosylated proteins with therapeutic potential. However, glycosylated proteins are not produced by bacteria, whereas many eucaryotic cells have the synthetic capability to glycosylate proteins. Thus, a means to efficiently transfect eucaryotic cells such that genetic instructions are provided to produce specific proteins at a high level while controlling the glycosylation pattern of the protein of interest is under active investigation. The progress and challenges associated with transfecting eucaryotic cells are discussed in another chapter in this section.

Another motivation for perfecting eucaryotic cell transformation is driven by many diseases that are now known to have specific genetic determinants. For example, as noted earlier, sickle cell anemia is the result of a missense mutation. Therefore, some envision that the genes within humans can be repaired or replaced to eliminate disease-driving mutations. Gene therapy is the practice of transfecting cells within the human body for the purpose of remedying genetic-based diseases and pathologies. Researchers are either attempting to harness the infecting properties of viruses or they are developing particle-based DNA delivery systems.

To understand further the technology and medical impacts of transfecting eucaryotic cells, an interesting example of fusing tissue engineering with molecular biology technology to demonstrate a means for treating human disease was reported by Stephen et al. (2001). Tissue engineers typically seek to replace diseased tissue with a functional replacement that integrates with the host. In this example, the somewhat altered goal was to implant cells that integrate with host tissue, *and* because of the engineered genetic "programming," substances are produced by the implanted cells that alter the course of a disease, such as ovarian cancer.

Mullerian Inhibiting Substance (MIS) was the substance of interest. MIS is a glycoslylated protein that normally fosters regression of the ducts in the human embryo. MIS has also been found to promote the regression of ovarian tumor cells; hence, some researchers view MIS as a potentially useful chemotherapeutic. However, purifying MIS and then targeting delivery to a particular location within the body are not easy tasks.

The alternative investigated was to implant genetically modified, MIS-producing cells proximal to the therapeutic's tissue target. Stephen et al. (2001) explored this strategy in mice with compromised immune systems. The transfected MIS-producing cells that were implanted into the mice were Chinese Hamster

Ovary (CHO) cells. CHO cells are commonly used in studies that require transfected cells because much is known on how to successfully transfect them. Because the immune systems of normal mice would normally attack CHO cells, mice with suppressed immune systems were used to demonstrate the concept.

Transfected CHO cells were first seeded and grown on polyglycolic acid (PGA) scaffolds. After implant preparation, the effect of different size implants was investigated. A correspondence was found between implant size and MIS blood level. Thereafter, human tumor tissue was implanted into different mice, and the subsequent tumor mass that developed in MIS-producing and untreated mice was measured. The results were encouraging; tumor proliferation was statistically less significant in MIS-producing mice.

Overall, molecular biology has generated an array of diverse and more effective therapeutics, which biomedical and biochemical engineers now help to produce and develop administration technologies. Many new applications await to be developed that can vanquish animal and human diseases in novel ways.

1.7 Computerized Storage and Use of DNA Sequence Information

The base sequences of the chromosomes of many organisms including humans have been sequenced, yet, the process of extracting useful information is ongoing. Inferring a functional product encoded by the sequence of a newly characterized organism requires rapid access to all known sequence information and the means to make rigorous comparisons. Consequently, a number of resources exist today that enable the work of scientists and technologists.

The Internet provides a gateway to numerous databases for nucleic acid and protein information. Available data includes both sequence information and structural details. Listed here are the most prominent databases used today:

Nucleic Acid Sequences
- National Center for Biotechnology Information
  http://www.ncbi.nlm.nih.gov/
- European Bioinformatics Institute
  http://www.ebi.ac.uk/
- Center for Information Biology and DNA Data Bank of Japan
  http://www.cib.nig.ac.jp/
  http://www.ddbj.nig.ac.jp/

Nucleic Acid Structure
- Nucleic Acid Database
  http://ndbserver.rutgers.edu/

Protein Sequences
- Swiss-Prot and TrEMBL
  http://us.expasy.org/sprot/

Protein Structures
- RCSB Protein Data Bank
  http://www.rcsb.org/pdb/
- Swiss-3DImage
  http://us.expasy.org/sw3d/

Protein Families and Domains
- Prosite
  http://us.expasy.org/prosite/

Software used to analyze data extracted from databases is ever changing and improving. Current applications are often described on the Web sites of the databases themselves. Descriptions of additional resources may be found in the literature.

1.8   Probing Gene Expression

As reviewed above, we now know how many mechanisms of gene expression operate. Moreover, we have made major progress on being able to manipulate the genetic inventory of cells as well as which genes are expressed. Consequently, interest has turned to fathoming how the collection of all gene expression events relate to each other and corresponds to particular disease conditions or behavioral traits. For example, some genes may be involved in interactive circuits where gene products interact with each other or expression occurs when a common set of external stimuli is present. Additionally, some genes may have alterations that lead to diseases or the loss of circuit function. Elucidating the operating gene circuits is important for yielding more predictable outcomes for metabolic and tissue engineering. For example, modifying a gene or inserting a new gene may either have a positive effect or there may be no effect because an alteration to one component in a circuit is overridden by the imbedded control mechanisms.

An obvious method for probing gene expression profiles and interrelationships is to analyze for the product(s) of each gene's expression. When a given gene encodes for an enzyme, then the protein isolated from a cell can be analyzed to determine what enzyme activities are present. This traditional method has significantly contributed to our current knowledge. However, it is labor intensive, and clues on when genes with unknown function are expressed and thus suggestions on their potential function cannot be obtained. A global view of how gene expression networks function is also difficult to construct with the single measurement approach.

1.8.1   DNA Microarrays Profile Many Gene Expression Events

Recall that when a gene is expressed, mRNA is first produced. This working copy of mRNA is then translated to yield a protein. If one could obtain a "snapshot" of all the mRNAs that are present in a cell as well as their relative abundance, then one would possess a profile of what genes are currently expressed and to what extent. The latter assumes that particular mRNA's abundance is proportional to the extent a particular gene is expressed. Additionally, if a baseline profile is established for a particular environmental situation, then one can determine which genes are "up regulated" or "down regulated" when environmental conditions are changed.

The apparatus for obtaining the mRNA profile described above is commonly referred to as either a DNA microarray, biochip, or gene array. Different segments of a cell's DNA are first attached to a surface, such as a glass slide. A slide can contain thousands of different "spots," where a different DNA sequence is present at each spot location, or multiples are used to permit replication. The cells subjected to analysis under a particular biological or environmental state contain many different mRNAs of varying abundances. DNA copies of the mRNAs are made using the activity of the enzyme, reverse transcriptase, which is viral in origin; the enzyme's activity reverses the Central Dogma in that mRNA $\rightarrow$ DNA occurs. When the mRNA-derived DNA copies (complementary DNAs, cDNAs) are introduced to a gene chip, a given cDNA will bind to surface-bound segment via base-pairing when a significant base-pairing opportunity is present. The cDNAs are also labeled with a fluorescent dye. Wherever a binding event occurs on the gene array, a fluorescent spot will appear. Nonfluorescent spots indicate that no match existed between the surface-bound DNA and mRNA-derived, copy DNA. One interpretation is that the gene encoded by the surface-bound segment was not expressed under the particular conditions used to propagate the cells.

There are many experimental designs used. Often, two treatments are applied to a DNA array. In this case, the cDNAs are obtained from cells grown under two different conditions. The cDNAs obtained from cells growing in two different conditions are also labeled with different fluorescent dyes. For example, a bacterium such as *E. coli* can be grown on two different carbon sources. When grown on one carbon source, the cDNAs are labeled red. When grown on a different carbon source, the cDNAs of the mRNAs are labeled green. When the red- and green-labeled cDNAs are applied to DNA arrays, there are four "spot" coloration results (1) bright spots absent, (2) red spots, (3) green spots, and (4) spots that vary in yellow coloration. The first case indicates that some particular genes are not expressed when either carbon source is used. The second and third cases indicate that different groups of genes are expressed depending on the carbon source metabolized. The fourth case suggests that some genes are coexpressed. The procedure just outlined is used for expression analysis because it is the level of mRNA that is analyzed, although indirectly due to the use of the mRNA → fluorescent DNA copying step. To enable quantification, the fluorescent intensities are measured with a scanner. Lasers are used to excite the fluorescence and the image is digitized. Digitization allows for the calculation of intensity ratios.

Another useful application is genome typing. As before, DNA fragments are first spotted on a glass slide or another surface. However, instead of determining mRNA levels, genomic DNA fragments from a cell are directly used after they have been tagged with a fluorescent dye. One use of genome typing is to determine if an organism possesses a gene similar to different, yet more completely characterized organism. A gene inventory can be built for the less characterized organism because a binding event suggests that the less characterized organism possesses a gene found in the well-characterized organism.

An example of the output from a gene array experiment is best viewed in color. Examples can be found, for example, at the Web site managed by the National Center for Biotechnology Information (NCBI) (http://www.ncbi.nlm.nih.gov/geo/info/print_stats.cgi), which is one archive for genomic and expression data. It is suggested that an example be viewed while reading this and other explanatory texts. Other databases have been developed where researchers archive their array results; other sources are provided in the reference list.

Ongoing work aims to improve the "chip" technology further. For example, depending on how the DNA is processed prior to binding to the surface, different false positive and negative results can occur. Thus, it is important to understand the details of DNA binding reactions in order to minimize confounding results. Another active research direction is to improve how data from such large-scale screening experiments is processed such that relationships between genes and environmental conditions are clearly extracted. One basic challenge is represented by the size of the dataset; hundreds or thousands of signals cannot be interpreted by the unaided human mind; hence, computer-aided statistical methods are used. Thresholding techniques are often used to include or exclude particular signals from a gene chip and if done incorrectly, false positive and negatives can result. Finally, the analysis of time series data is of high interest. Such data can reveal the temporal sequence of how gene circuits operate. Again, large datasets are used, which presents challenges, and tools used in other fields for model identification from data with potential inherent uncertainty are being explored for use in this context.

References and Recommended Further Reading

Alberts, B., Bray, D., Lewis, J., Raff, M., Roberts, K., and Watson, J.D. *Molecular Biology of the Cell.* Garland Publishing, New York, 1994.

Dieffenbach, C.W. and Dveksler, G.S., eds. *PCR Primer: A Laboratory Manual.* Cold Spring Harbor Laboratory Press, Cold Spring Harbor, New York, 2003.

McPherson, M.J. and Møller, S.G. *PCR.* BIOS Scientific Publishers Limited, Oxford, 2001.

Stephen, A.E., Masiakos, P.T., Segev, D.L., Vacanti, J.P., Donahoe, P.K., and MacLaughlin, D.T. "Tissue-engineered cells producing complex recombinant proteins inhibit ovarian cancer *in vivo*." *Proc. Natl Acad. Sci. USA,* 98, 3214–3219, 2001.

Backgrounds on Some Molecular Biology Pioneers

Jacques Monod, François Jacob, & André Lwoff http://www.nobel.se/medicine/laureates/1965/

The Oswald T. Avery Collection from the National Library of Medicine http://profiles.nlm.nih.gov/CC/

Herbert Boyer http://www.accessexcellence.com/AB/BC/Herbert_Boyer.html

Theodor Svedberg http://www.nobel.se/chemistry/laureates/1926/svedberg-bio.html

James Sumner http://www.nobel.se/chemistry/laureates/1946/

Data Bases and Other Supplementary Materials on Basic Molecular Biology

The Comparative RNA Web (CRW) Site: an online database of comparative sequence and structure information for ribosomal, intron, and other RNAs. Jamie J. Cannone, Sankar Subramanian, Murray N. Schnare, James R. Collett, Lisa M. D'Souza, Yushi Du, Brian Feng, Nan Lin, Lakshmi V. Madabusi, Kirsten M. Müller, Nupur Pande, Zhidi Shang, Nan Yu, and Robin R. Gutell. *BMC Bioinformatics*, 2002; 3: 2. Copyright© 2002, Cannone et al.; licensee BioMed Central Ltd. Verbatim copying and redistribution of this article are permitted in any medium for any purpose, provided this notice is preserved along with the article's original URL.
   http://www.pubmedcentral.nih.gov/articlerender.fcgi?artid=65690&rendertype=abstract

Science Magazine Guide to On-Line Life Science Glossaries (The glossaries also talk to you).
   http://www.sciencemag.org/feature/plus/sfg/education/glossaries.shtml

General Glossary of Molecular Life Science Terms and Concepts from National Human Genome Research Institute (The glossaries also talk to you). http://www.genome.gov/10002096

Pictorial Dictionary of Protein Structural Levels from the National Human Genome Research Institute (The glossaries also talk to you).
   http://www.genome.gov/Pages/Hyperion//DIR/VIP/Glossary/Illustration/protein.shtml

Genentech Corporate Web Site http://www.gene.com/gene/index.jsp

A Journal Devoted to *Archaea http://archaea.ws/*

A Page on *Archaea* Sponsored by the American Society for Microbiology
   http://www.microbe.org/microbes/archaea.asp

Alternate Page on *Archaea* Sponsored by the American Society for Microbiology
   http://www.microbeworld.org/htm/aboutmicro/microbes/types/archaea.htm

The American Society for Microbiology http://www.asm.org/

Survey of DNA Crime Laboratories, 2001 from the U.S. Department of Justice
   http://www.ojp.usdoj.gov/bjs/pub/pdf/sdnacl01.pdf

Human Genome Project Information: DNA Forensics
   http://www.ornl.gov/TechResources/Human_Genome/elsi/forensics.html

Report and Recommendations of The Panel to Assess the NIH Investment in Research On Gene Therapy.
   http://www.nih.gov/news/panelrep.html

Prions are an Issue in Colorado and Elsewhere. Informative reports and an example of a monitoring study are provided in
   (http://resourcescommittee.house.gov/107cong/forests/2002may16/miller.htm
   http://www.nrel.colostate.edu/projects/cwd/

Information and Three-Dimensional Displays of Proteins and Enzymes (Protein Data Bank)
   http://www.rcsb.org/pdb/

More Information and Archives Regarding DNA Arrays

National Center for Biotechnology Information (NCBI)
   http://www.ncbi.nlm.nih.gov/geo/info/print_stats.cgi

Stanford Microarray Data Base. http://genome-www5.stanford.edu/

A Commercial Site with a lot of Background. http://www.gene-chips.com/

2

Systems and Technology Involving Bacteria

Nicole Bleckwenn
William Bentley
*University of Maryland
Biotechnology Institute*

2.1 Introduction

Bacteria are unicellular, relatively simple, and can double in very short times. These attributes can be exploited for technological advantage. They are useful for the expression of large quantities of products, such as proteins and enzymes, as well as small molecules that are not efficiently synthesized in the laboratory via bio-organic chemistry. Since bacteria lack the posttranslational machinery endogenous to eukaryotic cells (e.g., glycosylation; see Chapter 1), they are unable to process very complex proteins. However, a number of proteins with therapeutic value, such as insulin can be readily produced using bacteria. We will describe the molecular basis, from a systems viewpoint, for the many technological achievements already realized using bacteria, as well as those that are likely to see continued research and development.

2.2 Elements for Expression

In order to utilize bacterial culture as a production system for recombinant products, the cells must be "genetically engineered" to contain the genes for the products that are desired and the proper control elements that will allow expression of those products under the chosen conditions. Chapter 1 described some basic background information on the genetic elements and their function. As previously stated, *plasmid vectors* are generally the method-of-choice for inserting a gene of interest into the bacterial cells. The plasmid DNA is altered to contain the gene for the protein of interest with upstream cognate control

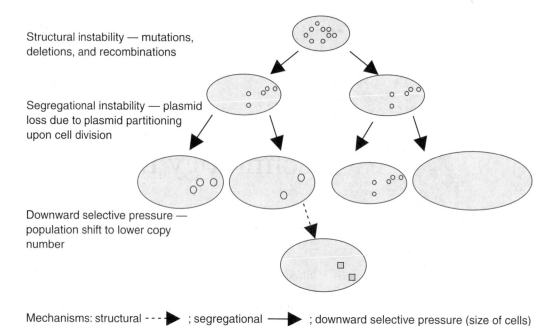

Structural instability — mutations, deletions, and recombinations

Segregational instability — plasmid loss due to plasmid partitioning upon cell division

Downward selective pressure — population shift to lower copy number

Mechanisms: structural - - - ▶ ; segregational ⟶ ; downward selective pressure (size of cells)

FIGURE 2.1 Mechanisms for plasmid loss (instability). Structural instability can lead to plasmid defects; segregational instability is caused by uneven distribution of plasmids to daughter cells; downward selective pressure is the combination of segregational and structural instability and the observation that plasmid-free cells grow (and divide) more quickly (denoted by large cells).

sequences. This plasmid is then inserted or "transformed" into "competent" bacteria. The most common methods to transform these cells are either through electrical or chemical means. These processes make the cells competent, which in a sense, open pores in the bacterial membranes big enough to allow entry of plasmid DNA. Because plasmids are naturally occurring among the *Eubacteria*, they are readily accepted by the cells. However, since plasmids are redistributed among the daughter cells upon cell division, there is a finite probability that the transformed cells are capable of losing or transferring plasmids. Some plasmids are thought to be randomly distributed to the daughter cells and in these cases, mother cells with few plasmids will generate daughter cells with no plasmids at a relatively high frequency. For example, if a dividing cell has just one plasmid, then one of the daughter cells will be born without a plasmid. Once that cell divides, it begins a process where its own progeny overtake cells with plasmids. Typically, cells that have more plasmids redirect more of the cellular machinery to functions encoded by the plasmid, and the cells grow more slowly. A schematic of this process is shown in Figure 2.1.

The loss of the recombinant plasmid must thus be prevented. This can be accomplished by inserting genetic stability elements, such as genes that encode antibiotic resistance, into the same plasmid as the gene of interest, and then provide antibiotics in the growth medium. In Chapter 1, the selection marker was used to identify positive clones. Here the same marker can serve to maintain a productive bioreactor. If the culture is grown under conditions of selection for a marker, such as in the presence of an antibiotic, only those cells retaining the plasmid with the resistance gene product will grow and proliferate in the culture. Another technique to minimize this problem is to use an inducible promoter so that resources are directed to protein production only after the culture has grown sufficiently. When product expression is *inducible*, the cells are less stressed because they are not producing product. Hence, they will be less likely to lose their plasmids, as reallocated resources are only needed for plasmid DNA replication. Also important for the expression of our gene of interest is the plasmid *copy number*, or the number of plasmid copies per cell or per chromosome. Generally, the higher the copy number, the more product is made, but there can be a trade-off in that high copy number cells may become overburdened and not grow properly.

In addition to maintaining the gene of interest on the plasmid, one needs to incorporate genetic switches that "turn on" or "turn off" expression. *Operons* are the natural molecular switches used by prokaryotic organisms to control expression of genes (see Figure 1.3). These natural segments can be "cut" and "pasted" into plasmids using restriction enzymes and ligases (biomolecular scissors and glue, respectively) to control expression of specific gene sequences that are desired, leading to the expression of recombinant products. The reconstruction of "controllable" promoters upstream (5′) of a gene of interest creates an *inducible expression system*. The best understood operon is the lactose or *lac* operon (see http://web.mit.edu/esgbio/www/pge/lac.html). It consists of genes for the repressor protein, promoter, operator, and three enzyme genes, *lacZ*, *lacY*, and *lacA*, which code for β-galactosidase, lactose permease, and galactoside transacetylase, respectively. Incidentally, genes are italicized and lowercase when written; proteins are capitalized and not italicized (e.g., *LacZ* for β-galactosidase). Lactose, as the inducer, binds the repressor preventing binding of the repressor to the operator, allowing transcription by RNA polymerase.

In the prior chapter, it was noted that sometimes more than inducer or repressor binding to an operator can be involved with turning genes on or off. *Catabolite repression* is one classic example that occurs at the *lac* promoter site. In the absence of the preferred carbon source, such as glucose, the intracellular cyclic AMP (cAMP) level rises. The rise reflects a deficiency in the usual molecular source of energy used to drive biosynthetic reactions, ATP. The cAMP complexes with CAP ("catabolite gene activator protein" or also called "cAMP Repressor Protein," CRP) to bind to the promoter, which further enhances RNA polymerase binding, and amplifies transcription and translation of the three enzymes. This can be a problem in industrial fermentations where glucose is used as the principal carbon source: when glucose is present there is little production of the desired protein.

Industrial utilization of the *lac* operon has been tailored, therefore, for controlled expression of proteins. Part of the *lac* promoter sequence (-10 region), which provides for *lac* induction is included; but the -35 region is taken from the tryptophan operon because it is not subject to catabolite repression. The combination, *tac*, is reportedly ten times stronger than the native *lac* sequence. A gratuitous (nonmetabolized) inducer, IPTG (isopropyl-β-D-thiogalactopyranoside), has been shown to act as an effective inducer for this hybrid system.

2.3   A Cell-to-Cell Communications Operon

Many operons have been studied that take queues from the environment or other parts of the cell and modulate protein expression at the level of transcription. Some of these are simple sugars, such as lactose for the *lac* operon, but other operons involve different small molecules in their control architectures. Another example has to do with all out cell warfare: survival of microbes that live in a symbiotic relationship with squid [1,2]. It turns out that the nocturnal Hawaiian bobtail squid emits light downwards through its mantle cavity and, by matching the intensity of the moon- and starlight above, the squid becomes invisible to other predators below. The adult squid is ~2 cm long and some very interesting photos are found in Fuqua and Greenberg [1]. How does this squid make light? There is a *Vibrio fischeri* light organ close to the ink sac within the mantle cavity of the animal. This light organ contains ~10^{11} *Vibrio fischeri* cells per milliliter, and these *Vibrio* actually make the light by the expressing light emitting genes denoted *lux* (as per the Latin saying "*fiat lux*: let there be light"). So, in the absence of the *Vibrio*, the squid (and the *Vibrio*) would be swallowed up by large fish.

The *lux* genes are transcribed in an operon that responds to another small molecule, 3-oxo-C6-HSL (which is an acylated homoserine lactone [HSL]), one of a family of HSLs that stimulate gene expression in many different bacteria. The interesting part of this phenomenon is that as the cells accumulate (like in the mantle cavity of the bobtail squid), they secrete HSLs that act as autoinducers (AI), which in turn, accumulate in concentration. As the autoinducer concentration reaches a critical point, the bacteria all respond in a multicellular coordinated fashion: they emit light! To accomplish this, the HSLs bind to cognate transcriptional activators, which then stimulate expression of the *lux* genes. The *lux* gene products use ATP and luciferin to produce small quantities of light. This process was given the name "quorum sensing" by Greenberg, who recognized that a certain number of bacteria (or, more appropriately, a certain concentration of its secreted autoinducer), was needed for a formal "vote."

The *lux* genes proved interesting from the perspective of the operon structure and the need to elucidate mechanisms by which bacteria respond to queues from their microenvironment. They are also interesting because they serve as *markers* of gene expression. That is, because the protein products of *lux* genes are easily seen (quantified), they are used as reporters of gene transcription. LacZ, from the *lac* operon, is another often used marker of gene expression. In order to delineate the function of gene sequences that putatively serve as promoters, operators, initiation sites, etc., marker genes are often included downstream of the DNA regulatory sequence in question. Then, expression of the marker is quantitatively compared, reflecting the strength of the promoter region under study.

2.4   Marker Proteins

Marker proteins have been used as vital tool in the study of bacterial systems and have also been used to evaluate the production of recombinant products from them. These markers make use of nature's diversity for specific purposes. Marker proteins are easily detected and measured. Markers allow us to assess what's happening in cells at the protein level. They also provide a measure of localized gene expression. They are inserted in series or in parallel in plasmid expression vectors to monitor the level of expression from the system and promoter. Common markers include β-galactosidase, green fluorescent protein (GFP), and dsRed. The use of protein markers accelerated during the late 1990s due, in large part, to the exquisite attributes of green fluorescent protein (reviewed in March et al. [3]). GFP requires no cofactors (such as ATP for *lux* genes) and no substrates (such as X-gal for *lacZ*). GFP can be readily visualized from within cells and tissues because it absorbs light in the UV/blue/violet range and emits it back at a longer wavelength, green. This is the basic premise of fluorescence. In the case of GFP, a simple photodiode detector can be used to quantify the level of its fluorescence [4].

Green fluorescent protein has been used to study gene regulation. It has been used to evaluate localization of proteins within cells. It has been used to visualize phagocytosis, where big cells (such as white blood cells in humans) devour little cells, such as microbes, swimming around in our blood stream. GFP has also been used to mark product protein synthesis in a host of organisms, from bacteria to insect larvae. Some interesting photos are available at www.chesapeakeperl.com, a company that makes proteins in caterpillars.

In the bacterial systems world, GFP has also been used to indicate both high and low oxygen tension in bioreactors. That is, the bacteria are transformed into mini cell-based sensors. In the case of high oxygen, DNA and protein damage can result due to the elicitation of oxygen radicals and reactive oxygen species (ROS), such as hydrogen peroxide. By inserting the *gfp* gene downstream of an ROS sensitive promoter, cells that become exposed to ROS synthesize GFP. This is readily detected by a GFP-specific optical probe that can be inserted into the fermentor. In this way, one can use the fluorescence measurement as an indicator of the cell's physiology.

It is common in industrial fermentations to use hardwired analytical instrumentation to monitor reactor conditions, such as temperature, pH, and oxygen. But, it is only in the most recent years, that bioprocess engineers have begun to examine the responses of the cells as indicators of their own microenvironments. Thus, one might typically equip a bioreactor with one (or several) oxygen probes, but this indicates the oxygen level in the liquid at the precise location of the probe. The cells, however, are constantly circulating in and out of spatially restricted areas like those near baffles, or areas of high shear rate like near the impellers. They might also pass by a feed tube, or the oxygenating air sparging ring (see Figure 2.2). By measuring their physiological response to oxygen, we learn more about the actual environment they experience. Hence we can develop more sophisticated process control schemes, tank and impeller designs, and even tailor host cells and protein expression vectors, that are designed to meet the physiological demands of the cells when they produce products.

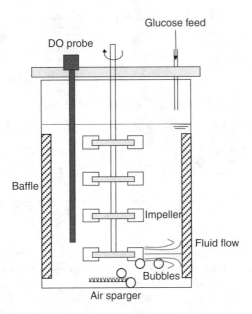

FIGURE 2.2 Schematic of a bioreactor. Oxygen is introduced to reactor at the air sparger. Bubbles are sheared at the impellers and entrained in the liquid, which impinges on the vessel walls and then is forced to circulate vertically. A well-mixed reactor has few "dead" or "stagnant" regions where circulation is minimal.

2.5 Growth of Bacterial Cultures

One of the advantages of using bacteria to make products is their rapid doubling time. Bacteria reproduce by binary fission: one becomes two, two become four, etc. The time over which the cells undergo a generation is also known as the doubling time. The number of cells, growing under binary fission, continually increases in an exponential manner. Thus, if a cell is making a protein and the cell grows exponentially, one can get copious quantities of protein in a short time.

Bacterial cultures are typically grown in liquid medium. Once inoculation occurs, the cells' growth can generally be described by a set of growth phases (see Figure 2.3). These begin with the lag phase, where the cells are adapting to the new environment and the cell number does not increase significantly. The next phase, called exponential or logarithmic growth phase, occurs when the cells are dividing rapidly and the cell mass and cell number are increasing exponentially. Here, the doubling time (τ_D), or time it takes the cell mass to double, is about 20 min for rapidly growing *E. coli*. The growth rate of exponentially growing cultures can be determined mathematically using the equation $\ln(X/X_0) = \mu(t - t_0)$ where X and X_0 are the cell concentrations at time t and time t_0, and μ is the *specific growth rate* in units of inverse time. The growth rate can also be determined graphically by plotting the logarithm (natural log scale) of the cell number data during this phase against time, the slope of the straight line will be the growth rate. The third phase of growth in a bacterial cell culture is the *stationary phase* where either nutrients become limiting or waste products become inhibiting. Here, the net growth rate becomes zero as the growth and death rates equal each other. Secondary metabolism may occur during this time, where nongrowth associated products and building blocks for survival in the changing environment are produced. When the cells finally succumb to the nutrient depleted conditions, they enter the *death phase*, where the cell number and optical density (measured as light absorbance in the visible region) actually decline.

The environment for growth of bacterial cultures must be carefully controlled to minimize the lag and stationary phases. This can be accomplished by increasing the inoculum size to increase the initial cell number and reduce the amount of time it takes for doubling of the culture to become apparent. If a low inoculum size is used, an extended "apparent" lag phase may just be due to the small number of cells which may be doubling, but do not register as a significant increase by the methods used to

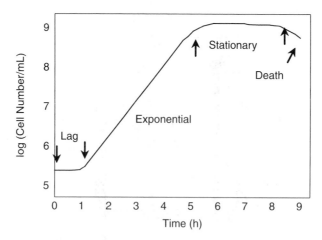

FIGURE 2.3 Phases of bacterial cell growth. After inoculation, cells adapt to their new environment during the *lag phase*, grow rapidly by regular binary fission during the *exponential phase*, stop growing from nutrient limitation during the *stationary phase*, then eventually die (*death phase*).

measure cell number. One can also ensure that the cells used in the inoculum are themselves growing exponentially. Then they will adapt more quickly to their new environment. The stationary phase can also be delayed, to maintain a longer exponential growth phase, by ensuring the culture environment through precise control of culture parameters, such as dissolved oxygen, pH, and temperature and also through appropriate medium exchange, which will provide all the necessary nutrients and remove any harmful waste products which may inhibit growth of the cells.

When growing bacteria to produce recombinant proteins, one of the most critical aspects is *oxygen transfer*. Typically this is a problem because the solubility of oxygen in water (or growth media) is very low. Cells utilize what is dissolved in the liquid and bacterial cells (which grow rapidly) use this oxygen at a very high rate. Hence, it is vital to deliver oxygen to the liquid phase at a rate that at least matches the bacterial consumption rate. The transport of oxygen is proportional to the *driving force* for mass transfer (concentration difference between the level of O_2 in the water at saturation and current O_2 level). The proportionality constant, the volumetric oxygen transfer coefficient from the gas to liquid interface, is denoted $k_L a$. This constant contains both a liquid film intrinsic rate constant, k_L (e.g., h^{-1}), and an interfacial area per unit volume, a (e.g., $cm^2/cm^3 = cm^{-1}$), over which the transport from the gas to liquid phases occurs. Aeration is most commonly achieved by sparging the liquid medium through tubing and other distribution devices having small orifices. Bubbles are generated in the liquid medium providing surface area for mass transfer surface. The impeller is typically located just above the sparger, this is the main distributor of oxygen because it shreds bubbles into tiny droplets of high surface area to volume ratio, a parameter that needs to be maximized for effective transfer. Hence, bubble creation, sizing, and distribution are all key to oxygen mass transfer in any given bioreactor.

Importantly, as the scale of a fermentation process increases (from lab to production), the height to diameter ratio of the bioreactor is often kept constant in the range of 1:2 to 1:3, and this means that the surface area to volume ratio of the entire reactor dramatically decreases at higher volumes. It then becomes even more important to understand the physical reactor system and the methods used to attain high levels of dissolved oxygen, as well as the interplay between the physical reactor and the cell physiology. Oxygen is important because bacterial metabolism is exquisitely controlled, as noted with respect to ROS. At times cell responses can so dramatically influence physiology, that the cells become completely nonproductive from a product standpoint. That is, depending on the insult, a cell response can influence many cellular activities.

The *heat shock response*, for example, is a well characterized physiological response in that many molecules have been identified that are either *upregulated* or *downregulated* due to the specific environmental insult (a rapidly increased temperature). The players that are changed include *proteases* (enzymes that digest proteins), *chaperones* (proteins that help fold proteins), transcription factors, as well as components of cell synthesis machinery [5]. In general, the cells rearrange or adapt their physiology for enhanced survival in the new condition. One of the key upregulated elements is the *heat shock transcription factor, sigma 32* (σ^{32}). As noted previously (e.g., bacterial autoinducers, HSLs), transcription is modulated by small molecule *effectors* that bind to cognate transcription factors, such as repressors and activators. One of the other vital components of bacterial transcription is the *sigma factor*, a protein that helps the polymerase bind to the specific initiation sites in order to carry out transcription. *E. coli* have seven sigma factors, each responsible for a specific regulatory domain. The sigma factor is thus a part of the transcriptional polymerase *holoenzyme*. Under normal conditions, bacteria use sigma factor 70 (σ^{70}) to target transcription of normal *housekeeping genes*. Under heat shock, σ^{32} overrides σ^{70}, and serves to amplify transcription of heat shock genes. The protein products of these genes are collectively known as *heat shock proteins (hsps)*, and are coordinately regulated by (σ^{32}). When cells overexpress recombinant protein, a "stress" response results, similar but not identical to the heat shock response. When genes are coordinately regulated, they constitute a *regulon*, which will be described in more detail in Section 2.6.

2.6 Regulons

The regulon consists of genes that are not necessarily located near each other in the genome nor do they necessarily have the same promoter/operator elements. The heat shock response regulon is a primary example whereby, in response to a sudden stress, such as a rise in temperature, the regulon initiates production of certain proteins at a higher (or lower) level than normal. Another regulon is associated with HSL-mediated quorum sensing: a series of proteins are up or downregulated in direct response to a particular queue. Understanding regulons, and how they interact, is an emerging area of *systems biology*. For example, a sigma factor associated with nutrient limitation, σ^S, is known to influence levels of proteins that also play a role in the heat shock response.

An effective way to characterize operons, regulons, and their role within the stoichiometry of bacterial metabolism is to refer to the interactions as *genetic circuits*. For example, in *Salmonella*, Bassler and coworkers [6] recently discovered that the uptake mechanism of the quorum sensing autoinducer was itself regulated by AI-2. Thus, the cells make autoinducer AI-2 in one biosynthesis pathway and they use this autoinducer to regulate its own uptake from the extracellular media by modulating transcription of the uptake genes. This constitutes a small genetic circuit. Interestingly, glucose (which plays a huge role in physiology) seems to play a direct role in quorum sensing. That is, CRP directly binds to the promoter region of *lsr* genes and modulates their transcription. Previous researchers had already shown that the bacterial autoinducer AI-2 regulates genes in other bacteria. Thus, it has become apparent that quorum circuitry and glucose circuitry intersect, and these intersections are not confined to *E. coli*, but rather are conserved among many bacteria.

Understanding the underpinning regulation of gene transcription in bacteria is important if we are to exploit their tremendous biosynthetic potential. Understanding the mapping of regulation onto metabolic pathways is important for generating microbial and eukaryotic systems that produce products. Manipulating metabolic flow using recombinant DNA techniques, as pointed out in Chapter 1, is now commonly referred to as *metabolic engineering* [7]. By altering existing pathways and augmenting cells with nonnative enzymatic capabilities, metabolic engineers have created microbes that make new products, including even plastics.

In bioreactors, cells damaged by high doses of oxygen that form radicals, peroxide, etc., upregulate stress related proteins that, in turn, have been exquisitely tailored and designed to deal with the high oxygen. Among the proteins that deal with oxygen transfer are peroxide scavengers, such as *superoxide dismutase* (SOD) and oxygen carriers, such as bacterial *hemoglobin*. In a metabolic engineering application, Stark and coworkers [8] transformed *E. coli* with hemoglobin from *Vitreoscilla* and after cultivating them at high cell density in an environment not noted for good oxygen transfer, they found increased product production. By metabolically engineering the cells, they transformed the oxygen genetic circuit into a positive regulatory element for increasing protein production when the cells were grown deprived of oxygen.

As noted above, some physiological and metabolic elements are tightly coordinated. This is not always the case. In fact, it is more likely that any two given elements are only loosely linked, even when they are directly connected by biochemical pathways. In this way, Nature's regulatory and control mechanisms can fine-tune systems to meet widely varied conditions that are typically experienced by the cells. Glycolysis, for example, is only loosely tied to the *tricarboxylic acid cycle* (TCA cycle), even though they are directly linked biochemically (see http://web.mit.edu/esgbio/www/glycolysis/dir.html). In glycolysis, glucose is brought into the cell and *catabolized* into three carbon sugars, such as *pyruvate*. Pyruvate is then converted to acetyl-CoA, which is brought into the TCA cycle. This circular pathway yields many compounds including CO_2, ATP, and chemical reducing potential in the form of NADH. The NADH is recycled to NAD^+, with concomitant generation of ATP, during *respiration (oxidative phosphorylation)*. Glucose uptake can actually exceed the electron transfer capacity of respiration, particularly if cells are grown in a rich growth medium containing high amounts of glucose. A result is the overflow of semi-oxidized sugars, such as acetate [9]. Metabolic engineering efforts to direct control of glycolysis and respiration have led to reduced acetate and higher product yields.

The desire to understand rates of material flow through metabolic pathways has received the attention of many researchers seeking to quantitatively describe cell physiology. *Metabolic Flux Analysis* [10,11], *Metabolic Control Analysis* [12], and several other mathematical techniques have been successfully applied to bacterial systems for the external manipulation of metabolic activities, including synthesis of nonnative compounds of commercial interest.

2.7   Engineering the System

As might be inferred from above, altering pathways for specific purposes requires first, a preliminary understanding of the interconnectedness of the pathway in question with other pathways. Then, one needs to understand the regulation of the flux through the pathway. Neither of these is trivial. Databases, such as KEGG (http://www.genome.ad.jp/kegg/), EcoCyc (http://ecocyc.org/), and NRCAM (http://www.nrcam.uchc.edu/) can help. Ultimately, one needs molecular tools to appropriately engineer the system.

Suppose material A moves down a path where it will be converted to either B or C, the specific direction decided by access to one of two enzymes (e_1 or e_2) (see Figure 2.4). In chemical reaction engineering, it is common to explain reaction kinetics by referring to reactants and products as "A," "B," or "C," etc. In the biochemical pathway for autoinducer AI-2 synthesis, "A," "B," and "C," might represent *S*-adenosylmethionine (SAM), *S*-adenosylhomocysteine (SAH), and *S*-ribosylhomocysteine (SRH), respectively. By incorporating the gene for enzyme, e_1, on a plasmid and by transforming the plasmid into the host bacteria, one can increase the level of enzyme, e_1, with the hope that it will increase the flux of material through that enzymatic pathway. This is, by far, the most common route for metabolically engineering the system. Another tack is to mutate the gene for e_2 (using one or more of the techniques from the last chapter) so that it is either of diminished activity or completely ablated. Under this scenario, the flux must proceed along enzyme, e_1. Again, this technique works extremely well, particularly for systems where there are few target enzymes or proteins that need to be mutated. Many examples have been developed for altering small molecule synthesis, such as decreased acetate production from *E. coli*. Another excellent example, that has to do with macromolecule synthesis, is the mutation of proteases that degrade recombinant proteins [13], so that overexpression of proteins is met with a less severe cell response (at least one devoid of product degrading proteases!). In general, however, this seemingly simple manipulation is met with unexpected cell responses. Such *pleiotropy* is common and is beginning to be elucidated, in large part because of the emerging experimental techniques that are used to understand cell physiology at the systems level (e.g., DNA microarrays from Chapter 1).

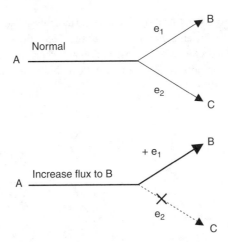

FIGURE 2.4 Pathway engineered to increase yield of compound "B." Normally (upper panel), flux of A proceeds through both enzymes e_1 and e_2, to produce B and C, respectively. By augmenting cells with additional e_1, or by deleting or downregulating e_2, one can increase yield of B (lower panel).

In summary, bacterial systems are the workhorse of modern biotechnology. The tools exist for their genetic manipulation. Also, industrial bioreactors attempt to create microenvironments suitable for bacterial growth and product expression. Through the exploitation of their rapid growth rates and biosynthetic capabilities, bacteria have served as miniature cell "factories" for the synthesis of many products and processes that are already on the market. With a more comprehensive understanding of their biosynthetic and biodegradative pathways (as well as their regulation!), next generation processes and products will certainly come to fruition.

References

[1] Fuqua, C. and E.P. Greenberg. 2002. Listening in on bacteria: acyl-homoserine lactone signalling. *Nat. Rev. Mol. Cell Biol.* **3:** 685–695.

[2] Lupp, C., M. Urbanowski, E.P. Greenberg, and E.G. Ruby. 2003. The *Vibrio fischeri* quorum-sensing systems *ain* and *lux* sequentially induce luminescence gene expression and are important for persistence in the squid host. *Mol. Microbiol.* **50:** 319–331.

[3] March, J.C., G. Rao, and W.E. Bentley. 2003. Biotechnological applications of green fluorescent protein. *Appl. Microbiol. Biotechnol.* **62:** 303–315.

[4] Kostov, Y., C.R. Albano, and G. Rao. 2000. All solid-state GFP sensor. *Biotechnol. Bioeng.* **70:** 473–477.

[5] Bukau, B. 1993. Regulation of the *Escherichia coli* heat-shock response. *Mol. Microbiol.* **9:** 671–680.

[6] Taga, M.E., S.T. Miller, and B.L. Bassler. 2003. Lsr-mediated transport and processing of AI-2 in *Salmonella typhimurium. Mol. Microbiol.* **50:** 1411–1427.

[7] Bailey, J.E. 1991. Toward a science of metabolic engineering. *Science* **252:** 1668–1675.

[8] Khosravi, M., D.A. Webster, and B.C. Stark. 1990. Presence of the bacterial hemoglobin gene improves alpha-amylase production of a recombinant *Escherichia coli* strain. *Plasmid* **24:** 190–194.

[9] Majewski, R.A. and M.M. Domach. 1990. Simple constrained-optimization view of acetate overflow in *Escherichia coli. Biotechnol. Bioeng.* **35:** 732–738.

[10] Hofmeyr, J.H. 1989. Control-pattern analysis of metabolic pathways. Flux and concentration control in linear pathways. *Eur. J. Biochem.* **186:** 343–354.

[11] Holms, H. 1996. Flux analysis and control of the central metabolic pathways in *Escherichia coli. FEMS Microbiol. Rev.* **19:** 85–116.

[12] Fell, D.A. and H.M. Sauro. 1985. Metabolic control and its analysis. Additional relationships between elasticities and control coefficients. *Eur. J. Biochem.* **148:** 555–561.

[13] Meerman, H.J. and G. Georgiou. 1994. Construction and characterization of a set of *E. coli* strains deficient in all known loci affecting the proteolytic stability of secreted recombinant proteins. *Biotechnology (NY)* **12:** 1107–1110.

3

Recombinant DNA Technology Using Mammalian Cells

Tina Sauerwald
Centocor R&D Inc.

Michael Betenbaugh
Johns Hopkins University

3.1 Expression in Mammalian Cells

3.1.1 Introduction

Mammalian cells, like bacterial hosts, can be engineered to produce various types of recombinant proteins including secreted proteins, such as monoclonal antibodies or growth factors; intracellular proteins such as enzymes; and membrane proteins such as growth factor receptors. Mammalian expression systems offer numerous advantages over the use of bacteria, yeast, or insect cells for the production of complex recombinant proteins of human or mammalian origin. Mammalian cells can generate fully functional mammalian recombinant proteins including correct folding and proper posttranslational modifications such as disulfide bond formation, prenylation, carboxylation, and phosphorylation. Of special note is the capacity for certain mammalian cell lines to perform glycosylational modifications very similar to those obtained in humans. As a result, secreted and membrane glycoproteins generated by mammalian cells are not recognized as foreign by the human immune system and will remain in the circulatory system for extended periods. In addition, mammalian cells readily secrete some recombinant proteins, allowing for ease of isolation of the product from the surrounding culture medium. In contrast, many bacterial systems require intracellular expression and the attendant purification and refolding of proteins from cell lysates. Regardless of the type of recombinant protein being produced, expression is dependent upon multiple factors. These include factors at the level of the DNA, including gene copy number or insertion site in the genome, at the level of RNA , such as mRNA processing and stability, and polypeptide considerations, such as folding, transport, processing, and stability. In order to generate the product of interest, many facets of cell line development can be considered, including vector design, the use of inducible systems, type of mammalian cell lines, transfection methods, transient vs. stable transfection, selection, and single cell cloning. These facets are discussed in greater detail later.

3.1.2 Vector Design

Mammalian expression vectors can be classified into two main categories: viral vectors and plasmid vectors. Viral vectors are usually inactivated viruses engineered to code for a foreign gene of interest, whereas plasmids are circular DNA elements containing prokaryotic, eukaryotic, and viral DNA. The initial gene manipulation steps with plasmid vectors are performed in bacteria due to the ease of performing genetic engineering techniques in these hosts. Prokaryotic sequences are necessary for replication of the plasmid in the bacterial hosts, but, the target gene of interest is not expressed. Instead, viral and eukaryotic sequences control transcription of a selectable marker gene and the gene encoding the product of interest once the vector is inserted into the mammalian host. The vectors are generally classified with respect to the viral backbone used as the basis for construction. Some examples of viral backbones include adeno, herpes simplex, SV40, and vaccinia, all of which are useful in a broad array of mammalian cell types.

Viral vectors allow for efficient transfer of foreign DNA into the host cell through the production of infectious virus particles. The viral delivery system is typically a defective virus, which contains the sequence for the gene of interest under the control of a viral promoter. The defective virus is incapable of replicating without the aid of a helper cell line containing the genes coding for the structural proteins that allow for the packaging of the recombinant progeny virus. Recombinant vaccinia virus and alphaviruses, of which Sindbis virus and Semliki Forest virus are the most common, are examples of viral expression systems useful for high-level transient expression. Both vaccinia virus and alphavirus systems are operative in a broad range of cell lines; however, cell death is rapidly observed following infection. Adenovirus, adeno-associated virus, and retrovirus all provide longer-term, lower-level expression. Adeno-associated virus will infect a more versatile range of cells while randomly integrating into the host cell's genome in contrast to adenovirus, which displays site-specific integration into chromosome 19. The multiplicity of infection, the condition of the cells and culture at the time of infection, and the promoter driving the foreign gene all play an important role in protein production regardless of the type of viral vector used. In addition, although viral vectors provide a convenient method for production in many cell types, the use of this system for the generation of commercial production cell lines may raise serious regulatory concerns.

Plasmid vectors are composed of multiple elements as shown in Figure 3.1. These components typically include a strong promoter located upstream of the 5′ ATG start codon for the DNA coding for a foreign gene of interest and a polyadenylation sequence (poly A tail) located downstream from the 3′ stop codon

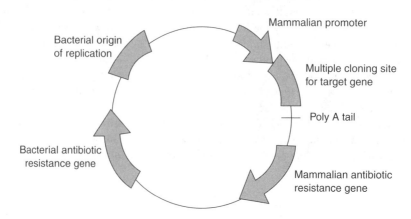

FIGURE 3.1 Typical mammalian expression vector.

of the foreign gene. A polylinker sequence comprising numerous restriction enzyme sites is present in many plasmids allowing for ease of insertion of different target DNA sequences in between the promoter and polyadenylation sequence. A second promoter and polyadenylation sequence is present to control transcription of a selectable marker such as an antibiotic resistance gene. Promoters may be derived from either viruses or cellular genes. Some of the most common constitutive viral promoters are SV40 early, cytomegalovirus (CMV) immediate early, and adenovirus major late (AdMLP). In addition, promoters have originated from such cellular genes as heat shock protein (HSP) and immunoglobulins (Ig). Polyadenylation sequences, which are necessary for the termination and polyadenylation of the transcribed mRNA, also have been derived from the SV40 genome and Ig genes. Numerous selectable markers, discussed in detail later in the text, exist that either offer cytotoxic drug resistance or encode for a metabolic gene. Additional components that may be added to plasmids include Kozak sequences, which promote efficient translation of the adjoining foreign DNA; enhancers, which are *cis*-acting DNA sequences to promote transcription; and introns, which may increase the expression level of the foreign DNA. In addition to the above eukaryotic expression components, plasmids also include an origin of replication (ori) and a bacterial selection marker, such as ampicillin or kanamycin, in order to allow for propagation and cloning in a bacterial host, usually *Escherichia coli*.

Sometimes it is desirable to coexpress multiple genes in a mammalian cell line, in which case cells may be transfected with either multiple plasmids, each coding for a different foreign gene, a single plasmid containing multiple promoters and gene insertion sites, or a polycistronic plasmid. A polycistronic plasmid contains two (dicistronic), three (tricistronic), or four (quatrocistronic) genes under the control of one promoter. In this system, a single mRNA transcript is produced with only the first cistron, or gene, translated in a cap-dependent manner. Prior to each subsequent gene, an internal ribosome entry site (IRES) is inserted. Consequently, the IRES element initiates translation of each subsequent cistron. The most common IRES elements used are those derived from encephalomyocarditis virus or poliovirus. Variations in the expression level among the coexpressed genes are observed in this system and may be attributed to the foreign gene and the IRES element used. In those instances when the final gene is a selection marker, weakening of translation initiation allows for an elevation in expression level of the gene of interest. In addition, upon the creation of a stable cell line, the use of a selectable marker $3'$ to the foreign gene should result in foreign gene expression in all surviving selected colonies. For example, when neomycin phosphotransferase selection was used downstream of the gene coding for human 5-HTI1Da serotonin receptor and the encephalomyocarditis IRES, all clonal cell lines expressed similar levels of the receptor [1].

Most plasmids will integrate randomly into the host chromosome. However, a key problem that arises to restrict gene expression is the insertion of the foreign DNA into an inactive region of the chromosome. To combat this dilemma, site-specific recombinases have been studied to target the integration of foreign DNA into specific, active chromosomal areas. The family of site-specific recombinases, which catalyzes the inclusion or exclusion of DNA fragments in a chromosome, comprises several members including Cre, Flp, HP1, and XerD. All four of these enzymes recognize unique nucleic acid sequences composed of two palindromic sequences sandwiched around a DNA core. However, the recognition sites generally do not occur naturally in eukaryotes; therefore, the host cell's genome must be altered to include the recognition site. Then transfection of the recombinase and foreign gene may be performed, resulting in site-specific recombination.

Although the majority of plasmid vectors have the capability to insert into the genome of the host cell posttransfection, there are instances in which integration is not desired. For these applications, a type of vector called the episomal vector may be used. An episomal vector has been developed based on the Epstein–Barr virus (EBV) that allows for production of a foreign gene while being maintained within the nucleus separate from the host cell's genome. Advantages of this type of system include the insertion of large stretches of foreign DNA into the vector and the consequent production of protein independent from integration site variability. In one example, an episomal vector was generated with a tricistronic system that provided for the expression of blue, green, and yellow fluorescent proteins simultaneously in a stably transfected 293 cell line [2].

3.1.3 Inducible Systems

The ability to regulate foreign gene expression in a cell offers the capability to express proteins that are cytotoxic to the cell and alternatively to study the function of a particular foreign gene in a mammalian cell line. An ideal inducible system should possess the following characteristics (1) minimal or no expression of the foreign gene in the absence of inducer, (2) high gene expression in the presence of inducer, (3) a rapid response rate to the addition and removal of inducer, (4) a repeatable response to the addition and removal of inducer, and (5) no pleiotropic effects upon induction. Numerous inducible vector systems are used that exploit endogenous or modified cellular promoters that respond to exogenous stresses or signals, such as metal ions, steroid hormones, cytokines, hypoxia, and heat shock. The problem with many of these systems is that they are of mammalian origin; consequently, there are pleiotropic effects in which other cellular genes also will be induced, confounding experimental results. This lack of selectivity of these promoters has been addressed through mutation of the cellular elements or the use of nonmammalian systems. Examples of improved inducible systems include the RU486/mifepristone inducible system, the FK506/rapamycin inducible system, the tetracycline inducible system, and the ecdysone inducible system. The ecdysone inducible expression system, as shown in Figure 3.2, is described in detail as an example of inducible promoters.

Ecdysone, a *Drosophila melanogaster* steroid hormone, targets its respective ecdysone receptor (EcR). Upon dimerization of this receptor to the product of the *Drosophila* ultraspiracle gene (USP), the heterodimer functions as an ecdysone-dependent transcriptional activator. In order to create an ecdysone inducible system, the EcR and USP genes are transfected into a mammalian cell line of interest. Next, or in concert, a foreign gene of interest is introduced into the mammalian cells under the control of an EcR-USP sensitive transcriptional activator (Figure 3.2, Part I). In the absence of any inducer, transcription is repressed (Part IIa). However, addition of the inducer, ecdysone, or analogs such as muristerone A, results in binding of the inducer to the EcR-USP complex and subsequent activation of transcription (Part IIb) [3,4]. Improvements to the 3-fold induction observed in the original system have been made that have successfully increased foreign gene expression following induction. The use of the retinoic X receptor (RXR), the mammalian homolog to USP, in the heterodimer with EcR improved responsiveness of induction 34-fold and creating an EcR/GR hybrid by replacing EcR's N-terminal transactivation domain with the corresponding domain of the glucocorticoid receptor led to a 3- to 11-fold induction [5]. However, the most potent induction observed by these researchers involved the use of another EcR hybrid containing the VP16 activation domain in conjunction with RXR giving a 212-fold induction [5]. Since this early work, even greater improvements have been made including a 8900-fold induction observed in a two-hybrid system at 48 h postinduction [6]. Benefits of the ecdysone inducible system include the lack of toxicity of ecdysone, minimal basal expression by the promoter when not induced, and lack of EcR homologs in mammalian cell lines.

3.1.4 Cell Lines

Numerous cell lines have been developed for the purpose of recombinant protein expression; however, several cell lines have dominated the field. Chinese hamster ovary (CHO), NSO and SP2/0 murine myeloma, human embryonic kidney (HEK293), and COS cell lines are popular choices. HeLa, BHK, YB2/0, and PerC6 are several other available options that are not discussed in detail here. Several of these cell lines can be grown in attachment-dependent monolayers or suspension cultures. For large-scale culture, cell suspension is preferred.

Generally, Chinese hamster ovary cells are used as either CHO-K1 cells or as *dhfr⁻* cells for the generation of stable cell lines. The original *dhfr⁻* cell line was developed by Dr. Lawrence Chasin through the mutagenesis and selection of the CHO-K1 line [7]. Cells were selected based on their inability to produce dihydrofolate reductase, an enzyme necessary for the conversion of folate to tetrahydrofolate. From this early work, the CHO *dhfr*-deficient cell lines, DG44 and DXB11, have been generated as expression systems that take advantage of the lack of endogenous *dhfr* expression in conjunction with sequential

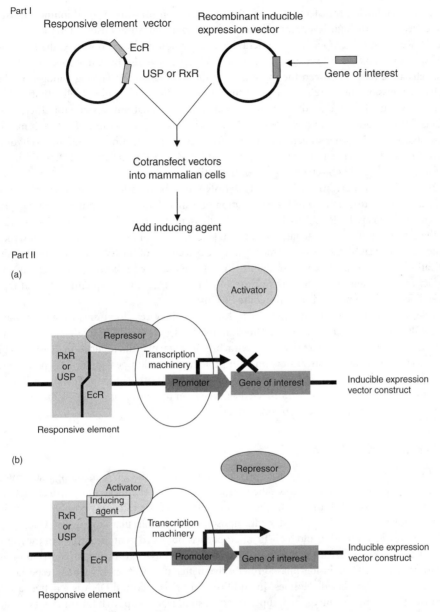

FIGURE 3.2 Ecdysone inducible mammalian expression system. Part I: Components of the transfection system. Part II(a): Uninduced system, (b): Induction of gene expression by addition of inducing agent.

methotrexate selection following transfection to amplify the copy number of the foreign gene of interest. Gene amplification is a survival tactic for the mammalian cells since the transfected and incorporated plasmid also contains the DHFR gene to overcome methotrexate selection by a mechanism described in detail in a later section. Because inhibition of the cytotoxic agent, methotrexate, occurs stoichiometrically, the cells will increase their copy numbers to overcome the effects of the drug.

Expression in NSO cells gained importance with the discovery that because NSO cells express exceedingly low levels of glutamine synthetase (GS), the GS gene used in combination with glutamine-free medium and the GS inhibitor, methionine sulfoximine, can be used to generate cell lines expressing high levels of foreign proteins [8]. GS is an enzyme responsible for the production of glutamine from ammonia and glutamate. Following transfection and increasing selection pressure of methionine sulfoximine in glutamine-free medium, high-level expression of a chimeric antibody was observed in the resultant stable cell line. However, in this amplification system, lower copy numbers were observed than that normally obtained with the CHO-DHFR system [8]. A similar GS system has also been developed in CHO as well.

SP2/0 cells are a fusion between the myeloma cell line P3X63Ag8.653 lacking endogenous light and heavy-chain expression and BALB/c spleen cells that possess anti-sheep red blood cell activity [9]. This cell line is commonly used for the production of antibodies due to its natural capacity for efficient secretion of proteins. Introduction of antibody DNA can be done by one of two methods. First, cells may be fused to mouse spleen cells in order to generate a hybridoma cell line that produces an antibody of interest. Otherwise, a transfectoma cell line may be generated by transfecting cells with a plasmid or plasmids coding for the heavy- and light-chain regions of the antibody.

HEK293 cells and its derivatives, 293T and 293EBNA, may be used for transient or stable expression [10]. HEK293 cells were generated by transformation of primary cultures of human embryogenic kidney (HEK) cells with sheared adenovirus DNA, 293T cells were generated by modification of HEK293 to express the activating protein, SV40 large T-antigen. For expression in HEK293 or 293T cells, the foreign gene generally is driven by the CMV promoter and the placement of the SV40 ori on the plasmid allows for replication in 293T cells. In contrast, 293EBNA cells were derived following modification to express another activating protein, Epstein–Barr nuclear antigen (EBNA)–1. Consequently, plasmid replication in this cell line requires a plasmid containing the EBV ori.

COS cells originated from the African Green Monkey kidney cell line transformed with an origin-defective SV40 genome [11]. Because the cell lines are able to express the SV40 large T-antigen, transfection with a plasmid containing an SV40 ori leads to extrachromosomal plasmid replication. Plasmid replication reaches a maximum at 48 h posttransfection with protein production peaking at 72 h posttransfection. After this point, the transfected cells will begin to undergo cell death, consequently, this cell line is used primarily for transient expression. A transfected COS cell can produce tens of thousands of copies of the desired protein at maximum expression conditions.

3.1.5 Transfection Methods

In order for a mammalian cell to produce a recombinant protein, the DNA encoding that protein must be transferred into the cell in a process called transfection. Both chemical and physical methods have been developed to accomplish this goal. Chemical methods include calcium phosphate coprecipitation and cationic polymers such as DEAE-dextran, liposomes, and molecular conjugates, whereas physical methods include electroporation and biolistic microparticle bombardment. Regardless of the transfection protocol, the cells' rate of growth and the condition of the DNA are principal contributors to high transfection efficiency. Cells in log-phase growth give better transfection efficiencies especially for the generation of stably transfected cell lines. In addition, linearized plasmid DNA is a better facilitator of stable transfections, whereas undigested, supercoiled plasmid DNA is optimal for transient transfections.

Calcium phosphate coprecipitation was one of the first chemical methods widely used to transfer DNA into cells in culture. To accomplish this, calcium chloride and a phosphate buffer such as HEPES-buffered saline or BES-buffered saline is mixed with DNA. The result is a precipitate that distributes throughout the cell culture. Uptake of the precipitate, and consequently the DNA, is believed to be achieved through phagocytosis [12]. An important issue affecting transfection efficiency for this method is the pH of the phosphate buffer solution. The pH of the buffer should be maintained between 6.95 as in BES-buffered saline and 7.1 as in HEPES-buffered saline. In addition, the quality of the precipitate must be uniform and removed after incubation. Calcium phosphate coprecipitation works for both transient and stable transfections in numerous cell lines, both adherent and suspension.

The cationic polymer, DEAE-dextran, is another widely used transfection method. DEAE-dextran is a positively charged polymer that binds to the negatively charged DNA when mixed. Upon exposure of the cells to the mixture, the negatively charged cellular membranes will adhere to the mixture allowing for endocytosis of the DNA. Limits of this system are its usefulness in transient transfections only and its cytotoxicity to the cell culture. Other cationic polymers used for transfection include polyamidoamine dendrimer, protamine, and polyethyleneimine.

Liposome-mediated delivery of DNA is a highly efficient transfection technique suitable for those cell lines that experience toxicity from calcium phosphate coprecipitation or DEAE-dextran. Upon encapsulation of the DNA, the DNA enters the cell either through endocytosis of the vesicle or by fusion with the cell membrane. The essential component of the liposome is a synthetic cationic lipid composed of a positively charged hydrophilic head region, which binds to the negatively charged phosphate group of DNA, and a lipid tail. Thus the charge of the DNA is neutralized, which allows for its transfer through the negatively charged cell membrane. Other lipids, such as dioleoylphosphatidyl-ethanolamine, may be mixed with the cationic lipid to form the liposome. Benefits of liposome-mediated delivery include no restriction on the size of the DNA, the ability to use both attachment and suspension cells, and success in both transient and stable systems. However, optimization of experimental parameters including the duration of transfection and the ratio of DNA to lipid must be performed in order to achieve efficient transfection.

Molecular conjugates are yet another cationic-based transfection technique. The conjugation of DNA to a cationic amino acid such as polylysine allows for the effective transfer of DNA into the cell due to its ability to condense the DNA. The conjugate's size is a critical parameter and can be altered by changing the salt solution in which it is made. Advantages to this approach include the ability to modify the conjugate itself to enhance cellular specificity by the addition of components such as a nuclear localization signal.

Electroporation is a physical transfection technique involving the application of a controlled electrical pulse to the cell in order to create a temporary localized permeabilization of it's membrane. The most commonly employed electrical pulses are the capacitance discharge or exponential decay pulse and the square or rectangular-wave pulse. The exponential decay pulse is generated when a charged capacitor is discharged into a mixture of cells and DNA. In comparison, the square-wave pulse is produced by a temporary application of a high voltage. Numerous parameters affecting electroporation include the temperature of the cells during and immediately postelectroporation, the buffer, which is an important determinant due to its electrical resistance, the growth rate of the cells, and the plasmid. The use of supercoiled plasmid results in higher gene expression transiently, whereas the use of linearized plasmid is more effective for the production of stable cell lines. Overall, electroporation is a more rapid transfection method in comparison to the chemical methods described herein. It is especially applicable to suspension cultures and cell lines that are difficult to transfect by other methods.

Biolistic microparticle bombardment, commonly called the gene gun, involves the physical forced entry into the cell through the acceleration of DNA coated with gold particles or other metals. Less DNA and fewer cells are required for this method as compared to the other physical transfection method of electroporation. In addition, both transient and stable transfections may be performed using the same experimental conditions. One of the advantages to this system is that cellular damage is minimized; however, a disadvantage is that the penetration of the DNA into the cell can be limiting as well.

While these approaches represent many of the most common transfection techniques, this is certainly not an exhaustive list. Other methods, such as microinjection and protoplast fusion not discussed here, are also currently available.

3.1.6   Transient vs. Stable Transfection

Upon transfection of a vector into a cell, two options exist for expression. The protein product may be expressed either transiently or stably. Transient transfection is a rapid protein expression technique that may last from several days to approximately 2 weeks with the maximum level of production occurring anywhere from 12 to 96 h posttransfection. When using plasmids, the plasmid and the resulting encoded protein are rapidly reproduced by the cell, then over time, the DNA and its resultant expression disappear. Viral vectors are typically transient in nature in which the expression vector takes control of the cell's protein expression machinery for a limited period prior to cell death and eventual lysis. Transient expression is a convenient method used to produce milligram quantities of protein quickly for experiments and to test the functionality of a newly created vector prior to the generation of a stable cell line. A common method for testing a new vector is to clone into it a reporter gene as the gene of interest. The reporter gene used should be a gene that is not exogenously expressed by the cell. The most common reporter genes used are green fluorescent protein (GFP), firefly luciferase (Luc), chloramphenical acetyltransferase (CAT), and β-galactosidase (β-gal).

Stable expression is used when larger quantities of product or longer-term production is derived. Stable expression also is preferable for generating proteins with more consistent product quality characteristics including glycosylation and other posttranslational modifications. Stable transfection is a more laborious procedure in which a selectable marker is added to the culture 24 to 48 h after transfection. Those cells that do not express a foreign protein to combat the effects of the selection agent will succumb to death within several days. Depending upon the vector used, continuous selection will allow for the vector to be either integrated into the genome of the cell or episomal, meaning that is will be sustained external to the chromosome. During this time of selection, the cultures are subjected to limited dilutions such that over a several week period, a colony of cells will result from each single cell or clone. These colonies then may be assayed for production of the target gene of interest, which is typically different from the gene responsible for resistance against the selection agent. In this way, a stably expressing cell line is generated over a period of several weeks to months.

3.1.7 Selectable Markers

Vectors used for stable transfection may incorporate genes for one of two types of selection: the conferring of resistance to cytotoxic drugs added to the culture medium or expression of genes involved in nucleotide biosynthesis.

Numerous cytotoxic drug and gene combinations are in use. These include G418 (geneticin), hygromycin B, puromycin, and blasticidin. G418 inhibits eukaryotic protein synthesis. However, expression of the bacterial neomycin resistance gene, aminoglycoside 3′ phosphotransferase (*aph*), will phosphorylate G418 thus inactivating it. Hygromycin B, also an inhibitor of eukaryotic protein synthesis through the inhibition of ribosome translocation, is neutralized by expression of hygromycin B phosphotransferase from the *E. coli hph* gene. Puromycin results in translation termination unless puromycin acetyltransferase is produced from the *S. alboniger pac gene*. Alternatively, the presence of blasticidin, an inhibitor of translational elongation, is combated by expression of the *B. cereus bsr* gene that codes for blasticidin S deaminase. Several other cytotoxic drug and gene combinations are in existence and have a similar mode of action, either through the inhibition of DNA, RNA, or protein synthesis.

A second class of cytotoxic drugs and gene combinations exist that involve either negative or positive selection of genes implicated in nucleotide metabolism. Nucleotides may be produced in the cell by de novo synthesis, which uses basic compounds such as sugars and amino acids to produce IMP and UMP, the first precursor nucleotides in the de novo pathway. Alternatively, when the de novo pathway is blocked, a salvage pathway may be used. The salvage pathway synthesizes nucleotides from exogenously added thymidine or purines. For example, in the de novo pathway, tetrahydrofolate derivatives are necessary for IMP and TMP synthesis. When the cytotoxic agent methotrexate is added to the culture media, nucleotide synthesis is inhibited unless DHFR, coded for by the dihydrofolate reductase gene, is present. This form of selection is used in cell lines that have had endogenous DHFR production deleted, such as CHO DG44.

In comparison, several salvage pathway enzymes exist, such as xanthine-guanine phosphoribosyltransferase (XGPRT). The bacterial *gpt* gene that codes for the enzyme XGPRT is the counterpart to the mammalian hypoxanthine-guanine phosphoribosyltransferase (HGPRT) salvage enzyme. However, XGPRT and not HGPRT can utilize the purine xanthine to produce XMP and ultimately GMP. Therefore, the presence of the cytotoxic agent mycophenolic acid, an inhibitor of the IMP to XMP reaction, will be counteracted by the expression of XGPRT when xanthine is supplemented in the culture medium.

Because every cell line will display different death kinetics upon exposure to a cytotoxic drug, the initial use of the drug as a selectable agent necessitates the need for a dose response curve to determine the optimal concentration to obtain selection. The dose response curve will enable the identification of the concentration of selectable marker that allows only those cell lines expressing a desirable level of the resistance marker to survive. When several vectors are incorporated into a cell line for the expression of multiple genes in a cell line, each vector should contain a different selectable marker. In this instance, the cytotoxic drug against each marker is added to the culture medium to select only for those cells incorporating all the desired vectors.

3.1.8   Single Cell Cloning Methods

The standard method for obtaining stable cell lines involves cloning by limiting dilution. In this technique, transfected cells that have been selected for stable expression are plated at low density in tissue culture plates so that colonies resulting from single cells or clones are obtained. These colonies then are expanded for testing of expression of the transfected foreign gene. An alternative to limiting dilution cloning involves the use of cell sorting by flow cytometry. In this approach, as cells are sorted, 96 well tissue culture plates are seeded at one cell per well. Several criteria, such as viability and cell morphology, are used as sort parameters. In the instance of the subcloning of an established stable cell line, these parameters are used to seed a 96 well plate at one cell per well. Because expression of the foreign gene is not a parameter in this type of single cell sorting, this is a random approach to subcloning. However, if the foreign gene is tagged with a fluorescent marker, such as GFP, then fluorescence intensity will become the most critical sort criterion in what is called fluorescence activated cell sorting (FACS). Other uses of fluorescence include the fluorescent tagging of a cell surface protein, or in some instances, a secreted protein such as an antibody. Although antibodies are secreted by the cell into the surrounding culture medium, antigen-coupled fluorescent microspheres or fluorescently conjugated secondary antibodies will bind to those antibodies transiently passing through the plasma membrane at the cell's surface. This approach will allow for sorting of those single cells with the greatest cell surface fluorescence. Although cloning by limiting dilution is a somewhat rudimentary approach involving screening of many clones that may or may not express the foreign gene, it is an inexpensive and relatively straightforward method to use. In contrast, the use of a sorting flow cytometer can be prohibitively expensive for some smaller laboratories and operator error is a reality for inexperienced users. If used by an experienced cytometrist, this approach tends to be more effective for isolating desirable single cell clones especially when foreign protein expression is used as one of the sorting parameters.

References

[1] Rees, S., Coote, J., Stables, J., Goodson, S., Harris, S., and Lee, M.G. (1996) Bicistronic vector for the creation of stable mammalian cell lines that predisposes all antibiotic-resistant cells to express recombinant protein. *Biotechniques* **20**, 102–104, 106, 108–110.

[2] Zhu, J., Musco, M.L., and Grance, M.J. (1999) Three-color flow cytometry analysis of tricistronic expression of eBFP, eGFP, and eYFP using EMCV-IRES linkages. *Cytometry* **37**, 51–59.

[3] Yao, T.P., Segraves, W.A., Oro, A.E., McKeown, M., and Evans, R.M. (1992) Drosophila ultraspiracle modulates ecdysone receptor function via heterodimer formation. *Cell* **2**, 63–72.

[4] Yao, T.P., Forman, B.M., Jiang, Z., Cherbas, L., Chen, J.D., McKeown, M., Cherbas, P., and Evans, R.M. (1993) Functional ecdysone receptor is the product of the EcR and Ultraspiracle genes. *Nature* **366**, 476–479.

[5] No, D., Yao, T.-P., and Evans, R.M. (1996) Ecdysone-inducible gene expression in mammalian cells and transgenic mice. *Proc. Natl Acad. Sci. USA* **93**, 3346–3351.

[6] Palli, S.R., Kapitskaya, M.Z., Kumar, M.B., and Cress, D.E. (2003) Improved ecdysone receptor-based inducible gene regulation system. *Eur. J. Biochem.* **270**, 1308–1315.

[7] Urlaub, G. and Chasin, L.A. (1980) Isolation of Chinese hamster cell mutants deficient in dihydrofolate reductase activity. *Proc. Natl Acad. Sci. USA* **77**, 4216–4220.

[8] Bebbington, C.R., Renner, G., Thompson, S., King, D., Abrams, D., and Yarronton, G.T. (1992) High level expression of a recombinant antibody from myeloma cells using a glutamine synthetase gene as an amplifiable selectable marker. *BioTechnology* **10**, 169–175.

[9] Kearney, J.F., Radbruch, A., Liesegang, B., and Rajewsky, K. (1979) A new mouse myeloma cell line that has lost immunoglobulin expression but permits the construction of antibody-secreting hybrid cell lines. *J. Immunol.* **123**, 1548–1550.

[10] Graham, F.L., Smiley, J., Russell, W.C., and Nairn, R. (1977) Characteristics of a human cell line transformed by DNA from human adenovirus type 5. *J. Gen. Virol.* **36**, 59–74.

[11] Gluzman, Y. (1981) SV40-transformed simian cells support the replication of early SV40 mutants. *Cell* **23**, 175–182.

[12] Loyter, A., Scangos, G.A., and Ruddle, F.H. (1982) Mechanisms of DNA uptake by mammalian cells: fate of exogenously added DNA monitored by the use of fluorescent dyes. *Proc. Natl Acad. Sci. USA* **79**, 422–426.

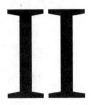

Transport Phenomena and Biomimetic Systems

Robert J. Fisher
The SABRE Institute and Massachusetts Institute of Technology

THE INTENTION OF THIS SECTION is to couple the concepts of transport phenomena with chemical reaction kinetics and thermodynamics to introduce the field of reaction engineering. This is essential information needed to design and control engineering devices, particularly flow reactor systems. Through extension of these concepts, combined with materials design, to mimic biological systems in form and function, the field of biomimicry has evolved. The development of Biomimetic Systems is a rapidly emerging technology with expanding applications. Specialized journals devoted to exploring both the analysis of existing biological materials and processes, and the design and production of synthetic analogs that mimic biological properties are now emerging. These journals blend a biological approach with a materials/engineering science viewpoint covering topics that include: analysis of the design criteria used by organisms in the selection of specific biosynthetic materials and structures; analysis of the optimization criteria used in natural systems; development of systems modeled on biological analogs; and applications of "intelligent" or "smart" materials in areas such as biosensors, robotics, and aerospace. This biomimicry theme is prevalent throughout all the chapters in this section, including one specifically devoted to these concepts with explicit examples of applications to reacting and transport processes.

The field of transport phenomena traditionally encompasses the subjects of momentum transport (viscous flow), energy transport (heat conduction, convection, and radiation), and mass transport (diffusion). In this section the media in which the transport occurs is regarded as continua; however, some molecular explanations are discussed. The continuum approach is of more immediate interest to engineers, but both approaches are required to thoroughly master the subject. The current emphasis in engineering education is on understanding basic physical principles vs. "blind" use of empiricism. Consequently, it is imperative that the reader seek further edification in classical transport phenomena texts; general [Bird et al., 1960; Deen, 1996], with chemically reactive systems [Rosner, 1986], and more specifically, with a biologically oriented approach [Lightfoot, 1974; Fournier, 1999]. The laws (conservation principles, etc.) governing such transport will be seen to influence (1) the local rates at which reactants encounter one another; (2) the temperature field within body regions (or compartments in pharmacokinetics modeling); (3) the volume (or area) needed to accomplish the desired turnover or transport rates; and (4) the amount and fate of species involved in mass transport and metabolic rates. For biomedical systems such as dialysis, in which only physical changes occur, the same general principles, usually with more simplifications, are used to design and analyze these devices. The transport laws governing nonreactive systems can often be used to make rational predictions of the behavior of "analogous" reacting systems. The importance of relative time scales will be discussed throughout this section by all authors. It is particularly important to establish orders-of-magnitude and to make realistic limiting calculations. Dimensional analysis and pharmacokinetic modeling techniques are especially attractive for these purposes; in fact, they may permit unifying the whole of biological transport [see other sections of this handbook and Enderle et al., 1999; Fisher, 1999]. As the reader progresses, the importance of transport phenomena in applied biology becomes steadily more apparent. "In all living organisms, but most especially the higher animals, diffusional and flow limitations are of critical importance; moreover, we live in a very delicate state of balance with respect to these two processes" [Lightfoot, 1974].

Each chapter in this section is somewhat self-contained. Similar concepts are brought forth and reinforced through applications and discussions. However, to further enhance the benefits obtained by the reader, it is prudent to first discuss some elementary concepts; the most relevant being control volume selection and flow reactors.

When applying the conservation laws to fluid matter treated as a continuum, the question arises as to the amount of matter to be considered. Typically this decision is based on convenience and/or level of detail required. There is no single choice. Many possibilities exist that can lead to the same useful predictions. The conservation laws of continuum dynamics can be applied to the fluid contained in a volume of arbitrary size, shape, and state of motion. The volume selected is termed a "control volume." The simplest is one where every point on its surface moves with the local fluid velocity. It is called a "material" control volume since, in the absence of diffusion across its interface, it retains the material originally present within its control surface. Although conceptually simple, they are not readily used since they move through space, change their volume, and deform. An analysis of the motion of material control volumes is usually termed "Legrangian" and time derivatives are termed "material" or "substantial" derivatives.

Another simple class of control volumes is defined by surfaces fixed in physical space, through which the fluid flows. These "fixed" control volumes are termed "Eularian" and may be either macroscopic or differential in any or all directions. The fluid contained within a Eularian control volume is said to be, in thermodynamic terms, an "open" (flow) system.

The most general type of control volume is defined by surfaces that move "arbitrarily," that is, not related to the local fluid velocity. Such control volumes are used to analyze the behavior of nonmaterial "waves" in fluids, as well as moving phase boundaries in the presence of mass transfer across the interface [Crank, 1956; Fisher, 1989].

Characterization of the mass transfer processes in bioreactors, as used in cell or tissue culture systems, is essential when designing and evaluating their performance. Flow reactor systems bring together various reactants in a continuous fashion while simultaneously withdrawing products and excess reactants. These reactors generally provide optimum productivity and performance [Levenspiel, 1989; Freshney, 2000; Shuler and Kargi, 2001]. They are classified as either tank or tube type reactors. Each represents extremes in the behavior of the gross fluid motion. Tank type reactors are characterized by instant and complete mixing of the contents and are therefore termed perfectly mixed, or backmixed, reactors. Tube type reactors are characterized by the lack of mixing in the flow direction and are termed plug flow, or tubular, reactors. The performance of actual reactors, though not fully represented by these idealized flow patterns, may match them so closely that they can be modeled as such with negligible error. Others can be modeled as combinations of tank and tube type over various regions.

An idealized backmixed reactor is analyzed as follows. Consider a stirred vessel containing a known fluid volume, into which multiple streams may be flowing that contain reactants, enzymes (biocatalysts), nutrients, reaction medium, and so on. When all these components are brought together in the vessel, under properly controlled conditions such as temperature, pressure, and concentrations of each component, the desired reactions occur. The vessel is well mixed to promote good contacting of all components and hence an efficient reaction scheme can be maintained. The well-mixed state is achieved when samples withdrawn from different locations, including the exit, at the same instance in time are indistinguishable. The system is termed "lumped" vs. "distributed," as in a plug flow system where location matters. The response characteristics of a backmixed reactor are significantly different from those of a plug flow reactor. How reaction time variations affect performance and how quickly each system responds to upsets in the process conditions are key factors. The backmixed system is far more sluggish than the plug flow system. To evaluate the role of reaction time variations, the concept of residence time and how it is determined must be discussed. A brief analysis of a batch reactor will be useful in understanding the basic principles involved.

In batch systems, there is no flow in or out. The feed (initial charge) is placed in the reactor at the start of the process and the products are withdrawn all at once at some time later. The time-for-reaction is thus readily determined. This is significant since the conversion of reactants to products is a function of time, and can be obtained from knowledge of the reaction rate and its dependence upon composition and process variables. Since these other factors are typically controlled at a constant value, the-time-for-reaction is the key parameter in the reactor design process. In a batch reactor, the concentration of reactants is time-dependent and, therefore, the rate of reaction as well. Conversion is now related to reaction time through the use of calculus. For this system, residence time, equal to the processing time, is the time for reaction.

In a backmixed reactor, the conversion of reactants is controlled by the average length of time fluid elements remain in the reactor (their residence time). The ratio of the volume of fluid in the tank to the volumetric flow rate of the exit stream determines the residence time. Recall that in an ideal system of this type, operating at steady state, concentrations in the vessel are uniform and equal to those in the exit stream and thus the reaction rate is maintained at a constant value. Conversion of individual reactants and yield of specific products can be determined simply by multiplying the appropriate rate of interest by the residence time. With imperfect mixing, fluid elements have a distribution of residence times and the performance of the reactor is clearly altered.

Analysis of the plug flow reactor system is based on the premise that there is no mixing in the flow direction and thus no interaction between neighboring fluid elements as they traverse the length of the reactor. This idealization permits use of the results obtained from the analysis of the batch reactor system. Each fluid element in the tubular reactor functions as a small batch reactor, undisturbed by its neighboring elements, and its reaction time is well defined as the ratio of tube length to the volume averaged fluid velocity. Concentration varies along the length of the reactor (also, rate), and can be simply related to reaction time. The mathematical analysis and prediction of performance is similar to that for a batch reactor. This analysis shows that the plug flow configuration yields higher conversions than the backmixed vessel, given equal residence times and the same processing conditions. However, the plug flow reactor responds more quickly to system upsets and is more difficult to control.

Most actual reactors deviate from these idealized systems primarily because of nonuniform velocity profiles, channeling and bypassing of fluids, and the presence of stagnant regions caused by reactor shape and internal components such as baffles, heat transfer coils, and measurement probes. Disruptions to the flow path are common when dealing with heterogeneous systems, particularly when solids are present. To model these actual reactors, various regions are compartmentalized and represented as combinations of plug flow and backmixed elements. For illustration, a brief discussion of recycle, packed bed, and fluidized bed reactor systems follows.

Recycle reactors are basically plug flow reactors with a portion of the exit stream recycled to the inlet, which provides multiple passes through the reactor to increase conversion. It is particularly useful in biocatalytic reactor designs, in which the use of a packed bed is desired because of physical problems associated with contacting and subsequent separation of the phases. The recycle reactor provides an excellent means to obtain backmixed behavior from a physically configured tubular reactor. Multiple reactors of various types, combined in series or parallel arrangements, can improve performance and meet other physical requirements. Contact patterns using multiple entries into a single reactor can emulate these situations. A system demonstrating this characteristic is a plug flow reactor with uniform side entry. If these entry points are distributed along the length with no front entry, the system will perform as a single backmixed system. The significance is that backmixed behavior is obtained without continual stirring or the use of recycle pumps. Furthermore, if these side entry points are limited to only a portion of the reactor length, then the system functions as backmixed reactors in series with plug flow reactors.

Special consideration needs to be given to heterogeneous reactors, in which interaction of the phases is required for the reactions to proceed. In these situations, the rate of reaction may not be the deciding factor in the reactor design. The rate of transport of reactants and products from one phase to another can limit the rate at which products are obtained. For example, if reactants cannot get to the surface of a solid catalyst faster than they would react at the surface, then the overall (observed) rate of the process is controlled by this mass transfer step. To improve the rate, the mass transfer must be increased. It would be useless to make changes that would affect only the surface reaction rate. Furthermore, if products do not leave the surface rapidly, they may block reaction sites and thus limit the overall rate. Efficient contacting patterns need to be utilized. Hence, fluidized bed reactors (two-phase backmixed emulator), trickle-bed systems (three-phase packed bed emulator), and slurry reactors (three-phase backmixed emulator) have evolved as important bioreactors. They are readily simulated, designed, scaled up, and modified to meet specific contacting demands in cell and tissue culture systems [Shuler and Kargi, 2001].

Flow reactors of all shapes, sizes, and uses are encountered in all phases of life. Examples of interest to bioengineers include: the pharmaceutical industry, to produce aspirin, penicillin, and other drugs; the biomass processing industry, to produce alcohol, enzymes and other specialty proteins, and value added products; and the biotechnologically important tissue and cell culture systems. The type of reactor used depends on the specific application and on the scale desired. The choice is based on a number of factors. The primary ones are the reaction rate (or other rate-limiting process), the product distribution specifications, and the catalyst or other material characteristics, such as chemical and physical stability.

Using living systems require more thorough discussions because, in these systems, the solid phase may change its dimensions as the reaction proceeds. Particles that increase in size, such as growing cell clusters, can fall out of the reaction zone and alter flow patterns within the vessel. This occurs when gravity overcomes fluid buoyancy and drag forces. In some instances, this biomass growth is the desired product; however, the substances produced by reactions catalyzed by the cellular enzymes are usually the desired products. By reproducing themselves, these cells provide more enzymes and thus productivity increases are possible. Note, however, that there are both advantages and disadvantages to using these whole cell systems versus the enzymes directly. The cell membrane can be a resistance for transport; the consumption of reactant as a nutrient for cell processes reduces the efficiency of raw material usage; and special precautions must be taken to maintain a healthy environment and thus productivity [Freshney, 2000; Lewis and Colton, 2004]. The payoff, however, is that the enzymes within their natural environment are generally more active and safer from poisons or other factors that could reduce their effectiveness. Interesting examples are microbial fermentation processes, as discussed earlier. Backmixed flow reactors are used in these applications. They are best suited to maintain the cell line at a particular stage in its life cycle to obtain the desired results. The uniform and constant environment provided for the cells minimizes the adjustments that they need to make concerning nutrient changes, metabolic wastes, and so forth, such that production can proceed at a constant rate. The term "chemostat" is used when referring to backmixed reactors used in biotechnology applications. These are typically tank type systems with mechanical agitation. All the reactor types discussed earlier, however, are applicable. Recall that mixed flow characteristics can be obtained in tubular reactors if recycle or side entry or both is employed. Thus, air lift systems using a vertical column with recycle and side entry ports is a popular design.

The design, analysis, and simulation of reactors thus becomes an integral part of the bioengineering profession. The study of chemical kinetics, particularly when coupled with complex physical phenomena, such as the transport of heat, mass, and momentum, is required to determine or predict reactor performance. It thus becomes imperative to uncouple and unmask the fundamental phenomenological events in reactors and to subsequently incorporate them in a concerted manner to meet the objectives of specific applications. This need further emphasizes the role played by the physical aspects of reactor behavior in the stability and controllability of the entire process. The following chapters in this section demonstrate the importance of all the concepts presented in this introduction.

References

Bird, R.B., Stewart, W.E., and Lightfoot, E.N. (1960), *Transport Phenomena*, John Wiley & Sons, New York.

Crank, J. (1956), *The Mathematics of Diffusion*, Oxford University Press, Oxford.

Deen, W.M. (1996), *Analysis of Transport Phenomena*, Oxford Press, New York.

Enderle, J., Blanchard, S., and Bronzino, J.D., Eds. (1999), *Introduction to Biomedical Engineering*, Academic Press, New York.

Fisher, R.J. (1989), Diffusion with immobilization in membranes: Part II, in *Biological and Synthetic Membranes*, Butterfield, A., Ed., Alan R. Liss, Inc., New York, pp. 138–151.

Fisher, R.J. (1999), Compartmental analysis, in *Introduction to Biomedical Engineering*, Academic Press, New York, Chap. 8.

Fournier, R.L. (1999), *Basic Transport Phenomena in Biomedical Engineering*, Taylor & Francis, Philadelphia.

Freshney, R.I. (2000), *Culture of Animal Cells*, 4th ed., Wiley-Liss, New York.

Levenspiel, O. (1989), *The Chemical Reactor Omnibook*, Oregon State University Press, Corvallis, OR.

Lewis, A.S. and Colton, C.K. (2004), Tissue engineering for insulin replacement in diabetes, in Ma, P.X. and Elisseeff, J. Eds. *Scaffolding in Tissue Engineering*, Marcel Dekker, New York (in press).

Lightfoot, E.N. (1974), *Transport Phenomena and Living Systems*, John Wiley & Sons, New York.

Rosner, D.E. (1986), *Transport Processes in Chemically Reacting Flow Systems*, Butterworth Publishers, Boston, MA.

Shuler, M.L. and Kargi, F. (2001), *Bioprocess Engineering: Basic Concepts*, 2nd ed., Prentice-Hall, Englewood Cliffs, NJ.

4

Biomimetic Systems

Robert J. Fisher
*The SABRE Institute and
Massachusetts Institute
of Technology*

Humans have always been fascinated by the phenomenological events, both biological and physical in nature, that are revealed to us by our environment. Our innate curiosity drives us to study these observations and understand the fundamental basis of the mechanisms involved. Practical outcomes are the development of predictive capabilities of occurrence and the control of these events and their subsequent consequences; our safety and comfort being major incentives. Furthermore, we wish to design processes that mimic the beneficial aspects associated with their natural counterparts. Experience has taught us that these natural processes are complex and durable and that adaptability with multifunctionality is a must for biological systems to survive. Evolution, aiding these living systems to adapt to new environmental challenges, occurs at the molecular scale. Our need to be molecular scientists and engineers is thus apparent. Knowledge of the molecular building blocks used in the architectural configurations of both living and nonliving systems, along with an understanding of their design and the processes used for implementation, is essential for control and utilization. The ability to mimic demonstrates a sufficient knowledge base to design systems requiring controlled functionality. To perfect this approach, a series of sensor/reporter systems must be available. A particularly attractive feature of living systems is their unique ability to diagnose and repair localized damages through a continuously distributed sensor network with inter- and intracellular communication capabilities. Mimicry of these networks is an integral component of many emerging research thrust areas, in particular, tissue engineering. Significant emphasis has been toward the development of intelligent membranes, specifically using sensor/reporter technology. A successful approach has been to couple transformation and separation technologies with detection and control systems.

The concept of intelligent barriers and substrates, such as membranes, arises from the coupling of this sensor/reporter technology with controlled chemistry and reaction engineering, selective transport phenomena, and innovative systems design. Engineered membrane mimetics are required to respond and adapt to environmental stresses, whether intentionally imposed or stochastic in nature. These intelligent membranes may take the form of polymeric films, composite materials, ceramics, supported liquid membranes, or as laminates. Their important feature is specific chemical functionality, engineered to provide selective transport, structural integrity, controlled stability and release, and sensor/reporter capabilities. Applications as active transport and electron transfer chain mimics and their use in studying the consequences of environmental stresses on enzymatic functions create valuable insights into cellular mechanisms.

Advanced materials, designed through knowledge gained from analysis of biological systems, have been instrumental in the progression and success of many tissue engineering applications. Their biocompatibility, multifunctionality, and physio-chemical properties are essential attributes. When incorporated with living cells, for example in organ/tissue constructs, integrated systems biology behavioral mimicry can be accomplished. This is particularly useful for drug efficacy and toxicity screening tests and thus minimizing the use of animals for these studies. For example, having an effective blood brain barrier mimetic, a realistic blood substitute, and cell culture analogs for the various organs needed for a useful animal surrogate system promotes more rapid development of therapeutic drugs. These biomimetic studies influence all phases, that is, the design, development, and delivery characteristics, of this effort. The design, applicability, and performance of these systems are briefly discussed in subsequent paragraphs in this chapter and in greater depth in other locations throughout this handbook.

4.1 Concepts of Biomimicry

Discoveries that have emerged from a wide spectrum of disciplines, ranging from biotechnology and genetics to polymer and molecular engineering, are extending the design and manufacturing possibilities for mimetic systems that were once incomprehensible. Understanding of the fundamental concepts inherent in natural processes has led to a broad spectrum of new processes and materials modeled on these systems [Srinivasan et al., 1991]. Natural processes, such as active transport systems functioning in living systems, have been successfully mimicked and useful applications in other fields, such as pollution prevention, have been demonstrated [Thoresen and Fisher, 1995]. Understanding the mechanisms at the molecular level, which living systems utilize, is needed before success at the macroscale can be assured. Multifunctionality, hierarchical organization, adaptability, reliability, self-regulation, and reparability are the key elements that living systems rely upon and that we must mimic to develop "intelligent systems." Successes to date have been based on the use of techniques associated with research advances made in areas such as molecular engineering of thin films and nanocapsules, neural networks, reporter/sensor technology, morphology and properties developments in polymer blends, transport phenomena in stationary and reacting flow systems, cell culture and immobilization technologies, controlled release and stability mechanisms for therapeutic agents, and environmental stress analyses. A few examples in the bioengineering field are molecular design of supported liquid membranes to mimic active transport of ions, noninvasive sensors to monitor *in vivo* glucose concentrations, detection of microbial contamination by bioluminescence, immunomagnetic capture of pathogens, improved encapsulation systems, carrier molecules for targeting, imaging and controlled release of pharmaceutics, *in situ* regeneration of coenzymes electrochemically, and measurement of transport and failure mechanisms in "smart" composites. All these successes were accomplished through interdisciplinary approaches, essentially using three major impact themes: Morphology and Properties

Development; Molecular Engineering of Thin Films and Nanocapsules; and Biotechnology, Bioreaction Engineering, and Systems Development.

4.1.1 Morphology and Properties Development

Polymer blends are a major focus of this research area [Weiss et al., 1995]. Technology, however, has outpaced a detailed understanding of many facets of this science, which impedes the development and application of new materials. The purpose of this research is to develop the fundamental science that influences the phase behavior, phase architecture, and morphology and interfacial properties of polymer blends. The main medical areas where polymers and composites (polymeric) have found wide use are artificial organs, the cardiovascular system, orthopedics, dental sciences, ophthalmology, and drug delivery systems. Success has been related to the wide range of mechanical properties, transformation processes (shape possibilities), and low production costs. The limitation has been their interaction with living tissue. To overcome the biological deficiencies of synthetic polymers and enhance mechanical characteristics, a class of bioartificial polymeric materials has been introduced based on blends, composites, and interpenetrating polymer networks of both synthetic and biological polymers. Preparations from biopolymers such as fibrin, collagen, and hyaluronic acid with synthetic polymers such as polyurethane, poly(acrylic acid), and poly(vinyl alcohol) are available [Giusti et al., 1993; Luo and Prestwich, 2001].

4.1.2 Molecular Engineering of Thin Films and Nanocapsules

The focus in the thin film research impact area is to develop a fundamental understanding of how morphology can be controlled in (1) organic thin film composites prepared by Langmuir–Blodgett (LB) monolayer and multilayer techniques and (2) the molecular design of membrane systems using ionomers and selected supported liquids. Controlled structures of this nature will find immediate application in several aspects of smart materials development, particularly in microsensors.

The ability to form nano-sized particles and emulsions that encapsulate active ingredients is an essential skill applicable to many facets of the engineering biosciences. Nanotechnologies have a major impact on drug delivery, molecular targeting, medical imaging, biosensor development, and in the cosmetic, personal care products, and nutraceutics industries, to mention only a few. New techniques utilize high shear fields to obtain particle sizes in the range 50 to 100 nm; about the size of the turbulent eddies developed. Stable emulsions can be formed with conventional mixing equipment where high shear elongation flow fields are generated near the tip of high-speed blades, but only in the range 500 nm and larger. High shear stresses can also be generated by forcing the components of the microemulsion to flow through a microporous material. The resultant solution contains average particle sizes as small as 50 nm. Units that incorporate jet impingement on a solid surface or with another jet also perform in this size range. Molecular self-assembly systems using novel biocompatible synthetic polymer compounds are also under development. These have been used successfully to encapsulate chemotherapeutic drugs and perflourocarbons (PFC) [Kumar et al., 2004]. The high oxygen solubility of PFC's makes them attractive as blood surrogates and also as additives in immunoisolation tissue encapsulation systems to enhance gas transport. Using nanoencapsulation techniques, these compounds can be dispersed throughout microencapsulating matrices and in tissue extracellular matrix scaffold systems.

Surfaces, interfaces, and microstructures play an important role in many research frontiers. Exploration of structural property relationships at the atomic and molecular level, investigating elementary chemical and physical transformations occurring at phase boundaries, applying modern theoretical methods for predicting chemical dynamics at surfaces, and integration of this knowledge into models that can be used in process design and evaluation are within the realm of surface and interfacial engineering. The control of surface functionality by proper selection of the composition of the LB films and the self-assembling (amphiphatic) molecular systems can mimic many functions of a biologically active membrane. An informative comparison is that between inverted erythrocyte ghosts [Dinno et al., 1991; Matthews et al., 1993] and their synthetic mimics when environmental stresses are imposed on both systems. These model systems can assist in mechanistic studies to understand the functional alterations that result from ultrasound, EM fields, and UV radiation. The behavior of carrier molecules and receptor site functionality must be mimicked properly along with simulating disturbances in the Proton Motive Force of viable cells. Use of ion/electron transport ionomers in membrane-catalyst preparations is beneficial for programs such as electroenzymatic synthesis and metabolic pathway emulation [Fisher et al., 2000; Chen et al., 2004]. Development of new membranes used in artificial organs and advances in micelle reaction systems have resulted from these efforts.

4.1.3 Biotechnology, Bioreaction Engineering, and Systems Development

Focus for this research area is on (1) sensor/receptor reporter systems and detection methods; (2) transport processes in biological and synthetic membranes; (3) biomedical and bioconversion process development; and (4) smart film/intelligent barrier systems. These topics require coupling with the previously discussed areas and the use of biochemical reaction engineering techniques. Included in all of these areas is the concept of metabolic engineering — the modification of the metabolism of organisms to produce useful products. Extensive research in bioconversion processes is currently being directed to producing important pharmaceutics. Expanded efforts are also needed in the field of cell and tissue engineering, that is, the manipulation or reconstruction of cell and tissue function using molecular approaches.

4.2 Biomimicry and Tissue Engineering

Before we can develop useful *ex vivo* and *in vitro* systems for the numerous applications in tissue engineering, we must have an appreciation of cellular function *in vivo*. Knowledge of the tissue microenvironment and communication with other organs is essential. The key questions that must therefore be addressed in the realm of tissue engineering thus are, how can tissue function be built, reconstructed, and modified? To answer these we develop a standard approach based on the following axioms [Palsson, 2000] (1) in organogenesis and wound healing, proper cellular communications, with respect to each others activities, are of paramount concern since a systematic and regulated response is required from all participating cells; (2) the function of fully formed organs is strongly dependent on the coordinated function of multiple cell types with tissue function based on multicellular aggregates; (3) the functionality of an individual cell is strongly affected by its microenvironment (within 100 μm of the cell, i.e., the characteristic length scale); (4) this microenvironment is further characterized by (i) neighboring cells, that is, cell–cell contact and presence of molecular signals (soluble growth factors, signal transduction, trafficking, etc.), (ii) transport processes and physical interactions with the extracellular matrix (ECM), and (iii) the local geometry, in particular its effects on microcirculation. The importance of the microcirculation is that it connects all microenvironments to the whole body environment. Most metabolically active cells in the body are located within a few hundred micrometers from a capillary. This high degree of vascularization is necessary to provide the perfusion environment that connects every cell to a source and sink for respiratory gases, a source of nutrients from the small intestine, the hormones from the pancreas, liver, and glandular system, clearance of waste products via the kidneys and liver, delivery of immune system respondents and so forth. The engineering of these functions *ex vivo* is the domain of bioreactor design, a topic discussed briefly in the introduction to this section and elsewhere in this handbook. These cell culture devices must appropriately simulate and provide these macroenvironmental functions while respecting the need for the formation of microenvironments. Consequently, they must possess perfusion characteristics that allow for uniformity down to the 100 μm length scale. These are stringent design requirements that must be addressed with a high priority to properly account for the role of neighboring cells, the extracellular matrix, cyto-/chemokine and hormone trafficking, geometry, the dynamics of respiration, and transport of nutrients and metabolic by-products for each tissue system considered. These dynamic, chemical, and geometric variables must be duplicated as accurately as possible to achieve proper mimicry. Since this is a difficult task, a significant portion of another chapter in this section is devoted to developing methods to describe the microenvironment. Using the tools discussed there, we can develop systems to control microenvironments for *in vivo*, *ex vivo*, or *in vitro* applications.

The approach taken here to achieve the desired microenvironments is through use of novel membrane systems. They are designed to possess unique features for the specific application of interest and in many cases to exhibit stimulant/response characteristics. These so-called intelligent or smart membranes are the result of biomimicry, that is, having biomimetic features. Through functionalized membranes, typically in concerted assemblies, these systems respond to external stresses (chemical and physical in nature) to eliminate the threat either by altering stress characteristics or by modifying and protecting the cell/tissue microenvironment. An example is a microencapsulation motif for beta cell islet clusters to perform as pancreas. This system uses multiple membrane materials, each with its unique characteristics and performance requirements, coupled with nanospheres dispersed throughout the matrix, which contain additional materials for enhanced transport and barrier properties and respond to specific stimuli.

The communication of every cell with its immediate environment and other tissues is a key requisite for successful tissue function. This need establishes important spatial–temporal characteristics and a significant signaling/information processing network [Lauffenburger and Linderman, 1993]. Understanding this network and the information it contains is what the tissue engineer wishes to express and manage. For example, to stimulate the beginning of a specific cellular process appropriate signals to the nucleus are delivered at the cell membrane and transmitted through the cytoplasm by a variety of signal transduction mechanisms. Some signals are delivered by soluble growth factors that may originate from the circulating blood or from neighboring cells. The signal networking process is initiated after these molecules bind to selective receptors. The microenvironment is also characterized by cellular composition, the ECM, molecular dynamics (nutrients, metabolic waste products, and respiratory gases traffic in and out of the microenvironment in a highly dynamic manner), and local geometry (size scale of approximately 100 μm). Each of these can also provide the cell with important signals (dependent upon a characteristic time and length scale) to initiate specific cell functions for the tissue system to perform in a coordinated manner. If this arrangement is disrupted, cells that are unable to provide tissue function are obtained. Further discussions on this topic are presented in other chapters in this handbook devoted to cellular communications.

4.2.1 Integrated Systems

The interactions brought about by communications between tissue microenvironments and the whole body system, via the vascular network, provide a basis for the Systems Biology approach taken to understand the performance differences observed *in vivo* vs. *in vitro*. The response of one tissue system to changes in another (due to signals generated, such as metabolic products or hormones) must be properly mimicked by coupling individual cell culture analog (CCA) systems through a series of microbioreactors if whole body *in vivo* responses are to be meaningfully predicted. The need for microscale reactors is obvious when we consider the limited amount of tissue/cells available for these *in vitro* studies. This is particularly true when dealing with the pancreatic system where intact islets must be used (vs. individual beta cells) for induced insulin production by glucose stimulation. Their supply is extremely limited and maintaining viability and functionality is quite complex since the islet clusters *in vivo* are highly vascularized and this feature is difficult to maintain in preservation protocols or reproduce in mimetic systems. Therefore, the time scale for their usefulness is limited. Furthermore, one needs to minimize the amount of serum used (the communication fluid flowing through and between these biomimetic reactors), since in many cases, the serum obtained from actual patients must be used for proper mimicry. An animal surrogate system, primarily for drug toxicity studies, is currently being developed using this CCA concept [Shuler et al., 1996; also see Shuler et al., Chapter 8]. A general CCA system is one of three topics selected to illustrate these system interaction concepts in the following subsections. Another is associated with use of compartmental analysis in understanding the distribution and fate of molecular species, particularly pharmaceutics, and the third is the need for facilitated transport across the blood brain barrier, due to its complexities, when these species are introduced into the whole body by systemic administration.

Compartmental analysis and modeling was first formalized in the context of isotropic tracer kinetics to determine distribution parameters for fluid-borne species in both living and inert systems; particularly useful for determining flow patterns in reactors and tissue uptake parameters [Fisher, 2000]. Over time it has evolved and grown as a formal body of theory [Cobelli et al., 1979]. Models developed using compartmental analysis techniques are a class of dynamic, that is, differential equation, models derived from mass balance considerations. These compartmental models are widely used for quantitative analysis of the kinetics of "materials" in physiologic systems. These materials can be either exogenous, such as a drug or a tracer, or endogenous, such as a reactant (substrate) or a hormone. Kinetics include processes such as production, distribution, transport, utilization, and substrate–hormone control interactions.

4.2.2 Blood Brain Barrier

Many drugs, particularly water-soluble or high molecular weight compounds, do not enter the brain following traditional systemic administration methods because their permeation rate through blood capillaries is very slow. This blood brain barrier (BBB) severely limits the number of drugs that are candidates for treating brain disease. New strategies for increasing the permeability of brain capillaries to drugs are constantly being tested and are discussed elsewhere (see Saltzman; Chapter 11). A seemingly effective technique, of particular interest for this section is to utilize specific nutrient transport systems in brain capillaries to facilitate drug transport. For example, certain metabolic precursors are transported across endothelial cells by the neutral amino acid transport system and therefore, analog compounds could be used as both chaperones and targeting species. Also, direct delivery into the brain tissue by infusion, implantation of a drug releasing matrix, and transplantation of drug secreting cells are being considered. These approaches provide sustained drug delivery that can be confined to specific sites, localizing therapy to a given region. Because they provide a localized and continuous source of active drug molecules, the total drug dosage can be less than that with systemic administration. Polymeric implants, for controlled drug release, can also be designed to protect unreleased drug from degradation in the body and to permit localization of extremely high doses at precisely defined locations in the brain. Infusion systems require periodic refilling. This usually requires the drug to be stored in a liquid reservoir at body temperature and therefore many drugs are not suitable for this application since they are not stable under these conditions.

Coupling of these approaches, using nanosphere technologies to entrap the drug (sometimes modified for enhanced encapsulation stability) along with surface modifications of the spheres for specific targeting, has a higher probability of success to enhance transport into the brain. Proof of concept experiments can be conducted using a valid BBB model as an effective biomimetic. An *in vitro* coculture system composed of porcine brain capillary endothelial cells (BCEC) with porcine astrocytes is widely accepted as a valid BBB model. Using standard cell culturing techniques the astrocytes are seeded on the bottom of permeable membrane filters with BCEC seated on the top. This configuration permits communication between the two cell lines without disruption of the endothelial cell monolayer. The filters are suspended in a chamber of fluid such that an upper chamber is formed analogous to the lumen of a brain capillary blood vessel. BBB permeability is determined from measurement of transendothelial electrical resistance (TEER); a standard technique that measures the cell layer's ability to resist passage of a low electrical current. It essentially represents the passages of small ions and is the most sensitive measure of BBB integrity. The nanospheres can be used to encapsulate the radioactive labeled drug and tested for their toxicity to the BBB using TEER and noting if loss of barrier properties are observed. Inulin (5200 Da) is used as a marker species to represent potential pharmaceutical drug candidates and when used without nanosphere encapsulation provides a reasonable control. For example, its transport across the BBB is quite slow; <2% after 4 h of exposure. In proof of concept experiments, for the same time period and drug concentrations, more than 16% of the Inulin within nanospheres crossed the BBB [Kumar et al., 2004]. Although mechanistic details are lacking, this greater than eightfold increase in rate represents a dramatic increase and supports the premise that nanosphere encapsulation can facilitate drug delivery across the BBB and further illustrates the usefulness of this BBB biomimetic system.

4.2.3 Vascular System

Nutrient supply and gas exchange can become limiting in high cell density situation, as in tissue emulation *in vitro*, due to lack of an effective vasculature mimetic system to provide *in vivo* perfusion conditions. Many different system configurations/designs have been considered to overcome these deficiencies, such as cellulose and gel-foam sponge matrix materials, filter-well inserts, and mimetic membranes in novel bioreactor systems [Freshney, 2000]. Of particular interest here is the use of synthetic polymer capillary fibers (hollow fibers) in perfusion chambers where they can support cell growth on their outer surfaces and are gas and nutrient permeable. Medium, saturated with 5% CO_2 in air, is pumped through the lumen of the capillary fibers (in a bundle configuration) and cells attached and growing on the outer surface of the fibers, fed by diffusion from the perfusate, can reach tissue-like cell densities. Different polymers and ultrafiltration properties provide molecular cutoffs at 10 to 100 kDa, regulating macromolecule diffusion. It is now possible for the cells to behave as they would *in vivo*. For example, in such cultures, choriocarcinoma cells release more human chorionic gonadotrophin than they would in conventional monolayer culture and colonic carcinoma cells produce elevated levels of carcinoembryonic antigen (CEA) [Freshney, 2000]. Unfortunately, sampling cells and determining cell density are difficult from these commercially available chambers. New configurations are presently being designed and tested to overcome these limitations and are discussed in the chapter on microenvironment control (in this section of the handbook).

4.2.4 Implants

The transport of mass to and within a tissue is determined primarily by convection and diffusion processes that occur throughout the whole body system. The design of systems, for example, in cellular therapy, must consider methods to promote this integrated process and not just deal with the transport issues of the devise itself. An encapsulated tissue system implant must develop an enhanced localized vasculature. This may be accomplished by (1) recruiting vessels from the preexisting network of the host vasculature and (2) stimulating new vessel growth resulting from an angiogenic response of host vessels to the implant [Jain, 1994; Peattie et al., 2004]. Therefore, when considering implantation of encapsulated tissue/cells it would be prudent to design the implant to have this biomimetic characteristic, namely, to elicit an angiogenic response from a component of and in the matrix itself. For example, it is known that hyaluronic hydrogels can be synthesized to be biodegradable and that these degradation products stimulate microvessel growth. Also, any biocompatible matrix could be loaded with cytokines that would diffuse out on their own and be released via degradation mechanisms. A resent study [Peattie et al., 2004] demonstrated these facts and identified synergistic behaviors. In summary, cross-linked hyaluronic acid (HA) hydrogels were evaluated for their ability to elicit new microvessel growth *in vivo* when loaded with one of two cytokines, vascular endothelial growth factor (VEGF) or basic fibroblast growth factor (bFGF). HA film samples were surgically implanted in the ear pinnas of mice, and the ears retrieved 7 or 14 days post-implantation. Histologic analysis showed that all groups receiving an implant demonstrated significantly more microvessel density than control ears undergoing surgery but receiving no implant. Moreover, aqueous administration of either growth factor produced substantially more vessel growth than an HA implant with no cytokine. However, the most striking result obtained was a dramatic synergistic interaction between HA and VEGF. New vessel growth was quantified by a metric developed during that study; that is, a dimensionless neovascularization index (NI). This index is defined to represent the number of additional vessels present postimplant in a treatment group, minus the additional number due to the surgical procedure alone, normalized by the contralateral count. Presentation of VEGF in cross-linked HA generated vessel density of NI = 6.7 at day 14. This was more than twice the effect of the sum of HA alone (NI = 1.8) plus VEGF alone (NI = 1.3). This was twice the vessel density generated by coaddition of HA and bFGF (NI = 3.4). New therapeutic approaches for numerous pathologies could be notably enhanced by this localized, synergistic angiogenic response produced by release of VEGF from cross-linked HA films.

4.3 Biomimetic Membranes for Ion Transport

Cells must take nutrients from their extracellular environment to grow and maintain metabolic activity. The selectivity and rate that these molecular species enter can be important in regulatory processes. The mechanisms involved depend upon the size of the molecules to be transported across the cell membrane. These biological membranes consist of a continuous double layer of lipid molecules in which various membrane proteins are imbedded. Individual lipid molecules are able to diffuse rapidly within their own monolayer; however, they rarely "flip-flop" spontaneously between these two monolayers. These molecules are amphoteric and assemble spontaneously into bilayers when placed in water. Sealed compartments are thus formed, which reseal if torn.

The topic of membrane transport is discussed in detail in many texts [Lehninger, 1988; Alberts et al., 1989]. The following discussion is limited to membrane transport of small molecules, hence excluding macromolecules such as polypeptides, polysaccharides, and polynucleotides. The lipid bilayer is a highly impermeable barrier to most polar molecules and thus prevents the loss of the water soluble contents of the cell interior. Consequently, cells have developed special means to transport these species across their membranes. Specialized transmembrane proteins accomplish this, each responsible for the transfer of a specific molecule or group of closely related molecules. The mechanism can be either energy independent, as in passive and facilitated diffusion, or energy dependent, as in active transport and group translocation.

In passive diffusion, molecules are transported with (or "down") a concentration gradient that is thermodynamically favorable and can occur spontaneously. Facilitated diffusion utilizes a carrier molecule, imbedded in the membrane, that can combine specifically and reversibly with the molecule to be transported. This carrier protein undergoes conformational changes when the target molecule binds and again when it releases that molecule on the transverse side of the membrane. This binding is dependent on favorable thermodynamics related to the concentration of free vs. bound species. An equilibrium is established, as in a Langmuir isotherm, on both sides of the membrane. Thus, the rate of transport is proportional to concentration differences maintained on each side of the membrane and the direction of flow is down this gradient. Active transport is similar to facilitated transport in that a carrier protein is necessary; however, it occurs against (up) a concentration gradient, which is thermodynamically unfavorable and thus requires energy. Group translocation requires chemical modification of the substance during the process of transport. This conversion process traps the molecule on a specific side of the membrane due to its asymmetric nature and the essential irreversibility of the transformation. These complexities lead to difficulties in mimicry; thus, research in this area is slow in developing.

Several energy sources are possible for active transport, including electrostatic or pH gradients of the proton motive force (PMF), secondary gradients derived from the PMF by other active transport systems, and by the hydrolysis of ATP. The development of these ion gradients enables the cell to store potential energy in the form of these gradients.

It is essential to realize that simple synthetic lipid bilayers, that is, protein-free, can mimic only passive diffusion processes since they are impermeable to ions but freely permeable to water. Thermodynamically, virtually any molecule should diffuse across a protein-free, synthetic lipid bilayer down its concentration gradient. However, it is the rate of diffusion that is of concern, which is highly dependent upon the size of the molecule and its relative solubility in oil (i.e., the hydrophobic interior of the bilayer). Consequently, small nonpolar molecules such as O_2 readily diffuse. If small enough, uncharged polar molecules such as CO_2, ethanol, and urea can diffuse rapidly, whereas glycerol is more difficult and glucose is essentially excluded. Water, because it has such a small volume and is uncharged, diffuses rapidly even though it is polar and relatively insoluble in the hydrophobic phase of the bilayer. Charged particles, on the other hand, no matter how small, such as Na^+ and K^+, are essentially excluded. This is due to the charge and the high degree of hydration preventing them from entering the hydrocarbon phase. Quantitatively, water permeates the bilayer at a rate 10^3 faster than urea, 10^6 faster than glucose, and 10^9 faster than small ions such as K^+. Thus, only nonpolar molecules and small uncharged polar molecules can cross the cellular lipid membrane directly by simple (passive) diffusion; others require specific membrane transport proteins, as either carriers or channels. Synthetic membranes can be designed for specific biomedical applications that can mimic the transport processes discussed earlier [Michaels, 1988]. Membrane selectivity and transport are enhanced with the aid of highly selective complexing agents, impregnated as either fixed site or mobile carriers. To use these membranes to their full potential, the mechanism of this diffusion needs to be thoroughly understood.

4.3.1 Active Transport Biomimetics

Extensive theoretical and experimental work has previously been reported for supported liquid membrane systems (SLMS) as effective mimics of active transport of ions [Cussler et al., 1989; Kalachev et al., 1992; Thoresen and Fisher, 1995; Stockton and Fisher, 1998]. This was successfully demonstrated using di-(2 ethyl hexyl)-phosphoric acid as the mobile carrier dissolved in n-dodecane, supported in various inert hydrophobic microporous matrices (e.g., polypropylene), with copper and nickel ions as the transported species. The results showed that a pH differential between the aqueous feed and strip streams, separated by the SLMS, mimics the PMF required for the active transport process that occurred. The model for transport in an SLMS is represented by a five-step resistance-in-series approach, as follows (1) diffusion of the ion through a hydrodynamic boundary layer; (2) desolvation of the ion, where it expels the water molecules in its coordination sphere and enters the organic phase via ion exchange with the mobile carrier at the feed/membrane interface; (3) diffusion of the ion-carrier complex across the SLMS to the strip/membrane interface; (4) solvation of the ion as it enters the aqueous strip solution via ion exchange; and (5) transport of the ion through the hydrodynamic boundary layer to the bulk stripping solution. A local Peclet number is used to characterize the hydrodynamics and the mass transfer occurring at the fluid/SLMS interface. The SLMS itself is modeled as a heterogeneous surface with mass transfer and reaction occurring only at active sites; in this case, the transverse pores. Long-term stability and toxicity problems limit their application, as configured above, in the biomedical arena. Use in combination with fixed site carrier membranes as entrapping barriers has great potential and is an active research area. Some success has been obtained using (1) reticulated vitreous carbon as the support matrix and Nafion, for the thin film "active barrier"; and (2) an ethylene-acrylic acid ionomer, utilizing the carboxylic acid groups as the fixed site carriers. The most probable design for biomedical applications appears to be a laminate composite system that incorporates less toxic SLMSs and highly selective molecularly engineered thin film entrapping membranes. Use of fixed site carrier membranes in these innovative designs requires knowledge of transport characteristics. Cussler et al. [1989] have theoretically predicted a jumping mechanism for these systems. Kalachev et al. [1992] have shown that this mechanism can also occur in an SLMS at certain carrier concentrations. This mechanism allows for more efficient transport than common facilitated diffusion. Stability over time and a larger range of carrier concentrations where jumping occurs make fixed-carrier membranes attractive for biomedical applications. A brief discussion of these jumping mechanisms follows.

4.3.2 Mechanism for Facilitated Diffusion in Fixed-Carrier Membranes

A theory for the mechanism of diffusion through a membrane using a fixed carrier covalently bound to the solid matrix, was developed previously [Cussler et al., 1989]. The concept is that the solute molecule jumps from one carrier to the next in sequence. Facilitated diffusion can occur only if these "chained" carriers are reasonably close to each other and have some limited mobility. The advantages of using a chained carrier in a solid matrix vs. a mobile carrier in a liquid membrane are that the stability is improved, there is no potential for solvent loss from the system, and the transport may actually be enhanced. Their theory is compared to that for the mobile carriers in the SLMS. For the fixed-carrier (chained) system, the assumptions of fast reactions and that they take place only at the interface are also used. The major difference is that the complex formed cannot diffuse across the membrane since the carrier is covalently bound to the polymer chain in the membrane. Although the complex does not diffuse in the classical random walk concept, it can "jiggle" around its equilibrium position. This movement can bring it into contact range with an uncomplexed carrier also "jiggling," and result in a reversible interaction typical to normal receptor/ligand surface motion. It is assumed that no uncomplexed solute can pass through the membrane; it would be immobilized and taken from the diffusion process. The transport process that is operable is best explained by viewing the chained-carrier membrane as a lamella structure where each layer is of thickness L. Every carrier can move a distance X around its neutral position and is a length L away from its neighbors. Diffusion can occur only over the distance X. Therefore, there is a specific concentration where a solute flux is first detected, termed percolation threshold, occurring when $L = X$. This threshold concentration is estimated as $C = 1/L^3 N_a$, where C is the average concentration, L is the distance between carrier molecules, and N_a is Avogadro's number. In summary, the mechanism is that of intramolecular diffusion; each chained carrier having limited mobility within the membrane. A carrier at the fluid–membrane interface reacts with the species to be transported and subsequently comes in contact with an uncomplexed carrier and reacts with it, repeating this transfer process across the entire width of the membrane.

4.3.3 Jumping Mechanism in Immobilized Liquid Membranes

Facilitated diffusion was studied in immobilized liquid membranes using a system composed of a microporous nitrocellulose film impregnated with tri-n-octylamine (TOA) in n-decane [Kalachev et al., 1992]. Experiments were monitored by measuring the conductivity of the feed and strip streams. The transport of ions (cobalt and iron) from an acidic feed (HCl) to a basic strip solution (NH_4OH) was accomplished. Their results suggest that there are three distinct transport regimes operable in the membrane. The first occurs at short times and exhibits very little ion transport. This initial time is termed the ion penetration time and is simply the transport time across the membrane. At long times, a rapid increase in indiscriminate transport is observed. At this critical time and beyond, there are stability problems; that is, loss of solvent from the pores leading to the degradation of the membrane and the formation of channels that compromise the ion selective nature of the system and its barrier properties.

Recall that their experiments were for a selective transport with (not against) the ion gradient. It is only in the intermediate time regime that actual facilitated transport occurs. In this second region, experiments were conducted using a cobalt feed solution for various times and carrier concentrations; all experiments showed a peak in flux. The velocity of the transported species can be obtained from these results and the penetration time vs. carrier concentration is available. At the threshold carrier concentration these researchers claim that the mechanism of transport is by jumping, as proposed earlier, for fixed site carriers. The carrier molecules are now close enough to participate in a "bucket brigade" transport mechanism. The carrier molecules use local mobility, made possible by a low viscous solution of n-decane, to oscillate, passing the transported species from one to another. This motion results in faster transport than common facilitated transport, which relies on the random walk concept and occurs at lower TOA concentrations. It is in this low concentration region that the carrier molecules are too far apart to participate in the jumping scheme. At higher concentrations, well above the threshold value, the increased viscosity interferes with carrier mobility; the jumping is less direct or does not occur because of the increased bonding sites and hence removal of the species from the transport process.

4.4 Assessing Mass Transfer Resistances in Biomimetic Reactors

4.4.1 Uncoupling Resistances

Characterization of mass transfer limitations in biomimetic reactors is essential when designing and evaluating their performance. When used in Cell Culture Analog (CCA) systems, the proper mimicry of the role of intrinsic kinetics and transport phenomena cannot be overemphasized. Lack of the desired similitude will negate the credibility of the phenomenological observations as pertaining to toxicity and pharmaceutical efficacy. The systems must be designed to allow manipulation, and thus control, of all interfacial events. The majority of material transfer studies for gaseous substrates are based on the assumption that the primary resistance is at the gas/liquid interface. Studies examining the use of hollow fiber membranes to enhance gas/liquid transport have been successfully conducted [Grasso et al., 1995]. The liquid/cell interfacial resistance is thus uncoupled from that of the gas/liquid interface and they can now be examined separately to evaluate their potential impacts. A reduction in the mean velocity gradient, while maintaining a constant substrate flux into the liquid, resulted in a shift in the limiting resistance from the gas/liquid to the liquid/cell interface. This shift manifested itself as an increase in the Monad apparent half-saturation constant for the chemoautotrophic methanogenic microbial system selected as a convenient analog. The result of these studies significantly influences the design and evaluation of reactors used in the biomedical engineering (BME) research area, especially for the animal surrogate or CCA systems. Although a reactor can be considered as well mixed based on spatial invariance in cell density, it was demonstrated that significant mass transfer resistance may remain at the liquid/cellular boundary layer.

There are three major points to be stressed. First, the liquid/cellular interface may contribute significantly to mass transfer limitations. Second, when mass transfer limitations exist the intrinsic biokinetics parameters cannot be determined. In biochemical reactor design, intrinsic parameters are essential to model adequately the system performance. Furthermore, without an understanding of the intrinsic biokinetics, one cannot accurately study transport mechanisms across biological membranes. The determination of passive or active transport across membranes is strongly affected by the extent of the liquid/cellular interfacial resistance.

4.4.2 Use in Physiologically Based Pharmacokinetics Models and Cell Culture Analog Systems

The potential toxicity of, and the action of, a pharmaceutical is tested primarily using animal studies. Since this technique can be problematic from both a scientific and ethical basis [Gura, 1997], alternatives have been sought. *In vitro* methods using isolated cells [Del Raso, 1993] are inexpensive, quick, and generally present no ethical issues. However, the use of isolated cell cultures does not fully represent the full range of biochemical activity as in the whole organism. Tissue slices and engineered tissues have also been studied but not without their inherent problems, such as the lack of interchange of metabolites among organs and the time dependent exposure within the animal. An alternative to both *in vitro* and animal studies is the use of computer models based on physiologically based pharmacokinetics (PBPK) models [Connolly and Anderson, 1991]. These models mimic the integrated, multi-compartment nature of animals and thus can predict the time-dependent changes in blood and tissue concentrations of the parent chemical and its metabolites. The obvious limitations lie in that a response is based on assumed mechanisms; therefore, secondary and "unexpected" effects are not included. Furthermore, parameter estimation is difficult. Consequently, the need for animal surrogates or CCA systems is created. The pioneering work of M.L. Shuler's group at Cornell University [Sweeney et al., 1995; Shuler et al., 1996; Mufti and Shuler, 1998; also a chapter in this section of the handbook) and many others has led to the following approach.

These CCA systems are physical representations of the PBPK structure where cells or engineered tissues are used in organ compartments. The fluid medium that circulates between compartments acts as a "blood surrogate." Small scale bioreactors housing the appropriate cell types are the physical compartments that represent organs or tissues. This concept combines attributes of PBPK and *in vitro* systems. Furthermore, it is an integrated system that can mimic dose-release kinetics, conversion into specific metabolites from each organ, and the interchange of these metabolites between compartments. Since the CCA system permits dose-exposure scenarios that can replicate those of animal studies, it works in conjunction with a PBPK as a tool to evaluate and modify proposed mechanisms. Thus, bioreactor design and performance evaluation testing is crucial to the success of this animal surrogate concept. Efficient transfer of substrates, nutrients, stimulants, etc. from the gas phase across all interfaces may be critical for the efficacy of certain biotransformation processes and in improving blood compatibility of biosensors monitoring the compartments. Gas/liquid mass transfer theories are well established for microbial processes [Cussler, 1984]. However, biotransformation processes also involve liquid/cellular interfacial transport. In these bioreactor systems, a gaseous species is transported across two interfaces. Each could be a rate-determining step and can mask intrinsic kinetics modeling studies associated with cellular growth and substrate conversion and product formation.

A methanogenic chemoautotrophic process was selected for study because of its relative simplicity and strong dependence on gaseous nutrient transport, thus establishing a firm quantitative base case [Grasso et al., 1995]. The primary objective was to compare the effect of fluid hydrodynamics on mass transfer across the liquid/cellular interface of planktonic cells and the subsequent impact upon growth kinetics. Standard experimental protocol to measure the gas/liquid resistance was employed [Cussler, 1984; Grasso et al., 1995]. The determination of the liquid/cellular resistance is more complex. The thickness of the boundary layer was calculated under various hydrodynamic conditions and combined with molecular diffusion and mass action kinetics to obtain the transfer resistance. Microbial growth kinetics associated with these hydrodynamic conditions can also be examined. Since Monad models are commonly applied to describe chemoautotrophic growth kinetics [Ferry, 1993] the half-saturation constant can be an indicator of mass transfer limitations. The measured (apparent) value will be greater than the intrinsic value, as demonstrated in these earlier studies and mentioned previously.

4.5 Electroenzymatic Membrane Reactors as Electron Transfer Chain Biomimetics

4.5.1 Mimicry of *In Vivo* Coenzyme Regeneration Processes

In many biosynthesis processes, a coenzyme is required in combination with the base enzymes to function as high-efficiency catalysts. A regeneration system is needed to repeatedly recycle the coenzyme to reduce operating costs in continuous *in vitro* synthesis processes, mimicking the *in vivo* regenerative process involving an electron transfer chain system. Multiple reaction sequences are initiated as in metabolic cycles. NAD(H) is one such coenzyme. Because of its high cost, much effort has focused on improving the NAD(H) regeneration process [Chenault and Whitesides, 1987], with electrochemical methods receiving increased attention. The direct regeneration on an electrode has proven to be extremely difficult [Paxinos et al., 1991]. Either acceleration of protonation or inhibition of intermolecular coupling of NAD^+ is required. Redox mediators have permitted the coupling of enzymatic and electrochemical reactions; the mediator accepts the electrons from the electrode and transfers them to the coenzyme via an enzymatic reaction, and thus regeneration/recycling of the coenzyme during a biosynthesis reaction can be accomplished [Hoogvliet et al., 1988]. The immobilization of mediator and enzyme on electrodes can reduce the separation procedure, increase the selectivity, and stabilize the enzyme activity [Fry et al., 1994]. Various viologen mediators and electrodes have been investigated for the NADH system in batch configurations [Kunugi et al., 1990]. The mechanism and kinetics were investigated by cyclic voltammetry, rotating disk electrode, and impedance measurement techniques. The performance of electrochemical regeneration of NADH on an enzyme immobilized electrode for the biosynthesis of lactate in a packed bed flow reactor [Fisher et al., 2000; Chen et al., 2004] is selected as a model system to illustrate an electron transfer chain biomimetic.

4.5.2 Electroenzymatic Production of Lactate from Pyruvate

The reaction scheme is composed of a three-reaction sequence: (1) the NADH-dependent enzymatic (lactate dehydrogenase: LDH) synthesis of lactate from pyruvate; (2) the regeneration of NADH from NAD^+ and enzymatic (lipoamide dehydrogenase: LipDH) reaction with the mediator (methyl viologen);

and (3) the electrochemical (electrode) reaction. The methyl viologen (MV^{2+}) accepts electrons from the cathode and donates them to the NAD^+ via the LipDH reaction. The regenerated NADH in solution is converted to NAD^+ in the enzymatic (LDH) conversion of pyruvate to lactate. A key feature of this system is the *in situ* regeneration of the coenzyme NADH. A flow-by porous reactor utilizes the immobilized enzyme system (LipDH and methyl viologen as a mediator) within the porous graphite cathodes, encapsulated by a cation exchange membrane (Nafion, 124). The free-flowing fluid contains the pyruvate/lactate reaction mixture, the LDH, and the NADH/NAD^+ system. Lactate yields up to 70% have been obtained when the reactor system was operated in a semi-batch (i.e., recirculation) mode for 24 h, as compared to only 50% when operated in a simple batch mode for 200 h. The multi-pass, dynamic input operating scheme permitted optimization studies to be conducted on system parameters. This includes concentrations of all components in the free solution (initial and dynamic input values could be readily adjusted through recycle conditioning), flow rates, and electrode composition and their transport characteristics. By varying the flow rates through this membrane reactor system, operating regimes can be identified that determine the controlling mechanism for process synthesis (i.e., mass transfer vs. kinetics limitations). Procedures for operational map development are thus established.

References

Alberts, B., D. Bray, J. Lewis, M. Raff, K. Roberts, and J.D. Watson (1989). *Molecular Biology of the Cell*, 2nd ed., Garland, New York.

Chen, X., J.M. Fenton, R.J. Fisher, and R.A. Peattie (2004). Evaluation of *in-situ* electro-enzymatic regeneration of co-enzyme NADH in packed bed membrane reactors: biosynthesis of lactate, *J. El. Chem. Soc.*, 151, 236–242.

Chenault, H.K. and G.H. Whitesides (1987). Electrochemical methods for NAD(H) regeneration, *Appl. Biochem. Biotechnol.*, 14, 147.

Cobelli, C., A. Lepschy, and J.G. Romanin (1979). Identifiability results on some constrained compartmental systems. *Math. Biosci.*, 47, 173–196.

Connolly, R.B. and M.E. Anderson (1991). Biologically based pharmacodynamic models: tool for toxicological research and risk assessment. *Annu. Rev. Pharmacol. Toxicol.*, 31, 503.

Cussler, E.L. (1984) *Diffusion: Mass Transfer in Fluid Systems*, Cambridge University Press, New York.

Cussler, E., R. Aris, and A. Bhown (1989). On the limits of facilitated diffusion, *J. Membr. Sci.*, 43, 149–164.

Del Raso, N.J. (1993). *In vitro* methodologies for enhanced toxicity testing. *Toxicol. Lett.* 68, 91.

Dinno, M.A., R.J. Fisher, J.C. Matthews, L.A. Crum, and W. Kennedy (1991). Effects of ultrasound on membrane bound ATPase activity, *J. Acous. Soc. AM.*, 90, No. 4, 2358.

Ferry, J.G. (1993). *Methanogenesis*, Chapman & Hall, New York.

Fisher, R.J. (2000) Compartmental analysis, in *Introduction to Biomedical Engineering*, J. Enderle, S. Blanchard, and J. Bronzino (Eds), Academic Press, Orlando, FL.

Fisher, R.J., J.M. Fenton, and J. Iranmahboob (2000). Electro-enzymatic synthesis of lactate using electron transfer chain biomimetic membranes, *J. Membr. Sci.*, 177, 17–24.

Freshney, R.I. (2000). *Culture of Animal Cells*, 4th ed., Wiley-Liss, New York.

Fry, A.J., S.B. Sobolov, M.D. Leonida, and K.I. Viovodov (1994). *Denki Kagaku*, 62, 1260.

Giusti, P., L. Lazzeri, and L. Lelli (1993). Bioartificial polymeric materials, *TRIP*, 1, 352.

Grasso, K., K. Strevett, and R. Fisher (1995). Uncoupling mass transfer limitations of gaseous substrates in microbial systems. *Chem. Eng. J.*, 59, 2, 195–204.

Gura, T. (1997). Systems for identifying new drugs are faulty, *Science*, 273, 1041.

Hoogvliet, J.C., L.C. Lievense, C.V. Kijk, and C. Veeger (1998). Redox mediators coupling enzymatic and electrochemical reactions for coenzyme regeneration. *Eur. J. Biochem.*, 174, 273.

Jain, R.K.(1994). Transport phenomena in tumors, *Adv. Chem. Eng.*, 19, 129–194.

Kalachev, A.A., L.M. Kardivarenko, N.A. Plate, and V.V. Bargreev (1992). Facilitated diffusion in immob-
    ilized liquid membranes: experimental verification of the jumping mechanism and percolation
    threshold in membrane transport, *J. Membr. Sci.*, 75, 1–5.

Kumar, R., M.H. Chien, V.S. Parmar, L.A. Sameulson, J. Kumar, R. Nicolosi, S. Yoganathan, and
    A.C. Watterson (2004) Design and synthesis of surpa molecular assemblies for drug delivery
    applications. *J. Am. Chem. Soc.*, 126, 10640–10644.

Kunugi, S., K. Ikeda, T. Nakashima, and H. Yamada (1990). Viologen mediators for NADH systems. *Polym.
    Bull.*, 24, 247.

Lauffenburger, D.A. and J.J. Linderman (1993). *Receptors: Models for Binding, Trafficking, and Signaling*,
    Oxford University Press, New York.

Lehninger, A.I. (1988). *Principles of Biochemistry*, Worth Publishers, New York.

Luo, Y. and G.D. Prestwich (2001). Hyaluronic acid-N-hydroxysuccinimide: a useful intermediate for
    bioconjugation. *Bioconjugate Chem.*, 12, 1085–1088.

Michaels, A.L. (1988). Membranes, membrane processes and their applications: needs, unsolved problems,
    and challenges of the 1990s. *Desalination*, 77, 5–34.

Matthews, J.C., W.L. Harder, W.K. Richardson, R.J. Fisher, A.M. Al-Karmi, L.A. Crum, and M.A. Dinno
    (1993). Inactivation of firefly luciferase and rat erythrocyte ATPase by ultrasound. *Membr. Biochem.*,
    10, 213–220.

Mufti, N.A. and M.L. Shuler (1998). Different *in vitro* systems affect cypia1 activity in response to
    2,3,78-tetrachlorodibenzo-p-dioxin. *Toxicol. In Vitro*, 12, 259.

Palsson, B. (2000). Tissue engineering, in *Introduction to Biomedical Engineering*, J. Enderle, S. Blanchard,
    and J. Bronzino (Eds), Academic Press, Orlando, FL, Chap. 12.

Paxinos, A.S., H. Gunther, D.J.M. Schmedding, and H. Simon (1995). *Bioelectro. Bioenerg.*, 25, 425.

Peattie, R.A., A.P. Nayate, M.A. Firpo, J. Shelby, R.J. Fisher, and G.D. Prestwich (2004). Stimulation
    of *in vivo* angiogenesis by cytokine-loaded hyaluronic acid hydrogel implants. *Biomaterials*, 25,
    2789–2798.

Shuler, M.L., A. Ghanem, D. Quick, M.C. Wang, and P. Miller (1996). A self-regulating cell culture analog
    device to mimic animal and human toxicological responses. *Biotechnol. Bioeng.*, 52, 45.

Srinivasan, A.V., G.K. Haritos, and F.L. Hedberg (1991). Biomimetics: advancing man-made materials
    through gruidance from nature, *Appl. Mech. Rev.*, 44, 463–482.

Stockton, E. and R.J. Fisher (1998). Designing biomimetic membranes for ion transport, *Proc. NEBC/IEEE
    Trans.*, 24, 49–51.

Sweeney, L.M., M.L. Shuler, J.G. Babish, and A. Ghanem (1995). A cell culture analog of rodent physiology:
    application to naphthalene toxicology. *Toxicol. In Vitro*, 9, 307.

Thoresen, K. and R.J. Fisher (1995). Use of supported liquid membranes as biomimetics of active transport
    processes, *Biomimetics*, 3, 31–66.

Weiss, R.A., C. Beretta, S. Sasonga, and A. Garton (1995). Polymer blends designed for interfacial transport.
    Appl. Polym. Sci., 41, 491.

5

Diffusional Processes and Engineering Design

E.N. Lightfoot
University of Wisconsin

Mass transport and diffusional processes play key roles in biomedical engineering at several levels, both within the body and in extracorporeal circuits. The roles of mass transfer in tissue function are discussed in Chapter 115 (Lightfoot and Duca), and here we will concentrate on external processes and design of therapeutic regimens. Moreover, we will depend heavily upon major references [Bird et al., 1960; Ho and Sirkar, 1992; Noble and Stern, 1995; Lightfoot and Lightfoot, 1997; Schmidt-Nielsen, 1997; Welling, 1997; Bassingthwaighte et al., 1998] and seek understanding rather than detailed descriptions.

All mass transport processes, which can be defined as the technology for moving one species in a mixture relative to another, depend ultimately upon diffusion as the basis for the desired selective motion. Diffusion takes many forms, and a general description is provided in Table 115.7 of Chapter 115 of previous edition. However, a great deal of information can often be obtained by carefully written statements of simple constraints, and that of conservation of mass is the most useful for our purposes. We shall begin with examples where this suffices and show how one can determine the validity of such a simple approach. We then proceed to situations where more detailed analysis is needed.

5.1 Applications of Allometry

Much of biomedical engineering requires transferring information obtained from animal experiments to humans, and here interspecies similarities have proven quite useful. Many properties of living systems scale simply with body mass according to the simple allometric equation [Schmidt-Nielsen, 1997]:

$$P = aM^b \tag{5.1}$$

Here P is any property, M is average species mass, and a and b are species independent constants. Among the most important of such relations is that of basal metabolic rate of warm blooded animals, for which the total rate of oxygen consumption is given by

$$R_{O_2,\text{tot}} \approx 3.5M^{3/4} \tag{5.2}$$

Here $R_{O_2,\text{tot}}$ is ml O_2 (STP) consumed per hour, and M is body mass in grams. Other important properties, for example blood volume per unit mass and decrease of total oxygen content per unit volume of blood on passing through the arterial system, are invariant: b is zero. It follows that average blood circulation time

$$T_{\text{circ}} \propto M^{1/4} \tag{5.3}$$

This is an important result because it means that flow limited body processes scale with the 1/4-power of body mass. Moreover, T_{circ} is the first of the time constants which we shall find to govern most diffusional processes.

An important application is the prediction of human drug elimination kinetics from animal experiments. For many it is found that

$$cV/m_0 = f(t/T_{\text{circ}}) \tag{5.4}$$

where c is blood concentration of the drug, V is body volume, and m_0 is the initial drug dose. The function f can be quite complex but, to a first order, it is independent of species [see Dedrick et al., 1970; also Lightfoot, 1974]. Moreover, V can be calculated from mass assuming a species independent density close to 1 g/ml. Success of Equation 5.4 requires that drug distribution between blood and body tissues be independent of drug concentration and that elimination be assumed flow limited. We now ask when this last assumption can be justified.

5.2 Flow Limited Processes

Processes in which diffusion and reaction rates are fast relative to mean solute residence times are said to be flow limited because change in diffusion or kinetic rates has little effect on the process under investigation. Although very few biomedically interesting processes are flow limited in this sense at a detailed level of description, it is often found that the global behavior of a complex system can be so described with little error. To understand this we look briefly at Figure 5.1a a closed system of constant volume V with a single inlet and single outlet. Blood or other fluid is flowing through this system at a constant flow rate Q and with a decaying inlet solute concentration

$$c_{\text{in}}(t) = c_0 e^{-t/T_{\text{BC}}} \tag{5.5}$$

We now calculate the difference between this inlet concentration and the outlet concentration $c_{\text{out}}(t)$, for two quite different situations: plug flow in our system (PF), and perfect mixing (CSTR for continuous stirred tank reactor). In both cases the mean residence time is $T_{\text{m}} \equiv V/Q$. The results are:

PF: Here, there is just a time delay without other change, so that

$$t < T_{\text{m}}: c_{\text{out}} - c_{\text{in}} = -c_0 e^{-t/T_{\text{BC}}} \tag{5.6a}$$

$$t > T_{\text{m}}: c_{\text{out}} - c_{\text{in}} = c_0 e^{-t/T_{\text{BC}}}[e^{T_{\text{M}}/T_{\text{BC}}} - 1] \tag{5.6b}$$

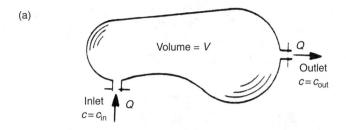

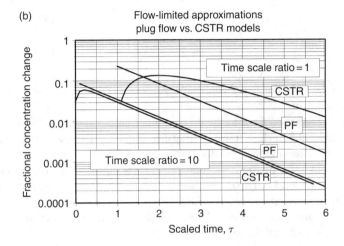

FIGURE 5.1   (a) A simple flow system and (b) flow limited approximations.

CSTR: Here the internal concentration is uniform at the outlet level, and

$$c_{out} - c_{in} = \left(\frac{R}{R-1}\right)[e^{-\tau} - e^{-R\tau}] - e^{-\tau t}; \quad R = T_{BC}/T_M \tag{5.7}$$

These results are plotted in Figure 5.1b for two time-constant ratios, $T_{BC}/T_M = 1$ and $T_{BC}/T_M = 10$. The two flow conditions are seen to produce very different behavior for equal time constants, but these differences quickly become minor when $T_M \ll T_{BC}$. More specifically, the effect of our system flow conditions on the inlet concentration becomes insensitive to these conditions when two criteria are met:

$$T_m \ll T_{BC} \tag{5.8a}$$

$$t = T_{OBS} \geq T_m \tag{5.8b}$$

Here T_{OBS} is the observer time, that is, the time before which there is no interest in the system behavior. These are the conditions of time constant separation, of great practical importance in all engineering design calculations. Usually "much less than" can be taken to be less than a third, and vice versa, and one tenth is almost always sufficient. Thus, using time constant separation to simplify process descriptions is usually referred to as an order-of-magnitude approximation. Returning to Figure 5.1a we may now write a macroscopic mass balance [Bird et al., 1960, Ch. 22) of the form

$$V dc/dt \approx Q(c_m - c) + V\langle R \rangle \tag{5.9}$$

where c is both average internal and exit concentration, and $\langle R \rangle$ is the average rate of solute formation by chemical reaction. Here we have used the CSTR approximation as the simplest to handle mathematically.

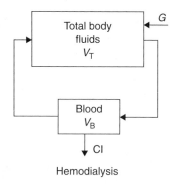

FIGURE 5.2 Modeling hemodialysis.

This expression is valid only under the constraints of Equation 5.8, but these are commonly met in conditions of medical interest.

The major utility of Equation 5.9 is in the description of networks such as the organ network of the human body, and applications include transient drug distribution, anaesthesia, and the study of metabolic processes [Welling, 1997; Bassingthwaighte et al., 1998]. Here an equation similar to Equation 5.8 must be written for each element of the network, but individual organs can be combined, so long as the resulting element conforms to Equation 5.8. These processes are often lumped under the heading of pharmacokinetics, and a large literature has developed [Welling, 1997]. An example of great economic importance is hemodialysis for the treatment of end stage kidney disease. Here the body can be approximated by the simple diagram of Figure 5.2, and the defining equations reduce to

$$V_T dc_T/dt = Q_B(c_B - c_T) + G \tag{5.9a}$$

$$V_B dc_B/dt = -Q_B(c_B - c_T) - Cl \cdot c_B \tag{5.9b}$$

Here the subscript B and T refer to the blood and (whole body) tissue respectively; G is the rate of toxin generation, and Cl is the clearance of the dialyzer. Comparison of prediction with observation is shown for creatinine in Figure 5.3. Here the parameters of Equation 5.9 were determined for the first day's treatment. It may be seen that the pharmacokinetic approximation permits accurate extrapolation for four additional days.

5.3   Extracorporeal Systems

Next we look at the problem of designing extracorporeal systems, and these can normally be classified into a small number of categories. We shall consider steady-state membrane separators, chromatographic devices, and flow reactors.

5.3.1   Membrane Separators

The purpose of these devices is to transfer solute from one flowing steam to another, and there are two subcategories distinguished by the ratio of transmembrane flow induced (convective) and diffusional solute. This ratio in turn is defined by a Péclet number,

$$Pe \equiv \langle v \rangle / P \tag{5.10}$$

$$P \equiv N_i / \Delta c_i \tag{5.11}$$

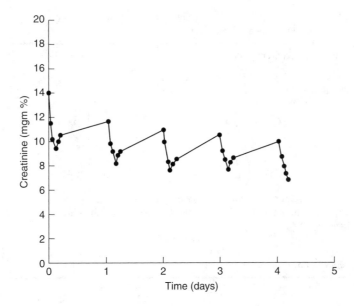

FIGURE 5.3   Actual creatinine dynamics compared to prediction.

Here $\langle v \rangle$ is the observable transmembrane solvent velocity, and P is the membrane solute diffusional permeability. The permeability in turn is defined as the ratio of the molar flux of solute transport, moles/area-time, to the solute concentration difference causing this transport. The most familiar examples of low-Pe devices are blood oxygenators and hemodialyzers. High-Pe systems include micro-, ultra-, and nano-filtration and reverse osmosis. The design and operation of membrane separators is discussed in some detail in standard references [Ho and Sirkar, 1992; Noble and Stern, 1995], and a summary of useful predictions is provided in Section 5.4.

Low-Pe devices are by far the simpler. Solute transport in dialyzers is essentially unaffected by the small amount of transmembrane water flow, and one may therefore use standard design techniques based on membrane permeabilities, usually supplied by the vendor, and mass transfer coefficients in the adjacent fluids. Local fluxes can be described by the simple expression

$$N_i = K_c(c_{ib} - c_{ie}) \tag{5.12}$$

where N_i is the molar flux of the solute "i" across the membrane, moles/area-time, K_c is the overall mass transfer coefficient, c_i is molar solute concentration while the subscripts "b" and "e" refer to blood and the external fluid, respectively. The overall mass transfer coefficient must be calculated from the two fluid phase coefficients and membrane permeability. Hemodialysis solutes tend to distribute uniformly between blood (on a cell-free basis), and one may use the simple approximation

$$1/K_c = (1/k_b) + (1/P) + (1 + k_e) \tag{5.13}$$

Here k_b and k_e are the mass transfer coefficients for the blood and external fluid, here dialysate, respectively. These phase mass transfer coefficients can usually be estimated to an acceptable accuracy from simple asymptotic formulas [Lightfoot and Lightfoot, 1997]. Examples of the latter are given in Table 5.1. For unequally distributed solutes, Equation 5.3 must be appropriately modified [Lightfoot and Lightfoot, 1997], and, for blood this can be something of a problem [Popel, 1989].

Equipment performance for dialyzers is normally expressed in terms of clearance

$$Cl = f c_{i,in} Q \tag{5.14}$$

TABLE 5.1 Asymptotic Nusselt Numbers for Laminar Duct Flow
(With Fully Developed Velocity Profiles)

Constant wall concentration	Constant wall mass flux

Thermal entrance region

Plug flow:

$$\mathrm{Nu_{loc}} = \frac{1}{\sqrt{\pi}} \left(\frac{vD^2}{Ðz} \right)^{1/2} \qquad\qquad \mathrm{Nu_{loc}} = \frac{\sqrt{\pi}}{2} \left(\frac{vD^2}{Ðz} \right)^{1/2}$$

Parabolic velocity profile:

$$\mathrm{Nu_{loc}} = \frac{1}{9^{1/3}\Gamma(4/3)} \left(\frac{gD^3}{Ðz} \right)^{1/3} \qquad\qquad \mathrm{Nu_{loc}} = \frac{\Gamma(2/3)}{9^{1/3}} \left(\frac{gD^3}{Ðz} \right)^{1/3}$$

Here z is distance in the flow direction and g is the rate of change of velocity with
distance from the wall, evaluated at the wall. Nusselt numbers are local values,
evaluated at z.

Fully developed region

| Plug flow: | $\mathrm{Nu_{loc}} = 5.783$ | $\mathrm{Nu_{loc}} = 8$ |
| Parabolic flow: | $\mathrm{Nu} = 3.656$ | $\mathrm{Nu} = 48/11$ |

where f is the fraction of incoming solute "i" removed from the blood, $c_{i,\mathrm{in}}$ is concentration of solute
"i" in the entering blood, and Q is volumetric blood flow rate. Clearance is a convenient measure as it
is independent of solute concentration, and it is easily determined experimentally. Prediction is useful
for device design, but in operation, clearance is usually determined along with effective blood flow rates
and tissue water volumes from numerical analysis of a test dialysis procedure. The efficiency of blood
oxygenators can be dominated by either membrane permeability or mass transfer in the flowing blood,
and it is complicated by the kinetics and thermodynamics of the oxygen/hemoglobin system. These aspects
are discussed in detail by Popel [1989].

High-Pe devices are dominated by transmembrane water transport, and detailed discussion must be
left to the above cited references. However, it is important to recognize their primary function is to remove
water and undesired solutes while retaining one solute which is desired. Rejection of the desired product
increases toward an asymptote as water flux increases, and one should operate near this asymptote if at
all possible. The relation between water flux and rejection is perhaps best determined experimentally.
However, as water flux increases the rejected solute concentration at the interface between the feed stream
and the membrane also increases. This process, usually known as concentration polarization, typically
produces a significant increase in osmotic pressure which acts to reduce the flow. Polarization is a complex
process, but to a good approximation the trans-membrane water velocity is given by

$$\langle v \rangle \approx \ln(c_{s\delta}/c_{s0}) \cdot (\rho_\delta/\rho_0) \cdot \Theta \cdot k_c \tag{5.15}$$

Here c_s is concentration of the rejected solute, r is solution density, k_c is the concentration-based mass
transfer coefficient in the absence of water flux, and the subscripts δ and 0 refer to conditions at the
membrane surface and bulk of the fed solution, respectively. The factor Θ is a correction for variable
viscosity and diffusivity, approximated at least for some systems by

$$\Theta \equiv \langle Ð^\star \rangle^{2/3} \langle 1/\mu^\star \rangle^{1/3} \tag{5.16}$$

and $\langle D^\star \rangle$ and $\langle 1/\mu^\star \rangle$ are the averages of solute diffusivity and reciprocal solution viscosity at the membrane
surface and bulk solution divided by these quantities in the bulk solution. These equations are reasonable
once appreciable polarization has occurred, if rejection is high, and they are a modification of earlier
boundary-layer analyses of Kozinski and Lightfoot [1972]. They are more accurate than the more recent
results made using simple film theory discussed in Ho and Sirkar [1992] and Noble and Stern [1995],

both in incorporating the coefficient 1.4 and in the corrections for variable diffusivity and viscosity. The coefficient of 1.4 is a correction to account for boundary-layer compression accompanying transmembrane flow, not allowed for in film theory. Typical geometry insensitive boundary layer behavior is assumed, and these equations are not restricted to any given rejected solute or equipment configuration. However, in order to calculate the pressure drop required to obtain this flow, one must use the expression

$$\Delta p = \pi + v/k_h \tag{5.17}$$

where Δp is transmembrane pressure drop, π is solute osmotic pressure at the membrane surface, and k_h is the hydraulic permeability of the membrane. The osmotic pressure in turn is a function of solute concentration at the membrane surface, and thus is different for each rejected solute.

5.3.2 Chromatographic Columns

Chromatography is very widely used in biomedical analyses and to a significant extent for extracorporeal processing of blood and other body fluids. Recovery of proteins from blood is of particular importance, and these applications can be expected to grow. Good basic texts are available for underlying dynamic theory [Guiochon et al., 1994] and chemistry [Snyder et al., 1997], and a series of design papers is recommended [Athalye et al., 1992; Lightfoot et al., 1997; Lode et al., 1998; Yuan et al., in press]. Differential chromatography, in which small mixed-solute pulses are separated by selective migration along a packed column, is the simplest, and much of the chromatographic literature is based on concepts developed for this basic process.

In differential chromatography, the individual solutes do not interact, and the effluent curve for each is usually close to a Gaussian distribution:

$$c_f(L, t) = c_0 \exp\left[-\left(\frac{t}{\bar{t}} - 1\right)^2\right] \bigg/ (2\pi)^{t/2}(\sigma/\bar{t}) \tag{5.18}$$

where $c_f(L, t)$ is the fluid phase concentration leaving a column of length L at time t, $\bar{t}$ is the mean solute residence time, and σ is the standard deviation of the distribution; c_0 is the maximum effluent concentration. Degree of separation is defined in terms of the resolution, R_{12} defined as in Figure 5.4

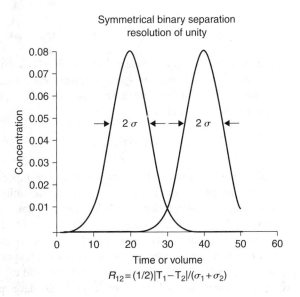

FIGURE 5.4 Resolution in differential chromatography.

where separation with a resolution of unity is shown. Here the distance between the two mean residence times $(\bar{t}_1 - \bar{t}_2)$, 40 and 20 in Figure 5.4, increase in direct proportion to column length, while the standard deviations increase with its square root. Thus resolution is proportional to the square root of column length. Column performance is normally rated in terms of the number of equivalent theoretical plates, N defined by

$$N \equiv (\bar{t}/\sigma)^2 \tag{5.19}$$

Methods of predicting N from column design and operating conditions are described in the above mentioned references [see Athalye et al., 1992].

5.3.3 Flow Reactors

Development of small flow reactors for diagnostic purposes is a fast growing field. Patient monitoring of blood glucose is probably the largest current example, but new applications for a wide variety of purposes are rapidly being developed. These are essentially miniaturized variants of industrial reactors and normally consist of channels and reservoirs with overall dimensions of centimeters and channel diameters of millimeters or even tenths of millimeters. The key elements in their description are convective mass transfer, dispersion, and reaction, and they differ from larger systems only in parameter magnitudes. In particular, flow is almost invariably laminar and Schmidt numbers

$$Sc \equiv \mu/\rho\mathcal{D} \tag{5.20}$$

are always high, never less than 10^5. Here μ is solvent viscosity, ρ is its density, and $\mathcal{D}$ is effective solute diffusivity through the solution. These aspects are briefly described in the next section.

5.4 Useful Correlations

5.4.1 Convective Mass Transfer

Mass transfer coefficients k_c are best correlated in the dimensionless form of mass transfer Nusselt numbers defined as

$$Nu \equiv k_c D/\mathcal{D} \tag{5.21}$$

where D is any convenient characteristic length, typically diameter for tubes. For the high-Sc systems considered above, these Nusselt numbers are functions only of a dimensionless ratio L^*, system geometry, and boundary conditions [Lightfoot and Lightfoot, 1997]. The scaled length L^* in turn is just the ratio of mean solvent residence time to lateral diffusion time:

$$L^* \equiv (L/\langle v \rangle)/(D^2/24\mathcal{D}) \tag{5.22}$$

For all geometries these functions have the same three characteristics: an entrance region solution for L^* "much" less than unity, a constant asymptotic value for L^* "much" greater than unity (the "fully developed" region), and a relatively unimportant transition region for L^* close to unity. Normally the entrance region is of most practical importance and can be used without great error up to L^* of unity. Typical results are shown in Table 5.1. The entrance region results are valid for both tubes (circular cross-section) and between parallel plates; it may be noted that the reference length D cancels. It appears to the same power on both sides of the equations. The correlations for laminar flow are also valid for non-Newtonian fluids if the appropriate wall velocity gradients are used. The solutions for fully developed flow are, however, only useful for round tubes and either plug or Poiseuille flow as indicated. These are much less important as they result in very low transfer rates. Plug and Poiseuille (parabolic) flows are limiting situations, and most real situations will be between them. Plug flow is approximated in ultrafiltration where the high solute concentrations produce a locally high viscosity. Poiseuille flow is a good approximation for dialysis.

5.4.2 Convective Dispersion and the One-Dimensional Convective Diffusion Equation

Non-uniform velocity profiles tend to reduce axial concentration gradients, a result which is qualitatively similar to a high axial diffusivity. As a result, it is common practice to approximate the diffusion equation for duct flow as

$$\partial \bar{c}/\partial t + \langle v \rangle \partial \bar{c}/\partial z \equiv Ð_{\text{eff}} \partial^2 \bar{c}/\partial z^2 \langle R_{i,\text{eff}} \rangle \qquad (5.23)$$

Here the overline indicates an average over the flow cross-section, usually further approximated as the cup-mixing or bulk concentration [Bird et al., 1960], $\langle v \rangle$ is the flow average velocity, $Ð_{\text{eff}}$ is an effective diffusivity, and $\langle R_{i,\text{eff}} \rangle$ is the rate of solute addition per unit volume by reaction plus mass transfer across the wall:

$$\langle R_{i,\text{eff}} \rangle = \langle R_{i,\text{chem}} \rangle + (C/S)K_c(c_e - \bar{c}) \qquad (5.24)$$

Here $\langle R_{i,\text{chem}} \rangle$ is the average volumetric rate of formation of species "i," moles/volume-time, C is the duct circumference, S is its cross-sectional area, and c_e is the solute concentration outside the duct wall, that is, in the surrounding fluid.

For Newtonian tube flow at $L*$ greater than unity, it is reasonable to write

$$Ð_{\text{eff}}/D \approx 1 + (1/192)(D\langle v \rangle/Ð^2) \qquad (5.25)$$

The restrictions on this result and some additional useful approximations are widely discussed in the mass transfer literature [see Ananthkrishnan et al., 1965]. For flow in packed beds, one often sees

$$Ð_{\text{eff}}/D \approx 0.4(Dv_2/Ð) \qquad (5.26)$$

but more accurate expressions are available [Athalye et al., 1992]. Convective dispersion is a very complex subject with a large literature, and successful application requires careful study [Brenner, 1962; Ananthkrishnan et al., 1965; Edwards et al., 1991].

References

Ananthakrishnan, V., W.N. Gill, and A.J. Barduhn, 1965, Laminar dispersion in capillaries, *AIChEJ*, 11, 1063–1072.

Athalye, A.M., S.J. Gibbs, and E.N. Lightfoot, 1992, Predictability of chromatographic separations: study of size exclusion media with narrow particle size distributions, *J. Chromatogr. A*, 589, 71–85.

Bassingthwaighte, J.B., C.A. Goresky, and J.H. Linehan, 1998, *Whole Organ Approaches to Cellular Metabolism*, Springer-Verlag, New York.

Bird, R.B., W.E. Stewart, and E.N. Lightfoot, 1960, *Transport Phenomena*, John Wiley & Sons, New York.

Brenner, H., 1962, The diffusion model of longitudinal mixing in beds of finite length, *CES*, 17, 229–243.

Dedrick, R.L., K.B. Bischoff, and D.S. Zaharko, 1970, Interspecies correlation of plasma concentration history of methotrexate (NSC-740), *Cancer Ther. Rep.*, Part I, 54, 95.

Edwards, D.A., M. Shapiro, H. Brenner, and M. Shapira, 1991, *Transport in Porous Media*, Wiley, New York.

Guiochon, G., S.G. Shirazi, and A.M. Katti, 1994, *Fundamentals of Preparative and Non-Linear Chromatography*, Academic Press, New York.

Ho, W.S.W. and K.K. Sirkar, 1992, *Membrane Handbook*, Van Nostrand Reinhold, New York.

Kozinski, A.A. and E.N. Lightfoot, 1972, Protein ultrafiltration, *AIChEJ*, 18, 1030–1040.

Lightfoot, E.N., 1974, *Transport Phenomena and Living Systems*, Wiley-Interscience, New York.

Lightfoot, E.N. and E.J. Lightfoot, 1997, *Mass Transfer in Kirk–Othmer Encyclopedia of Separation Technology*.

Lightfoot, E.N. and K.A. Duca, 2000, The roles of mass transfer in tissue function, in *The Biomedical Engineering Handbook*, 2nd ed., Bronzino, J., Ed., CRC Press, Boca Raton, FL, chap. 115.

Lightfoot, E.N., J.L. Coffman, F. Lode, T.W. Perkins, and T.W. Root, 1997, Refining the description of protein chromatography, *J. Chromatgr. A*, 760, 130.

Lode, F., A. Rosenfeld, Q.S. Yuan, T.W. Root, and E.N. Lightfoot, 1998, Refining the scale-up of chromatographic separations, *J. Chromatogr. A*, 796, 3–14.

Noble, R.D. and S.A. Stern, 1995, *Membrane Separations Technology*, Elsevier, London.

Popel, A.S. 1989, Theory of oxygen transport to tissue, *Clin. Rev. Biomed. Eng.*, 17, 257.

Schmidt-Nielsen, 1997, *Animal Physiology*, 5th ed., Cambridge University Press, Cambridge.

Snyder, L.R., J.J. Kirkland, and J.L. Glajch, 1997, John Wiley & Sons, New York.

Welling, P.G. 1997, *Pharmacokinetics*, American Chemical Society.

Yuan, Q.S., A. Rosenfeld, T.W. Root, D.J. Klingenberg, and E.N. Lightfoot, Flow distribution in chromatographic columns, *J. Chromatogr. A*.

6

Microvascular Heat Transfer

James W. Baish
Bucknell University

6.1   Introduction and Conceptual Challenges

Models of microvascular heat transfer are useful for optimizing thermal therapies such as hyperthermia treatment, for modeling thermoregulatory response at the tissue level, for assessing environmental hazards that involve tissue heating, for using thermal means of diagnosing vascular pathologies and for relating blood flow to heat clearance in thermal methods of blood perfusion measurement. For example, the effect of local hyperthermia treatment is determined by the length of time that the tissue is held at an elevated temperature, nominally 43°C or higher. Since the tissue temperature depends on the balance between the heat added by artificial means and the tissue's ability to clear that heat, an understanding of the means by which the blood transports heat is essential. This section of the handbook outlines the general problems associated with such processes while more extensive reviews and tutorials on microvascular heat transfer may be found elsewhere [1–4].

The temperature range of interest for all of these applications is intermediate between freezing and boiling, making only sensible heat exchange by conduction and convection important mechanisms of heat transfer. At high and low temperatures such as those present during laser ablation or electrocautery and cryopreservation or cryosurgery the change of phase and accompanying mass transport present problems beyond the scope of this section [see Reference 5].

Whereas the equations that govern heat transport are formally similar to those that govern diffusive mass transport, heat and diffusing molecules interact with the microvasculature in fundamentally different ways because the thermal diffusivity of most tissues is roughly two orders of magnitude greater than the diffusivity for mass transport of most mobile species (1.5×10^{-7} m^2/sec for heat vs. 1.5×10^{-9} m^2/sec for O_2). Mass transport is largely restricted to the smallest blood vessels, the capillaries, arterioles, and venules, whereas heat transport occurs in somewhat larger, so-called thermally significant blood vessels with diameters in the range from 80 μm to 1 mm. The modes of heat transport differ from those of mass transport, not simply because these vessels are larger, but because they are have a different geometrical arrangement than the vessels primarily responsible for mass transport. Many capillary beds approximate a uniformly spaced array of parallel vessels that can be well modeled by the Krogh cylinder model. In contrast, the **thermally significant vessels** are in a tree-like arrangement that typically undergoes several generations of branching within the size range of interest and are often found as countercurrent pairs in which the artery and vein may be separated by one vessel diameter or less. Moreover, the vascular architecture of the thermally significant vessels is less well characterized than that of either the primary mass exchange vessels or the larger, less numerous supply vessels that carry blood over large distances in the body. There are too few supply vessels to contribute much to the overall energy balance in the tissue, but they are often far from thermal equilibrium with the surroundinig tissue producing large local perturbations in the tissue temperature. Much of the microvascular heat exchange occurs as blood flows from the larger supply vessels into the more numerous and densely spaced, thermally significant vessels.

Although the details of the vascular architecture for particular organs have been well characterized in individual cases, variability among individuals makes the use of such published data valid only in a statistical sense. Current imaging technology can be used to map and numerically model thermally significant blood vessels larger than 600 μm diameter [6], but smaller vessels must be analyzed by other approaches as illustrated below.

An additional challenge arises from the spatial and temporal variability of the blood flow in tissue. The thermoregulatory system and the metabolic needs of tissues can change the blood perfusion rates by a factor as great as 15 to 25.

6.2 Basic Concepts

For purposes of thermal analysis, vascular tissues are generally assumed to consist of two interacting subvolumes, a solid tissue subvolume and a blood subvolume which contains flowing blood. These subvolumes thermally interact through the walls of the blood vessels where heat, but little mass is exchanged. Because the tissue subvolume can transport heat by conduction alone, it may be modeled by the standard heat diffusion equation [7]

$$\nabla k_t \nabla T_t(\vec{r}, t) + \dot{q}_t'''(\vec{r}, t) = \rho_t c_t \frac{\partial T_t(\vec{r}, t)}{\partial t} \qquad (6.1)$$

where T_t is the local tissue temperature, k_t is the **thermal conductivity** of the tissue, $\dot{q}_t'''$ is the rate of volumetric heat generation from metabolism or external source, ρ_t is the tissue density and c_t is the tissue **specific heat**. The properties used in Equation 6.1 may be assumed to be bulk properties that average over the details of the interstitial fluid, extracellular matrix, and cellular content of the tissue. In the blood subvolume heat may also be transported by advection which adds a blood velocity dependent term as given by [7]

$$\nabla k_b \nabla T_b(\vec{r}, t) - \rho_b c_b \vec{u}_b(\vec{r}, t) \cdot \nabla T_b(\vec{r}, t) + \dot{q}_b'''(\vec{r}, t) = \rho_b c_b \frac{\partial T_b(\vec{r}, t)}{\partial t} \qquad (6.2)$$

where $\vec{u}_b$ is the local blood velocity and all other parameters pertain to the local properties of the blood. Potential energy, kinetic energy, and viscous dissipation effects are typically neglected.

At the internal boundary on the vessel walls we expect a continuity of heat flux $k_b \nabla T_b(\vec{r}_w, t) = k_t \nabla T_t(\vec{r}_w, t)$ and temperature $T_b(\vec{r}_w, t) = T_t(\vec{r}_w, t)$ where $\vec{r}_w$ represents points on the vessel wall. Few attempts have been made to solve Equation 6.1 and Equation 6.2 exactly, primarily due to the complexity of the vascular architecture and the paucity of data on the blood velocity field in any particular instance. The sections that follow present approaches to the problem of microvascular heat transport that fall broadly into the categories of vascular models that consider the response of one or a few blood vessels to their immediate surroundings and continuum models that seek to average the effects of many blood vessels to obtain a single field equation that may be solved for a local average of the tissue temperature.

6.3 Heat Transfer to Blood Vessels

6.3.1 Vascular Models

Most vascular models are based on the assumption that the behavior of blood flowing in a blood vessel is formally similar to that of a fluid flowing steadily in a roughly circular tube (see Figure 6.1), that is [8],

$$\pi r_a^2 \rho_b c_b \bar{u} \frac{d\bar{T}_a(s)}{ds} = q'(s) \tag{6.3}$$

where $\bar{T}_a(s)$ is the mixed mean temperature of the blood for a given vessel cross section, r_a is the vessel radius, $\bar{u}$ is mean blood speed in the vessel, $q'(s)$ is the rate at which heat conducts into the vessel per unit length, and s is the spatial coordinate along the vessel axis. For a vessel that interacts only with a cylinder of adjacent tissue we have

$$q'(s) = U' 2\pi r_a (\bar{T}_t(s) - \bar{T}_a(s)) \tag{6.4}$$

where U' is the overall heat transfer coefficient between the tissue and the blood. Typically, the thermal resistance inside the blood vessel is much smaller than that in the tissue cylinder so to a first approximate we have $U' 2\pi r_a \approx k_t \sigma$ where the **conduction shape factor** σ relating local tissue temperature $\bar{T}_t(s)$ to the blood temperature may be estimated from

$$\sigma \approx \frac{2\pi}{\ln(r_t/r_a)} \tag{6.5}$$

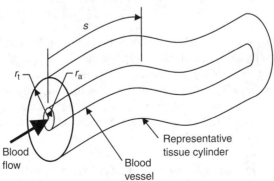

FIGURE 6.1   Representative tissue cylinder surrounding a blood vessel showing the radial and axial position coordinates.

6.3.2 Equilibration Lengths

One of the most useful concepts that arises from the simple vascular model presented above is the **equilibration length** L_e, which may be defined as the characteristic length over which the blood at an inlet temperature $\bar{T}_{a_o}$ equilibrates with surrounding tissue at a constant temperature $\bar{T}_t$. The solution for Equation 6.3 and Equation 6.4 under these conditions is given by

$$\frac{\bar{T}_a(s) - \bar{T}_t}{\bar{T}_{a_o} - \bar{T}_t} = \exp\left(-\frac{s}{L_e}\right) \tag{6.6}$$

where the equilibration length is given by

$$L_e = \frac{\pi r_a^2 \rho_b c_b \bar{u}}{k_t \sigma} \tag{6.7}$$

Chen and Holmes [9] found that vessels with diameters of about 175 μm have an anatomical length comparable to their thermal equilibration length, thus making vessels of this approximate size the dominant site of tissue–blood heat exchange. Accordingly, these vessels are known as the *thermally significant blood vessels*. Much smaller vessels, while more numerous, carry blood that has already equilibrated with the surrounding tissue and much larger vessels, while not in equilibrium with the surrounding tissue are too sparsely spaced to contribute significantly to the overall energy balance [8]. Even though the larger vessels do not exchange large quantities of heat with the tissue subvolume they cannot be ignored, because these vessels produce large local perturbations to the tissue temperature and form a source of blood for tissues that is at a much different temperature than the local tissue temperature.

6.3.3 Countercurrent Heat Exchange

Thermally significant blood vessels are frequently found in closely spaced countercurrent pairs. Only a slight modification to the preceding formulas is needed for heat exchange between adjacent arteries and veins with countercurrent flow [10]

$$q'(s) = k_t \sigma_\Delta (\bar{T}_v(s) - \bar{T}_a(s)) \tag{6.8}$$

where $\bar{T}_v(s)$ is the mixed mean temperature in the adjacent vein and the conduction shape factor is given approximately by [7]

$$\sigma_\Delta \approx \frac{2\pi}{\cosh^{-1}[(w^2 - r_a^2 - r_v^2)/(2r_a r_v)]} \tag{6.9}$$

where w is the distance between the vessel axes and r_v is the radius of the vein. The blood temperatures in the artery and vein must be obtained simultaneously, but still yield an equilibration length of the form given in Equation 6.7. Substitution of representative property values, blood speeds and vessel dimensions reveals that countercurrent vessels have equilibration lengths that are about one third that of isolated vessels of similar size [10]. Based on this observation, the only vessels that participate significantly in the overall energy balance in the tissue are those larger than about 50 μm in diameter. Countercurrent exchange is sufficiently vigorous that venous blood has been observed to recapture up to 41% of that lost from artery [11].

The shape factors given above are only rough analytical approximations that do not include the effects of finite thermal resistance within the blood vessels and other geometrical effects. The reader is referred to Table 6.1 for references that address these issues. A careful review of the effects of the boundary condition at the vessel wall is given by Roemer [12].

TABLE 6.1 Shape Factors for Various Vascular Geometries

Geometry	Ref.
Single vessel to skin surface	[10]
Single vessel to tissue cylinder	[9]
Countercurrent vessel to vessel	[10,51]
Countercurrent vessels to tissue cylinder	[29]
Countercurrent vessels with a thin tissue layer	[52]
Multiple parallel vessels	[53]
Vessels near a junction of vessels	[54]

Typical Dimension of blood vessels are available in Tables 1.3 and 1.4 of this handbook.

6.3.4 Heat Transfer Inside of a Blood Vessel

A detailed analysis of the steady-state heat transfer between the blood vessel wall and the mixed mean temperature of the blood can be done using standard heat transfer methods

$$q'(s) = h\pi d(T_w(s) - T_b) \tag{6.10}$$

where d is the vessel diameter, $T_w(s)$ is the vessel wall temperature and the convective heat transfer coefficient h may be found from Victor and Shah's [13] recommendation that the Nusselt number may be obtained from

$$\bar{N}u_D = \frac{hd}{k_b} = 4 + 0.155 \exp(1.58 \log_{10} \text{Gz}) \quad \text{Gz} < 10^3 \tag{6.11}$$

where Gz is the Graetz number defined as

$$\text{Gz} = \frac{\rho_b c_b \bar{u} d^2}{k_b L} \tag{6.12}$$

where L is the vessel length (see also Barozzi and Dumas [14]).

In the larger blood vessels, pulsatility may have pronounced effects on blood velocity and pressure. Such transient flow effects have little impact on average heat transfer rates. The Nusselt number averaged over a cycle of pulsation differs no more than 11% from the steady-state value [15]. Since the resistance to heat flow is greater in the surrounding tissue than it is in within the blood vessel, the net effect of pulsatility on tissue–vessel heat transfer is generally negligible except when transients on the time scale of a cycle of pulsation are of interest.

6.4 Models of Perfused Tissues

6.4.1 Continuum Models

Continuum models of microvascular heat transfer are intended to average over the effects of many vessels so that the blood velocity field need not be modeled in detail. Such models are usually in the form of a modified heat diffusion equation in which the effects of blood perfusion are accounted for by one or more additional terms. These equations then can be solved to yield a local average temperature that does not include the details of the temperature field around every individual vessel, but provides information on

TABLE 6.2 Representative Thermal Property Values

Tissue	Thermal conductivity (W/m-K)	Thermal diffusivity (m^2/sec)	Perfusion (m^3/m^3-sec)
Aorta	0.461 [20]	1.25×10^{-7} [20]	—
Fat of spleen	0.3337 [55]	1.314×10^{-7} [55]	
Spleen	0.5394 [55]	1.444×10^{-7} [55]	0.023 [56]
Pancreas	0.5417 [55]	1.702×10^{-7} [55]	0.0091 [56]
Cerebral cortex	0.5153 [55]	1.468×10^{-7} [55]	0.0067 [57]
Renal cortex	0.5466 [55]	1.470×10^{-7} [55]	0.077 [58]
Myocardium	0.5367 [55]	1.474×10^{-7} [55]	0.0188 [59]
Liver	0.5122 [55]	1.412×10^{-7} [55]	0.0233 [60]
Lung	0.4506 [55]	1.307×10^{-7} [55]	
Adenocarcinoma of breast	0.5641 [55]	1.436×10^{-7} [55]	
Resting muscle	0.478 [61]	1.59×10^{-7} [61]	0.0007 [59]
Bone			
Whole blood (21°C)	0.492 [61]	1.19×10^{-7} [61]	—
Plasma (21°C)	0.570 [61]	1.21×10^{-7} [61]	—
Water	0.628 [7]	1.5136×10^{-7} [7]	—

the broad trends in the tissue temperature (Table 6.2). The temperature they predict may be defined as

$$\bar{T}_t(\vec{r}, t) = \frac{1}{\delta V} \int_{\delta V} T_t(\vec{r}', t) \mathrm{d}V' \tag{6.13}$$

where δV is a volume that is assumed to be large enough to encompass a reasonable number of thermally significant blood vessels, but much smaller than the scale of the tissue as a whole. Much of the confusion concerning the proper form of the bioheat equation stems from the difficulty in precisely defining such a length scale. Unlike a typical porous medium such as water percolating through sand where the grains of sand fall into a relatively narrow range of length scales, blood vessels form a branching structure with length scales spanning many orders of magnitude.

6.4.1.1 Formulations

6.4.1.1.1 Pennes Heat Sink Model
In 1948, physiologist Harry Pennes modeled the temperature profile in the human forearm by introducing the assumptions that the primary site of equilibration was the capillary bed and that each volume of tissue has a supply of arterial blood that is at the core temperature of the body. The Pennes' Bioheat equation has the form [16]

$$\nabla k \nabla \bar{T}_t(\vec{r}, t) + \dot{\omega}_b(\vec{r}, t) \rho_b c_b (T_a - \bar{T}_t(\vec{r}, t)) + \dot{q}'''(\vec{r}, t) = \rho c \frac{\partial \bar{T}_t(\vec{r}, t)}{\partial t} \tag{6.14}$$

where $\dot{\omega}_b$ is taken to be the blood **perfusion rate** in volume of blood per unit volume of tissue per unit time and T_a is an arterial supply temperature which is generally assumed to remain constant and equal to the core temperature of the body, nominally 37°C. The other thermal parameters are taken to be effective values that average over the blood and tissue subvolumes. Major advantages of this formulation are that it is readily solvable for constant parameter values, requires no anatomical data, and in the absence of independent measurement of the actual blood rate and heat generation rate gives two adjustable parameters ($\dot{\omega}_b(\vec{r}, t)$ and T_a) that can be used to fit the majority of the experimental results available. On the downside, the model gives no prediction of the actual details of the vascular temperatures, the actual blood perfusion rate is usually unknown and not exactly equal to the value of $\dot{\omega}_b$ that best fits the thermal data, the assumption of constant arterial temperature is not generally valid and, based on the equilibration length studies presented in the previous section, thermal equilibration occurs prior to the capillary bed. Despite these weaknesses, the Pennes formulation is the primary choice of modelers. Equilibration prior to the capillary bed does not invalidate the model provided that the averaging volume is large enough to encompass many vessels of the size in which equilibration actually occurs and that the venous return does not exchange significant quantities of heat after leaving the equilibrating vessels. As long as $\dot{\omega}_b$ and T_a are taken as adjustable, curve-fitting parameters rather than literally as the perfusion rate and arterial blood temperature the model may be used fruitfully, provided that the results are interpreted accordingly.

6.4.1.1.2 Directed Perfusion
Some of the shortcomings of the Pennes model were addressed by Wulff [17] in a formulation that is essentially the same as used for common porous media

$$\nabla k \nabla \bar{T}_t(\vec{r}, t) - \rho c \vec{u}(\vec{r}, t) \cdot \nabla \bar{T}_t(\vec{r}, t) + \dot{q}'''(\vec{r}, t) = \rho c \frac{\partial \bar{T}_t(\vec{r}, t)}{\partial t} \tag{6.15}$$

where $\vec{u}$ is a velocity averaged over both the tissue and blood subvolumes. Among the difficulties with this model are that it is valid only when the tissue and blood are in near-thermal equilibrium and when the averaging volume is small enough to prevent adjacent arteries and veins from canceling out their contributions to the average velocity, thus erroneously suggesting that the blood perfusion has no net effect on the tissue heat transfer. Equation 6.15 is rarely applied in practical situations, but served as an important conceptual challenge to the Pennes formulation in the 1970s and 1980s.

6.4.1.1.3 Effective Conductivity Model
The oldest continuum formulation is the effective conductivity model

$$\nabla k_{\text{eff}} \nabla \bar{T}_t(\vec{r}, t) + \dot{q}'''(\vec{r}, t) = \rho_t c_t \frac{\partial \bar{T}_t(\vec{r}, t)}{\partial t} \tag{6.16}$$

where the **effective conductivity** is comprised of the intrinsic thermal conductivity of the tissue and a perfusion dependent increment. In principle, an effective conductivity can be defined from any known heat flow and temperature difference, that is,

$$k_{\text{eff}} = \frac{q}{\Delta T} f\left(\frac{L}{A}\right) \tag{6.17}$$

where $f(L/A)$ is a function of geometry with dimensions length^{-1} (e.g., $\Delta x/A$ in a slab geometry). Originally introduced as an empirical quantity [18], the effective conductivity has been linked to the Pennes formulation in the measurement for blood perfusion rates via small, heated, implanted probes [19–21]. And in 1985, Weinbaum and Jiji [22] theoretically related the effective conductivity to the blood flow and anatomy for a restricted class of tissues and heating conditions which are dominated by a closely space artery–vein architecture and which can satisfy the constraint [23]

$$\frac{d\bar{T}_t}{ds} \approx \frac{1}{2} \frac{d(\bar{T}_a + \bar{T}_v)}{ds} \tag{6.18}$$

Here the effective conductivity is a tensor quantity related to the flow and anatomy according to [22]

$$k_{\text{eff}} = k_t \left(1 + \frac{\pi^2 \rho_b^2 c_b^2 n r_a^4 \bar{u}^2 \cos^2 \phi}{k_t^2 \sigma_\Delta}\right) \tag{6.19}$$

where the enhancement is in the direction of the vessel axes and where n is the number of artery–vein pairs per unit area and ϕ is the angle of the vessel axes relative to the temperature gradient. The near equilibrium required by Equation 6.18 is likely to be valid only in tissues in which all vessels are smaller than 200 μm diameter such as the outer few millimeters near the skin and in the absence of intense heat sources. Closely spaced, artery–vein pairs have been shown to act like highly conductive fibers even when the near equilibrium condition in Equation 6.18 is violated [24]. The radius of the thermally equivalent fiber is given by

$$r_{\text{fiber}} = (wr_a)^{1/2} \tag{6.20}$$

and its conductivity is given by

$$k_{\text{fiber}} = \frac{(\rho_b c_b \bar{u})^2 r_a^3 \cosh^{-1}(w/r_a)}{wk_t} \tag{6.21}$$

Under these nonequilibrium conditions the tissue–blood system acts like a fiber-composite material, but cannot be well-modeled as a single homogeneous material with effective properties.

6.4.1.2 Combination

Recognizing that several mechanism of heat transport may be at play in tissue, Chen and Holmes [9] suggested the following formulation which incorporates the effects discussed above:

$$\nabla k_{\text{eff}}(\vec{r}, t)\nabla \bar{T}_t(\vec{r}, t) + \dot{\omega}_b(\vec{r}, t)\rho_b c_b(T_a^* - \bar{T}_t(\vec{r}, t)) - \rho_b c_b \vec{u}_b(\vec{r}, t) \cdot \nabla \bar{T}_t(\vec{r}, t) + \dot{q}'''(\vec{r}, t) = \rho_t c_t \frac{\partial \bar{T}_t(\vec{r}, t)}{\partial t} \tag{6.22}$$

where T_a^* is the temperature exiting the last artery that is individually modeled. The primary value of this formulation is its conceptual generality. In practice, this formulation is difficult to apply because it requires knowledge of a great many adjustable parameters, most of which have not been independently measured to date.

6.4.1.2.1 Heat Sink Model with Effectiveness

Using somewhat different approaches, Brinck and Werner [25] and Weinbaum et al. [26] have proposed that the shortcomings of the Pennes model can be overcome by introducing a heat transfer effectiveness factor ε to modify the heat sink term as follows:

$$\nabla k_t \nabla \bar{T}_t(\vec{r}, t) + \varepsilon(\vec{r}, t)\dot{\omega}_b(\vec{r}, t)\rho_b c_b(\bar{T}(\vec{r}, t)_t - T_a) + \dot{q}'''(\vec{r}, t) = \rho_t c_t \frac{\partial \bar{T}_t(\vec{r}, t)}{\partial t} \tag{6.23}$$

where $0 \leq \varepsilon \geq 1$. In Brinck and Werner [25] formulation ε is a curve-fitting parameter that allows the actual (rather than the thermally equivalent) perfusion rate to be used. Weinbaum et al. [26] provide an analytical result for ε that is valid for blood vessels smaller than 300 μm diameter in skeletal muscle. In both formulations $\varepsilon < 1$ arises from the countercurrent heat exchange mechanism that shunts heat directly between the artery and vein without requiring the heat-carrying blood to first pass through the smaller connecting vessels. A correction factor of 0.58 is recommended for human limbs [27]. Theory predicts that the correction factor is independent of the perfusion rate.

6.4.2 Multi-Equation Models

The value of the continuum models is that they do not require a separate solution for the blood subvolume. In each continuum formulation, the behavior of the blood vessels is modeled by introducing assumptions that allow solution of only a single differential equation. But by solving only one equation, all detailed information on the temperature of the blood in individual blood vessels is lost. Several investigators have introduced multiequation models that typically model the tissue, arteries, and veins as three separate, but interacting, subvolumes [10,28–31]. As with the other nonPennes formulations, these methods are difficult to apply to particular clinical applications, but provide theoretical insights into microvascular heat transfer.

6.4.3 Vascular Reconstruction Models

As an alternative to the three-equation models, a more complete reconstruction of the vasculature may be used along with a scheme for solving the resulting flow, conduction and advection equations [6,32–41]. Since the reconstructed vasculature is similar to the actual vasculature only in a statistical sense, these models provide the mean temperature as predicted by the continuum models, as well as insight into the mechanisms of heat transport, the sites of thermal interaction and the degree of thermal perturbations produced by vessels of a given size, but they cannot provide the actual details of the temperature field in a given living tissue. These models tend to be computationally intensive due to the high spatial resolution needed to account for all of the thermally significant blood vessels.

6.5 Parameter Values

6.5.1 Thermal Properties

The intrinsic thermal properties of tissues depend strongly on their composition. Cooper and Trezek [42] recommend the following correlations for the thermal conductivity

$$k = \rho \times 10^{-3}(0.628 f_{\text{water}} + 0.117 f_{\text{proteins}} + 0.231 f_{\text{fats}}) \text{ W/m-K} \qquad (6.24)$$

specific heat

$$c_p = 4{,}200 f_{\text{water}} + 1{,}090 f_{\text{proteins}} + 2{,}300 f_{\text{fats}} \text{ J/kg-K} \qquad (6.25)$$

and density

$$\rho = \frac{1}{f_{\text{water}}/1{,}000 + f_{\text{proteins}}/1{,}540 + f_{\text{fats}}/815} \text{ kg/m}^3 \qquad (6.26)$$

where f_{water}, f_{proteins}, and f_{fats} are the mass fractions of water, proteins, and fats, respectively.

6.5.2 Thermoregulation

Humans maintain a nearly constant core temperature through a combination of physiological and behavior responses to the environment. For example, heat loss or gain at the skin surface may be modified by changes in the skin blood flow, the rate of sweating, or clothing. In deeper tissues, the dependence of the blood perfusion rate, the metabolic heat generation rate and vessel diameters depend on the environmental and physiological conditions in a complex, organ-specific manner. The blood perfusion varies widely among tissue types and for some tissues can change dramatically depending on the metabolic or thermoregulatory needs of the tissue. The situation is further complicated by the feedback control aspects of the thermoregulatory systems that utilize a combination of central and peripheral temperature sensors as well as local and more distributed actuators.

The following examples are provided to illustrate some of the considerations, not to exhaustively explore this complicated issue. A model of the whole body is typically needed even for a relatively local stimulus, especially when the heat input represents a significant fraction of the whole body heat load. The reader is referred to extensive handbook entries on environmental response for more information [43,44]. Whole body models of the thermoregulatory system are discussed in Wissler [45].

Chato [1] suggests that the temperature dependence of the blood perfusion effect can be approximated by a scalar effective conductivity

$$k_{\text{eff}} = 4.82 - 4.44833[1.00075^{-1.575^{(T_t - 25)}}] \text{ W/m-K} \tag{6.27}$$

which is intended for used in Equation 6.16.

Under conditions of local hyperthermia, where the heated volume is small compared to the body as a whole, the blood perfusion rate may undergo complex changes. Based on experimental data the following correlations have been suggested [46,47] for muscle

$$\dot{\omega}_b \rho = \begin{cases} 0.45 + 3.55 \exp\left(-\dfrac{(T - 45.0)^2}{12.0}\right) & T \leq 45.0 \\ 4.00 & T > 45.0 \end{cases} \tag{6.28}$$

for fat

$$\dot{\omega}_b \rho = \begin{cases} 0.36 + 0.36 \exp\left(-\dfrac{(T - 45.0)^2}{12.0}\right) & T \leq 45.0 \\ 0.72 & T > 45.0 \end{cases} \tag{6.29}$$

and for tumor

$$\dot{\omega}_b \rho = \begin{cases} 0.833 & T < 37.0 \\ 0.833 - (T - 37.0)^{4.8}/5.438 \times 10^3 & 37.0 \leq T \leq 42.0 \\ 0.416 & T > 42.0 \end{cases} \tag{6.30}$$

Chronic heating over a period of weeks has been observed to increase vascular density and ultimately to reduce tissue temperature under constant heating conditions [48,49]. The rate and extent of adaptation are tissue specific.

The metabolic rate may also undergo thermoregulatory changes. For example, the temperature dependence of the metabolism in the leg muscle and skin may be modeled with [50]

$$\dot{q}_m''' = 170(2)^{[(T_0 - T_t)/10]} \text{ W/m}^3 \tag{6.31}$$

The metabolic rate and blood flow may also be linked through processes that reflect the fact that sustained increased metabolic activity generally requires increased blood flow.

6.5.3 Clinical Heat Generation

Thermal therapies such as hyperthermia treatment rely on local heat generation rates several orders of magnitude greater than produced by the metabolism. Under these circumstances, the metabolic heat generation is often neglected with little error.

6.6 Solutions of Models

The steady-state solution with spatially and temporally constant parameter values including the rate of heat generation for a tissue half space with a fixed temperature on the skin T_{skin} is given by

$$\bar{T}_t(x) = T_{\text{skin}} \exp\left[-\left(\frac{\dot{\omega}_b \rho_b c_b}{k_t}\right)^{1/2} x\right] + \left(T_a + \frac{\dot{q}'''}{\dot{\omega}_b \rho_b c_b}\right)\left\{1 - \exp\left[-\left(\frac{\dot{\omega}_b \rho_b c_b}{k_t}\right)^{1/2} x\right]\right\} \tag{6.32}$$

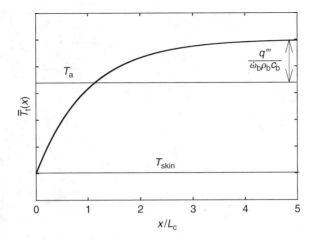

FIGURE 6.2   One-dimensional steady-state solution of Pennes bioheat equation for constant parameter values.

This solution reveals that perturbations to the tissue temperature decay exponentially with a characteristic length of

$$L_c = \left(\frac{k_t}{\dot{\omega}_b \rho_b c_b} \right)^{1/2} \tag{6.33}$$

which for typical values of the perfusion rate $\dot{\omega}_b = 0.1 \times 10^{-3}$ to 3.0×10^{-3} m³/m³-sec yields $L_c = 6.5 \times 10^{-3}$ to 36×10^{-3} m (Figure 6.2).

The transient solution of Pennes' bioheat equation with constant perfusion rate for an initial uniform temperature of T_0, in the absence of any spatial dependence is

$$\bar{T}_t(t) = T_0 \exp\left[-\left(\frac{\dot{\omega}_b \rho_b c_b}{\rho_t c_t} \right) t \right] + \left(T_a + \frac{\dot{q}'''}{\dot{\omega}_b \rho_b c_b} \right) \left\{ 1 - \exp\left[-\left(\frac{\dot{\omega}_b \rho_b c_b}{\rho_t c_t} \right) t \right] \right\} \tag{6.34}$$

Here the solution reveals a characteristic time scale

$$t_c = \frac{\rho_t c_t}{\dot{\omega}_b \rho_b c_b} \tag{6.35}$$

that has typical values in the range of $t_c = 300$ to 10,000 sec (Figure 6.3). This solution is valid only when thermoregulatory changes in the perfusion rate are small or occur over a much longer time than the characteristic timescale t_c.

Numerical solution of the heat sink model is readily obtained by standard methods such as finite differences, finite element, boundary element, and Green's functions provided that the parameter values and appropriate boundary conditions are known.

Defining Terms

Conduction shape factor: Dimensionless factor used to account for the geometrical effects in steady-state heat conduction between surfaces at different temperatures.

Effective conductivity: An modified thermal conductivity that includes the intrinsic thermal conductivity of the tissue as well as a contribution from blood perfusion effects.

Equilibration length: Characteristic length scale over which blood in a blood vessel will change temperature in response to surrounding tissue at a different temperature.

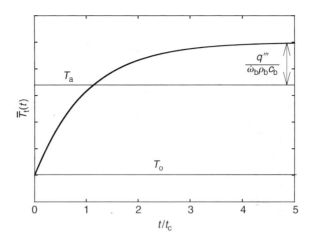

FIGURE 6.3 Transient solution of Pennes bioheat equation for constant parameter values in the absence of spatial effects.

Perfusion rate: Quantity of blood provided to a unit of tissue per unit time.
Specific heat: Quantity of energy needed to increase for a unit temperature increase for a unit of mass.
Thermal conductivity: Rate of energy transfer by thermal conduction for a unit temperature gradient per unit of cross-sectional area.
Thermally significant vessel: Blood vessels large enough and numerous enough to contribute significantly to overall heat transfer rates in tissue.

All conductivities and diffusivities are from humans at 37°C except the value for skeletal muscle which is from sheep at 21°C. Perfusion values are from various mammals as noted in the references. Significant digits do not imply accuracy. The temperature coefficient for thermal conductivity ranges from −0.000254 to 0.0039 W/m-K-°C with 0.001265 W/m-K-°C typical of most tissues as compared to 0.001575 W/m-K-°C for water [55]. The temperature coefficient for thermal diffusivity ranges from −4.9 × 10^{-10} m^2/sec-°C to 8.4 × 10^{-10} m^2/sec-°C with 5.19 × 10^{-10} m^2/sec-°C typical of most tissues as compared to 4.73 × 10^{-10} m^2/sec-°C for water [55]. The values are provided in this table are representative values presented for tutorial purposes. The reader is referred to the primary literature for values appropriate for specific design applications.

References

[1] Chato, J.C., Fundamentals of bioheat transfer, in *Thermal Dosimetry and Treatment Planning*, M. Gautherie, Ed., 1990, Springer-Verlag: New York, pp. 1–56.
[2] Charny, C.K., Mathematical models of bioheat transfer, in *Bioengineering Heat Transfer: Advances in Heat Transfer*, Y.I. Cho, Ed., 1992, Academic Press: Boston, pp. 19–155.
[3] Arkin, M., L.X. Xu, and K.R. Holmes, Recent developments in modeling heat transfer in blood perfused tissues. *IEEE Trans. Biomed. Eng.*, 1994, 41: 97–107.
[4] Eto, T.K. and B. Rubinsky, Bioheat transfer, in *Introduction to Bioengineering*, S.A. Berger, W. Goldsmith, and E.R. Lewis, Eds, 1996, Oxford University Press: Oxford, pp. 203–227.
[5] Diller, K.R., Modeling of bioheat transfer processes at high and low temperatures, in *Bioengineering Heat Transfer: Advances in Heat Transfer*, Y.I. Cho, Ed., 1992, Academic Press: Boston, pp. 157–357.
[6] Craciunescu, O.I. et al., Discretizing large traceable vessels and using DE-MRI perfusion maps yields numerical temperature contours that match the MR noninvasive measurements. *Med. Phys.*, 2001, 28: 2289–2296.

[7] Incropera, F.P. and D.P. DeWitt, *Fundamentals of Heat and Mass Transfer*. 4th ed., 1996, John Wiley & Sons: New York.

[8] Chato, J.C., Heat transfer to blood vessels. *J. Biomech. Eng.*, 1980, 102: 110–118.

[9] Chen, M.M. and K.R. Holmes, Microvascular contributions in tissue heat transfer. *Ann. N. Y. Acad. Sci.*, 1980, 325: 137–150.

[10] Weinbaum, S., L.M. Jiji, and D.E. Lemons, Theory and experiment for the effect of vascular microstructure on surface tissue heat transfer — part I: anatomical foundation and model conceptualization. *J. Biomech. Eng.*, 1984, 106: 321–330.

[11] He, Q., D. Lemons, and S. Weinbaum, Experimental measurements of the temperature variation along artery–vein pairs from 200 to 1000 μm diameter in rat hind limb. *J. Biomech. Eng.*, 2002, 124: 656–661.

[12] Roemer, R.B., Conditions for equivalency of countercurrent vessel heat transfer formulations. *J. Biomech. Eng.*, 1999, 121: 514–520.

[13] Victor, S.A. and V.L. Shah, Steady state heat transfer to blood flowing in the entrance region of a tube. *Int. J. Heat Mass Transfer*, 1976, 19: 777–783.

[14] Barozzi, G.S. and A. Dumas, Convective heat transfer coefficients in the circulation. *J. Biomech. Eng.*, 1991, 113: 308–313.

[15] Craciunescu, O.I. and S. Clegg, Pulsatile blood flow effects on temperature distribution and heat transfer in rigid blood vessels. *J. Biomech. Eng.*, 2001, 123: 500–505.

[16] Pennes, H.H., Analysis of tissue and arterial blood temperatures in the resting forearm. *J. Appl. Physiol.*, 1948, 1: 93–122.

[17] Wulff, W., The energy conservation equation for living tissue. *IEEE Trans. Biomed. Eng.*, 1974, 21: 494–495.

[18] Bazett, H.C. and B. McGlone, Temperature gradients in tissues in man. *Am. J. Physiol.*, 1927, 82: 415–428.

[19] Perl, W., Heat and matter distribution in body tissues and the determination of tissue bloodflow by local clearance methods. *J. Theor. Biol.*, 1962, 2: 201–235.

[20] Valvano, J.W. et al., Thermal conductivity and diffusivity of arterial walls. ASME, 1984, 8, 1–29.

[21] Arkin, H., K.R. Holmes, and M.M. Chen, A technique for measuring the thermal conductivity and evaluating the "apparent conductivity" concept in biomaterials. *J. Biomech. Eng.*, 1989, 111: 276–282.

[22] Weinbaum, S. and L.M. Jiji, A new simplified bioheat equation for the effect of blood flow on local average tissue temperature. *J. Biomech. Eng.*, 1985, 107: 131–139.

[23] Weinbaum, S. and L.M. Jiji, The matching of thermal fields surrounding countercurrent microvessels and the closure approximation in the Weinbaum-Jiji equation. *J. Biomech. Eng.*, 1989, 111: 271–275.

[24] Baish, J.W., Heat transport by countercurrent blood vessels in the presence of an arbitrary temperature gradient. *J. Biomech. Eng.*, 1990, 112: 207–211.

[25] Brinck, H. and J. Werner, Efficiency function: improvement of classical bioheat approach. *J. Appl. Physiol.*, 1994, 77: 1617–1622.

[26] Weinbaum, S. et al., A new fundamental bioheat equation for muscle tissue — part I: blood perfusion term. *J. Biomech. Eng.*, 1997, 119: 278–288.

[27] Zhu, L. et al., A new fundamental bioheat equation for muscle tissue — part II: temperature of SAV vessels. *J. Biomech. Eng.*, 2002, 124: 121–132.

[28] Jiji, L.M., S. Weinbaum, and D.E. Lemons, Theory and experiment for the effect of vascular microstructure on surface tissue heat transfer — part II: model formulation and solution. *J. Biomech. Eng.*, 1984, 106: 331–341.

[29] Baish, J.W., P.S. Ayyaswamy, and K.R. Foster, Small-scale temperature fluctuations in perfused tissue during local hyperthermia. *J. Biomech. Eng.*, 1986, 108: 246–250.

[30] Baish, J.W., P.S. Ayyaswamy, and K.R. Foster, Heat transport mechanisms in vascular tissues: a model comparison. *J. Biomech. Eng.*, 1986, 108: 324–331.

[31] Charny, C.K. and R.L. Levin, Bioheat transfer in a branching countercurrent network during hyperthermia. *J. Biomech. Eng.*, 1989, 111: 263–270.

[32] Baish, J.W., Formulation of a statistical model of heat transfer in perfused tissue. *J. Biomech. Eng.*, 1994, 116: 521–527.

[33] Huang, H.W., Z.P. Chen, and R.B. Roemer, A counter current vascular network model of heat transfer in tissues. *J. Biomech. Eng.*, 1996, 118: 120–129.

[34] Van der Koijk, J.F. et al., The influence of vasculature on temperature distributions in MECS interstitial hyperthermia: importance of longitudinal control. *Int. J. Hyperthermia*, 1997, 13: 365–386.

[35] van Leeuwen, G.M.J. et al., Tests of the geometrical description of blood vessels in a thermal model using counter-current geometries. *Phys. Med. Biol.*, 1997, 42: 1515–1532.

[36] van Leeuwen, G.M.J. et al., Accuracy of geometrical modelling of heat transfer from tissue to blood vessels. *Phys. Med. Biol.*, 1997, 42: 1451–1460.

[37] Van Leeuwen, G.M.J., A.N.T.J. Kotte, and J.J.W. Lagendijk, A flexible algorithm for construction of 3-D vessel networks for use in thermal modeling. *IEEE Trans. Biomed. Eng.*, 1998, 45: 596–605.

[38] Kotte, A.N.T.J., G.M.J. Van Leeuwen, and J.J.K. Lagendijk, Modelling the thermal impact of a discrete vessel tree. *Phys. Med. Biol.*, 1999, 44: 57–74.

[39] Van Leeuwen, G.M.J. et al., Temperature simulations in tissue with a realistic computer generated vessel network. *Phys. Med. Biol.*, 2000, 45: 1035–1049.

[40] Raaymakers, B.W., A.N.T.J. Kotte, and J.J.K. Lagendijk, How to apply a discrete vessel model in thermal simulations when only incomplete vessel data are available. *Phys. Med. Biol.*, 2000, 45: 3385–3401.

[41] Kou, H.-S., T.-C. Shih, and W.-L. Lin, Effect of the directional blood flow on thermal distribution during thermal therapy: an application of a Green's function based on the porous model. *Phys. Med. Biol.*, 2003, 48: 1577–1589.

[42] Cooper, T.E. and G.J. Trezek, Correlation of thermal properties of some human tissue with water content. *Aerospace Med.*, 1971, 42: 24–27.

[43] ASHRAE, Physiological Principles and Thermal Comfort, in *ASHRAE Handbook: Fundamentals*, 1993, ASHRAE Inc.: Atlanta, GA, pp. 8.1–8.29.

[44] Fregly, M.J. and C.M. Blatteis, Eds., Section 4: Environmental physiology, in *Handbook of Physiology*, Vol. I, 1996, American Physiological Society: New York.

[45] Wissler, E.H., Mathematical simulation of human thermal behavior using whole body models, in *Heat Transfer in Medicine and Biology: Analysis and Applications*, A. Shitzer and R.C. Eberhart, Eds., 1985, Plenum Press: New York, pp. 325–373.

[46] Erdmann, B., J. Lang, and M. Seebass, Optimization of temperature distributions for regional hyperthermia based on a nonlinear heat transfer model. *Ann. N.Y. Acad. Sci.*, 1998, 858: 36–46.

[47] Lang, J., B. Erdmann, and M. Seebass, Impact of nonlinear heat transfer on temperature control in regional hyperthermia. *IEEE Trans. Biomed. Eng.*, 1999, 46: 1129–1138.

[48] Seese, T.M. et al., Characterization of tissue morphology, angiogenesis, and temperature in the adaptive response of muscle tissue to chronic heating. *Lab. Invest.*, 1998, 78: 1553–1562.

[49] Saidel, G.M. et al., Temperature and perfusion responses of muscle and lung tissue during chronic heating *in vivo*. *Med. Biol. Eng. Computing*, 2001, 39: 126–133.

[50] Mitchell, J.W. et al., Thermal response of human legs during cooling. *J. Appl. Physiol.*, 1970, 29: 859–856.

[51] Wissler, E.H., An analytical solution of countercurrent heat transfer between parallel vessels with a linear axial temperature gradient. *J. Biomech. Eng.*, 1988, 110: 254–256.

[52] Zhu, L. and S. Weinbaum, A model for heat transfer from embedded blood vessels in two-dimensional tissue preparations. *J. Biomech. Eng.*, 1995, 117: 64–73.

[53] Cousins, A., On the Nusselt number in heat transfer between multiple parallel blood vessels. *J. Biomech. Eng.*, 1997, 119: 127–129.

[54] Baish, J.W., J.K. Miller, and M.J. Zivitz, Heat transfer in the vicinity of the junction of two blood vessels, in *Advances in Bioheat and Mass Transfer: Microscale Analysis of Thermal Injury Processes, Instrumentation, Modeling and Clinical Applications*, R.B. Roemer, Ed., 1993, ASME: New York, pp. 95–100.

[55] Valvano, J.W., J.R. Cochran, and K.R. Diller, Thermal conductivity and diffusivity of biomaterials measured with self-heated thermistors. *Int. J. Thermophys.*, 1985, 6: 301–311.

[56] Kapin, M.A. and J.L. Ferguson, Hemodynamic and regional circulatory alterations in dog during anaphylactic challenge. *Am. J. Physiol.*, 1985, 249: H430–H437.

[57] Haws, C.W. and D.D. Heistad, Effects of nimodipine on crebral vasoconstrictor responses. *Am. J. Physiol.*, 1984, 247: H170–H176.

[58] Passmore, J.C., R.E. Neiberger, and S.W. Eden, Measurement of intrarenal anatomic distribution of krypton-85 in endotoxic shock in dogs. *Am. J. Physiol.*, 1977, 232: H54–H58.

[59] Koehler, R.C., R.J. Traystman, and J. Jones, Regional blood flow and O_2 transport during hypoxic and CO hypoxia in neonatal and sheep. *Am. J. Physiol.*, 1985, 248: H118–H124.

[60] Seyde, W.C. et al., Effects of anesthetics on regional hemodynamics in normovolemic and hemorrhaged rats. *Am. J. Physiol.*, 1985, 249: H164–H173.

[61] Balasubramaniam, T.A. and H.F. Bowman, Thermal conductivity and thermal diffusivity of biomaterials: a simultaneous measurement technique. *Trans. ASME, J. Biomech. Eng.*, 1977, 99: 148–154.

7

Perfusion Effects and Hydrodynamics

Robert A. Peattie
Oregon State University

Robert J. Fisher
*The SABRE Institute and
Massachusetts Institute
of Technology*

7.1 Introduction

Biological processes within living systems are significantly influenced by the flow of liquids and gases. Biomedical engineers must therefore understand hydrodynamic phenomena [1] and their vital role in the biological processes that occur within the body [2]. In particular, engineers are concerned with perfusion effects in the cellular microenvironment, and the ability of the circulatory and respiratory systems to provide a whole body communication network with dynamic response capabilities. Understanding the fundamental principles of fluid flow involved in these processes is also essential for describing transport of mass and heat through the body, as well as to know how tissue function can be built, reconstructed, and if need be modified for clinical applications.

From a geometric and flow standpoint, the body may be considered a network of highly specialized and interconnected organ systems. The key elements of this network for transport and communication are its pathway (the circulatory system) and its fluid (blood). Of interest for engineering purposes are the ability of the circulatory system to transport oxygen and carbon dioxide, glucose, other nutrients and metabolites, and signal molecules to and from the tissues, as well as to provide an avenue for stress-response agents from the immune system, including cytokines, antibodies, leukocytes, and macrophages and system repair agents such as stem cells and platelets. The bulk transport capability provided by convective flow helps to overcome the large diffusional resistance that would otherwise be offered by such a large entity as the human body. At rest, the mean blood circulation time is of the order of 1 min. Therefore, given that the total amount of blood circulating is about 76 to 80 ml/kg (5.3 to 5.6 l for a 70 kg "standard male"), the flow from the heart to this branching network is about 95 ml/sec. This and other order of magnitude estimates for the human body are available elsewhere, for example, References 2 to 4.

Although the fluids most often considered in biofluid mechanics studies are blood and air, other fluids such as urine, perspiration, tears, ocular aqueous and vitreous fluids, and the synovial fluid in the joints can also be important in evaluating tissue system behavioral responses to induced chemical and physical stresses. For purposes of analysis, these fluids are often assumed to exhibit Newtonian behavior, although the synovial fluid and blood under certain conditions can be non-Newtonian. Since blood is a suspension it has interesting properties; it behaves as a Newtonian fluid for large shear rates, but is highly non-Newtonian for low shear rates. The synovial fluid exhibits viscoelastic characteristics that are particularly suited to its function of joint lubrication, for which elasticity is beneficial. These viscoelastic characteristics must be accounted for when considering tissue therapy for joint injuries.

Further complicating analysis is the fact that blood, air, and other physiologic fluids travel through three-dimensional passageways that are often highly branched and distensible. Within these pathways, disturbed or turbulent flow regimes may be mixed with stable, laminar regions. For example, blood flow is laminar in many parts of a healthy circulatory system in spite of the potential for peak Reynolds numbers (defined below) of the order of 10,000. However, "bursts" of turbulence are detected in the aorta during a fraction of each cardiac cycle. An occlusion or stenosis in the circulatory system, such as the stenosis of a heart valve, will promote such turbulence. Airflow in the lung is normally stable and laminar during inspiration, but is less so during expiration and heavy breathing, coughing, or an obstruction can result in fully turbulent flow, with Reynolds numbers of 50,000 a possibility.

Although elasticity of vessel walls can significantly complicate fluid flow analysis, biologically it provides important homeostatic benefits. For example, pulsatile blood flow induces accompanying expansions and contractions in healthy elastic-wall vessels. These wall displacements then influence the flow fields. Elastic behavior maintains the norm of laminar flow that minimizes wall stress, lowers flow resistance, and thus energy dissipation and fosters maximum life of the vessel. In combination with pulsatile flow, distensibility permits strain relaxation of the wall tissue with each cardiac cycle, which provides an exercise routine promoting extended "on-line" use.

The term *perfusion* is used in engineering biosciences to identify the rate of blood supplied to a unit quantity of an organ or tissue. Clearly, perfusion of *in vitro* tissue systems is necessary to maintain cell viability along with functionality to mimic *in vivo* behavior. Furthermore, it is highly likely that cell viability and normoperative metabolism are dependent on the three-dimensional structure of the microvessels distributed through any tissue bed, which establishes an appropriate microenvironment through both biochemical and biophysical mechanisms. This includes transmitting both intracellular and long-range signals along the scaffolding of the extracellular matrix.

The primary objective of this chapter is to summarize the most important ideas of fluid dynamics, as hydrodynamic and hemodynamic principles have many important applications in physiology, pathophysiology, and tissue engineering. In fact, the interaction of fluids and supported tissue is of paramount importance to tissue development and viability, both *in vivo* and *in vitro*. The strength of adhesion and dynamics of detachment of mammalian cells from engineered biomaterials and scaffolds are important subjects of ongoing research [5], as are the effects of shear on receptor–ligand binding at the cell–fluid interface. Flow-induced stress has numerous critical consequences for cells, altering transport across the cell membrane, receptor density and distribution, binding affinity and signal generation with subsequent trafficking within the cell [6]. In addition, design and use of perfusion systems such as membrane biomimetic reactors and hollow fibers is most effective when careful attention is given to issues of hydrodynamic similitude. Similarly, understanding the role of fluid mechanical phenomena in arterial disease and subsequent therapeutic applications is clearly dependent on appreciation of hemodynamics.

A thorough treatment of the mathematics needed for model development and analysis is beyond the scope of this volume, and is presented in numerous sources [1,2]. Herein, the goal is to provide a physical understanding of the important issues relevant to hemodynamic flow and transport. Solution methods are summarized, and the benefits associated with use of computational fluid dynamics (CFD) packages are described. In particular, quantifying hemodynamic events can require invasive experimentation and extensive model and computational analysis.

7.2 Elements of Theoretical Hydrodynamics

It is essential that engineers understand both the advantages and the limitations of mathematical theories and models of biological phenomena, as well as the assumptions underlying those models. Mechanical theories often begin with Newton's second law ($\mathbf{F} = m\mathbf{a}$). When applied to continuous distributions of Newtonian fluids, Newton's second law gives rise to the *Navier–Stokes equations*. In brief, these equations provide an expression governing the motion of fluids such as air and water for which the rate of motion is linearly proportional to the applied stress producing the motion. Later in this chapter, the basic concepts from which the Navier–Stokes equations have been developed are summarized along with a few general ideas about boundary layers and turbulence. Applications to the vascular system are then treated in the context of pulsatile flow. It is hoped that this very generalized approach will allow the reader to appreciate the complexities involved in an analytic solution to pulsatile phenomena, a necessity for properly describing vascular hemodynamics for clinical evaluations.

7.2.1 Elements of Continuum Mechanics

The theory of fluid flow, together with the theory of elasticity, makes up the field of continuum mechanics, which is the study of the mechanics of continuously distributed materials. Such materials may be either solid or fluid, or may have intermediate viscoelastic properties. Since the concept of a continuous medium, or continuum, does not take into consideration the molecular structure of matter, it is inherently an idealization. However, as long as the smallest length scale in any problem under consideration is very much larger than the size of the molecules making up the medium and the mean free path within the medium, for mechanical purposes all mass may safely be assumed to be continuously distributed in space. As a result, the density of materials can be considered to be a continuous function of spatial position and time.

7.2.1.1 Constitutive Equations

The response of any fluid to applied forces and temperature disturbances can be used to characterize the material. For this purpose, functional relationships between applied stresses and the resulting rate of strain field of the fluid are needed. Fluids that are homogeneous and isotropic, and for which there is a linear relationship between the state of stress within the fluid s_{ij} and the rate of strain tensor ξ_{ij}, where i and j denote the Cartesian coordinates x, y, and z, are called *Newtonian*. In physiologic settings, Newtonian fluids normally behave as if incompressible. For such fluids, it can be shown that

$$s_{ij} = -P\delta_{ij} + 2\mu\xi_{ij} \tag{7.1}$$

with μ the dynamic viscosity of the fluid and $P = P(x, y, z)$ the fluid pressure.

7.2.1.2 Conservation (Field) Equations

In vector notation, conservation of mass for a continuous fluid is expressed through

$$\frac{\partial \rho}{\partial t} + \nabla \bullet \rho\mathbf{u} = 0 \tag{7.2}$$

where ρ is the fluid density and $\mathbf{u} = \mathbf{u}(x, y, z)$ is the vector velocity field. When the fluid is incompressible, density is constant and Equation 7.2 reduces to the well-known *continuity condition*, $\nabla \bullet \mathbf{u} = 0$. The continuity condition can also be expressed in terms of Cartesian velocity components (u, v, w) as $\partial u/\partial x + \partial v/\partial y + \partial w/\partial z = 0$.

The basic equation of Newtonian fluid motion, the Navier–Stokes equations, can be developed by substitution of the constitutive relationship for a Newtonian fluid, P-1, into the Cauchy principle of momentum balance for a continuous material [7]. In writing the second law for a continuously distributed fluid, care must be taken to correctly express the acceleration of the fluid particle to which the forces are being applied through the *material derivative* Du/Dt, where $Du/Dt = \partial \mathbf{u}/\partial t + (\mathbf{u} \bullet \nabla)\mathbf{u}$. That is, the velocity of a fluid particle may change for either of two reasons, because the particle accelerates or decelerates with time (*temporal acceleration*) or because the particle moves to a new position, at which the velocity has different magnitude and direction (*convective acceleration*).

A flow field for which $\partial/\partial t = 0$ for all possible properties of the fluid and its flow is described as *steady*, to indicate that it is independent of time. However, the statement $\partial \mathbf{u}/\partial t = 0$ does not imply $Du/Dt = 0$, and similarly $Du/Dt = 0$ does not imply that $\partial \mathbf{u}/\partial t = 0$.

Using the material derivative, the Navier–Stokes equations for an incompressible fluid can be written in vector form as

$$\frac{D\mathbf{u}}{Dt} = \mathbf{B} - \frac{1}{\rho}\nabla P + \nu \nabla^2 \mathbf{u} \tag{7.3}$$

where ν is the fluid kinematic viscosity $= \mu/\rho$.

Expanded in full, the Navier–Stokes equations are three simultaneous, nonlinear scalar equations, one for each component of the velocity field. In Cartesian coordinates, Equation 7.3 takes the form

$$\frac{\partial u}{\partial t} + u\frac{\partial u}{\partial x} + v\frac{\partial u}{\partial y} + w\frac{\partial u}{\partial z} = B_x - \frac{1}{\rho}\frac{\partial P}{\partial x} + \nu\left(\frac{\partial^2 u}{\partial x^2} + \frac{\partial^2 u}{\partial y^2} + \frac{\partial^2 u}{\partial z^2}\right) \tag{7.4a}$$

$$\frac{\partial v}{\partial t} + u\frac{\partial v}{\partial x} + v\frac{\partial v}{\partial y} + w\frac{\partial v}{\partial z} = B_y - \frac{1}{\rho}\frac{\partial P}{\partial y} + \nu\left(\frac{\partial^2 v}{\partial x^2} + \frac{\partial^2 v}{\partial y^2} + \frac{\partial^2 v}{\partial z^2}\right) \tag{7.4b}$$

$$\frac{\partial w}{\partial t} + u\frac{\partial w}{\partial x} + v\frac{\partial w}{\partial y} + w\frac{\partial w}{\partial z} = B_z - \frac{1}{\rho}\frac{\partial P}{\partial z} + \nu\left(\frac{\partial^2 w}{\partial x^2} + \frac{\partial^2 w}{\partial y^2} + \frac{\partial^2 w}{\partial z^2}\right) \tag{7.4c}$$

Flow fields may be determined by solution of the Navier–Stokes equations, provided $\mathbf{B}$ is known. This is generally not a difficulty, since the only body force normally significant in hemodynamic applications is gravity. For an incompressible flow, there are then four unknown dependent variables, the three components of velocity and the pressure P, and four governing equations, the three components of the Navier–Stokes equations and the continuity condition. It is important to emphasize that this set of equations is *not* sufficient to calculate the flow field when the flow is compressible or involves temperature changes, since pressure, density, and temperature are then interrelated, which introduces new dependent variables to the problem.

Solution of the Navier–Stokes equations also requires that boundary conditions and sometimes initial conditions as well be specified for the flow field of interest. By far the most common boundary condition in physiologic and other engineering flows is the so-called *no-slip condition*, requiring that the layer of fluid elements in contact with a boundary have the same velocity as the boundary itself. For an unmoving, rigid wall, as in a pipe, this velocity is zero. However, in the vasculature, vessel walls expand and contract during the cardiac cycle.

Flow patterns and accompanying flow field characteristics depend largely on the values of governing dimensionless parameters. There are many such parameters, each relevant to specific types of flow settings, but the principle parameter of steady flows is the *Reynolds number*, Re, defined as $Re = \rho UL/\mu$, where U is a characteristic velocity of the flow field and L is a characteristic length. Both U and L must be selected for the specific problem under study and, in general, both will have different values in different problems. For pipe flow, U is most commonly selected to be the mean velocity of the flow with L the pipe diameter.

It can be shown that the Reynolds number represents the ratio of inertial forces to viscous forces in the flow field. Flows at sufficiently low Re therefore behave as if highly viscous, with little to no fluid acceleration possible. At the opposite extreme, high Re flows behave as if lacking viscosity. One consequence of this distinction is that very high Reynolds number flow fields may, at first thought, seem to contradict the no-slip condition, in that they seem to "slip" along a solid boundary exerting no shear stress. This dilemma was first resolved in 1905 with Prandtl's introduction of the *boundary layer*, a thin region of the flow field adjacent to the boundary in which viscous effects are important and the no slip condition is obeyed [8–10].

7.2.1.3 Turbulence and Instabilities

Flow fields are broadly classified as either *laminar* or *turbulent* to distinguish between smooth and irregular motion, respectively. Fluid elements in laminar flow fields follow well-defined paths indicating smooth flow in discrete layers or "laminae," with minimal exchange of material between layers due to the lack of macroscopic mixing. The transport of momentum between system boundaries is thus controlled by molecular action, and is dependent on the fluid viscosity.

In contrast, many flows in nature as well as engineered applications are found to fluctuate randomly and continuously, rather than streaming smoothly, and are classified as turbulent. Turbulent flows are characterized by a vigorous mixing action throughout the flow field, which is caused by *eddies* of varying size within the flow. Since these eddies fluctuate randomly, the velocity field in a turbulent flow is not constant in time. Although turbulent flows therefore do not meet the above definition for steady, the velocity at any point presents a statistically distinct time-average value that is constant. Turbulent flows are therefore described as *stationary*, rather than truly unsteady.

Physically, the two flow states are linked, in the sense that any flow can be stable and laminar if the ratio of inertial to viscous forces is sufficiently small. Turbulence results when this ratio exceeds a *critical value*, above which the flow becomes unstable to perturbations and breaks down into fluctuations.

Fully turbulent flow fields have four defining characteristics [10,11]: they fluctuate *randomly*, they are *three-dimensional*, they are *dissipative*, and they are *dispersive*. The *turbulence intensity I* of any flow field is defined as the ratio of velocity fluctuations u' to time-average velocity $\bar{u}$, $I = u'/\bar{u}$.

Steady flow in straight, rigid pipes is characterized by only one dimensionless parameter, the Reynolds number. It was shown by Osborne Reynolds that for Re < 2000, incidental disturbances in the flow field are damped out and the flow remains stable and laminar. For Re < 2000, brief bursts of fluctuations appear in the velocity separated by periods of laminar flow. As Re increases, the duration and intensity of these bursts increases until they merge together into full turbulence. Laminar flow may be achieved with Re as large as 20,000 or greater in extremely smooth pipes, but it is unstable to flow disturbances and rapidly becomes turbulent if perturbed.

Since the Navier–Stokes equations govern all the behavior of any Newtonian fluid flow, it follows that turbulent flow patterns should be predictable through analysis based on those equations. However, although turbulent flows have been investigated for more than a century and the equations of motion analyzed in great detail, no general approach to the solution of problems in turbulent flow has been found. Statistical studies invariably lead to a situation in which there are more unknown variables than equations, which is called the *closure problem* of turbulence. Efforts to circumvent this difficulty have included phenomenologic concepts such as *eddy viscosity* and *mixing length*, as well as analytical methods including dimensional analysis and asymptotic invariance studies.

7.2.2 Flow in Tubes

Flow in a tube is the most common fluid dynamic phenomenon in the physiology of living organisms, and is the basis for transport of nutrient molecules, respiratory gases, hormones, and a variety of other important solutes throughout the body of all complex living plants and animals. Only single-celled organisms, and multicelled organisms with small numbers of cells, can survive without a mechanism for transporting such molecules, although even these organisms exchange materials with their external environment through fluid-filled spaces. Higher organisms, needing to transport molecules and materials over larger distances, rely on organized systems of directed flows through networks of tubes to carry fluids and solutes. In human physiology, the circulatory system, which consists of the heart, the blood vessels of the vascular tree, and the fluid, blood and which serves to transport blood throughout the body tissues, is perhaps the most obvious example of an organ system dedicated to creating and sustaining flow in a network of tubes. However, flow in tubes is also a central characteristic of the respiratory, digestive, and urinary systems. Furthermore, the immune system utilizes systemic circulatory mechanisms to facilitate transport of antibodies, white blood cells, and lymph throughout the body, while the endocrine system is critically dependent on blood flow for delivery of its secreted hormones to the appropriate target organs or tissues. In addition, reproductive functions are also based on fluid flow in tubes. Thus, seven of the ten major organ systems depend on flow in tubes to fulfill their functions.

7.2.2.1 Steady Poiseuille Flow

The most basic state of motion for fluid in a pipe is one in which the motion occurs at a constant rate, independent of time. The pressure–flow relation for laminar, steady flow in round tubes is called *Poiseuille's Law*, after J.L.M. Poiseuille, the French physiologist who first derived the relation in 1840 [12]. Accordingly, steady flow through a pipe or channel that is driven by a pressure difference between the pipe ends of just sufficient magnitude to overcome the tendency of the fluid to dissipate energy through the action of viscosity is called *Poiseuille flow*.

Strictly speaking, Poiseuille's Law applies only to steady, laminar flow through pipes that are straight, rigid, and infinitely long with uniform diameter, so that effects at the pipe ends may be neglected without loss of accuracy. However, although neither physiologic vessels nor industrial tubes fulfill all those conditions exactly, Poiseuille relationships have proven to be of such widespread usefulness that they are often applied even when the underlying assumptions are not met. As such, Poiseuille flow can be taken as the starting point for analysis of cardiovascular, respiratory, and other physiologic flows of interest.

A straight, rigid round pipe is shown in Figure 7.1, with x denoting the pipe axis and a the pipe radius. Flow in the pipe is governed by the Navier–Stokes equations, which for these conditions reduce to $d^2 u/dr^2 + (1/r)(du/dr) = -\kappa/\mu$, with the conditions that the flow field must be symmetric about the pipe center line, that is, $du/dr|_{r=0} = 0$, and the no-slip boundary condition applies at the wall, $u = 0$ at $r = a$. Under these conditions, the velocity field solution is $u(r) = (\kappa/4\mu)(a^2 - r^2)$.

The velocity profile described by this solution has the familiar parabolic form known as Poiseuille flow (Figure 7.1). The velocity at the wall ($r = a$) is clearly zero, as required by the no-slip condition, while as expected on physical grounds, the maximum velocity occurs on the axis of the tube ($r = 0$) where $u_{max} = \kappa a^2/4\mu$. At any position between the wall and the tube axis, the velocity varies smoothly with r, with no step change at any point.

From physical analysis, it can be shown that the parabolic velocity profile results from a *balance* of the forces on the fluid in the pipe. The pressure gradient along the pipe accelerates fluid in the forward direction through the pipe, while at the same time, viscous shear stress retards the fluid motion. A parabolic profile is created by the balance of these effects.

Although the velocity profile is important and informative, in practice one is apt to be more concerned with measurement of the *discharge rate*, or total rate of flow in the pipe, Q, which can be accessed far more

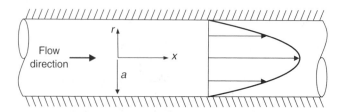

FIGURE 7.1 Parabolic velocity profile characteristic of Poiseuille flow in a round pipe of radius a. x, r-coordinate system with origin on the pipe centerline.

easily. The volume flow rate is given by area-integration of the velocity across the tube cross section:

$$Q = \int_A \mathbf{u} \bullet d\mathbf{A} = \frac{\partial P}{\partial x} \frac{\pi a^4}{8\mu} \tag{7.5}$$

which is Poiseuille's Law.

For convenience, the relation between pressure and flow rate is often reexpressed in an Ohm's Law form, driving force = flow × resistance, or $\partial P/\partial x = Q \cdot (8\mu/\pi a^4)$, from which the resistance to flow, $8\mu/\pi a^4$, is seen to be inversely proportional to the fourth power of the tube radius.

A further point about Poiseuille flow concerns the area-average velocity, U. Clearly, $U = Q/$ cross-sectional area $= (\pi \kappa a^4/8\mu)/\pi a^2 = \kappa a^2/8\mu$. But, as was pointed out, the maximum velocity in the tube is $u_{max} = \kappa a^2/4\mu$. Hence $U = u_{max}/2 = (1/2)u|_{r=0} = (1/2)u_{CL}$.

Finally, the shear stress exerted by the flow on the wall can be a critical parameter, particularly when it is desired to control the wall's exposure to shear. From the solution for $u(r)$, it can be shown that wall shear stress, τ_w, is given by

$$\tau_w = -\mu \frac{du}{dr}\bigg|_{r=a} = \frac{\partial P}{\partial x} \frac{a}{2} = \frac{4\mu Q}{\pi a^3} \tag{7.6}$$

To summarize, Poiseuille's Law, Equation 7.5, provides a relation between the pressure drop and net laminar flow in any tube, while Equation 7.6 provides a relation between the flow rate and wall shear stress. Thus, physical forces on the wall may be calculated from knowledge of the flow fields.

7.2.2.2 Entrance Flow

It can be shown that a Poiseuille velocity profile is the velocity distribution that minimizes energy dissipation in steady laminar flow through a rigid tube. Consequently, it is not surprising that if the flow in a tube encounters a perturbation that alters its profile, such as a branch vessel or a region of stenosis, immediately downstream of the perturbation the velocity profile will be disturbed away from a parabolic form, perhaps highly so. However, if the Reynolds number is low enough for the flow to remain stable as it convects downstream from the site of the original distribution, a parabolic form is gradually recovered. Consequently, at a sufficient distance downstream, a fully developed parabolic velocity profile again emerges.

Both blood vessels and bronchial tubes of the lung possess enormous number of branches, each of which produces its own flow disturbance. As a result, many physiologic flows may not be fully developed over a significant fraction of their length. It therefore becomes important to ask, what length of tube is required for a perturbed velocity profile to recover its parabolic form, that is, how long is the entrance length in a given tube? This question can be formally posed as, if x is the coordinate along the tube axis, for what value of x does $u|_{r=0} = 2U$? Through dimensional analysis it can be shown that $x/d = $ const $\times (\rho dU/\mu) = $ const $\times$ Re, where d is the tube diameter. Thus, the length of tube over which the flow develops is const $\times$ Re $\times d$. The constant must be determined by experiment, and is found to be in the range 0.03 to 0.04.

Since the entrance length, in units of tube diameters, is proportional to the Reynolds number and the mean Reynolds number for flow in large tubes such as the aorta and trachea is of the order of 500 to 1000, the entrance length in these vessels can be as much as 20 to 30 diameters. In fact, there are few segments of these vessels even close to that length without a branch or curve that perturbs their flow. Consequently, flow in them can be expected to almost never be fully developed. In contrast, flow in the smallest bronchioles, arterioles, and capillaries may take place with Re < 1. As a result, their entrance length is $\ll 1$ diameter, and flow in them will virtually always be nearly or fully developed.

7.2.2.3 Mechanical Energy Equation

Flow fields in tubes with more complex shapes than simple straight pipes, such as those possessing bends, curves, orifices, and other intricacies, are often analyzed with an *energy balance* approach, since they are not well described by Poiseuille's Law. Understanding such flow fields is significant for *in vitro* studies and perfusion devices, to establish dynamic similitude parameters, as well as for *in vivo* studies of curved as well as branched vessel flows. For any system of total energy E, the *first law of thermodynamics* states that any change in the energy of the system ΔE must appear as either heat transferred to the system in unit time Q or as work done by the system W, so that $\Delta E = Q - W$. Here a sign convention is taken such that Q, when positive, represents heat transferred *to* the system and W, when positive, is the work done *by* the system on its surroundings. The general form of the energy equation for a fluid system is

$$\dot{Q} - \dot{W}_s = \frac{d}{dt} \int_V \left(\frac{U^2}{2} + gz + e \right) \rho \, dV + \int_S \left(\frac{p}{\rho} + \frac{U^2}{2} + gz + e \right) \rho \mathbf{u} \cdot d\mathbf{S} \qquad (7.7)$$

where W_s, the "shaft work," represents work done on the fluid contained within a volume V bounded by a surface S by pumps, turbines, or other external devices through which power is often transmitted by means of a shaft, $U^2/2$ is the kinetic energy per unit mass of the fluid within V, gz is its potential energy per unit mass, with z the vertical coordinate and g gravitational acceleration, e is its internal energy per unit mass, and the density ρ is assumed to be constant.

The general equation can be simplified greatly when the flow is steady, since the total energy contained within any prescribed volume is then constant, and $d/dt = 0$. Applying Equation 7.7 to steady flow through a control volume whose end faces are denoted 1 and 2 respectively, then gives

$$\frac{p_1}{\gamma} + \beta_1 \frac{U_1^2}{2g} + z_1 + h_P = \frac{p_2}{\gamma} + \beta_2 \frac{U_2^2}{2g} + z_2 + h_L \qquad (7.8)$$

where p_1 and p_2 are the pressures at faces 1 and 2, z_1 and z_2 are the vertical positions of those faces, $\gamma = \rho g$, h_p represents head supplied by a pump, and the coefficients β_1 and β_2 are kinetic energy correction factors introduced to simplify notation. Calculations show that $\beta = 1$ when the velocity is uniform across the section, and $\beta = 2$ for laminar Poiseuille flow. Mechanical energy lost from the system is lumped together as a single term called *head loss*, h_L. For flow in a rigid pipe of length L and diameter d, h_L is well represented by $h_L = f(L/d)(U^2/2g)$, where f is called the *friction factor* of the pipe, and depends on both the pipe roughness and the flow Reynolds number. It can be shown that for laminar flow, $f = 64/\text{Re}$. Then $h_L = (32 \mu L U / \gamma d^2)$. Forms that h_L can take on in turbulent flows are given in a variety of texts [13,14].

It is worth repeating that Equation 7.8 is only correct when the fluid density is constant, as is normally the case in tissue and engineering applications and even for air flow in the lung. Compressibility effects require separate energy considerations.

7.3 Pulsatile Flow

Flow in a straight, round tube driven by an axial pressure gradient that varies in time is the basis for blood transport in the arterial tree as well as respiratory gas transport in the trachea and bronchi. When the flow is confined within a tube of *rigid*, undeformable walls, its direction will always be parallel to the tube axis, so that there will only be an axial component of velocity $\mathbf{u} = (u(r, t), 0, 0)$ (Figure 7.2). Since all the fluid elements in the tube will then respond to any change in the pressure magnitude instantaneously and in unison, regardless of axial position, the velocity profile will be the same at all positions along the tube. It is as if all the fluid in the tube moves as a single rigid body.

As a result of the flow field accelerations and decelerations in pulsatile flows, a special type of boundary layer known as the *Stokes layer* develops. When the pressure gradient varies sinusoidally in time, as the pressure increases to its maximum, the flow increases, and as the pressure decreases, the flow does too.

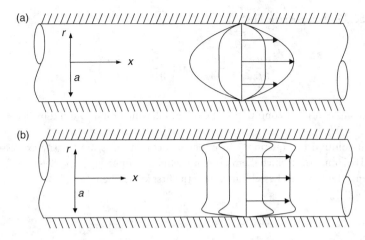

FIGURE 7.2 Representative velocity profiles of laminar, oscillatory flow in a straight, rigid tube, at four phases of the flow cycle. (a) $\alpha = 3$, (b) $\alpha = 13$.

If the oscillations are of very low frequency, the velocity field will essentially be in phase with the pressure gradient and the boundary layers will have adequate time to grow into the tube core region. In the limit of very low frequency, the velocity field must therefore approach that of a steady Poiseuille flow. As frequency increases, however, the pressure gradient changes more rapidly and the flow begins to lag behind due to the inertia of the fluid. The Stokes layers then become confined to a region near the wall, lacking the time required for further growth. In addition, the flow amplitude decreases with increasing oscillation frequency as pressure gradient reversals occur more and more rapidly. In the limit of very high frequency, fluid in the tube center hardly moves at all and the Stokes layers are confined to very thin region along the wall.

Because of the inertia of the fluid, the Stokes layer thickness, δ, is inversely related to the flow frequency, with $\delta \propto (v/\omega)^{1/2}$, where ω is the flow angular frequency (in rad/sec).

7.3.1 Hemodynamics in Rigid Tubes: Womersley's Theory

The rhythmic contractions of the heart produce a pressure distribution in the arterial tree that includes both a steady component, P_s, and a purely oscillatory component, P_{osc}, as does the velocity field. In contrast, flow in the trachea and bronchi has no steady component, and thus is purely oscillatory. It is common practice to refer to these components of pressure and flow as *steady* and *oscillatory*, respectively, and to use the term *pulsatile* to refer to the superposition of the two. A very useful feature of these flows, when they occur in rigid tubes, is that the governing equation (Equation 7.10) is linear, since the flow field is unidirectional and independent of axial position. The steady and oscillatory components can therefore be decoupled from each other, and analyzed separately. This gives

$$P(x, t) = P_s(x) + P_{osc}(x, t)$$

$$u(r, t) = u_s(r) + u_{osc}(r, t)$$

(7.9)

The oscillatory component of this flow may be analyzed assuming the flow to be fully developed, so that entrance effects may be neglected, and to be driven by a purely oscillatory pressure gradient, $-(1/\rho)(\partial P/\partial x) = K \cos(\omega t) = \mathrm{Re}(Ke^{i\omega t})$, where $i = \sqrt{-1}$ and here "Re" indicates the Real part of $Ke^{i\omega t}$. It is also convenient to introduce a new dimensionless parameter, the Womersley number, α [15], defined as $\alpha = a(\omega/v)^{1/2}$. Thus defined, α represents the ratio of the tube radius to the Stokes layer thickness.

The velocity field is then governed by

$$\frac{\partial u}{\partial t} = -\frac{1}{\rho}\frac{\partial P}{\partial x} + \upsilon\left(\frac{\partial^2 u}{\partial r^2} + \frac{1}{r}\frac{\partial u}{\partial r}\right) \tag{7.10}$$

subject to the no-slip boundary condition at the tube wall, which for a round tube takes the form $\mathbf{u} = 0$ for $r = a$.

The particular solution to Equation 7.10 under this condition is most easily expressed in terms of complex ber and bei functions, which themselves are defined through [16] $\mathrm{ber}(r) + i \cdot \mathrm{bei}(r) = J_0(r \cdot i\sqrt{i})$, where J_0 represents the complex Bessel function of the first kind. Then

$$u(r,t) = \frac{K}{\omega}(B\cos\omega t + (1-A)\sin\omega t) \tag{7.11}$$

where

$$A = \frac{\mathrm{ber}\alpha \cdot \mathrm{ber}\alpha(r/a) + \mathrm{bei}\alpha \cdot \mathrm{bei}\alpha(r/a)}{\mathrm{ber}^2\alpha + \mathrm{bei}^2\alpha} \tag{7.12a}$$

and

$$B = \frac{\mathrm{bei}\alpha \cdot \mathrm{ber}\alpha(r/a) - \mathrm{ber}\alpha \cdot \mathrm{bei}\alpha(r/a)}{\mathrm{ber}^2\alpha + \mathrm{bei}^2\alpha} \tag{7.12b}$$

Representative velocity profiles derived from these expressions are shown in Figure 7.2 for two values of α at four phases of the flow cycle. In these figures the radial position, r, has been normalized by the tube radius, a. At $\alpha = 3$ (Figure 7.2a), a value that under resting conditions can occur in the smallest arteries and larger arterioles as well as the middle airways, Stokes layers can occupy a significant fraction of the tube radius. The velocity at the wall is zero, as required by the no-slip condition, and as in steady flow the velocity varies smoothly with r, with no step change at any point. However, even at this low α, the velocity profile resembles a parabola only during peak flow rates. At other flow phases, a more uniform profile forms across the tube core.

In contrast, at $\alpha = 13$ (Figure 7.2b), which characterizes rest state flow in the aorta and trachea, the velocity profile of the pipe core is nearly uniform at all flow phases. Flow in the boundary layer is out of phase with that in the core, and flow reversals are possible in the Stokes layer. These changes in the velocity fields result from the inertia of the fluid, since as the flow frequency increases, less time is available in each flow cycle to accelerate the fluid.

To these flow fields, of course, must be added a steady component if the flow field is pulsatile rather than purely oscillatory.

As with steady flows, it is important to be able to use these expressions for the velocity field to determine the instantaneous total volume flow rate, Q_{inst}, or equivalently the instantaneous mean velocity, U_{inst}, since $Q_{\mathrm{inst}} = U_{\mathrm{inst}} \times$ pipe area. It can be shown that the mean velocity is [17]

$$
\begin{aligned}
U(t) &= \frac{K}{\omega}\left(\frac{2D}{\alpha}\cos\omega t + \left(\frac{1-2C}{\alpha}\right)\sin\omega t\right) \\
&= \frac{K}{\omega}\sigma\cos(\omega t - \delta)
\end{aligned}
\tag{7.13}
$$

where

$$C = \frac{\mathrm{ber}\alpha \cdot \mathrm{bei}'\alpha - \mathrm{bei}\alpha \cdot \mathrm{ber}'\alpha}{\mathrm{ber}^2\alpha + \mathrm{bei}^2\alpha} \tag{7.14a}$$

$$D = \frac{\mathrm{ber}\alpha \cdot \mathrm{ber}'\alpha + \mathrm{bei}\alpha \cdot \mathrm{bei}'\alpha}{\mathrm{ber}^2\alpha + \mathrm{bei}^2\alpha} \tag{7.14b}$$

$$\sigma^2 = \left(\frac{1-2C}{\alpha}\right)^2 + \left(\frac{2D}{\alpha}\right)^2 \tag{7.14c}$$

$$\tan\delta = \frac{(1-2C/\alpha)}{(2D/\alpha)} \tag{7.14d}$$

The oscillatory shear stress at the wall, $\tau_{w,osc}$, is given by $\tau_{w,osc} = -\mu(\partial u_{osc}/\partial r)|_{r=a}$. This results in

$$\tau_{w,osc} = \mathrm{Re}\left(\frac{\rho K a \sqrt{i}}{\alpha} \frac{J_1(a\sqrt{-i\omega/\upsilon})}{J_0(a\sqrt{-i\omega/\upsilon})} \cdot e^{i\omega t}\right) \tag{7.15}$$

As with the oscillatory flow rate, the oscillatory wall shear stress lags the pressure gradient, reaching a maximum during peak flow.

7.3.2 Hemodynamics in Elastic Tubes

Because of the mathematical complexity of analysis of pulsatile flows in elastic tubes, and the variety of physical phenomena associated with them, space does not permit a full description of this topic. The reader is instead referred to a number of excellent references for a more complete treatment [18–20]. Here we only briefly summarize the most important features of these flows, to give the reader a sense of the richness of the physics underlying them.

In brief, in a tube with a nonrigid wall, any pressure change within the tube will lead to localized bulging of the tube wall in the high-pressure region (Figure 7.3). Fluid can then flow in the radial direction into the bulge. Hence, not only is the radial velocity v no longer zero, but both u and v can no longer be independent of x even far from the tube ends. Thus the flow field is governed by the continuity condition

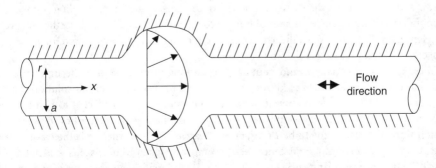

FIGURE 7.3 Local bulging of the tube wall at regions of high pressure in pulsatile flow in an elastic tube.

along with the full Navier–Stokes equations. Assuming axial symmetry of the tube, these become

$$\frac{\partial u}{\partial x} + \frac{\partial v}{\partial r} + \frac{v}{r} = 0 \tag{7.16}$$

$$\frac{\partial u}{\partial t} + u\frac{\partial u}{\partial x} + v\frac{\partial u}{\partial r} = -\frac{1}{\rho}\frac{\partial P}{\partial x} + \nu\left(\frac{\partial^2 u}{\partial x^2} + \frac{\partial^2 u}{\partial r^2} + \frac{1}{r}\frac{\partial u}{\partial r}\right)$$

$$\frac{\partial v}{\partial t} + u\frac{\partial v}{\partial x} + v\frac{\partial v}{\partial r} = -\frac{1}{\rho}\frac{\partial P}{\partial r} + \nu\left(\frac{\partial^2 v}{\partial x^2} + \frac{\partial^2 v}{\partial r^2} + \frac{1}{r}\frac{\partial v}{\partial r} - \frac{v}{r^2}\right) \tag{7.17}$$

The most important consequence of this is that even if the inlet pressure gradient depends only on t, within the tube the pressure gradient depends on x as well as t. An oscillatory pressure gradient applied at the tube entrance therefore propagates down the tube in a wave motion. Both the pressure and the velocity fields therefore take on wave characteristics.

The speed with which these waves travel down the tube can be expected to depend on the fluid inertia, that is, on its density and on the wall stiffness. If the wall thickness is small compared to the tube radius and the effect of viscosity is neglected, the wave speed c_0 is given by the Moen–Korteweg formula $c_0 = (Eh/\rho d)^{1/2}$, where E is the stiffness, or Young's modulus, of the tube wall and h is its thickness. As can be expected on physical grounds, the wave speed increases as the wall stiffness rises until when E becomes infinite, the wall is rigid. Thus oscillatory motion in a *rigid* tube, in which all the fluid moves together in bulk, may be thought of as resulting from a wave traveling with infinite speed, so that any change in the pressure gradient is felt throughout the whole tube instantaneously. In an *elastic* tube, by contrast, pressure changes are felt locally at first and then propagate downstream at finite speed.

Because of the action of the pressure and shear stress on the wall position and displacement, oscillatory flow in an elastic tube is inherently a *coupled* problem, in the sense that it is not possible in general to determine the fluid motion without also determining the resulting wall motion; the two are intrinsically linked. It can be shown [18] that the motion of the *wall* is governed by

$$\frac{\partial^2 \varsigma}{\partial t^2} = \frac{E}{(1-\sigma^2)\rho_w}\left(\frac{\partial^2 \varsigma}{\partial x^2} + \frac{\sigma}{a}\frac{\partial^2 \eta}{\partial x}\right) - \frac{\tau_w}{\rho_w h} \tag{7.18a}$$

$$\frac{\partial^2 \eta}{\partial t^2} = \frac{P_w}{\rho_w h} - \frac{E}{(1-\sigma^2)\rho_w a}\left(\frac{\eta}{a} + \sigma\frac{\partial \varsigma}{\partial x}\right) \tag{7.18b}$$

where ς and η are the axial and radial displacement of the wall, respectively (both of which may vary with axial position x), P_w and τ_w are the fluid pressure and shear stress at the wall, ρ_w is the wall density and σ is Poisson's ratio, a wall material property. Equation 7.18(a) and Equation 7.18(b) indicate the coupling of the wall and fluid motions, since they explicitly describe ς and η, which are properties of the *wall*, in terms of P_w and τ_w, which are themselves properties of the *flow*. In addition, coupling is imposed by the no-slip boundary condition, since the layer of fluid in contact with the wall must have the same velocity as the wall. Hence, $\partial \varsigma/\partial t = u(x, a, t)$, the axial component of velocity at the wall, and $\partial \eta/\partial t = v(x, a, t)$, the radial component of velocity at the wall.

With these governing equations and boundary conditions in place, and if the input pressure distribution that drives the flow field is known, it is possible to develop a formal solution for the axial velocity. For an oscillatory flow, the input pressure would normally be expected to be of a sinusoidal form $P(x, r, t) = \text{const} \cdot e^{i\omega t}$. Following Reference 18, the method of characteristics shows the pressure distribution throughout the tube to be $P(x, r, t) = A(x, r)e^{i\omega(t-x/c)}$, where c is the wave speed in the fluid and A is the pressure amplitude. Since the fluid must be taken to be viscous, c is not equal to c_0, the inviscid fluid wave speed. Instead, $c = c_0(2/(1 - \sigma^2)z)^{1/2}$, with z a parameter of the problem that depends on a, ω, ν, σ, ρ, ρ_w, and h. It can also be shown that the pressure amplitude A depends on x, but not on r, and therefore the pressure is uniform across any axial position in the tube [18]. Under these conditions, the solution for u, the principal velocity component of interest, can be stated as

$$u(x, r, t) = \mathrm{Re}\left(\frac{A}{\rho c} \left\{ 1 - G \frac{J_0\left(r\sqrt{-i\omega/\upsilon}\right)}{J_0\left(a\sqrt{-i\omega/\upsilon}\right)} \right\} \cdot e^{i\omega(t - x/c)} \right) \qquad (7.19)$$

with G a factor that modifies the velocity profile shape compared to that in a rigid tube due to the wall elasticity. G is given by

$$G = \frac{2 + z(2\nu - 1)}{z(2\nu - g)} \qquad (7.20)$$

with

$$g = \frac{2J_1(a\sqrt{-i\omega/\upsilon})}{(a\sqrt{-i\omega/\upsilon})J_0(a\sqrt{-i\omega/\upsilon})} \qquad (7.21)$$

It is apparent from inspection of Equation 7.19 that the difference between the velocity field in a rigid tube and that in an elastic tube is contained in the factor G. However, since G is complex, and both its real and imaginary parts depend on the flow frequency ω, the difference is by no means readily evident. The reader is referred to Reference 18 for detailed depiction of representative velocity profiles. Nevertheless, it is important to note here that because the pressure distribution in an elastic tube takes the form of a traveling wave, *two separate* periodic oscillations can be derived from Equation 7.19. The first is that at any given axial position in the tube, the velocity profile varies sinusoidally with time, just as it does in a rigid tube. The second, however, is that at any instant of time during the flow cycle, the velocity field also varies sinusoidally in space. Fluid flows *away* from regions in which the pressure is greatest and *toward* regions in which it is least. In a rigid tube, there is only one region of maximum pressure, the upstream tube end, and only one region of minimum pressure, the downstream end. Between them, the pressure varies linearly with axial position x. In contrast, in an elastic tube the pressure varies *sinusoidally* with x, so that many high-pressure regions can exist along the tube and these lead to a series of flow reversals at any specific time.

A final word about oscillatory flow in an elastic tube concerns the possibility of *wave reflections*. In a rigid tube, there is no wave motion as such, and flow arriving at an obstruction or branch is disturbed in some way, but otherwise progresses through the obstruction. In contrast, the wave nature of flow in an elastic tube leads to entirely different behavior at an obstacle. At an obstruction such as a bifurcation or a branch, some of the energy associated with pressure and flow is transmitted through the obstruction, while the remainder is *reflected*. This leads to a highly complex pattern of superposing primary and reflected pressure and flow waves, particularly in the arterial tree since blood vessels are elastic and vessel branchings are ubiquitous throughout the vascular system. Such wave reflections may be analyzed in terms of transmission line theory [7,18].

7.3.3 Turbulence in Pulsatile Flow

Transition to turbulence in oscillatory pipe flows occurs through fundamentally different mechanisms than transition in steady flows, for two reasons. The first is that the oscillatory nature of the flow leads to a unique base state, the most important feature of which is the formation of an oscillatory Stokes layer on the tube wall. This layer has its own stability characteristics, which are not comparable to the stability characteristics of the boundary layer of steady flow. The second reason is that temporal deceleration destabilizes the whole flow field, so that perturbations of the Stokes layer can cause the flow to break down into unstable, random fluctuations. Instability often occurs during the deceleration phase of the flow cycle, and is immediately followed by relaminarization as the net flow decays to zero prior to reversal.

Because of these characteristics, during deceleration phases of the flow cycle instabilities are observable in the Stokes layer even at much lower Reynolds numbers than those for which they would be found in steady flow [21].

Since the Stokes layer thickness δ itself depends on the flow frequency, transition to turbulence depends on the Womersley number as well as the Reynolds number. Experimental measurements of the velocity made in rigid tubes by noninvasive optical techniques [21] have shown that over a range of values of $\alpha \geq 8$, the flow was found to be fully laminar for $Re_\delta \leq 500$, where Re_δ is the Reynolds number based on the Stokes layer thickness rather than tube diameter. That is, $Re_\delta = U\delta/\nu$. For $500 < Re_\delta < 1300$, the core flow remained laminar while the Stokes layer became unstable during the deceleration phase of fluid motion. This turbulence was most intense in an annular region near the tube wall. These results are in accord with theoretical predictions of instabilities in Stokes layers [22,23]. For higher values of Re_δ, instability can be expected to spread across the tube core.

7.4   Models and Computational Techniques

7.4.1   Approximations to the Navier–Stokes Equations

The Navier–Stokes equations, Equation 7.3 and Equation 7.4, together with the continuity condition, provide a complete set of governing equations for the motion of an incompressible Newtonian fluid. If appropriate boundary and initial conditions can be specified for the motion of such a fluid in a given flow system, in principle a full set of governing equations and conditions for the system will be known. It may then be expected that the fluid motion can be deduced simply by solution of the resulting boundary value problem. Unfortunately, however, the mathematical difficulties resulting from the nonlinear character of the acceleration terms $D\mathbf{u}/Dt$ in the Navier–Stokes equations are so great that only a very limited number of exact solutions have ever been found. The simplest of these pertain to cases in which the velocity has the same direction at every point in the flow field, as in the steady and pulsatile pipe flows discussed earlier.

Accordingly, there is a strong incentive to seek conditions under which one or more of the terms in Equation 7.3 are negligible or nearly so, and therefore an approximate and much simpler governing equation can be generated by neglecting them altogether. For example, the Reynolds number represents the ratio of inertial to viscous forces in the flow field. Accordingly, in flows for which $Re \gg 1$, it can be shown that the viscous term $\nu\nabla^2\mathbf{u}$ is very much smaller than the acceleration $D\mathbf{u}/Dt$. Consequently, it can be omitted from the governing equation, which leads to solutions that are approximately valid at least outside the boundary layer. Conversely, when $Re \ll 1$, the viscous term $\nu\nabla^2\mathbf{u}$ is much larger than the acceleration $D\mathbf{u}/Dt$.

In summary, these approximations show that viscosity is important in three situations:

1. When the overall Reynolds number is *low*, since then viscous effects act over the full flow field
2. When the overall Reynolds number is *high*, viscosity is important in thin boundary layers
3. When the flow is *enclosed*, as in a pipe flow, since then the available diffusion time is very large and viscous effects can become important in the whole flow after some initial region or time

An alternative approach to seeking simplifications to the Navier–Stokes equations is to accept the full set of equations, but approximate each term in the equation with a simpler form that permits solutions to be developed. Although the resulting equations are only *approximately* correct, the advent of modern digital computers has allowed them to be written with great fineness, so that highly accurate solutions are achieved. These techniques are called CFD.

7.4.2   Computational Fluid Dynamics

The steady improvement in computer speed and memory capabilities since the 1950s has made it possible for CFD to become a very powerful and versatile tool for the analysis of complex problems of interest in the engineering biosciences. By providing a cost-effective means to simulate real flows in detail,

CFD permits studying complex problems combining thermodynamics, chemical reaction kinetics, and transport phenomena with fluid flow aspects. In addition, such problems often arise in highly complex geometries. Consequently, they may be far too difficult to study accurately without computational model approaches.

Furthermore, CFD offers a means for testing flow conditions that are unachievable or prohibitively expensive to test experimentally. For example, most flow loops and wind tunnels are limited to a fixed range of flow rates and governing parameter values. Such limits generally do not apply to CFD analyses. Moreover, flow under a wide range of parameter values may be tested with far less cost than performing repeated experiments.

A representative example of widespread interest to biomedical engineers is the analysis of hemodynamics in blood vessel models. When analyzing biologic responses to flow or before employing newly developed surgical procedures, characterization studies need to be conducted to substantiate applicability. Cellular metabolic rates in encapsulated and free states, as well as pertinent transport phenomena, can be evaluated in anatomically realistic vessel configurations. These data, coupled with computational fluid dynamics modeling, provide the basis for redesign/reconfigurations as apropos. CFD is a very powerful and versatile tool for an analysis of this type.

At present, computational fluid dynamics methods are finding many new and diverse applications in bioengineering and biomimetics. For example, CFD techniques can be used to predict (1) velocity and stress distribution maps in complex reactor performance studies as well as in vascular and bronchial models; (2) strength of adhesion and dynamics of detachment for mammalian cells; (3) transport properties for nonhomogeneous materials and nonideal interfaces; (4) multicomponent diffusion rates using the Maxwell–Stefan transport model, as opposed to the limited traditional Fickian approach, incorporating interactive molecular immobilizing sites; and (5) materials processing capabilities useful in encapsulation technology and designing functional surfaces.

Although a full description of CFD techniques is beyond the scope of this chapter, thorough descriptions of the methods and procedures may be found in many texts, for example, References 24–26.

References

[1] Bird, R.B., Stewart, W.E., and Lightfoot, E.N. (2002) *Transport Phenomena*, 2nd ed. John Wiley & Sons, New York.

[2] Lightfoot, E.N. (1974) *Transport Phenomena and Living Systems*. Wiley-Interscience, New York.

[3] Cooney, D.O. (1976) *Biomedical Engineering Principles*. Dekker, New York.

[4] Lightfoot, E.N. and Duca, K.A. (2000) The roles of mass transfer in tissue function. In Bronzino, J.D. (Ed.) *The Biomedical Engineering Handbook*, 2nd ed. CRC Press, Boca Raton, FL, Chap. 115.

[5] Goldstein, A.S. and DiMilla, P.A. (1997) *Biotechnol. Bioeng.* 55: 616.

[6] Lauffenburger, D.A. and Linderman, J.J. (1993) *Receptors: Models for Binding, Trafficking, and Signaling*. Oxford University Press, New York.

[7] Fung, Y.C. (1997) *Biomechanics: Circulation*. Springer-Verlag, New York.

[8] Lamb, H. (1945) *Hydrodynamics*. Dover Publishing, Inc., New York.

[9] Schlichting, H. (1979) *Boundary Layer Theory*, 7th ed. McGraw-Hill, New York.

[10] Hinze, J.O. (1986) *Turbulence* (Reissued). McGraw-Hill, New York.

[11] Tennekes, H. and Lumley, J.L. (1972) *A First Course in Turbulence*. MIT Press, Cambridge, MA.

[12] Poiseuille, J.L.M. (1840) *Comptes Rendus* 11: 961.

[13] Fox, R.W. and McDonald, A.T. (1992) *Introduction to Fluid Mechanics*, 4th ed. John Wiley & Sons, New York.

[14] Roberson, J.A. and Crowe, C.T. (1997) *Engineering Fluid Mechanics*, 6th ed. John Wiley & Sons, New York.

[15] Womersley, J.R. (1955) *J. Physiol.* 127: 553.

[16] Dwight, H.B. (1961) *Tables of Integrals and Other Mathematical Data*. McMillan Publishing Co., New York.

[17] Gerrard, J.H. (1971) *J. Fluid Mech.* 46: 43.

[18] Zamir, M. (2000) *The Physics of Pulsatile Flow*. AIP Press, Springer-Verlag, New York.

[19] Womersley, J.R. (1955) *Phil. Mag.* 46: 199.

[20] Atabek, S.C. and Lew, H.S. (1966) *Biophys. J.* 6: 481.

[21] Eckmann, D.M. and Grotberg, J.B. (1991) *J. Fluid Mech.* 222: 329.

[22] Davis, S.H. and von Kerczek, C. (1973) *Arch. Ration. Mech. Anal.* 188: 112.

[23] von Kerczek, C. and Davis, S.H. (1974) *J. Fluid Mech.* 62: 753.

[24] Fletcher, C.A. (1991) *Computational Techniques for Fluid Dynamics*, Vol. I, 2nd ed. Springer-Verlag, Berlin.

[25] Fletcher, C.A. (1991) *Computational Techniques for Fluid Dynamics*, Vol. II, 2nd ed. Springer-Verlag, Berlin.

[26] Chung, T.J. (2002) *Computational Fluid Dynamics*. Cambridge University Press, Cambridge.

8

Animal Surrogate Systems

Michael L. Shuler
Sarina G. Harris
Xinran Li
Cornell University

8.1 Background

Animal surrogate or cell culture analog (CCA) systems mimic the biochemical response of an animal or human when challenged with a chemical or drug. A true animal surrogate is a device that replicates the circulation, metabolism, or adsorption of a chemical and its metabolites using interconnected multiple compartments to represent key organs. These compartments make use of **engineered tissues** or cell cultures. **Physiologically based pharmacokinetic models (PBPK)** guide the design of the device. The animal surrogate, particularly a human surrogate, can provide important insights into toxicity and efficacy of a drug or chemical when it is impractical or imprudent to use living animals (or humans) for testing. The combination of a CCA and PBPK provides a rational basis to relate molecular mechanisms to whole animal response.

8.1.1 Limitations of Animal Studies

The primary method used to test the potential toxicity of a chemical or action of a pharmaceutical is to use animal studies, predominantly with rodents. Animal studies are problematic. The primary difficulties are that the results may not be meaningful to the assessment of human response [Gura, 1997]. Because of the intrinsic complexity of a living organism and the inherent variability within a species, animal studies are difficult to use to identify unambiguously the underlying molecular mechanism for action of a chemical. The lack of a clear relationship among all of the molecular mechanisms to whole animal response makes extrapolation across species difficult. This factor is particularly crucial when extrapolation of rodent data to humans is an objective. Further, without a good mechanistic model it is difficult to rationally extrapolate from high doses to low doses. However, this disadvantage due to complexity can be an advantage; the animal is a "black box" and provides response data even when the mechanism of action is unknown. Further disadvantages reside in the high cost of animal studies, the long period of time often necessary to secure results, and the potential ethical problems in animal studies.

8.1.2 Alternatives to Animal Studies

In vitro methods using isolated cells [Del Raso, 1993] are inexpensive, quick, and have almost no ethical constraints. Because the culture environment can be specified and controlled, the use of isolated cells facilitates interpretation in terms of a biochemical mechanism. Since human cells can be used as well as animal cells, cross-species extrapolation is facilitated.

However, these techniques are not fully representative of human or animal response. Typical *in vitro* experiments expose isolated cells to a static dose of a chemical or drug. It is difficult to relate this static exposure to specific doses in a whole animal. The time-dependent change in the concentration of a chemical in an animal's organ cannot be replicated. If one organ modifies a chemical or prodrug, which acts elsewhere, these situations would not be revealed by the normal *in vitro* test. Another related approach is the use of isolated cell cultures in a flow system such as a microphysiometer (McConnell et al., 1992; Cooke and O'Kennedy, 1999). Cells are cultured in a microscale (2.8 μl) flow cell and changes in pH, measured electronically, report changes in cell physiology. An important use of this technology is the analysis or response of membrane-bound receptors in mammalian cells. The flow system allows a signal to be applied and then removed.

A major limitation on the use of cell cultures is that isolated cells do not fully represent the full range of biochemical activity of the corresponding cell type when in a whole animal. Engineered tissues, especially cocultures [Bhatia et al., 1998], can provide a more "natural" environment, which can improve (i.e., make normal) cell function. Another alternative is the use of **tissue slices**, typically from the liver [Olinga et al., 1997]. Tissue slices require the sacrifice of the animal; there is intrinsic variability, and biochemical activities can decay rapidly after harvest. The use of isolated tissue slices also does not reproduce interchange of metabolites among organs and the time-dependent exposure that occurs within an animal.

An alternative to both animal and *in vitro* studies is the use of computer models based on PBPK models [Connolly and Anderson, 1991]. PBPK models can be applied to both humans and animals. Because PBPK models mimic the integrated, multicompartment nature of animals, they can predict the time-dependent changes in blood and tissue concentrations of a parent chemical or its metabolites. Although construction of a robust, comprehensive PBPK is time-consuming, once the PBPK is in place many scenarios concerning exposure to a chemical or treatment strategies with a drug can be run quickly and inexpensively. Since PBPKs can be constructed for both animals and humans, cross-species extrapolation is facilitated. There are, however, significant limitations in relying solely on PBPK models. The primary limitation is that a PBPK can only provide a response based on assumed mechanisms. Secondary and unexpected effects are not included. A further limitation is the difficulty in estimating parameters, particularly kinetic parameters.

None of these alternatives satisfactorily predicts human response to chemicals or drugs.

8.2 The Cell Culture Analog Concept

A CCA is a physical replica of the structure of a PBPK where cells or engineered tissues are used in organ compartments to achieve the metabolic and biochemical characteristics of the animal. Cell culture medium circulates between compartments and acts as a "blood surrogate." Small-scale bioreactors with the appropriate cell types in the physical device represent organs or tissues.

The CCA concept combines attributes of a PBPK and other *in vitro* systems. Unlike other *in vitro* systems, the CCA is an integrated system that can mimic dose dynamics and allows for conversion of a parent compound into metabolites and the interchange of metabolites between compartments. A CCA system allows dose exposure scenarios that can replicate the exposure scenarios of animal studies.

A CCA is intended to work in conjunction with a PBPK as a tool to test and refine mechanistic hypotheses. A molecular model can be embedded in a tissue model which is embedded in the PBPK. Thus, the molecular model is related to the overall metabolic response. The PBPK can be made an exact replica of the CCA; the predicted response and measured CCA, response should exactly match if the PBPK contains a complete and accurate description of the molecular mechanisms. In the CCA, all flow rates, the number of cells in each compartment, and the levels of each enzyme can be measured independently, so no adjustable parameters are required. If the PBPK predictions and CCA results disagree, then the description of the molecular mechanisms is incomplete. The CCA and PBPK can be used in an iterative manner to test modifications in the proposed mechanism. When the PBPK is extended to describe the whole animal, failure to predict animal response would be due to inaccurate description of transport (particularly within an organ), inability to accurately measure kinetic parameters (e.g., *in vivo* enzyme levels or activities), or the presence *in vivo* or metabolic activities not present in the cultured cells or tissues. Advances in tissue engineering will provide tissue constructs to use in a CCA that will display more authentic metabolism than isolated cell cultures.

The goal is predicting human pharmacological response to drugs or assessing risk due to chemical exposure. A PBPK that can make an accurate prediction of both animal CCA and animal experiments would be "validated." If we use the same approach to constructing a human PBPK and CCA for the same compound, then we would have a rational basis to extrapolate animal response to predict human response when human experiments would be inappropriate. Also, since the PBPK is mechanistically based, it would provide a basis for extrapolation to low doses. The CCA/PBPK approach complements animal studies by potentially providing an improved basis for extrapolation to humans.

Further, PBPKs validated as described previously provide a basis for prediction of human response to mixtures of drugs or chemicals. Drug and chemical interactions may be synergistic or antagonistic. If a PBPK for compound A and a PBPK for compound B are combined, then the response to any mixture of A and B should be predictable since the mechanisms for response to both A and B are included.

8.3   Prototype CCA

A simple three-component CCA mimicking rodent response to a challenge by naphthalene has been tested by Sweeney et al. [1995]. While this prototype system did not fulfill the criteria for a CCA of physically realistic organ residence times or ratio of cell numbers in each organ, it did represent a multicompartment system with fluid recirculation. The three components were liver, lung, and other perfused tissues. These experiments used cultured rat hepatoma (H4IIE) cells for the liver and lung (L2) cells for the lung compartment. No cells were required in "other tissues" in this model since no metabolic reactions were postulated to occur elsewhere for naphthalene or its metabolites. The H4IIE cells contained enzyme systems for activation of naphthalene (cytochrome P450IA1) to the epoxide form and conversion to dihydrodiol (epoxide hydrolase) and conjugation with glutathione (glutathione-S-transferase). The L2 cells had no enzymes for naphthalene activation. Cells were cultured in glass vessels as monolayers. Experiments with this system using lactate dihydrogenase release (LDH) and glutathione levels as dependent parameters supported a hypothesis where naphthalene is activated in the "liver" and reactive metabolites circulate to the "lung" causing glutathione depletion and cell death as measured by LDH release. Increasing the level of cytochrome p450 activity in the "liver" by increasing cell numbers or by preinducing H4IIE cells led to increased death of L2 cells. Experiments with "liver"–blank; "lung"–"lung," and "lung"–blank combinations all supported the hypothesis of a circulating reactive metabolite as the cause of L2 cell death.

This prototype system [Sweeney et al., 1995] was difficult to operate, very nonphysiologic, and made time course experiments very difficult. An alternative system using packed bed reactors for the "liver" and "lung" compartments has been tested [Ghanem and Shuler, 2000a]. This system successfully allowed time course studies, was more compact and simpler to operate, and was physiological with respect to the ratio of "liver" to "lung" cells. While liquid residence times improved in this system, they still were not physiologic (i.e., 114 sec vs. an *in vivo* value of 21 sec in the liver and 6.6 sec vs. *in vivo* lung value of about 1.5 sec) due to physical limitations on flow through the packed beds. Unlike the prototype system, no response to naphthalene was observed.

This difference in response of the two CCA designs was explained through the use of PBPK models of each CCA [Ghanem and Shuler, 2000b]. In the prototype system, the large liquid residence times in the liver and the lung allowed formation of large amounts of naphthol from naphthalene oxide and presumably the conversion of napthol into quinones that were toxic. In the packed bed system, liquid residence times were sufficiently small so that the predicted naphthol level was negligible. Thus, the PBPK provided a mechanistic basis to explain the differences in response of the two experimental configurations.

Using a very simple CCA, Mufti and Shuler [1998] demonstrated that response of human hepatoma (HepG2) to exposure to dioxin (2,3,7,8-tetrachlorodibenzo-*p*-dioxin) is dependent on how the dose is delivered. The induction of cytochrome p450IA1 activity was used as a model response for exposure to dioxin. Data were evaluated to estimate dioxin levels giving cytochrome P450IA1 activity 0.01% of maximal induced activity. Such an analysis mimics the type of analysis used to estimate risk due to chemical exposure. The "allowable" dioxin concentration was 4×10^{-3} nM using a batch spinner flask, 4×10^{-4} nM using a one-compartment system with continuous feed, and 1×10^{-5} nM using a simple two-compartment CCA. Further, response could be correlated to an estimate of the amount of dioxin bound to the cytosolic Ah receptor with a simple model for two different human hepatoma cell lines. This work illustrates the potential usefulness of a CCA approach in risk assessment.

Ma et al. [1997] have discussed an *in vitro* human placenta model for drug testing. This was a two-compartment perfusion system using human trophoblast cells attached to a chemically modified polyethylene terephthalate fibrous matrix as a cell culture scaffold. This system is a CCA in the same sense as the two-compartment system used to estimate response to dioxin.

Integration of cell culture and microfabrication to form CCA or CCA-like systems has advanced rapidly in the last four years. The use of microfabricated devices should allow relatively high throughput studies that are inexpensive, conserve scarce reagents and tissues, and facilitate automated collection and processing of data. One example is the device built by Takayama and coworkers to imitate the behavior of the vascular system. They have fabricated a device with 320 mechanical actuators to maintain and control automated cell culture within microfabricated channels (Sharchi Takayama, personal communication). While this system mimics aspects of the whole body, it does not use multiple cell types with recirculating flow.

The construction of simple microscale CCAs with multiple cell types and recirculating flow has been accomplished. A simple three-compartment system ("liver"–"lung"–other tissue) using monolayer cultures of HepG2-C3A for "liver" and L2 for "lung" has been microfabricated onto a silicon chip (2.5 cm × 2.5 cm) [Sin et al., 2004]. While monolayer cultures are a poor representation of the physiology of real tissues, this system demonstrates that an "animal-on-a-chip" model is possible. A dissolved oxygen sensor using a fluorescent ruthenium complex was integrated into the system, demonstrating the potential to build real-time sensors into such a device.

The use of a microscale CCA for toxicity studies has been demonstrated using naphthalene as a model toxicant for proof-of-concept studies. A silicon-based, microfabricated CCA with four chambers was used: a "liver"–"lung"–"fat"–other tissue model. In an initial study, the "fat" chamber was left blank [Viravaidya et al., 2004a] and in a subsequent study [Viravaidya et al., 2004b], the "fat" chamber held a monolayer of 3T3-LI cells differentiated to mimic adipocytes. These studies demonstrated that naphthalene is converted in the liver by P4501A1 into a reactive metabolite that circulates to the lung compartment. Further, the experiments show that 1,2-naphthalenediol and 1,2-naphthoquinone are the primary reactive metabolites that cause reduction in glutathione levels and cell death in the lung. Excess levels of 1-naphthol are converted to 1,2-naphthalenediol, which is consistent with the prior study on the macroscale packed bed CCA [Ghanem and Shuler, 2000b]. Naphthaquinone and naphthalenediol can be intraconverted through redox cycling generating reactive oxygen species. Naphthaquinone addition is toxic by itself. The addition of fat modulates toxicity providing significant, but partial, protection. These studies, together, demonstrate the utility of this approach.

The above examples are the first that attempt to mimic circulation and metabolic response to model an animal as an integrated system. However, others have used engineered tissues as a basis for testing the efficacy of drugs or toxicity of chemicals. These tissues are important in themselves and could become elements in an integrated CCA.

8.4 Use of Engineered Tissues or Cells for Toxicity/Pharmacology

The primary use of engineered tissues for toxicity testing has been with epithelial cells that mimic the barrier properties of the skin or gut or endothelial cells that mimic the blood-brain barrier (BBB). The use of isolated cell cultures has been of modest utility due to artifacts introduced by dissolving test agents in medium and due to the extreme sensitivity of isolated cells to these agents compared to *in vivo* tissue.

One of the first reports on the use of engineered cells is that by Gay et al. [1992] reporting on the use of a living skin equivalent as an *in vitro* dermatotoxicity model. The living skin equivalent consists of a coculture of human dermal fibroblasts in a collagen-containing matrix overlaid with human keratinocytes that have formed a stratified epidermis. This *in vitro* model used a measurement of mitrochondrial function (i.e., the colorimetric thiazolyl blue assay) to determine toxicity. Eighteen chemicals were tested. Eleven compounds classified as nonirritating had minimal or no effect on mitochondrial activity. For seven known human skin irritants, the concentration that inhibited mitochondrial activity by 50% corresponded to the threshold value for each of these compounds to cause irritation on human skin. However, living skin equivalents did not fully mimic the barrier properties of human skin; water permeability was 30-fold greater in the living skin equivalent than in human skin. Kriwet and Parenteau [1996] report the permeabilities of 20 different compounds in *in vitro* skin models. Skin cultures are slightly more permeable (two- or threefold) for highly lipophilic substances and considerably more permeable (about tenfold) for polar substances than human-cadaver or freshly excised human skin. Validation of four *in vitro* tests for skin corrosion by the European Center for the Validation of Alternative Methods (ECVAM) has led to a combination of *in vitro* tests becoming mandatory for determining skin corrosion of chemicals in the European Union [Fentem and Botham, 2002]. These *in vitro* tests include a combination of rat skin electrical resistance measurements and commercial reconstituted skin equivalents (EpiDerm^{TM} and EPISKIN^{TM}). Similarly, after a series of prevalidation studies, both EpiDerm^{TM} and EPISKIN^{TM} have entered a two-phase validation study led by ECVAM, scheduled to be completed by 2005, to assess the model(s) acceptability for predicting skin irritation [Botham, 2004]. Both of the commercial reconstituted skin equivalents are based on human skin resections; a skin model based on a cell line would be cheaper and more readily available to a larger number of labs. Suhonen et al. [2003] measured permeability coefficients of eighteen test compounds across a stratified rat epidermal keratinocyte cell line grown on a collagen gel at an air–liquid interface. The permeabilities were on average twofold greater than for human cadaver epidermis (range 0.3- to 5.2-fold difference); this cell culture model tended to overpredict the permeability of lipophilic solutes.

The above tests are static. Pasternak and Miller [1996] have tested a system to predict eye irritation combining perfusion and a tissue model consisting of MDCK (Madin-Darby canine kidney) epithelial cells cultured on a semiporous cellulose ester membrane filter. The system could be fully automated using measurement of transepithelial electrical resistance (TER) as an end point. A decrease in TER is an indicator of cell damage. The system was tested using nonionic surfactants and predicted the relative ocular toxicity of these compounds. The perfusion system mimics some dose scenarios (e.g., tearing) more easily than a static system and provides a more consistent environment for the cultured cells. The authors cite as a major advantage that the TER can be measured throughout the entire exposure protocol without physically disturbing the tissue model and introducing artifacts in the response.

Probably the most used cell-based assay is the Caco-2 model of the intestine to determine oral availability of a drug or chemical. The Caco-2 cell cultures are derived from a human colon adenocarcinoma cell line. The use of the Caco-2 cell line for prediction of drug permeability was reviewed by Artursson et al. [2001]. Artursson concludes that Caco-2 monolayers best predict the permeabilities of drugs which exhibit passive transcellular transport. For drug molecules transported by carrier proteins, the expression of the specific transport system in the Caco-2 monolayer needs to be characterized. The cell line, C2Bbel, is a clonal isolate of Caco-2 cells that is more homogeneous in apical brush border expression than the Caco-2 cell line. These cells form a polarized monolayer with an apical brush border morphologically comparable to the human colon. Tight junctions around the cells act to restrict passive diffusion by the paracellular route mimicking the transport resistance in the intestine. Hydrophobic solutes pass primarily by the transcellular route and hydrophilic compounds by the paracellular route. Yu and Sinko [1997] have demonstrated that the substratum (e.g., membrane) properties upon which the monolayer forms can become important in estimating the barrier properties of such *in vitro* systems. The barrier effects of the substratum need to be separated from the intrinsic property of the monolayers. Further, Anderle et al. [1998] have shown that the chemical nature of substratum and other culture conditions can alter transport properties. Sattler et al. [1997] provide one example (with hypericin) of how this model system can be used to evaluate effects of formulation (e.g., use of cyclodextrin or liposomes) on oral bioavailability. Another example is the application of the Caco-2 system to transport of paclitaxel across the intestine [Walle and Walle, 1998]. Rapid passive transport was partially counter-balanced by an efflux pump (probably P-glycoprotein) limiting oral bioavailability.

To study adhesion and invasion of Candida albicans, Dieterich et al. [2002] mixed fibroblasts into a liquid collagen solution and then solidified the collagen into a gel on a cell culture insert. Caco-2 were cocultured on top of the fibroblast/collagen gel matrix to model interactions in the human intestinal lining. In another coculture system, Caco-2 cells cocultured with mouse lymphocytes reproduced characteristics of Peyer's patches, regions of the intestinal lining specialized to present antigens and microorganisms to the immune system [Kerneis et al., 1997, 2000]. This Caco-2/lymphocyte model exhibited temperature-sensitive transport of latex beads and *Vibrio cholerae*. Such a model could help to design oral vaccines and other drug delivery platforms.

Another barrier of intense interest for drug delivery is the BBB. The BBB is formed by the endothelial cells of the brain capillaries. Primary characteristics are the high resistance of the capillary due to the presence of complex tight junctions inhibiting paracellular transport and the low endocytic activity of this tissue. Several *in vitro* models of the BBB have been developed, and there are many reviews of these models and their possible uses as permeability and toxicity screens (see Reinhardt and Gloor, 1997; Gumbleton and Audus, 2001; Lundquist and Renftel, 2002). The most common *in vitro* BBB model consists of a monolayer of either primary isolated brain capillary endothelial cells, primary isolated endothelial cells from elsewhere in the body, or an endothelial cell line cultured on a membrane insert. The endothelial cells are often cocultured with astrocyte or astroglial cells (another brain cell type), which has been shown to increase the barrier properties of the model. An interesting model with endothelial cells and astrocytes cocultured on opposite sides of "capillaries" in a hollow-fiber reactor incorporates continuous physiological perfusion of the endothelial cells [Stanness et al., 1996]. Harris and Shuler present a unique membrane, an order of magnitude thinner than those available commercially, for close contact coculture of endothelial and astrocytes [Harris and Shuler, 2003; Harris Ma, 2004]. The biggest challenge with *in vitro* BBB models is obtaining endothelial cell cultures, which display extensive tight junctions as observed *in vivo*. According to de Boer et al. [1999], the large number of *in vitro* models and the accompanying diversity in laboratory techniques, makes quantitative comparisons between models quite difficult. An example of an *in vitro* BBB system applied to a toxicological study is described by Glynn and Mehran [1998] who used bovine brain microvessel endothelial cells grown on porous polycarbonate filters to compare the transport of nevirapine, a reverse transcriptase inhibitor to other HIV antiretroviral agents. Nevirapine was the most permeable antiretroviral agent and hence may have value in HIV treatment in reducing levels of HIV in the brain.

Besides the skin, gut, and BBB, there are other coculture models exhibiting crosstalk between the cocultured cell types that were developed for measuring toxicity. For example, an epithelial/fibroblast [Lang et al., 1998] coculture model of the bronchial epithelial was used to examine ozone toxicity. Bone resorption caused by Pasteurella multocida toxin was studied in an osteoclast/osteoblast direct contact coculture model [Mullan and Lax, 1998]. Brana et al. [1999] cultured 400-μm thick rat brain (hippocampal) slices on a membrane insert and cultured the murine macrophage cell line (RAW 264.7) underneath. When challenged with the HIV-1 derived Tat protein, neuronal cell death in the brain slice occurred only when cocultured with the macrophage cell line. This model could be used to identify neurotoxic soluble molecules released by macrophages.

These isolated cultures mimic an important aspect of cell physiology (oral uptake or transport into the brain). In principle, they could be combined with other tissue mimics of nonbarrier tissues to form a CCA that would be especially useful in testing pharmaceuticals.

Recently, advances in engineering of nonbarrier tissues have led to the possibility of using these tissues for toxicological testing. These advances have primarily been with three-dimensional (3D) cell constructs. Unlike conventional two-dimensional systems, 3D cell cultures can represent the specific morphological and biochemical properties of the corresponding *in vivo* tissue, and are able to remain in a differentiated and functionally active state for many weeks.

One type of 3D systems is based on the guided self-formation of multicellular spheroids. Such spheroids have been used primarily with liver and renal cells. One example of the use of such cultures is the study of gliadin toxicity [Elli et al., 2003]. In addition, Goodwin et al. [2000] have constructed a 3D model for assessment of *in vitro* toxicity in *Balaena mysticetus* renal tissue.

In vitro cell culture models with human liver cells have shown great potential in predicting studies on drug toxicity and metabolism in the pharmaceutical industry. Zeilinger et al. [2002] developed a bioreactor culture model that permits the 3D coculture of liver cells under continuous medium perfusion with decentralized mass exchange and integral oxygenation. Powers and Domansky [2002] designed a microfabricated array bioreactor for perfused 3D liver culture. The 3D scaffolds were constructed by deep reactive ion etching of silicon wafers to create channels with cell-adhesive walls. A cell-retaining filter was used in these scaffolds. The reactor housing was designed to deliver a continuous perfusate across the top of the channels and through the 3D tissue cultures in the channels. The perfusate flow rates were designed to meet estimated values of cellular oxygen demands and fluid shear stress at or below the physiological shear range (<2 dyne/cm^2). Primary rat liver cells cultured for two weeks in the channels rearranged themselves to form tissue-like structures.

Such 3D cell cultures could be incorporated into a CCA device. Of particular interest may be 3D hydrogels, which are relatively easy to produce and are adaptable to cocultures. While extensive work has been done with hydrogel cultures [Drury and Mooney, 2003], these studies have not focused on applications to toxicity testing. Hydrogels are easy to make and it can be used to study cocultures. The hydrogel must be biocompatible, bioresorbable, and nontoxic such that it does not bias the experiments.

A CCA based on the concepts described here and incorporating these advanced engineered tissues could become a powerful tool for preclinical testing of pharmaceuticals. While drug leads are expanding rapidly in number, the capacity to increase animal and human clinical studies is limited. It is imperative that preclinical testing and predictions for human response become more accurate. A CCA should become an important tool in preclinical testing.

8.5 Future Prospects

The most serious bottleneck in pharmaceutical development is the ability to complete ADMET (adsorption-distribution-metabolism-elimination-toxicity) studies early enough in the development process to focus resources on the best drug candidates. Of particular importance will be human surrogates that can improve the probability that a drug will be successful in clinical trials. Such trials may cost more than a 100 million dollars and success at the rate of one in three rather than current values (about one in eight) would offer significant economic advantage.

Over the last four years, the development of integrated devices that combine cell culture and microfabrication make the possibility of commercial applications to pharmaceutical evaluation a real possibility (see Freedman [2004], Griffith et al. [1997] for discussion). However, the authenticity of engineered tissues remains a hurdle. While tissue with low levels of vascularization (e.g., skin and cartilage) can be mimicked reasonably well, vascularized tissues (e.g., liver) are still quite challenging. As improvements in tissue engineering occur, one of the first applications will be in testing of chemicals and pharmaceuticals. Over the next five years, we expect CCA type systems to become industrially important in preclinical testing of pharmaceuticals and in evaluating chemicals (and chemical mixtures) for toxicity.

Defining Terms

Animal surrogate: A physiologically based cell or tissue multicompartmented device with fluid circulation to mimic metabolism and fate of a drug or chemical.

Engineered tissues: Cell culture mimic of a tissue or organ; often combines a polymer scaffold and one or more cell types.

Physiologically-based pharmacokinetic model (PBPK): A computer model that replicates animal physiology by subdividing the body into a number of anatomical compartments, each compartment interconnected through the body fluid systems; used to describe the time-dependent distribution and disposition of a substance.

Tissue slice: A living organ is sliced into thin sections for use in toxicity studies; one primary organ can provide material for many tests.

References

Anderle, P., Niederer, E., Werner, R., Hilgendorf, C., Spahn-Langguth, H., Wunderu-Allenspach, H., Merkle, H.P., and Langguth, P. (1998). P-glycoprotein (P-gp) mediated efflux in Caco-2 cell monolayers: the influence of culturing conditions and drug exposure on P-gp expression levels. *J. Pharm. Sci.* 87: 757.

Artursson, P., Palm, K., and Luthman, K. (2001). Caco-2 monolayers n experimental and theoretical predictions of drug transport. *Adv. Drug Del. Rev.* 46: 2001.

Bhatia, S.N., Balis, U.J., Yarmush, M.L., and Toner, M. (1998). Microfabrication of hepatocyte/fibroblast co-cultures: role of homotypic cell interactions. *Biotechnol. Prog.* 14: 378.

Botham, P. (2004). The validation of *in vitro* methods for skin irritation. *Toxicol. Lett.* 149: 387.

Brana, C., Biggs, T.E., Mann, D.A., and Sundstrom, L.E. (1999). A macrophage hippocampal slice co-culture system: application to the study of HIV-induced brain damage. *J. Neurosci. Meth.* 90: 7.

Connolly, R.B. and Andersen, M.E. (1991). Biologically based pharmacodynamic models: tool for toxicological research and risk assessment. *Annu. Rev. Pharmacol. Toxicol.* 31: 503.

Cooke, D. and O'Kennedy, R. (1999). Comparison of the detrazolium salt assay for succinate dehydrogenase with the cytosensor microphysiometer in the assessment of compound toxicities. *Anal. Biochem.* 274: 188–194.

de Boer, A.G., Gaillard, P.J., and Breimer, D.D. (1999). The transference of results between blood–brain barrier cell culture systems. *Eur. J. Pharm. Sci.* 8: 1.

Del Raso, N.J. (1993). *In vitro* methodologies for enhanced toxicity testing. *Toxicol. Lett.* 68: 91

Dieterich, C., Schandar, M., Noll, M., Johannes, F.-J., Brunner, H., Graeve, T., and Rupp, S. (2002). *In vitro* reconstructed human epithelia reveal contributions of *Candida albicans EFG1* and *CPH1* to adhesion and invasion. *Microbiology* 148: 497.

Drury, J.L. and Mooney, D.J. (2003). Hydrogels for tissue engineering: scaffold design variables and applications. *Biomaterials* 24: 4337–4351.

Elli, L., Dolfini, E., and Bardella, M.T. (2003). Gliadin cytotoxicity and *in vitro* cell cultures. *Toxicol. Lett.* 146: 1.

Fentem, J.H. and Botham, P.A. (2002). ECVAM's activities in validating alternative tests for skin corrosion and irritation. *Altern. Lab. Anim.* 30: 61.

Freedman, D.H. (2004). The silicon guinea pig. *Technol. Rev.* 107: 62.

Gay, R., Swiderek, M., Nelson, D., and Ernesti, A. (1992). The living skin equivalent as a model *in vitro* for ranking the toxic potential of dermal irritants. *Toxic. In Vitro* 6: 303.

Ghanem, A. and Shuler, M.L. (2000a). Characterization of a perfusion reactor utilizing mammalian cells on microcarrier beads. *Biotechnol. Prog.* 16: 471–479.

Ghanem, A. and Shuler, M.L. (2000b). Combining cell culture analogue reactor designs and PBPK models to probe mechanisms of naphthalene toxicity. *Biotechnol. Prog.* 16: 334.

Glynn, S.L. and Mehran, Y. (1998). *In vitro* blood–brain barrier permeability of nevirapine compared to other HIV antiretroviral agents. *J. Pharm. Sci.* 87: 306.

Goodwin, T.J., Coate-Li, L., Linnehan, R.M., and Hammond, T.G. (2000). Cellular responses to mechanical stress selected contribution: a three-dimensional model for assessment of *in vitro* toxicity in *Balaena mysticetus* renal tissue. *J. Appl. Physiol.* 89: 2508.

Griffith, L.G., Wu, B., Cima, M.J., Powers, M., Chaignaud, B., and Vacanti, J.P. (1997). *In vitro* organogenesis of vascularized liver tissue. *Ann. N.Y. Acad. Sci.* 831: 382.

Gura, T. (1997). Systems for identifying new drugs are often faulty. *Science* 273: 1041.

Gumbleton, M. and Audus, K.L. (2001). Progress and limitations in the use of *in vitro* cell cultures to serve as a permeability screen for the blood–brain barrier. *J. Pharm. Sci.* 90: 1681.

Harris, S. and Shuler, M.L. (2003). Growth of endothelial cells on microfabricated silicon nitride membranes for an *in vitro* model of the blood–brain barrier. *Biotechnol. Bioprocess Eng.* 8: 246.

Harris Ma, S. (2004). A physiologically based *in vitro* model of the blood–brain barrier utilizing a nanofabricated membrane. Ph.D. Thesis. Cornell University, Ithaca, New York.

Kerneis, S., Bogdanova, A., Kraehenbuhl, J.-P., and Pringualt, E. (1997). Conversion by Peyer's patch lymphocytes of human enterocytes into M cells that transport bacteria. *Science* 277: 949.

Kerneis, S., Caliot, E., Stubbe, H., Bogdanova, A., Karaehenbuhl, J.-P., and Pringault, E. (2000). Molecular studies of the intestinal mucosal barrier physiopathology using cocultures of epithelial and immune cells: a technical update. *Microbes Infect.* 2: 1119.

Kriwet, K. and Parenteau, N.L. (1996). *In vitro* skin models. *Cosmetics Toiletries* 111: 93.

Lang, D.S., Jorres, R.A., Mucke, M., Siegfried, W., and Magnussen, H. (1998). Interactions between human bronchoepithelial cells and lung fibroblasts after ozone exposure *in vitro*. *Toxicol. Lett.* 96, 97: 13.

Lundquist, S. and Renftel, M. (2002). The use of *in vitro* cell culture models for mechanistic studies and as permeability screens for the blood–brain barrier in the pharmaceutical industry — background and current status in the drug discovery process. *Vasc. Pharmacol.* 38: 335.

Ma, T., Yang, S.-T., and Kniss, D.A. (1997). Development of an *in vitro* human placenta model by the cultivation of human trophoblasts in a fiber-based bioreactor system. *Am. Inst. Chem. Eng. Ann. Mtg.*, Los Angeles, CA, Nov. 16–21.

McConnell, H.M., Owicki, J.C., Parce, J.W., Miller, D.L., Baxter, G.T., Wada, H.G., and Pitchford, S. (1992). The cytometer microphysiometer: biological applications of silicon technology. *Science* 257: 1906.

Mufti, N.A. and Shuler, M.L. (1998). Different *in vitro* systems affect CYPIA1 activity in response to 2,3,7,8-tetrachlorodibenzo-p-dioxin. *Toxicol. In Vitro* 12: 259.

Mullan, P.B. and Lax, A.J. (1998). *Pasteurella multocida* toxin stimulates bone resorption by osteoclasts via interaction with osteoblasts. *Calcif. Tissue Int.* 63: 340.

Olinga, P., Meijer, D.K.F., Slooff, M.J.H., and Groothuis, G.M.M. (1997). Liver slices in *in vitro* pharmacotoxicology with special reference to the use of human liver tissue. *Toxicol. In Vitro* 12: 77.

Pasternak, A.S. and Miller, W.M. (1996). Measurement of trans-epithelial electrical resistance in perfusion: potential application for *in vitro* ocular toxicity testing. *Biotechnol. Bioeng.* 50: 568.

Powers, M.J. and Domansky, K. (2002). A microfabricated array bioreactor for perfused 3D liver culture, *Biotechnol. Bioeng.* 78: 257.

Reinhardt, C.A. and Gloor, S.M. (1997). Co-culture blood–brain barrier models and their use for pharmatoxicological screening. *Toxicol. In Vitro* 11: 513.

Sattler, S., Schaefer, U., Schneider, W., Hoelzl, J., and Lehr, C.-M. (1997). Binding, uptake, and transport of hypericin by Caco-2 cell monolayers. *J. Pharm. Sci.* 86: 1120.

Sin, A., Chin, K.C., Jamil, M.F., Kostov, Y., Rao, G., and Shuler, M.L. (2004). The design and fabrication of three-chamber microscale cell culture analog devices with integrated dissolved oxygen sensors. *Biotechnol. Prog.* 20: 338.

Stanness, K.A., Guatteo, E., and Janigro, D. (1996). A dynamic model of the blood–brain barrier "*in vitro.*" *NeuroToxicology* 17: 481.

Suhonen, T.M., Pasonen-Seppanen, S., Kirjavainen, M., Tammi, M., Tammi, R., and Urtti, A. (2003). Epidermal cell culture model derived from rat keratinocytes with permeability characteristics comparable to human cadaver skin. *Eur. J. Pharm. Sci.* 20: 107.

Sweeney, L.M., Shuler, M.L., Babish, J.G., and Ghanem, A. (1995). A cell culture analog of rodent physiology: application to naphthalene toxicology. *Toxicol. In Vitro* 9: 307.

Walle, U.K. and Walle, T. (1998). Taxol transport by human intestinal epithelial Caco-2 cells. *Drug Metabol. Disposit.* 26: 343.

Yu, H. and Sinko, P.J. (1997). Influence of the microporous substratum and hydrodynamics on resistances to drug transport in cell culture systems: calculation of intrinsic transport parameters. *J. Pharm. Sci.* 86: 1448.

Viravaidya, K., Sin, A., and Shuler, M.L. (2004a). Development of a microscale cell culture analog to probe naphthalene toxicity. *Biotechnol. Prog.* 20: 316.

Viravaidya, K. and Shuler, M.L. (2004b). Incorporation of 3T3-L1 cells to mimic bioaccumulation in a microscale cell culture analog device for toxicity studies. *Biotechnol. Prog.* 20: 590.

Zeilinger, K., Sauer, I.M., Pless, G., Strobel, C., Rudzitis, J., Wang, A., Nussler, A.K., Grebe, A., Mao, L., Auth, S.H.G., Unger, J., Neuhaus, P., and Gerlach, J.C. (2002). Three-dimensional co-culture of primary human liver cells in bioreactors for *in vitro* drug studies: effects of the initial cell quality on the long-term maintenance of hepatocyte-specific functions. *ATLA* 30: 525.

9

Arterial Wall Mass Transport: The Possible Role of Blood Phase Resistance in the Localization of Arterial Disease

John M. Tarbell
The City College of New York

Yuchen Qui
Cordis Corporation

Atherosclerosis is a disease of the large arteries which involves a characteristic accumulation of high molecular weight lipoprotein in the arterial wall [1]. The disease tends to be localized in regions of curvature and branching in arteries where fluid shear stress (shear rate) is altered from its normal patterns in straight vessels [2]. The possible role of fluid mechanics in the localization of atherosclerosis has been debated for many years [3,4]. One possibility considered early on was that the blood phase resistance to lipid transport, which could be affected by local fluid mechanics, played a role in the focal accumulation of lipid in arteries. Studies by Caro and Nerem [5], however, showed that the uptake of lipid in arteries could not be correlated with fluid phase mass transport, leading to the conclusion that the wall (endothelium) and not the blood, was the limiting resistance to lipid transport. This suggested that fluid mechanical effects on macromolecular transport were the result of direct mechanical influences on the transport characteristics of the endothelium.

While the transport of large molecules such as low density lipoprotein (LDL) and other high molecular weight materials, which are highly impeded by the endothelium, may be limited by the wall and not the fluid (blood), other low molecular weight species which undergo rapid reaction on the endothelial surface (e.g., adenosine triphosphate — ATP) or which are consumed rapidly by the underlying tissue (e.g., oxygen) may be limited by the fluid phase. With these possibilities in mind, the purpose of this short review is to compare the rates of transport in the blood phase to the rates of reaction on the endothelial surface, the rates of transport across the endothelium, and the rates of consumption within the wall of several important biomolecules. It will then be possible to assess quantitatively the importance of fluid phase transport; to determine which molecules are likely to be affected by local fluid mechanics; to determine where in blood vessels these influences are most likely to be manifest; and finally, to speculate about the role of fluid phase mass transport in the localization of atherosclerosis.

9.1 Steady-State Transport Modeling

9.1.1 Reactive Surface

Referring to Figure 9.1, we will assume that the species of interest is transported from the blood vessel lumen, where its bulk concentration is C_b, to the blood vessel surface, where its concentration is C_s, by a convective–diffusive mechanism which depends on the local fluid mechanics and can be characterized by a fluid-phase mass transfer coefficient k_L (see Reference 6 for further background). The species flux in the blood phase is given by

$$J_s = k_L(C_b - C_s) \tag{9.1}$$

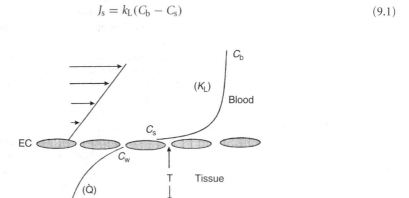

FIGURE 9.1   Schematic diagram of arterial wall transport processes showing the concentration profile of a solute which is being transported from the blood, where its bulk concentration is C_b, to the surface of the endothelium, where its concentration is C_s, then across the endothelium, where the subendothelial concentration is C_w, and finally to a minimum value within the tissue, C_{min}. Transport of the solute in the blood phase is characterized by the mass transport coefficient, k_L; consumption of the solute at the endothelial surface is described by a first-order reaction with rate constant, k_r; movement of the solute across the endothelium depends on the permeability coefficient, Pe; and reaction of the solute within the tissue volume is quantified by a zeroeth order consumption rate, $\dot{Q}$.

At the endothelial surface, the species may undergo an enzyme-catalyzed surface reaction (e.g., the hydrolysis of ATP to ADP) which can be modeled using classical Michaelis-Menten kinetics with a rate given by

$$V = \frac{V_{\max} C_s}{k_m + C_s} \tag{9.2}$$

where $V_{\max}$ is the maximum rate (high C_s) and k_m is the Michaelis constant. When $C_s \ll k_m$, as is often the case, then the reaction rate is pseudo-first order

$$V = k_r C_s \tag{9.3}$$

with the rate constant for the surface reaction given by $k_r = V_{\max}/k_m$.

At steady state, the transport to the surface is balanced by the consumption at the surface so that

$$k_L(C_b - C_s) = k_r C_s \tag{9.4}$$

It will be convenient to cast this equation into a dimensionless form by multiplying it by d/D, where d is the vessel diameter and D is the diffusion coefficient of the transported species in blood, or the media of interest. Equation 9.4 then becomes

$$\text{Sh}(C_b - C_s) = \text{Da}_r C_s \tag{9.5}$$

where

$$\text{Sh} \equiv \frac{k_L d}{D} \tag{9.6}$$

is the Sherwood number (dimensionless mass transfer coefficient), and

$$\text{Da}_r \equiv \frac{k_r d}{D} \tag{9.7}$$

is the Damköhler number (dimensionless reaction rate coefficient). Solving Equation 9.5 for the surface concentration one finds

$$\frac{C_s}{C_b} = \frac{1}{1 + \text{Da}_r/\text{Sh}} \tag{9.8}$$

When $\text{Da}_r \ll \text{Sh}$,

$$C_s = C_b \tag{9.9}$$

and the process is termed "wall-limited" or "reaction-limited." On the other hand, when $\text{Da}_r \gg \text{Sh}$,

$$C_s = \left(\frac{\text{Sh}}{\text{Da}_r}\right) C_b \tag{9.10}$$

and the process is termed "transport-limited" or "fluid phase-limited." It is in this transport-limited case that the surface concentration, and in turn the surface reaction rate, depend on the fluid mechanics which determines the Sherwood number. It will therefore be useful to compare the magnitudes of Da_r and Sh to determine whether fluid mechanics plays a role in the overall transport process of a surface reactive species.

9.1.2 Permeable Surface

Many species will permeate the endothelium without reacting at the luminal surface (e.g., albumin, LDL) and their rate of transport (flux) across the surface layer can be described by

$$J_s = \text{Pe}(C_s - C_w) \tag{9.11}$$

where Pe is the endothelial permeability coefficient and C_w is the wall concentration beneath the endothelium. If the resistance to transport offered by the endothelium is significant, then it will be reasonable to assume

$$C_w \ll C_s \tag{9.12}$$

so that at steady state when the fluid and surface fluxes balance,

$$k_L(C_b - C_s) = \text{Pe}C_s \tag{9.13}$$

Multiplying Equation 9.13 by d/D to introduce dimensionless parameters and then solving for the surface concentration leads to

$$\frac{C_s}{C_b} = \frac{1}{1 + \text{Da}_e/\text{Sh}} \tag{9.14}$$

where Sh was defined in Equation 9.6 and

$$\text{Da}_e \equiv \frac{\text{Pe}d}{D} \tag{9.15}$$

is a Damkhöler number based on endothelial permeability. Equation 9.14 shows that when $\text{Da}_e \ll \text{Sh}$, the transport process is again "wall-limited." When $\text{Da}_e \gg \text{Sh}$, fluid mechanics again becomes important through the Sherwood number.

9.1.3 Reactive Wall

Oxygen is transported readily across the endothelium (Hellums), but unlike most proteins, is rapidly consumed by the underlying tissue. In this case it is fair to neglect the endothelial transport resistance (assume $C_w = C_s$), and then by equating the rate of transport to the wall with the (zeroeth-order) consumption rate within the wall we obtain

$$K_L(C_b - C_s) = \mathring{Q}T \tag{9.16}$$

where $\mathring{Q}$ is the tissue consumption rate and T is the tissue thickness (distance from the surface to the minimum tissue concentration, see Figure 9.1). For the specific case of O_2 transport, it is conventional to replace concentration (C) with partial pressure (P) through the Henry's law relationship $C = KP$, where K is the Henry's law constant. Invoking this relationship and rearranging Equation 9.16 into a convenient dimensionless form, we obtain

$$\frac{P_s}{P_b} = 1 - \frac{\text{Da}_w}{\text{Sh}} \tag{9.17}$$

where Sh was defined in Equation 9.6, and Da_w is another Damköhler number based on the wall consumption rate

$$Da_w = \frac{\mathring{Q}Td}{KDP_b} \tag{9.18}$$

Clearly when $Da_w \ll Sh$, the process is wall limited. But, as $Da_w \rightarrow Sh$, the process becomes limited by transport in the fluid phase ($P_s \rightarrow 0$), and fluid mechanics plays a role. Because we are treating the tissue consumption rate as a zeroeth order reaction, the case $Da_w > Sh$ is not meaningful ($P_s < 0$). In reality, as Sh is reduced, the tissue consumption rate must be reduced due to the lack of oxygen supply from the blood.

9.2   Damköhler Numbers for Important Solutes

A wide range of Damköhler numbers characterize the transport of biomolecular solutes in vessel walls of the cardiovascular system, and in this section we focus on four important species as examples of typical biotransport processes: adenosine triphosphate (ATP), a species that reacts vigorously on the endothelial surface, albumin, and LDL, species which are transported across a permeable endothelial surface; and oxygen, which is rapidly consumed within the vessel wall. Since most vascular disease (atherosclerosis) occurs in vessels between 3 and 10 mm in diameter, we use a vessel of 5 mm diameter to provide estimates of typical Damköhler numbers.

9.2.1   Adenosine Triphosphate

The ATP is degraded at the endothelial surface by enzymes (ectonucleotidases) to form adenosine diphosphate (ADP). The Michaelis–Menten kinetics for this reaction have been determined by Gordon et al. [7] using cultured porcine aortic endothelial cells: $k_m = 249\ \mu M$, $V_{max} = 22$ nmol/min/10^6 cells. V_{max} can be converted to a molar flux by using a typical endothelial cell surface density of 1.2×10^5 cells/cm^2, with the result that the pseudo-first order rate constant (Equation 9.3) is $k_r = 1.77 \times 10^{-4}$ cm/sec. Assuming a diffusivity of 5.0×10^{-6} cm^2/sec for ATP [8], and a vessel diameter of 5 mm, we find

$$Da_r = 17.7$$

9.2.2   Albumin and LDL

These macromolecules are transported across the endothelium by a variety of mechanisms including nonspecific and receptor-mediated trancytosis, and paracellular transport through normal or "leaky" inter-endothelial junctions [9,10]. In rabbit aortas, Truskey et al. [11] measured endothelial permeability to LDL and observed values on the order of $Pe = 1.0 \times 10^{-8}$ cm/sec in uniformly permeable regions, but found that permeability increased significantly in punctate regions associated with cells in mitosis to a level of $Pe = 5 \times 10^{-7}$ cm/sec. Using this range of values for Pe, assuming a diffusivity of 2.5×10^{-7} cm^2/sec for LDL, and a vessel diameter of 5 mm, we find

$$Da_e = 0.02{-}1.0 \quad (LDL)$$

For albumin, Truskey et al. [12] reported values of the order $Pe = 4.0 \times 10^{-8}$ cm/sec in the rabbit aorta. This presumably corresponded to regions of uniform permeability. They did not report values in punctate regions of elevated permeability. More recently, Lever et al. [13] reported Pe values of similar magnitude in the thoracic and abdominal aorta as well as the carotid and renal arteries of rabbits. In the ascending aorta and pulmonary artery, however, they observed elevated permeability to albumin on the order of

Pe $= 1.5 \times 10^{-7}$ cm/sec. Assuming a diffusivity of 7.3×10^{-7} cm^2/sec for albumin, a vessel diameter of 5 mm, and the range of Pe values described above, we obtain

$$Da_e = 0.027{-}0.10 \quad \text{(albumin)}$$

9.2.3 Oxygen

The first barrier encountered by oxygen after being transported from the blood is the endothelial layer. Although arterial endothelial cells consume oxygen [14], the pseudo-first order rate constant for this consumption is estimated to be an order of magnitude lower than that of ATP, and it is therefore reasonable to neglect the endothelial cell consumption relative to the much more significant consumption by the underlying tissue. Liu et al. [15] measured the oxygen permeability of cultured bovine aortic and human umbilical vein endothelial cells and obtained values of 1.42×10^{-2} cm/sec for bovine cell monolayers and 1.96×10^{-2} cm/sec for human cell monolayers. Because the endothelial permeability to oxygen is so high, it is fair to neglect the transport resistance of the endothelium and to direct attention to the oxygen consumption rate within the tissue.

To evaluate the Damkhöler number based on the tissue consumption rate (Equation 9.17), we turn to data of Buerk and Goldstick [16] for $\mathring{Q}/(KD)$ measured both *in vivo* and *in vitro* in dog, rabbit, and pig blood vessels. The values of $\mathring{Q}/(KD)$ reported by Buerk and Goldstick are based on tissue properties for KD. To translate these tissue values into blood values, as required in our estimates (Equation 9.17), we use the relationship $(KD)_{\text{tissue}} = N(KD)_{\text{water}}$ suggested by Paul et al. [17] and assume $(KD)_{\text{blood}} = (KD)_{\text{water}}$. In the thoracic aorta of dogs, $\mathring{Q}/(KD)$ ranged from 1.29×10^5 to 5.88×10^5 torr/cm^2 in the tissue. The thickness (distance to the minimum tissue O$_2$ concentration) of the thoracic aorta was 250 μm and the diameter is estimated to be 0.9 cm [18]. PO$_2$ measured in the blood (P_b) was 90 torr. Introducing these values into Equation 9.17 we find:

$$Da_w = 10.8{-}49.0 \quad \text{(thoracic aorta)}$$

In the femoral artery of dogs, $\mathring{Q}/(KD)$ ranged from 35.2×10^5 to 46.9×10^5 torr/cm^2 in the tissue. The thickness of the femoral artery was 50 μm and the estimated diameter is 0.4 cm [18]. PO$_2$ measured in the blood was about 80 torr. These values lead to the following estimates:

$$Da_w = 29.3{-}39.1 \quad \text{(femoral artery)}$$

9.3   Sherwood Numbers in the Circulation

9.3.1 Straight Vessels

For smooth, cylindrical tubes (a model of straight blood vessels) with well-mixed entry flow, one can invoke the thin concentration boundary layer theory of Lévêque [6] to estimate the Sherwood number in the entry region of the vessel where the concentration boundary is developing. This leads to

$$Sh = 1.08x^{\star-1/3} \quad \text{(constant wall concentration)} \tag{9.19a}$$

$$1.30x^{\star-1/3} \quad \text{(constant wall flux)} \tag{9.19b}$$

where

$$x^{\star} = \frac{x/d}{\text{Re} \cdot \text{Sc}} \tag{9.20}$$

is a dimensionless axial distance which accounts for differing rates of concentration boundary layer growth due to convection and diffusion. In Equation 9.20, Re $= vd/\nu$ is the Reynolds number, Sc $= \nu/D$

TABLE 9.1 Transport Characteristics in a Straight
Aorta

Species	Sc	$x^\star$	Sh	Da
O_2	2,900	4.1×10^{-5}	31.1	10.8–49.0
ATP	7,000	1.7×10^{-5}	41.8	17.7
Albumin	48,000	2.5×10^{-6}	79.2	0.027–0.100
LDL	140,000	8.6×10^{-7}	114	0.02–1.00

Note: $d = 1$ cm, $x = 60$ cm, $Re = 500$, $v = 0.035$ cm^2/sec.

is the Schmidt number, and their product is the Péclet number. Equation 9.19 is quite accurate for distances from the entrance satisfying $x^\star < 0.001$. Sh continues to drop with increasing axial distance as the concentration boundary layer grows, as described by the classical Graetz solution of the analogous heat transfer problem [19]. When the concentration boundary layer becomes fully developed, Sh approaches its asymptotic minimum value,

$$Sh = 3.66 \quad \text{(constant wall concentration)} \tag{9.21a}$$

$$Sh = 4.36 \quad \text{(constant wall flux)} \tag{9.21b}$$

For a straight vessel, Sh cannot drop below these asymptotic values. Equation 9.19 and Equation 9.21 also indicate that the wall boundary condition has little effect on the Sherwood number.

It is instructive to estimate Sh at the end of a straight tube having dimensions and flow rate characteristics of the human aorta (actually a tapered tube). Table 9.1 compares Sh and Da (for O_2, ATP, albumin, and LDL) at the end of a 60-cm long model aorta having a diameter of 1 cm and a flow characterized by $Re = 500$.

Table 9.1 clearly reveals that for a straight aorta, transport is in the entry or Lévêque regime ($x^\star < 10^{-3}$). For albumin and LDL, Da $\ll$ Sh, and transport is expected to be "wall-limited." For O_2 and ATP, Da $\sim$ Sh, and the possibility of "fluid phase-limited" transport exists. At the lowest possible rates of wall mass transport in a straight vessel (Sh $= 3.66-4.36$), transport is still expected to be "wall-limited" for albumin and LDL, whereas it would be "fluid-phase limited" for oxygen and ATP.

9.4 Nonuniform Geometries Associated with Atherogenesis

9.4.1 Sudden Expansion

Flow through a sudden expansion (Figure 9.2) at sufficiently high Reynolds number induces flow separation at the expansion point followed by reattachment downstream. This is a simple model of physiological flow separation. The separation zone is associated with low wall shear stress since this quantity is identically zero at the separation and reattachment points.

An experimental study of oxygen transport in saline and blood for an area expansion ratio of 6.7 and Reynolds numbers in the range 160 to 850 [20] displayed the general spatial distribution of Sh displayed in Figure 9.2. The minimum value of Sh was observed near the separation point and the maximum value appeared near the reattachment point. The maximum Sh ranged between 500 and several thousand depending on the conditions and the minimum value was approximately 50. A numerical study of the analogous heat transfer problem by Ma et al. [21] at a lower area expansion ratio (4.42) and Schmidt number (Sc $= 105$) showed the same qualitative trends indicated in Figure 9.2, but the Sherwood numbers were considerably lower (between 4 and 40) due to the lower expansion ratio, lower Schmidt number, and different entrance conditions. In both of these studies, Sh did not drop below its fully developed tube flow value at any axial location.

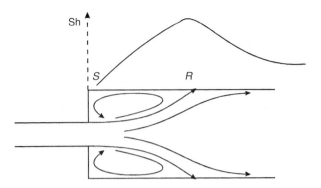

FIGURE 9.2   Schematic diagram showing the spatial distribution of the Sherwood number downstream of a sudden expansion. The flow separates (S) from the wall at the expansion point and reattaches (R) downstream. The Sherwood number is reduced near the separation point (radial velocity away from the wall) and elevated near the reattachment point (radial velocity toward the wall).

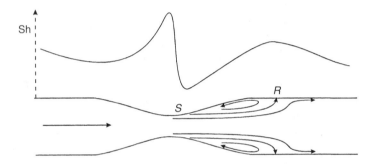

FIGURE 9.3   Schematic diagram showing the spatial distribution of the Sherwood number around a symmetric stenosis. The flow converges upstream of the stenosis where the Sherwood number is elevated (radial velocity toward the wall). The flow separates (S) from the wall just downstream of the throat, if the Reynolds number is high enough, and reattaches (R) downstream. The Sherwood number is reduced near the separation point (radial velocity away from the wall) and elevated near the reattachment point (radial velocity toward the wall).

The sudden expansion flow field provides insight into the mechanism controlling the spatial distribution of the Sherwood number in separated flows. Near the reattachment point, the radial velocity component convects solute toward the wall (enhancing transport), whereas near the separation point, the radial velocity component convects solute away from the wall (diminishing transport). The net result of this radial convective transport superimposed on diffusive transport (toward the wall) is a maximum in Sh near the reattachment point and a minimum in Sh near the separation point.

9.4.2 Stenosis

Flow through a symmetric stenosis at sufficiently high Reynolds number (Figure 9.3) will lead to flow separation at a point downstream of the throat and reattachment further downstream. Again, because the wall shear stress is identically zero at the separation and reattachment points, the separation zone is a region of low wall shear stress. Conversely, converging flow upstream of the stenosis induces elevated wall shear stress.

Schneiderman et al. [22] performed numerical simulations of steady flow and transport in an axisymmetric, 89% area restriction stenosis with a sinusoidal axial wall contour at various Reynolds numbers for a Schmidt number typical of oxygen transport. Relative to a uniform tube, Sh was always elevated in the converging flow region upstream of the stenosis, and when Re was low enough to suppress flow separation, transport remained elevated downstream of the stenosis as well. At high Re (Figure 9.3), flow separation produced a region of diminished transport (relative to a uniform tube) while reattachment induced elevated transport. The lowest value of Sh in the diminished transport regime was approximately 10. This occurred at Re = 16, a flow state for which separation was incipient. At high Re, the minimum Sh was elevated above 10, and the region of diminished transport was reduced in axial extent.

More recent numerical simulations by Rappitsch and Perktold [23,24] for a 75% stenosis in steady flow (Re = 448, Sc = 2,000 [oxygen]) and sinusoidal flow (Re = 300, Sc = 46,000 [albumin]) show the same basic trends depicted in Figure 9.3. Again, Sh was reduced in a narrow region around the separation point, but did not drop below approximately 10.

Moore and Ethier [25] also simulated oxygen transport in a symmetric stenosis, but they accounted for the binding of oxygen to hemoglobin and solved for both the oxygen and oxyhemoglobin concentrations. They determined axial Sh profiles throughout the stenosis, which showed the same basic tendencies indicated in Figure 9.3. However, because hemoglobin has a much higher molecular weight and Schmidt number than oxygen (about 100 times higher Sc), the local values of Sh were higher than computed on the basis of free oxygen transport alone. This is expected since simple transport considerations (Lévêque solution) suggest $Sh \propto Sc^{1/3}$.

The Sh profile for the stenosis (Figure 9.3) reflects the same underlying mechanisms that were operative in the sudden expansion (Figure 9.2): radial flow directed toward the wall enhances transport near the reattachment point, while radial flow directed away from the wall diminishes transport near the separation point.

9.4.3 Bifurcation

A few numerical studies of flow and transport in the carotid artery bifurcation have been reported recently as summarized in Figure 9.4. The carotid artery bifurcation is a major site for the localization of atherosclerosis, predominantly on the outer wall (away from the flow divider) in the flow separation zone which is a region of low and oscillating wall shear stress [26]. Perktold et al. [27] simulated O_2 transport in a realistic pulsatile flow through an anatomically realistic three-dimensional carotid bifurcation geometry using a constant wall concentration boundary condition. Ma et al. [28] simulated oxygen transport in steady flow through a realistic, three-dimensional, carotid bifurcation with a constant wall concentration boundary condition.

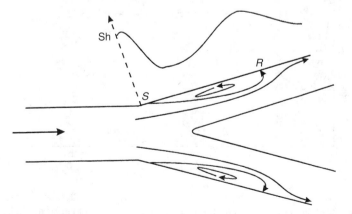

FIGURE 9.4 Schematic diagram showing the spatial distribution of the Sherwood number along the outer wall of a bifurcation. The flow separates (S) if the Reynolds number is high enough and there is an increase in cross-sectional area through the bifurcation, and reattaches (R) downstream. The Sherwood number is reduced near the separation point (radial velocity away from the wall) and elevated near the reattachment point (radial velocity toward the wall).

As in the sudden expansion and stenosis geometries, the bifurcation geometry can induce flow separation on the outer wall with reattachment downstream. Again there is a region of attenuated transport near the separation point and amplified transport near the reattachment point. Perktold et al. [27] predicted minimum Sherwood numbers close to zero in the flow separation zone. Ma et al. [28] predicted the same general spatial distribution, but the minimum Sherwood number was approximately 25. Differences in the minimum Sherwood number may be due to differing entry lengths upstream of the bifurcation as well as differences in flow pulsatility.

9.4.4 Curvature

Localization of atherosclerosis has also been associated with arterial curvature [2]. For example, the inner curvature of proximal coronary arteries as they bend over the curved surface of the heart has been associated with plaque localization [29]. Qiu [30] carried out three-dimensional, unsteady flow computations in an elastic (moving wall) model of a curved coronary artery for O_2 transport with a constant wall concentration boundary condition. He obtained the results shown in Figure 9.5. Because

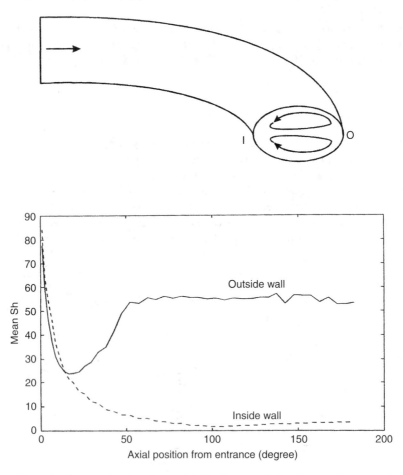

FIGURE 9.5 Schematic diagram showing the spatial distribution of the Sherwood number along the inner (I — toward the center of curvature) and outer (O — away from the center of curvature) walls of a curved vessel. In the entry region, before the secondary flow has developed, the Sherwood number follows a Lévêque distribution. As the secondary flow evolves, the Sherwood number becomes elevated on the outer wall where the radial velocity of the secondary flow is toward the wall, and diminished on the inner wall where radial velocity of the secondary flow is away from the wall.

Qiu assumed uniform axial velocity and concentration profiles (with no secondary flow) at the curved tube entrance ($0°$), there is an entrance region ($\sim25°$) where Sh essentially follows a Lévêque boundary layer development. Eventually ($\sim50°$), the secondary flow effects become manifest, and marked differences in transport rates between the inside wall (low transport: Sh $\sim$ 2) and the outside wall (high transport: Sh $\sim$ 55) develop. The regions of high and low transport in the curved vessel geometry cannot be associated with axial flow separation (as in the expansion, stenosis, and bifurcation) because flow separation does not occur at the modest curvature levels in the coronary artery simulation.

The secondary flow (in the plane perpendicular to the axial flow, see Figure 9.5) determines, in large measure, the differences in transport rates between the inside and outside walls. The radial velocity is directed toward the wall at the outside, leading to enhancement of transport by a convective mechanism. At the inside of the curvature, the radial velocity is directed away from the wall, and transport is impeded by the convective mechanism. This secondary flow mechanism produces transport rates that are 25 times higher on the outside wall than the inside wall. This is to be contrasted with wall shear stress values which, for the coronary artery condition, are less than two times higher on the outside wall than on the inside wall [31]. Earlier studies of fully developed, steady flow and transport in curved tubes [32] are consistent with the above observations.

9.5   Discussion

The considerations of mass transport in the fluid (blood) phase and consumption by the vessel wall described in the preceding sections indicate that only highly reactive species such as O_2 and ATP can be "transport-limited." Larger molecules such as albumin and LDL, which are not rapidly transformed within the vessel wall, are not likely to be transport-limited.

For O_2, ATP, and other molecules characterized by large values of the Damkhöler number, transport limitation will occur in regions of the circulation where the Sherwood number is low (Sh < Da). Localized regions of low Sh arise in nonuniform geometries around flow separation points (not reattachment points) where radial flow velocities are directed away from the wall, and in secondary flow regions where the secondary velocity is directed away from the wall (inside wall of a curved vessel).

Considerable supporting experimental evidence for the above conclusions is available, and a few representative studies will be mentioned here. Santilli et al. [33] measured transarterial wall oxygen tension gradients at the dog carotid bifurcation. Oxygen tensions at the carotid sinus (outer wall in Figure 9.4) were significantly decreased in the inner 40% of the artery wall compared to an upstream control location. Oxygen tensions at the flow divider (inner wall in Figure 9.4) were increased significantly throughout the artery wall compared with control locations. These observations are consistent with fluid phase-limited oxygen transport at the outer wall of the carotid bifurcation.

Dull et al. [8] measured the response of intracellular free calcium in cultured bovine aortic endothelial cells (BAECs) after step changes in flow rate, using media containing either ATP or a non-reactive analog of ATP. In the presence of ATP, which is rapidly degraded by enzymes on the endothelial cell surface, step changes in flow rate induced rapid changes in intracellular calcium which were not apparent when the inactive ATP analog was used in place of ATP. The interpretation of these experiments was that increases in flow increased the rate of mass transport of ATP to the cell surface and exceeded the capacity of the surface enzymes to degrade ATP. This allowed ATP to reach surface receptors and stimulate intracellular calcium. This study thus provided evidence that ATP transport to the endothelium could be fluid phase (transport)-limited.

Caro and Nerem [5] measured the uptake of labeled cholesterol bound to serum lipoprotein in excised dog arteries under well-defined conditions in which the Lévêque solution (Equation 9.19) described the fluid phase mass transport process. If the transport of lipoprotein to the surface had been controlled by the fluid phase, they should have observed a decrease in uptake with distance from the vessel entrance following a $x^{-1/3}$ law (Equation 9.19). They did not, however, observe any significant spatial variation of uptake of lipoprotein over the length of the blood vessel. This observation is consistent with "wall-limited" transport of lipoprotein as we have suggested in the preceding sections.

9.6 Possible Role of Blood Phase Transport in Atherogenesis

Accumulation of lipid in the arterial intima is a hallmark of atherosclerosis, a disease that tends to be localized on the outer walls of arterial bifurcations and the inner walls of arterial curvatures [2]. The outer walls of bifurcations and the inner walls of curvatures may have localized regions characterized by relatively low blood phase transport rates (low Sh in Figure 9.4 and Figure 9.5). But, how can low transport rates lead to high accumulation of lipid in the wall? If, as we have argued in this review, LDL transport is really not affected by the blood phase fluid mechanics, but is limited by the endothelium, how can local fluid mechanics influence intimal lipid accumulation? There are several possible scenarios for a fluid mechanical influence which are reviewed briefly.

9.6.1 Direct Mechanical Effects on Endothelial Cells

The outerwalls of bifurcations and the inner walls of curved vessels are characterized by low mean wall shear stress, and significant temporal oscillations in wall shear stress direction (oscillatory shear stress) [2]. Endothelial cells in this low, oscillatory shear environment tend to assume a polyhedral, cobblestone enface morphology, whereas endothelial cells in high shear regions tend to be elongated in the direction of flow. It has been suggested that these altered morphologies, which represent chronic adaptive responses to altered fluid mechanical environments, are characterized by distinct macromolecular permeability characteristics [2,10] as direct responses of the endothelial layer to altered mechanical environments. In addition, a number of studies have shown that fluid shear stress on the endothelial surface can have an acute influence on endothelial transport properties both *in vitro* [34–37] and *in vivo* [38,39].

9.6.2 Hypoxic Effect on Endothelial Cells

Hypoxia (low oxygen tension), which can be induced by a blood phase transport limitation, can lead to a breakdown of the endothelial transport barrier either by a direct effect on the endothelial layer or by an indirect mechanism in which hypoxia up-regulates the production of hyperpermeabilizing cytokines from other cells in the arterial wall. A number of recent studies have shown that hypoxia increases macromolecular transport across endothelial monolayers in culture due to metabolic stress [40–42]. These studies describe direct effects on the endothelial layer since other cells present in the vessel wall were not present in the cell culture systems.

9.6.3 Hypoxia Induces VEGF

Many cell lines express increased amounts of vascular endothelial growth factor (VEGF) when subjected to hypoxic conditions as do normal tissues exposed to hypoxia, functional anemia, or localized ischemia [43]. VEGF is a multifunctional cytokine that acts as an important regulator of angiogenesis and as a potent vascular permeabilizing agent [43,44]. VEGF is believed to play an important role in the hyperpermeability of microvessels in tumors, the leakage of proteins in diabetic retinopathy, and other vascular pathologies [45,46]. Thus, a plausible scenario for the increase in lipid uptake in regions of poor blood phase mass transport is the following: Hypoxia up-regulates the production of VEGF by cells within the vascular wall and the VEGF in turn permeabilizes the endothelium, allowing increased transport of lipid into the wall. This mechanism can be depicted schematically as follows:

$$O_2 \downarrow \rightarrow VEGF \uparrow \rightarrow Pe \uparrow$$

In support of this view, several recent studies have shown that VEGF is enriched in human atherosclerotic lesions [47,48]. Smooth muscle cells and macrophages appear to be the predominant sources of VEGF in such lesions. Thus, a mechanism in which hypoxia induces VEGF and hyperpermeability is plausible, but at the present time it must only be considered a hypothesis relating fluid phase transport limitation and enhanced macromolecular permeability.

References

[1] Ross, R., Atherosclerosis: a defense mechanism gone awry, *Am. J. Pathol.*, 143, 987, 1993.

[2] Nerem, R., Atherosclerosis and the role of wall shear stress, in *Flow-Dependent Regulation of Vascular Function*, Bevan, J.A., Kaley, G., and Rubany, G.M., Eds., Oxford University Press, New York, 1995.

[3] Caro, L.G., Fitz-Gerald, J.M., and Schroter, R.C., Atheroma and arterial wall shear: observation, correlation and proposal of a shear dependent mass transfer mechanism for atherogenesis, *Proc. R. Soc. London (Biol.)*, 177, 109, 1971.

[4] Fry, D.L., Acute vascular endothelial changes associated with increased blood velocity gradients, *Circ. Res.*, 22, 165, 1968.

[5] Caro, C.G. and Nerem, R.M., Transport of 14C-4-cholesterol between serum and wall in the perfused dog common carotid artery, *Circ. Res.*, 32, 187, 1973.

[6] Basmadjian, D., The effect of flow and mass transport in thrombogenesis, *Ann. Biomed. Eng.*, 18, 685, 1990.

[7] Gordon, E.L., Pearson, J.D., and Slakey, L.L., The hydrolysis of extra cellular adenine nucleotides by cultured endothelial cells from pig aorta, *J. Biol. Chem.*, 261, 15496, 1986.

[8] Dull, R.O., Tarbell, J.M., and Davies, P.F., Mechanisms of flow-mediated signal transduction in endothelial cells: kinetics of ATP surface concentrations, *J. Vasc. Res.*, 29, 410, 1992.

[9] Lin, S.J., Jan, K.M., Schuessler, G., Weinbaum, S., and Chien, S., Enhanced macromolecular permeability of aortic endothelial cells in association with mitosis, *Atherosclerosis*, 17, 71, 1988.

[10] Weinbaum, S. and Chien, S., Lipid transport aspects of atherogensis, *J. Biomech. Eng.*, 115, 602, 1993.

[11] Truskey, G.A., Roberts, W.L., Herrmann, R.A., and Malinauskas, R.A., Measurement of endothelial permeability to 125I-low density lipoproteins in rabbit arteries by use of en face preparations, *Circ. Res.*, 71, 883, 1992.

[12] Truskey, G.A., Colton, C.K., and Smith, K.A., Quantitative analysis of protein transport in the arterial wall, in *Structure and Function of the Circulation*, Vol. 3, Schwarts, C.J., Werthessen, N.T., and Wolf, S., Eds., Plenum Publishing Corp., 1981, p. 287.

[13] Lever, M.J., Jay, M.T., and Coleman, P.J., Plasma protein entry and retention in the vascular wall: possible factors in atherogenesis, *Can. J. Physiol. Pharmacol.*, 74, 818, 1996.

[14] Motterlini, R., Kerger, H., Green, C.J., Winslow, R.M., and Intaglietta, M., Depression of endothelial and smooth muscle cell oxygen consumption by endotoxin. *Am. J. Physiol.*, 275, H776, 1998.

[15] Liu, C.Y., Eskin, S.G., and Hellums, J.D., The oxygen permeability of cultured endothelial cell monolayers, paper presented at the *20th International Society of Oxygen Transport to Tissue Conference*, August 26–30, Mianz, Germany, 1992.

[16] Buerk, D.G. and Goldstick, T.K., Arterial wall oxygen consumption rate varies spatially, *Am. J. Physiol.*, 243, H948, 1982.

[17] Paul, R.J., Chemical energetics of vascular smooth muscle, in *Handbook of Physiology. The Cardiovascular System. Vascular Smooth Muscle*, Vol. 2, The American Physiological Society, Bethesda, MD, 1980, p. 201.

[18] Caro, C.G., Pedley, T.J., Schroter, R.C., and Seed, W.A., *The Mechanics of the Circulation*, Oxford University Press, Oxford, 1978.

[19] Bennett, C.O. and Meyers, J.E., *Momentum, Heat and Mass Transfer*, McGraw-Hill, New York, 1962.

[20] Thum, T.F. and Diller, T.E., Mass transfer in recirculating blood flow, *Chem. Eng. Commun.*, 47, 93, 1986.

[21] Ma, P., Li, X., and Ku, D.N., Heat and mass transfer in a separated flow region of high Prandtl and Schmidt numbers under pulsatile conditions, *Int. J. Heat Mass Transfer*, 1994.

[22] Schneiderman, G., Ellis, C.G., and Goldstick, T.K., Mass transport to walls of stenosed arteries: variation with Reynolds number and blood flow separation, *J. Biomech.*, 12, 869, 1979.

[23] Rappitsch, G. and Perktold, K., Computer simulation of convective diffusion processes in large arteries, *J. Biomech.*, 29, 207, 1996.

[24] Rappitsch, G. and Perktold, K., Pulsatile albumin transport in large arteries: a numerical simulation study, *J. Biomech. Eng.*, 118, 511, 1996.

[25] Moore, J.A. and Ethier, C.R., Oxygen mass transfer calculations in large arteries, *J. Biomech. Eng.*, 119, 469, 1997.

[26] Ku, D.N., Giddens, D.P., Zarins, C.K., and Glagov, S., Pulsatile flow and atherosclerosis in the human carotid bifurcation: positive correlation between plaque location and low and oscillating shear stress, *Arteriosclerosis*, 5, 293, 1985.

[27] Perktold, K., Rappitsch, G., Hofer, M., and Karner, G., Numerical simulation of mass transfer in a realistic carotid artery bifurcation model, *Proceedings of the Bioengineering Conference (ASME), BED*, 35, 85, 1997.

[28] Ma, P., Li, X., and Ku, D.N., Convective mass transfer at the carotid bifurcation, *J. Biomech.*, 30, 565, 1997.

[29] Chang, L.J. and Tarbell, J.M., A numerical study of flow in curved tubes simulating coronary arteries, *J. Biomech.*, 21, 927, 1988.

[30] Qiu, Y., Numerical simulation of oxygen transport in a compliant curved tube model of a coronary artery, *Ann. Biomed. Eng.*, 28, 26–38, 2000.

[31] Qiu, Y. and Tarbell, J., Numerical simulation of pulsatile flow in a compliant curved tube model of a coronary artery, *J. Biomech. Eng.*, 122, 77–85, 2000.

[32] Kalb, C.E. and Seader, J.D., Heat and mass transfer phenomena for viscous flow in curved circular tubes, *Int. J. Heat Mass Transfer*, 15, 801, 1972.

[33] Santilli, S.M., Stevens, R.B., Anderson, J.G., Payne, W.D., and Caldwell, M.D.-F., Transarterial wall oxygen gradients at the dog carotid bifurcation, *Am. J. Physiol.*, 268, H155, 1995.

[34] Jo, H., Dull, R.O., Hollis, T.M., and Tarbell, J.M., Endothelial permeability is shear-dependent, time-dependent, and reversible, *Am. J. Physiol.*, 260, H1992, 1991.

[35] Chang, Y.S., Yaccino, J., Lakshminarayanan, S., Frangos, J.A., and Tarbell, J.M., Shear-induced increase in hydraulic conductivity in endothelial cells is mediated is by a nitric oxide-dependent mechanism. *Arterioscler. Thromb. Vasc. Biol.*, 20, 35–42, 2000.

[36] DeMaio, L., Gardner, T.G., Tarbell, J.M., and Antonetti, D.A., Shear stress-induced increase in hydraulic conductivity is correlated with increased occludin phosphorylation and decreased occulin expression in cultured endothelial monolayers, *Am. J. Physiol.*, 281, H105–H113, 2001.

[37] Hillsley, M.V. and Tarbell, J.M., Oscillatory shear stress alters endothelial hydraulic conductivity by a nitric oxide-dependent mechanism, *Biochem. Biophys. Res. Commun.*, 293, 1466–1471, 2002.

[38] Williams, D.A., Thipakorn, B., and Huxley, V.H., *In situ* shear stress related to capillary function, *FASEB J.*, 8, M17, 1994.

[39] Yuan, Y., Granger, H.J., Zawieja, D.C., and Chilian, W.M., Flow modulates coronary venular permeability by a nitric oxide-related mechanism, *Am. J. Physiol.*, 263, H641, 1992.

[40] Fischer, S., Renz, D., Schaper, W., and Karliczek, G.F., Effects of barbiturates on hypoxic cultures of brain derived microvascular endothelial cells, *Brain Res.*, 707, 47, 1996.

[41] Kondo, T., Kinouchi, H., Kawase, M., and Yoshimoto, T., Astroglial cells inhibit the increasing permeability of brain endothelial cell monolayer following hypoxia/reoxygeneration, *Neurosci. Lett.*, 208, 101, 1996.

[42] Plateel, M., Teissier, E., and Cecchelli, R., Hypoxia dramatically increases the nonspecific transport of blood-borne proteins to the brain, *J. Neurochem.*, 68, 874, 1997.

[43] Brown, L., Detmer, M., Claffey, K., Nagy, J., Peng, D., Dvorak, A., and Duorak, H., Vascular permeability factor/vascular endothelial growth factor: a multifunctional angiogenic cytokine, in *Regulation*

of Angiogenesis, Goldberg, I.D. and Rosen, E.M., Eds., Birkhäuser Verlag, Basel, Switzerland, 1997.

[44] Ferrara, N. and Davis-Smyth, T., The biology of vascular endothelial growth factor, *Endocrine Rev.*, 18, 4, 1997.

[45] Chang, Y., Munn, L., Hillsley, M., Dull, R., Yuan, J., Lakshminarayanan, S., Gardner, T., Jain, R., and Tarbell, J.M., Effect of vascular endothelial growth factor on cultured endothelial cell monolayer transport properties. *Microvasc. Res.*, 59, 265–277, 2000.

[46] Lakshminarayaman, S., Antonetti, D., Gardner, T., and Tarbell, J.M., Effect of VEGF on hydraulic conductivity of retinal microvascular endothelial monolayers the role of NO. *Invest. Ophth. Vis. Sci.*, 41, 4256–4261, 2000.

[47] Couffinhal, T., Kearney, M., Witxzenbichler, B., Chen, D., Murohara, T., Losordo, D.W., Symes, J., and Isner, J.M., Vascular endothelial growth factor/vascular permeability factor (VEGF/VPF) in normal and atherosclerotic human arteries, *Am. J. Pathol.*, 150, 1673, 1997.

[48] Ramos, M.A., Kuzuya, M., Esaki, T., Miura, S., Satake, S., Asai, T., Kanda, S., Hayashi, T., and Iguchi, A., Induction of macrophage VEGF in response to oxidized LDL and VEGF accumulation in human atherosclerotic lesions, *Arterioscler. Thromb. Vasc. Biol.*, 18, 1188, 1998.

10

Control of the Microenvironment

Robert J. Fisher
The SABRE Institute and Massachusetts Institute of Technology

Robert A. Peattie
Oregon State University

10.1 Introduction

The evolving technologies and advances in the engineering biosciences are expected to have significant impact in the fields of pharmaceutical engineering (drug production, delivery, targeting, and metabolism), molecular engineering (biomaterial design and biomimetics), biomedical reaction engineering (microreactor design, animal surrogate systems, artificial organs, and extracorporeal devices), and metabolic process control (receptor–ligand binding, signal transduction, and trafficking). Since understanding of the cell/tissue environment will help produce major developments in all of these areas, the ability to characterize, control, and ultimately manipulate the microenvironment is critical. The key challenges, as identified by many sources [Palsson, 2000], are (1) proper reconstruction of the microenvironment for the development of tissue function, (2) scale-up to generate a significant amount of properly functioning microenvironments to be of clinical importance, (3) automating cellular therapy systems/devices to operate and perform at clinically meaningful scales, and (4) implementation in the clinical setting in concert with all the cell handling and preservation procedures required to administer cellular therapies. The direction of this chapter is toward supporting efforts to address these issues. Thus, the primary objective is to introduce the fundamental concepts needed to reconstruct tissues *ex vivo* and produce cells of sufficient quantity that maintain stabilized performance for extended time periods of clinical relevance. The delivery of cellular therapies, as a goal, was selected as one representative theme for illustration.

Before we can develop useful *ex vivo* and *in vitro* systems for the numerous applications sought, we must first have an appreciation of cellular function *in vivo*. Knowledge of the tissue microenvironment and communication with other organs is essential. We need to understand how tissue function can be built, reconstructed, and modified. Our approach is based on the following axioms [Palsson, 2000] (1) in organogenesis and wound healing, proper cellular communications with respect to each others activities are of paramount concern since a systematic and regulated response is required from all participating cells; (2) the function of fully formed organs is strongly dependent on the coordinated function of multiple cell types with tissue function based on multicellular aggregates; (3) the functionality of an individual cell is strongly affected by its microenvironment (within 100 μm of the cell, i.e., the characteristic length scale); (4) this microenvironment is further characterized by (i) neighboring cells, that is, cell–cell contact and presence of molecular signals (soluble growth factors, signal transduction, trafficking, etc.), (ii) transport processes and physical interactions with the extracellular matrix (ECM), and (iii) the local geometry, in particular its effects on microcirculation.

The importance of the microcirculation is that it connects all the microenvironments in every tissue to their larger whole body environment. Most metabolically active cells in the body are located within a few hundred micrometers from a capillary. This high degree of vascularity is necessary to provide the perfusion environment that connects every cell to a source and sink for respiratory gases, a source of nutrients from the small intestine, the hormones from the pancreas, liver, and glandular system, clearance of waste products via the kidneys and liver, delivery of immune system respondents, and so forth [Jain, 1994]. Further, the three-dimensional arrangement of microvessels in any tissue bed is critical for efficient functioning. This *in vivo* network develops in response to physical and chemical (molecular) clues and thus reproduction of the microenvironment with its attendant signal molecule capabilities is an essential feature of an engineered tissue system.

The engineering of these functions *ex vivo* is within the domain of bioreactor design [Freshney, 2000; Shuler, 2000]; a topic discussed briefly in this chapter and elsewhere in this handbook. Cell culture devices must possess perfusion characteristics that allow for uniformity down to the 100 μm length scale. These are stringent design requirements that must be addressed with a high priority to properly account for the role of neighboring cells, the ECM, cyto-/chemokine and hormone trafficking, cell-ECM geometric factors, respiratory dynamics, and transport of nutrients and metabolic by-products for each tissue system considered. To achieve proper reconstitution of the cellular microenvironment these dynamic, chemical, and geometric variables must be duplicated as accurately as possible. Since this is a difficult task, significant effort is devoted to developing quantitative methods to describe the cell-scale microenvironment. Once available, these methods can be used to develop an understanding of the key problems associated with any given phenomenological event, formulate solution strategies, and analyze experimental results. It is important to stress that most useful analyses in tissue engineering are performed with approximate calculations based on physiological and cell biological data; basically, determining tissue "specification sheets." Such calculations are useful for interpreting organ physiology, and providing a starting point for more extensive experimental and computational programs needed to identify the specific needs of a given tissue system (examples are given later in this chapter). Using the tools obtained from studying subjects such as biomimetics (materials behavior, membrane development, and similitude/simulation techniques), transport phenomena (mass, heat, and momentum transfer), reaction kinetics, and reactor performance/design systems that control microenvironments for *in vivo, ex vivo,* or *in vitro* applications can be developed.

The emphasis taken here to achieve these desired tissue microenvironments is through use of novel membrane systems designed to possess unique features for the specific application of interest, and in many cases to exhibit stimulant/response characteristics. These so-called intelligent or smart membranes are the result of biomimicry, that is, they have biomimetic features. Through functionalized membranes, typically in concerted assemblies, these systems respond to external stresses (chemical and physical in nature) to eliminate the threat either by altering stress characteristics or by modifying and protecting the cell/tissue microenvironment. An example (discussed further later in this chapter), is a microencapsulation motif for beta cell islet clusters to perform as an artificial pancreas. This system uses multiple membrane materials, each with its unique characteristics and performance requirements, coupled with nanospheres dispersed throughout the matrix, which contain additional materials to enhance transport and barrier properties, and initiate as well as respond to specific stimuli. This chapter is structured to develop an understanding of the technologies required to design systems of this nature and to ensure their stable performance.

10.2 Tissue Microenvironments

The communication of every cell with its immediate environment and other tissues establishes important spatial–temporal characteristics and develops a significant signaling/information processing network. The microenvironment is further characterized by cellular composition, the ECM, molecular dynamics (nutrients, metabolic waste products, respiratory gases traffic in and out of the microenvironment in a highly dynamic manner), and local geometric factors (size scale of $\sim$100 μm). Each of these can also provide the cell with important signals (dependent upon a characteristic time and length scale) to initiate specific cell functions for the tissue system to perform in a coordinated manner. If this arrangement is disrupted, cells that are unable to provide tissue function are obtained. Further discussions on this topic are presented in later sections devoted to cellular communications.

10.2.1 Specifying Performance Criteria

Each tissue or organ undergoes its own unique and complex developmental program. There are, however, a number of common features of each component of the microenvironment that is discussed in subsequent sections. The idea is to establish general criteria to guide the design of systems possessing these requisite global characteristics and functionality. Two representative tissue microenvironments (blood and bone) are selected here for a brief comparison to illustrate common features and distinctions.

10.2.2 Estimating Tissue Function

10.2.2.1 Blood

Interpretation of the physiological respiratory function of blood has been aided by insightful, yet straight-forward approximating calculations to establish basic functionalities and biologic design specifications. For example, blood needs to deliver about 10 mM of oxygen per minute to the body. Given a gross circulation rate of about 5 l/min, the delivery rate to tissues is about 2 mM oxygen per liter during each pass through its circulatory system. The basic requirements that circulating blood must meet to deliver adequate oxygen to tissues are determined by the following; blood leaving the lungs has a partial pressure of oxygen between 90 and 100 mmHg and drops to about 35–40 mmHg in the venous blood at rest and to about 27 mmHg during strenuous exercise. Thus, the required oxygen delivered to the tissues is accomplished through a partial pressure drop of about 55 mmHg, on average. Unfortunately, the solubility of oxygen in aqueous media is low; its solubility is given by Henry's law relationship, where the liquid phase concentration is linearly proportional to its partial pressure. This equilibrium coefficient is about 0.0013 mM/mmHg. Consequently, the amount of oxygen that can be delivered by this mechanism is limited to roughly 0.07 mM; significantly below the required 2 mM. The solubility of oxygen in blood must therefore be enhanced by some other mechanism; by a factor to about 30 at rest and 60 during strenuous exercise. This, of course, is accomplished by hemoglobin within red blood cells. However, to see how this came about, let's probe a little further. Enhancement could be obtained by putting an oxygen binding protein into the perfusion fluid. To stay within the vascular bed this protein would have to be 50 to 100 kDa in size. With only a single binding site, the required protein concentration is 500 to 1000 g/l, which is too concentrated from both an osmolarity and viscosity (ten times) standpoint and clearly impractical. Furthermore, circulating proteases will lead to a short plasma half-life for these proteins. By increasing to four sites per oxygen carrying molecule, the protein concentration is reduced to 2.3 mM and confining it within a protective cell membrane solves the escape, viscosity, and proteolysis problems. Obviously, nature has solved these problems since these are characteristics of hemoglobin within red blood cells. Furthermore, a more elaborate kinetics study of the binding characteristics of hemoglobin shows that a positive cooperativity exists and can provide the desired oxygen transfer capabilities both at rest and under strenuous exercise.

These functions of blood establish standards that are difficult to mimic. When designing systems for *in vivo* applications promoting angiogenesis and minimizing diffusion lengths help alleviate oxygen delivery problems. Attempting to mimic this behavior in perfusion reactors, whether as extracorporeal devises or as production systems, is more complex since a blood substitute (e.g., perflouorocarbons in microemulsions) is typically needed. Performance, functionality, toxicity, and transport phenomena issues must be addressed. In summary, to maintain tissue viability and function within devices and microcapsules, methods are being developed to enhance mass transfer, especially that of oxygen. These methods include use of vascularizing membranes, *in situ* oxygen generation, use of thinner encapsulation membranes, and enhancing oxygen carrying capacity in encapsulated materials. All these topics are addressed in subsequent sections throughout this chapter.

10.2.2.2 Bone Marrow Microenvironment

Perfusion rates in human bone marrow cultures are set by determining how often the media should be replenished. A dynamics similarity analysis with the *in vivo* situation is therefore appropriate. With a cell density of about 500 million cells/ml, blood perfusion through bone marrow *in vivo* is about 0.08 ml/cc/min, that is, a cell specific perfusion rate of about 2.3 ml/10 million cells/day. Cell densities on the order of 1 million cells/ml are typical for starting cultures; 10 million cells would be placed in 10 ml of culture media containing about 20% serum (vol/vol). To accomplish a full daily media exchange would correspond to replacing the serum at 2 ml/10 million cells/day, which is similar to the number calculated previously. These conditions were used in the late 1980s and led to the development of prolific cell cultures of human bone marrow. Subsequent scale-up produced a clinically meaningful number of cells that are currently undergoing clinical trials.

10.2.3 Communication

Tissue development is regulated by a complex set of events in which cells of the developing organ interact with each other and with other organs and tissue microenvironments. The vascular system connects all the microenvironments in every tissue to their larger whole body environment. As discussed previously, a high degree of vascularity is necessary to transport signal molecules through this communication network at the rate and quantity required.

10.2.3.1 Cellular Communication Within Tissues

Cells within tissues communicate with each other for a variety of important reasons, such as localizing cells within the microenvironment, directing cellular migration, and initiating growth factor mediated developmental programs [Long, 2000]. This communication is accomplished via three primary methods (1) cells secrete a wide variety of soluble signal and messenger molecules including Ca^{++}, hormones, paracrine and autocrine agents, catecholamines, growth and inhibitory factors, eicosanoids, chemokines, and many other types of cytokines, (2) via direct cell–cell contact, and (3) secreted proteins that alter the EMC chemical milieu. Each of these communication techniques differ in terms of their specificity, and their characteristic time and length scales; thus suitable to convey a particular type of message. These information exchanges are mediated by well-defined, highly specific receptor–ligand interactions that stimulate or control cell activities. For example, the appearance of specific growth factors leads to proliferation of cells expressing receptors for these growth factors. Further, chemical gradients exist, which signal cells to move along tracts of molecules into a defined tissue area. High concentrations of the attractant or other signals then serve to localize cells by stopping their sojourn.

10.2.3.2 Soluble Growth Factors

Growth factors are a critical component of the tissue microenvironment inducing multifunctional behavior [Freshney, 2000]. Their role in the signal processing network is particularly important for this chapter. They are small proteins in the size range of 15 to 20 kDa with a relatively high chemical stability. Initially, growth factors were discovered as active factors that originated in biological fluids and were known as colony stimulating factors. It is now known that growth factors are produced by a signaling cell and secreted to reach target cells through autocrine and paracrine mechanisms. They bind to their receptors found in cellular membranes, with high affinities and trigger a complex signal transduction process. Typically the receptor complex changes in such a way that its intracellular components take on catalytic activities. These receptor-ligand complexes are internalized in some cases with a typical time constant for internalization of the order 15 to 30 min. It has been shown that 10,000 to 70,000 growth factor molecules need to be consumed to stimulate cell division in complex cell cultures. Growth factors propagate a maximum distance of about 200 μm from their secretion source. Minimum time constants for the signaling processes are about 20 min. However, much longer times are encountered if the growth factor is sequestered. The kinetics of these processes are complex and detailed analyses can be found elsewhere [Lauffenburger and Linderman, 1993] since they are beyond the scope of this chapter.

10.2.3.3 Direct Cell-to-Cell Contact

Direct contact between adjacent cells is common in epithelially derived tissues, and can also occur with osteocytes and both smooth and cardiac myocytes. Contact is maintained through specialized membrane structures including desmosomes, tight junctions, and gap junctions, each of which incorporates cell adhesion molecules, surface proteins, cadherins, and connexins. Tight junctions and desmosomes are thought to bind adjacent cells cohesively, preventing fluid flow between cells. *In vivo* they are found, for example, in intestinal mucosal epithelium, where their presence prevents leakage of the intestinal contents through the mucosa. In contrast, gap junctions form direct cytoplasmic bridges between adjacent cells. The functional unit of a gap junction, called a connexon, is approximately 1.5 nm in diameter, and thus will allow molecules below about 1 kDa to pass between cells.

These cell-to-cell connections permit mechanical forces to be transmitted through tissue beds. A rapidly growing body of literature details how fluid mechanical shear forces influence cell and tissue adhesion functions (a topic discussed more thoroughly in other chapters), and it is known that signals are transmitted to the nucleus by cell stretching and compression. Thus, the mechanical role of the cytoskeleton in affecting tissue function by transducing and responding to mechanical forces is becoming better understood.

10.2.3.4 Extracellular Matrix and Cell–Tissue Interactions

The ECM is the chemical microenvironment that interconnects all the cells in the tissue and their cytoskeletal elements. The multifunctional behavior of the ECM is an important faucet of tissue performance since it provides tissue with mechanical support. The ECM also provides cells with a substrate in which to migrate, as well as serving as a storage site for signal and communications molecules. A number of adhesion and ECM receptor molecules located on the cell surface play a major role in facilitating cell–ECM communications by transmitting instructions for migration, replication, differentiation, and apoptosis. Consequently, the ECM is composed of a large number of components that have varying mechanical and regulatory capabilities that provide its structural, dynamic, and informational functions. It is constantly being modified. For instance, ECM components are degraded by metalloproteases. About 3% of the matrix in cardiac muscle is turned over daily.

The composition of the ECM determines the nature of the signals being processed and in turn can be governed or modified by the cells comprising the tissue. The ECM can direct all cellular fate processes, providing a means for cells to communicate with signals that are more stable and may be more specific and stronger than those delivered by the diffusion process needed with growth factors. A summary of the components of the ECM and their functions for various tissues is given in Palsson [2000].

Many research groups are attempting to construct artificial ECMs. The scaffolding for these matrices has taken the form of polymer materials that can be surface modified for desired functionalities. In some cases they are designed to be biodegradable allowing the cells to replace this material with its natural counterpart as they establish themselves and their tissue function. The major obstacle is that the properties of this matrix are difficult to specify since the properties of natural ECMs are complex and not fully known. Furthermore, two-way communication between cells is difficult to mimic since the information contained within these conversations is also not fully known. At this time, the full spectrum of ECM functionalities can only be provided by the cells themselves.

10.2.3.5 Communication with the Whole Body Environment

The importance of the vascular system and in particular, the microcirculation, cannot be over emphasized. This network is needed to connect all the microenvironments in every tissue to their larger whole body environment. A complex vascular morphology is established such that most metabolically active cells in the body are located within a few hundred micrometers from a capillary. This high degree of vascularity is necessary to provide the perfusion environment that connects every cell to a source and sink for respiratory gases, a source of nutrients from the small intestine, the hormones from the pancreas, liver, and glandular system, clearance of waste products via the kidneys and liver, delivery of immune system respondents and so forth [Jain, 1994; Freshney, 2000; other chapters in this section of the handbook]. Transport of mass (and heat) in normal and neoplastic tissues, occurs primarily by convection and diffusion processes that take place throughout the whole circulatory system and ECM [Jain, 1994; Fournier, 1999]. The design of *in vivo* systems therefore must consider methods to promote this communication process, not only deal with the transport issues of the devise itself. The implanted tissue system vasculature must therefore consist of (1) vessels recruited from the preexisting network of the host vasculature and (2) vessels resulting from the angiogenic response of host vessels to implanted cells [Jain, 1994; Peattie et al., 2004]. Although the implant vascular originates from the host vasculature, its organization may be completely different depending on the tissue type, its growth rate, and its location. The architecture may be different not only among varying tissue types but also between an implant and any spontaneous tissue outgrowth originating from growth factor stimuli, from the implant, or as a whole body response.

A blood borne molecule or cell that enters the vasculature reaches the tissue microenvironment and individual cells via (i) distribution through the vascular tree, (ii) convection and diffusion across the microvascular wall, (iii) convection and diffusion through the interstitial fluid and ECM, and (iv) transport across the cell membrane [Lightfoot, 1974]. The sojourn of molecules through the vasculature is governed by the morphology of that network (i.e., the number, length, diameter, and geometrical arrangement of various blood vessels) and the blood flow rate (determining perfusion performance). Transport across vessel walls to interstitial space and across cell membranes depends on the physical properties of the molecules (e.g., size, charge, and configuration), physiological properties of these barriers, (e.g., transport pathways), and driving force (e.g., concentration and pressure gradients). Furthermore, specific or nonspecific binding to tissue components can alter the transport rate of molecules through a barrier by hindering the species and changing the transport parameters [Fisher, 1989].

Since the convective component of the transport processes via blood depends primarily on local blood flow in the tissue, coupled with vascular morphology of the tissue, hydrodynamics must be considered in designing for performance. In addition, perfusion rate requirements must take into account diffusional boundary layers along with the geometric factors of tissues and implants. In general, implant volume changes as a function of time more rapidly than for normal tissue due to tissue outgrowth, fibrotic tissue formation, and macrophage attachment. All these effects contribute to increased diffusion paths and nutrient consumption. Even with these distinctions among different tissues, the mathematical models of transport in normal, neoplastic, and implanted tissues both with and without barriers, whether in *vivo*, *ex vivo*, or *in vitro*, are identical. The only differences lie in the selection of physiological, geometric, and transport parameters. Furthermore, similar transport analyses can be applied to extracorporeal and novel bioreactor systems and their associated scale-up studies. Examples include artificial organs, animal surrogate systems, and the coupling of compartmental analysis with cell culture analogs in drug delivery and efficacy testing. Designing appropriate bioreactor systems for these applications is a challenge for tissue engineering teams collaborating with reaction engineering experts.

10.2.4 Cellularity

The number of cells found in the tissue microenvironment can be estimated as follows. The packing density of cells is in the order of a billion cells/cc; tissues typically form with a porosity of between 0.5 and 0.7 and therefore have a cell density of approximately 100 to 500 million cells/cc. Thus an order of magnitude estimate for a cube with a 100 μm edge, the mean intercapillary length scale, is about 500 cells. For comparison, simple multicellular organisms have about 1000 cells. Of course, the cellularity of the tissue microenvironment is dependent upon the tissue and the cell types composing it. At the extreme, ligaments, tendons, aponeuroses, and their associated dense connective tissue are acellular. Fibrocartilage is at the low end of cell-containing tissues, with about 1 million cells/cc or about 1 cell per characteristic cube. This implies that the microenvironment is simply one cell maintaining its ECM.

In most tissue microenvironments, many cell types are found in addition to the predominate cells that characterize that tissue. Leukocytes and immune system cells, including lymphocytes, monocytes, macrophages, plasma cells, and mast cells, can be demonstrated in nearly all tissues and organs, particularly during periods of inflammation. Precursor cells and residual undifferentiated cell types are present in most tissues as well, even in adults. Such cell types include mesenchymal cells (connective tissues), satellite cells (skeletal muscle), and pluripotential stem cells (hematopoietic tissues). Endothelial cells make up the wall of capillary microvessels and thus are present in all perfused tissues.

10.2.5 Dynamics

In most tissues and organs, the microenvironment is constantly in change due to the transient nature of the multitude of events occurring. Matrix replacement, cell motion, perfusion, oxygenation, metabolism, and cell signaling all contribute to a continuous turnover. Each of these events has its own characteristic time constant. It is the relative magnitude of these time constants that dictate which processes can be considered in a pseudosteady state with respect to the others. Determining the dynamic parameters of the major events (estimates available in Lightfoot [1974]; Long [2000]; Palsson [2000]) is imperative for successful modeling and design studies.

Timescaling of the systemic differential equations governing the physicochemical behavior of any tissue is extremely valuable in reducing the number of dependent variables needed to predict responses to selected perturbations and to evaluate system stability. In many cell-based systems, overall dynamics are controlled by transport and reaction rates. Controlling selected species transport then becomes the major issue since, under certain conditions, transport resistances may be beneficial. For example, when substrate inhibition kinetics is observed, performance is enhanced as the substrate transport rate is restricted. Furthermore, multiple steady states, with subsequent hysteresis problems, have been observed in these encapsulated systems as well as in continuous, suspension cell cultures [Bruns et al., 1973; Europa et al., 2000; Fisher et al., 2000]. Consequently, perturbations in the macroenvironment of an encapsulated cell/tissue system can force the system to a new, less desired, steady state where cellular metabolism as measured by, for example, glucose consumption and amino acid synthesis, is altered. Simply returning the macroenvironment to its original state may not be effective in returning the cellular system to its original (desired) metabolic state. The perturbation magnitudes that force a system to seek a new steady state, and subsequent hysteresis lags, are readily estimated from basic kinetics and mass transfer studies [Bruns et al., 1973; Europa et al., 2000]. However, incorporation of intelligent behavior into an encapsulation system permits mediation of this behavior. This may be accomplished by controlling the cell/tissue microenvironment through the modification of externally induced chemical, biological (as in a macrophage or T-cell), or physical stresses and through selectively and temporally releasing therapeutic agents or signal compounds to modify cellular metabolism. Various novel bioreactor systems that are currently available as "off the shelf" items can be modified to perform these tasks in appropriate hydrodynamic flow fields, with controlled transport and contacting patterns, and at a microscale of relevance.

10.2.6 Geometry

Geometric similitude is important in attempting to mimic *in vivo* tissue behavior in engineered devises. The shape and size of any given tissue bed must be known to aid in the design of these devises since geometric parameters help establish constraints for both physical and behavioral criteria. Many microenvironments are effectively 2D surfaces [Palsson, 2000]. Bone marrow has a fractal cellular arrangement with an effective dimensionality of 2.7, whereas the brain is a 3D structure. These facts dictate the type of culture technique (high density, as obtained with hollow fiber devises, vs. the conventional monolayer culture) to be used for best implant performance. For example, choriocarcinoma cells release more human chorionic gonadotrophin when using this type of high density culture [Freshney, 2000].

10.2.7 System Interactions: Reaction and Transport Processes

The interactions brought about by communications between tissue microenvironments and the whole body system, via the vascular network, provide a basis for the systems biology approach taken to understand the performance differences observed *in vivo* vs. *in vitro*. The response of one tissue system to changes in another due to signals generated, metabolic product accumulation, or hormone appearances must be properly mimicked by coupling individual cell culture analog systems through a series of microbioreactors if whole body *in vivo* responses are to be meaningfully predicted. The need for microscale reactors is obvious given the limited amount of tissue or cells available for many *in vitro* studies. This is particularly true when dealing with the pancreatic system [Galletti et al., 2000; Lewis and Colton, 2004] where intact Langerhans islets must be used rather than individual beta cells for induced insulin production by glucose stimulation. Their supply is extremely limited and maintaining viability and functionality is quite complex since the islet clusters *in vivo* are highly vascularized and this feature is difficult to reproduce in preservation protocols.

The coupling of reaction kinetics with transport processes is necessary to develop effective bioreactor systems. Further discussion of this topic is given later in this chapter (see "Reacting Systems and Bioreactors" and "Illustrative Example" for reactor design specifications and mass transfer analysis in encapsulation motifs, respectively). Heat and momentum transport are major topics discussed in other chapters in this section of the handbook. Brief comments on the necessity for these studies are presented as here.

In all living organisms, but especially the higher animals, diffusion and flow limitations are of critical importance. In adapting problem solving strategies for mathematical analysis and modeling of specific physiologic transport problems, it becomes particularly important to establish orders of magnitude and to make realistic limiting calculations. Especially attractive for these purposes are dimensional analysis and pharmacokinetic modeling; it seems in fact that these may permit unifying the whole of biological mass transport. Distributed-parameter transport modeling is also helpful. To obtain useful models one must set very specific goals and work toward them by systematically comparing theory and experiment. Particularly important are the estimation of transport properties and the development of specialized conservation equations, as for ultrathin membranes, about which only limited information is known. Thus analysis of physiologic transport stands in strong contrast to classical areas of transport phenomena [Lightfoot, 1974; Rosner, 1986; Brodkey and Hershey, 1988; Deen, 1996; Fournier, 1999; Bird et al., 2002].

Mass transfer lies at the heart of physiology and provides major constraints on the metabolic rates and anatomy of living organisms, from the organization of organ networks to molecular intracellular structures. Limitations on mass transfer rates are major constraints for nutrient supply, waste elimination, and information transmission. The primary functional units of metabolically active muscle and brain, liver lobules, and kidney nephrons have evolved to just eliminate significant mass transfer limitations in the physiological state [Lightfoot, 1974]. Turnover rates of highly regulated enzymes are just less than diffusion limitations. Signal transmission rates are frequently mass transport limited [Lauffenburger and

Linderman, 1993] and very ingenious mechanisms have evolved to speed these processes [Palsson, 2000]. Consequently, understanding tissue mass transport is important to accurately interpret transport-based experiments that involve complex interactions of transport and reaction processes, and further, our ability to design effective devices and biosensors.

Models for microvascular heat transfer are useful for understanding tissue thermoregulation, for optimizing thermal therapies such as hypothermia treatment, for modeling thermal regulatory response at the tissue level, for assessing microenvironment hazards that involve tissue heating, for using thermal means of diagnosing vascular pathologies, and for relating blood flow to heat clearance in thermal methods of blood perfusion measurement [Jain, 1994]. For example, the effect of local hypothermia treatment is determined by the length of time that the tissue is held at an elevated temperature, normally 43°C or higher. Since the tissue temperature depends on the balance between the heat added by artificial means and the tissue's ability to clear that heat, an understanding of the means by which the blood transports heat is essential for assessing the tissue's response to any thermal perturbation. The thermal regulatory system and the metabolic needs of tissues can change the blood perfusion rates in some tissues by a factor 25 [Baish, 2000]. More expensive reviews and tutorials on microvascular heat transfer may be found elsewhere [Cooney, 1976; Jain, 1994; Baish, 2000].

Biological processes within living systems are significantly influenced by the flow of liquids and gases. Consequently, understanding the basic pressure and flow mechanisms involved in biofluid processes is essential for our ability to design biomimetic systems. Simulations using Computational Fluid Dynamics (CFD) models to develop the necessary similitude and performance predictions and the experimental evaluations of prototype devices are crucial for successful *in vivo* implantation applications. Even for systems intended to remain *in vitro*, the effects of physiological fluids must be anticipated. Other complex devices, such as the development of bioreactors as surrogate systems, also need design guidance from CFD methods. The interaction of fluids and supported tissue is paramount in tissue engineering and the control of the microenvironment. The strength of adhesion and dynamics of detachment of mammalian cells from engineered biomaterials scaffolds is important ongoing research, as is the effects of shear on receptor–ligand binding at cell–fluid interfaces. In addition to altering transport across the cell membrane, and possibly more important, receptor location, binding affinity and signal generation, with subsequent trafficking within the cell [Lauffenburger and Linderman, 1993], can be changed.

Furthermore, the analysis and design of reactors is highly dependent upon knowing the nonideal flow patterns that exist within the vessel. In principle, if we have a complete velocity distribution map for the fluid, then we are able to predict the behavior of any given vessel as a reactor. Once considered an impractical approach, this is now obtainable by computing the velocity distribution using CFD-based procedures in which the full conservation equations are solved for the reactor geometry of interest. Both the nonlinear nature of these equations themselves and appropriate nonlinear constitutive relationships can readily be taken into consideration.

10.3   Reacting Systems and Bioreactors

Chemical reactions, usually closely coupled with transport phenomena, sustain and support life processes. Combining these with thermodynamics identifies the area of reaction engineering. Knowledge of the fundamentals involved is essential for our understanding of these reacting systems and ability to design and control engineering devices, such as the novel flow reactor systems needed by tissue engineers. These systems provide the required experimental conditions, that is, appropriate flow fields, with controlled transport and contacting patterns, and at a microscale of relevance.

The coupling of encapsulation technologies with cell culture techniques permits the extended use of these bioreactors with complex tissue systems such as islet clusters. Existing reactor systems are also useful in obtaining the basic transport and reaction kinetics parameters necessary to design the novel devices required for biomedical applications. In summary, the relevance of this work to the biotechnology and health care-based industries is in the development, of artificial organ systems, extra-corporeal devices to bridge transplantation, biosensors, drug design, discovery, development, and controlled delivery systems. Furthermore, the control and stabilization of metabolic processes has a major impact on many research programs including the development of animal surrogate systems for toxicity testing and biotechnological processes for the production of pharmaceuticals.

10.3.1 Reactor Types

Characterization of the mass transfer processes in bioreactors, as used in cell/tissue culture systems is essential when designing and evaluating their performance. Flow reactor systems bring together various reactants in a continuous fashion while simultaneously withdrawing products and excess reactants. These reactors generally provide optimum productivity and performance. They are classified as either tank- or tube-type reactors. Each represents extremes in the behavior of the gross fluid motion within the vessel. Tank-type reactors are characterized by instant and complete mixing of the contents and are therefore termed perfectly mixed or back-mixed reactors. Tube-type reactors are characterized by lack of mixing in the flow direction and are called plug flow or tubular reactors. The performance of actual reactors, though not fully represented by these idealized flow patterns, may match them so closely that they can be modeled as such with negligible error. Others can be modeled as combinations of tank and tube type over various regions.

Also in use are batch systems, where there is no flow in or out. The feed (initial charge) is placed in the reactor at the start of the process and the products are withdrawn (all at once) some time later. Reaction time is thus readily determined. This is significant since conversion is a function of time and can be obtained from knowledge of the reaction rate and its dependence upon concentration and process variables. Since operating conditions such as temperature, pressure, and concentration are typically controlled at a constant value, the time for reaction is the key parameter in the reactor design process. In a batch reactor, the concentration of reactants change with time and, therefore, the rate of reaction does as well.

Most actual reactors deviate from these idealized systems primarily because of nonuniform velocity profiles, channeling and bypassing of fluids, and the presence of stagnant regions caused by reactor shape and internal components such as baffles, heat transfer coils, and measurement probes. Disruptions to the flow path are common when dealing with heterogeneous systems, particularly when solids are present, as when using encapsulated systems. To model these actual reactors, various regions are compartmentalized and represented as combinations of plug flow and back-mixed elements. The study of biochemical kinetics, particularly when coupled with complex physical phenomena, such as the transport of heat, mass, and momentum, is required to determine or predict reactor performance. It is imperative to uncouple and unmask fundamental phenomenological events in reactors and to subsequently incorporate them in a concerted manner to meet objectives of specific applications. This need further emphasizes the role played by the physical aspects of reactor operation in process stability and controllability.

10.3.2 Design of Microreactors

Microscale reaction systems are often desirable for biomedical and biotechnological applications, in which the component substrates may be expensive or available only in very small quantities. This is particularly true when it is desired to conduct reactions with living cells. The advantages of microreactors are briefly summarized here. An important point to bear in mind is that these microscale systems, by their very nature, are differential reactors, that is, very low single pass conversions. Although this single pass analysis is quite beneficial when intermediate species kinetics studies are required, multiple passes, and subsequent reservoir dynamics, may be needed for higher conversion experimental programs. A few of the intrinsic qualities of microreactors are as follows:

- Minimizes reactant (serum) requirements
- Minimizes the quantity of cells or biocatalysts and support material
- Short contact time reactions can be studied more reliably at reduced flow rate

- Extend duration of experimental times, that is, longer continuous operation with small resource consumption
- "Aging" studies, both accelerated and long term, are more easily conducted
- Minimizes transport effects
- Coping with both mixing and flow distribution problems is less formidable and the data is more amenable to analysis
- Compatibility with spectroscopic systems
- *In situ* studies utilizing advanced spectroscopic techniques are easier to conduct since size restrictions are reduced
- Control of aseptic environment, operation in a biohazard/laminar flow hood is easily implemented, as is the optimum placement of ancillary equipment

10.3.3 Scale-up and Operational Maps

These are complex topics requiring a thorough background in chemical reaction engineering. An extensive literature has been published on the art and technology of scale-up. Here our objective is only to direct readers to some of the sources most pertinent to bioreactors; works worthy of attention are textbooks on biomedical engineering [Fournier, 1999; Palsson, 2000] and cell culture methods [Freshney, 2000].

The use of various membrane configurations coupled with bioreactors has lead to multiple functionality improvements and innovations. Implementation as guard beds, recycle conditioning vessels (with solids separations capabilities), *in situ* extraction systems, and slipstream (and bypass) reactors for "biocatalyst" activity maintenance, are but a few important examples representing successful applications when using living systems operating in controlled microenvironments.

The biosynthesis of lactate from pyruvate [Chen et al., 2004] is an illustrative example of the use of reactor hydrodynamic characterization and mass transport studies to improve performance through identification of operating regimes in which selected mechanisms dominate. Exploitation of this knowledge can then enhance the contribution from the desired phenomena. The operational protocols to enter these regimes, once they are documented, are termed operational maps. The multi-pass, dynamic input operating scheme used in that study permitted system parameter optimization studies to be conducted; including concentrations of all components in the free solution, flow rates, and electrode composition and their transport characteristics. Operating regimes that determined the controlling mechanism for process synthesis (e.g., mass transfer vs. kinetics limitations) were readily identified by varying system variables and operating conditions. Thus, procedures for developing operational maps were established and implemented.

10.4 Illustrative Example: Control of Hormone Diseases via Tissue Therapy

The treatment of autoimmune disorders with cell/tissue therapy has shown significant promise. A successful implant comprises cells or tissue surrounded by a biocompatible matrix permitting the entry of small molecules such as oxygen, nutrients, and electrolytes and exit of toxic metabolites, hormones, and other small bioactive compounds, while excluding antibodies and T-cells, thus protecting the encapsulated cells/tissue. Systems of this type are currently being evaluated for the treatment of a variety of disorders including type I diabetes mellitus, Hashimoto's disease (thyroiditis), and kidney failure. Several key issues need to be addressed before the clinical use of this technology can be realized, such as, tissue supply, maintenance of cell viability and functionality, and protection from immune rejection. Viability and metabolic functionality are controlled by the transport of essential biochemical signal molecules, nutrients, and respiratory gases. In particular, maintenance of sufficient oxygen levels in the encapsulation device is critical to avoid local domains of necrotic and hypometabolic cells. Oxygen transport can be enhanced through several means including the selection of optimal encapsulation configurations, promotion of vascularization at the implantation site, and seeding at an optimal cell density. Despite research efforts directed in these areas, oxygen transport remains one of the major limitations in maintaining cell viability and functionality. To improve this situation resent efforts have focused on the design of a novel nanotechnology-based encapsulation motif containing specific oxygen carriers. Such a motif will ensure complete metabolic functionality of the encapsulated cells and allow the cells to retain functionality over extended time, that is, months as opposed to weeks.

10.4.1 Transport Considerations

Our emphasis here is to describe the issues relevant to development of encapsulation motifs for tissue/cellular systems that help control their microenvironments. The objective is to discuss and utilize mechanisms by which molecular transport occurs through complex media. Experimental protocols focus on the selective transport of solute molecules to evaluate proposed mechanisms and establish performance criteria. Numerous models have been postulated to explain these phenomenological observations and to develop methodologies to predict performance, thereby facilitating the design of successful encapsulation systems. Issues that need to be incorporated into these models include (1) interfacial phenomena between the bulk fluid and the outer membrane surfaces and along a pore wall, (2) sorption into the membrane matrix itself with diffusion possibly affected by immobilization at specific interactive sites, (3) free and fixed site diffusion within the matrix and if appropriate, through the porous regions, whether as distinct pores, microchannels, or other nonhomogeneous discrete areas, and (4) any chemical reactions that could alter the nature of the diffusing species or the media itself.

Two models developed previously from the analysis of transport in hydrogel membranes [Yasuda and Lamaze, 1971; Fang et al., 1998] describe the various aspects of importance to us. Both pore and sorption mechanisms may be active but their classification, and thus characterization, is based upon which, if either, dominates. When considering a pore mechanism, the solute is envisioned as passing through fluid filled micropores (or channels) in the membrane. For molecules and their mean free path much smaller than these opening, a simple Fickian diffusion model will suffice. Knudsen diffusion will be considered when the pore size is smaller than the mean free path yet still larger than molecular diameter. As the pore and molecular sizes approach each other, hindered diffusion occurs where physical/chemical interactions of significant magnitude, not simply elastic collisions, play a dominate role in transport rates. It is in this region that interactions at the molecular level, such as surface adsorption (physical or chemisorption), absorption into the matrix (solubility), and molecular transformation become major phenomenological factors. Consideration must now be given to rate events, extent of reaction, equilibrium partitioning, irreversibility, site proximity, degree of saturation, and desorption. Migration rates along fiber or crystalline components in the matrix (and pore surface) are dependent upon energetics as well as site proximity, where a shunt pathway could be established to enhance transport if close enough. Otherwise, random adsorption events could hinder the transport process, analogous to diffusion with immobilization [Fisher, 1989]. However, once reaction sites are fully saturated, a normal diffusive zone can be established. The influence of chemical reactive sites can be determined following prior analyses [Cussler, 1984] when appropriate, as in functionalized surfaces and sites distributed throughout a membrane. In contrast, in porous materials possessing microchannels, but lacking a well-defined pore structure, the dominant phase is the fluid that fills these voids. This situation is analogous to that in a swollen fibrous media, in which solute can diffuse readily but encounters fibers in its sojourn through the membrane. These encounters have a random aspect due to the nonhomogeneous nature of the membrane. They could be passive, as in elastic collisions, or active through affinity interactions as in the pore concept described earlier.

Transport through nonporous materials requires solute to be absorbed (solubilized) in the matrix material. Solute molecules are thus subject to thermodynamic equilibrium factors at the fluid–solid interfaces, as well as the nature of the fluid and solid phases themselves. These include ion strength, degree of solute hydration, and other interactive forces. Once the solute is within the membrane, a simple Fickian diffusion mechanism may take place. Furthermore, all the other affinity events, as discussed for the pore model, could occur at interactive sites establishing a more complex transport process.

Combinations of these mechanisms may be observed in any membrane system that has distinct fluid, amorphous, crystalline, and functionalized regions, whether classified as porous or nonporous. Membranes may be characterized with respect to these mechanistic events, as modeled, based on experimental transport measurements. The analysis tools used to interpret these results are briefly discussed later in the context of this example case study.

10.4.2 Selection of Diabetes as Representative Case Study

The National Institute of Diabetes and Digestive and Kidney Diseases (NIDDKD) estimates that there are 16 million people (nearly 1 in 17) that have diabetes in the United States alone. It is one of the most common and wide-spread diseases, with as high as 6% of the world population suffering from diabetes. In addition to the primary symptom, loss of blood glucose regulation, complications, and sequelae of diabetes include blindness, cardiovascular disease, and loss of peripheral nerve function. When including these complications, diabetes is the fourth most important cause of mortality in the United States and the main cause of permanent blindness. The American Diabetes Association estimates that diabetics consume 15% of U.S. health-care costs (more than twice their percentage of the population), that is, the total cost of diabetic morbidity and mortality to be more than $90 billion per year. At least 50% of that figure attributed to direct medical costs for the care of diabetic patients. Although most of the affected individuals are not dependent upon interventional insulin replacement, NIDDKD estimates that 800,000 diabetics do require this treatment to manage blood glucose regulation. However, insulin delivery is not a cure. Restoration of normal glucose regulation by improved insulin therapy techniques that regulate insulin delivery offers the hope of circumventing the need for injection treatments and eliminating the serious debilitating secondary complications. Consequently, many research paths are being followed to determine how normal pancreatic functions can be returned to the body. These include whole pancreas transplants, human and animal islet transplantation, fetal tissue exchange, and creation of artificial beta cells, each with its pros and cons. The two major problems are the lack of sufficient organs or cells to transplant and the rejection of transplants. Since there is a severe shortage of adult pancreases, that is, 1,000 patients per available organ, alternatives such as islet cell transplantation are being sought. Cell transplantation, if it could be successfully achieved, would help with both of these major problems. Use of either "artificial" islets, potentially grown from stem or beta cells themselves, or xenogenic islet clusters, in combination with designed materials for immunoisolation functionality could lead to restoration of normoperative glycemic control without the need for insulin therapy.

10.4.3 Encapsulation Motif: Specifications, Design, and Evaluation

The goal of ongoing research programs is to improve the success rate of pancreatic islet cell transplantation and thus provide a better means to regulate glucose levels for diabetic patients. This is being accomplished through immunoisolation and immunoalteration technologies implemented using intelligent membrane encapsulation systems. These systems exist as multilayered microcapsules that utilize semipermeable membranes that permit transport of nutrients, insulin, and metabolic waste products while excluding antibody and T-cell transport [Lewis and Colton, 2004].

The immunoisolative capabilities of the encapsulation motif are based upon a size-exclusion principle whereby antibodies (primarily IgM and IgG) and complement proteins of the immune system are unable to reach the implanted cells. In order to activate the complement pathway in which antibodies bind specific complement proteins and ultimately destroy the implanted cells through lysis, one IgM molecule (MW = 800 kDa; ~30 nm diameter) and one molecule of complement protein C1q (MW = 410 kDa, ~30 nm diameter) must bind together. Alternatively, two IgG molecules (MW = 150 kDa each, ~20 nm total diameter) bind in concert with C1q to destroy the implant cells. Encapsulating cells in materials with a molecular weight cutoff of roughly 200 kDa therefore shields cell surface antigens from exposure to these antibodies.

It is important to also consider the ability of implanted cells to shed antigens into the surrounding host tissues, triggering another type of immune response. Many such shed antigens are composed of major histocompatibility complex (MHC) antigens, which are too small (57 to 61 kDa) to be retained by the encapsulation motif. Activation of the immune system in this manner recruits macrophages, which release reactive oxygen species in an attempt to destroy the implanted cells. The inclusion of reactive sites within the matrix that function as free radical scavengers is thus desirable to protect the cells from these toxic compounds. This may be possible using nanosphere technologies, whether active ingredient loaded or by their own characteristics, dispersing them throughout the microsized beads. Simultaneously, nanosphere technology may also be designed to augment respiratory gas exchange. The solubility of O_2 in water or blood plasma is approximately 2 ml O_2 per 100 ml of solution at standard temperature and pressure, which is at least an order of magnitude low for encapsulation purposes. Thus, selected O_2 carriers, such as perfluorocarbons, could be incorporated into the nanospheres or as microemulsions into the matrix of the encapsulating motif.

Transport to and from encapsulated cells of nutrients, respiratory gases, and similar small molecules is not affected by pore sizes commonly found in encapsulation motifs. However, transport of desired proteins, synthesized by the cells, out of the encapsulation matrix can be limited by the pore size of the material. Large secreted proteins (e.g., MW ~660 kDa) will be blocked by the MW cutoffs needed to shield the implanted cells from antibodies, whereas the diffusion of MW = 28 kDa and smaller proteins will not. Consequently, the molecular weight cutoff of the encapsulation material must be carefully chosen when transport of a secreted natural compound such as insulin is desired.

The hypothesis underlying this effort is that macromolecular biomaterial encapsulation materials can be engineered that would promote islet cluster viability while simultaneously facilitating desirable biologic responses. For encapsulation materials to be physiologically functional for metabolite transport and hormone secretion, their most important properties need to be biocompatibility and selective semipermeability. However, to promote implant longevity as well as augment tissue interstitium transport and exchange characteristics, an equally important sub-characteristic is the ability to stimulate neovascularization and vascular ingrowth *in situ*. Approaches, such as biodegradation of a sacrificial outer layer that either releases or "generates" growth factors to promote angiogenesis, are currently being studied [Peattie et al., 2004]. Thus, a single encapsulating material will not in general possess the spectrum of properties for a successful implantation. The design of a multilayer motif, in which each layer is selected to contribute specific functions, must be considered.

One must also account for the possibility that in certain situations increased transport resistances may be beneficial. For example, when substrate inhibition kinetics behavior is observed, performance is improved as the substrate transport rate is restricted. Mammalian cells can establish multiple steady states, with subsequent hysteresis effects, while in continuous culture at the same dilution rate and feed medium. Consequently, perturbations in the macroenvironment of an encapsulated cell/tissue system can force the system to a new, less desired, steady state with altered cellular metabolism. Simply returning the macroenvironment to its original state may not be effective in returning the cellular system to its original metabolic state, and hence predicted performance is unfavorable. The magnitudes of the macroenvironment perturbations forcing the system to seek a new steady state may be estimated from models developed simulating experimentally measured metabolism. Such behavior can be mediated by the encapsulation motif through its control of the cell/tissue microenvironment. In principle, the intelligent behavior of a proposed encapsulation system will allow the maintenance of the desired microenvironment through modification of stresses and release of necessary compounds. Characterization of the required materials in this motif and subsequent efficacy testing with appropriate cell/tissue systems is an integral component of these efforts. Fortunately, the majority of materials that must meet these objectives (desired functionalities) are currently available. A thorough discussion of the techniques used to characterize these materials can be found in many sources [Crank, 1956; Cussler, 1984; Deen, 1996; Sokolnicki, 2004; Sokolnicki et al., 2004]. The key points are summarized as follows.

10.4.3.1 Physical and Transport Parameters

A variety of physical parameters may be measured or calculated as necessary for the analysis and interpretation of transport measurements. The hydrated encapsulation matrix or membrane volume is obtained using a water displacement technique. The porosity can be estimated through a simple mass balance. Membrane morphology studies are usually conducted using scanning electron microscopy (SEM); an available, simple and straightforward method to determine physical characteristics of the membranes. Along with the equilibrium weight swelling ratio porosity measurement technique, surface morphology can be examined by SEM to determine the type and structure of the void space. System dimensions are obtained by direct measurement and simple calculations.

The membrane permeability is determined using a pseudosteady state analysis based on Fick's law, equilibrium partitioning to the membrane surface, and the observed concentration difference across the membrane. The instantaneous flux, j, through the matrix or membrane (in a diffusion cell apparatus) is then given by:

$$-j = \frac{[P]}{l}(C_D - C_R) \tag{10.1}$$

where l is the total length of the membrane and C_D and C_R are the concentrations within the donor cell and the receptor cell, respectively [Cussler, 1984]. The parameter P is the membrane permeability and is defined as: $P = D \cdot H$, where the partition coefficient, H, is the ratio of solute at/on the membrane surface to that free in solution, and D is the effective diffusion coefficient in the membrane. Using a time variant mass balance for each compartment and subject to the initial condition, $(C_{0,D} - C_{0,R}) = (C_{1,D} - C_{1,R})$ at $t = 0$, the solution obtained provides a method to interpret transport measurements and calculate the permeability:

$$P = \frac{1}{\beta t} \cdot \ln \frac{(C_{0,\text{Donor}} - C_{0,\text{Receptor}})}{(C_{1,\text{Donor}} - C_{1,\text{Receptor}})} \tag{10.2}$$

The parameter β is a physical constant containing the dimensions of the diffusion cell and the membrane.

Measurements of dextran transport can be used to validate the effectiveness of a pore model for a given motif. Investigation of the relation between molecular size and rate of transport can establish whether diffusion is hindered due to pore walls or simply due to collisions with fibers in the diffusion path. To determine the unhindered diffusion rate of dextran molecules in water, the diffusivity at infinite dilution [Davidson and Deen, 1988; Labraun and Junter, 1994], must be calculated using the Stokes–Einstein equation:

$$D_o = \frac{kT}{6\pi \eta_w r_H} \tag{10.3}$$

where r_H, the hydrodynamic radii of the dextran molecules, is obtained using the Stokes–Einstein correlation based on molecular weight, k is Boltzman's constant, T is the absolute temperature, and η_w is the viscosity of water at that temperature. Calculated diffusion coefficients of various molecular weight dextrans in water at dilute and semidilute concentrations are reported in the literature [Callaghan and Pinder, 1983]. A ratio of D_{eff} to D_o less than one indicates that a hindered diffusion process is present. If this ratio is dependent on molecular size, then pore (or microchannel) dimensions dominate vs. collisions with individual fibers.

When using a horizontal diffusion cell, the diffusivity of a solute through a particular membrane can only be determined directly from these experimental transport measurements under select conditions, that is, if the partition coefficient and all physical parameters of the membrane and apparatus are known. Although membrane external dimensions can often be measured with reasonable accuracy, pore characteristics are typically lumped into an apparatus parameter that must be determined by calibration experiments and is accordingly subject to experimental error. Consequently, permeability determination is not a fundamental process. Its usefulness is restricted to applications within a data collection regime. Extensions to predict performance and provide better design protocols for novel applications requires that the fundamental parameters, diffusivity, and partition coefficients, be known. Both can be obtained from desorption experiments, but data analysis from such experiments is more complicated, particularly when the motif geometry is nonspherical. One can use this technique to estimate both parameters, and then conduct adsorption tests to provide a direct measure of the partition coefficients, thereby providing redundancy checks for all three parameters, P, D, and H. Even with this more extensive data analysis program, one can only obtain effective diffusivities since the internal membrane structure is usually quite complex.

Marker species, such as vitamin B12, bovine serum albumin (BSA), and lysozyme, are generally selected to provide a reasonable range in size and properties for the solutes in desorption experiments. Membranes are initially saturated with one solute, then immersed in a buffer solution of known volume. Mathematical analysis of the resulting desorption is based on an infinite sheet of uniform thickness placed in a solution, allowing solute to diffuse from the sheet. Since membrane diameters are more than 100 times greater than the thickness, assumption of an infinite sheet is appropriate. The solution to this model system was developed by Crank [1956] in a form expressing the total amount of solute, M_t, in the solution at time t as a fraction of the amount after infinite time, M_∞. An infinite series form is obtained where D_{eff} appears in the exponential terms and can be recovered using a nonlinear fitting routine. The number of terms retained in the summation is dependent on the magnitude of time and the relative spacing of the system eigenvalues. The calculated diffusion coefficients are then compared to those in pure solvent and establish a basis to identify a hindered diffusion mechanism. An analysis of the adsorption behavior of the marker molecules in the membranes assists in the investigation of the mass transport phenomena by identifying if solute–matrix (fiber) interactions are significant.

The ability to execute a research program to obtain the requisite data to evaluate and implement designed encapsulation motifs, for example, develop a prototype from experimental data for clinical testing, is dependent upon coordinating all the efforts described so far. This includes using the various novel bioreactor systems discussed earlier to perform these tasks in appropriate flow fields, with controlled transport and contacting patterns, and at a microscale of relevance. Concerted programs will help in attaining the goal of understanding the microenvironment of encapsulated systems to control and optimize tissue function.

References

Baish, J.W. (2000). Microvascular heat transfer. In *The Biomedical Engineering Handbook*, Bronzino, J.D. (Ed.) 2nd ed. CRC Press, Boca Raton, FL, Chapter 98.

Bird, R.B., Stewart, W.E., and Lightfoot, E.N. (2002). *Transport Phenomena*, 2nd ed. John Wiley & Sons, New York.

Brodkey R.S. and Hershey, H.C. (1988). *Transport Phenomena: A Unified Approach*. McGraw-Hill, New York.

Bruns, D.D., Bailey, J.E., and Luss, D. (1973). *Biotechnol. Bioeng.* 15: 1131.

Chen, X., Fenton, J.M., Fisher, R.J., and Peattie, R.A., (2004). *J. Electochem. Soc.*, 151: 2.

Cooney, D.O. (1976). *Biomedical Engineering Principles*. Dekker, New York.

Crank, J. (1956). *The Mathematics of Diffusion*. Oxford University Press, London.

Cussler, E.L. (1984). *Diffusion: Mass Transfer in Fluid Systems*. Cambridge University Press, New York.

Davidson, M.G. and Deen, W.M. (1988). Hindered diffusion of water-soluble macromolecules in membranes, *Macromolecules* 21, 3474.

Deen, W.M. (1996). *Analysis of Transport Phenomena*. Oxford Press, New York.

Europa, A.F., Grambhir, A., Fu, P.C., and Hu, W.S. (2000). *Biotechnol. Bioeng.* 67: 25.

Fang, Y., Cheng, Q., and Lu, X.-B. (1998). Kinetics of *in vitro* drug release from chitosan/gelatin hybrid membranes, *J. Appl. Polym. Sci.*, 68: 1751.

Fisher, R.J. (1989). Diffusion with immobilization in membranes: transport and failure mechanisms; part II — transport mechanisms. In *Biological and Synthetic Membranes*, Butterfield, A. (Ed.), Alan R. Liss Co., New York.

Fisher, R.J. (2000). Compartmental analysis. In *Introduction to Biomedical Engineering*, Enderle, J., Blanchard, S., and Bronzino, J., (Eds), Academic Press, Orlando, FL, Chapter 8.

Fisher, R.J., Roberts, S.C., and Peattie, R.A. (2000). *Ann. Biomed. Eng.* 28: 39.

Fournier, R.L. (1999). *Basic Transport Phenomena in Biomedical Engineering*. Taylor & Francis, Philadelphia, PA.

Freshney, R.I. (2000). *Culture of Animal Cells: A Manual of Basic Technique*, 4th ed. Wiley-Liss, New York.

Callaghan, P.T. and Pinder, D.N. (1983). A pulsed field gradient NMR study of self-diffusion in a polydisperse polymer system: dextran in water. *Macromolecules* 16: 968.

Galletti, P.M., Colton, C.K., Jaffrin, M., and Reach, G. (2000). Artifical pancreas. In *The Biomedical Engineering Handbook*, 2nd ed., Bronzino, J.D. (Ed.), CRC Press, Boca Raton, FL, Chapter 134.

Jain, R.K. (1994). *Transport Phenomena in Tumors, Advances in Chemical Engineering*, Vol. 19, pp. 129–194, Academic Press, Inc.

Labraum, L. and Junter, G.A. (1994). Diffusion of dextrans through microporous membrane fibers, *J. Membr. Sci.* 88, 253.

Lauffenburger, D.A. and Linderman, J.J. (1993). *Receptors: Models for Binding, Trafficking, and Signaling*. Oxford University Press, New York.

Lewis, A.S. and Colton, C.K. (2004). Tissue engineering for insulin replacement in diabetes. In *Scaffolding in Tissue Engineering*, Ma, P. and Elisseeff, J. (Eds), Marcel Dekker, New York (in press).

Lightfoot, E.N. (1974). *Transport Phenomena and Living Systems*. John Wiley & Sons, New York.

Long, M.W. (2000). Tissue microenvironments, In *The Biomedical Engineering Handbook*, 2nd ed., Vol. II, Bronzino, J.D. (Ed.), CRC Press, Boca Raton, FL, Chapter 118.

Palsson, B. (2000). Tissue engineering. In *Introduction to Biomedical Engineering*, Enderle, J., Blanchard, S., and Bronzino, J. (Eds) Academic Press, Orlando, FL, Chapter 12.

Peattie, R.A., Nayate, A.P., Firpo, M.A., Shelby, J., Fisher, R.J., and Prestwich, G.D. (2004). Stimulation of *in vivo* angiogenesis by cytokine-loaded hyaluronic acid hydrogel implants. *Biomaterials* 25: 2789–2798.

Rosner, D.E. (1986). *Transport Processes in Chemically Reacting Flow Systems*. Butterworth Publishers, Boston.

Shuler, M.J. (2000). *Animal Surrogate Systems*. In *The Biomedical Engineering Handbook*, 2nd ed., Vol. II, Bronzino, J.D. (Ed.) CRC Press, Boca Raton, FL, Chapter 97.

Sokolnicki, A.M., Fisher, R.J., Harrah, T.P., and Kaplan, D.L. (2005). Permeability of bacterial cellulose membranes. *J. Membr. Sci.* 6793, 1–13.

Yasuda, H. and Lamaze, C.E. (1971). *J. Macromol. Sci. Phys.* B5: 111.

11

Interstitial Transport in the Brain: Principles for Local Drug Delivery

W. Mark Saltzman
Yale University

11.1 Introduction

Traditional methods for delivering drugs to the brain are inadequate. Many drugs, particularly water-soluble or high molecular weight compounds, do not enter the brain following systemic administration because they permeate through blood capillaries very slowly. This blood–brain barrier (BBB) severely limits the number of drugs that are candidates for treating brain disease.

Several strategies for increasing the permeability of brain capillaries to drugs have been tested. Since the BBB is generally permeable to lipid soluble compounds which can dissolve and diffuse through endothelial cell membranes [1,2], a common approach for enhancing brain delivery of compounds is chemical modification to enhance lipid solubility [3]. Unfortunately, lipidization approaches are not useful for drugs with molecular weight larger than 1000. Another approach for increasing permeability is the entrapment of drugs in liposomes [4], but delivery may be limited by liposome stability in the plasma and uptake at other tissue sites.

Specific nutrient transport systems in brain capillaries can be used to facilitate drug entry into the brain. L-dopa (L-3,4-dihydroxyphenylalanine), a metabolic precursor of dopamine, is transported across endothelial cells by the neutral amino acid transport system [5]. L-dopa permeates through capillaries into the striatal tissue, where it is decarboxylated to form dopamine. Therefore, systemic administration of L-dopa is often beneficial to patients with Parkinson's disease. Certain protein modifications, such as cationization [6] and anionization [7], produce enhanced uptake in the brain. Modification of drugs [8,9] by linkage to an antitransferrin receptor antibody also appears to enhance transport into the brain. This approach depends on receptor-mediated transcytosis of transferrin–receptor complexes by brain endothelial cells; substantial uptake also occurs in the liver.

The permeability of brain capillaries can be transiently increased by intra-arterial injection of the hyperosmolar solutions, which disrupt interendothelial tight junctions [10]. But BBB disruption affects capillary permeability throughout the brain, enhancing permeability to all compounds in the blood, not just the agent of interest. Intraventricular therapy, where agents are administered directly into the CSF of the ventricles, results in high concentrations within the brain tissue, but only in regions immediately surrounding the ventricles [11,12]. Because the agent must diffuse into the brain parenchyma from the ventricles, and because of the high rate of clearance of agents in the CNS into the peripheral circulation, this strategy cannot be used to deliver agents deep into the brain.

Because of the difficulty in achieving therapeutic drug levels by systemic administration, methods for direct administration of drugs into the brain parenchyma have been tested. Drugs can be delivered directly into the brain tissue by infusion, implantation of a drug-releasing matrix, or transplantation of drug-secreting cells [13]. These approaches provide sustained drug delivery that can be limited to specific sites, localizing therapy to a brain region. Because these methods provide a localized and continuous source of active drug molecules, the total drug dose can be less than needed with systemic administration. With polymeric controlled release, the implants can also be designed to protect unreleased drug from degradation in the body and to permit localization of extremely high doses (up to the solubility of the drug) at precisely defined locations in the brain. Infusion systems require periodic refilling; the drug is usually stored in a liquid reservoir at body temperature and many drugs are not stable under these conditions.

This chapter describes the transport of drug molecules that are directly delivered into the brain. For purposes of clarity, a specific example is considered: polymeric implants that provide controlled release of chemotherapy. The results can be extended to other modes of administration [13,14] and other types of drug agents [15].

11.2 Implantable Controlled Delivery Systems for Chemotherapy

The kinetics of drug release from a controlled release system are usually characterized *in vitro*, by measuring the amount of drug released from the matrix into a well-stirred reservoir of phosphate buffered water or saline at 37°C. Controlled release profiles for some representative anticancer agents are shown in Figure 11.1. All of the agents selected for these studies — 1,3-bis(2-chloroethyl)-1-nitrosourea (BCNU), 4-HC, cisplatin, and taxol — are used clinically for chemotherapy of brain tumors. The controlled release period can vary from several days to many months, depending on properties of the drug, the polymer, and the method of formulation. Therefore, the delivery system can be tailored to the therapeutic situation by manipulation of implant properties.

The release of drug molecules from polymer matrices can be regulated by diffusion of drug through the polymer matrix or degradation of the polymer matrix. In many cases (including the release of BCNU, cisplatin, and 4HC from the degradable matrices shown in Figure 11.1), drug release from biodegradable polymers appears to be diffusion-mediated, probably because the time for polymer degradation is longer than the time required for drug diffusion through the polymer. In certain cases linear release, which appears to correlate with the polymer degradation rate, can be achieved; this might be the case for taxol

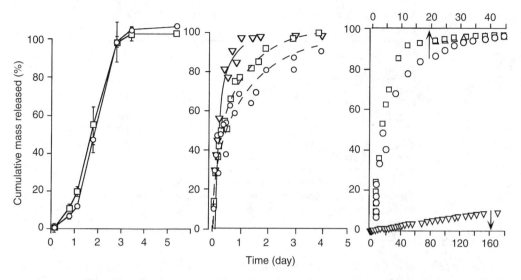

FIGURE 11.1 Controlled release of anticancer compounds from polymeric matrices. (a) Release of cisplatin (circles) from a biodegradable copolymer of fatty acid dimers and sebacic acid, p(FAD:SA), initially containing 10% drug (see References 32 and 33 for details). (b) Release of BCNU from EVAc matrices (circles), polyanhydride matrices p(CPP:SA) (squares), and p(FAD:SA) (triangles) matrices initially containing 20% drug. (c) Release of BCNU (squares), 4HC (circles), and taxol (triangles) from p(CPP:SA) matrices initially containing 20% drug. Note that panel (c) has two time axes: the lower axis applies to the release of taxol and the upper axis applies to the release of BCNU and 4HC.

release from the biodegradable matrix (Figure 11.1) although the exceedingly low solubility of taxol in water may also contribute substantially to the slowness of release.

For diffusion-mediated release, the amount of drug released from the polymer is proportional to the concentration gradient of the drug in the polymer. By performing a mass balance on drug molecules within a differential volume element in the polymer matrix, a conservation equation for drug within the matrix is obtained:

$$\frac{\partial C_p}{\partial t} = D_p \nabla^2 C_p \tag{11.1}$$

where C_p is the local concentration of drug in the polymer and D_p is the diffusion coefficient of the drug in the polymer matrix. This equation can be solved, with appropriate boundary and initial conditions, to obtain the cumulative mass of drug released as a function of time; the details of this procedure are described elsewhere [16]. A useful approximate solution, which is valid for the initial 60% of release, is:

$$M_t = 4M_o \sqrt{\frac{D_{i:p} t}{\pi L^2}} \tag{11.2}$$

where M_t is the cumulative mass of drug released from the matrix, M_o is the initial mass of drug in the matrix, and L is the thickness of the implant. By comparing Equation 11.2 to the experimentally determined profiles, the rate of diffusion of the agent in the polymer matrix can be estimated (Table 11.1).

11.3   Drug Transport After Release from the Implant

Bypassing the BBB is necessary, but not sufficient for effective drug delivery. Consider the consequences of implanting a delivery system, such as one of the materials characterized above, within the brain. Molecules released into the interstitial fluid in the brain extracellular space must penetrate into the brain tissue to

TABLE 11.1   Diffusion Coefficients for Chemotherapy Drug Release from Biocompatible Polymer Matrices[a]

Drug	Polymer	Initial loading (%)	D_p (cm^2/sec)
Cisplatin	P(FAD:SA)	10	6.8×10^{-9}
BCNU	EVAc	20	1.6×10^{-8}
BCNU	P(FAD:SA)	20	6.9×10^{-8}
BCNU	P(CPP:SA)	20	2.3×10^{-8} (panel b)
			2.0×10^{-8} (panel c)
4HC	P(CPP:SA)	20	3.1×10^{-10}
Taxol	P(CPP:SA)	20	n.a.

[a] Diffusion coefficients were obtained by comparing the experimental data show in Figure 11.1 to Equation 11.2 and determining the best value of the diffusion coefficient to represent the data.
Abbreviations: not applicable (n.a.).

reach tumor cells distant from the implanted device. Before these drug molecules can reach the target site, however, they might be eliminated from the interstitium by partitioning into brain capillaries or cells, entering the cerebrospinal fluid, or being inactivated by extracellular enzymes. Elimination always accompanies dispersion; therefore, regardless of the design of the delivery system, one must understand the dynamics of both processes in order to predict the spatial pattern of drug distribution after delivery.

The polymer implant is surrounded by biological tissue, composed of cells and an extracellular space (ECS) filled with extracellular fluid (ECF). Immediately following implantation, drug molecules escape from the polymer and penetrate the tissue. Once in the brain tissue, drug molecules (1) diffuse through the tortuous ECS in the tissue, (2) diffuse across semipermeable tissue capillaries to enter the systemic circulation and, therefore, are removed from the brain tissue, (3) diffuse across cell membranes by passive, active, or facilitated transport paths, to enter the intracellular space, (4) transform, spontaneously or by an enzyme-mediated pathway, into other compounds, and (5) bind to fixed elements in the tissue. Each of these events influence drug therapy: diffusion through the ECS is the primary mechanism of drug distribution in brain tissue; elimination of the drug occurs when it is removed from the ECF or transformed; and binding or internalization may slow the progress of the drug through the tissue.

A mass balance on a differential volume element in the tissue [17] gives a general equation describing drug transport in the region near the polymer [18]:

$$\frac{\partial C_i}{\partial t} + \bar{v} \cdot \nabla C_t = D_b \nabla^2 C_i + R_e(C_i) - \frac{\partial B}{\partial t} \tag{11.3}$$

where C is the concentration of the diffusible drug in the tissue surrounding the implant (g/cm^3 tissue), v is the fluid velocity (cm/sec), D_b is the diffusion coefficient of the drug in the tissue (cm^2/sec), $R_e(C)$ is the rate of drug elimination from the ECF (g/sec cm^3 tissue), B is the concentration of drug bound or internalized in cells (g/cm^3 tissue), and t is the time following implantation. In deriving this equation, the conventions developed by Nicholson [20], based on volume-averaging in a complex medium, and Patlak and Fenstermacher [18] were combined. In this version of the equation, the concentrations C and B and the elimination rate $R_e(C)$ are defined per unit volume of tissue. D_b is an effective diffusion coefficient, which must be corrected from the diffusion coefficient for the drug in water to account for the tortuosity of the ECS.

When the binding reactions are rapid, the amount of intracellular or bound drug can be assumed to be directly proportional, with an equilibrium coefficient K_{bind}, to the amount of drug available for internalization or binding:

$$B = K_{bind} C \tag{11.4}$$

Substitution of Equation 11.4 into Equation 11.3 yields, with some simplification:

$$\frac{\partial C_t}{\partial t} = \frac{1}{1 + K_{bind}} (D_b \nabla^2 C_t + R_e(C_t) - \bar{v} \cdot \nabla C_t) \tag{11.5}$$

The drug elimination rate, $R_e(C)$, can be expanded into the following terms:

$$R_e(C_t) = k_{bbb} \left(\frac{C_t}{\varepsilon_{ecs}} - C_{plasma} \right) + \frac{V_{max} C_t}{K_m + C_t} + k_{ne} C_t \tag{11.6}$$

where k_{bbb} is the permeability of the BBB (defined based on concentration in the ECS), C_{plasma} is the concentration of drug in the blood plasma, V_{max} and K_m are Michaelis–Menton constants, and k_{ne} is a first order rate constant for drug elimination due to nonenzymatic reactions. For any particular drug, some of the rate constants may be very small, reflecting the relative importance of each mechanism of drug elimination. If it is assumed that the permeability of the BBB is low ($C_{pl} \ll C$) and the concentration of drug in the brain is sufficiently low so that any enzymatic reactions are in the first order regime ($C \ll K_m$), Equation 11.6 can be reduced to:

$$-R_e(C_t) = \frac{k_{bbb}}{\varepsilon_{ecs}} C_t + \frac{V_{max}}{K_m} C_t + k_{ne} C_t = k_{app} C_t \tag{11.7}$$

where k_{app} is a lumped first order rate constant. With these assumptions, Equation 11.4 can be simplified by definition of an apparent diffusion coefficient, D^*, and an apparent first order elimination constant, k^*:

$$\frac{\partial C_t}{\partial t} = D^* \nabla^2 C_t + k^* C_t - \frac{\bar{v} \cdot \nabla C_t}{1 + K_{bind}} \tag{11.8}$$

where $k^* = k_{app}/(1 + K_{bind})$ and $D = D_b/(1 + K_{bind})$.

Boundary and initial conditions are required for solution of differential Equation 11.8. If a spherical implant of radius R is implanted into a homogeneous region of the brain, at a site sufficiently far from anatomical boundaries, the following assumptions are reasonable:

$$C_t = 0 \quad \text{for } t = 0; \ r > R \tag{11.9}$$

$$C_t = C_i \quad \text{for } t > 0; \ r = R \tag{11.10}$$

$$C_t = 0 \quad \text{for } t > 0; \ r \to \infty \tag{11.11}$$

In many situations, drug transport due to bulk flow can be neglected. This assumption (v is zero) is common in previous studies of drug distribution in brain tissue [18]. For example, in a previous study of cisplatin distribution following continuous infusion into the brain, the effects of bulk flow were found to be small, except within 0.5 mm of the site of infusion [21]. In the cases considered here, since drug molecules enter the tissue by diffusion from the polymer implant, not by pressure-driven flow of a fluid, no flow should be introduced by the presence of the polymer. With fluid convection assumed negligible, the general governing equation in the tissue, Equation 11.8, reduces to:

$$\frac{\partial C_i}{\partial t} = D^* \nabla^2 C_t + k^* C_t \tag{11.12}$$

The no-flow assumption may be inappropriate in certain situations. In brain tumors, edema and fluid movement are significant components of the disease. In addition, some drugs can elicit cytotoxic edema.

Certain drug/polymer combinations can also release drugs in sufficient quantity to create density-induced fluid convection.

Equation 11.12, with conditions 11.9 through 11.11, can be solved by Laplace transform techniques [13] to yield:

$$\frac{C_t}{C_i} = \frac{1}{2\zeta}\left\{\exp[-\phi(\zeta-1)]\mathrm{erfc}\left[\frac{\zeta-1}{2\sqrt{\tau}}-\phi\sqrt{\tau}\right]+\exp[\phi(\zeta-1)]\mathrm{erfc}\left[\frac{\zeta-1}{2\sqrt{\tau}}+\phi\sqrt{\tau}\right]\right\} \quad (11.13)$$

where the dimensionless variables are defined as follows:

$$\zeta = \frac{r}{R}; \quad \tau = \frac{D^*t}{R^2}; \quad \phi = R\sqrt{\frac{k^*}{D^*}} \quad (11.14)$$

The differential equation also has a steady-state solution, which is obtained by solving Equation 11.12 with the time derivative set equal to zero and subject to the boundary conditions 11.9 and 11.10:

$$\frac{C_t}{C_i} = \frac{1}{\zeta}\exp[-\phi(\zeta-1)] \quad (11.15)$$

Figure 11.2 shows concentration profiles calculated using Equation 11.13 and Equation 11.15. In this situation, which was obtained using reasonable values for all of the parameters, steady-state is reached approximately 1 h after implantation of the delivery device. The time required to achieve steady-state depends on the rate of diffusion and elimination, as previously described [22], but will be significantly less than 24 h for most drug molecules.

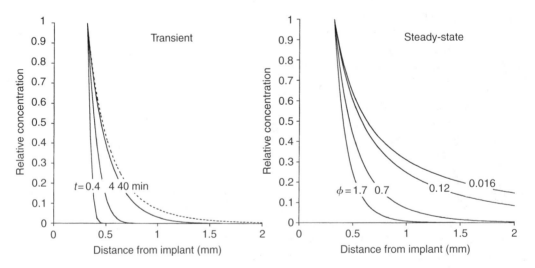

FIGURE 11.2 Concentration profiles after implantation of a spherical drug-releasing implant. (Panel a, Transient) Solid lines represent the transient solution to Equation 11.12 (i.e., Equation 11.13) with the following parameter values: $D^* = 4 \times 10^{-7}$ cm^2/sec; $R = 0.032$ cm; $k^* = 1.9 \times 10^{-4}$ sec^{-1} ($t^{1/2} = 1$ h). The dashed line represents the steady-state solution (i.e., Equation 11.15) for the same parameters. (Panel b, Steady-state) Solid lines in this plot represent Equation 11.15 with the following parameters: $D^* = 4 \times 10^{-7}$ cm^2/sec; $R = 0.032$ cm. Each curve represents the steady-state concentration profile for drugs with different elimination half-lives in the brain, corresponding to different dimensionless moduli, f: $t^{1/2} = 10$ min ($f = 1.7$); 1 h (0.7); 34 h (0.12); and 190 h (0.016).

11.4 Application of Diffusion–Elimination Models to Intracranial BCNU Delivery Systems

The preceding mathematical analysis, which assumes diffusion and first-order elimination in the tissue, agrees well with experimental concentration profiles obtained after implantation of controlled release polymers (Figure 11.3). At 3, 7, and 14 d after implantation of a BCNU-releasing implant, the concentration profile at the site of the implant was very similar. The parameter values (obtained by fitting Equation 11.15 to the experimental data) were consistent with parameters obtained using other methods [19], suggesting that diffusion and first-order elimination were sufficient to account for the pattern of drug concentration observed during this period. Parameter values were similar at 3, 7, and 14 d, indicating that the rates of drug release, drug dispersion, and drug elimination did not change during this period. This equation has been compared to concentration profiles measured for a variety of molecules delivered by polymer implants to the brain — dexamethasone [22], molecular weight fractions of dextran [23], nerve growth factor in rats [24,25], BCNU in rats [19], rabbits [26], and monkeys [27]. In each of these cases, the steady-state diffusion-elimination model appears to capture most of the important features of drug transport.

This model can be used to develop guidelines for the design of intracranial delivery systems. Table 11.2 lists some of the important physical and biological characteristics of a few compounds that have been considered for interstitial delivery to treat brain tumors. When the implant is surrounded by tissue, the maximum rate of drug release is determined by the solubility of the drug, C_s, and the rate of diffusive transport through the tissue:

$$\left(\frac{dM_t}{dt}\right)_{max} = (\text{Maximum flux}) \times (\text{Surface area}) = -D^* \frac{\partial C_t}{\partial r}\bigg|_R 4\pi R^2 \qquad (11.16)$$

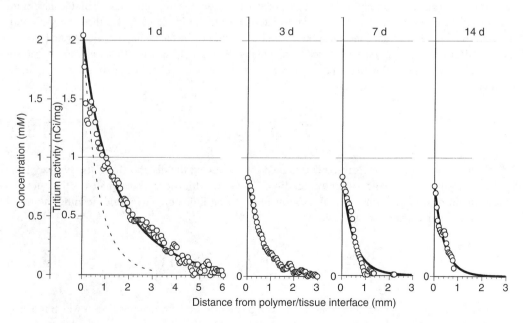

FIGURE 11.3 Concentration profiles after implantation of a BCNU-releasing implant. Solutions to Equation 11.15 were compared to experimental data obtained by quantitative autoradiographic techniques. The solid lines in the three panels labeled 3, 7, and 14 d were all obtained using the following parameters: $R = 0.15$ cm; $f = 2.1$; and $C_I = 0.81$ mM. The solid line in the panel labeled 1 d was obtained using the following parameters: $R = 0.15$ cm; $f = 0.7$; and $C_I = 1.9$ mM. Modified from Fung et al., *Pharm. Res.*, 1996, 13: 671–682.

TABLE 11.2   Implant Design Applied to Three Chemotherapy Compounds[a]

	BCNU	4HC	Methotrexate
Molecular weight (D_a)	214	293	454
Solubility (mM)	12	100	100
$\log_{10}K$	1.53	0.6	−1.85
k^* (h)	70	70	1
D^* (10^{-7} cm^2/sec)	14	14	5
Toxic concentration in culture (μM)	25	10	0.04
Maximum re;ease rate (mg/d)	1.2	14	17
Implant lifetime at max rate (d)	0.85	0.07	0.06
Maximum concentration in tissue for 1-week-releasing implant (mM)	1.5	1.1	1.8
RT (mm)	1.3	2.5	5

[a] K is the octanol : water partition coefficient, k is the rate of elimination due to permeation through capillaries, D_b is the diffusion coefficient of the drug in the brain. The following values are assumed, consistent with our results from polymer delivery to rats and rabbits: radius of spherical implant, $R = 1.5$ mm; mass of implant, $M = 10$ mg; drug loading in implant, Load = 10%.

Evaluating the derivative in Equation 11.16 from the steady-state concentration profile (Equation 11.15) yields:

$$\left(\frac{dM_i}{dt}\right)_{max} = 8\pi \dot{D}^* C_s R \qquad (11.17)$$

Regardless of the properties of the implant, it is not possible to release drug into the tissue at a rate faster than determined by Equation 11.17. If the release rate from the implant is less than this maximum rate, C_i (the concentration in the tissue immediately outside the implant) is less than the saturation concentration, C_s. The actual concentration C_i can be determined by balancing the release rate from the implant (dMt/dt, which can be determined from Equation 11.2 provided that diffusion is the mechanism of release from the implant) with the rate of penetration into the tissue obtained by substituting C_I for C_s in Equation 11.17:

$$C^* = \frac{dM_i}{dt}\left(\frac{1}{8\pi D^* R}\right) \qquad (11.18)$$

The effective region of therapy can be determined by calculating the distance from the surface of the implant to the point where the concentration drops below the cytotoxic level (estimated as the cytotoxic concentration determined from *in vitro* experiments). Using Equation 11.15, and defining the radial distance for effective treatment as R_T, yields:

$$\frac{C_{cytotoxic}}{C_i} = \frac{R}{R_T}\exp\left\{-R\sqrt{\frac{k^*}{D^*}}\left(\frac{R_T}{R}-1\right)\right\} \qquad (11.19)$$

Alternately, an effective penetration distance, d_P, can be defined as the radial position at which the drug concentration has dropped to 10% of the peak concentration:

$$0.10 = \frac{R}{d_P}\exp\left\{-R\sqrt{\frac{k^*}{D^*}}\left(\frac{d_P}{R}-1\right)\right\} \qquad (11.20)$$

These equations provide quantitative criteria for evaluating the suitability of chemotherapy agents for direct intracranial delivery (Table 11.2).

11.5 Limitations and Extensions of the Diffusion–Elimination Model

11.5.1 Failure of the Model in Certain Situations

The previous section outlined one method for analysis of drug transport after implantation of a drug-releasing device. A simple pseudo-steady-state equation (Equation 11.15) yielded simple guidelines (Equation 11.16 to Equation 11.19) for device design. Because the assumptions of the model were satisfied over a substantial fraction of the release period (days 3 to 14, based on the data shown in Figure 11.3), this analysis may be useful for predicting the effects of BCNU release from biodegradable implants. Pseudo-steady-state assumptions are reasonable during this period of drug release, presumably because the time required to achieve steady-state (which is on the order of minutes) is much less than the characteristic time associated with changes in the rate of BCNU release from the implant (which is on the order of days).

But experimental concentration profiles measured 1 d after implantation were noticeably different: the peak concentration was substantially higher and the drug penetration into the surrounding tissue was deeper (see the left-hand panel of Figure 11.3). This behavior cannot be easily explained by the pseudo-steady-state models described above. For example, if the difference observed at 1 d represents transient behavior, the concentration observed at a fixed radial position should increase with time (Figure 11.2); in contrast, the experimental concentration at any radial position on Day 1 is higher than the concentration measured at that same position on subsequent days.

11.5.2 Effect of Drug Release Rate

Alternately, the observed difference at 1 d might be due to variability in the rate of BCNU release from the polymer implant over this period, with transport characteristics in the tissue remaining constant. When similar BCNU-releasing implants are tested in vitro, the rate of drug release did decrease over time (Figure 11.1). Equation 11.18 predicts the variation in peak concentration with release rate; the twofold higher concentration observed at the interface on Day 1 (as compared to Days 3 to 14) could be explained by a twofold higher release rate on Day 1. But the effective penetration distance, d_P, does not depend on release rate. Experimentally measured penetration distances are ~1.4 mm on Days 3, 7, and 14 and ~5 mm on Day 1. This difference in penetration is shown more clearly in the Day 1 panel of Figure 11.3: the dashed line shows the predicted concentration profile if k^* and D^* were assumed equal to the values obtained for Days 3, 7, and 14. Changes in the rate of BCNU release are insufficient to explain the differences observed experimentally.

11.5.3 Determinants of Tissue Penetration

Penetration of BCNU is enhanced at Day 1 relative to penetration at Days 3, 7, and 14. For an implant of fixed size, penetration depends only on the ratio of elimination rate to diffusion rate: k^*/D^*. Increased penetration results from a decrease in this ratio (Figure 11.2), which could occur because of either a decreased rate of elimination (smaller k^*) or an increased rate of diffusion (larger D^*). But there are no good reasons to believe that BCNU diffusion or elimination are different on Day 1 than on Days 3 through 14. With its high lipid solubility, BCNU can diffuse readily through brain tissue. In addition, elimination of BCNU from the brain occurs predominantly by partitioning into the circulation; since BCNU can permeate the capillary wall by diffusion, elimination is not a saturable process. Perhaps the enhanced penetration of BCNU is due to the presence of another process for drug dispersion, such as bulk fluid flow, which was neglected in the previous analysis.

The diffusion/elimination model compares favorably with available experimental data, but the assumptions used in predicting concentration profiles in the brain may not be appropriate in all cases. Deviations from the predicted concentration profiles may occur due to extracellular fluid flows in the brain, complicated patterns of drug binding, or multistep elimination pathways. The motion of interstitial fluid in the vicinity of the polymer and the tumor periphery may not always be negligible, as mentioned above. The interstitial fluid velocity is proportional to the pressure gradient in the interstitium; higher interstitial pressure in tumors — due to tumor cell proliferation, high vascular permeability, and the absence of functioning lymphatic vessels — may lead to steep interstitial pressure gradients at the periphery of the tumor [28]. As a result, interstitial fluid flows within the tumor may influence drug transport. A drug at the periphery of the tumor must overcome outward convection to diffuse into the tumor. Similarly, local edema after surgical implantation of the polymer may cause significant fluid movement in the vicinity of the polymer. More complete mathematical models that include the convective contribution to drug transport are required.

11.5.4   Effect of Fluid Convection

When bulk fluid flow is present ($v \neq 0$), concentration profiles can be predicted from Equation 11.8, subject to the same boundary and initial conditions (Equation 11.9 to Equation 11.11). In addition to Equation 11.8, continuity equations for water are needed to determine the variation of fluid velocity in the radial direction. This set of equations has been used to describe concentration profiles during microinfusion of drugs into the brain [14]. Relative concentrations were predicted by assuming that the brain behaves as a porous medium (i.e., velocity is related to pressure gradient by Darcy's law). Water introduced into the brain can expand the interstitial space; this effect is balanced by the flow of water in the radial direction away from the infusion source and, to a lesser extent, by the movement of water across the capillary wall.

In the presence of fluid flow, penetration of drug away from the source is enhanced (Figure 11.4). The extent of penetration depends on the velocity of the flow and the rate of elimination of the drug. These calculations were performed for macromolecular drugs, which have limited permeability across the brain capillary wall. The curves indicate steady-state concentration profiles for three different proteins with metabolic half-lives of 10 min, 1 or 33.5 h. In the absence of fluid flow, drugs with longer half-lives penetrate deeper into the tissue (solid lines in Figure 11.4 were obtained from Equation 11.15). This effect is amplified by the presence of flow (dashed lines in Figure 11.4).

During microinfusion, drug is introduced by pressure-driven fluid flow from a small catheter. Therefore, pressure gradients are produced in the brain interstitial space, which lead to fluid flow through the porous brain microenvironment. Volumetric infusion rates of 3 μl/min were assumed in the calculations reproduced in Figure 11.4. Since loss of water through the brain vasculature is small, the velocity can be determined as a function of radial position:

$$v_r = \frac{q}{4\pi r^2 \varepsilon} \tag{11.21}$$

where q is the volumetric infusion rate and e is the volume fraction of the interstitial space in the brain (~ 0.20). Fluid velocity decreases with radial distance from the implant (Table 11.3); but at all locations within the first 20 mm of the implant site, predicted velocity was much greater than the velocities reported previously during edema or tumor growth in the brain.

The profiles predicted in Figure 11.4 were associated with the introduction of substantial volumes of fluid at the delivery site. Flow-related phenomena are probably less important in drug delivery by polymer implants. Still, this model provides useful guidelines for predicting the influence of fluid flow on local rates of drug movement. Clearly, the effect of flow velocity on drug distribution is substantial (Figure 11.4). Even relatively low flows, perhaps as small as 0.03 μm/sec, are large enough to account for the enhancement in BCNU penetration observed at Day 1 in Figure 11.3.

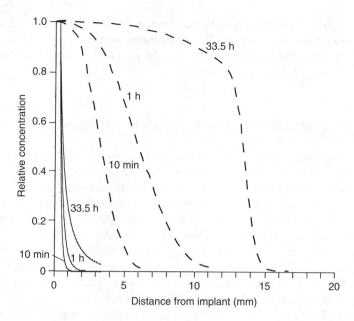

FIGURE 11.4 Concentration profiles predicted in the absence (solid lines) and presence (dashed lines) of interstitial fluid flow. Solid lines were obtained from Equation 11.15 with the following parameter values: $R = 0.032$ cm; $D = 4 \times 10^{-7}$ cm²/sec; and $k^* = \ln(2)/t^{1/2}$ where $t^{1/2}$ is either 10 min, 1 or 33.5 h as indicated on the graph. Dashed lines were obtained from Reference 14 using the same parameter values and an infusion rate of 3 μl/min. The dashed line indicating the interstitial flow calculation for the long-lived drug ($t^{1/2} = 33.5$ h) was not at steady-state, but at 12 h after initiation of the flow.

TABLE 11.3 Interstitial Fluid Velocity as a Function of Radial Position During Microinfusion[a]

Radial position (mm)	Interstitial velocity (μm/sec)
2	5.0
5	0.8
10	0.2
20	0.05

[a] Calculated by method reported in Morrison et al., *Am. J. Physiol.*, 1994, 266: R292–R305.

11.5.5 Effect of Metabolism

The metabolism, elimination, and binding of drug are assumed to be first order processes in our simple analysis. This assumption may not be realistic in all cases, especially for complex agents such as proteins. The metabolism of drugs in normal and tumor tissues is incompletely understood. Other cellular factors (e.g., the heterogeneity of tumor-associated antigen expression and multidrug resistance) that influence the uptake of therapeutic agents may not be accounted for by our simple first order elimination.

Finally, changes in the brain that occur during the course of therapy are not properly considered in this model. Irradiation can be safely administered when a BCNU-loaded polymer has been implanted in monkey brains, suggesting the feasibility of adjuvant radiotherapy. However, irradiation also causes necrosis in the brain. The necrotic region has a lower perfusion rate and interstitial pressure than tumor tissue; thus, the convective interstitial flow due to fluid leakage is expected to be smaller. Interstitial diffusion of macromolecules is higher in tumor tissue than in normal tissue, as the tumor tissue has larger interstitial spaces [29]. The progressive changes in tissue properties — due to changes in tumor size, irradiation, and activity of chemotherapy agent — may be an important determinant of drug transport and effectiveness of therapy in the clinical situation.

11.6 New Approaches to Drug Delivery Suggested by Modeling

Mathematical models, which describe the transport of drug following controlled delivery, can predict the penetration distance of drug and the local concentration of drug as a function of time and location. The calculations indicate that drugs with slow elimination will penetrate deeper into the tissue. The modulus f, which represents the ratio of elimination to diffusion rates in the tissue, provides a quantitative criterion for selecting agents for interstitial delivery. For example, high molecular weight dextrans were retained longer in the brain space, and penetrated a larger region of the brain than low molecular weight molecules following release from an intracranial implant [23]. This suggests a strategy for modifying molecules to improve their tissue penetration by conjugating active drug molecules to inert polymeric carriers. For conjugated drugs, the extent of penetration should depend on the modulus f for the conjugated compound as well as the degree of stability of the drug-carrier linkage.

The effects of conjugation and stability of the linkage between drug and carrier on enhancing tissue penetration in the brain have been studied in a model system [30]. Methotrexate (MTX)-dextran conjugates with different dissociation rates were produced by linking MTX to dextran (molecular weight 70,000) through a short-lived ester bond (half-life ≈ 3 d) and a longer-lived amide bond (half-life > 20 d). The extent of penetration for MTX-dextran conjugates was studied in three-dimensional human brain tumor cell cultures; penetration was significantly enhanced for MTX-dextran conjugates and the increased penetration was correlated with the stability of the linkage. These results suggest that modification of existing drugs may increase their efficacy against brain tumors when delivered directly to the brain interstitium.

11.7 Conclusion

Controlled release polymer implants are a useful new technology for delivering drugs directly to the brain interstitium. This approach is already in clinical use for treatment of tumors [31], and could soon impact treatment of other diseases. The mathematical models described in this paper provide a rational framework for analyzing drug distribution after delivery. These models describe the behavior of chemotherapy compounds very well and allow prediction of the effect of changing properties of the implant or the drug. More complex models are needed to describe the behavior of macromolecules, which encounter multiple modes of elimination and metabolism and are subject to the effects of fluid flow. In addition, variations on this approach may be useful for analyzing drug delivery in other situations.

References

[1] Lieb, W. and Stein, W., Biological membranes behave as non-porous polymeric sheets with respect to the diffusion of non-electrolytes. *Nature*, 1969, 224: 240–249.

[2] Stein, W.D., *The Movement of Molecules Across Cell Membranes.* 1967, New York: Academic Press.

[3] Simpkins, J., Bodor, N., and Enz, A., Direct evidence for brain-specific release of dopamine from a redox delivery system. *J. Pharmacol. Sci.*, 1985, 74: 1033–1036.

[4] Gregoriadis, G., The carrier potential of liposomes in biology and medicine. *N. Engl. J. Med.*, 1976, 295: 704–710.

[5] Cotzias, C.G., Van Woert, M.H., and Schiffer, L.M., Aromatic amino acids and modification of parkinsonism. *N. Engl. J. Med.*, 1967, 276: 374–379.

[6] Triguero, D., Buciak, J.B., Yang, J., and Pardridge, W.M., Blood–brain barrier transport of cationized immunoglobulin G: enhanced delivery compared to native protein. *Proc. Natl Acad. Sci. USA*, 1989, 86: 4761–4765.

[7] Tokuda, H., Takakura, Y., and Hashida, M., Targeted delivery of polyanions to the brain. *Proc. Int. Symp. Control. Rel. Bioact. Mat.*, 1993, 20: 270–271.

[8] Friden, P., Walus, L., Musso, G., Taylor, M., Malfroy, B., and Starzyk, R., Anti-transferrin receptor antibody and antibody-drug conjugates cross the blood–brain barrier. *Proc. Natl Acad. Sci. USA*, 1991, 88: 4771–4775.

[9] Friden, P.M., Walus, L.R., Watson, P., Doctrow, S.R., Kozarich, J.W., Backman, C., Bergman, H., Hoffer, B., Bloom, F., and Granholm, A.-C., Blood–brain barrier penetration and *in vivo* activity of an NGF conjugate. *Science*, 1993, 259: 373–377.

[10] Neuwelt, E., Barnett, P., Hellstrom, I., Hellstrom, K., Beaumier, P., McCormick, C., and Weigel, R., Delivery of melanoma-associated immunoglobulin monoclonal antibody and Fab fragments to normal brain utilizing osmotic blood–brain barrier disruption. *Cancer Res.*, 1988, 48: 4725–4729.

[11] Blasberg, R., Patlak, C., and Fenstermacher, J., Intrathecal chemotherapy: brain tissue profiles after ventriculocisternal perfusion. *J. Pharmacol. Exp. Therap.*, 1975, 195: 73–83.

[12] Yan, Q., Matheson, C., Sun, J., Radeke, M.J., Feinstein, S.C., and Miller, J.A., Distribution of intracerebral ventricularly administered neurotrophins in rat brain and its correlation with Trk receptor expression. *Exp. Neurol.*, 1994, 127: 23–36.

[13] Mahoney, M.J. and Saltzman, W.M., Controlled release of proteins to tissue transplants for the treatment of neurodegenerative disorders. *J. Pharm. Sci.*, 1996, 85: 1276–1281.

[14] Morrison, P.F., Laske, D.W., Bobo, H., Oldfield, E.H., and Dedrick, R.L., High-flow microinfusion: tissue penetration and pharmacodynamics. *Am. J. Physiol.*, 1994, 266: R292–R305.

[15] Haller, M.F. and Saltzman, W.M., Localized delivery of proteins in the brain: can transport be customized? *Pharm. Res.*, 1998, 15: 377–385.

[16] Wyatt, T.L. and Saltzman, W.M., Protein delivery from non-degradable polymer matrices, in *Protein Delivery — Physical Systems*, Saunders, L. and Hendren, W. (Eds.) 1997, New York: Plenum Press, pp. 119–137.

[17] Bird, R.B., Stewart, W.E., and Lightfoot, E.N., *Transport Phenomena*. 1960, New York: John Wiley & Sons, p. 780.

[18] Patlak, C. and Fenstermacher, J., Measurements of dog blood–brain transfer constants by ventriculocisternal perfusion. *Am. J. Physiol.*, 1975, 229: 877–884.

[19] Fung, L., Shin, M., Tyler, B., Brem, H., and Saltzman, W.M., Chemotherapeutic drugs released from polymers: distribution of 1,3-bis(2-chloroethyl)-1-nitrosourea in the rat brain. *Pharm. Res.*, 1996, 13: 671–682.

[20] Nicholson, C., Diffusion from an injected volume of a substance in brain tissue with arbitrary volume fraction and tortuosity. *Brain Res.*, 1985, 333: 325–329.

[21] Morrison, P. and Dedrick, R.L., Transport of cisplatin in rat brain following microinfusion: an analysis. *J. Pharm. Sci.*, 1986, 75: 120–128.

[22] Saltzman, W.M. and Radomsky, M.L., Drugs released from polymers: diffusion and elimination in brain tissue. *Chem. Eng. Sci.*, 1991, 46: 2429–2444.

[23] Dang, W. and Saltzman, W.M., Dextran retention in the rat brain following controlled release from a polymer. *Biotechnol. Prog.*, 1992, 8: 527–532.

[24] Krewson, C.E., Klarman, M., and Saltzman, W.M., Distribution of nerve growth factor following direct delivery to brain interstitium. *Brain Res.*, 1995, 680: 196–206.

[25] Krewson, C.E. and Saltzman, W.M., Transport and elimination of recombinant human NGF during long-term delivery to the brain. *Brain Res.*, 1996, 727: 169–181.

[26] Strasser, J.F., Fung, L.K., Eller, S., Grossman, S.A., and Saltzman, W.M., Distribution of 1,3-bis(2-chloroethyl)-1-nitrosourea (BCNU) and tracers in the rabbit brain following inter-stitial delivery by biodegradable polymer implants. *J. Pharmacol. Exp. Therap.*, 1995, 275: 1647–1655.

[27] Fung, L.K., Ewend, M.G., Sills, A., Sipos, E.P., Thompson, R., Watts, M., Colvin, O.M., Brem, H., and Saltzman, W.M., Pharmacokinetics of interstitial delivery of carmustine, 4-hydroperoxycyclophosphamide, and paclitaxel from a biodegradable polymer implant in the monkey brain. *Cancer Res.*, 1998, 58: 672–684.

[28] Jain, R.K., Barriers to drug delivery in solid tumors. *Sci. Am.*, 1994, 271: 58–65.

[29] Clauss, M.A. and Jain, R.K., Interstitial transport of rabbit and sheep antibodies in normal and neoplastic tissues. *Cancer Res.*, 1990, 50: 3487–3492.

[30] Dang, W.B., Colvin, O.M., Brem, H., and Saltzman, W.M., Covalent coupling of methotrexate to dextran enhances the penetration of cytotoxicity into a tissue-like matrix. *Cancer Res.*, 1994, 54: 1729–1735.

[31] Brem, H., Piantadosi, S., Burger, P.C., Walker, M., Selker, R., Vick, N.A., Black, K., Sisti, M., Brem, S., Mohr, G., Muller, P., Morawetz, R., Schold, S.C., and Group, P.-B.T.T., Placebo-controlled trial of safety and efficacy of intraoperative controlled delivery by biodegradable polymers of chemotherapy for recurrent gliomas. *Lancet*, 1995, 345: 1008–1012.

[32] Dang, W. and Saltzman, W.M., Controlled release of macromolecules from a biodegradable polyanhydride matrix. *J. Biomater. Sci., Polym. Ed.*, 1994, 6: 291–311.

[33] Dang, W., *Engineering Drugs and Delivery Systems for Brain Tumor Therapy*. 1993, The Johns Hopkins University.

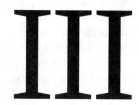

Biotechnology

Martin L. Yarmush and Mehmet Toner
Massachusetts General Hospital, Harvard Medical School, and the Shriners Burns Hospital

T HE TERM *BIOTECHNOLOGY* HAS UNDERGONE significant change over the past 50 years or so. During the period prior to the 1980s, biotechnology referred primarily to the use of microorganisms for large-scale industrial processes such as antibiotic production. Since the 1980s, with the advent of recombinant DNA technology, monoclonal antibody technology, and new technologies for studying and handling cells and tissues, the field of biotechnology has undergone a tremendous resurgence in a wide range of applications pertinent to industry, medicine, and science in general. It is some of these new ideas, concepts, and technologies that will be covered in this section. We have assembled a set of chapters that covers most topics in biotechnology that might interest the practicing biomedical engineer. Absent by design is coverage of agricultural, bioprocess, and environmental biotechnology, which is beyond the scope of this handbook.

Chapter 14 deals with our present ability to manipulate genetic material. This capability, which provides the practitioner with the potential to generate new proteins with improved biochemical and physico-chemical properties, has led to the formation of the field of protein engineering. Chapter 12 describes applications of nucleic acid chemistry. The burgeoning field of antisense technology is introduced with emphasis on basic techniques and potential applications to AIDS and cancer, and Chapter 12 is dedicated toward identifying the computational, chemical, and machine tools which are being developed and refined for genome analysis. Applied virology is the implied heading for Chapters 13 and 18, in which viral vaccines and viral-mediated gene therapy are the main foci.

Finally, Chapter 15 focus on important aspects of cell structure and function. These topics share a common approach toward quantitative analysis of cell behavior in order to develop the principles for cell growth and function. By viewing the world of biomedical biotechnology through our paradigm of proteins and nucleic acids to viruses to cells, today's biomedical engineer will hopefully be prepared to meet the challenge of participating in the greater field of biotechnology as an educated observer at the very least.

12

Tools for Genome Analysis

Robert Kaiser
University of Washington

The development of sophisticated and powerful recombinant techniques for manipulating and analyzing genetic material has led to the emergence of a new biologic discipline, often termed molecular biology. The tools of molecular biology have enabled scientists to begin to understand many of the fundamental processes of life, generally through the identification, isolation, and structural and functional analysis of individual or, at best, limited numbers of genes. Biology is now at a point where it is feasible to begin a more ambitious endeavor — the complete genetic analysis of entire genomes. Genome analysis aims not only to identify and molecularly characterize all the genes that orchestrate the development of an organism but also to understand the complex and interactive regulatory mechanisms of these genes, their organization in the genome, and the role of genetic variation in disease, adaptability, and individuality. Additionally, the study of homologous genetic regions across species can provide important insight into their evolutionary history.

As can be seen in Table 12.1, the genome of even a small organism consists of a very large amount of information. Thus the analysis of a complete genome is not simply a matter of using conventional techniques that work well with individual genes (comprised of perhaps 1,000 to 10,000 base pairs) a sufficient (very large) number of times to cover the genome. Such a brute-force approach would be too slow and too expensive, and conventional data-handling techniques would be inadequate for the task of cataloging, storing, retrieving, and analyzing such a large amount of information. The amount of manual labor and scientific expertise required would be prohibitive. New technology is needed to provide high-throughput, low-cost automation and reduced reliance on expert intervention at intermediate levels in the processes required for large-scale genetic analysis. Novel computational tools are required to deal

TABLE 12.1   DNA Content of Various Genomes in Monomer
Units (Base Pairs)

Organism	Type	Size
Phage T4	Bacteriophage (virus)	160,000
Escherichia coli	Bacterium	4,000,000
Saccharomyces	Yeast	14,000,000
Arabidopsis thaliana	Plant	100,000,000
Caenorhabditis elegans	Nematode	100,000,000
Drosophila melanogaster	Insect (fruit fly)	165,000,000
Mouse	Mammal	3,000,000,000
Human	Mammal	3,500,000,000

Source: Adapted from Watson, J.D., Gilman, M., Witkowski, J.,
and Zoller, M. (Eds) (1992). *Recombinant DNA*; Lewin, B.
(1987). *Genes III*, With permission.

with the large volumes of genetic information produced. Individual tools must be integrated smoothly to produce an analytical system in which samples are tracked through the entire analytical process, intermediate decisions and branch points are few, a stable, reliable and routine protocol or set of protocols is employed, and the resulting information is presented to the biologic scientist in a useful and meaningful format. It is important to realize that the development of these tools requires the interdisciplinary efforts of biologists, chemists, physicists, engineers, mathematicians, and computer scientists.

Genome analysis is a complex and extended series of interrelated processes. The basic processes involved are diagrammed in Figure 12.1. At each stage, new biologic, chemical, physical (mechanical, optical), and computational tools have been developed within the last 10 years that have begun to enable large-scale (megabase) genetic analysis. These developments have largely been spurred by the goals of the Human Genome Project, a worldwide effort to decipher the entirety of human genetics. However, biologists are still a significant ways away from having a true genome analysis capability [3], and as such, new technologies are still emerging.

This chapter cannot hope to describe in depth the entire suite of tools currently in use in genome analysis. Instead, it will attempt to present the basic principles involved and to highlight some of the recent enabling technological developments that are likely to remain in use in genome analysis for the foreseeable future. Some fundamental knowledge of biology is assumed; in this regard, an excellent beginning text for individuals with a minimal background in molecular biology is that by Watson et al. [1].

12.1   General Principles

The fundamental blueprint for any cell or organism is encoded in its genetic material, its deoxyribonucleic acid (DNA). DNA is a linear polymer derived from a four-letter biochemical alphabet — A, C, G, and T. These four letters are often referred to as nucleotides or bases. The linear order of bases in a segment of DNA is termed its DNA sequence and determines its function. A gene is a segment of DNA whose sequence directly determines its translated protein product. Other DNA sequences are recognized by the cellular machinery as start and stop sites for protein synthesis, regulate the temporal or spatial expression of genes, or play a role in the organization of higher-order DNA structures such as chromosomes. Thus a thorough understanding of the DNA sequence of a cell or organism is fundamental to an understanding of its biology.

Recombinant DNA technology affords biologists the capability to manipulate and analyze DNA sequences. Many of the techniques employed take advantage of a basic property of DNA, the molecular complementarity of the two strands of the double helix. This complementarity arises from the specific hydrogen-bonding interactions between pairs of DNA bases, A with T and C with G. Paired double strands of DNA can be denatured, or rendered into the component single strands, by any process that disrupts

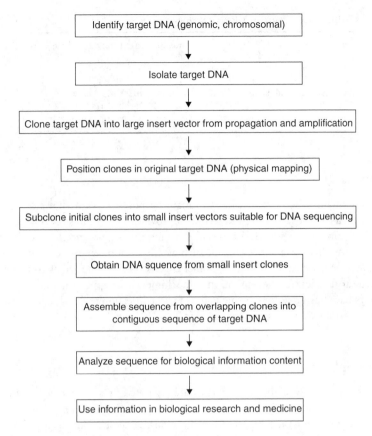

FIGURE 12.1   Basic steps in genome analysis.

TABLE 12.2   Enzymes Commonly Used in Genome Analysis

Enzyme	Function	Common use
Restriction endonuclease	Cleave double-stranded DNA at specific sites	Mapping, cloning
DNA polymerase	Synthesize complementary DNA strand	DNA sequencing, amplification
Polynucleotide kinase	Adds phosphate to 5′ end of single-stranded DNA	Radiolabeling, cloning
Terminal transferase	Adds nucleotides to the 3′ end of single-stranded DNA	Labeling
Reverse transcriptase	Makes DNA copy from RNA	RNA sequencing, cDNA cloning
DNA ligase	Covalently joins two DNA fragments	Cloning

these hydrogen bonds — high temperature, chaotropic agents, or pH extremes. Complementary single strands also can be renatured into the duplex structure by reversing the disruptive element; this process is sometimes referred to as hybridization or annealing, particularly when one of the strands has been supplied from some exogenous source.

Molecular biology makes extensive use of the DNA-modifying enzymes employed by cells during replication, translation, repair, and protection from foreign DNA. A list of commonly used enzymes, their functions, and some of the experimental techniques in which they are utilized is provided in Table 12.2.

12.2   Enabling Technologies

The following are broadly applicable tools that have been developed in the context of molecular biology and are commonly used in genome analysis.

TABLE 12.3 Common Cloning Vectors

Vector	Approximate insert size range (base pairs)
Bacteriophage M13	100–5000
Plasmid	100–10,000
Bacteriophage lambda	10,000–15,000
Cosmid	25,000–50,000
Yeast artificial chromosome (YAC)	100,000–1,000,000

12.2.1 Cloning

Cloning is a recombinant procedure that has two main purposes: First, it allows one to select a single DNA fragment from a complex mixture, and second, it provides a means to store, manipulate, propagate, and produce large numbers of identical molecules having this single ancestor. A cloning vector is a DNA fragment derived from a microorganism, such as a bacteriophage or yeast, into which a foreign DNA fragment may be inserted to produce a chimeric DNA species. The vector contains all the genetic information necessary to allow for the replication of the chimera in an appropriate host organism. A variety of cloning vectors have been developed which allow for the insertion and stable propagation of foreign DNA segments of various sizes; these are indicated in Table 12.3.

12.2.2 Electrophoresis

Electrophoresis is a process whereby nucleic acids are separated by size in a sieving matrix under the influence of an electric field. In free solution, DNA, being highly negatively charged by virtue of its phosphodiester backbone, migrates rapidly toward the positive pole of an electric field. If the DNA is forced instead to travel through a molecularly porous substance, such as a gel, the smaller (shorter) fragments of DNA will travel through the pores more rapidly than the larger (longer) fragments, thus effecting separation. Agarose, a highly purified derivative of agar, is commonly used to separate relatively large fragments of DNA (100 to 50,000 base pairs) with modest resolution (50 to 100 base pairs), while cross-linked polyacrylamide is used to separate smaller fragments (10 to 1,000 base pairs) with single base-pair resolution. Fragment sizes are generally estimated by comparison with standards run in another lane of the same gel. Electrophoresis is used extensively as both an analytical and a preparative tool in molecular biology.

12.2.3 Enzymatic DNA Sequencing

In the late 1970s, Sanger and coworkers [4] reported a procedure employing DNA polymerase to obtain DNA sequence information from unknown cloned fragments. While significant improvements and modifications have been made since that time, the basic technique remains the same: DNA polymerase is used to synthesize a complementary copy of an unknown single-stranded DNA (the template) in the presence of the four DNA monomers (deoxynucleotide triphosphates, or dNTPs). DNA polymerase requires a double-stranded starting point, so a single-stranded DNA (the primer) is hybridized at a unique site on the template (usually in the vector), and it is at this point that DNA synthesis is initiated. Key to the sequencing process is the use of a modified monomer, a dideoxynucleotide triphosphate (ddNTP), in each reaction. The ddNTP lacks the 3′-hydroxyl functionality (it has been replaced by a hydrogen) necessary for phosphodiester bond formation, and its incorporation thus blocks further elongation of the growing chain by polymerase. Four reactions are carried out, each containing all four dNTPs and one of the four ddNTPs. By using the proper ratios of dNTPs to ddNTP, each reaction generates a nested set of fragments, each fragment beginning at exactly the same point (the primer) and terminating with a particular ddNTP

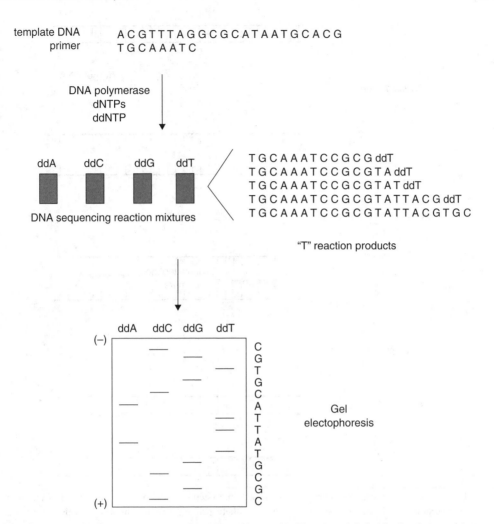

template DNA   A C G T T T A G G C G C A T A A T G C A C G
      primer   T G C A A A T C

DNA polymerase
dNTPs
ddNTP

ddA   ddC   ddG   ddT   T G C A A A T C C G C G ddT
                                        T G C A A A T C C G C G T A ddT
                                        T G C A A A T C C G C G T A T ddT
                                        T G C A A A T C C G C G T A T T A C G ddT
DNA sequencing reaction mixtures   T G C A A A T C C G C G T A T T A C G T G C

                                             "T" reaction products

                  ddA   ddC   ddG   ddT
           (−)   C
                                            G
                                            T
                                            G
                                            C
                                            A   Gel
                                            T   electophoresis
                                            T
                                            A
                                            T
                                            G
                                            C
                                            G
           (+)   C

FIGURE 12.2 Enzymatic DNA sequencing. A synthetic oligonucleotide primer is hybridized to its complementary site on the template DNA. DNA polymerase and dNTPs are then used to synthesize a complementary copy of the unknown portion of the template in the presence of a chain-terminating ddNTP (see text). A nested set of fragments beginning with the primer sequence and ending at every ddNTP position is produced in each reaction (the ddTTP reaction products are shown). Four reactions are carried out, one for each ddNTP. The products of each reaction are then separated by gel electrophoresis in individual lanes, and the resulting ladders are visualized. The DNA sequence is obtained by reading up the set of four ladders, one base at a time, from smallest to largest fragment.

at each base complementary to that ddNTP in the template sequence. The products of the reactions are then separated by electrophoresis in four lanes of a polyacrylamide slab gel. Since conventional sequencing procedures utilize radiolabeling (incorporation of a small amount of ^{32}P- or ^{35}S-labeled dNTP by the polymerase), visualization of the gel is achieved by exposing it to film. The sequence can be obtained from the resulting autoradiogram, which appears as a series of bands (often termed a ladder) in each of the four lanes. Each band is composed of fragments of a single size, the shortest fragments being at the bottom of the gel and the longest at the top. Adjacent bands represent a single base pair difference, so the sequence is determined by reading up the ladders in the four lanes and noting which lane contains the band with the next largest sized fragments. The enzymatic sequencing process is diagrammed in Figure 12.2. It should be noted that although other methods exist, the enzymatic sequencing technique is currently the most commonly used DNA sequencing procedure due to its simplicity and reliability.

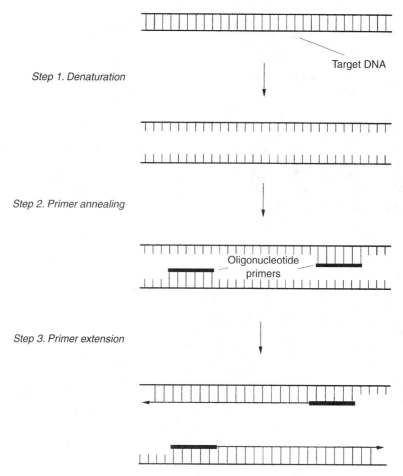

FIGURE 12.3 The first cycle in the polymerase chain reaction. In step 1, the double-stranded target DNA is thermally denatured to produce single-stranded species. A pair of synthetic primers, flanking the specific region of interest, are annealed to the single strands to form initiation sites for DNA synthesis by polymerase (step 2). Finally, complementary copies of each target single strand are synthesized by polymerase in the presence of dNTPs, thus doubling the amount of target DNA initially present (step 3). Repetition of this cycle effectively doubles the target population, affording one million-fold or greater amplification of the initial target sequence.

12.2.4   Polymerase Chain Reaction (PCR)

PCR [5] is an *in vitro* procedure for amplifying particular DNA sequences up to 108-fold that is utilized in an ever-increasing variety of ways in genome analysis. The sequence to be amplified is defined by a pair of single-stranded primers designed to hybridize to unique sites flanking the target sequence on opposite strands. DNA polymerase in the presence of the four dNTPs is used to synthesize a complementary DNA copy across the target sequence starting at the two primer sites. The amplification procedure is performed by repeating the following cycle 25 to 50 times (see Figure 12.3). First, the double-stranded target DNA is denatured at high temperature (94 to 96°C). Second, the mixture is cooled, allowing the primers to anneal to their complementary sites on the target single strands. Third, the temperature is adjusted for optimal DNA polymerase activity, initiating synthesis. Since the primers are complementary to the newly synthesized strands as well as the original target, each cycle of denaturation/annealing/synthesis effectively doubles the amount of target sequence present in the reaction, resulting in a 2^n amplification (n = number of cycles). The initial implementation of PCR utilized a polymerase that was unstable at the high temperatures required for denaturation, thus requiring manual addition of polymerase prior to the synthesis step of every cycle. An important technological development was the isolation of DNA polymerase from a thermophilic bacterium, Thermus aquaticus (Taq), which can withstand the high denaturation temperatures [6]. Additionally, the high optimal synthesis temperature (70 to 72°C) of Taq polymerase improves the specificity of the amplification process by reducing spurious priming from annealing of the primers to nonspecific secondary sites in the target.

While PCR can be performed successfully manually, it is a tedious process, and numerous thermal cycling instruments have become commercially available. Modern thermal cyclers are programmable and capable of processing many samples at once, using either small plastic tubes or microtiter plates, and are characterized by accurate and consistent temperature control at all sample positions, rapid temperature ramping, and minimal temperature over/undershoot. Temperature control is provided by a variety of means (Peltier elements, forced air, water) using metal blocks or water or air baths. Speed, precise temperature control, and high sample throughput are the watchwords of current thermal cycler design.

PCR technology is commonly used to provide sufficient material for cloning from genomic DNA sources, to identify and characterize particular DNA sequences in an unknown mixture, to rapidly produce templates for DNA sequencing from very small amounts of target DNA, and in cycle sequencing, a modification of the enzymatic sequencing procedure that utilizes Taq polymerase and thermal cycling to amplify the products of the sequencing reactions.

12.2.5 Chemical Synthesis of Oligodeoxynucleotides

The widespread use of techniques based on DNA polymerase, such as enzymatic DNA sequencing and the PCR, as well as of numerous other techniques utilizing short, defined-sequence, single-stranded DNAs in genome analysis, is largely due to the ease with which small oligodeoxynucleotides can be obtained. The chemical synthesis of oligonucleotides has become a routine feature of both individual biology laboratories and core facilities. The most widely used chemistry for assembling short (<100 base pair) oligonucleotides is the phosphoramidite approach [7], which has developed over the past 15 years or so. This approach is characterized by rapid, high-yield reactions and stable reagents. Like modern peptide synthesis chemistry, the approach relies on the tethering of the growing DNA chain to a solid support (classically glass or silica beads, more recently cross-linked polystyrene) and is cyclic in nature. At the end of the assembly, the desired oligonucleotide is chemically cleaved from the support, generally in a form that is sufficiently pure for its immediate use in a number of applications. The solid phase provides two significant advantages: It allows for the use of large reagent excesses, driving the reactions to near completion in accord with the laws of mass action while reducing the removal of these excesses following the reactions to a simple matter of thorough washing, and it enables the reactions to be performed in simple, flow-through cartridges, making the entire synthesis procedure easily automatable. Indeed, a number of chemical DNA synthesis instruments ("gene machines") are commercially available, capable of synthesizing one to several oligonucleotides at once. Desired sequences are programmed through a keyboard or touchpad, reagents are installed, and DNA is obtained a few hours later. Improvements in both chemistry and instrument design have been aimed at increasing synthesis throughput (reduced cycle times, increased number of simultaneous sequence assemblies), decreasing scale (most applications in genome analysis require subnanomole quantities of any particular oligonucleotide), and concomitant with these two, reducing cost per oligonucleotide.

12.3 Tools for Genome Analysis

12.3.1 Physical Mapping

In the analysis of genomes, it is often useful to begin with a less complex mixture than an entire genome DNA sample. Individual chromosomes can be obtained in high purity using a technology known as chromosome sorting [8], a form of flow cytometry. A suspension of chromosomes stained with fluorescent dye is flowed past a laser beam. As a chromosome enters the beam, appropriate optics detect the scattered and emitted light. Past the beam, the stream is acoustically broken into small droplets. The optical signals are used to electronically trigger the collection of droplets containing chromosomes by electrostatically charging these droplets and deflecting them into a collection medium using a strong electric field. Chromosomes can be differentiated by staining the suspension with two different dyes that bind in differing amounts to the various chromosomes and looking at the ratio of the emission intensity of each dye as it passes the laser/detector. Current commercial chromosome sorting instrumentation is relatively slow, requiring several days to collect sufficient material for subsequent analysis.

As mentioned previously, whole genomes or even chromosomes cannot yet be analyzed as intact entities. As such, fractionation of large nucleic acids into smaller fragments is necessary to obtain the physical material on which to perform genetic analysis. Fractionation can be achieved using a variety of techniques: limited or complete digestion by restriction enzymes, sonication, or physical shearing through a small orifice. These fragments are then cloned into an appropriate vector, the choice of which depends on the size range of fragments involved (see Table 12.3). The composite set of clones derived from a large nucleic acid is termed a library. In general, it is necessary to produce several libraries in different cloning vectors containing different-sized inserts. This is necessary because the mapping of clones is facilitated by larger inserts, while the sequencing of clones requires shorter inserts.

The library-generating process yields a very large number of clones having an almost random distribution of insert endpoints in the original fragment. It would be very costly to analyze all clones in a library, and unnecessary as well. Instead, a subset of overlapping clones is selected whose inserts span the entire starting fragment. These clones must be arrayed in the linear order in which they are found in the starting fragment; the process for doing this is called physical mapping. The conventional method for physically mapping clones uses restriction enzymes to cleave each clone at enzyme-specific sites, separating the products of the digestion by electrophoresis, and comparing the resulting patterns of restriction fragment sizes for different clones to find similarities. Clones exhibiting a number of the same-sized fragments likely possess the same subsequence and thus overlap. Clearly, the longer the inserts contained in the library, the faster a large genetic region can be covered by this process, since fewer clones are required to span the distance. Physical mapping also provides landmarks, the enzyme cleavage sites in the sequence, that can be used to provide reference points for the mapping of genes and other functional sequences. Mapping by restriction enzyme digestion is simple and reliable to perform; however, manual map assembly from the digest data is laborious, and significant effort is currently being expended in the development of robust and accurate map assembly software.

Normal agarose gel electrophoresis can effectively separate DNA fragments less than 10,000 base pairs and fragments between 10,000 and 50,000 base pairs less effectively under special conditions. However, the development of very large insert cloning vectors, such as the yeast artificial chromosome [9], necessitated the separation of fragments significantly larger than 10,000 base pairs to allow for use in physical mapping. In order to address this issue, a technology called pulsed-field gel electrophoresis (PFGE) was developed. Unlike conventional electrophoresis, in which the electric field remains essentially constant, homogeneous, and unidirectional during a separation, PFGE utilizes an electric field that periodically changes its orientation. The principle of PFGE is thought to be as follows: When DNA molecules are placed in an electric field, the molecules elongate in the direction of the field and then begin to migrate through the gel pores. When the field is removed, the molecules relax to a more random coiled state and stop moving. Reapplication of the field in another orientation causes the DNA to change its conformation in order to align in that direction prior to migration. The time required for this conformational change to occur has been found to be very dependent on the size of the molecules, with larger molecules reorienting more slowly than small ones. Thus longer DNAs move more slowly under the influence of the constantly switching electric field than shorter ones, and size-based separation occurs. PFGE separations of molecules as large as 10 million base pairs have been demonstrated. Numerous instruments for PFGE have been constructed, differing largely in the strategy employed to provide electric field switching [10].

Physical maps based on restriction sites are of limited long-term utility, since they require the provision of physical material from the specific library from which the map was derived in order to be utilized experimentally. A more robust landmarking approach based on the PCR has been developed recently [11], termed sequence-tagged site (STS) content mapping. An STS is a short, unique sequence in a genome that can be amplified by the PCR. Clones in a library are screened for the presence of a particular STS using PCR; if the STS is indeed unique in the genome, then clones possessing that STS are reliably expected to overlap. Physical mapping is thus reduced to choosing and synthesizing pairs of PCR primers that define unique sequences in the genome. Additionally, since STSs are defined by pairs of primer sequences, they can be stored in a database and are thus universally accessible.

12.3.2 DNA Sequencing

Early in the development of tools for large-scale DNA analysis, it was recognized that one of the most costly and time-consuming processes was the accumulation of DNA sequence information. Two factors, the use of radioisotopic labels and the manual reading and recording of DNA sequence films, made it impossible to consider genome-scale (106 to 109 base pairs) sequence analysis using the conventional techniques. To address this, several groups embarked on the development of automated DNA sequencing instruments [12–14]. Today, automated DNA sequencing is one of the most highly advanced of the technologies for genome analysis, largely due to the extensive effort expended in instrument design, biochemical organization, and software development.

Key to the development of these instruments was the demonstration that fluorescence could be employed in the place of autoradiography for detection of fragments in DNA sequencing gels and that the use of fluorescent labels enabled the acquisition of DNA sequence data in an automated fashion in real time. Two approaches have been demonstrated: the "single-color, four-lane" approach and the "four-color, single-lane" approach. The former simply replaces the radioisotopic label used in conventional enzymatic sequencing with a fluorescent label, and the sequence is determined by the order of fluorescent bands in the four lanes of the gel. The latter utilizes a different-colored label for each of the four sequencing reactions (thus A might be "blue," C, "green," G, "yellow," and T, "red"). The four base-specific reactions are performed separately and upon completion are combined and electrophoresed in a single lane of the gel, and the DNA sequence is determined from the temporal pattern of fluorescent colors passing the detector. For a fixed number of gel lanes (current commercial automated DNA sequencers have 24 to 36), the four-color approach provides greater sample throughput than the single-color approach. Instruments employing the four-color technology are more widely used for genome analysis at present, and as such, this strategy will be discussed more fully.

In order to utilize fluorescence as a detection strategy for DNA sequencing, a chemistry had to be developed for the specific incorporation of fluorophores into the nested set of fragments produced in the enzymatic sequencing reactions. The flexibility of chemical DNA synthesis provided a solution to this problem. A chemistry was developed for the incorporation of an aliphatic primary amine in the last cycle of primer synthesis (i.e., at the $5'$ terminus) using standard DNA synthesis protocols [15,16]. This amine was then conjugated with any of several of readily available amine-reactive fluorochromes that had been developed previously for the labeling of proteins to produce the desired labeled sequencing primers. The purified dye-primer was demonstrated to perform well in DNA sequencing, exhibiting both efficient extension by the polymerase and the necessary single-base resolution in the electrophoretic separation [12]. A set of four spectrally discriminable, amine-reactive fluorophores has been developed [16] for DNA sequencing.

While dye-primers are relatively easy to obtain by this method, they are costly to prepare in small quantities and require sophisticated chromatographic instrumentation to obtain products pure enough for sequencing use. Thus they are generally prepared in large amounts and employed as vector-specific "universal" primers, as in situations in which a very large number of inserts cloned in a given vector need to be sequenced [17]. For occasions where small amounts of sample-specific primers are needed, as in the sequencing of products from the PCR, a simpler and more economical alternative is the use of dideoxynucleotides covalently coupled to fluorescent dyes (so-called dye-terminators), since these reagents allow the use of conventional unlabeled primers [18].

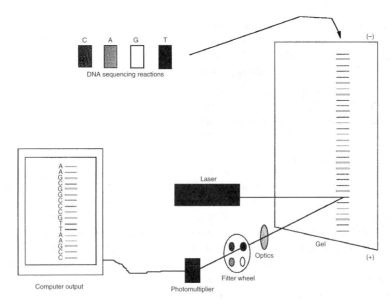

FIGURE 12.4 Schematic illustration of automated fluorescence-based DNA sequencing using the "four-color, single-lane" approach. The products of each of the four enzymatic sequencing reactions are "color-coded" with a different fluorescent dye, either through the use of dye-labeled primers or dye-terminators. The four reaction mixtures are then combined and the mixture separated by gel electrophoresis. The beam of an argon ion laser is mechanically scanned across the width of the gel near its bottom to excite the labeled fragments to fluorescence. The emitted light is collected through a four-color filter wheel onto a photomultiplier tube. The color of each fluorescing band is determined automatically by a computer from the characteristic four-point spectrum of each dye, and the order of colors passing the detector is subsequently translated into DNA sequence information.

Special instrumentation (Figure 12.4) has been developed for the fluorescence-based detection of nucleic acids in DNA sequencing gels. An argon ion laser is used to excite the fluorescent labels in order to provide sufficient excitation energy at the appropriate wavelength for high-sensitivity detection. The laser beam is mechanically scanned across the width of the gel near its bottom in order to interrogate all lanes. As the labeled DNA fragments undergoing electrophoresis move through the laser beam, their emission is collected by focusing optics onto a photomultiplier tube located on the scanning stage. Between the photomultiplier tube and the gel is a rotating four-color filter wheel. The emitted light from the gel is collected through each of the four filters in the wheel in turn, generating a continuous four-point spectrum of the detected radiation. The color of the emission of the passing bands is determined from the characteristic four-point spectrum of each fluorophore, and the identified color is then translated into DNA sequence using the associated dye/base pairings. Sequence acquisition and data analysis are handled completely by computer; the system is sufficiently sophisticated that the operator can load the samples on the gel, activate the electrophoresis and the data acquisition, and return the next day for the analyzed data. The current commercial implementation of this technology produces about 450 to 500 bases per lane of analyzed DNA sequence information at an error rate of a few percent in a 12- to 14-h period.

The rate of data production of current DNA sequencers is still too low to provide true genome-scale analytical capabilities, although projects in the few hundred kilobase pair range have been accomplished. Improvements such as the use of gel-filled capillaries [19] or ultrathin slab gels (thicknesses on the order of 50 to 100 mm as opposed to the conventional 200 to 400 mm) [20,21] are currently being explored. The improved heat dissipation in these thin-gel systems allows for the use of increased electric field strengths during electrophoresis, with a concomitant reduction in run time of fivefold or so.

The greatly increased throughput of the automated instruments over manual techniques has resulted in the generation of a new bottleneck in the DNA sequencing process that will only be exacerbated by higher-throughput systems: the preparation of sufficient sequencing reaction products for analysis. This encompasses two preparative processes, the preparation of sequencing templates and the performance of sequencing reactions. Automation of the latter process has been approached initially through the development of programmable pipetting robots that operate in the 96-well microtiter plate format commonly used for immunoassays, since a 96-well plate will accommodate sequencing reactions for 24 templates. Sequencing robots of this sort have become important tools for large-scale sequencing projects. Template preparation has proven more difficult to automate. No reliable system for selecting clones, infecting and culturing bacteria, and isolating DNA has been produced, although several attempts are in progress. It is clear that unlike in the case of the sequencing robots, where instrumentation has mimicked manual manipulations with programmable mechanics, successful automation of template preparation will require a rethinking of current techniques with an eye toward process automation. Furthermore, in order to obtain true genome-scale automation, the entire sequencing procedure from template preparation through data acquisition will need to be reengineered to minimize, if not eliminate, operator intervention using the principles of systems integration, process management, and feedback control.

12.3.3 Genetic Mapping

Simply stated, genetic mapping is concerned with identifying the location of genes on chromosomes. Classically, this is accomplished using a combination of mendelian and molecular genetics called linkage analysis, a complete description of which is too complex to be fully described here (but see Watson et al. [1]). However, an interesting approach to physically locating clones (and the genes contained within them) on chromosomes is afforded by a technique termed fluorescence in situ hybridization (FISH) [22]. Fluorescently labeled DNA probes derived from cosmid clones can be hybridized to chromosome spreads, and the location of the probe-chromosome hybrid can be observed using fluorescence microscopy. Not only can clones be mapped to particular chromosomes in this way, but positions and distances relative to chromosomal landmarks (such as cytogenetic bands, telomere, or centromere) can be estimated to as little as 50,000 base pairs in some cases, although 1 million base pairs or larger is more usual. The technique is particularly useful when two or more probes of different colors are used to order sequences relative to one another.

12.3.4 Computation

Computation plays a central role in genome analysis at a variety of levels, and significant efforts has been expanded on the development of software and hardware tools for biologic applications. A large effort has been expended in the development of software that will rapidly assemble a large contiguous DNA sequence from the many smaller sequences obtained from automated instruments. This assembly process is computationally demanding, and only recently have good software tools for this purpose become readily available. Automated sequencers produce 400 to 500 base pairs of sequence per template per run. However, in order to completely determine the linear sequence of a 50,000-base-pair cosmid insert (which can be conceptually represented as a linear array of 100 adjacent 500-base-pair templates), it is necessary to assemble sequence from some 300 to 1,000 clones to obtain the redundancy of data needed for a high-accuracy finished sequence, depending on the degree to which the clones can be preselected for sequencing based on a previously determined physical map. Currently, the tools for acquiring and assembling sequence information are significantly better than those for physical mapping; as such, most large-scale projects employ strategies that emphasize sequencing at the expense of mapping [23]. Improved tools for acquiring and assembling mapping data are under development, however, and it remains to be seen what effect they will have on the speed and cost of obtaining finished sequence on a genome scale relative to the current situation.

Many software tools have been developed in the context of the local needs of large-scale projects. These include software for instrument control (data acquisition and signal processing), laboratory information-management systems, and local data-handling schemes. The development of process approaches to the automation of genome analysis will necessitate the continued development of tools of these types.

The final outcome of the analysis of any genome will be a tremendous amount of sequence information that must be accessible to researchers interested in the biology of the organism from which it was derived. Frequently, the finished genomic sequence will be the aggregate result of the efforts of many laboratories. National and international information resources (databases) are currently being established worldwide to address the issues of collecting, storing, correlating, annotating, standardizing, and distributing this information. Significant effort is also being expended to develop tools for the rapid analysis of genome sequence data that will enable biologists to find new genes and other functional genetic regions, compare very large DNA sequences for similarity, and study the role of genetic variation in biology. Eventually, as the robust tools for predicting protein tertiary structure and function from primary acid sequence data are developed, genome analysis will extend to the protein domain through the translation of new DNA sequences into their functional protein products.

12.4   Conclusions

Genome analysis is a large-scale endeavor whose goal is the complete understanding of the basic blueprint of life The scale of even the smallest genomes of biologic interest is too large to be effectively analyzed using the traditional tools of molecular biology and genetics. Over the past 10 years, a suite of biochemical techniques and bioanalytical instrumentation has been developed that has allowed biologists to begin to probe large genetic regions, although true genome-scale technology is still in its infancy. It is anticipated that the next 10 years will see developments in the technology for physical mapping, DNA sequencing, and genetic mapping that will allow for a 10- to 100-fold increase in our ability to analyze genomes, with a concomitant decrease in cost, through the application of process-based principles and assembly-line approaches. The successful realization of a true genome analysis capability will require the close collaborative efforts of individuals from numerous disciplines in both science and engineering.

Acknowledgments

I would like to thank Dr. Leroy Hood, Dr. Maynard Olson, Dr. Barbara Trask, Dr. Tim Hunkapiller, Dr. Deborah Nickerson, and Dr. Lee Rowen for the useful information, both written and verbal, that they provided me during the preparation of this chapter.

References

[1] Watson, J.D., Gilman, M., Witkowski, J., and Zoller, M. (Eds) (1992). *Recombinant DNA*, 2d ed. New York, Scientific American Books, WH Freeman.

[2] Lewin, B. (1987). *Genes III*, 3rd ed. New York, Wiley.

[3] Olson, M.V. (1993). The human genome project. *Proc. Natl. Acad. Sci. U.S.A.* 90: 4338.

[4] Sanger, F., Nicklen, S., and Coulson, A.R. (1977). DNA sequencing with chain-terminating inhibitors. *Proc. Natl Acad. Sci USA* 74: 5463.

[5] Saiki, R.K., Scharf, S.J., and Faloona, F. et al. (1985). Enzymatic amplification of betaglobin sequences and restriction site analysis for diagnosis of sickle cell anemia. *Science* 230: 1350.

[6] Saiki, R.K., Gelfand, D.H., and Stoffel, S. et al. (1988). Primer-directed enzymatic amplification of DNA with a thermostable DNA polymerase. *Science* 239: 487.

[7] Gait, M.J. (Ed.) (1984). *Oligonucleotide Synthesis: A Practical Approach.* Oxford, England, IRL Press.

[8] Engh, Gvd. (1993). New applications of flow cytometry. *Curr. Opin. Biotechnol.* 4: 63.

[9] Burke, D.T., Carle, G.F., and Olson, M.V. (1987). Cloning of large segments of exogenous DNA into yeast by means of artificial chromosome vectors. *Science* 236: 806.

[10] Lai, E., Birren, B.W., Clark, S.M., and Hood, L. (1989). Pulsed field gel electrophoresis. *Biotechniques* 7: 34.

[11] Olson, M., Hood, L., Cantor, C., and Botstein, D. (1989). A common language for physical mapping of the human genome. *Science* 245: 1434.

[12] Smith, L.M., Sanders, J.Z., Kaiser, R.J. et al. (1986). Fluorescence detection in automated DNA sequence analysis. *Nature* 321: 674.

[13] Prober, J.M., Trainor, G.L., Dam, R.J. et al. (1987). A system for rapid DNA sequencing with fluorescent chain terminating dideoxynucleotides. *Science* 238: 336.

[14] Ansorge, W., Sproat, B., Stegemann, J. et al. (1987). Automated DNA sequencing: ultrasensitive detection of fluorescent bands during electrophoresis. *Nucleic Acids Res.* 15: 4593.

[15] Smith, L.M., Fung, S., Hunkapiller, M.W. et al. (1985). The synthesis of oligonucleotides containing an aliphtic amino group at the 5′ terminus: synthesis of fluorescent DNA primers for use in DNA sequencing. *Nucleic Acids Res.* 15: 2399.

[16] Connell, C., Fung, S., Heiner, C. et al. (1987). *Biotechniques* 5: 342.

[17] Kaiser, R., Hunkapiller, T., Heiner, C., and Hood, L. (1993). Specific primer-directed DNA sequence analysis using automated fluorescence detection and labeled primers. *Meth. Enzymol.* 218: 122.

[18] Lee, L.G., Connell, C.R., Woo, S.L. et al. (1992). DNA sequencing with dye-labeled terminators and T7 DNA polymerase: effect of dyes and dNTPs on incorporation of dye-terminators and probability analysis of termination fragments. *Nucleic Acids Res.* 20: 2471.

[19] Mathies, R.A. and Huang, X.C. (1992). Capillary array electrophoresis: an approach to high-speed, high-throughput DNA sequencing. *Nature* 359: 167.

[20] Brumley, R.L. Jr. and Smith, L.M. (1991). Rapid DNA sequencing by horizontal ultrathin gel electrophoresis. *Nucleic Acids Res.* 19: 4121.

[21] Stegemann, J., Schwager, C., Erfle, H. et al. (1991). High speed on-line DNA sequencing on ultrathin slab gels. *Nucleic Acids Res.* 19: 675.

[22] Trask, B.J. (1991). Gene mapping by in situ hybridization. *Curr. Opin. Genet. Dev.* 1: 82.

[23] Hunkapiller, T., Kaiser, R.J., Koop, B.F., and Hood, L. (1991). Large-scale and automated DNA sequencing. *Science* 254: 59.

13

Vaccine Production

John G. Aunins
Ann L. Lee
David B. Volkin
Merck Research Laboratories

Vaccines are biologic preparations that elicit immune system responses that protect an animal against pathogenic organisms. The primary component of the vaccine is an **antigen**, which can be a weakened (**attenuated**) version of an infectious **pathogen** or a purified molecule derived from the pathogen. Upon oral administration or injection of a vaccine, the immune system generates humoral (antibody) and cellular (cytotoxic, or killer T cell) responses that destroy the antigen or antigen-infected cells. When properly administered, the immune response to a vaccine has a long-term memory component, which protects the host against future infections. Vaccines often contain **adjuvants** to enhance immune response, as well as formulation agents to preserve the antigen during storage or upon administration, to provide proper delivery of antigen, and to minimize side reactions.

Table 13.1 presents a simple classification scheme for vaccines according to the type of organism and antigen, Live, attenuated whole-organism vaccines have been favored for simplicity of manufacture and for the strong immune response generated when the organism creates a subclinical infection before being overwhelmed. These are useful when the organism can be reliably attenuated in pathogenicity (while maintaining immunogenicity) or when the organism is difficult to cultivate *ex vivo* in large quantities and hence large amounts of antigen cannot be prepared. Conversely, subunit antigen vaccines are used when it is easy to generate large amounts of the antigen or when the whole organisms is not reliably attenuated. Since there is no replication *in vivo*, subunit vaccines rely on administrating relatively large amounts of antigen mass and are almost always adjuvanted to try to minimize the antigen needed. Subunit preparations have steadily gained favor, since biologic, engineering, and analytical improvements make them easily manufactured and characterized to a consistent standard. Passive vaccines are antibody

TABLE 13.1   Classification Scheme for Vaccines

Types of organism	Live attenuated cells/particles	Killed, inactivated cells/particles	Subcellular/parallel vaccines	Passive immunization
Virus	Measles, mumps, rubella, polio, yellow fever, varicella*, rotavirus*	Polio, hepatitis B, rabies, yellow fever, Japanese encephalitis, influenza, hepatitis A*	*Virus-like particles* Hepatitis B, HIV gp120-vaccinia* *Characterized single/combined antigens* Influenza HA+NA, herpes simplex gD*	*Immune serum globulin* Rabis, hepatitis B, cytomegalovirus *Monoclonal antibody* Anti-HIV gp120*
Bacterium	Tuberculosis (BCG), typhoid	Pertussis, cholera, plague bacillus	Toxoids Tetanus, diphtheria *Characterized single/combined antigens* Pertussis PT + FHA + LPF + PSA + 69kD, *Pneumococcus polysaccharides (23)*, *Menningococcus polysaccharides* Polysaccharide-protein conjugates Haemophilus b, Pneumococcus*	Immune serum globulin Tetanus, Nonspecific Ig

* Denotes vaccines in development.

preparations from human blood serum. These substitute for the patient's humoral response for immune-suppressed persons, for postexposure prophylaxis of disease, and for high infection risk situations where immediate protection is required, such as for travelers or medical personnel. Even more so than subunit vaccines, large amounts of antibodies are required. These vaccines do not provide long-term immune memory.

The organism and the nature of the antigen combine to determine the technologies of manufacture for the vaccine. Vaccine production generally involves growing the organism or its antigenic parts (cultivation), treating it to purify and detoxify the organism and antigen (downstream processing), and in many cases further combining the antigen with adjuvants to increase its antigenicity and improve storage stability (formulation). These three aspects of production will be discussed, in addition to future trends in vaccine technology. This chapter does not include vaccines for parasitic disease [Barbet, 1989], such as malaria, since such vaccines are not yet commercially available.

13.1   Antigen Cultivation

13.1.1   Microbial Cultivation

13.1.1.1   Bacterial Growth

As far as cultivation is concerned, the fundamental principles of cell growth are identical for the various types of bacterial vaccines. Detailed aspects of bacterial growth and metabolism can be found in Ingraham et al. [1983]. In the simplest whole-cell vaccines, obtaining cell mass is the objective of cultivation. Growth is an autocatalytic process where the cell duplicates by fission; growth is described by the differential equation

$$\frac{dX}{dt} = \mu X_v \tag{13.1}$$

where X is the total mass concentration of cells, X_v is the mass concentration of living, or viable cells, and μ is the specific growth rate in units of cells per cell time. In this equation, the growth rate of the cell is a function of the cells' physical and chemical environment:

$$\mu = f(\text{temperature, pH, dissolved oxygen, } C_1, C_2, C_3, \ldots, C_n) \qquad (13.2)$$

All bacteria have a narrow range of temperatures permissive to growth; for human pathogens, the optimal temperature is usually 37°C; however, for attenuated strains, the optimal temperature may be purposefully lowered by mutation. At the end of culture, heat in excess of 50°C is sometimes used to kill pathogenic bacteria. Dissolved oxygen concentration is usually critical, since the organism will either require it or be inhibited by it. Cultivation of *Clostridium tetani*, for example, is conducted completely anaerobically.

In Equation 13.2, C_i is the concentration of nutrient i presented to the cells. Nutrient conditions profoundly affect cell growth rate and the ultimate cell mass concentration achievable. At a minimum, the cells must be presented with a carbon source, a nitrogen source, and various elements in trace quantities. The carbon source, usually a carbohydrate such as glucose, is used for energy metabolism and as a precursor for various anabolites, small chemicals used to build the cell. The nitrogen source, which can be ammonia, or a complex amino acid mix such as a protein hydrolysate, also can be used to produce energy but is mainly present as a precursor for amino acid anabolites for protein production. The elements K, Mg, Ca, Fe, Mn, Mo, Co, Cu, and Zn are cofactors required in trace quantities for enzymatic reactions in the cell. Inorganic phosphorus and sulfur are incorporated into proteins, polysaccharides, and polynucleotides.

Historically, bacterial vaccines have been grown in a batchwise fashion on complex and ill-defined nutrient mixtures, which usually include animal and vegetable protein digests. An example is *Bordetella pertussis* cultivation on Wheeler and Cohen medium [World Health Organization, 1977c], which contains corn starch, an acid digest of bovine milk, casein, and a dialyzed lysate of brewer's yeast cells. The starch serves as the carbon source. The casein digest provides amino acids as a nitrogen source. The yeast extract provides amino acids and vitamins, as well as some trace elements, nucleotides, and carbohydrates. Such complex media components make it difficult to predict the fermentation performance, since their atomic and molecular compositions are not easily analyzed, and since they may contain hidden inhibitors of cell growth or antigen production. More recently, defined media have been used to better reproduce cell growth and antigen yield. In a defined medium, pure sugars, amino acids, vitamins, and other antibodies are used. When a single nutrient concentration limits cell growth, the growth rate can be described by Monod kinetics

$$\mu = \frac{\mu_{\max} C_i}{C_i + K} \qquad (13.3)$$

Here $\mu_{\max}$ is the maximum specific rate, and K is the Monod constant for growth on the nutrient, an empirically determined number. It is seen from this equation that at high nutrient concentrations, the cell grows at maximum rate, as if the substrate were not limiting. At low concentration as the nutrient becomes limiting, the growth rate drops to zero, and the culture ends.

13.1.1.2 Antigen Production

Cultivation of microbes for subunit vaccines is similar to that of whole-cell vaccines, but here one is concerned with the production of the antigenic protein, polysaccharide, or antigen-encoding polynucleotide as opposed to the whole cell; thus cell growth is not necessarily the main objective. The goal is to maintain the proper environmental and nutritional factors for production of the desired product. Similar to Equation 13.1 and Equation 13.2 above, one can describe antigen production by

$$\frac{dP}{dt} = q_p X_v - k_d P \quad \text{where } q_p \text{ and } k_d = f(\text{temperature, pH, dissolved O}_2, C_1, \ldots, C_n) \qquad (13.4)$$

where P is the product antigen concentration, q_p is the cell-specific productivity, and k_d is a degradation rate constant. For example, the production of pertussis toxin occurs best at slightly alkaline pH, about 8.0 [Jagicza et al., 1986]. *Corynebacterium diphtheriae* toxin production is affected by the concentration of iron [Reylveld, 1980]. Nutrient effects on degradation can be found for hepatitis B virus vaccine, whose production is actually a microbial cultivation. Here, recombinant DNA inserted into *Saccharomyces cerevisiae* yeast cells produces the hepatitis B surface antigen protein (HBsAg), which spontaneously assembles into virus-like particles (about 100 protein monomers per particle) within the cell. Prolonged starvation of the yeast cells can cause production of cellular proteases that degrade the antigen protein to provide nutrition. Consequently, maximum production of antigen is accomplished by not allowing the yeast culture to attain maximum cell mass but by harvesting the culture prior to nutrient depletion.

13.1.1.3 Cultivation Technology

Cultivation vessels for bacterial vaccines were initially bottles containing stagnant liquid or agar-gelled medium, where the bacteria grew at the liquid or agar surface. These typically resulted in low concentrations of the bacteria due to the limited penetration depth of diffusion-supplied oxygen and due to the limited diffusibility of nutrients through the stagnant liquid or agar. Despite the low mass, growth of the bacteria at the gas–liquid interface can result in cell differentiation (pellicle formation) and improved production of antigen (increased q_p). For the past several decades, however, glass and stainless steel fermentors have been used to increase production scale and productivity. Fermentors mix a liquid culture medium via an impeller, thus achieving quicker growth and higher cell mass concentrations than would be achievable by diffusive supply of nutrients. For aerobic microbe cultivations, fermenters oxygenate the culture by bubbling air directly into the medium. This increases the oxygen supply rate dramatically over diffusion supply. Due to the low solubility of oxygen in water, oxygen must be continuously supplied to avoid limitation of this nutrient.

13.1.2 Virus Cultivation

Virus cultivation is more complex than bacterial cultivation because viruses are, by themselves, nonreplicating. Virus must be grown on a host cell substrate, which can be animal tissue, embryo, or *ex vivo* cells; the host substrate determines the cultivation technology. In the United States, only Japanese encephalitis virus vaccine is still produced from infected mature animals. Worldwide, many vaccines are produced in chicken embryos, an inexpensive substrate. The remainder of vaccines are produced from *ex vivo* cultivated animal cells. Some virus-like particle vaccines are made by recombinant DNA techniques in either microbial or animal cells, for example, hepatitis B virus vaccine, which is made in yeast as mentioned above, or in Chinese hamster ovary cells. An interesting synopsis of the development of rabies vaccine technology from Pasteur's use of animal tissues to modern use of *ex vivo* cells can be found in Sureau [1987].

13.1.2.1 *In Vivo* Virus Cultivation

Virus cultivation *in vivo* is straightforward, since relatively little control can be exercised on the host tissue. Virus is simply inoculated into the organ, and after incubation, the infected organ is harvested. Influenza virus is the prototypical *in vivo* vaccine; the virus is inoculated into the allantoic sac of 9- to 11-day-old fertilized chicken eggs. The eggs are incubated at about 33°C for 2 to 3 days, candled for viability and lack of contamination from the inoculation, and then the allantoic fluid is harvested. The process of inoculating, incubating, candling, and harvesting hundreds of thousands of eggs can be highly automated [Metzgar and Newhart, 1977].

13.1.2.2 *Ex Vivo* Virus Cultivation

Use of *ex vivo* cell substrates is the most recent technique in vaccine cultivation. In the case of measles and mumps vaccines, the cell substrate is chicken embryo cells that have been generated by trypsin enzyme treatment that dissociates the embryonic cells. Similarly, some rabies vaccines use cells derived from fetal rhesus monkey kidneys. Since the 1960s, cell lines have been generated that can be characterized, banked, and cryopreserved. Cryopreserved cells have been adopted to ensure reproducibility and freedom from contaminating viruses and microorganisms and to bypass the ethical problem of extensive use of animal tissues. Examples of commonly used cell lines are WI-38 and MRC-5, both human embryonic lung cells, and Vero, an African green monkey kidney cell line.

Ex vivo cells must be cultivated in a bioreactor, in liquid nutrient medium, with aeration. The principles of cell growth are the same as for bacterial cells described above, with some important additions. First, *ex vivo* animal cells cannot synthesize the range of metabolites and hormones necessary for survival and growth and must be provided with these compounds. Second, virus production is usually fatal to the host cells. Cells also become more fragile during infection, a process that is to an extent decoupled from cell growth. Virus growth and degradation and cell death kinetics can influence the choice of process or bioreactor. Third, all *ex vivo* cells used for human vaccine manufacture require a surface to adhere to in order to grow and function properly. Finally, animal cells lack the cross-linked, rigid polysaccharide cell wall that gives physical protection to microorganisms. These last three factors combine to necessitate specialized bioreactors.

Cell Growth. Supplying cells with nutrients and growth factors is accomplished by growing the cells in a complex yet defined medium, which is supplemented with 2 to 10% (v/v) animal blood serum. The complex medium will typically contain glucose and L-glutamine as energy sources, some or all of the 20 predominant L-amino acids, vitamins, nucleotides, salts, and trace elements. For polio virus, productivity is a function of energy source availability [Eagle and Habel, 1956] and may depend on other nutrients. For polio and other viruses, the presence of the divalent cations Ca^{2+} and Mg^{2+} promotes viral attachment and entry into cells and stabilizes the virus particles. Serum provides growth-promoting hormones, lipids and cholesterol, surface attachment-promoting proteins such as fibronectin, and a host of other functions. The serum used is unusually of fetal bovine origin, since this source is particularly rich in growth-promoting hormones and contains low levels of antibodies that could neutralize virus. After cell growth, and before infection, the medium is usually changed to serum-free or low-serum medium. This is done both to avoid virus neutralization and to reduce the bovine protein impurities in the harvested virus. These proteins are **immunogenic** and can be difficult to purify away, especially for live-virus vaccines.

13.1.2.2.1 Virus Production Kinetics
An intriguing aspect of *ex vivo* virus cultivation is that each process depends on whether the virus remains cell-associated, is secreted, or lyses the host cells and whether the virus is stable in culture. With few exceptions, a cell produces a finite amount of virus before dying, as opposed to producing the virus persistently. This is because the host cell protein and DNA/RNA synthesis organelles are usually commandeered by virus synthesis, and the host cannot produce its own proteins, DNA, or RNA. The goal then becomes to maximize cell concentration, as outlined above for bacterial vaccines, while maintaining the cells in a competent state to produce virus. Since infection is transient and often rapid, cell-specific virus productivity is not constant, and productivity is usually correlated with the cell state at inoculation. Specific productivity can be a function of the cell growth rate, since this determines the available protein and nucleic acid synthetic capacity. Although virus production can be nutrient-limited, good nutrition is usually ensured by the medium exchange at inoculation mentioned above. For viruses that infect cells slowly, nutrition is supplied by exchanging the medium several times, batchwise or by continuous perfusion.

For many viruses, the degradation term in Equation 13.4 can be significant. This can be due to inherent thermal instability of the virus, oxidation, or proteases released from lysed cells. For an unstable virus, obtaining a synchronized infection can be key to maximizing titers. Here, the multiplicity of infection (MOI), the number of virus inoculated per cell, is an important parameter. An MOI greater than unity results in most cells being infected at once, giving the maximum net virus production rate.

13.1.2.2.2 Cultivation Technology
The fragility of animal cells during infection and the surface attachment requirement create a requirement for special reactors [Prokop and Rosenberg, 1989]. To an extent, reactor choice and productivity are determined by the reactor surface area. Small, simple, and uncontrolled vessels, such as a flat-sided

T-flask or Roux bottle, made of polystyrene or glass, can be used for small-scale culture. With these flasks the medium is stagnant, so fragile infected cells are not exposed to fluid motion forces during culture. Like bacterial cultures, productivity can be limited due to the slow diffusion of nutrients and oxygen. To obtain larger surface areas, roller bottles or Cell Factories are used, but like egg embryo culture, robotic automation is required to substantially increase the scale of production. Even larger culture scales (≥ 50 l) are accommodated in glass or stainless steel bioreactors, which are actively supplied with oxygen and pH controlled. The growth surface is typically supplied as a fixed bed of plates, spheres, or fibers or, alternately, as a dispersion of about 200-mm spherical particles known as microcarriers [Reuveny, 1990]. Microcarrier bioreactors are used for polio and rabies production [Montagnon et al., 1984]. The stirred-tank microcarrier reactors are similar to bacterial fermentors but are operated at much lower stirring speeds and gas sparging rates so as to minimize damage to the fragile cells. Packed-bed reactors are used for hepatitis A virus vaccine production [Aboud et al., 1994]. These types of reactors can give superior performance for highly lytic viruses because they subject the cells to much lower fluid mechanical forces. Design considerations for animal cell reactors may be found in Aunins and Henzler [1993].

13.2   Downstream Processing

Following cultivation, the antigen is recovered, isolated in crude form, further purified, and/or inactivated to give the unformulated product; these steps are referred to collectively as the downstream process. The complexity of a downstream process varies greatly depending on whether the antigen is the whole organism, a semipurified subunit, or a highly purified subunit. Although the sequence and combination of steps are unique for each vaccine, there is a general method to purification. The first steps reduce the volume of working material and provide crude separation from contaminants. Later steps typically resolve molecules more powerfully but are limited to relatively clean feed streams. Some manufacturing steps are classic small laboratory techniques, because many vaccine antigens are quite potent, requiring only micrograms of material; historically, manufacturing scale-up has not been a critical issue.

13.2.1   Purification Principles

13.2.1.1   Recovery

Recovery steps achieve concentration and liberation of the antigen. The first recovery step consists of separating the cells and/or virus from the fermentation broth or culture medium. The objective is to capture and concentrate the cells for cell-associated antigens or to clarify the medium of particulates for extracellular antigens. In the first case, the particle separation simultaneously concentrates the antigen. The two methods used are centrifugation and filtration. Batch volume and feed solids content determine whether centrifugation or filtration is appropriate; guidelines for centrifugation are given by Datar and Rosen [1993] and Atkinson and Mavituna [1991]. Filtration is used increasingly as filter materials science improves to give filters that do not bind antigen. Filtration can either be dead-end or cross-flow. Dead-end filters are usually fibrous depth filters and are used when the particulate load is low and the antigen is extracellular. In cross-flow filtration, the particles are retained by a microporous (≥ 0.1 mm) or ultrafiltration (≤ 0.1 mm) membrane. The feed stream is circulated tangential to the membrane surface at high velocity to keep the cells and other particulates from forming a filter cake on the membrane [Hanisch, 1986].

   If the desired antigen is subcellular and cell-associated, the next recovery step is likely to be cell lysis. This can be accomplished by high-pressure valve homogenization, bead mills, or chemical lysis with detergent or chaotropic agents, to name only a few techniques. The homogenate or cell lysate may subsequently be clarified, again using either centrifugation or membrane filtration.

13.2.1.2 Isolation

Isolation is conducted to achieve crude fractionation from contaminants that are unlike the antigen; precipitation and extraction are often used here. These techniques rely on large differences in charge or solubility between antigen and contaminants. Prior to isolation, the recovered process stream may be treated enzymatically with nucleases, proteases, or lipases to remove DNA/RNA, protein, and lipids, the major macromolecular contaminants. Nonionic detergents such as Tween and Triton can serve a similar function to separate components, provided they do not denature the antigen. Subsequent purification steps must be designed to remove the enzyme(s) or detergent, however.

Ammonium sulfate salt precipitation is a classic method used to concentrate and partially purify various proteins, for example, diphtheria and tetanus toxins. Alcohol precipitation is effective for separating polysaccharides from proteins. Cohn cold alcohol precipitation is a classic technique used to fractionate blood serum for antibody isolation. Both techniques concentrate antigen for further treatment.

Liquid–liquid extraction, either aqueous–organic or aqueous–aqueous, is another isolation technique suitable for vaccine purification. In a two-phase aqueous polymer system, the separation is based on the selective partitioning of the product from an aqueous liquid phase containing, for example, polyethylene glycol (PEG), into a second, immiscible aqueous liquid phase that contains another polymer, for example, dextran, or containing a salt [Kelley and Hatton, 1992].

13.2.1.3 Final Purification

Further purification of the vaccine product is to remove contaminants that have properties closely resembling the antigen. These sophisticated techniques resolve molecules with small differences in charge, hydrophobicity, density, or size.

Density-gradient centrifugation, although not readily scalable, is a popular technique for final purification of viruses [Polson, 1993]. Either rate-zonal centrifugation, where the separation is based on differences in sedimentation rate, or isopycnic equilibrium centrifugation, where the separation is based solely on density differences, is used. Further details on these techniques can be found in Dobrota and Hinton [1992].

Finally, different types of chromatography are employed to manufacture highly pure vaccines; principles can be found in Janson and Ryden [1989]. Ion-exchange chromatography (IEC) is based on differences in overall charge and distribution of charge on the components. Hydrophobic-interaction chromatography (HIC) exploits differences in hydrophobicity. Affinity chromatography is based on specific stereochemical interactions common only to the antigen and the ligand. Size-exclusion chromatography (SEC) separates on the basis of size and shape. Often, multiple chromatographic steps are used, since the separation mechanisms are complementary. IEC and HIC can sometimes be used early in the process to gain substantial purification; SEC is typically used as a final polishing step. This technique, along with ultrafiltration, may be used to exchange buffers for formulation at the end of purification.

13.2.1.4 Inactivation

For nonattenuated whole organisms or for toxin antigens, the preparation must be inactivated to eliminate pathogenicity. This is accomplished by heat pasteurization, by cross-linking using formaldehyde or glutaraldehyde, or by alkylating using agents such as b-propiolactone. The agent is chosen for effectiveness without destruction of antigenicity. For whole organisms, the inactivation abolishes infectivity. For antigens such as the diphtheria and tetanus toxins, formaldehyde treatment removes the toxicity of the antigen itself as well as killing the organism. These detoxified antigens are known as toxoids.

The placement of inactivation in the process depends largely on safety issues. For pathogen cultures, inactivation traditionally has been immediately after cultivation to eliminate danger to manufacturing personnel. For inactivation with cross-linking agents, however, the step may be placed later in the process in order to minimize interference by contaminants that either foil inactivation of the organism or cause carryover of antigen-contaminant cross-linked entities that could cause safety problems, that is, side-reactions in patients.

13.2.2 Purification Examples

Examples of purification processes are presented below, illustrating how the individual techniques are combined to create purification processes.

13.2.2.1 Bacterial Vaccines

Salmonella typhi Ty21, a vaccine for typhoid fever, and BCG (bacille Calmette-Guérin, a strain of *Mycobacterium bovis*) vaccine against *Myobacterium tuberculosis*, are the only vaccines licensed for human use based on live, attenuated bacteria. Downstream processing consists of collecting the cells by continuous-flow centrifugation or using cross-flow membrane filtration. For M. bovis that are grown in a liquid submerged fermenter culture, Tween 20 is added to keep the cells from aggregating, and the cultures are collected as above. Tween 20, however, has been found to decrease virulence. In contrast, if the BCG is grown in stagnant bottles as a surface pellicle, the downstream process consists of collecting the pellicle sheet, which is a moist cake, and then homogenizing the cake using a ball mill. Milling time is critical, since prolonged milling kills the cells and too little milling leaves clumps of bacteria in suspension.

Most current whooping cough vaccines are inactivated whole B. pertussis. The cells are harvested by centrifugation and then resuspended in buffer, which is the supernate in some cases. This is done because some of the filamentous hemagglutinin (FHA) and pertussis toxin (PT) antigens are released into the supernate. The cell concentrate is inactivated by mild heat and stored with thimerosal and/or formaldehyde. The inactivation process serves the dual purpose of killing the cells and inactivating the toxins.

C. diphtheria vaccine is typical of a crude protein toxoid vaccine. Here the 58 kDa toxin is the antigen, and it is converted to a toxoid with formaldehyde and crudely purified. The cells are first separated from the toxin by centrifugation. Sometimes the pathogen culture is inactivated with formaldehyde before centrifugation. The supernate is treated with formaldehyde to 0.75%, and it is stored for 4 to 6 weeks at 37°C to allow complete detoxification [Pappenheimer, 1984]. The toxoid is then concentrated by ultrafiltration and fractionated from contaminants by ammonium sulfate precipitation. During detoxification of crude material, reactions with formaldehyde lead to a variety of products. The toxin is internally cross-linked and also cross-linked to other toxins, beef peptones from the medium, and other medium proteins. Because detoxification creates a population of molecules containing antigen, the purity of this product is only about 60 to 70%.

Due to the cross-linking of impurities, improved processes have been developed to purify toxins before formaldehyde treatment. Purification by ammonium sulfate fractionation, followed by ion-exchange and/or size-exclusion chromatography, is capable of yielding diphtheria or tetanus toxins with purities ranging from 85 to 95%. The purified toxin is then treated with formaldehyde or glutaraldehyde [Relyveld and Ben-Efraim, 1983] to form the toxoid. Likewise, whole-cell pertussis vaccine is being replaced by subunit vaccines. Here, the pertussis toxin (PT) and the filamentous hemagglutinin (FHA) are purified from the supernate. These two antigens are isolated by ammonium sulfate precipitation, followed by sucrose density-gradient centrifugation to remove impurities such as endotoxin. The FHA and PT are then detoxified with formaldehyde [Sato et al., 1984].

Bacterial components other than proteins also have been developed for use as subunit vaccines. One class of bacterial vaccines is based on capsular polysaccharides. Polysaccharides from Meningococcus, Pneumococcus, and *Haemophilus influenzae* type b are used for vaccines against these organisms. After separating the cells, the polysaccharides are typically purified using a series of alcohol precipitations. As described below, these polysaccharides are not antigenic in infants. As a consequence, the polysaccharides are chemically cross-linked, or conjugated, to a highly purified antigenic protein carrier. After conjugation, there are purification steps to remove unreacted polysaccharide protein, and small-molecular-weight cross-linking reagents. Several manufacturers have introduced pediatric conjugate vaccines against *H. influenzae* type b (Hib-conjugate).

13.2.2.2   Viral Vaccines

Live viral vaccines have limited downstream processes. For secreted viruses such as measles, mumps, and rubella, cell debris is simply removed by filtration and the supernate frozen. In many cases it is necessary to process quickly and at refrigerated temperatures, since live virus can be unstable [Cryz and Gluck, 1990].

For cell-associated virus such as herpesviruses, for example, *Varicella zoster* (chickenpox virus), the cells are washed with a physiologic saline buffer to remove medium contaminants and are harvested. This can be done by placing them into a stabilizer formulation (see below) and then mechanically scraping the cells from the growth surface. Alternately, the cells can be harvested from the growth surface chemically or enzymatically. For the latter, the cells are centrifuged and resuspended in stabilizer medium. The virus is then liberated by disrupting the cells, usually by sonication, and the virus-containing supernate is clarified by dead-end filtration and frozen.

Early inactivated influenza virus vaccines contained relatively crude virus. The allantoic fluid was harvested, followed by formaldehyde inactivation of the whole virus, and adsorption to aluminum phosphate (see below), which may have provided some purification as well. The early vaccines, however, were associated with reactogenicity. For some current processes, the virus is purified by rate-zonal centrifugation, which effectively eliminates the contaminants from the allantoic fluid. The virus is then inactivated with formaldehyde or b-propiolactone, which preserves the antigenicity of both the hemagglutinin (HA) and neuraminidase (NA) antigens. Undesirable side reactions have been even further reduced with the introduction of split vaccines, where the virus particle is disrupted by an organic solvent or detergent and then inactivated. By further purifying the split vaccine using a method such as zonal centrifugation to separate the other virion components from the HA and NA antigens, an even more highly purified HA + NA vaccine is available. These antigens are considered to elicit protective antibodies against influenza [Tyrrell, 1976].

Recently, an extensive purification process was developed for hepatitis A vaccine, yielding a >90% pure product [Aboud et al., 1994]. The intracellular virus is released from the cells by Triton detergent lysis, followed by nuclease enzyme treatment for removal of RNA and DNA. The virus is concentrated and detergent removed by ion-exchange chromatography. PEG precipitation and chloroform solvent extraction purify away most of the cellular proteins, and final purification and polishing are achieved by ion-exchange and size-exclusion chromatography. The virus particle is then inactivated with formaldehyde. In this case, inactivation comes last for two reasons. First, the virus is attenuated, so there is no risk to process personnel. Second, placing the inactivation after the size-exclusion step ensures that there are no contaminants or virus aggregates that may cause incomplete inactivation.

The first hepatitis B virus vaccines were derived from human plasma [Hilleman, 1993]. The virus is a 22-nm-diameter particle, much larger than most biologic molecules. Isolation was achieved by ammonium sulfate or PEG precipitation, followed by rate zonal centrifugation and isopycnic banding to take advantage of the large particle size. The preparation was then treated with pepsin protease, urea, and formaldehyde or heat. The latter steps ensure inactivation of possible contaminant viruses from the blood serum. More recently, recombinant DNA-derived hepatitis B vaccines are expressed as an intracellular noninfectious particle in yeast and use a completely different purification process. Here, the emphasis is to remove the yeast host contaminants, particularly high levels of nucleic acids and polysaccharides. Details on the various manufacturing processes have been described by Sitrin et al. [1993].

13.2.2.3   Antibody Preparations

Antibody preparation starts from the plasma pool prepared by removing the cellular components of blood. Cold ethanol is added in increments to precipitate fractions of the blood proteins, and the precipitate containing IgG antibodies is collected. This is further redissolved and purified by ultrafiltration, which also exchanges the buffer to the stabilizer formulation. Sometimes ion-exchange chromatography is used for further purification. Although the plasma is screened for viral contamination prior to pooling, all three purification techniques remove some virus.

13.3 Formulation and Delivery

Successful vaccination requires both the development of a stable dosage form for *in vitro* storage and the proper delivery and presentation of the antigen to elicit a vigorous immune response *in vivo*. This is done by adjuvanting the vaccine and/or by formulating the adjuvanted antigen. An adjuvant is defined as an agent that enhances the immune response against an antigen. A formulation contains an antigen in a delivery vehicle designed to preserve the (adjuvenated) antigen and to deliver it to a specific target organ or over a desired time period. Despite adjuvanting and formulation efforts, most current vaccines require multiple doses to create immune memory.

13.3.1 Live Organisms

Live viruses and bacteria die relatively quickly in liquid solution (without an optimal environment) and are therefore usually stored in the frozen state. Preserving the infectivity of frozen live-organism vaccines is typically accomplished by lyophilization or freeze-drying. The freeze-drying process involves freezing the organism in the presence of stabilizers, followed by sublimation of both bulk water (primary drying) and more tightly bound water (secondary drying). The dehydration process reduces the conformational flexibility of the macromolecules, providing protection against thermal denaturation. Stabilizers also provide conformational stability and protect against other inactivating mechanisms such as amino acid deamidation, oxidation, and light-catalyzed reaction.

Final water content of the freeze-dried product is the most important parameter for the drying process. Although low water content enhances storage stability, overdrying inactivates biologic molecules, since removal of tightly bound water disrupts antigen conformation. Influenza virus suspensions have been shown to be more stable at 1.7% (w/w) water than either 0.4 to 1% or 2.1 to 3.2% [Greiff and Rightsel, 1968]. Other lyophilization parameters that must be optimized pertain to heat and mass transfer, including (1) the rate of freezing and sublimation, (2) vial location in the freeze-drier, and (3) the type of vial and stopper used to cap the vial. Rates of freezing and drying affect phase transitions and compositions, changing the viable organism yield on lyophilization and the degradation rate of the remaining viable organisms on storage.

Stabilizers are identified by trial-and-error screening and by examining the mechanisms of inactivation. They can be classified into four categories depending on their purpose: specific, nonspecific, competitive, and pharmaceutical. Specific stabilizers are ligands that naturally bind biologic macromolecules. For example, enzyme antigens are often stabilized by their natural substrates or closely related compounds. Antigen stabilizers for the liquid state also stabilize during freezing. Nonspecific stabilizers such as sugars, amino acids, and neutral salts stabilize proteins and virus structures via a variety of mechanisms. Sugars and polyols act as bound water substitutes, preserving conformational integrity without possessing the chemical reactivity of water. Buffer salts preserve optimal pH. Competitive inhibitors outcompete the organism or antigen for inactivating conditions, such as gas-liquid interfaces, oxygen, or trace-metal ions [Volkin and Klibanov, 1989]. Finally, pharmaceutical stabilizers may be added to preserve pharmaceutical elegance, that is, to prevent collapse of the lyophilized powder during the drying cycle, which creates difficult redissolution. Large-molecular-weight polymers such as carbohydrates (dextrans or starch) or proteins such as albumin or gelatin are used for this purpose. For example, a buffered sorbitol-gelatin medium has been used successfully to preserve the infectivity of measles virus vaccine during lyophilized storage for several years at 2 to 8°C [Hilleman, 1989]. An example of live bacterium formulation to preserve activity on administration is typhoid fever vaccine, administered orally, *S. typhi* bacteria are lyophilized to a powder to preserve viability on the shelf, and the powder is encapsulated in gelatin to preserve bacterial viability when passing through the low-pH stomach. The gelatin capsule dissolves in the intestine to deliver the live bacteria.

Oral polio vaccine is an exception to the general rule of lyophilization, since polio virus is inherently quite stable relative to other viruses. It is formulated as a frozen liquid and can be used for a limited time after thawing [Melnick, 1984]. In the presence of specific stabilizers such as $MgCl_2$, extended 4°C stability can be obtained.

13.3.2 Subunit Antigens

Inactivated and/or purified viral and bacterial antigens inherently offer enhanced stability because whole-organism infectivity does not need to be preserved. However, these antigens are not as immunogenic as live organisms and thus are administered with an adjuvant. They are usually formulated as an aqueous liquid suspension or solution, although they can be lyophilized under the same principles as above. The major adjuvant recognized as safe for human use is alum. Alum is a general term referring to various hydrated aluminum salts; a discussion of the different alums can be found in Shirodkar et al. [1990]. Vaccines can be formulated with alum adjuvants by two distinct methods: adsorption to performed aluminum precipitates or precipitation of aluminum salts in the presence of the antigen, thus adsorbing and entrapping the antigen. Alum's adjuvant activity is classically believed to be a "depot" effect, slowly delivering antigen over time *in vivo*. In addition, alum particles are believed to be phagocytized by macrophages.

Alum properties vary depending on the salt used. Adjuvants labeled aluminum hydroxide are actually aluminum oxyhydroxide, AlO(OH). This material is crystalline, has a fibrous morphology, and has a positive surface charge at neutral pH. In contrast, aluminum phosphate adjuvants are networks of platelike particles of amorphous aluminum hydroxyphosphate and possess a negative surface charge at neutral pH. Finally, alum coprecipitate vaccines are prepared by mixing an acidic alum solution of $KAl(SO_4)_2 \cdot 12H_2O$ with an antigen solution buffered at neutral pH, sometimes actively pH-controlled with base. At neutral pH, the aluminum forms a precipitate, entrapping and adsorbing the antigen. The composition and physical properties of this alum vary with processing conditions and the buffer anions. In general, an amorphous aluminum hydroxy(buffer anion)sulfate material is formed.

Process parameters must be optimized for each antigen to ensure proper adsorption and storage stability. First, since antigen adsorption isotherms are a function of the antigen's isoelectric point and the type of alum used [Seeber et al., 1991], the proper alum and adsorption pH must be chosen. Second, the buffer ions in solution can affect the physical properties of alum over time, resulting in changes in solution pH and antigen adsorption. Finally, heat sterilization of alum solutions and precipitates prior to antigen adsorption can alter their properties. Alum is used to adjuvant virtually all the existing inactivated or formaldehyde-treated vaccines, as well as purified subunit vaccines such as HBsAg and Hib-conjugate vaccines. The exception is for some bacterial polysaccharide vaccines and for new vaccines under development (see below).

An interesting vaccine development challenge was encountered with Hib-conjugate pediatric vaccines, which consist of purified capsular polysaccharides. Although purified, unadjuvanted polysaccharide is used in adults, it is not sufficiently immunogenic in children under age 2, the population is greatest risk [Ellis, 1992; Howard, 1992]. Chemical conjugation, or cross-linking, of the PRP polysaccharide to an antigenic protein adjuvant elicits T-helper cell activation, resulting in higher antibody production. Variations in conjugation chemistry and protein carriers have been developed; example proteins are the diphtheria toxoid (CRM 197), tetanus toxoid, and the outer membrane protein complex of N. meningitidis [Ellis, 1992; Howard, 1992]. The conjugated polysaccharide is sometimes adsorbed to alum for further adjuvant action.

13.4 Future Trends

The reader will have noted that many production aspects for existing vaccines are quite archaic. This is so because most vaccines were developed before the biotechnology revolution, which is creating a generation of highly purified and better-characterized subunit vaccines. As such, for older vaccines "the process defines the product," and process improvements cannot readily be incorporated into these poorly characterized vaccines without extensive new clinical trials. With improved scientific capabilities, we can understand the effects of process changes on the physicochemical properties of new vaccines and on their behavior *in vivo*.

13.4.1 Vaccine Cultivation

Future cultivation methods will resemble existing methods of microbial and virus culture. Ill-defined medium components and cells will be replaced to enhance reproducibility in production. For bacterial and *ex vivo* cultivated virus, analytical advances will make monitoring the environment and nutritional status of the culture more ubiquitous. However, the major changes will be in novel product types — single-molecule subunit antigens, virus-like particles, monoclonal antibodies, and gene-therapy vaccines, each of which will incorporate novel processes.

Newer subunit vaccine antigens will be cultivated via recombinant DNA in microbial or animal cells. Several virus-like particle vaccines are under development using recombinant baculovirus (nuclear poly-hedrosis virus) to infect insect cells (spodoptera frugipeeda or trichoplusia ni). Like the hepatitis B vaccine, the viral antigens spontaneously assemble into a noninfectious capsid within the cell. Although the meta-bolic pathways of insect cells differ from vertebrates, cultivation principles are similar. Insect cells do not require surface attachment and are grown much like bacteria. However, they also lack a cell wall and are larger and hence more fragile than vertebrate cells.

Passive antibody vaccines have been prepared up to now from human blood serum. Consequently, there has been no need for cultivation methods beyond vaccination and conventional harvest of antibody-containing blood from donors. Due to safety concerns over using human blood, passive vaccines will likely be monoclonal antibodies or cocktails thereof prepared *in vitro* by the cultivation of hybridoma or myeloma cell lines. This approach is under investigation for anti-HIV-1 antibodies [Emini et al., 1992]. Cultivation of these cell lines involves the same principles of animal cell cultivation as described above, with the exception that hybridomas can be less fastidious in nutritional requirements, and they do not require surface attachment for growth. These features will allow for defined serum-free media and simpler cultivation vessels and procedures.

For the gene-therapy approach, the patient actually produces the antigen. A DNA polynucleotide encoding protein antigen(s) is injected intramuscularly into the patient. The muscle absorbs the DNA and produces the antigen, thereby eliciting an immune response [Ulmer et al., 1993]. For cultivation, produc-tion of the DNA plasmid is the objective, which can be done efficiently by bacteria such as Escherichia coli. Such vaccines are not sufficiently far along in development to generalize the factors that influence their production; however, it is expected that producer cells and process conditions that favor high cell mass, DNA replication, and DNA stability will be important. A potential beauty of this vaccination approach is that for cultivation, purification, and formulation, many vaccines can conceivably be made by identical processes, since the plasmids are inactive within the bacterium and possess roughly the same nucleotide composition.

13.4.2 Downstream Processing

Future vaccines will be more highly purified in order to minimize side effects, and future improvements will be to assist this goal. The use of chemically defined culture media will impact favorably on downstream processing by providing a cleaner feedstock. Advances in filtration membranes and in chromatographic support binding capacity and throughput will improve ease of purification. Affinity purification methods that rely on specific "lock and key" interactions between a chromatographic support and the antigen will see greater use as well. Techniques amenable to larger scales will be more important to meet increased market demands and to reduce manufacturing costs. HPLC and other analytical techniques will provide greater process monitoring and control throughout purification.

As seen during the evolution of diphtheria and tetanus toxoid vaccines, the trend will be to purify toxins prior to inactivation to reduce their cross-linking with other impurities. New inactivating agents such as hydrogen peroxide and ethyl dimethylaminopropyl carbodiimide have been investigated for pertussis toxin, which do not have problems of cross-linking or reversion of the toxoid to toxin status.

Molecular biology is likely to have an even greater impact on purification. Molecular cloning of proteins allows the addition of amino acid sequences that can facilitate purification, for example, polyhistidine or polyalanine tails for metal ion, or ion-exchange chromatography. Recent efforts also have employed genetic manipulation to inactivate toxins, eliminating the need for the chemical treatment step.

13.4.3 Vaccine Adjuvants and Formulation

Many new subunit antigens lack the inherent immunogenicity found in the natural organism, thereby creating the need for better adjuvants. Concomitantly, the practical problem of enhancing worldwide immunization coverage has stimulated development of single-shot vaccine formulations in which booster doses are unnecessary. Thus future vaccine delivery systems will aim at reducing the number of doses via controlled antigen release and will increase vaccine efficacy by improving the mechanism of antigen presentation (i.e., controlled release of antigen over time or directing of antigen to specific antigen-presenting cells). Major efforts are also being made to combine antigens into single-shot vaccines to improve immunization rates for infants, who currently receive up to 15 injections during the first 2 years of life. Coadministration of antigens presents unique challenges to formulation as well.

Recent advances in the understanding of *in vivo* antigen presentation to the immune system has generated considerable interest in developing novel vaccine adjuvants. The efficacy of an adjuvant is judged by its ability to stimulate specific antibody production and killer cell proliferation. Developments in biology now allow analysis of activity by the particular immune cells that are responsible for these processes. Examples of adjuvants currently under development include saponin detergents, muramyl dipeptides, and lipopolysaccharides (endotoxin), including lipid A derivatives. As well, cytokine growth factors that stimulate immune cells directly are under investigation.

Emulsion and liposome delivery vehicles are also being examined to enhance the presentation of antigen and adjuvant to the immune system [Allison and Byars, 1992; Edelman, 1992]. Controlled-release delivery systems are also being developed that encapsulate antigen inside a polymer-based solid microsphere. The size of the particles typically varies between 1 and 300 mm depending on the manufacturing process. Microspheres are prepared by first dissolving the biodegradable polymer in an organic solvent. The adjuvanted antigen, in aqueous solution or lyophilized powder form, is then emulsified into the solvent-polymer continuous phase. Microspheres are then formed by either solvent evaporation, phase-separation, or spray-drying, resulting in entrapment of antigen [Morris et al., 1994]. The most frequently employed biodegradable controlled-released delivery systems use FDA-approved poly(lactide-co-glycolide) copolymers (PLGA), which hydrolyze *in vivo* to nontoxic lactic and glycolic acid monomers. Degradation rate can be optimized by varying the microsphere size and the monomer ratio. Antigen stability during encapsulation and during *in vivo* release from the microspheres remains a challenge. Other challenges to manufacturing include encapsulation process reproducibility, minimizing antigen exposure to denaturing organic solvents, and ensuring sterility. Methods are being developed to address these issues, including the addition of stabilizers for processing purposes only. It should be noted that microsphere technology may permit vaccines to be targeted to specific cells; they can potentially be delivered orally or nasally to produce a mucosal immune response.

Other potential delivery technologies include liposomes and alginate polysaccharide and poly(dicarboxylatophenoxy)phosphazene polymers. The latter two form aqueous hydrogels in the presence of divalent cations [Khan et al., 1994]. Antigens can thus be entrapped under aqueous conditions with minimal processing by simply mixing antigen and soluble aqueous polymer and dripping the mixture into a solution of $CaCl_2$. The particles erode by Ca^{2+} loss, mechanical and chemical degradation, and macrophage attack. For alginate polymers, monomer composition also determines the polymer's immunogenicity, and thus the material can serve as both adjuvant and release vehicle.

For combination vaccines, storage and administration compatibility of the different antigens must be demonstrated. Live-organism vaccines are probably not compatible with purified antigens, since the former usually require lyophilization and the latter are liquid formulas. Within a class of vaccines, formulation is challenging. Whereas it is relatively straightforward to adjuvant and formulate a single antigen, combining antigens is more difficult because each has its own unique alum species, pH, buffer ion, and preservative optimum. Nevertheless, several combination vaccines have reached the market, and others are undergoing clinical trials.

13.5 Conclusions

Although vaccinology and manufacturing methods have come a considerable distance over the past 40 years, much more development will occur. There will be challenges for biotechnologists to arrive at safer, more effective vaccines for an ever-increasing number of antigen targets. If government interference and legal liability questions do not hamper innovation, vaccines will remain one of the most cost-effective and logical biomedical technologies of the next century, as disease is prevented rather than treated.

Challenges are also posed in bringing existing vaccines to technologically undeveloped nations, where they are needed most. This problem is almost exclusively dominated by the cost of vaccine manufacture and the reliability of distribution. Hence it is fertile ground for engineering improvements in vaccine production.

Defining Terms

Adjuvant: A chemical or biologic substance that enhances immune response against an antigen. Used here as a verb, the action of combining an antigen and an adjuvant.

Antigen: A macromolecule or assembly of macromolecules from a pathogenic organism that the immune system recognizes as foreign.

Attenuation: The process of mutating an organism so that it no longer causes disease.

Immunogen: A molecule or assembly of molecules with the ability to invoke an immune system response.

Pathogen: A disease-causing organism, either a virus, mycobacterium, or bacterium.

References

Aboud R.A., Aunins J.G., Buckland B.C. et al. 1994. Hepatitis A Virus Vaccine. International patent application, publication number WO 94/03589, Feb. 17, 1994.

Allison A.C. and Byars N.E. 1992. Immunologic adjuvants and their mode of action. In R.W. Ellis (Ed.), *Vaccines: New Approaches to Immunological Problems*, p. 431. Reading, MA, Butterworth-Heinemann.

Atkinson B. and Mavituna F. 1991. *Biochemical Engineering and Biotechnology Handbook*, 2nd ed. London, Macmillan.

Aunins J.G. and Henzler H.-J. 1993. Aeration in cell culture bioreactors. In H.-J. Rehm et al. (Eds.), *Biotechnology*, 2nd ed., vol. 3, p. 219. Weinheim, Germany, VCH Verlag.

Bachmayer H. 1976. Split and subunit vaccines. In P. Selby (Ed.), *Influenza Virus, Vaccines, and Strategy*, p. 149. New York, Academic Press.

Barbet A.F. 1989. Vaccines for parasitic infections. *Adv. Vet. Sci. Comp. Med.* 33: 345.

Cryz S.J. and Reinhard G. 1990. Large-scale production of attenuated bacterial and viral vaccines. In G.C. Woodrow and M.M. Levine (Eds.), *New Generation Vaccines*, p. 921. New York, Marcel Dekker.

Datar R.V. and Rosen C.-G. 1993. Cell and cell debris removal: centrifugation and crossflow filtration. In H.-J. Rehm et al. (Eds.), *Biotechnology*, 2nd ed., vol. 3, p. 469. Weinheim, Germany, VCH Verlag.

Dobrota M. and Hinton R. 1992. Conditions for density gradient separations. In D. Rickwood (Ed.), *Preparative Centrifugation: A Practical Approach*, p. 77. New York, Oxford University Press.

Eagle H. and Habel K. 1956. The nutritional requirements for the propagation of poliomyelitis virus by the HeLa cell. *J. Exp. Med.* 104: 271.

Edelman R. 1992. An update on vaccine adjuvants in clinical trial. *AIDS Res. Hum. Retrovir* 8: 1409.

Ellis R.W. 1992. Vaccine development: progression from target antigen to product. In J.E. Ciardi et al. (Eds.), *Genetically Engineered Vaccines*, p. 263. New York, Plenum Press.

Emini E.A., Schleif W.A., Nunberg J.H. et al. 1992. Prevention of HIV-1 infection in chimpanzees by gp120 V3 domain-specific monoclonal antibodies. *Nature* 355: 728.

Greiff D. and Rightsel W.A. 1968. Stability of suspensions of influenza virus dried to different contents of residual moisture by sublimation in vacuo. *Appl. Microbiol.* 16: 835.

Hanisch W. 1986. Cell harvesting. In W.C. McGregor (Ed.), *Membrane Separations in Biotechnology*, p. 66. New York, Marcel Dekker.

Hewlett E.L. and Cherry J.D. 1990. New and improved vaccines against pertussis. In G.C. Woodrow and M.M. Levine (Eds.), *New Generation Vaccines*, p. 231. New York, Marcel Dekker.

Hilleman M.R. 1989. Improving the heat stability of vaccines: problems, needs and approaches. *Rev. Infect. Dis.* 11: S613.

Hilleman M.R. 1993. Plasma-derived hepatitis B vaccine: a breakthrough in preventive medicine. In R. Ellis (Ed.), *Hepatitus B Vaccines in Clinical Practice*, p. 17. New York, Marcel Dekker.

Howard A.J. 1992. Haemophilus influenzae type-b vaccines. *Br. J. Hosp. Med.* 48: 44.

Ingraham J.L., Maaløe O., and Neidhardt F.C. 1983. *Growth of the Bacterial Cell.* Sunderland, MA, Sinauer.

Jagicza A., Balla P., Lendvai N. et al. 1986. Additional information for the continuous cultivation of *Bordetella pertussis* for the vaccine production in bioreactor. *Ann. Immunol. Hung.* 26: 89.

Janson J.-C. and Ryden L. (Eds.) 1989. *Protein Purification Principles, High Resolution Methods, and Applications.* Weinheim, Germany, VCH Verlag.

Kelley B.D. and Hatton T.A. 1993. Protein purification by liquid–liquid extraction. In H.-J. Rehm et al. (Eds.), *Biotechnology*, 2nd ed, vol. 3, p. 594. Weinheim, Germany, VCH Verlag.

Khan M.Z.I., Opdebeeck J.P., and Tucker I.G. 1994. Immunopotentiation and delivery systems for antigens for single-step immunization: recent trends and progress. *Pharmacol. Res.* 11: 2.

Melnick J.L. 1984. Live attenuated oral poliovirus vaccine. *Rev. Infect. Dis.* 6: S323.

Metzgar D.P. and Newhart R.H. 1977. U.S. patent no. 4,057,626, Nov. 78, 1977.

Montagnon B., Vincent-Falquet J.C., and Fanget B. 1984. Thousand litre scale microcarrier culture of vero cells for killed polio virus vaccine: promising results. *Dev. Biol. Stand.* 55: 37.

Morris W., Steinhoff M.C., and Russell P.K. 1994. Potential of polymer microencapsulation technology for vaccine innovation. *Vaccine* 12: 5.

Pappenheimer A.M. 1984. Diphtheria. In R. Germanier (Ed.), *Bacterial Vaccines*, p. 1. New York, Academic Press.

Polson A. 1993. *Virus Separation and Preparation.* New York, Marcel Dekker.

Prokop A. and Rosenberg M.Z. 1989. Bioreactor for mammalian cell culture. In A. Fiechter (Ed.), *Advances in Biochemical Engineering, Vol. 39: Vertebrate Cell Culture II and Enzyme Technology*, p. 29. Berlin, Springer-Verlag.

Rappuoli R. 1990. New and improved vaccines against diphtheria and tetanus. In G.C. Woodrow and M.M. Levine (Eds.), *New Generation Vaccines*, p. 251. New York, Marcel Dekker.

Relyveld E.H. 1980. Current developments in production and testing of tetanus and diphtheria vaccines. In A. Mizrahi et al. (Eds.), *Progress in Clinical and Biological Research, Vol. 47: New Developments with Human and Veterinary Vaccines*, p. 51. New York, Alan R. Liss.

Relyveld E.H. and Ben-Efraim S. 1983. Preparation of vaccines by the action of glutaraldehyde on toxins, bacteria, viruses, allergens and cells. In S.P. Colowic and N.O. Kaplan (Eds.), *Methods in Enzymology*, vol. 93, p. 24. New York, Academic Press.

Reuveny S. 1990. Microcarrier culture systems. In A.S. Lubiniecki (Ed.), *In Large-Scale Mammalian Cell Culture Technology*, p. 271. New York, Marcel Dekker.

Sato Y., Kimura M., and Fukumi H. 1984. Development of a pertussis component vaccine in Japan. *Lancet* 1: 122.

Seeber S.J., White J.L., and Helm S.L. 1991. Predicting the adsorption of proteins by aluminum-containing adjuvants. *Vaccine* 9: 201.

Shirodkar S., Hutchinson R.L., Perry D.L. et al. 1990. Aluminum compounds used as adjuvants in vaccines. *Pharmacol. Res.* 7: 1282.

Sitrin R.D., Wampler D.E., and Ellis R. 1993. Survey of licensed hepatitis B vaccines and their product processes. In R. Ellis (Ed.), *Hepatitus B Vaccines in Clinical Practice*, p. 83. New York, Marcel Dekker.

Sureau P. 1987. Rabies vaccine production in animal cell cultures. In A. Fiechter (Ed.), *Advances in Biochemical Engineering and Biotechnology*, vol. 34, p. 111. Berlin, Springer-Verlag.

Tyrrell D.A.J. 1976. Inactivated whole virus vaccine. In P. Selby (Ed.), *Influenza, Virus, Vaccines and Strategy*, p. 137. New York, Academic Press.

Ulmer J.B., Donnelly J.J., Parker S.E. et al. 1993. Heterologous protection against influenza by injection of DNA encoding a viral protein. *Science* 259: 1745.

Volkin D.B. and Klibanov A.M. 1989. Minimizing protein inactivation. In T.E. Creighton (Ed.), *Protein Function: A Practical Approach*, pp. 1–12. Oxford, IRL Press.

Further Information

A detailed description of all the aspects of traditional bacterial vaccine manufacture may be found in the World Health Organization technical report series for the production of whole-cell pertussis, diphtheria, and tetanus toxoid vaccines:

World Health Organization. 1997a. BLG/UNDP/77.1 Rev. 1. Manual for the Production and Control of Vaccines: Diphtheria Toxoid.

World Health Organization. 1997b. BLG/UNDP/77.2 Rev. 1. Manual for the Production and Control of Vaccines: Tetanus Toxoid.

World Health Organization. 1997c. BLG/UNDP/77.3 Rev. 1. Manual for the Production and Control of Vaccines: Pertussis Vaccine.

A description of all the aspects of cell culture and viral vaccine manufacture may be found in Spier R.E. and Griffiths J.B. 1985. *Animal Cell Biotechnology*, vol. 1 to 3. London, Academic Press.

For a review of virology and virus characteristics, the reader is referred to Fields B.N. and Knipe D.M. (Eds.). 1990. *Virology*, 2nd ed, vol. 1 and 2. New York, Raven Press.

14

Protein Engineering

Scott Banta
Columbia University

Proteins are the workhorses of the cell. With different combinations of the 20 common amino acids (and some modification of these amino acids), proteins have been evolved with a staggering array of functions and capabilities including: the specific binding of ligands, catalysis of complex chemical reactions, functionality in extreme environments, transportation of valuable molecules, and the exhibition of diverse structural and material properties. Therefore, there has been a long and rich body of research aimed at the investigation of proteins and their abilities, which has been partially motivated due to their widespread participation in disease processes.

The main thrusts in the field of protein engineering can be loosely divided into two areas. Originally, protein engineering evolved as (1) a powerful method for the investigation and verification of hypotheses during the study of protein functions. For example, theories that arose about the mechanisms of enzymatic catalysis could be proven or debunked through the mutation of key amino acid side chains. This approach has greatly enhanced our understanding and appreciation of a wide variety of protein structures and functions.

Out of this academic pursuit, it was soon realized that these same techniques could also be used to (2) engineer proteins for desired improvements. Proteins are generally optimized to function in their native environments. As enzymes are to be increasingly employed in new situations, and in novel therapeutic applications, methods for the rapid and targeted improvements of proteins are required. This chapter will focus on the latter focus of protein engineering, and an attempt will be made to provide an overview of the state of the art of protein engineering, especially as it pertains to the field of biomedical engineering.

14.1   Protein Engineering Goals

When protein engineering is used to attempt to improve proteins, there are often many traits that can be targeted for improvements. These traits can be roughly divided into four categories (Table 14.1).

Many proteins of interest are enzymes, and the most obvious trait of an enzyme to alter is its *activity*. This can involve improving the native activity of the enzyme toward a substrate, or trying to coax the enzyme to have an activity toward an alternative substrate or to produce an alternative product. Often natural enzymes are regulated in some way, through either feedback control or some other mechanism, and often it is of interest to modulate this effect.

In many applications, the activity of the enzyme may be adequate, but it may be desirable to have the enzyme function in a nonnatural environment. When these proteins are utilized in a foreign environment, they are no longer optimized to function there. Therefore, efforts have been aimed at improving the *stability* and functionality of the enzyme in the new environment. This new environment may differ from the natural environment in temperature, pH, ionic strength, solvent chemistry, or combinations of these.

Another area of active research is the engineering of protein *expression* and quality. Generally, proteins that are subjected to protein engineering are no longer being expressed in their native organism. These changes can result in low protein yields, or proteins of poor quality. For example, many proteins from higher life forms often undergo posttranslational modifications during their production, and these modifications may not be performed properly in the new expression system. Therefore, many researchers have attempted to alter and improve the yield and quality of the recombinant protein product.

Finally, there are several other *miscellaneous* protein engineering goals that do not fit into the above categories. For example, it is clear that protein purification can be an expensive and complex procedure, and therefore some projects are designed to simplify these steps. Another area of active research is aimed at "humanizing" engineered proteins to decrease their tendency to illicit an immune response in therapeutic applications.

TABLE 14.1   Traits that can be Altered Through Protein Engineering

Activity	Improved catalysis with natural substrate or cofactor
	Improved catalysis with nonnatural substrate or cofactor
	Increased catalysis in nonnatural solvent
	Improved ligand binding
	Decreased effects of inhibition
Stability	Increased thermostability
	Increased activity in alternative pH
	Increased activity in different ionic strength
	Improved protein folding
	Decreased susceptibility to proteolysis
	Pharmacokinetics
Expression	Improved expression levels in nonnatural host
	Targeted expression to different cellular location
	Added tags to detect protein expression
	Altered posttranslational modifications
Other traits	Added tags to facilitate purification
	Altered tendency for polymerization
	Added tags to visualize localization
	Engineered allosteric binding sites
	Altered isoelectric point
	Decreased immunogenicity

14.2 Preliminary Requirements

Before a protein engineering project can begin, a certain amount of information is required about the protein of interest. First, the amino acid sequence of the protein is required. Second, the DNA sequence that encodes the amino acid sequence is needed, as most protein engineering work is done at the DNA level (Figure 14.1). There are several methods that can be used to obtain the DNA sequence from a source organism, including the powerful polymerase chain reaction (PCR) [1].

Regardless of the source organism of the protein, most protein engineering work uses bacterial systems. Therefore, once a DNA sequence is obtained, it is usually inserted into a bacterial plasmid, which is a double-stranded circular DNA element. The plasmid generally has an origin of replication, so that the bacterial strain can propagate the plasmid, as well as a gene encoding resistance to an antibiotic drug, such as ampicillin. By growing the cells in the presence of the drug, they are forced to harbor the plasmid in order to survive. The plasmid can also contain regulatory sequences to direct the expression of the target protein.

Although not required, a third tool that can aid in the engineering of a protein is 3-dimensional (3-D) structural information. If the protein is similar in structure to other well-studied proteins, it may be possible to infer basic structural information through its homology to other known structures. However, the determination of the 3-D structure of the actual protein, either using x-ray crystallography or nuclear magnetic resonance (NMR) techniques, is ideal. This information can then be used to attempt to guide the protein engineering effort.

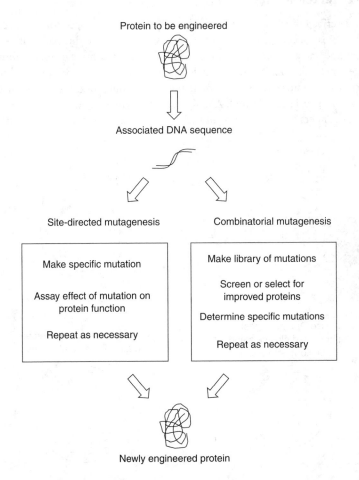

FIGURE 14.1 Overview of protein engineering.

The final requirement for the engineering of a protein is a method for assaying whether the trait(s) of the protein have been improved. At times, this requirement can be a rate-limiting step in protein engineering. For example, if it is desired to improve the kinetic parameters of an enzyme, it may be necessary to purify each new mutant enzyme and perform extensive kinetic characterizations to determine the results of the mutation.

14.3 Rational Mutagenesis

In order to actually make alterations to proteins, two main approaches have been developed and described (1) rational mutagenesis, and (2) combinatorial methods (Figure 14.1). In rational mutagenesis, a "top-down" approach is taken, where a hypothesis is made about mutations at a specific location, which is often guided by 3-D structural information, and the hypothesis is tested through the mutation of specific amino acids and assays of the subsequent mutant proteins. This is in contrast to the combinatorial paradigms, which are described in the next section, where a "bottom-up" approach is taken. In this approach, a library of different mutant proteins is produced. A method is then developed to screen or select members of the library that have an improved trait, and then the mutations that caused the improvement are determined later. Both of these methods have been extensively used in the literature for the successful engineering of a wide variety of important proteins.

14.3.1 Site-Directed Mutagenesis

Since it was first described in 1978 [2], many methods have been developed for the specific alteration of a DNA sequence to create a change in a protein, which is known as site-directed mutagenesis. Currently, one of the fastest and most flexible ways to perform site-directed mutagenesis is through the use of the QuickChange® method from Stratagene (La Jolla, CA) (Figure 14.2). This protocol requires a pair of complementary DNA oligonucleotides that contain the desired mutation(s) along with flanking sequences that will hybridize to the original plasmid. A high-fidelity polymerase enzyme is added that can use the oligonucleotides as primers to create a copy of the rest of the original plasmid. The original unmutated

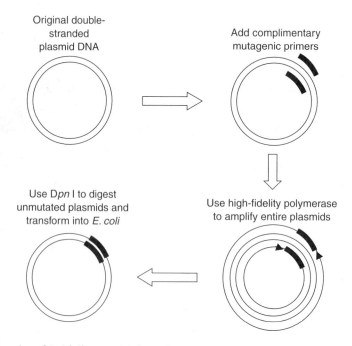

FIGURE 14.2   Overview of QuickChange® site-directed mutagenesis from Stratagene.

plasmid is then digested away, and the new mutant plasmid can be inserted back into a bacterial host. This and other methods have reduced the chore of site-directed mutagenesis to an almost trivial laboratory exercise.

14.3.2 Other Methods

Site-directed mutagenesis can be used to rapidly change amino acids, insert amino acids, and delete amino acids in almost any plasmid construct. However, it is not capable of making large changes, such as dramatic insertions, deletions, or significant rearrangements. In order to do this type of work, restriction endonucleases can be used. These enzymes have the ability to cleave DNA at very specific recognition sequences, and a DNA ligase can be used to reconnect the DNA sequences together. Due to the degeneracy of the amino acid code, site-directed mutagenesis can often be used to introduce recognition sequences for different restriction endonucleases into the plasmid, without altering the associated protein sequence. Using these tools, it is possible to cut and paste DNA sequences in almost any way, and thus it is possible to make fusion proteins, to swap domains of proteins, and to remove entire sections of proteins. These techniques are also often used in the creation of libraries of mutant proteins, as described in the next section.

14.3.3 An Example: Insulin

Rational protein engineering has been successfully used in a variety of problems of interest in biomedical engineering. One of the first, and perhaps the most widely used examples can be found with the protein engineering of human insulin for the treatment of diabetes [3]. Native insulin has evolved to form dimers and hexamers, so that it can be produced and stockpiled in the pancreas before it is needed for release in the body. When purified insulin is injected subcutaneously following a meal as a treatment for diabetes, only the active monomer form is desired, and thus the formation of dimers and hexamers can slow absorption. This has been addressed using site-directed mutagenesis to introduce repulsive charges and steric hindrances at the dimer interface, in order to reduce the tendency of human insulin to self-assemble. This work has led to insulin monomers that have an increased rate of absorption, and thus a produce a preferable postprandial plasma concentration profile [4].

14.4 Combinatorial Methods

Site-directed mutagenesis has been a valuable method for the engineering of many proteins, but a significant limitation on this technique is that it can be difficult to know what mutations should be made in order to obtain a desired functionality. For example, in order to increase the thermostability of a protein, it is not clear by looking at a 3-D structure which amino acid side chains will affect this trait. In addition, improvements made in the thermostability of the enzyme may adversely affect other properties of the protein, such as enzymatic activity. Therefore, there has been a good deal of interest in combinatorial methods for protein engineering, which can be used to sample a large area of the protein solution space, and thus rapidly identify proteins with desired functionalities.

The combinatorial methods generally require two separate protocols. First, a method is designed to generate a combinatorial library, such that it is diverse enough to include the desired protein solutions. Second, a method is chosen to isolate the best solutions from this library and identify the resulting mutations.

14.4.1 Library Construction

There are several methods available for the generation of the mutant libraries. If the protein or peptide is very small, or if it is desired to randomize only a small part of a protein, then it can be possible to produce a library with random combinations of the 20 amino acids at specific locations [5]. Of course,

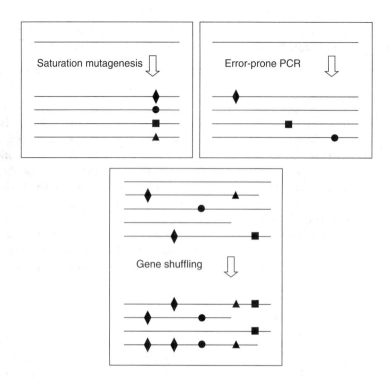

FIGURE 14.3 Comparison of methods used to generate mutant protein libraries. Symbols represent different codons.

this procedure, known as *saturation mutagenesis* (Figure 14.3), is not possible with large numbers of amino acids, as the possible members of library will grow unmanageable very rapidly.

Alternative methods have been described which aim to mimic the process of natural evolution. One way to accomplish this is to repeatedly amplify the native DNA sequence using PCR, but under suboptimal conditions [6]. This will cause the polymerase enzyme to make mistakes at a known error-rate, and thus a library with small random changes throughout the protein will be created (Figure 14.3). One of the significant limitations of this *error-prone PCR* approach is that the mutations are often conservative, and that amino acid insertions and deletions cannot occur.

Probably the most interesting protocol for library construction is modeled after sexual homologous recombination. In this method, the native DNA sequence is combined with similar DNA sequences. These other sequences can encode for similar proteins found in alternative organisms, proteins that have slightly different activities, and even proteins that were already created through other protein engineering methods (like error-prone PCR). The sequences are then randomly fragmented and allowed to reassemble, such that pieces of the different parent sequences are combined together to make random chimeras. This process, known as *gene shuffling*, allows for a greater sampling of the possible sequence space, and it can permit large amino acid changes, insertions, and deletions [7,8] (Figure 14.3). Following the first reports of gene shuffling, other techniques have been developed to extend and improve the methods for making random chimeras from even distantly related DNA sequences [9].

14.4.2 Screening and Selection Methods

Once a strategy is chosen for the construction of the library, a method must be employed in order to determine which proteins (and ultimately which mutations) exhibit an improvement in the desired trait(s). This can be accomplished in two ways, either through a (1) screening method, where members of the library are randomly interrogated for desired improvements, or (2) a selection method, where the library is enriched to only contain members that display improvements which are then screened.

TABLE 14.2   Methods for Associating Protein Libraries with
Their Cognate DNA Sequences

Replicate libraries	Stamped copies of agar plates
	Duplicates of multi-welled plates
Physical linkages	Phage display
	Bacterial cell surface display
	Yeast cell surface display
	Mammalian cell surface display
	Ribosomal display
	Plasmid display
Compartmentalization	Cellular pathways
	In vitro emulsions
	n-Hybrid systems

Source: From Lin, H. and Cornish, V.K. *Angew Chem. Int. Ed.
Engl.* 41: 4402–4425, 2002. With permission.

This decision will depend on the nature of the trait that is to be improved, as well as the format of the protein library.

Once a newly improved peptide or protein is identified from the library, by either a selection or a screen, the sequence of the new protein will be desired. Since it can be difficult or impossible to amplify and sequence the protein directly, it is generally preferred to use the DNA for amplification and sequencing. Therefore, several methods have been described for use in selection or screening where the mutant protein libraries are somehow associated with their cognate DNA sequences (Table 14.2) [10].

In the simplest case, the protein and DNA are *compartmentalized* together naturally in a cell. If the desired trait can be assessed through phenotypic selection, without disrupting the cell, then it can be fairly straightforward to select for cells exhibiting the desired improvements, and then sequence the DNA for the responsible mutations.

If the cell needs to be destroyed in order to assay the performance of the new proteins, then *replicate libraries* of cells with assigned addresses can be constructed, so that one copy can be used for a functional assay and the other copy can be used for sequence identification. In this approach, a selection is often not possible, and screening techniques are used.

Finally, if the trait to be altered needs to be measured outside of the cell, like the binding of a ligand, then there are several methods available to physically link the expressed mutant proteins to their mutant DNA sequences. This can be accomplished using *display techniques*, where the mutant proteins are displayed on the surface of a DNA carrying vehicle, such as a virus (phages), bacteria, yeast, mammalian cell, ribosome, and even the plasmid DNA itself. These methods are very amenable to a selection protocol, and then the attached vehicle can be used to retrieve the DNA sequence of the displayed proteins.

14.4.3 Some Examples

In order to perform combinatorial mutagenesis, the final protocol will depend on the nature of the trait chosen for improvement. In one of the earliest examples of combinatorial mutagenesis, error-prone PCR was used to generate a library of mutant subtilisin E proteases. A replicated library method was used to screen colonies that secreted enzymes with improved activity in an organic solvent [11]. More recently, by using both error-prone PCR and gene shuffling, combined with yeast cell surface display, it was possible to select single-chain antibodies with femtomolar binding affinities [12].

As these techniques have been improved, reports have started to appear describing the evolution of enzymes with medical applications. A recent paper has reported the gene shuffling of over 20 human interferon-α genes and the use of phage display, which was used to select mutant cytokines that demonstrated superior antiviral and antiproliferation activities in a mouse cell assay [13]. In an other recent work, a butyrylcholinesterase (BChE) enzyme has been evolved using a mammalian cell expression system to improve its natural ability to metabolize cocaine, which could be used as a treatment for both acute cocaine overdose and addiction [14].

14.5 Assessment of Improvements and Cycle Repetition

Once mutant proteins are produced, either rationally or combinatorially, the new proteins need to be characterized in order to determine the full effects of the underlying mutations. It has been repeatedly shown that improvements in one trait can come at the cost of another trait. This can be especially true in combinatorial methods, where "you get what you screen for." Once the effects of the mutations are understood, the process is repeated in order to produce further improvements in the protein of interest. In some cases, it may also be useful to combine the methods or protein engineering. For example, combinatorial methods may suggest an area in the protein that should be further investigated using site-directed mutagenesis.

14.6 Conclusions

In the past 25 years, protein engineering has evolved as a powerful tool for the study and manipulation of proteins, and this young field has already produced many important results in the basic sciences, as well as in the applied disciplines [15]. With the completion of the human genome project, there is an intensified interest in the elucidation of new protein structures and functions, and protein engineering will play an important role in these efforts. In addition, as combinatorial methods are improved and possibly combined with traditional site-directed mutagenesis, it seems likely that proteins displaying even greater deviations from nature's palette will be constructed. A powerful example of this potential can be seen in the recent report of the use of saturation mutagenesis and phage display to use the lipocalin protein as a scaffold for the generation of completely *de novo* binding proteins [16,17]. The creation of new proteins, with new functionalities, will undoubtedly lead to novel and improved proteins for therapeutic uses, as well as novel proteins that will play pivotal roles in other medical advances. The combination of protein engineering with metabolic engineering (Chapter 15) also presents the intriguing possibility of designing and creating new proteins as participants in synthetic metabolic pathways.

References

[1] Saiki, R.K., Scharf, S., Faloona, F., Mullis, K.B., Horn, G.T. et al. Enzymatic amplification of beta-globin genomic sequences and restriction site analysis for diagnosis of sickle cell anemia. *Science* 230: 1350–1354, 1985.

[2] Hutchison, C.A., 3rd, Phillips, S., Edgell, M.H., Gillam, S., Jahnke, P. et al. Mutagenesis at a specific position in a DNA sequence. *J. Biol. Chem.* 253: 6551–6560, 1978.

[3] Brange, J. The new era of biotech insulin analogues. *Diabetologia* 40 (Suppl 2): S48–S53, 1997.

[4] Brange, J., Ribel, U., Hansen, J.F., Dodson, G., Hansen, M.T. et al. Monomeric insulins obtained by protein engineering and their medical implications. *Nature* 333: 679–682, 1988.

[5] Wells, J.A., Vasser, M., and Powers, D.B. Cassette mutagenesis: an efficient method for generation of multiple mutations at defined sites. *Gene* 34: 315–323, 1985.

[6] Leung, D.W., Chen, E., and Goeddel, D.V. A method for random mutagenesis of a defined DNA segment using a modified polymerase chain reaction. *Technique* 1: 11–15, 1989.

[7] Stemmer, W.P. Rapid evolution of a protein *in vitro* by DNA shuffling. *Nature* 370: 389–391, 1994.

[8] Stemmer, W.P. DNA shuffling by random fragmentation and reassembly: *in vitro* recombination for molecular evolution. *Proc. Natl Acad. Sci. USA* 91: 10747–10751, 1994.

[9] Neylon, C. Chemical and biochemical strategies for the randomization of protein encoding DNA sequences: library construction methods for directed evolution. *Nucleic Acids Res.* 32: 1448–1459, 2004.

[10] Lin, H. and Cornish, V.W. Screening and selection methods for large-scale analysis of protein function. *Angew Chem. Int. Ed. Engl.* 41: 4402–4425, 2002.

[11] Chen, K. and Arnold, F.H. Tuning the activity of an enzyme for unusual environments: sequential random mutagenesis of subtilisin E for catalysis in dimethylformamide. *Proc. Natl Acad Sci. USA* 90: 5618–5622, 1993.

[12] Boder, E.T., Midelfort, K.S., and Wittrup, K.D. Directed evolution of antibody fragments with monovalent femtomolar antigen-binding affinity. *Proc. Natl Acad. Sci. USA* 97: 10701–10705, 2000.

[13] Chang, C.C., Chen, T.T., Cox, B.W., Dawes, G.N., Stemmer, W.P. et al. Evolution of a cytokine using DNA family shuffling. *Nat. Biotechnol.* 17: 793–797, 1999.

[14] Vasserot, A.P., Dickinson, C.D., Tang, Y., Huse, W.D., Manchester, K.S. et al. Optimization of protein therapeutics by directed evolution. *Drug Discov. Today* 8: 118–126, 2003.

[15] Brannigan, J.A. and Wilkinson, A.J. Protein engineering 20 years on. *Nat. Rev. Mol. Cell Biol.* 3: 964–970, 2002.

[16] Beste, G., Schmidt, F.S., Stibora, T., and Skerra, A. Small antibody-like proteins with prescribed ligand specificities derived from the lipocalin fold. *Proc. Natl Acad. Sci. USA* 96: 1898–1903, 1999.

[17] Schlehuber, S., Beste, G., and Skerra, A. A novel type of receptor protein, based on the lipocalin scaffold, with specificity for digoxigenin. *J. Mol. Biol.* 297: 1105–1120, 2000.

Further Information

Several books have been published on the classical techniques and applications of protein engineering, including: Wrede, P. and Schneider, G. (Eds.), 1994, *Concepts in Protein Engineering and Design*, Walter de Gruyter, Berlin; and Cleland, J.L. and Craik, C.S. (Eds.), 1996, *Protein Engineering Principles and Practice*, Wiley-Liss, New York. Two recent books on directed evolution methods and protocols are also of interest: Arnold, F.H. and Georgiou, G. (Eds.), 2003, *Directed Evolution Library Creation Methods and Protocols*, Humana Press, New Jersey; and Arnold, F.H. and Georgiou, G. (Eds.), 2003, *Directed Enzyme Evolution Screening and Selection Methods*, Humana Press, New Jersey.

15

Metabolic Engineering

Scott Banta
Columbia University

Craig Zupke
Amgen Corporation

Cellular metabolism is an intricate and highly evolved chemical network that allows a cell or organism to extract and utilize material from its environment to make useful products including primary metabolites, secondary metabolites, and high-energy molecules. The study of the metabolic capabilities of different cells has been an active area of inquiry for many years. Recently, the field of Metabolic Engineering has evolved, which allows for (a) the quantitative modeling and characterization of metabolic networks, and (b) the engineering of metabolic networks to bring about a desired new goal. Metabolic engineering was originally developed and applied for use in prokaryotic systems, but recently it has been increasingly applied to eukaryotic systems and problems of biomedical interest.

Metabolic engineering is a relatively young field, and as it has evolved, some general principles and techniques have emerged. In particular, several mathematical modeling techniques have been developed, including Metabolic Flux Analysis (MFA) and Metabolic Control Analysis (MCA). These techniques allow for the quantitative characterization of the cellular metabolism in either normal or perturbed states. These approaches can be used to both suggest strategies for, and interpret the results of, metabolic pathway engineering.

Advances in the field of molecular biology have resulted in a set of highly effective tools for the rational alteration of metabolic pathways. Using these tools and techniques, including recombinant DNA technology, gene therapy, and antisense DNA techniques, it is possible to add, remove, and fundamentally alter metabolic pathways in almost any cell type. These approaches can be used to create cells and organisms with nonnatural metabolic abilities, which can be used in both biotechnology and biomedicine.

Metabolic engineering is inherently multidisciplinary, combining knowledge and techniques from cellular and molecular biology, biochemistry, chemical engineering, mathematics, computer science, and physiology. The purpose of this chapter is to provide an overview of the main themes in metabolic engineering, as well as to describe the state of the art of metabolic engineering as it pertains to biomedical engineering.

15.1   Metabolic Engineering Goals

The first goal of metabolic engineering is the quantitative modeling of metabolic pathways. For simple metabolic networks, sophisticated mathematical modeling of the network can yield a platform that can be used to predict the behavior of the system under different conditions. For example, an elaborate kinetic model of red blood cell metabolism has been constructed that can be used to explore the response of the cells to different environments [1]. For more complex metabolic systems, this approach may prove to be prohibitively difficult due to the extensive experimental work required to thoroughly characterize the kinetic behavior of the enzymes in the network. Therefore, other modeling techniques have been developed to provide insights into different metabolic states, as well as levels of control in metabolic networks. For example, several of these alternative approaches have been used to study hepatic metabolism under different physiological conditions [2–4].

The second goal of metabolic engineering is the directed improvement of existing metabolic pathways to reach a desired goal. This generally involves adding, changing, or deleting a reaction in a metabolic network to overcome potential bottlenecks and improve the production of a desired product. For biomedical applications, this approach has been generally applied for two reasons: for the introduction of metabolic pathways that are missing for genetic reasons (inborn errors of metabolism) and for the creation of new metabolic pathways in order to advance a cure for a disease. The expression of liver phenylalanine hydroxylase in the muscles of mice as a potential cure for genetic phenylketonouria represents a combination of these approaches [5].

15.2   Metabolic Networks and Flux Measurements

Before the goals of metabolic engineering can be pursued, basic information about the metabolic network is required as well as the experimental measurements of metabolic fluxes through the network.

15.2.1   Network Construction

The metabolic network in a cell is a complex and nonlinear system that has evolved for specific functions. This network generally includes central carbon metabolism, energy conversion, secondary metabolite production, transport reactions, regulatory mechanisms, etc. The metabolic networks for many important cell types are well understood and available in the literature [6]. However, sometimes a cell or organ system has extensive metabolic capabilities, but only a subset of these functions is active under different conditions. For example, a hepatocyte is capable of both gluconeogenesis and glycolysis, but only one of these metabolic pathways is dominant at any given time. Therefore, the metabolic network is often tailored to best reflect the expected network behavior.

In some cases, only limited information is available about the metabolic network in the cell. This can occur when exotic organisms are employed in biotechnology applications, or when exotic pathogens are studied, and this may require extensive network characterizations before the capabilities of the network can be investigated. Recently, genome sequencing has been used as a tool to assist in these efforts [7]. It may be possible to use genomic data to help to identify enzymes that participate in a new metabolic pathway.

15.2.2   Flux Measurements

In order to begin the modeling and eventual improvement of a metabolic network, experimental measurements of the fluxes through the network are required. The flux through a given pathway is a central concept

TABLE 15.1   Techniques of Metabolic Engineering

Metabolic flux measurements
  Measurement of external metabolite fluxes
  In vivo NMR
  Isotopomer analysis

Metabolic pathway modeling
  Metabolic flux analysis
  Extreme pathway analysis and elementary mode analysis
  Metabolic control analysis
  Kinetic modeling
  Biochemical systems theory
  Cybernetic modeling

Metabolic pathway alterations
  Cellular transfection
  Viral gene delivery
  Antisense technology
  RNA interference

in metabolic engineering, and it is defined as the amount of material that moves between metabolic pools per unit time. Some of these metabolic fluxes occur strictly inside of the cell, and others occur across the cellular boundary. Several tools and techniques haven been developed to assist in the measurement of metabolic fluxes (Table 15.1).

The simplest method for obtaining flux data is to directly measure the uptake or release of selected metabolites by the cells or tissue systems. For example, it is fairly easy to measure the uptake of glucose by cells in a bioreactor. Once the external metabolite fluxes are obtained, the modeling techniques described in the following sections can be used to estimate the associated internal metabolic fluxes.

The measurement of internal metabolic fluxes is more difficult. The direct measurement of intracellular fluxes is possible with *in vivo* nuclear magnetic resonance (NMR) spectroscopy. However, the inherent insensitivity of NMR limits its applicability. An improvement over this approach can be found with isotopic tracer techniques [8]. In isotope tracer methods the cells to be studied are provided with a substrate specifically labeled with a detectable isotope (usually ^{14}C or ^{13}C). The incorporation of label into cellular material and by-products is governed by the fluxes through the biochemical pathways. The quantity and distribution of label is measured and combined with knowledge of the metabolic network to estimate some of the intracellular fluxes. The choices of substrate labeling patterns, as well as which by-products to measure, are guided by careful analysis of the assumed biochemical network. These experiments are usually performed at isotopic steady state so that the flow of isotope into each atom of a metabolite equals the flux out. For the nth atom of the kth metabolite the flux balance is [9]:

$$\sum_i V_{i,k} S_i(m) = S_k(n) \sum_o V_{o,k} \tag{15.1}$$

where $S_i(m)$ is the specific activity of the mth atom of the ith metabolite, which contributes to the labeling of the nth atom of the kth metabolite, $S_k(n)$. $V_{i,k}$ and $V_{o,k}$ are the input and output fluxes of the kth metabolite, respectively. The system of equations represented by Equation 15.1 can be solved for the fluxes ($V_{i,k}$, $V_{o,k}$) from measurements of the specific activities. A similar analysis can be applied to the isotope isomers, or isotopomers, yielding more information from a single experiment. Isotopomer analysis is not just concerned with the average enrichment of individual atoms. Instead, it involves quantifying the amounts of the different isotopomers, which occur at a specific metabolic state. The isotopomer distribution contains more information than that obtained from positional enrichments, making it generally a more powerful technique. Both mass spectrometry and NMR can be used to analyze isotopomer distributions.

15.3   Modeling of Metabolic Networks

Once a metabolic network has been defined and some metabolic fluxes (either external and internal) have been measured, several mathematical modeling tools have been developed to advance our understanding of the metabolic network (Table 15.1) [10]. The applications of these tools can provide valuable insights into the operation of the metabolic network as well as to generate targets for directed pathway improvements.

15.3.1   Metabolic Flux Analysis

If enough fluxes are measured at a metabolic steady state, MFA [11,12] can be used to estimate the fluxes through the remainder of the metabolic reaction network (Figure 15.1). This analysis is powerful because only the stoichiometry of the biochemical reaction network is required, and no knowledge of the chemical reaction kinetics is needed. MFA is usually formulated as a matrix equation:

$$\frac{dX}{dt} = S^T M = 0 \qquad (15.2)$$

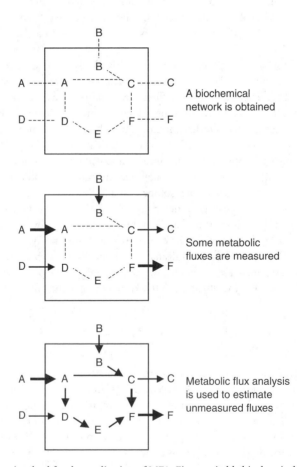

FIGURE 15.1   The steps involved for the application of MFA. First a suitable biochemical network is obtained from the literature or from direct experimentation. Some metabolic fluxes are measured, either directly or by isotopomer techniques. MFA is then used to estimate the values of the unmeasured fluxes in the network based upon the measured metabolic fluxes in a manner analogous to Kirchoff's current law.

where X is a vector of metabolite concentrations, S^T is the matrix of stoichiometric coefficients for the biochemical network, and M is a vector of the metabolic fluxes. A pseudo steady state is assumed, so that the metabolic pool sizes are not significantly changing, and thus the equation can be set to zero. The equation can then be decomposed into the measured ($_M$) and unmeasured ($_C$) metabolic fluxes (Equation 15.3).

$$0 = S^T M = S_M^T M_M + S_C^T M_C \qquad (15.3)$$

And this equation can be used to solve for the vector of unmeasured metabolic fluxes (Equation 15.4).

$$M_C = -(S_C^T)^{-1} S_M^T M_M^T \qquad (15.4)$$

In order to obtain a unique solution to this system, a minimal number of measured fluxes are required. If the system is underdetermined, it is possible to gain insight into the behavior of the system using linear programming and objective functions [13].

In order to extract more information from the steady-state flux model, extreme pathway analysis (EPA) and elementary mode analysis (EMA) have been developed [14,15]. In these approaches, the metabolic reaction network is decomposed into a collection of small irreversible functional pathways. When these pathways are weighted and superimposed back together, they are able to form the original metabolic flux network. By examining the elementary pathways, and using linear optimization tools, it is possible to better explore the metabolic capabilities of a network, and this can also be used to suggest useful metabolic pathway alterations.

15.3.2 Metabolic Control Analysis

MFA and related techniques are able to provide insight into the steady-state behavior of the biochemical network, but it is often of interest to explore levels of control within the network. Metabolic control analysis (MCA) grew from the work originally presented by Kacser and Burns [16] and Heinrich and Rapoport [17]. MCA provides a framework for analyzing and quantifying the distributed control that enzymes exert in biochemical networks.

In the discussion that follows, a metabolic network consists of enzymes (e), metabolites (X), substrates (S), and products (P). For simplicity, we assume that the reaction rate, v_i, is proportional to the enzyme concentration, e_i. If this is not true then some modifications of the analysis are required [18]. The concentrations of the products and substrates are fixed but the metabolite concentrations are free to change in order to achieve a steady state flux, J. An example of a simple, unbranched network is:

$$S \xrightarrow{e_1} X_1 \xrightarrow{e_2} X_2 \xrightarrow{e_3} X_3 \xrightarrow{e_4} P$$

MCA is essentially a sensitivity analysis, which determines how perturbations in a particular parameter (usually enzyme concentration) affect a variable (like steady-state flux). The measures of the sensitivities are control coefficients defined as follows:

$$C_{e_i}^J \equiv \frac{e_i}{J} \frac{\partial J}{\partial e_i} = \frac{\partial \ln |J|}{\partial \ln e_i} \qquad (15.5)$$

The flux control coefficient, $C_{e_i}^J$, is a measure of how the flux J changes in response to small perturbations in the concentration or activity of enzyme i. The magnitude of the control coefficient is a measure of how important a particular enzyme is in the determination of the steady-state flux. The summation theorem relates the individual flux control coefficients:

$$\sum_i C_{e_i}^J = 1 \tag{15.6}$$

A large value for $C_{e_i}^J$ indicates that an increase in the activity of enzyme i (e_i) should result in a large change in the metabolic flux. Thus, enzymes with large flux control coefficients may be good targets for metabolic pathway alterations. Often, there are several enzymes in a network with comparably large C values indicating that there is no single rate-limiting enzyme.

The challenge in analyzing a metabolic network is the determination of the flux control coefficients. It is possible to determine them directly by "enzyme titration" combined with the measurement of the new steady-state flux. For *in vivo* systems this would require alteration of enzyme expression through an inducible promoter and is not very practical for a moderately sized network. A more common method of altering enzyme activities involves titration with a specific inhibitor. However, this technique can be complicated by nonspecific effects of the added inhibitor and unknown inhibitor kinetics.

Although the control coefficients are properties of the network, they can be related to individual enzyme kinetics through elasticity coefficients. If a metabolite concentration, X, is altered, there will be an effect on the reaction rates in which X is involved. The elasticity coefficient, $\varepsilon_X^{v_i}$, is a measure of the effect changes in X has on v_i, the rate of reaction catalyzed by enzyme e_i:

$$\varepsilon_X^{v_i} \equiv \frac{X}{v_i}\frac{\partial v_i}{\partial X} = \frac{\partial \ln v_i}{\partial \ln X} \tag{15.7}$$

The flux control connectivity theorem relates the flux control coefficients to the elasticity coefficients:

$$\sum_i C_{e_i}^J \varepsilon_{X_k}^{v_i} = 0 \quad \text{for all } k \tag{15.8}$$

In principle, if the enzyme kinetics and steady-state metabolite concentrations are known, then it is possible to calculate the elasticities and through Equation 15.8 determine the flux control coefficients.

This traditional approach of MCA can be considered to be "bottom up" since all of the individual enzyme flux control coefficients are determined in order to describe the control structure of a large network. A "top down" approach has also been described, which makes extensive use of lumping of reactions together to determine group flux control coefficients [19]. These can give some information about the overall control of a metabolic network, without its complete characterization.

Consider a simple, multi-reaction pathway:

$$S \rightarrow \rightarrow \rightarrow X \rightarrow \rightarrow \rightarrow P$$

$$\text{produces } X \quad \text{consumes } X$$

$$J_1 \qquad\qquad J_2$$

The reactions of a metabolic network are divided into two groups, those that produce a particular metabolite, X, and those that consume it. By manipulating the concentration of X, and measuring the resulting fluxes, J_1 and J_2, "group" or "overall" elasticities, $*\varepsilon$, of the X producers and X consumers can be determined. Application of the connectivity theorem (Equation 15.8) then permits the calculation of the group control coefficient for both groups of reactions. Each pathway can subsequently be divided into smaller groups centered around different metabolites and the process repeated. The advantage of the top-down approach is that useful information about the control architecture of a metabolic network can be obtained more quickly. This approach is particularly appropriate for highly complex systems like organs or even whole body metabolism [20].

15.3.3 Kinetic Models

Both MFA and MCA can provide detailed insights into the behavior of a metabolic network, but neither of these techniques requires kinetic information about the enzymes in the metabolic network, and thus they cannot be predictive. For simple metabolic networks, containing a few enzymes, it may be possible to measure the enzyme kinetics and then produce a predictive model of metabolism [21]. But for large network systems, this would be prohibitively difficult. Therefore, simplifying approaches have been suggested. In Biochemical Systems Theory (BST), metabolic reaction rates are modeled as power-law expressions [22]. In the Cybernetic approach, some kinetic information is combined with cybernetic variables, which are used to regulate the metabolic network according to objective functions [23]. These techniques require large assumptions about the behavior of the metabolic network, but the predictive power of the models can be highly useful in the design of metabolic pathway improvements.

15.3.4 Examples

The modeling techniques developed for metabolic engineering have been used in several cases to yield valuable information about the metabolic states of different cells, tissues, and organ systems of biomedical interest. For example, MFA has been used to characterize the metabolic response exhibited by the liver several days following a moderate burn injury [3,24]. MCA has been applied to the study of a variety of physiological conditions including cardiac function during reduced coronary blood flow (hibernating myocardium) [25], mitochondrial diseases [26], and even whole body metabolism [20]. EPA and BST have both been used to study erythrocyte metabolism [27,28]. Although these different modeling techniques have predominantly been used in biotechnology applications, it is becoming clear that these techniques will enjoy increased application in biomedical research as metabolic engineering is utilized to investigate medically relevant problems.

15.4 Metabolic Pathway Engineering

The second goal of metabolic engineering is to create new metabolic pathways that are able to perform desired new functions. This process can involve the insertion of new enzymes or changes in expression and regulation of existing enzymes in a metabolic pathway.

The diversity of biochemical reactions found in nature for use in pathway additions is quite extensive, with many enzymes being unique to particular organisms. Pathways can be constructed that are similar to those found in alternative organisms or it is possible to construct metabolic networks that perform a specific transformation not found anywhere in nature. The possibilities are even further increased when enzymes that have been engineered to have nonnatural abilities (protein engineering) are used. When exploring the possibility of synthesizing new biochemical pathways, there are several key issues that may need to be addressed. Given a database of possible enzymatic activities and a choice of substrate and product, one must first generate a complete set of possible biochemical reactions that can perform the desired conversion. Once they are generated, the set of possible biochemical pathways must be checked for thermodynamic feasibility and evaluated in terms of yields, cofactor requirements, and other constraints that might be present.

The addition of new biochemical pathways, or the modification of existing pathways, is likely to affect the rest of the cellular metabolism. The new or altered pathways may compete with other reactions for intermediates or cofactors. To precisely predict the impact of the manipulation of a metabolic network is virtually impossible since it would require a perfect model of all enzyme kinetics and of the control of gene expression. However, attempts have been made to develop modeling techniques to predict the behavior of altered organisms [29].

The tremendous growth in molecular biology in the last several decades has produced a host of tools and techniques that have greatly simplified the process of metabolic pathway construction (Table 15.1).

There have been many examples of creating new metabolic pathways in bacterial systems, but more recently there has been an increase in the examples of pathway manipulation for medical applications.

15.4.1 Recombinant DNA

Traditional recombinant DNA techniques are very flexible and are powerful tools for implementing specific metabolic changes. The first step is the isolation of the DNA that encodes an enzyme of interest. The cloning of the genes encoding specific enzymes from host cells has become a relatively routine procedure, and a description of this procedure lies outside of the scope of this chapter. Once new genes are cloned, they can easily be combined with different promoter sequences, which can then direct the regulation and expression of the new enzyme in the new cellular host.

Once a gene and promoter are obtained, the recombinant gene must be inserted into the new host cell [30]. This is a straightforward procedure when working with prokaryotic systems, but it becomes more complex in eukaryotic applications. Traditional techniques for genetic manipulation generally require the host cells to be cultured *in vitro*. The foreign DNA can then be introduced into the cultured cells through different transfection protocols, including Ca_2PO_4 precipitation, electroporation, and lipofection. The foreign DNA sequence also generally contains a selectable marker, so that the few cells that incorporate the new DNA stably into the genome are retained through selection of the marker. Once a cell line is produced that permanently contains the desired new metabolic alterations, it can be reinserted into its proper environment as part of a therapeutic advance.

15.4.2 Viral Gene Delivery

A major drawback in the use of the traditional recombinant DNA techniques is the inability to insert foreign DNA *in vivo*. This problem has been addressed through the development of viral gene delivery techniques. In these approaches, viral-based vectors are used (retrovirus, adenovirus, adeno associated virus, etc.), which are able to infect targeted cells, and stably insert foreign DNA into the cells. This has tremendous advantages in that it can be used *in vivo*, and it is especially well suited to the correction of inborn errors of metabolism. As the safety and efficacy of these approaches are improved, it is quite likely that it will be possible to use this approach to manipulate other valuable metabolic pathways [31].

15.4.3 Genetic Interference

The previous techniques are mostly used for the addition of metabolic pathways to cells, but sometimes it is desirable to decrease the activity of an enzyme in a pathway. One way this can be accomplished is through the use of antisense technology [32,33]. This can be accomplished in a transient fashion, through the introduction of antisense DNA sequences that are complimentary to the mRNA sequence of the targeted gene. This forms an RNA/DNA hybrid that will stall the translation of the targeted gene. This effect can also be obtained in a permanent fashion through the transfection of the antisense DNA under the control of a promoter. This will result in the production of antisense RNA that will also bind to the targeted mRNA to halt gene expression.

Recently, there has been a great deal of interest in RNA interference (RNAi) [32,34]. In this technique, short double stranded RNA is introduced into cells, or hairpin RNA sequences are stably expressed in cells (Figure 15.2). The double stranded RNA is then processed by the Dicer enzyme to produce short interfering RNAs (siRNAs). These are incorporated into an enzymatic RNA-induced silencing complex (RISC) that is activated with ATP and is able to mediate the cleavage of the target mRNA. This technique has already been used in a high-throughput screen to explore the loss of function of genes in mammalian cells [35] and it is clear that this technique will soon have a large impact on the engineering of metabolic pathways.

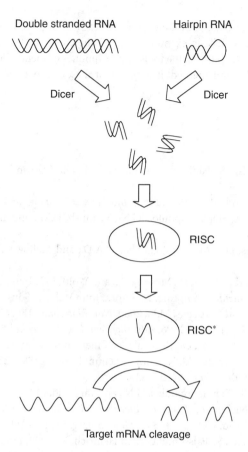

FIGURE 15.2 The mechanism of RNA interference (RNAi). Exogenous double stranded RNA or endogenous hairpin RNA is cleaved by Dicer to make short interfering RNAs (siRNAs). These are incorporated into the RNA-induced silencing complex (RISC). Upon activation with ATP, the siRNA unwinds and the RISC* complex mediates the cleavage of the target mRNA.

15.4.4 Examples

Metabolic pathway engineering has been applied to several medically relevant problems. A good deal of work has been aimed at creating a metabolic pathway capable of dopamine production as a cure for Parkinson's disease. In one approach, fibroblasts have been cultured *in vitro*, a portion of the pathway for dopamine production has been introduced into the cells, and the cells have been implanted in an animal model of Parkinson's [36]. In an alternative approach, viral gene delivery has been used to introduce three enzymes required for dopamine production directly into the brains of a Parkinson's animal model [37]. Metabolic pathway engineering has also been used to attempt alternative treatments for Diabetes. Insulin expression has been engineered into non-insulin-producing cells [38], and glucose sensitivity has been engineered into insulin-producing cells [39]. As the tools and techniques for metabolic pathway engineering are improved, it is likely that these approaches will be expanded in order to attempt to bring new treatments to other diseased states.

15.5 Summary

Metabolic engineering has evolved rapidly in the past few years as an exciting and multidisciplinary field that allows for the quantitative characterization of cellular metabolism as well as the directed manipulation of cellular metabolism. With these techniques, it has already been possible to insert novel biochemical pathways into simple cells. A striking example of this is the creation of a yeast cell line that functions with an expanded genetic code [40]. As the tools and techniques of metabolic engineering are expanded, improved, and more widely implemented, it is clear that these approaches will increasingly impact the biomedical community.

References

[1] Jamshidi, N., Edwards, J.S., Fahland, T., Church, G.M., and Palsson, B.O., 2001, *Bioinformatics* 17: 286–287.

[2] Ainscow, E.K. and Brand, M.D., 1999, *Eur. J. Biochem.* 265: 1043–1055.

[3] Lee, K., Berthiaume, F., Stephanopoulos, G.N., Yarmush, D.M., and Yarmush, M.L., 2000, *Metab. Eng.* 2: 312–327.

[4] Carvalho, R.A., Jones, J.G., McGuirk, C., Sherry, A.D., and Malloy, C.R., 2002, *NMR Biomed.* 15: 45–51.

[5] Harding, C.O., Wild, K., Chang, D., Messing, A., and Wolff, J.A., 1998, *Gene Ther.* 5: 677–683.

[6] Michal, G. 1999, *Biochemical Pathways*. New York: John Wiley & Sons.

[7] Cornish-Bowden, A. and Cardenas, M.L., 2000, *Nat. Biotechnol.* 18: 267–268.

[8] Wiechert, W. and de Graaf, A.A., 1996, *Adv. Biochem. Eng. Biotechnol.* 54: 109–154.

[9] Blum, J.J. and Stein, R.B., 1982, On the analysis of metabolic networks, in *Biological Regulation and Development*, K.R. Yamamoto, Ed. New York: Plenum Press, pp. 99–125.

[10] Wiechert, W., 2002, *J. Biotechnol.* 94: 37–63.

[11] Lee, K., Berthiaume, F., Stephanopoulos, G.N., and Yarmush, M.L., 1999, *Tissue Eng.* 5: 347–368.

[12] Christensen, B. and Nielsen, J., 2000, *Adv. Biochem. Eng. Biotechnol.* 66: 209–231.

[13] Edwards, J.S. and Palsson, B.O., 1998, *Biotechnol. Bioeng.* 58: 162–169.

[14] Schilling, C.H., Schuster, S., Palsson, B.O., and Heinrich, R., 1999, *Biotechnol. Prog.* 15: 296–303.

[15] Schuster, S., Fell, D.A., and Dandekar, T., 2000, *Nat. Biotechnol.* 18: 326–332.

[16] Kacser, H. and Burns, J.A., 1973, *Symp. Soc. Exp. Biol.* 27: 65–104.

[17] Heinrich, R. and Rapoport, T.A., 1974, *Eur. J. Biochem.* 42: 89–95.

[18] Liao, J.C. and Delgado, J., 1993, *Biotechnol. Prog.* 9: 221.

[19] Brown, G.C., Lakin-Thomas, P.L., and Brand, M.D., 1990, *Eur. J. Biochem.* 192: 355–362.

[20] Brown, G.C., 1994, *Biochem. J.* 297: 115–122.

[21] Schuster, R. and Holzhutter, H.G., 1995, *Eur. J. Biochem.* 229: 403–418.

[22] Savageau, M.A., 1991, *J. Theor. Biol.* 151: 509–530.

[23] Varner, J. and Ramkrishna, D., 1999, *Biotechnol. Prog.* 15: 407–425.

[24] Yamaguchi, Y., Yu, Y.M., Zupke, C., Yarmush, D.M., Berthiaume, F. et al., 1997, *Surgery* 121: 295–303.

[25] Vogt, A.M., Poolman, M., Ackermann, C., Yildiz, M., Schoels, W. et al., 2002, *J. Biol. Chem.* 277: 24411–24419.

[26] Letellier, T., Malgat, M., Rossignol, R., and Mazat, J.P., 1998, *Mol. Cell Biochem.* 184: 409–417.

[27] Wiback, S.J. and Palsson, B.O., 2002, *Biophys. J.* 83: 808–818.

[28] Ni, T.C. and Savageau, M.A., 1996, *J. Biol. Chem.* 271: 7927–7941.

[29] Liao, J.C. and Oh, M.K., 1999, *Metab. Eng.* 1: 214–223.

[30] Smith, K.R., 2002, *J. Biotechnol.* 99: 1–22.

[31] Wang, F., Raab, R.M., Washabaugh, M.W., and Buckland, B.C., 2000, *Metab. Eng.* 2: 126–139.

[32] Lee, L.K. and Roth, C.M., 2003, *Curr. Opin. Biotechnol.* 14: 505–511.

[33] Roth, C.M. and Yarmush, M.L., 1999, *Annu. Rev. Biomed. Eng.* 1: 265–297.

[34] Hannon, G.J., 2002, *Nature* 418: 244–251.

[35] Silva, J.M., Mizuno, H., Brady, A., Lucito, R., and Hannon, G.J., 2004, *Proc. Natl Acad. Sci. USA* 101: 6548–6552.

[36] Leff, S.E., Rendahl, K.G., Spratt, S.K., Kang, U.J., and Mandel, R.J., 1998, *Exp. Neurol.* 151: 249–264.

[37] Azzouz, M., Martin-Rendon, E., Barber, R.D., Mitrophanous, K.A., Carter, E.E. et al., 2002, *J. Neurosci.* 22: 10302–10312.

[38] Mitanchez, D., Chen, R., Massias, J.F., Porteu, A., Mignon, A. et al., 1998, *FEBS Lett.* 421: 285–289.

[39] Motoyoshi, S., Shirotani, T., Araki, E., Sakai, K., Kaneko, K. et al., 1998, *Diabetologia* 41: 1492–1501.

[40] Chin, J.W., Cropp, T.A., Anderson, J.C., Mukherji, M., Zhang, Z. et al., 2003, *Science* 301: 964–967.

Further Information

A pioneering discussion of the field of metabolic engineering can be found in: Bailey, J.E. (1991) "Toward a science of metabolic engineering," *Science* 252: 1668–1675. An excellent reference for the modeling aspects of metabolic engineering: *Metabolic Engineering*, Stephanopolous, G.N., Aristidou, A.A., and Nielsen, J., Eds. (1998) Academic Press, San Diego, CA. A recent review of the biomedical applications of metabolic engineering: Yarmush, M.L. and Banta, S. (2003) "Metabolic engineering: advances in modeling and intervention in health and disease," *Annu. Rev. Biomed. Eng.* 5: 349–381.

16

Monoclonal Antibodies and Their Engineered Fragments

Zaki Megeed
David M. Yarmush
Martin L. Yarmush
*Center for Engineering in
Medicine/Surgical Services
Massachusetts General Hospital
Shriners Burns Hospital for Children
Harvard Medical School*

Srikanth Sundaram
*Harvard Medical School
Rutgers University*

Since the publication of the second edition of the *Biomedical Engineering Handbook,* the use of monoclonal antibodies for research, diagnostic, and therapeutic applications has continued to increase at a rapid rate. The production of chimeric, humanized, and human antibodies for therapeutic applications is now the norm, and the fruits of these approaches are reflected in the increased rate of clinical success, in comparison to murine monoclonal antibodies. The objective of this chapter is to provide the reader with a fundamental understanding of monoclonal antibodies and their engineered fragments. In doing so, we have sought to maintain the historical perspective provided in the second edition, through references to the seminal works in the field, while further supplementing the text with the more recent therapeutic and diagnostic applications.

Antibodies are a class of topographically homologous multidomain glycoproteins produced by the immune system that displays a remarkably diverse range of binding specificities. The primary repertoire of antibodies consists of approximately 10^9 different specificities, each of which can be produced by an encounter with the appropriate antigen. This diversity is produced by a series of genetic events, each of which plays a role in determining the final function of the antibody molecule. After the initial exposure to the antigen, additional diversity occurs by a process of somatic mutation so that, for any selected antigen, about 10^4 new binding specificities are generated. Thus, the immunologic repertoire is the most diverse system of binding proteins in biology. Antibodies also display remarkable binding specificity. For example, it has been shown that antibodies are able to distinguish between *ortho-*, *meta-*, and *para-*forms of the same haptenic group [Landsteiner, 1945]. This exquisite specificity and diversity make antibodies ideal candidates for diagnostic and therapeutic applications.

Originally, the source of antibodies was antisera, which by their nature are limited in quantity and heterogeneous in quality. Antibodies derived from such sera are termed *polyclonal antibodies*. Polyclonal antibody production requires methods for the introduction of immunogen into animals, withdrawal of blood for testing the antibody levels, and finally exsanguination for collection of immune sera. These apparently simple technical requirements are complicated by the necessity of choosing a suitable species and immunization protocol that will produce a highly immune animal in a short time. Choice of animal is determined by animal housing facilities available, amount of antiserum required (a mouse will afford only 1.0 to 1.5 ml of blood; a goat can provide several liters), and the amount of immunogen available (mice will usually respond very well to 50 μg or less of antigen; goats may require several milligrams). Another consideration is the phylogenic relationship between the animal from which the immunogen is derived and that used for antibody production. In most cases, it is advisable to immunize a species phylogenetically unrelated to the immunogen donor, and for highly conserved mammalian proteins, nonmammals (e.g., chickens) should be used for antibody production. The polyclonal antibody elicited by an antigen facilitates the localization, phagocytosis, and complement-mediated lysis of that antigen; thus the usual polyclonal immune response has clear advantages *in vivo*. Unfortunately, the antibody heterogeneity that increases immune protection *in vivo* often reduces the usefulness of an antiserum for diagnostic and therapeutic applications. Conventional heterogeneous antisera vary from animal to animal and contain undesirable nonspecific or cross-reacting antibodies. Removal of unwanted specificities from a polyclonal antibody preparation is a time-consuming task, involving repeated adsorption techniques, which often results in the loss of much of the desired antibody and seldom is very effective in reducing the heterogeneity of an antiserum.

After the development of hybridoma technology [Kohler and Milstein, 1975], a potentially unlimited quantity of homogeneous antibodies, with precisely defined specificities and affinities (*monoclonal antibodies*), became available. This resulted in a step change in the utility of antibodies. Monoclonal antibodies (mAbs) have gained increasing importance as reagents in diagnostic and therapeutic medicine, in the identification and determination of antigen molecules, in biocatalysis (catalytic antibodies), and in affinity purification and labeling of antigens and cells.

16.1 Structure and Function of Antibodies

Antibody molecules are essentially required to carry out two principal roles in the immune response. First, they recognize and bind nonself or foreign material (antigen binding). In molecular terms, this generally means binding to structures on the surface of the foreign material (antigenic determinants) that differ from those on the host. Second, they trigger the elimination of foreign material (biologic effector functions). In molecular terms, this involves binding of effector molecules (such as complement) to the antibody–antigen complex to trigger elimination mechanisms such as the complement system and phagocytosis by macrophages and neutrophils.

In humans, five major immunoglobulin classes have been identified, which include immunoglobulins G (IgG), A (IgA), M (IgM), D (IgD), and E (IgE). With the exception of IgA (dimer) and IgM (pentamer), all other antibody classes are monomeric. The monomeric antibody molecule consists of a basic four-chain structure, as shown in Figure 16.1. There are two distinct types of chains: the light (L) and heavy chains (H). They are held together by interchain disulfides, and the two heavy chains are held together by numerous disulfides in the hinge region. The light chains have a molecular weight of about 25,000 Da, while the heavy chains have a molecular weight of 50,000 to 77,000 Da, depending on the isotope. The light

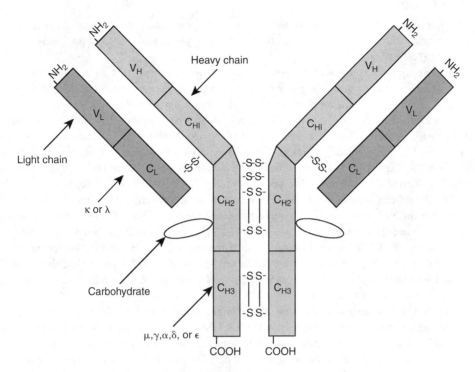

FIGURE 16.1 The structure of a monomeric antibody molecule.

chains can be divided into two subclasses, kappa (κ) and lambda (λ), based on their structures and amino acid sequences. In humans, about 65% of the antibody molecules have κ chains, whereas in rodents, they constitute over 95% of all antibody molecules. The light chain consists of two structural domains: the carboxy-terminal half of the chain is constant except for certain allotypic and isotype variations and is called the C_L (constant: light chain) region, whereas the amino-terminal half of the chain shows high sequence variability and is known as the V_L (variable: light chain) region. The heavy chains are unique for each immunoglobulin class and are designated by the Greek letter corresponding to the capital letter designation of the immunoglobulin class (α for the H chains of IgA, γ for the H chains of IgG). IgM and IgA have a third chain component, the J-chain, which joins the monomeric units. The heavy chain usually consists of four domains: the amino-terminal region ($\sim$110 amino acid residues) exhibits high sequence variability and is called the V_H (variable: heavy chain) region, whereas there are three domains called C_{H1}, C_{H2}, and C_{H3} in the constant part of the chain. The C_{H2} domain is glycosylated, and it has been shown that this glycosylation is important in some of the effector functions of antibody molecules. The extent of glycosylation varies with the antibody class and the method of its production. In some antibodies (i.e., IgE and IgM), there is an additional domain in the constant part of the heavy chain called the C_{H4} region. The hinge region of the heavy chain (found between the C_{H1} and C_{H2} domains) contains a large number of hydrophilic and proline residues and is responsible for the segmental flexibility of the antibody molecule.

All binding interactions with the antigen occur within the variable domains (V_H and V_L). Each variable domain consists of three regions of relatively greater variability, which have been termed *hypervariable* (HV) or *complementarity-determining regions* (CDRs) because they are the regions that determine specificity for a particular antigen. Each CDR is relatively short, consisting of 6 to 15 residues. In general, the topography of the six combined CDRs (three from each variable domain) produces a structure that is designed to accommodate the particular antigen. The CDRs on the light chain include residues 24–34 (Ll), 50–56 (L2), and 89–73 (L3), whereas those on the heavy chain include residues 31–35 (H1), 50–65 (H2), and 95–102 (H3) in the Kabat numbering system. The regions between the hypervariable regions are called the *framework regions* (FRs) because they are more conserved and play an important structural role. The effector functions are, on the other hand, mediated via the two C-terminal constant domains, namely, the C_{H2} and C_{H3}.

Each variable region is composed of several different genetic elements that are separate on the germ line chromosome but rearrange in the B-cell to produce a variable-region exon. The light chain is composed of two genetic elements, a variable (V) gene and a joining (J) gene. The V_κ gene generally encodes residues 1 to 95 in a kappa light chain, and the J_κ gene encodes residues 96 to 107, which is the carboxyl end of the variable region. Thus the kappa variable gene encodes all the first and second hypervariable regions (Ll and L2), and a major portion of the third hypervariable region (L3). In humans, there are approximately 76 different V_κ genes and about 5 functional J_κ genes [Kawasaki et al., 2001]; the potential diversity is increased by the imprecision of V–J joining. The heavy-chain variable region is similarly produced by the splicing together of genetic elements that are distant from each other in the germ line. The mature V_H region is produced by the splicing of a variable gene segment (V) to a diversity segment (D) and to a joining (J) segment. There are about 300 V_H genes, about 5 D_H genes, and 9 functional J_H genes [Tizard, 1992]. With respect to the CDRs of the heavy chain, H1 and H2 are encoded by the V_H gene, while the H3 region is formed by the joining of the V, D, and J genes. Additional diversity is generated by recombinational inaccuracies, light- and heavy-chain recombination, and N-region additions.

The three-dimensional structure of several monoclonal antibodies has been determined via x-ray crystallography and has been reviewed extensively [Padlan, 1994]. Each domain consists of a sandwich of 13 sheets with a layer of four and three strands making up the constant domains and a layer of four and five strands making up the variable domains. The CDRs are highly solvent exposed and are the loops at the ends of the variable-region β strands that interact directly with the antigen. The superimposition of several V_L and V_H structures from available x-ray crystallographic coordinates using the conserved framework residues shows that the framework residues of the antibody variable domains are spatially closely superimposable. The CDRs varied in shape, length, and sequence. Similarities in the structures of the CDRs from one antibody to another suggest that they are held in a fixed position in space, at least within a domain. In addition, the N- and C-termini of the CDRs were rigidly constrained by the framework residues. Among the CDRs, Ll, L2, H2, and H3 show the most conformational variability.

16.2 Monoclonal Antibody Cloning Techniques

The original method for cloning murine monoclonal antibodies is through the fusion of antibody-producing spleen B-cells and a myeloma cell line [Kohler and Milstein, 1975]. Subsequently, monoclonal antibodies have been cloned without resorting to hybridoma technology, via the expression of combinatorial libraries of antibody genes isolated directly from either immunized or naive murine spleens or human peripheral blood lymphocytes. In addition, the display of functional antibody fragments (Fab, sFv, Fv) on the surface of filamentous bacteriophage has further facilitated the screening and isolation of engineered antibody fragments directly from the immunologic repertoire. Repertoire cloning and phage display technology are now readily available in the form of commercial kits with complete reagents and protocols.

16.2.1 Hybridoma Technology

In 1975, Kohler and Milstein showed that mouse myeloma cells could be fused to B-lymphocytes from immunized mice to generate continuously growing, specific monoclonal antibody-secreting somatic cell hybrids, or *hybridoma* cells. In the fused hybridoma, the B-cell contributes the capacity to produce a specific antibody, and the myeloma cell confers longevity in culture and the ability to form tumors in animals.

The number of fusions obtained via hybridoma technology is small, and hence there is a need to select for fused cells. The selection protocol takes advantage of the fact that in normal cells there are two biosynthetic pathways to produce nucleotides and nucleic acids. The *de novo* pathway can be blocked with aminopterin, and the salvage pathway requires the presence of functional hypoxanthine guanine phosphoribosyl transferase (HGPRT). Thus, by choosing a myeloma cell line that is deficient in HGPRT as the "fusion partner," Kohler and Milstein devised a selection protocol. The hybrid cells are selected using hypoxanthine, aminopterin, and thymidine (HAT) medium, in which only myeloma cells that have fused to spleen cells are able to survive (since unfused myeloma cells are HGPRT). There is no need to select for unfused spleen cells because these die in culture.

Briefly, animals (mice or rats) are immunized by injecting them with soluble antigen or cells and an immunoadjuvant. Three or four weeks later, the animals receive a booster injection of the antigen without the adjuvant. Three to five days after this second injection, the spleens of those animals that produce the highest antibody titer to the antigen are excised. The spleen cells are mixed with an appropriate fusion partner, which is usually a nonsecreting hybridoma or myeloma cell (e.g., SP2/0 with 8-azaguanine selection) that is HGPRT. The cell suspension is briefly exposed to a solution of polyethylene glycol (PEG) to induce fusion by reversibly disrupting the cell membrane, and the hybrid cells are selected for in HAT medium. In general, mouse myelomas yield hybridization frequencies of about 1 to 100 clones per 10^7 lymphocytes. After 4 to 21 days, hybridoma cells are visible and culture supernatants are screened for antibody secretion by a number of techniques (e.g., radioimmunoassay, ELISA, and immunoblotting). Those culture wells that are positive for antibody production are then expanded and subcloned by limiting dilution or in soft agar, to ensure that they are derived from a single progenitor cell and to ensure stability of antibody production. The subclones are, in turn, screened for antibody secretion, and selected clones are expanded for antibody production *in vitro*, using culture flasks or bioreactors, or *in vivo* as ascites in mice. Reversion of hybridomas to nonsecreting forms can occur due to loss or rearrangement of chromosomes.

The most commonly used protocol is the PEG fusion technique, which, even under the most efficient conditions, results in the fusion of <0.5% of the spleen cells, with only about 1 in 10^5 cells forming viable hybrids. Several methods have been developed to enhance conventional hybrid formation that have led to incremental improvements in the efficiency of the fusion process (reviewed in Neil and Urnovitz, 1988). Methods that enhance conventional hybridoma formation include pretreatment of myeloma cells with colcemid and *in vitro* antigen stimulation of the spleen cells prior to fusion, addition of dimethyl sulfoxide (DMSO) or phytohemagglutinin (PHA) to PEG during fusion, and addition of insulin, growth factors, and human endothelial culture supernatants (HECS) to the growth medium after fusion. Other advances in fusion techniques include electrofusion, antigen bridging, and laser fusion. In electrofusion, cells in suspension are aligned using an ac current, resulting in cell–cell contact. A brief dc voltage is applied that induces fusion and has resulted in a 30- to 100-fold increase in fusion frequencies in some cases. Further improvement in electrofusion yields have been obtained by an antigen bridging, wherein avidin is conjugated with the antigen, and the myeloma cell membranes are treated with biotin. Spleen cells expressing immunoglobulins of correct specificity bind to the antigen–avidin complex and are in turn bound by the biotinylated cell membranes of the myeloma cells. Finally, laser-induced cell fusion in combination with antigen bridging has been used to circumvent the tedious and time-consuming screening process associated with traditional hybridoma techniques. Here, rather than performing the fusion process in "bulk," preselected B-cells, producing an antibody of desired specificity and affinity, are fused to myeloma cells by irradiating each target cell pair (viewed under a microscope) with laser pulses. Each resulting hybridoma cell is then identified, subcloned, and subsequently expanded.

In addition, improvements in immunization protocols such as suppression of dominant responses, *in vitro* or intrasplenic immunization, and antigen-targeting have also been developed. Suppression of dominant immune responses is used to permit the expression of antibody-producing cells with specificity for poor immunogens and is achieved using the selective ability of cyclophosphamide to dampen the immune response to a particular antigen, followed by subsequent immunization with a similar antigen.

In *in vitro* immunization, spleen cells from nonimmunized animals are incubated with small quantities of antigen in a growth medium that has been conditioned by the growth of thymocytes. This technique is used most commonly for the production of human hybridomas, where *in vivo* immunization is not feasible. Intrasplenic immunization involves direct injection of immunogen into the spleen and is typically used when only very small quantities of antigens are available. Other advantages include a shortened immunization time, ability to generate high-affinity antibodies, and improved diversity in the classes of antibodies generated. Finally, in antigen-targeting, the immune response is enhanced by targeting the antigen to specific cells of the immune system, for example, by coupling to anticlass II monoclonal antibodies.

Despite these improvements, many of the limitations of the hybridoma technique persist. First, it is slow and tedious, and labor- and cost-intensive. Second, only a few antibody-producing hybridoma lines are created per fusion, which does not provide a broad survey of the immunologic repertoire. Third, the actual antibody production rate is low. Fourth, it is not easy to control the class or subclass of the resulting antibodies, a characteristic that often determines their biological activity and usefulness.

16.2.2 Repertoire Cloning Technology

The shortcomings of hybridoma technology and the potential for improving the molecular properties of antibody molecules by a screening approach have led to the expression of the immunologic repertoire in *Escherichia coli* (*repertoire cloning*). Two advances were critical to the development of this technology. First, the identification of conserved regions at each end of the nucleotide sequences encoding the variable domains enabled the use of the PCRs to clone antibody Fv and Fab genes from both spleen genomic DNA and spleen messenger RNA [Orlandi et al., 1989; Sastry et al., 1989]. In the case of immunoglobulin variable-region genes, the J segments are sufficiently conserved to enable the design of universal "downstream" primers. In addition, by comparing the aligned sequences of many variable-region genes, it was found that 5′ ends of the V_H and V_L genes are also relatively conserved so as to enable the design of universal "upstream" primers, as well. These primers were then used to establish a repertoire of antibody variable-region genes. Second, the successful expression of functional antigen-binding fragments in bacteria using a periplasmic secretion strategy enabled the direct screening of libraries of cloned antibody genes for antigen binding [Better et al., 1988; Skerra and Pluckthun, 1988].

The first attempt at repertoire cloning resulted in the establishment of diverse libraries of V_H genes from spleen genomic DNA of mice immunized with either lysozyme or keyhole-limpet hemocyanin (KLH). From these libraries, V_H domains were expressed in *E. coli* [Ward et al., 1989]. Binding activities were detected against both antigens in both libraries; the first library, immunized against lysozyme, yielded 21 clones with antilysozyme activity and 2 with anti-KLH activity, while the second library, immunized against KLH, yielded 14 clones with anti-KLH activity and 2 with antilysozyme activity. Two V_H domains were characterized with affinities for lysozyme in the 20-nM range. The complete sequences of 48 V_H gene clones were determined and shown to be unique. The problems associated with this single-domain approach are (1) isolated V_H domains suffer from lower selectivity and poor solubility and (2) an important source of diversity arising from the combination of the heavy and light chains is lost.

In the so-called combinatorial approach, a bacteriophage λ vector system was used to express a combinatorial library of Fab fragments from the murine repertoire in *E. coli* [Huse et al., 1989]. The combinatorial expression library was constructed from spleen mRNA isolated from a mouse immunized with KLH-coupled *p*-nitrophenyl phosphonamidate (NPN) antigen in two steps. In the first step, separate heavy chain (Fd) and light chain (κ) libraries were constructed. These two libraries were then combined randomly, resulting in a combinatorial library in which each clone potentially co-expresses a heavy and a light chain. In this case, they obtained 25 million clones in the library, approximately 60% of which co-expressed both chains. One million of these were subsequently screened for antigen binding, resulting in approximately 100 antibody-producing, antigen-binding clones. The light- and heavy-chain libraries, when expressed individually, did not show any binding activity. In addition, the vector systems used also permitted the excision of a phagemid containing the Fab genes; when grown in *E. coli*, these permitted the production of functional Fab fragments in the periplasmic supernatants. While the study did not address the overall diversity of the library, it did establish repertoire cloning as a potential alternative to conventional hybridoma technology.

Repertoire cloning via the λ phage method has been used to generate antibodies to influenza virus hemagglutinin (HA) starting with mRNA from immunized mice [Caton and Koprowski, 1990]. A total of 10 antigen-binding clones were obtained by screening 125,000 clones from the combinatorial library consisting of 25 million members. Partial sequence analysis of the V_H and V_κ regions of five of the HA-positive recombinants revealed that all the HA-specific antibodies generated by repertoire cloning utilized a V_H region derived from members of a single B-cell clone in conjunction with one of two light chain variable regions. A majority of the HA-specific antibodies exhibited a common heavy–light-chain combination that was very similar to one previously identified among HA-specific hybridoma monoclonal antibodies. The relative representation of these sequences and the overall diversity of the library also were studied via hybridization studies and sequence analysis of randomly selected clones. It was determined that a single functional V_H sequence was present at a frequency of 1 in 50, while the more commonly occurring light chain sequence was present at a frequency of 1 in 275. This indicates that the overall diversity of the gene family representation in the library is fairly limited.

The λ phage method was also used to produce high-affinity human monoclonal antibodies specific for tetanus toxoid [Mullinax et al., 1990; Persson et al., 1991]. The source of the mRNA in these studies was peripheral blood lymphocytes (PBLs) from human donors previously immunized with tetanus toxoid and boosted with the antigen. Mullinax et al. [1990] estimated that the frequency of positive clones in the library was about 1 in 500, and their affinity constants ranged from 30×10^8 to 0.09×10^8 M^{-1}. However, the presence of a naturally occurring *Sac*I site (one of the restriction enzymes used to force clone PCR-amplified light-chain genes) in the gene for human C_κ may have resulted in a reduction in the frequency of positive clones. Persson et al. [1991] constructed three different combinatorial libraries using untreated PBLs, antigen-stimulated PBLs (cells cultured in the presence of the antigen), and antigen-panned PBLs (cells that were selected for binding to the antigen). Positive clones were obtained from the libraries with frequencies of 1 in 6000, 1 in 5000, and 1 in 4000, respectively. Apparent binding constants were estimated to be in the range of 10^7 to 10^9 M^{-1}. Sequence analysis of a limited number of clones isolated from the antigen-stimulated cell library indicated a greater diversity than that described for HA or NPN. For example, of the eight heavy chain CDR3 sequences examined, only two pairs appeared to be clonally related. The λ phage approach has also been used to rescue a functional human antirhesus D Fab from an Epstein-Barr Virus-transformed cell line [Burton, 1991].

In principle, repertoire cloning allows for the rapid and easy identification of monoclonal antibody fragments in a form suitable for genetic manipulation. It also provides for a much better survey of the immunologic repertoire than conventional hybridoma technology. However, repertoire cloning is not without its disadvantages. First, it allows for the production of only antibody fragments. This limitation can be overcome by mounting the repertoire cloned variable domains onto constant domains that possess the desired effector functions and using transfectoma technology to express the intact immunoglobulin genes in a variety of host systems. This has been demonstrated for the case of a human Fab fragment to tetanus toxoid, where the Fab gene fragment obtained via repertoire cloning was linked to an Fc fragment gene and successfully expressed in a CHO cell line [Bender et al., 1993]. The second limitation is the use of "immunized" repertoires, which has implications in the applicability of this technology for the production of human monoclonal antibodies. The studies reviewed earlier in this chapter have all used spleen cells or PBLs from immunized donors. This has resulted in a relatively high frequency of positive clones, eliminating the need for extensive screening. Generating monoclonal antibodies from "naive" donors (who have not had any exposure to the antigen) requires the screening of very large libraries. Third, the actual diversity of these libraries is still unclear. The studies reported above show a wide spectrum ranging from very limited (the HA studies) to moderate (NPN) to fairly marked diversity (tetanus toxoid). Finally, the combinatorial approach is disadvantageous in that it destroys the original pairing of the heavy and light chains selected for by immunization. Strategies for overcoming some of these limitations have already been developed and are reviewed in the following section.

16.2.3 Phage Display Technology

A critical requirement of the repertoire cloning approach is the ability to screen large libraries rapidly for clones that possess desired binding properties (e.g., binding affinity, specificity, catalysis). This is especially the case for naive human repertoires, wherein the host has not been immunized against the antigen of interest for ethical and safety reasons. In order to facilitate screening of large libraries of antibody genes, *phage display* of functional antibody fragments has been developed, which has resulted in an enormous increase in the utility of repertoire cloning technology. In phage display technology, functional antibody fragments (such as the sFv and Fab) are expressed on the surface of filamentous bacteriophage, which facilitates the selection of specific binders (or any other property such as catalysis) from a large pool of irrelevant antibody fragments. Typically, several hundred million phage particles (in a small volume of 50 to 100 ml) can be screened by allowing them to bind to the antigen of interest immobilized on a solid matrix, washing away the nonbinders, and eluting the binders.

Phage display of antibody fragments is accomplished by coupling of the antibody fragment to a coat protein of the filamentous bacteriophage. Two coat proteins have been used for this purpose, namely, the major coat protein encoded for by gene VIII and the adsorption protein encoded for by gene III. The system based on gene VIII displays several copies of the antibody fragment (theoretically there are 2000 copies of gene VIII product per phage) and is used for the selection of low-affinity binders. The gene III product is, on the other hand, present at approximately four copies per phage particle and leads to the selection of high-affinity binders. However, since the native gene III product is required for infectivity, at least one copy has to be a native one.

The feasibility of phage display of active antibody fragments was first demonstrated by McCafferty et al. [1990] when the single-chain Fv fragment (single-chain antibody) of the anti-hen egg white lysozyme (HEL) antibody was cloned into an fd phage vector at the *N*-terminal region of the gene III protein. This study showed that complete active sFv domains could be displayed on the surface of bacteriophage fd and that rare phage displaying functional sFv (1 in 106) can be isolated. Phage that bound HEL were unable to bind to turkey egg white lysozyme, which differs from HEL by only seven residues.

Similarly, active Fab fragments also have been displayed on phage surfaces using gene VIII [Kang et al., 1991]. In this method, assembly of the antibody Fab molecules in the periplasm occurs in concert with phage morphogenesis. The Fd chain of the antibody fused to the major coat protein VIII of phage M13 was co-expressed with κ chains, with both chains being delivered to the periplasmic space by the pelB leader sequence. Since the Fd chain is anchored in the membrane, the concomitant secretion of the κ chains results in the assembly of the two chains and hence the display of functional Fab on the membrane surface. Subsequent infection with helper phage resulted in phage particles that had incorporated functional Fab along their entire surface. Functionality of the incorporated Fab was confirmed by antigen-specific precipitation of phage, enzyme-linked immunoassays, and electron microscopy.

The production of soluble antibody fragments from selected phage can also be accomplished without subcloning [Hoogenboom et al., 1991]. The switch from surface display to soluble antibody is mediated via the use of an amber stop codon between the antibody gene and the phage gene. In a *supE* suppresser strain of *E. coli*, the amber codon is read as Glu and the resulting fusion protein is displayed on the surface of the phage. In nonsuppresser strains, however, the amber codon is read as a stop codon, resulting in the production of soluble antibody.

The combination of repertoire cloning and phage display was initially used to screen antibody fragments from repertoires produced from immunized animals, namely the production of Fv fragments specific for the hapten phenyloxazolone using immunized mice [Clackson et al., 1991], human Fab fragments to tetanus toxoid [Barbas et al., 1991], human Fab fragments to gp120 using lymphocytes isolated from HIV-positive individuals [Burton et al., 1991], and human Fab fragments to hepatitis B surface antigen from vaccinated individuals [Zebedee et al., 1992]. These studies established the utility of phage display as a powerful screening system for functional antibody fragments. For example, attempts to generate human Fab fragments against gp120 using the λ phage method failed to produce any binders. Phage display, on the other hand, resulted in 33 of 40 clones selected via antigen panning possessing clear reactivity with affinity constants of the order of 10^8 M^{-1}. In the case of the tetanus toxoid studies, phage display was used to isolate specific clones from a library that included known tetanus toxoid clones at a frequency of 1 in 170,000.

16.2.4 Bypassing Immunization

The next step was the application of phage display technology to generate antibodies from unimmunized donors (*naive repertoires*). Marks et al. [1992] constructed two combinatorial libraries starting from peripheral blood lymphocytes of unimmunized human donors, namely, an IgM library using γ-specific PCR primers and an IgG library using μ-specific primers. The libraries were screened using phage display and sFv fragments specific for nonself antigens such as turkey egg white lysozyme, bovine serum albumin, phenyloxazolone, and bovine thyroglobulin, as well as for self-antigens such as human thyroglobulin, human tumor necrosis factor α, cell surface markers, carcinoembryonic antigen, mucin, and human blood group antigens were isolated [Hoogenboom et al., 1992]. The binders were all isolated from the IgM library (with the exception of six clones for turkey egg white lysozyme isolated from the IgG library), and the affinities of the soluble antibody fragments were low to moderate (2×10^6 to 10^7 M^{-1}). These results are typical of the antibodies produced during a primary response.

The second stage of an immune response *in vivo* involves affinity maturation, in which the affinities of antibodies of the selected specificities are increased by a process of somatic mutation. Thus, one method by which the affinities of antibodies generated from naive repertoires may be increased is by mimicking this process. Random mutagenesis of the clones selected from naive repertoires has been accomplished by error-prone PCR [Gram et al., 1992]. In this study, low-affinity Fab fragments (10^4 to 10^5 M^{-1}) to progesterone were initially isolated from the library, and their affinities increased 13- to 30-fold via random mutagenesis. An alternative approach to improving the affinities of antibodies obtained from naive repertoires involves the use of chain shuffling. Marks et al. [1992] described the affinity maturation of a low-affinity antiphenyloxazolone antibody (3×10^7 M^{-1}). First, the existing light chain was replaced with a repertoire of *in vivo* somatically mutated light chains from unimmunized donors, resulting in the isolation of a clone with a 20-fold increase in affinity. Next, shuffling of the heavy chain in a similar manner, with the exception of retaining the original H3, resulted in a further increase in affinity of about 16-fold. The net increase in affinity (320-fold) resulted in a dissociation constant of 1 nM, which is comparable to the affinities obtained through hybridoma technology. Other approaches to bypassing human immunization involve the use of semisynthetic and synthetic combinatorial libraries [Barbas et al., 1992] and the immunization of SCID mice that have been populated with human peripheral blood lymphocytes [Duchosal et al., 1992].

16.3 Monoclonal Antibody Expression Systems

Several expression systems are currently available for *in vitro* production of antibodies such as bacteria, yeast, plants, baculovirus, and mammalian cells. In each of these systems, cloned antibody genes are the starting point for production. These are obtained either by traditional cloning techniques, starting with preexisting hybridomas, or by the more recent repertoire cloning techniques. Each of the aforementioned systems has its own advantages and disadvantages. For example, bacterial expression systems suffer from the following limitations: They cannot be used for producing intact antibodies nor can they glycosylate antibodies. Unglycosylated antibodies cannot perform many of the effector functions associated with normal antibody molecules. Proper folding may sometimes be a problem due to difficulty in forming disulfide bonds, and often, the expressed antibody may be toxic to the host cells. On the other hand, bacterial expression has the advantages that it is cheap, can potentially produce large amounts of the desired product, and can be easily scaled-up. In addition, for therapeutic products, bacterial sources are preferred over mammalian sources due to the potential for the contamination of mammalian cell lines with harmful viruses.

16.3.1 Bacterial Expression

Early attempts to express intact antibody molecules in bacteria were fairly unsuccessful. Expression of intact light and heavy chains in the cytoplasm resulted in the accumulation of the proteins as nonfunctional inclusion bodies. *In vitro* reassembly was very inefficient [Boss et al., 1984; Cabilly et al., 1984]. These results could be explained by the fact that the *E. coli* biosynthetic environment does not support protein folding that requires specific disulfide bond formation and posttranslational modifications, such as glycosylation.

The expression of antibody fragments has been much more successful. Bacterial expression of IgE "Fc-like" fragments has been reported [Kenten et al., 1984; Ishizaka et al., 1986]. These IgE fragments exhibited some of the biological properties characteristic of intact IgE molecules. The fragments constituted 18% of the total bacterial protein content but were insoluble and formed large inclusion bodies. Following reduction and reoxidation, more than 80% of the chains formed dimers. The fragment binds to the IgE receptor on basophils and mast cells and, when cross-linked, elicits the expected response (histamine release).

Cytoplasmic expression of a Fab fragment directed against muscle-type creatinine kinase, followed by *in vitro* folding, resulted in renaturation of about 40% of the misfolded protein, with a total active protein yield of 80 μg/ml at 10°C [Buchner and Rudolph, 1991]. Direct cytoplasmic expression of the so-called single-chain antibodies, which are novel recombinant polypeptides composed of an antibody V_L tethered to a V_H by a designed "linker" peptide, was the next important step. Various linkers have been used to join the two variable domains. Bird et al. [1988] used linkers of varying lengths (14 to 18 amino acids) to join the two variable domains. Huston et al. [1988] used a 15-amino acid "universal" linker with the sequence $(GGGGS)_3$. The single-chain protein accumulated in the cells as insoluble inclusion bodies and required *in vitro* refolding. However, after refolding, these proteins had both the affinity and specificity of the native Fabs.

In 1988, two groups reported the expression of functional antibody fragments (Fv and Fab, respectively) in *E. coli* [Better et al., 1988; Skerra and Pluckthun, 1988]. In both cases, the authors attempted to mimic the natural assembly and folding pathways of antibody molecules in bacteria. In eukaryotic cells, the two chains are expressed separately with signal sequences that direct their transport to the endoplasmic reticulum (ER), where the signal sequences are removed and correct folding, disulfide formation, and assembly of the two chains occur. By expressing the two chain fragments (V_L and V_H in the case of Fv expression and the Fd and κ chains in the case of Fab expression) separately with bacterial signal sequences, these workers were successful in directing the two precursor chains to the periplasmic space, where correct folding, assembly, and disulfide formation occurred along with the removal of the signal sequences, resulting in fully-functional antibody fragments. Skerra and Pluckthun [1988] reported the synthesis of the Fv fragment of MOPC 603, which had an affinity constant identical to that of the intact antibody. Better et al. [1988] reported the synthesis of the Fab fragment of an Ig that binds to a ganglioside antigen. While Skerra and Pluckthun obtained a yield of 0.2 mg/l after a periplasmic wash, Better et al. [1988] found that the Fab fragment was secreted into the culture medium with a yield of 2 mg/l. Previous attempts to synthesize an active, full-size Ig in *E. coli* by co-expression and secretion mediated by procaryotic signal sequences resulted in poor synthesis and secretion of the heavy chain.

Since these early reports, several additional reports have been published [for reviews, see Skerra and Pluckthun, 1988; Pluckthun, 1992; Maynard and Georgiou, 2000], which have established the two afore-mentioned strategies (namely, direct cytoplasmic expression of antibody fragments followed by *in vitro* refolding and periplasmic expression of functional fragments) as the standard procedures for bacterial expression of antibody fragments. Expression of the protein in the periplasmic space has the following advantages (1) the expressed protein is recovered in a fully functional form, thereby eliminating the need for *in vitro* refolding (as is required in the case of cytoplasmically expressed fragments) and (2) it greatly simplifies purification. On the other hand, direct cytoplasmic expression may, in some cases, reduce problems arising from toxicity of the expressed protein and may also increase the total yield of the protein.

Several improvements have been made in the past few years to simplify the expression and purification of antibody fragments in bacteria. These include the development of improved vectors with strong promoters for the high-level expression of antibody fragments, the incorporation of many different signal sequences, and the incorporation of cleavable affinity tags that simplify purification. Many of these systems are now commercially available, enabling rapid cloning, sequencing, and expression of immunoglobulin genes in bacteria within a matter of 2 to 3 weeks.

16.3.2 Expression in Lymphoid and Nonlymphoid Systems (Transfectoma Technology)

Expression of immunoglobulin genes by transfection into eukaryotic cells (*transfectoma technology*) such as myelomas and hybridomas is another approach for producing monoclonal antibodies [Morrison and Oi, 1989; Wright et al., 1992]. Myelomas and hybridomas are known to be capable of high-level expression of endogenous heavy- and light-chain genes and can glycosylate, assemble, and secrete functional antibody molecules and therefore are the most appropriate mammalian cells for immunoglobulin expression. Nonlymphoid expression in CHO and COS cells has also been used as a potential improvement over expression in lymphoid cells. The biological properties and effector functions, which are very important considerations for applications involving human therapy and diagnostics, are preserved in these methods of expression. However, transfectoma technology still involves working with eukaryotic cell lines with low antibody production rates and poor scale-up characteristics.

Transfectoma technology provides the ability to genetically manipulate immunoglobulin genes to produce antibody molecules with novel and improved properties. For example, production of *chimeric* and *humanized* antibodies, wherein the murine variable domains or CDRs are mounted onto a human antibody framework in an attempt to reduce the problem of immunogenicity in administering murine antibodies, was enabled by transfectoma technology. It is also possible to change the isotype of the transfectoma antibodies in order to change their biological activity. In addition, transfectoma technology has enabled the fusion of antibodies with nonimmunoglobulin proteins such as enzymes or toxins, resulting in novel antibody reagents used in industrial and medicinal applications.

In order to create the immunoglobulin molecules, the two genes encoding the heavy and light chains are transfected and both polypeptides must be synthesized and assembled. Several methods have been used to achieve this objective. Both the heavy- and light-chain genes have been inserted into a single vector and then transfected. This approach generates large, cumbersome expression vectors, and further manipulation of the vector is difficult. A second approach is to sequentially transfect the heavy- and light-chain genes. Alternatively, both genes may be introduced simultaneously into lymphoid cells using protoplast fusion.

Heavy and light-chain genes, when transfected together, produced complete, glycosylated, and assembled tetrameric antigen-binding antibody molecules with appropriate disulfide bonds. Under laboratory conditions, these transfected cells yield about 1 to 20 mg/l of secreted antibody. A persisting problem has been the expression levels of the transfected immunoglobulin genes. The expression of transfected heavy-chain genes frequently approaches the level obtained in myeloma cells; however, efficient expression of light chain genes is more difficult.

16.3.3 Expression in Yeast

Yeast is the simplest eukaryote capable of glycosylation and secretion, and has the advantages of rapid growth and ease of large-scale fermentation. It also does not harbor potentially harmful mammalian viruses. Initial attempts to express λ and μ immunoglobulin chains specific for the hapten NP in the yeast *Sacchromyces cerevisiae* under the control of the yeast 3-phosphoglycerate kinase (PGK) promoter resulted in the secretion into culture medium at moderate efficiency (5 to 40%), but the antibodies lacked antigen-binding activity [Wood et al., 1985]. Subsequent attempts to co-express heavy and light chains with the yeast invertase signal sequence, under the control of the yeast PGK promoter, were more successful, presumably due to differences in the efficiency of different yeast signal sequences in directing the secretion of mammalian proteins from yeast. Culture supernatants contained significant quantities of both light and heavy chains (100 and 50 to 80 mg/l, respectively) with about 50 to 70% of the heavy chain associated with the light chain. The yeast-derived mouse–human chimeric antibody L6 was indistinguishable from the native antibody in its antigen-binding properties [Horwitz et al., 1988; Better and Horwitz, 1989]. Furthermore, it was superior to the native antibody in mediating antibody-dependent cellular cytotoxicity (ADCC) but was incapable of eliciting complement-dependent cytolysis (CDC). Yeast-derived L6 Fab also was indistinguishable from proteolytically generated Fab as well as recombinant Fab generated from *E. coli.*

16.3.4 Expression in Baculovirus

The baculovirus expression system is potentially a very useful system for the production of large amounts of intact, fully functional antibodies for diagnostic and therapeutic applications. Foreign genes expressed in insect cell cultures infected with baculovirus can constitute as much as 50 to 75% of the total cellular protein, late in viral replication. Immunoglobulin gene expression is achieved by commercially available vectors that place the gene to be expressed under the control of the efficient promoter of the gene encoding the viral polyhedrin protein. The levels of expression seen in this system can be as much as 50- to 100-fold greater per cell than in procaryotes while retaining many of the advantages of eukaryotic expression systems, such as glycosylation and extracellular secretion. However, scale-up is not straightforward, since viral infection eventually results in cell death. There have been several reports of antibody secretion in a baculovirus system [reviewed in Potter et al., 1995].

16.3.5 Expression in Plants

The development of techniques for plant transformation has led to the expression of a number of foreign genes, including immunoglobulin genes, in transgenic plants [Hiatt and Ma, 1992]. A commonly used plant cell transformation protocol employs the ability of plasmid *Ti* of *Agrobacterium tumefaciens* to mediate gene transfer. The expression of a murine antiphosphonate ester catalytic antibody in transgenic plants was accomplished by first transforming the heavy- and light-chain genes individually into different tobacco plants [Hiatt et al., 1989]. These were then sexually crossed to obtain progeny that expressed both chains simultaneously. It was shown that leader sequences were necessary for the proper expression and assembly of the antibody molecules. The level of antibody expression was determined to be about 3 ng/mg of total protein, and the plant-derived antibody was comparable with ascites-derived antibody with respect to binding as well as catalysis.

16.4 Genetically Engineered Antibodies and Their Fragments

The modular structure of the antibody molecule allows the reshuffling of domains and the construction of functional antibody fragments. A schematic representation of such genetically engineered antibodies and their fragments is shown in Figure 16.2 and Figure 16.3.

Among intact engineered constructs are chimeric, humanized, human, and bifunctional antibodies [for reviews, see Sandhu, 1992; Wright et al., 1992; Kipriyanov and Le Gall, 2004]. A major issue in the long-term use of murine monoclonal antibodies for clinical applications is the immunogenicity of these molecules or the human anti-mouse antibody (HAMA) response. Chimeric antibodies are constructed by linking murine variable domains to human constant domains in order to reduce the immunogenicity of therapeutically administered murine monoclonals. The approach has been validated by several clinical trials, which show that chimeric antibodies are less likely to induce a HAMA response compared with their murine counterparts. In a more sophisticated approach, *CDR grafting* has been used to humanize murine monoclonal antibodies for human therapy by transplanting the CDRs of a murine monoclonal antibody of appropriate antigenic specificity onto a human framework.

Bifunctional antibodies that contain antigen-specific binding sites with two different specificities have been produced via genetic engineering as well as chemical techniques [Kufer et al., 2004]. The dual specificity of bispecific antibodies can be used to bring together the molecules or cells that mediate

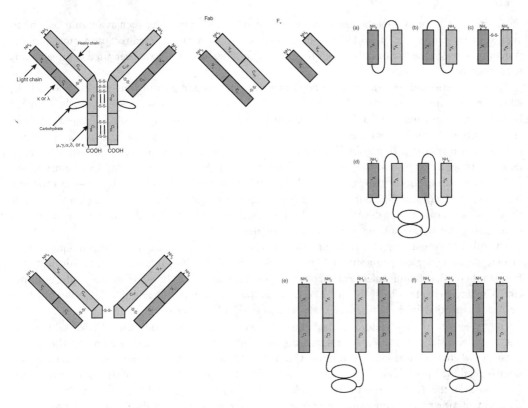

FIGURE 16.2 Schematic of an antibody molecule and its antigen-binding fragments. (a)–(e) Examples of the fragments expressed in *E. coli:* (a) single-chain Fv fragment in which the linking peptide joins the light and heavy Fv segments in the following manner: V_L (carboxyl terminus)–peptide linker–V_H (amino terminus); (b) single-chain Fv fragment with the following connection: V_L (amino terminus)–peptide linker–V_H (carboxyl terminus); (c) disulfide-linked Fv fragment; (d) "miniantibody" comprised of two helix-forming peptides each fused to a single-chain Fv; (e) Fab fragments linked by helix-forming peptide fused to heavy chain; (f) Fab fragments linked by helix-forming peptide to light chain.

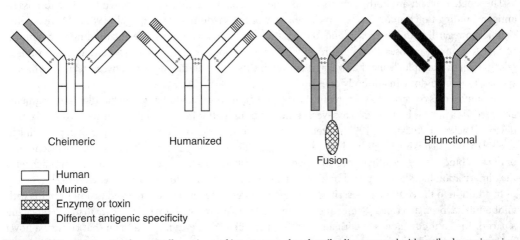

FIGURE 16.3 Schematic of genetically engineered intact monoclonal antibodies prepared with antibody-engineering techniques.

the desired effect. For example, a bispecific antibody that binds to target cells such as a tumor cell and to cytotoxic trigger molecules on host killer cells such as T cells has been used to redirect the normal immune system response to the tumor cells in question. Bispecific antibodies also have been used to target toxins to tumor cells.

The list of genetically engineered antibody fragments is a long and growing one [Brekke and Sandlie, 2003]. Of these, fragments such as the Fab, F(ab)$'_2$, Fv, and the Fc are not new and were initially produced by proteolytic digestion. The Fab fragment (fragment antigen binding) consists of the entire light chain and the two N-terminal domains of the heavy chain (V_H and C_{H1}, the so-called Fd chain) and was first generated by digestion with papain. The other fragment that is generated on papain digestion is the Fc fragment (fragment crystallizable), which is a dimeric unit composed of two C_{H2} and C_{H3} domains. The F(ab)$'_2$ fragment consists of two Fab arms held together by disulfide bonds in the hinge region and was first generated by pepsin digestion. Finally, the Fv fragment (fragment variable), which consists of just the two N-terminal variable domains, was also first generated by proteolytic digestion and is now more commonly generated via antigen-engineering techniques.

The other fragments depicted in Figure 16.2 are obtained by genetic engineering techniques. These include the sFv (single-chain antibody), the V_H domain (single-domain antibody), multivalent sFvs (miniantibodies), and multivalent Fabs. The multivalent constructs can be either monospecific or bispecific. The single-chain antibody (SCA, sFv) consists of the two variable domains linked together by a long flexible polypeptide linker [Bird et al., 1988; Huston et al., 1988]. The sFv is an attempt to stabilize the Fv fragment, which is known to dissociate at low concentrations into its individual domains due to the low-affinity constant for the V_H–V_L interaction. Two different constructs have been made: the V_L–V_H construct where the linker extends from the C terminus of the V_L domain to the N terminus of the V_H domain, and the V_H–V_L construct, where the linker runs from the C terminus of the V_H domain to the N terminus of the V_L. The linker is usually about 15-amino acids long and has no particular sequence requirements other than to minimize interference in the folding of the individual domains. The so-called universal linker used by many workers is (GGGGS)$_3$. Other strategies to stabilize the Fv fragment include chemical cross-linking of the two domains and disulfide-linked domains [Glockshuber et al., 1990]. Chemical cross-linking via glutaraldehyde has been demonstrated to be effective in stabilizing the Fv fragment in one instance; here, the cross-linking was carried out in the presence of the hapten (phosphorylcholine) to avoid modification of the binding site, an approach that may not be feasible with protein antigens. In the disulfide-linked sFv, Cys residues are introduced at suitable locations in the framework region of the Fv so as to form a natural interdomain disulfide bond. This strategy was shown to be much more effective in stabilizing the Fv fragment against thermal denaturation than either the single-chain antibody approach or chemical cross-linking for a case where all three approaches were tested [Glockshuber et al., 1990].

The single-domain antibody consists of just the V_H domain and has been shown by some to possess antigen-binding function on its own in the absence of the V_L domain [Ward et al., 1989]. There is some skepticism regarding this approach due to the rather high potential for nonspecific binding (the removal of the V_L domain exposes a very hydrophobic surface), poor solubility, and somewhat compromised selectivity. For example, while the Fv fragment retains its ability to distinguish between related antigenic species, the single-domain antibody does not.

Miniantibodies consist of sFv fragments held together by so-called dimerization handles. sFv fragments are fused via a flexible hinge region to several kinds of amphipathic helices, which then acts as dimerization devices [Pack and Pluckthun, 1992]. Alternately, the two sFvs can be fused via a long polypeptide linker, similar to the one linking the individual domains of each Fv but longer to maintain the relative orientation of the two binding sites. Multivalent Fabs have been constructed using a somewhat similar approach with the dimerization handles composed of zippers from transcription factors [Kostelny et al., 1992].

In addition to the constructs described above, a number of genetically engineered fusion proteins with antibodies has been described [Senter and Springer, 2001]. Antibody fusion proteins are made by replacing a part of the antibody molecule with a fusion partner, such as an enzyme or a toxin that confers a novel function to the antibody. In some cases, such as immunotoxins, the variable regions of the antibody are retained in order to retain antigen binding and specificity, while the constant domains are deleted and replaced by a toxin such as ricin or *Pseudomonas* exotoxin. Alternately, the constant regions are retained (thereby retaining the effector functions) and the variable regions replaced with other targeting proteins.

16.5 Applications of Monoclonal Antibodies and Fragments

The majority of applications for which monoclonal antibodies have been used can be divided into three general categories (1) purification, (2) diagnostic applications (whether for detecting cancer, analyzing for toxins in food, or monitoring substance abuse by athletes), and (3) therapeutic applications. From the time that monoclonal antibody technology was introduced almost 30 years ago, applications using whole antibodies have gradually been transformed into methodologies using antibody fragments such as the Fab_2, Fab', and Fv fragments, and even synthetic peptides of a CDR region. Antibody conjugates have come to include bound drugs, toxins, radioisotopes, lymphokines, and enzymes.

Table 16.1 lists the therapeutic monoclonal antibodies that are currently approved by the Food and Drug Administration (FDA) in the United States market. According to the Tufts Center for the Study of Drug Development, 311 therapeutic monoclonal antibodies had entered clinical trials by January 2004 [Reichert, 2004]. Thus far, the FDA has approved 17 therapeutic monoclonal antibodies. Three of these are murine antibodies, five chimeric, eight humanized, and one human [Reichert and Pavolu, 2004]. An analysis by Reichert and coworkers [2001] has shown that human, humanized, and chimeric antibodies have a higher probability of progression through each phase of clinical trials in comparison to their murine counterparts. This probability is reflected in the small number of approved murine monoclonal antibodies (3 of 17 total), despite the fact that these were the first monoclonal antibodies to be purified and characterized. As of May 2004, there were 132 monoclonal antibody products in various stages of development [Reichert and Pavolu, 2004]. Humanized antibodies comprised the largest fraction of the pipeline, with approximately 42%, while fully human antibodies accounted for 28%.

Since their discovery, there has been intense interest in using antibodies, or antibody-directed therapies, as "magic bullets" for the treatment of cancer, while minimizing the systemic toxicity of chemotherapeutics. However, this vision has encountered significant hurdles in its translation to practice. Successful therapeutic treatment of solid tumors with antibodies or antibody–drug conjugates must overcome the barriers to penetration within the tumor while maintaining conjugated drug potency, and releasing the drug inside the tumor cells. The rare case of complete remission for solid tumors is probably due to the inability of the antibody to penetrate the tumor. The barriers impeding the access of therapeutics to solid tumors have been characterized in detail [Jain, 2001]. These barriers include (1) the high interstitial fluid pressure in tumor nodules, (2) heterogeneous or poor vascularization of tumors, and (3) the long distances extravasated monoclonal antibodies must travel in the interstitial mesh of proteoglycans in the tumor. There also exists the possibility that tumor antigen shed from the surface limits antibody accumulation. In the case of bound toxins or drugs, there is the added concern that the liver and kidney are metabolizing and excreting the antibody conjugates. In this respect, immunoconjugates based on antibody fragments (such as the sFv) can be very advantageous. For example, it has been shown that the sFv exhibits rapid diffusion into the extravascular space, increased volume of distribution, enhanced tumor penetration, and improved renal elimination [Raag and Whitlow, 1995]. Nevertheless, antibody conjugate treatment of leukemia and lymphoma has generally resulted in a greater remission rate than that found in treatments of malignancies having solid tumors.

An alternative strategy to treat solid tumors is called antibody-directed enzyme prodrug therapy (ADEPT) [Senter and Springer, 2001]. ADEPT is a two-step approach, which involves using monoclonal antibodies to localize enzymes to tumor cell surface antigens. After the antibody–enzyme conjugate is bound to the cancer cells and cleared from systemic circulation, antitumor prodrugs are administered and converted to active drugs, only in the region of the tumor, by the antibody-conjugated enzyme. The activated small molecular weight drug is generally capable of penetratating deeper into the tumor mass than the corresponding antibody–drug conjugate, and the localized activation of the prodrug minimizes systemic toxicity.

TABLE 16.1 Therapeutic Monoclonal Antibodies Approved in the United States [Reichert and Pavolu, 2004]

Generic name	US trade name	Type	Antigen	Indication	Company
Abciximab	ReoPro	Chimeric	GP IIb/IIIa and vitronectin receptors	Inhibition of platelet aggregation	Centocor
Adalimumab	Humira	Human	TNF-α	Rheumatoid arthritis	Abbott
Alemtuzumab	Campath	Humanized	CD52	Leukemia	Millennium/ILEX
Basiliximab	Simulect	Chimeric	IL-2 receptor	Transplant rejection	Novartis
Bevacizumab	Avastin	Humanized	VEGF	Colorectal cancer	Genentech
Cetuximab	Erbitux	Chimeric	EGFR	Colorectal cancer	Imclone Systems
Daclizumab	Zenapax	Humanized	IL-2 receptor	Transplant rejection	Protein Design Labs
Efalizumab	Raptiva	Humanized	CD11a	Psoriasis	Genentech
Gemtuzumab ozogamicin	Mylotrarg	Humanized	CD33 (calichaemicin conjugate)	Leukemia	Wyeth
Ibritumomab tiuxetan	Zevalin	Murine	CD20 (chelate linker for ^{111}In or ^{90}Y	Lymphoma	Biogen IDEC
Infliximab	Remicade	Chimeric	TNF-α	Rheumatoid arthritis / Crohn's disease	Centocor
Muromonab-CD3	Orthoclone OKT3	Murine	CD3	Transplant rejection	Johnson and Johnson
Omalizumab	Xolair	Humanized	IgE	Allergic asthma	Genentech
Palivizumab	Synagis	Humanized	Respiratory syncytial virus (RSV)	RSV infection	MedImmune
Rituximab	Rituxan	Chimeric	CD20	Lymphoma	Biogen IDEC
Tositumomab-I131	BEXXAR	Murine	CD20 (also available linked to ^{131}I)	Lymphoma	Corixa
Trastuzumab	Herceptin	Humanized	HER2	Metastatic breast cancer	Genentech

TABLE 16.2   Diagnostic Monoclonal Antibodies Approved in the United States

Generic name	US trade name	Type	Antigen	Indication	Company
Arcitumomab	CEA-Scan	Murine	Carcinoembryonic antigen	Imaging colorectal cancer	Immunomedics
Imciromab pentetate	Myoscint	Murine	Cardiac myosin	Imaging cardiac necrosis	Centocor
Nofetumomab	Verluma	Murine	40 kDa glycoprotein	Imaging small cell lung cancer	Dr. Karl Thomae GmbH
Capromab pendetide	ProstaScint	Murnie	Prostate-specific membrane antigen	Imaging prostate Cancer	Cytogen

Antibodies have also gained widespread use as diagnostic agents, particularly in the imaging of tumors. Table 16.2 lists three monoclonal antibodies currently approved in the United States for tumor imaging, and one for the imaging of cardiac necrosis after myocardial infarction. The tumor imaging agents are directed toward antigens expressed on the surfaces of tumors, while the cardiac imaging agent binds exposed cardiac myosin in necrotic tissue. All four of the approved diagnostic monoclonal antibodies are murine. This reflects the fact that the HAMA response is less problematic when repeated administration and therapeutic efficacy are not required.

With regard to purification, the research literature is replete with examples of immunoaffinity purification of enzymes, receptors, peptides, and small organic molecules. In contrast, commercial applications of immunoaffinity chromatography, even for industrially or clinically relevant molecules, are far less widespread. Despite its potential utility, immunoadsorption is an expensive process. A significant portion of the high cost is the adsorbent itself, the cost of which is related to the cost of materials, preparation, and most importantly, the antibody. In addition, the binding capacity of the immunoadsorbent declines with repeated use, and a systematic study has shown that significant deactivation can typically take place over 40 to 100 cycles [Antonsen et al., 1991]. A number of factors can contribute to this degradation, including loss of antibody, structural change of the support matrix, nonspecific adsorption of contaminating proteins, incomplete antigen elution, and loss of antibody function. In most cases, this degradation results from repeated exposure to harsh elution conditions. Noteworthy commercial applications of immunoaffinity chromatography include the separation of factor VIII, used to treat hemophilia A, and factor IX, another coagulation factor in the blood-clotting cascade [Tharakan et al., 1992]. The immunoaffinity purification step for factor VIII was one of several additional steps added to the conventional preparation methodology in which plasma cryoprecipitates were heat-treated. The new method contains a virus-inactivation procedure that precedes the immunoaffinity column, followed by an additional chromatographic step (ion exchange). The latter step serves to eliminate the eluting solvent and further reduce virus-inactivating compounds. The often mentioned concern of antibody leakage from the column matrix did not appear as a problem. Furthermore, with the relatively mild elution conditions used (40% ethylene glycol), one would expect little change in the antibody-binding capacity over many elution cycles.

Immunoaffinity matrices often contain whole antibody as opposed to antibody fragments. Fragmentation of antibody by enzymatic means contributes additional steps to immunoadsorbent preparation, adding to the overall cost of the separation and is thus avoided. However, fragmentation can lead to a more efficient separation by enabling the orientation of antibody-binding sites on the surface of the immunomatrix [Prisyazhnoy et al., 1988; Yarmush et al., 1992]. Intact antibodies are bound in a random fashion, resulting in a loss of binding capacity upon immobilization. Recombinant antibody fragments can be more useful for immunoaffinity applications, due to the potential for production of large quantities of the protein at low cost and improved immobilization characteristics and stability [Blank et al., 2002]. In what one could consider the ultimate fragment of an antibody, some investigators have utilized a peptide based on the CDR region of one of the chains (termed *minimal recognition units*) to isolate the antigen.

Welling et al. [1990] synthesized and tested a 13-residue synthetic peptide having a sequence similar to one hypervariable region of an antilysozyme antibody.

In vitro diagnostic uses of antibodies are numerous and include the monitoring in clinical laboratories of the cardiac glycoside digoxin and the detection of the *Salmonella* bacteria in foods. These two examples highlight the fact that despite the exquisite specificity offered by monoclonal antibodies, detection is not failure-proof. Within digoxin immunoassays there are two possible interfering groups: endogenous digoxin-like substances and digoxin metabolites; moreover, several monoclonal antibodies may be necessary to avoid under- or overestimating digoxin concentrations. In the case of bacteria detection in food, at least two antibodies (MOPC 467 myeloma protein and 6H4 antibody) are needed to detect all strains of *Salmonella*.

16.6 Summary

The modular architecture of antibodies, both at the protein and gene levels, facilitates the manipulation of antibody properties via genetic engineering (*antibody engineering*). Antibody engineering has shown tremendous potential for basic studies and industrial and medical applications. It has been used to explore fundamental questions about the effect of structure on antigen binding and on the biologic effector functions of the antibody molecules. A knowledge of the rules by which the particular sequences of amino acids involved in the binding surface are chosen in response to an antigenic determinant would enable the production of antibodies with altered affinities and specificities. Understanding the structures and mechanisms involved in the effector function of antibodies has already resulted in the production of antibodies with novel biologic effector functions for use as diagnostic reagents and in therapeutic applications. In addition, the production of antibodies via immunoglobulin gene expression has enabled the engineering of chimeric, humanized, and human antibodies. These significant potential of these engineered antibodies is reflected in the number of clinical approvals in recent years.

References

Antonsen, K.P., C.K. Colton, and M.L. Yarmush (1991). Elution conditions and degradation mechanisms in long-term immunoadsorbent use. *Biotechnol. Prog.* **7**: 159–172.

Barbas, C.F., 3rd, J.D. Bain, D.M. Hoekstra, and R.A. Lerner (1992). Semisynthetic combinatorial antibody libraries: a chemical solution to the diversity problem. *Proc. Natl Acad. Sci. USA* **89**: 4457–4461.

Barbas, C.F., 3rd, A.S. Kang, R.A. Lerner, and S.J. Benkovic (1991). Assembly of combinatorial antibody libraries on phage surfaces: the gene III site. *Proc. Natl Acad. Sci. USA* **88**: 7978–7982.

Bender, E., J.M. Woof, J.D. Atkin, M.D. Barker, C.R. Bebbington, and D.R. Burton (1993). Recombinant human antibodies: linkage of an Fab fragment from a combinatorial library to an Fc fragment for expression in mammalian cell culture. *Hum. Antibodies Hybridomas* **4**: 74–79.

Better, M., C.P. Chang, R.R. Robinson, and A.H. Horwitz (1988). *Escherichia coli* secretion of an active chimeric antibody fragment. *Science* **240**: 1041–1043.

Better, M. and A.H. Horwitz (1989). Expression of engineered antibodies and antibody fragments in microorganisms. *Meth. Enzymol.* **178**: 476–496.

Bird, R.E., K.D. Hardman, J.W. Jacobson, S. Johnson, B.M. Kaufman, S.M. Lee, T. Lee, S.H. Pope, G.S. Riordan, and M. Whitlow (1988). Single-chain antigen-binding proteins. *Science* **242**: 423–426.

Blank, K., P. Lindner, B. Diefenbach, and A. Pluckthun (2002). Self-immobilizing recombinant antibody fragments for immunoaffinity chromatography: generic, parallel, and scalable protein purification. *Protein Expr. Purif.* **24**: 313–322.

Boss, M.A., J.H. Kenten, C.R. Wood, and J.S. Emtage (1984). Assembly of functional antibodies from immunoglobulin heavy and light chains synthesised in *E. coli. Nucleic Acids Res.* **12**: 3791–3806.

Brekke, O.H. and I. Sandlie (2003). Therapeutic antibodies for human diseases at the dawn of the twenty-first century. *Nat. Rev. Drug Discov.* **2**: 52–62.

Buchner, J. and R. Rudolph (1991). Renaturation, purification and characterization of recombinant Fab-fragments produced in *Escherichia coli. Biotechnology (N Y)* **9**: 157–162.

Burton, D.R. (1991). Human and mouse monoclonal antibodies by repertoire cloning. *Trends Biotechnol.* **9**: 169–175.

Burton, D.R., C.F. Barbas, 3rd, M.A. Persson, S. Koenig, R.M. Chanock, and R.A. Lerner (1991). A large array of human monoclonal antibodies to type 1 human immunodeficiency virus from combinatorial libraries of asymptomatic seropositive individuals. *Proc. Natl Acad. Sci. USA* **88**: 10134–10137.

Cabilly, S., A.D. Riggs, H. Pande, J.E. Shively, W.E. Holmes, M. Rey, L.J. Perry, R. Wetzel, and H.L. Heyneker (1984). Generation of antibody activity from immunoglobulin polypeptide chains produced in *Escherichia coli. Proc. Natl Acad. Sci. USA* **81**: 3273–3277.

Caton, A.J. and H. Koprowski (1990). Influenza virus hemagglutinin-specific antibodies isolated from a combinatorial expression library are closely related to the immune response of the donor. *Proc. Natl Acad. Sci. USA* **87**: 6450–6454.

Clackson, T., H.R. Hoogenboom, A.D. Griffiths, and G. Winter (1991). Making antibody fragments using phage display libraries. *Nature* **352**: 624–628.

Duchosal, M.A., S.A. Eming, P. Fischer, D. Leturcq, C.F. Barbas, 3rd, P.J. McConahey, R.H. Caothien, G.B. Thornton, F.J. Dixon, and D.R. Burton (1992). Immunization of hu-PBL-SCID mice and the rescue of human monoclonal Fab fragments through combinatorial libraries. *Nature* **355**: 258–262.

Glockshuber, R., M. Malia, I. Pfitzinger, and A. Pluckthun (1990). A comparison of strategies to stabilize immunoglobulin Fv-fragments. *Biochemistry* **29**: 1362–1367.

Gram, H., L.A. Marconi, C.F. Barbas, 3rd, T.A. Collet, R.A. Lerner, and A.S. Kang (1992). *In vitro* selection and affinity maturation of antibodies from a naive combinatorial immunoglobulin library. *Proc. Natl Acad. Sci. USA* **89**: 3576–3580.

Hiatt, A., R. Cafferkey, and K. Bowdish (1989). Production of antibodies in transgenic plants. *Nature* **342**: 76–78.

Hiatt, A. and J.K. Ma (1992). Monoclonal antibody engineering in plants. *FEBS Lett.* **307**: 71–75.

Hoogenboom, H.R., A.D. Griffiths, K.S. Johnson, D.J. Chiswell, P. Hudson, and G. Winter (1991). Multi-subunit proteins on the surface of filamentous phage: methodologies for displaying antibody (Fab) heavy and light chains. *Nucleic Acids Res.* **19**: 4133–4137.

Hoogenboom, H.R., J.D. Marks, A.D. Griffiths, and G. Winter (1992). Building antibodies from their genes. *Immunol. Rev.* **130**: 41–68.

Horwitz, A.H., C.P. Chang, M. Better, K.E. Hellstrom, and R.R. Robinson (1988). Secretion of functional antibody and Fab fragment from yeast cells. *Proc. Natl Acad. Sci. USA* **85**: 8678–8682.

Huse, W.D., L. Sastry, S.A. Iverson, A.S. Kang, M. Alting-Mees, D.R. Burton, S.J. Benkovic, and R.A. Lerner (1989). Generation of a large combinatorial library of the immunoglobulin repertoire in phage lambda. *Science* **246**: 1275–1281.

Huston, J.S., D. Levinson, M. Mudgett-Hunter, M.S. Tai, J. Novotny, M.N. Margolies, R.J. Ridge, R.E. Bruccoleri, E. Haber, R. Crea et al. (1988). Protein engineering of antibody binding sites: recovery of specific activity in an anti-digoxin single-chain Fv analogue produced in *Escherichia coli. Proc. Natl Acad. Sci. USA* **85**: 5879–5883.

Ishizaka, T., B. Helm, J. Hakimi, J. Niebyl, K. Ishizaka, and H. Gould (1986). Biological properties of a recombinant human immunoglobulin epsilon-chain fragment. *Proc. Natl Acad. Sci. USA* **83**: 8323–8327.

Jain, R.K. (2001). Delivery of molecular and cellular medicine to solid tumors. *Adv. Drug Deliv. Rev.* **46**: 149–168.

Kang, A.S., C.F. Barbas, K.D. Janda, S.J. Benkovic, and R.A. Lerner (1991). Linkage of recognition and replication functions by assembling combinatorial antibody Fab libraries along phage surfaces. *Proc. Natl Acad. Sci. USA* **88**: 4363–4366.

Kawasaki, K., S. Minoshima, E. Nakato, K. Shibuya, A. Shintani, S. Asakawa, T. Sasaki, H.G. Klobeck, G. Combriato, H.G. Zachau, and N. Shimizu (2001). Evolutionary dynamics of the human immunoglobulin kappa locus and the germline repertoire of the Vkappa genes. *Eur. J. Immunol.* **31**: 1017–1028.

Kenten, J., B. Helm, T. Ishizaka, P. Cattini, and H. Gould (1984). Properties of a human immunoglobulin epsilon-chain fragment synthesized in *Escherichia coli. Proc. Natl Acad. Sci. USA* **81**: 2955–2959.

Kipriyanov, S.M. and F. Le Gall (2004). Generation and production of engineered antibodies. *Mol. Biotechnol.* **26**: 39–60.

Kohler, G. and C. Milstein (1975). Continuous cultures of fused cells secreting antibody of predefined specificity. *Nature* **256**: 495–497.

Kostelny, S.A., M.S. Cole, and J.Y. Tso (1992). Formation of a bispecific antibody by the use of leucine zippers. *J. Immunol.* **148**: 1547–1553.

Kufer, P., R. Lutterbuse, and P.A. Baeuerle (2004). A revival of bispecific antibodies. *Trends Biotechnol.* **22**: 238–244.

Landsteiner, K. (1945). *The Specificity of Serological Reactions.* Cambridge, MA, Harvard University Press.

Marks, J.D., A.D. Griffiths, M. Malmqvist, T.P. Clackson, J.M. Bye, and G. Winter (1992). Bypassing immunization: building high-affinity human antibodies by chain shuffling. *Biotechnology* **10**: 779–783.

Maynard, J. and G. Georgiou (2000). Antibody engineering. *Annu. Rev. Biomed. Eng.* **2**: 339–376.

McCafferty, J., A.D. Griffiths, G. Winter, and D.J. Chiswell (1990). Phage antibodies: filamentous phage displaying antibody variable domains. *Nature* **348**: 552–554.

Morrison, S.L. and V.T. Oi (1989). Genetically engineered antibody molecules. *Adv. Immunol.* **44**: 65–92.

Mullinax, R.L., E.A. Gross, J.R. Amberg, B.N. Hay, H.H. Hogrefe, M.M. Kubitz, A. Greener, M. Alting-Mees, D. Ardourel, J.M. Short et al. (1990). Identification of human antibody fragment clones specific for tetanus toxoid in a bacteriophage lambda immunoexpression library. *Proc. Natl Acad. Sci. USA* **87**: 8095–8099.

Neil, G.A. and H.B. Urnovitz (1988). Recent improvements in the production of antibody-secreting hybridoma cells. *Trends Biotechnol.* **6**: 209–213.

Orlandi, R., D.H. Gussow, P.T. Jones, and G. Winter (1989). Cloning immunoglobulin variable domains for expression by the polymerase chain reaction. *Proc. Natl Acad. Sci. USA* **86**: 3833–3837.

Pack, P. and A. Pluckthun (1992). Miniantibodies: use of amphipathic helices to produce functional, flexibly linked dimeric FV fragments with high avidity in *Escherichia coli. Biochemistry* **31**: 1579–1584.

Padlan, E.A. (1994). Anatomy of the antibody molecule. *Mol. Immunol.* **31**: 169–217.

Persson, M.A., R.H. Caothien, and D.R. Burton (1991). Generation of diverse high-affinity human monoclonal antibodies by repertoire cloning. *Proc. Natl Acad. Sci. USA* **88**: 2432–2436.

Pluckthun, A. (1992). Mono- and bivalent antibody fragments produced in *Escherichia coli*: engineering, folding and antigen binding. *Immunol. Rev.* **130**: 151–188.

Potter, K.N., Y.C. Li, and J.D. Capra (1995). Antibody production in insect cells. *Antibody Expression and Engineering — ACS Symposium Series* **604**: 41–55.

Prisyazhnoy, V.S., M. Fusek, and Y.B. Alakhov (1988). Synthesis of high-capacity immunoaffinity sorbents with oriented immobilized immunoglobulins or their Fab' fragments for isolation of proteins. *J. Chromatogr.* **424**: 243–253.

Raag, R. and M. Whitlow (1995). Single-chain Fvs. *FASEB J.* **9**: 73–80.

Reichert, J. and A. Pavolu (2004). Monoclonal antibodies market. *Nat. Rev. Drug Discov.* **3**: 383–384.

Reichert, J.M. (2001). Monoclonal antibodies in the clinic. *Nat. Biotechnol.* **19**: 819–822.

Reichert, J.M. (2004). Trends in the development of therapeutic anti-cytokine antibodies. *Drug Discov. Today* **9**: 348.

Sandhu, J.S. (1992). Protein engineering of antibodies. *Crit. Rev. Biotechnol.* **12**: 437–462.

Sastry, L., M. Alting-Mees, W.D. Huse, J.M. Short, J.A. Sorge, B.N. Hay, K.D. Janda, S.J. Benkovic, and R.A. Lerner (1989). Cloning of the immunological repertoire in *Escherichia coli* for generation of monoclonal catalytic antibodies: construction of a heavy chain variable region-specific cDNA library. *Proc. Natl Acad. Sci. USA* **86**: 5728–5732.

Senter, P.D. and C.J. Springer (2001). Selective activation of anticancer prodrugs by monoclonal antibody-enzyme conjugates. *Adv. Drug Deliv. Rev.* **53**: 247–264.

Skerra, A. and A. Pluckthun (1988). Assembly of a functional immunoglobulin Fv fragment in *Escherichia coli. Science* **240**: 1038–1041.

Tharakan, J., F. Highsmith, D. Clark, and W. Drohan (1992). Physical and biochemical characterization of five commercial resins for immunoaffinity purification of factor IX. *J. Chromatogr.* **595**: 103–111.

Tizard, I.R. (1992). The genetic basis of antigen recognition. Immunology: an introduction. Orlando, Saunders College Publishing.

Ward, E.S., D. Gussow, A.D. Griffiths, P.T. Jones, and G. Winter (1989). Binding activities of a repertoire of single immunoglobulin variable domains secreted from *Escherichia coli. Nature* **341**: 544–546.

Welling, G.W., T. Geurts, J. van Gorkum, R.A. Damhof, J.W. Drijfhout, W. Bloemhoff, and S. Welling-Wester (1990). Synthetic antibody fragment as ligand in immunoaffinity chromatography. *J. Chromatogr.* **512**: 337–343.

Wood, C.R., M.A. Boss, J.H. Kenten, J.E. Calvert, N.A. Roberts, and J.S. Emtage (1985). The synthesis and *in vivo* assembly of functional antibodies in yeast. *Nature* **314**: 446–449.

Wright, A., S.U. Shin, and S.L. Morrison (1992). Genetically engineered antibodies: progress and prospects. *Crit. Rev. Immunol.* **12**: 125–168.

Yarmush, M.L., X.M. Lu, and D.M. Yarmush (1992). Coupling of antibody-binding fragments to solid-phase supports: site-directed binding of F(ab')2 fragments. *J. Biochem. Biophys. Meth.* **25**: 285–297.

Zebedee, S.L., C.F. Barbas, 3rd, Y.L. Hom, R.H. Caothien, R. Graff, J. DeGraw, J. Pyati, R. LaPolla, D.R. Burton, R.A. Lerner et al. (1992). Human combinatorial antibody libraries to hepatitis B surface antigen. *Proc. Natl Acad. Sci. USA* **89**: 3175–3179.

17

Biomolecular Engineering in Oligonucleotide Applications

S. Patrick Walton
Michigan State University

17.1 Introduction

As early as 1992, the possible contributions of engineering to the study of molecular processes in biology were being noted by the NIH [1]. At a conference entitled, "Research Opportunities in Biomolecular Engineering: The Interface Between Chemical Engineering and Biology," the term "biomolecular engineering" was defined as research and development at the interface of chemical engineering and biology with an emphasis at the molecular level [2]. However, due to the growth of biomedical and biochemical engineering and specific disciplines within those fields (e.g., metabolic, cell, and tissue engineering), a narrower definition is in order and will be applied here. In this chapter, biomolecular engineering will be defined as the use of experimental and theoretical information to identify controlling parameters that define the function of a biomolecule and then manipulation of the parameters through chemical and physical means to optimize the function of those biomolecules in the process of interest.

While proteins have traditionally been the platform utilized to enact cellular changes, it has become clear that the potential of nucleic acids as actors in the cellular milieu is significant and relevant in more ways than simply information flow. Unlike proteins where tertiary folding is critical to function and chemical changes to the molecules can greatly affect their activity, nucleic acids can easily and rapidly be modified in numerous ways to serve the potential needs of the researcher without sacrificing function. Nucleic acids, in particular synthetic oligonucleotides, can be modified on the backbone, on the sugar ring, or on the base to achieve a desired property. Oligonucleotides conjugated to active groups or noncovalently associated into complexes have also proven more active than their "naked" parent molecules. In each case, design decisions are motivated by constraints in tunable parameters, which must be identified for each specific application. Much early work in oligonucleotide modification was driven by the emergence of the field of antisense technology, for which the primary design variables are resistance to degradation by nucleases, cellular targeting and uptake, and oligonucleotide : RNA hybridization affinity. Modifications available to the scientist will be described from this historical basis. Subsequently, the contributions of biomolecular engineering to oligonucleotides used as aptamers and in RNA interference (RNAi; abbreviations listed at the end of the chapter) are discussed. The objective of this chapter is to highlight as exhaustively as possible the myriad possible options available when utilizing and modifying oligonucleotides, that is, the nucleic acid toolkit, so as to potentially provide inspiration in the development of new technologies and therapeutics. It is fully to be expected that optimization of a particular parameter will impact other parameters (examples in Table 17.1); these circumstances will be noted where relevant.

17.2 Antisense Principle

Antisense inhibition is based on the complementary hybridization of oligonucleotides with their target mRNAs. To achieve this effect, oligonucleotides must negotiate a complicated path to reach their targets. Oligonucleotides are typically administered to the extracellular medium and must diffuse to reach the cell surface. Serum-containing media for *in vitro* experiments contain nucleases, primarily 3′-exonucleases, that degrade oligonucleotides prior to reaching the cells [3]. Upon reaching the cell surface, oligonucleotides will bind to either scavenger receptors or to adsorbed bovine serum albumin [4–7]. The mode of internalization is either via adsorptive endocytosis or receptor-mediated endocytosis [8–10]. Regardless, oligonucleotides must then escape vesicular structures to reach the cytoplasm, though the mechanism for this process remains in doubt after years of investigation [11–14]. After finally accessing the cytoplasm, oligonucleotides then diffuse to locate their intracellular target from among the RNAs in the cell, with the majority of the effect occurring subsequent to accumulation of the oligonucleotides in the nucleus [15,16]. Having located their target mRNAs, oligonucleotides must then hybridize with sufficient affinity to exert an effect, whether through steric blockade of ribosomal progression or through RNase H-mediated RNA cleavage [17]. The activity of natural antisense oligonucleotides is limited by their degradation in the presence of nucleases and their relatively poor cellular uptake. In addition, oligonucleotides that successfully encounter their target mRNA must hybridize with sufficient affinity to exert a biological effect. These characteristics have been the primary focus of design improvements.

17.3 Design Parameters

17.3.1 Stability to Extracellular and Intracellular Nucleases

Nucleases are an important component in the regulation of cellular function and contribute to cellular defenses against bacterial and viral infections. However, when applying exogenous oligonucleotides in a therapeutic context, susceptibility to nucleases, of single-stranded molecules in particular, is a significant hurdle in achieving the desired function. The earliest modifications to nucleic acids focused on extending the half-life of oligonucleotides in serum and other biological fluids, both through chemical modification of oligonucleotides and through association of oligonucleotides with protective delivery vehicles. In many cases, ribose and nucleobase modifications have been applied in conjunction with backbone modifications providing a synergistic enhancement in half-life.

Natural phosphodiester (PO) oligonucleotides have a half-life as short as 5 min in the presence of single-strand endo- and exonucleases [18–22]. The earliest tested backbone-modified derivatives were

TABLE 17.1 Examples of Chemical Modifications Addressing Primary Design Parameters and Secondary Effects on Oligonucleotides

Primary design parameter	Example modification	Primary effect	Secondary effect(s)	Reference(s)
Nuclease stability	Natural PO	$t_{1/2}$ in serum $\approx$5 min		[18]
	PS (backbone)	$t_{1/2} \approx$ 4 h	Intermolecular affinity — → Nonspecific protein interactions — ↑ Immunological consequences *in vivo* — ↑	[18,27,202,203]
	2′-O-propyl (ribose)	$t_{1/2} \approx$ 1 h with PO	RNase H activity — →	[18,19]
	6-Methyl deoxyuridine (base)	$t_{1/2}$ > 24 h with PS	Intermolecular affinity — ↑	[64]
	3′-Dipyridophenazine (conjugate)	$t_{1/2} \approx$ 24 h with PO	Intermolecular affinity — →	[53]
Cellular uptake	Natural PO	$t_{1/2}$ > 2 h with PO Poor cytoplasmic access due to backbone charge		[204]
	Methylphosphonate (backbone)	Unchanged despite neutral backbone	Nuclease stability — ↑ Intermolecular affinity — →	[10,23,83]
Target affinity	3′-Cholesterol (conjugate)	Enhanced lipid association and uptake rate		[121]
	Natural PO	T_m of 15-mer for DNA complement $\approx$50–60°C	Nuclease resistance — ↑	[143,205]
	PNA (backbone)	ΔT_m/modification $\approx$1°C	RNase H activity — →	[206,207]
	LNA (ribose)	ΔT_m/modification up to 8°C	Nuclease stability — ↑ RNase H activation — →	[56,57,145]
	5-(1-Propynyl) cytosine/uracil (base)	ΔT_m/modification $\approx$2°C		[151]
	1-O-(1-pyrenylmethyl)glycerol (conjugate)	ΔT_m/modification $\approx$3–7°C (bulge) ΔT_m/modification $\approx$8–10°C (end)	RNA-DNA selectivity — ↑	[155]

methylphosphonate (MP) and phosphorothioate (PS) backbone oligonucleotides. Though receiving little current attention owing to other limitations [20,23], MP oligonucleotides have significant stability to nuclease digestion with half-lives in excess of 24 h for partially modified sequences [24]. PS oligonucleotides, with a sulfur atom substituted for a nonbridge backbone oxygen atom, have half-lives greater than 4 h [18,19], sufficient for most applications. PS oligonucleotides, however, have reduced target-binding affinity, increased nonspecific association with proteins, and greater toxicity and *in vivo* complications including complement activation [25–27]. These shortcomings in PS oligonucleotides have resulted in the examination of additional backbone modifications for nuclease resistance.

In phosphoramidate (PN) oligonucleotides, one backbone oxygen is replaced by an amino group. These can take two forms, where either the nonbridging oxygen in the backbone (nonbridging) or the 3′ oxygen of the ribose ring (N3′–P5′) is replaced by a nitrogen [28–33]. Though very stable to nuclease degradation [29], nonbridging PN molecules have lower affinity for their target mRNA molecules while N3′–P5′ PN oligonucleotides have similar nuclease resistance with increased target affinity [32]. Peptide nucleic acids (PNA) replace the PO backbone with an amide structure. These molecules are stable in response to nucleases as expected but are also stable in the presence of proteases [34]. Nuclease resistance through replacement of the backbone was achieved using another acyclic analogue, 1-[3-hydroxy-2-(hydroxymethyl) prop-1-enyl]thymine [35]. Oligonucleotides with only two of these modified nucleotides at the 3′ end showed markedly enhanced resistance to 3′-exonuclease [35].

A unique backbone modification replaces a nonbridging oxygen with a borane group (BH_3^-), maintaining backbone charge and conformation. In particular, nucleosides with this group are attractive as they are recognized by replication and transcription enzymes [36]. Boranophosphate (BP) oligonucleotides have twice the nuclease resistance of PS oligonucleotides [36]. Methylene(methylimino) (MMI) backbone linkages resist degradation while also conferring resistance to adjacent PO linkages, making them useful for the synthesis of chimeric backbone oligonucleotides [37,38]. 3′-Methylene-modified oligonucleotides also show significant nuclease resistance, though the specific contributions of the backbone modifications were not clear as the tested molecules also possessed other modifications [39].

A different approach to backbone modification was taken in the development of so-called dumbbell oligonucleotides [40]. These molecules are synthesized in a circular conformation, with an antisense DNA sequence conjugated to the complementary sense RNA sequence in antiparallel conformation by alkyl loops at each end. These molecules are "activated" by RNase H cleavage of the RNA portion of the stem, leaving the freed DNA to attack its complementary cellular target. Hence, until activation, these sequences do not have a free end to be attacked by exonucleases and are double-stranded to resist single-strand endonucleases. These molecules are protected from degradation through structure rather than chemical modification. An analogous approach used an artificial 3′–3′ linkage at the 3′ terminus of the oligonucleotide to prevent degradation [41].

Ribose modifications generate oligonucleotides that have RNA-like characters while not being as susceptible to nuclease degradation. Modifications to the sugar ring that have been tested have primarily focused on the 2′ position, though the 4′ position has received some minor attention (Figure 17.1a) [42]. Studies have investigated numerous atomic and molecular substitutions, such as 2′-amino, 2′-fluoro, 2′-O-methyl, 2′-O-propyl, 2′-O-butyl, 2′-O-pentyl, 2′-O-nonyl, 2′-O-allyl, 2′-O-3,3-dimethylallyl, 2′-O-methoxyethyl, 2′-O-aminopropyl, 2′-O-{2-[N,N-(dimethyl)aminooxy]ethyl} (2′-O-DMAOE), and 2′-O-{2-[N,N-(diethyl)aminooxy]ethyl} (2′-O-DEAOE) [17,43–52]. Half-lives of some 2′ modified oligonucleotides in the presence of nucleases have been found to approach or exceed that of PS oligonucleotides, in some cases with only four modified nucleotides at the 3′ end ($t_{1/2} > 24$ h) [50,51]. In connecting the 1′ carbon to the 2′ oxygen, oxetane constrained nucleotides were generated that almost completely protected against snake venom phosphodiesterase with only two 3′ modifications [53] Strangely, in serum, also thought to be primarily composed of 3′ exonucleases, the stability enhancement by this modification was only moderate at best.

A novel class of 2′ modified oligonucleotides called locked nucleic acids (LNAs) has recently received attention. These are also referred to as bridged nucleic acids (BNAs) as the modification locks the furanose

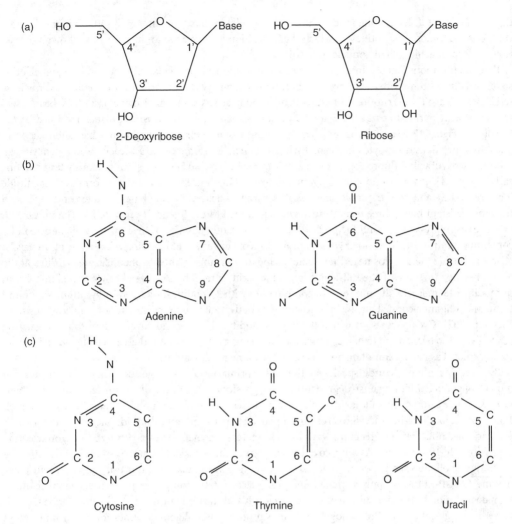

FIGURE 17.1 Components of natural nucleosides. (a) Deoxyribose and ribose sugars with labels. (b) Purine and pyrimidine nucleobases with labels. Base-pairing atoms are shown in bold text. Guanine and cytosine form three hydrogen bonds. Adenine forms two hydrogen bonds with either thymine (DNA) or uracil (RNA). Hydrogen atoms have not been explicitly displayed unless contributing to nucleic acid formation or structure.

ring into a C3′ *endo* conformation (typical for A-form helix) by forming a bridge between the 2′ oxygen and the 4′ carbon [54]. This covalent bond can be formed in either α or β conformation with either a methylene or ethylene linkage [55,56]. The nuclease resistance achieved using these nucleotides improves the half-life of natural nucleic acids by an order of magnitude [56,57]. Interestingly, oligonucleotides capped at both the 5′ and 3′ ends with LNA nucleotides are *less* nuclease resistant than those modified relatively uniformly throughout [57]. In morpholino oligonucleotides, the ribose sugar ring is replaced with a 6-membered morpholino ring in addition to using a phosphoramidate backbone. No cellular nuclease has been found that degrades these modified oligonucleotides [58,59].

Substitution of the natural chemical composition is not the only strategy for ribose modifications. Because natural nucleic acids are composed of many chiral centers, conformation has also been explored as a means of maximizing the natural chemistry of oligonucleotides while also protecting them from degradation. Natural ribose constituents are in D conformation, either C2′ *endo* (B-form helix) or C3′ *endo* with the 2′ constituents in *trans* to the nucleobase. Incorporating nine L-deoxycytidine modifications (vs. natural D-deoxycytidine) distributed evenly throughout a 19-mer oligonucleotide protected more than 50% of the full-length oligonucleotide from degradation in serum after 60 h [60]. Oligonucleotides containing arabinose nucleotides, in which the 2′ position is *cis* relative to the base, have shown nuclease resistance approaching PS oligonucleotides [61].

Base modifications that can interrupt nuclease progression are particularly valuable for oligonucleotide stability as they do not often compromise backbone chemistry or conformation for enhanced nuclease resistance. To avoid interruption of base-pairing, modifications to the nucleoside bases have been tested primarily with pyrimidines at the 5 and 6 positions, with some tests using purines modified at the 7 position (Figure 17.1b and c) [62–64]. The nuclease resistance for many pyrimidine base modifications, 6-azathymine; 6-azadeoxycytosine; 6-methyldeoxyuracil; 5,6-dimethyldeoxyuracil; 5-iododeoxyuracil; 5-bromodeoxyuracil; 5-fluorodeoxyuracil; and 5-methyldeoxycytosine, was simultaneously tested in one early study [64]. It was found that as compared to PO oligonucleotides at least an order of magnitude increase in the stability of the molecules in calf serum was achieved using base-modified end caps, with the most resistant being three 6-methyldeoxyuracils added to the 3′ end ($t_{1/2}$ = 24 h). The prevention of nuclease progression beyond the point of base modification has also been shown for oligonucleotides containing central 5-(N-aminoalkyl)carbamoyl-2′-deoxyuridines [65]. A single insertion of a tricyclic "G-clamp" analogue of cytosine, either phenoxazine or 9-(2-aminoethoxy)-phenoxazine cytosine, at the 3′ end resulted in 100% of the full-length oligonucleotide after 8 h as opposed to 0% remaining for an unmodified 19-mer after 20 min [66]. In combination with 2′ modifications, 2-thiothymidine was found to enhance oligonucleotide half-life but did not prevent degradation in the absence of a nuclease resistant backbone [67]. Cyclopurines, in which the base is modified by a second covalent link to the sugar ring (5′–8), have also been found to halt exonuclease progression [68]. However, these nucleotides can be more easily depicted as having simultaneous base and backbone modifications.

By attaching nonnucleotide species at the ends (primarily 3′) of oligonucleotides, conjugates can protect oligonucleotides against degradation through steric prevention of exonuclease initiation and progression. Examples include avidin–biotin complexes; hexanol; aminohexyl; acridine; cholesterol; 1,3 propanediol; 1-*O*-hexadecylglycerol; amino sugars; spermine, and dipyridophenazine [53,69–74]. An 8 nt 3′-terminal hairpin structure was shown to increase the half-life of a 19-mer PO oligonucleotide approximately 10-fold [75]. As with covalent conjugates, noncovalent complexes have shown effective protection of oligonucleotides against degradation. In the extracellular medium, asialoglycoprotein-poly-L-lysine (ASGP-PLL) and polyethyleneimine (PEI) electrostatic complexes protected oligonucleotides from degradation by steric repulsion of serum nucleases and encapsulation of the oligonucleotide [76,77]. Polyethylene glycol (PEG)–PEI nanogel complexes protected PO oligonucleotides for over 1 h in mouse serum [78].

17.3.2   Cellular Delivery and Uptake

In a therapeutic context, oligonucleotides must be delivered to the appropriate target tissue, associate with target cells, and be internalized. *In vitro* studies using chemical and mechanical permeabilization support the hypothesis that cellular uptake greatly limits oligonucleotide efficacy [79–82]. Achieving the necessary intracellular oligonucleotide concentration to enact an effect is limited by many factors, including protein adsorption and charge repulsion between the negatively charged oligonucleotide and the negatively charged cell surface. Issues of systemic and cellular delivery are being addressed by a number of different methods, including chemical modification of oligonucleotides to increase their hydrophobicity; conjugation of oligonucleotides to molecules that enhance biological half-life, cellular association, and endocytosis; and encapsulation of the oligonucleotide in various carriers, primarily cationic lipids or liposomes.

It was initially believed that increasing the hydrophobicity of oligonucleotides would enhance their association with lipid membranes as well as potentially allowing them to diffuse freely through the plasma membrane. This was accomplished using MP oligonucleotides. Despite their neutral backbone charge and their stability to nucleases [3], cellular uptake of fully MP oligonucleotides was shown to be very inefficient, with uptake primarily trapping the oligonucleotides in pinocytic vesicles with little or no nuclear accumulation after 4 h [10,83]. Similarly poor uptake has been described for noncharged PNA and morpholino oligonucleotides, which generally must be loaded by alternative chemical or physical strategies [84,85]. With limited available modifications and the significant enhancement of uptake via complexation with other molecules, direct backbone modifications for improvement of delivery have not received continued attention.

A standard *in vitro* means to deliver oligonucleotides is lipofection. Oligonucleotides are mixed with cationic lipids that condense around the negatively charged oligonucleotide forming a lipid vesicle (liposome), which interacts more easily with the lipophilic cellular membrane. The positively charged lipids also reduce the electrostatic repulsion between the oligonucleotide and the cell surface. Oligonucleotides separate from the liposomes following cellular internalization via adsorptive endocytosis [86–92]. Incorporation into liposomes has been shown to enhance efficacy by as much as 1000-fold in the inhibition of ICAM-1 and HIV-1 [93,94]. Targeted liposomes have also been examined as a method for enhancing specific, cellular delivery [6,95,96]. "Programmable" fusogenic vesicles are based on liposomes that can be destabilized to encourage fusion with cellular membranes to release contained oligonucleotides into the cytoplasmic compartment [97,98]. Liposomal preparations containing recombinant viral peptides have been proposed for virus-like transmission of encapsulated nucleic acid without viral complications [99].

Oligonucleotides conjugated with polycations such as poly-L-lysine (PLL) also have improved cellular uptake and efficacy [100,101]. Cationic "starburst" dendrimers showed modest enhancement of oligonucleotide uptake, though less than cationic lipid formations [102]. Morpholino and PNA oligonucleotides, having no backbone charge, cannot be complexed directly with cationic carriers for delivery; however efficient delivery was still achieved using a charged DNA molecule carrier complexed with polycationic species [103,104]. Condensation of oligonucleotides with protamine sulfate followed by incorporation in *anionic* lipid formulations, such that the overall charge ratio was 3/1 (+/−) showed enhanced nuclear localization in HepG2 cells [105]. Conjugation to proteins and carbohydrates can enhance the efficiency and specificity of delivery to a target organ, often the liver, while potentially mitigating the toxicity of the PLL moiety [106–108]. Oligonucleotide–PLL complexes have been conjugated to transferrin to utilize the transferrin receptor to mediate uptake in human leukemia (HL-60) cells [109]. This approach has also been used with specific ligands to other cellular receptors, such as the ASGP, EGF, and IGF1 receptors, with success [88,108–115]. This strategy has also been tested with noncovalent conjugates of oligonucleotide with PLL conjugated to the signal import peptide from Kaposi fibroblast growth factor with positive results [116]. Recent success at the lipofection of nondividing cells with plasmid using a nuclear localization signal suggests another potential conjugate for oligonucleotide delivery [117].

Early attempts at covalent conjugation focused on enhancing the oligonucleotide hydrophobicity. Oligonucleotides conjugated to cholesterol derivatives (chol-oligonucleotides) and other lipophilic compounds have improved association with cell membranes and internalization by cells, in some cases through interactions with cellular proteins [118–122]. Conjugation of poly(G) as a nonspecific ligand for the macrophage scavenger receptor showed order of magnitude enhancement in cellular accumulation of oligonucleotide in cell culture studies [123]. Peptide conjugates have also been used to mediate specific trafficking within cells. Peptides as simple as four lysines at the end of a PNA improved cellular uptake in transgenic mice [124]. PS and PNA oligonucleotides conjugated to HIV-1 Tat, transportan, and antennapedia homeodomain peptide showed enhanced cellular accumulation over free oligonucleotides [84,125,126]. Nuclear targeting peptide was conjugated to an oligonucleotide to enhance its nuclear localization in *Paramecium* [127].

For *in vivo* delivery, distinct issues of localization and persistence must be accounted for prior to cellular uptake and trafficking. One strategy for this utilizes biodegradable polymer microspheres to encapsulate oligonucleotides for site-specific delivery [128]. Distribution within the tissue, in this case rat brain, was improved. In addition, intracellular distribution, presumably due to enhanced extracellular concentration profile, was more even and longer lived [128]. In the particular case of delivery to the brain, fractional oligonucleotide uptake across the blood–brain barrier was also dramatically improved, approximately 8-fold increase, by positively charged PEG–PEI complexes [78].

17.3.3 Intermolecular Hybridization Affinity

The affinity of oligonucleotides for their target mRNA has been shown as a major determinant in antisense action [129,130]. The affinity of PO oligonucleotides for their complement varies greatly depending on both sequence, in particular GC content, and the folded structures of the oligonucleotide and the targeted strand [131,132]. Hybridization requires the delicate assembly of hydrogen bonds to overcome the innate repulsion of the two negatively charged nucleic acid backbones. Improvement of this interaction can be achieved through modifications to reduce electrostatic repulsion or enhance hydrogen bond formation/organization and base stacking (i.e., enthalpic enhancement) or through optimizing structure in the free strands to minimize change upon hybridization (entropic).

An early study catalogued numerous modifications and assessed their relative effects on the melting temperature (T_m) of duplexes of modified oligonucleotides with their RNA complement [133]. What is most striking about the study is that of 17 novel phosphorus-containing backbone modifications, including PS, none enhanced intermolecular T_m values. Likewise, for over 60 modified nonphosphorus backbones examined, none consistently enhanced the affinity of a modified oligonucleotide for its target RNA across a number of different sequence contexts with some achieving *destabilization* of up to 10°C per modification [133]. Modifications that caused significant destabilization of duplex formation also greatly reduced selectivity to mismatch sequences. Backbone modifications that enhance nuclease resistance generally reduce intermolecular affinity as seen with PS oligonucleotides (≈ -1°C per modification) and MP oligonucleotides (≈ -2°C per modification) [134].

Nonetheless, modified phosphate backbones have been identified that do improve hybridization. Replacement of the $3'$ oxygen with an amino group (N3'–P5' PN) or a methylene group increases T_m by approximately 1°C per modification relative to PO backbone molecules [39,135]. Incorporation of positive charges into the backbone using dimethyl aminopropyl PN linkages enhanced the binding of strands for their target and reduced the dependence of binding on salt concentration [136]. In addition, mismatch selectivity was extraordinary with an average of approximately −10°C per mismatch [136]. This hybridization is particularly unique in that it results from *parallel* strand interactions due to the α orientation of these modified nucleotides.

Additional success has been achieved through the use of nonphosphate backbones. Formacetal linkages, with the backbone phosphate ($5'$-OPO$_2$O-$3'$) replaced by methylene ($5'$-OCH$_2$O-$3'$) have lower affinity for their target RNA but $3'$-thioformacetal ($5'$-SCH$_2$O-$3'$) backbone nucleotides increase T_m by approximately 1°C per modification [137]. MMI backbone linkages marginally increase hybridization affinity but have been found to augment significantly the affinity increase provided by $2'$ ribose modifications [138]. Using an array of PNA 16-mer sequences, T_m values with DNA complement were measured at 70–80°C relative to 50–55°C for DNA:DNA hybrids [139]. An 11-mer PNA was shown to have sub-nanomolar affinity for its complementary target with single mismatches generating primarily enthalpic losses in excess of entropic gains [140].

Enhanced intermolecular affinity is most often achieved through ribose modifications, primarily those at the $2'$ position, in an attempt to approach most closely an A-form helix, which has been shown to be more energetically stable than B-form [141,142]. Through the synthesis of many modified nucleosides, it has been shown that, for single-chain groups, intermolecular affinity decreases with the size of the $2'$ group, the opposite trend from nuclease resistance [18,45]. Branched structures, however, can increase T_m for RNA while reducing DNA affinity and improving selectivity [50]. $2'$-O-anthraquinone-modified oligonucleotides had enhanced binding to complementary targets through intercalation of the anthraquinone group [143]. As this moiety intercalates into the helix structure, the relative enhancement for DNA is greater than that for RNA, due to the more pronounced grooves of the B-form helix.

Many $2'$ modifications seek to enhance affinity by reduced entropic cost through preorganization. A thorough review on this subject has been published [144]. This strategy led to the development of LNAs, which are conformationally locked in C3' *endo* conformation. The binding affinities of LNAs for their targets have been reported to be among the highest recorded with ΔT_m per modification values of up to 10°C in binding RNA [145]. The maximal increase in affinity per modification was achieved with mixed LNA–DNA oligonucleotides, suggesting that some compensation of the more flexible ribose for the constrained ring is required. However, the mechanism of affinity enhancement remains under debate; it is either enhanced preorganization of constrained nucleotides as originally postulated or improved nucleobase alignment [146,147]. In one study, stopped-flow kinetics results at 25°C showed that the dissociation rate constants primarily determined hybridization affinity and that the affinity increase due to incorporation of LNA nucleotides was enthalpic not entropic, indicating improved base-pairing [148]. Slower dissociation kinetics was also seen in triplex applications [149], lending credence to the observed behavior with duplexes.

Base modifications take advantage of improved hydrogen bonding or improved π electron sharing in base stacking. To enhance affinity, pyrimidine bases are most often modified as the single ring provides more flexibility in the size of the substituted groups. The earliest reported base modification that enhanced oligonucleotide affinity, C-5 propyne or in the current vernacular 5-(1-propynyl), showed an enhancement of the melting temperature of 1 to 2°C per modification [150,151]. Since then, many different modifications have been tested with varying affinity changes. Halides (F, Br, and I) at the 5 position alter T_m only slightly, ±0.3°C, while carbon chains at the 5 position most often proved destabilizing by at least 1°C per modification, with the notable exception of the 1-propynyl insertion [64,133]. Aminoglycoside substitution at the 5 position of cytidine created enhanced electrostatic interactions to increase T_m by 1.5°C per modification at 1 M NaCl and by 2.5°C per modification at 0.15 M NaCl, with RNA binding being preferentially enhanced over DNA, presumably due to enhanced sterics from the empty central axis of A-form helices [152].

While the majority of conjugates either reduce binding affinity due to sterics or have no effect since they do not interact with the nucleic acids (the notable exception being positively charged peptides [153]), some intercalating species have proven to greatly stabilize formed duplexes. Incorporation of a single acridine moiety increases T_m by an average of 5°C whether added at the 5′ terminus or at a central location [154]. Adding 1-O-(1-pyrenylmethyl)glycerol to the ends of short (6–8 mer) oligonucleotides increased affinity by ≈ 10°C per modification to its DNA complement [155]. Replacing an internal base by this group reduces affinity, but insertion as a bulge increases affinity beyond the fully matched sequence. Discrimination between DNA and RNA complements is also dramatically enhanced [155].

17.4 Other Applications

17.4.1 Aptamers

While primary sequence of oligonucleotides is critical to function in most nucleic acid applications, the simplicity of manipulation of nucleic acid secondary structure and the small "alphabet" of building blocks has led to the development of structure-based, functional oligonucleotides, termed aptamers. Both directed and combinatorial approaches have been used to generate oligonucleotides that effectively and specifically bind targeted molecules by means other than base-pairing. Initially, it was shown that small molecule targets could be bound by selected RNA molecules [156,157]. Selection and amplification strategies for protein targets (e.g., SELEX) soon yielded two protein-binding single-stranded aptamers for T4 DNA polymerase and one for human thrombin, each with nanomolar affinity for its target [158,159]. The sequence of the thrombin-binding oligonucleotide, GGTTGGTGTGGTTGG, makes clear why this oligonucleotide would have unique structure. Sequences with multiple guanines tend to arrange in planar G-quartet structures, and this was later confirmed [160,161]. The ability of these techniques to identify optimal structures was also noted by a subsequent mutation study in which no alterations in the center of the structured region provided gains in the stability of the selected structure [162]. The importance of the oligonucleotide structure rather than the sequence was confirmed through the use of 5-(1-pentynyl)-deoxyuridine nucleotides. New sequences were found in the presence of the modified nucleotides without a significant loss in binding affinity [163]. Similarly, replacement of PS aptamers with PO and 2′-O-methyl oligonucleotides of identical sequence markedly reduced the function of an aptamer targeting EGF receptor in cell culture [164].

Recognizing the importance of nuclease stability, aptamers targeting basic fibroblast growth factor incorporated 2'-amino modifications, the resulting aptamers being nonfunctional without the amino group [165]. It was found that incorporation of these moieties along the length of the aptamer also provided a framework for further modification and flexibility in the selection scheme [166]. A similar strategy involved providing a carbonyl group at the 5 position of uridine for downstream derivatization, in an attempt to enhance the "shape space" available to the oligonucleotides [167]. Nuclease resistant and *selection competent* aptamers with 2'-fluoro modifications were subsequently modified with 2'-*O*-methyl groups, enhancing their stability but rendering the oligonucleotides incompetent for further amplification [168]. Additional nuclease stability and improved cell and tissue uptake were achieved through 5' conjugation with diacylglycerol and noncovalent complex formation with cholesterol-containing liposomes [169]. The resulting complex produced the desired inhibition of cellular proliferation *in vivo*, while the naked aptamer could not. Subsequent *in vivo* studies showed that stable production of aptamers resulted in long-term inhibition of *Drosophila* B52 function in cell lines and adult animals, mitigating issues of delivery [170]. The protein binding of PS oligonucleotides, though a detriment for most applications, was found to be useful for the production of aptamers to prevent cell adhesion and cytokine stimulation [171,172]. Phosphorodithioate linkages (P-2S) have shown enhanced interactions with target proteins with similar nuclease stability to PS oligonucleotides [173].

A novel aptamer design method achieves nuclease stability through the use of mirror-image L-oligonucleotides. These molecules, termed "spiegelmers," cannot be generated using natural polymerases, necessitating development of an ingenious synthetic method [174]. The desire is to generate L-oligonucleotides (unnatural) to target proteins containing L-amino acids (natural). Taking advantage of chiral substrate specificity [175], SELEX is performed with D-oligonucleotides (natural) targeting peptides synthesized with mirror-image D-amino acids (unnatural). Once high affinity D-oligonucleotides are identified, the corresponding L-oligonucleotide, which is nuclease resistant and targets the natural proteins, is synthesized [174]. This strategy has been successfully applied in locating spiegelmers targeting multiple peptide and protein targets with K_D approximately 100 to 1000 nM [176–181]. Spiegelmers conjugated to 40 kDa PEG were found to have significantly longer biological half-lives than naked spiegelmers [177]. The technique is limited by the size of mirror-image target that can be easily synthesized, but recent work has shown that targeting stable protein domains may allow selection of aptamers against the full protein [178].

Aptamers can be designed to target nucleic acids with combined structural and complementarity interactions [182]. This type of aptamer has been developed successfully with DNA or RNA [182,183]. Standard selection methods isolated a stem–loop structure where the loop formed a complementary "kissing complex" with the targeted HIV-1 TAR RNA, in which the loop base-pairs with its complement and the stem provides additional structural stabilization. This type of loop–loop interaction is akin to the interaction of tRNA with mRNA in translation. The slight differences in the base composition between the RNA and DNA aptamers may reflect differences in the structures of RNA:RNA and RNA:DNA helices [184]. As in other cases, the natural RNA aptamer was ineffective in cell culture due to degradation, but a nuclease stable analogue that bound the TAR RNA with similar affinity successfully inhibited Tat-mediated transcription at submicromolar concentrations [185,186]. The importance of the structures formed by these aptamers was reinforced by the ablation of function due to alteration of the loop-closing base composition, a thermodynamically unfavorable alteration [186,187].

17.4.2 RNA Interference

RNA interference (RNAi) is a promising but relatively young technology that is being explored for highly specific gene expression inhibition. In RNAi, the presence of 21–23 nt double-stranded RNA (dsRNA) termed short interfering RNA (siRNA) in the cytoplasm of cells initiates recruitment of proteins to form the RNA-induced silencing complex (RISC), which cleaves the targeted mRNA [188,189]. Early work provided basic heuristic sequence design parameters for siRNAs [190,191], which has since been more thoroughly tested and revised by commercial siRNA providers [192]. siRNAs face some similar design issues to those of antisense oligonucleotides, being short nucleic acids that must enter cells, identify a target by Watson–Crick complementarity, and exert a biological function. However, modified siRNAs have three other significant constraints: they must be administered as double-stranded sequences, must form A-form helices when hybridized with the target mRNA, and must allow for the specific protein interactions required by the RNAi pathway [193]. In addition, the $5'$ end of the antisense strand siRNA must terminate in a hydroxyl group for efficient silencing [193,194]. The most common modification of siRNAs is to enhance stability with two $2'$-deoxythymidines at each $3'$ overhang [189]. Other chemical modifications have focused on further enhancement of nuclease resistance, improved inhibitory activity, and reduced nonspecific effects, though the number of published studies is currently small due to the relative youth of the field.

In general, RNA is highly susceptible to degradation by RNases leading to investigation of RNase resistant siRNA strands [195]. One strategy for extending the half-life of RNA is through the use of hairpins [196], which is a strategy used for simplified production of siRNAs [197]. The success of this approach in extending the time of RNAi has not been thoroughly studied. Fully and partially modified siRNAs containing either $2'$-fluoro, $2'$-deoxy, or $2'$-O-methyl ribose modifications; 5-bromo, 5-iodo, or 3-methyl uridine; or 2,6-diaminopurine (in place of adenine) modifications were examined for RNase resistance in cellular extracts, maximal inhibition of the target at more than 200 nM, the kinetics of inhibition, and the relative importance of the location of modifications on the activity of the molecules [195]. $2'$-Fluoro and $2'$-O-methyl-modified siRNAs showed enhanced nuclease resistance, maximally when both strands were modified, and sustained activity for approximately twice as long as unmodified duplexes (>120 h) but with reduced maximal inhibition [195,198]. Similar results were obtained with end-modified siRNAs [199], which were administered in serum-free conditions as serum seems to have predominantly double-stranded endonucleases [198]. Alternating $2'$-O-methyl modifications were sufficient to provide nuclease resistance, while five and ten nt consecutively modified stretches were not [198]. Curiously, highly resistant $2'$-O-methyl siRNAs showed no inhibitory activity, possibly due to interruption of protein interactions or excessive siRNA affinity preventing duplex unwinding [190,195]. The siRNAs containing two LNA modifications maintained the ability to inhibit caveolin expression from HeLa cells at similar concentration to the unmodified duplex, despite their high T_m values [200]. It remains to be seen if stabilizing modifications that enhance cell culture activity can translate to the *in vivo* situation, and recent data suggests that this may prove more troublesome than expected [201].

17.5 Summary

Oligonucleotides have proven to have great potential in a number of biotechnology and therapeutic applications. While the natural physical and chemical properties of oligonucleotides first drew the attention of researchers for the desired applications, it soon became clear that an oligonucleotide engineered specifically for the task would be more effective than an "off-the-rack" oligonucleotide. Beginning with enhancing the backbone for nuclease resistance, oligonucleotides are now engineered to meet every design constraint of the targeted application. The many functional groups available on the backbone, in the sugar moiety, and in the nucleobase provide a fertile basis from which to perform modifications. In concert, the analytical techniques available and the depth of knowledge of nucleic acid structures and interactions provide the scientist and engineer with the ability to fully understand the impact of the modifications not only on the intended design parameter but also on other oligonucleotide properties. The foundations of understanding derived from the development of antisense oligonucleotides for the lab and the clinic have begun to be applied to other oligonucleotide-based technologies, such as aptamers and siRNAs. While many similarities exist across these applications, the specific needs of each will be thoroughly examined and novel biomolecular engineering approaches applied in the synthesis of the next generation of designer oligonucleotides.

Abbreviations

ASGP   Asialoglycoprotein
BNA   Bridged nucleic acid
BP   Boranophosphate
DNase   Deoxyribonuclease
EGF   Epidermal growth factor
HIV   Human immunodeficiency virus
ICAM   Intracellular adhesion molecule
IGF   Insulin-like growth factor
LNA   Locked nucleic acid
MMI   Methylene(methylimino)
MP   Methylphosphonates
nt   Nucleotide
P-2S   Phosphorodithioate
PEG   Polyethyleneglycol
PEI   Polyethyleneimine
PLL   Poly-L-lysine
PN   Phosphoramidate
PNA   Peptide nucleic acid
PO   Phosphodiester
PS   Phosphorothioate
RISC   RNA-induced silencing complex
RNAi   RNA interference
RNase   Ribonuclease
SELEX   Systematic evolution of ligands by exponential enrichment
siRNA   Short, interfering RNA
T_m Melting temperature

References

[1] Veggeberg, S., At the interface of biology and chemical-engineering, *Scientist*, 7, 15, 1993.

[2] *Penn Engineering\\Chemical and Biomolecular Engineering\\Bio Opportunities for Chem Engrs.* http://www.seas.upenn.edu/cbe/biomolecular.html, 2004.

[3] Akhtar, S., Kole, R., and Juliano, R.L., Stability of antisense DNA oligodeoxynucleotide analogs in cellular extracts and sera, *Life Sci.*, 49, 1793, 1991.

[4] Geselowitz, D.A. and Neckers, L.M., Bovine serum albumin is a major oligonucleotide-binding protein found on the surface of cultured cells, *Antisense Res. Dev.*, 5, 213, 1995.

[5] Biessen, E.A. et al., Liver uptake of phosphodiester oligodeoxynucleotides is mediated by scavenger receptors, *Mol. Pharmacol.*, 53, 262, 1998.

[6] Chaudhuri, G., Scavenger receptor-mediated delivery of antisense mini-exon phosphorothioate oligonucleotide to Leishmania-infected macrophages. Selective and efficient elimination of the parasite, *Biochem. Pharmacol.*, 53, 385, 1997.

[7] Bijsterbosch, M.K. et al., *In vivo* fate of phosphorothioate antisense oligodeoxynucleotides: predominant uptake by scavenger receptors on endothelial liver cells, *Nucleic Acids Res.*, 25, 3290, 1997.

[8] Loke, S.L. et al., Characterization of oligonucleotide transport into living cells, *Proc. Natl Acad. Sci. USA*, 86, 3474, 1989.

[9] Yakubov, L.A. et al., Mechanism of oligonucleotide uptake by cells: involvement of specific receptors? *Proc. Natl Acad. Sci. USA*, 86, 6454, 1989.

[10] Shoji, Y. et al., Mechanism of cellular uptake of modified oligodeoxynucleotides containing methylphosphonate linkages, *Nucleic Acids Res.*, 19, 5543, 1991.

[11] Thierry, A.R. and Dritschilo, A., Intracellular availability of unmodified, phosphorothioated and liposomally encapsulated oligodeoxynucleotides for antisense activity, *Nucleic Acids Res.*, 20, 5691, 1992.

[12] Tam, R.C. et al., Biological availability and nuclease resistance extend the *in vitro* activity of a phosphorothioate-3′hydroxypropylamine oligonucleotide, *Nucleic Acids Res.*, 22, 977, 1994.

[13] Jensen, K.D., Kopeckova, P., and Kopecek, J., Antisense oligonucleotides delivered to the lysosome escape and actively inhibit the hepatitis B virus, *Bioconjug. Chem.*, 13, 975, 2002.

[14] Fattal, E., Couvreur, P., and Dubernet, C., "Smart" delivery of antisense oligonucleotides by anionic pH-sensitive liposomes, *Adv. Drug Deliv. Rev.*, 56, 931, 2004.

[15] Marcusson, E.G. et al., Phosphorothioate oligodeoxyribonucleotides dissociate from cationic lipids before entering the nucleus, *Nucleic Acids Res.*, 26, 2016, 1998.

[16] Stein, C.A., Two problems in antisense biotechnology: *in vitro* delivery and the design of antisense experiments, *Biochim. Biophys. Acta*, 1489, 45, 1999.

[17] Monia, B.P. et al., Evaluation of 2′-modified oligonucleotides containing 2′-deoxy gaps as antisense inhibitors of gene expression, *J. Biol. Chem.*, 268, 14514, 1993.

[18] Monia, B.P. et al., Nuclease resistance and antisense activity of modified oligonucleotides targeted to Ha-ras, *J. Biol. Chem.*, 271, 14533, 1996.

[19] McKay, R.A. et al., Enhanced activity of an antisense oligonucleotide targeting murine protein kinase C-alpha by the incorporation of 2′-O-propyl modifications, *Nucleic Acids Res.*, 24, 411, 1996.

[20] Nagel, K.M., Holstad, S.G., and Isenberg, K.E., Oligonucleotide pharmacotherapy: an antigene strategy, *Pharmacotherapy*, 13, 177, 1993.

[21] Iribarren, A.M., Cicero, D.O., and Neuner, P.J., Resistance to degradation by nucleases of (2′S)-2′-deoxy-2′-C-methyloligonucleotides, novel potential antisense probes, *Antisense Res. Dev.*, 4, 95, 1994.

[22] Agrawal, S. et al., Pharmacokinetics of antisense oligonucleotides, *Clin. Pharmacokinet.*, 28, 7, 1995.

[23] Milligan, J.F., Matteucci, M.D., and Martin, J.C., Current concepts in antisense drug design, *J. Med. Chem.*, 36, 1923, 1993.

[24] Quartin, R.S., Brakel, C.L., and Wetmur, J.G., Number and distribution of methylphosphonate linkages in oligodeoxynucleotides affect exo- and endonuclease sensitivity and ability to form RNase H substrates, *Nucleic Acids Res.*, 17, 7253, 1989.

[25] Crooke, S.T. et al., Pharmacokinetic properties of several novel oligonucleotide analogs in mice, *J. Pharmacol. Exp. Ther.*, 277, 923, 1996.

[26] Geary, R.S. et al., Pharmacokinetic properties of 2′-O-(2-methoxyethyl)-modified oligonucleotide analogs in rats, *J. Pharmacol. Exp. Ther.*, 296, 890, 2001.

[27] Galbraith, W.M. et al., Complement activation and hemodynamic changes following intravenous administration of phosphorothioate oligonucleotides in the monkey, *Antisense Res. Dev.*, 4, 201, 1994.

[28] Peyrottes, S. et al., Oligodeoxynucleoside phosphoramidates (P-NH2): synthesis and thermal stability of duplexes with DNA and RNA targets, *Nucleic Acids Res.*, 24, 1841, 1996.

[29] Heidenreich, O., Gryaznov, S., and Nerenberg, M., RNase H-independent antisense activity of oligonucleotide N3′–> P5′ phosphoramidates, *Nucleic Acids Res.*, 25, 776, 1997.

[30] Skorski, T. et al., Antileukemia effect of c-myc N3′–>P5′ phosphoramidate antisense oligonucleotides *in vivo*, *Proc. Natl Acad. Sci. USA*, 94, 3966, 1997.

[31] Hawley, P. et al., Comparison of binding of N3′–>P5′ phosphoramidate and phosphorothioate oligonucleotides to cell surface proteins of cultured cells, *Antisense Nucleic Acid Drug Dev.*, 9, 61, 1999.

[32] Gryaznov, S.M., Oligonucleotide N3′–>P5′ phosphoramidates as potential therapeutic agents, *Biochim. Biophys. Acta*, 1489, 131, 1999.

[33] Gryaznov, S. et al., Oligonucleotide N3′–>P5′ phosphoramidates as antisense agents, *Nucleic Acids Res.*, 24, 1508, 1996.

[34] Demidov, V.V. et al., Stability of peptide nucleic acids in human serum and cellular extracts, *Biochem. Pharmacol.*, 48, 1310, 1994.

[35] Boesen, T. et al., Oligonucleotides containing a new type of acyclic, achiral nucleoside analogue: 1-[3-hydroxy-2-(hydroxymethyl)prop-1-enyl]thymine, *Bioorg. Med. Chem. Lett.*, 13, 847, 2003.

[36] Shaw, B.R. et al., Reading, writing, and modulating genetic information with boranophosphate mimics of nucleotides, DNA, and RNA, *Ann. N.Y. Acad. Sci.*, 1002, 12, 2003.

[37] Bhat, B. et al., Synthesis of novel nucleic acid mimics via the stereoselective intermolecular radical coupling of 3′-iodo nucleosides and formaldoximes(1), *J. Org. Chem.*, 61, 8186, 1996.

[38] Yang, X. et al., NMR structure of an antisense DNA:RNA hybrid duplex containing a 3′-CH(2)N(CH(3))-O-5′ or an MMI backbone linker, *Biochemistry*, 38, 12586, 1999.

[39] An, H. et al., Synthesis of novel 3′-C-methylene thymidine and 5-methyluridine/cytidine H-phosphonates and phosphonamidites for new backbone modification of oligonucleotides, *J. Org. Chem.*, 66, 2789, 2001.

[40] Park, W.S. et al., Inhibition of HIV-1 replication by a new type of circular dumbbell RNA/DNA chimeric oligonucleotides, *Biochem. Biophys. Res. Commun.*, 270, 953, 2000.

[41] Boutorine, A.S. et al., Effect of derivatization of ribophosphate backbone and terminal ribophosphate groups in oligoribonucleotides on their stability and interaction with eukaryotic cells, *Biochimie*, 76, 23, 1994.

[42] Leydier, C. et al., 4′-Thio-RNA: synthesis of mixed base 4′-thio-oligoribonucleotides, nuclease resistance, and base pairing properties with complementary single and double strand, *Antisense Res. Dev.*, 5, 167, 1995.

[43] Pieken, W.A. et al., Kinetic characterization of ribonuclease-resistant 2′-modified hammerhead ribozymes, *Science*, 253, 314, 1991.

[44] Iribarren, A.M. et al., 2′-O-alkyl oligoribonucleotides as antisense probes, *Proc. Natl Acad. Sci. USA*, 87, 7747, 1990.

[45] Lesnik, E.A. et al., Oligodeoxynucleotides containing 2′-O-modified adenosine: synthesis and effects on stability of DNA:RNA duplexes, *Biochemistry*, 32, 7832, 1993.

[46] Kawasaki, A.M. et al., Uniformly modified 2′-deoxy-2′-fluoro phosphorothioate oligonucleotides as nuclease-resistant antisense compounds with high affinity and specificity for RNA targets, *J. Med. Chem.*, 36, 831, 1993.

[47] Boiziau, C. et al., Antisense 2′-O-alkyl oligoribonucleotides are efficient inhibitors of reverse transcription, *Nucleic Acids Res.*, 23, 64, 1995.

[48] Johansson, H.E. et al., Target-specific arrest of mRNA translation by antisense 2′-O-alkyloligoribonucleotides, *Nucleic Acids Res.*, 22, 4591, 1994.

[49] Brown-Driver, V. et al., Inhibition of translation of hepatitis C virus RNA by 2-modified antisense oligonucleotides, *Antisense Nucleic Acid Drug Dev.*, 9, 145, 1999.

[50] Prakash, T.P. et al., 2′-O-[2-[N,N-(dialkyl)aminooxy]ethyl]-modified antisense oligonucleotides, *Org. Lett.*, 2, 3995, 2000.

[51] Teplova, M. et al., Structural origins of the exonuclease resistance of a zwitterionic RNA, *Proc. Natl Acad. Sci. USA*, 96, 14240, 1999.

[52] Griffey, R.H. et al., 2′-O-aminopropyl ribonucleotides: a zwitterionic modification that enhances the exonuclease resistance and biological activity of antisense oligonucleotides, *J. Med. Chem.*, 39, 5100, 1996.

[53] Pradeepkumar, P.I., Amirkhanov, N.V., and Chattopadhyaya, J., Antisense oligonuclotides with oxetane-constrained cytidine enhance heteroduplex stability, and elicit satisfactory RNase H

response as well as showing improved resistance to both exo and endonucleases, *Org. Biomol. Chem.*, 1, 81, 2003.

[54] Kumar, R. et al., The first analogues of LNA (locked nucleic acids): phosphorothioate-LNA and 2′-thio-LNA, *Bioorg. Med. Chem. Lett.*, 8, 2219, 1998.

[55] Frieden, M. et al., Expanding the design horizon of antisense oligonucleotides with alpha-L-LNA, *Nucleic Acids Res.*, 31, 6365, 2003.

[56] Koizumi, M. et al., Triplex formation with 2′-O,4′-C-ethylene-bridged nucleic acids (ENA) having C3′-endo conformation at physiological pH, *Nucleic Acids Res.*, 31, 3267, 2003.

[57] Wahlestedt, C. et al., Potent and nontoxic antisense oligonucleotides containing locked nucleic acids, *Proc. Natl Acad. Sci. USA*, 97, 5633, 2000.

[58] Summerton, J., Morpholino antisense oligomers: the case for an RNase H-independent structural type, *Biochim. Biophys. Acta*, 1489, 141, 1999.

[59] Ekker, S.C., Morphants: a new systematic vertebrate functional genomics approach, *Yeast*, 17, 302, 2000.

[60] Damha, M.J., Giannaris, P.A., and Marfey, P., Antisense L/D-oligodeoxynucleotide chimeras: nuclease stability, base-pairing properties, and activity at directing ribonuclease H, *Biochemistry*, 33, 7877, 1994.

[61] Damha, M.J. et al., Hybrids of RNA and arabinonucleic acids (ANA and 2′ F-ANA) are substrates of ribonuclease h, *J. Am. Chem. Soc.*, 120, 12976, 1998.

[62] Seela, F. and Kehne, A., Oligomers with alternating thymidine and 2′-deoxytubercidin: duplex stabilization by a 7-deazapurine base, *Biochemistry*, 24, 7556, 1985.

[63] Wagner, R.W. et al., Potent and selective inhibition of gene expression by an antisense heptanucleotide, *Nat. Biotechnol.*, 14, 840, 1996.

[64] Sanghvi, Y.S. et al., Antisense oligodeoxynucleotides: synthesis, biophysical and biological evaluation of oligodeoxynucleotides containing modified pyrimidines, *Nucleic Acids Res.*, 21, 3197, 1993.

[65] Haginoya, N. et al., Nucleosides and nucleotides. Synthesis of oligodeoxyribonucleotides containing 5-(N-aminoalkyl)carbamoyl-2′-deoxyuridines by a new postsynthetic modification method and their thermal stability and nuclease-resistance properties, *Bioconjug. Chem.*, 8, 271, 1997.

[66] Maier, M.A. et al., Nuclease resistance of oligonucleotides containing the tricyclic cytosine analogues phenoxazine and 9-(2-aminoethoxy)-phenoxazine ("G-clamp") and origins of their nuclease resistance properties, *Biochemistry*, 41, 1323, 2002.

[67] Rajeev, K.G., Prakash, T.P., and Manoharan, M., 2′-modified-2-thiothymidine oligonucleotides, *Org. Lett.*, 5, 3005, 2003.

[68] Romieu, A., Gasparutto, D., and Cadet, J., Synthesis and characterization of oligonucleotides containing 5′,8-cyclopurine 2′-deoxyribonucleosides: (5′R)-5′,8-cyclo-2′-deoxyadenosine, (5′S)-5′,8-cyclo-2′-deoxyguanosine, and (5′R)-5′,8-cyclo-2′-deoxyguanosine, *Chem. Res. Toxicol.*, 12, 412, 1999.

[69] Boado, R.J. and Pardridge, W.M., Complete protection of antisense oligonucleotides against serum nuclease degradation by an avidin-biotin system, *Bioconjug. Chem.*, 3, 519, 1992.

[70] Gamper, H.B. et al., Facile preparation of nuclease resistant 3′ modified oligodeoxynucleotides, *Nucleic Acids Res.*, 21, 145, 1993.

[71] Herdewijn, P., Antisense oligonucleotides, *Verh. K. Acad. Geneeskd. Belg.*, 58, 359, 1996.

[72] Rait, A. et al., 3′-end conjugates of minimally phosphorothioate-protected oligonucleotides with 1-O-hexadecylglycerol: synthesis and anti-ras activity in radiation-resistant cells, *Bioconjug. Chem.*, 11, 153, 2000.

[73] Yokoyama, K. et al., Synthesis and biological properties of DNA-sugar conjugates, *Nucleic Acids Res. Suppl.*, 73, 2001.

[74] Kubo, T. et al., DNA conjugates as novel functional oligonucleotides, *Nucleosides Nucleotides Nucleic Acids*, 22, 1359, 2003.

[75] Mestre, B., Pratviel, G., and Meunier, B., Preparation and nuclease activity of hybrid "metal-lotris(methylpyridinium)porphyrin oligonucleotide" molecules having a 3'-loop for protection against 3'-exonucleases, *Bioconjug. Chem.*, 6, 466, 1995.

[76] Chiou, H.C. et al., Enhanced resistance to nuclease degradation of nucleic acids complexed to asialoglycoprotein–polylysine carriers, *Nucleic Acids Res.*, 22, 5439, 1994.

[77] Dheur, S. et al., Polyethylenimine but not cationic lipid improves antisense activity of 3'-capped phosphodiester oligonucleotides, *Antisense Nucleic Acid Drug Dev.*, 9, 515, 1999.

[78] Vinogradov, S.V., Batrakova, E.V., and Kabanov, A.V., Nanogels for oligonucleotide delivery to the brain, *Bioconjug. Chem.*, 15, 50, 2004.

[79] Bergan, R. et al., Electroporation enhances c-myc antisense oligodeoxynucleotide efficacy, *Nucleic Acids Res.*, 21, 3567, 1993.

[80] Schiedlmeier, B. et al., Nuclear transformation of Volvox carteri, *Proc. Natl Acad. Sci. USA*, 91, 5080, 1994.

[81] Lesh, R.E. et al., Reversible permeabilization. A novel technique for the intracellular introduction of antisense oligodeoxynucleotides into intact smooth muscle, *Circ. Res.*, 77, 220, 1995.

[82] Spiller, D.G. and Tidd, D.M., Nuclear delivery of antisense oligodeoxynucleotides through reversible permeabilization of human leukemia cells with streptolysin O, *Antisense Res. Dev.*, 5, 13, 1995.

[83] Zhao, Q. et al., Comparison of cellular binding and uptake of antisense phosphodiester, phosphorothioate, and mixed phosphorothioate and methylphosphonate oligonucleotides, *Antisense Res. Dev.*, 3, 53, 1993.

[84] Larsen, H.J., Bentin, T., and Nielsen, P.E., Antisense properties of peptide nucleic acid, *Biochim. Biophys. Acta*, 1489, 159, 1999.

[85] Schmajuk, G., Sierakowska, H., and Kole, R., Antisense oligonucleotides with different backbones. Modification of splicing pathways and efficacy of uptake, *J. Biol. Chem.*, 274, 21783, 1999.

[86] Zelphati, O. and Szoka, Jr., F.C., Mechanism of oligonucleotide release from cationic liposomes, *Proc. Natl Acad. Sci. USA*, 93, 11493, 1996.

[87] Ryser, J.-P. and Shen, W.-C., Drug-poly(lysine) conjugates: their potential for chemotherapy and for the study of endocytosis, in *Targeting of Drugs with Synthetic Systems*, Gregoriadis, G., Senior, J., and Poste, G., Eds., Plenum Press, New York, p. 103, 1986.

[88] Wu, G.Y. and Wu, C.H., Specific inhibition of hepatitis B viral gene expression *in vitro* by targeted antisense oligonucleotides, *J. Biol. Chem.*, 267, 12436, 1992.

[89] Wu-Pong, S., The role of multivalent cations in oligonucleotide cellular uptake, *Biochem. Mol. Biol. Int.*, 39, 511, 1996.

[90] Benimetskaya, L. et al., Mac-1 (CD11b/CD18) is an oligodeoxynucleotide-binding protein, *Nat. Med.*, 3, 414, 1997.

[91] Hawley, P. and Gibson, I., Interaction of oligodeoxynucleotides with mammalian cells, *Antisense Nucleic Acid Drug Dev.*, 6, 185, 1996.

[92] Vlassov, V.V., Balakireva, L.A., and Yakubov, L.A., Transport of oligonucleotides across natural and model membranes, *Biochim. Biophys. Acta*, 1197, 95, 1994.

[93] Bennett, C.F. et al., Inhibition of endothelial cell adhesion molecule expression with antisense oligonucleotides, *J. Immunol.*, 152, 3530, 1994.

[94] Lavigne, C. and Thierry, A.R., Enhanced antisense inhibition of human immunodeficiency virus type 1 in cell cultures by DLS delivery system, *Biochem. Biophys. Res. Commun.*, 237, 566, 1997.

[95] Leonetti, J.P. et al., Antibody-targeted liposomes containing oligodeoxyribonucleotides complementary to viral RNA selectively inhibit viral replication, *Proc. Natl Acad. Sci. USA*, 87, 2448, 1990.

[96] Wang, S. et al., Delivery of antisense oligodeoxyribonucleotides against the human epidermal growth factor receptor into cultured KB cells with liposomes conjugated to folate via polyethylene glycol, *Proc. Natl Acad. Sci. USA*, 92, 3318, 1995.

[97] Hu, Q. et al., Programmable fusogenic vesicles for intracellular delivery of antisense oligodeoxy-nucleotides: enhanced cellular uptake and biological effects, *Biochim. Biophys. Acta*, 1514, 1, 2001.

[98] Hu, Q., Bally, M.B., and Madden, T.D., Subcellular trafficking of antisense oligonucleotides and down-regulation of bcl-2 gene expression in human melanoma cells using a fusogenic liposome delivery system, *Nucleic Acids Res.*, 30, 3632, 2002.

[99] Haller, H. et al., Antisense oligodesoxynucleotide strategies in renal and cardiovascular disease, *Kidney Int.*, 53, 1550, 1998.

[100] Degols, G. et al., Poly(L-lysine)-conjugated oligonucleotides promote sequence-specific inhibition of acute HIV-1 infection, *Antisense Res. Dev.*, 2, 293, 1992.

[101] Leonetti, J.P. et al., Cell delivery and mechanisms of action of antisense oligonucleotides, *Prog. Nucleic Acid Res. Mol. Biol.*, 44, 143, 1993.

[102] Alahari, S.K. et al., Novel chemically modified oligonucleotides provide potent inhibition of P-glycoprotein expression, *J. Pharmacol. Exp. Ther.*, 286, 419, 1998.

[103] Doyle, D.F. et al., Inhibition of gene expression inside cells by peptide nucleic acids: effect of mRNA target sequence, mismatched bases, and PNA length, *Biochemistry*, 40, 53, 2001.

[104] Morcos, P.A., Achieving efficient delivery of morpholino oligos in cultured cells, *Genesis*, 30, 94, 2001.

[105] Welz, C. et al., Nuclear transport of oligonucleotides in HepG2-cells mediated by protamine sulfate and negatively charged liposomes, *Pharm. Res.*, 17, 1206, 2000.

[106] Lu, X.M. et al., Antisense DNA delivery *in vivo*: liver targeting by receptor-mediated uptake, *J. Nucl. Med.*, 35, 269, 1994.

[107] Akamatsu, K. et al., Disposition characteristics of glycosylated poly(amino acids) as liver cell-specific drug carrier, *J. Drug Target*, 6, 229, 1998.

[108] Biessen, E.A. et al., Targeted delivery of oligodeoxynucleotides to parenchymal liver cells *in vivo*, *Biochem. J.*, 340, 783, 1999.

[109] Citro, G. et al., Inhibition of leukemia cell proliferation by receptor-mediated uptake of c-myb antisense oligodeoxynucleotides, *Proc. Natl Acad Sci. USA*, 89, 7031, 1992.

[110] Deshpande, D. et al., Enhanced cellular uptake of oligonucleotides by EGF receptor-mediated endocytosis in A549 cells, *Pharm. Res.*, 13, 57, 1996.

[111] Bonfils, E. et al., Drug targeting: synthesis and endocytosis of oligonucleotide-neoglycoprotein conjugates, *Nucleic Acids Res.*, 20, 4621, 1992.

[112] Roth, C.M. et al., Targeted antisense modulation of inflammatory cytokine receptors, *Biotechnol. Bioeng.*, 55, 72, 1997.

[113] Basu, S. and Wickstrom, E., Synthesis and characterization of a peptide nucleic acid conjugated to a D-peptide analog of insulin-like growth factor 1 for increased cellular uptake, *Bioconjug. Chem.*, 8, 481, 1997.

[114] Rajur, S.B. et al., Covalent protein–oligonucleotide conjugates for efficient delivery of antisense molecules, *Bioconjug. Chem.*, 8, 935, 1997.

[115] Reinis, M., Damkova, M., and Korec, E., Receptor-mediated transport of oligodeoxynucleotides into hepatic cells, *J. Virol. Meth.*, 42, 99, 1993.

[116] Dokka, S. et al., Cellular delivery of oligonucleotides by synthetic import peptide carrier, *Pharm. Res.*, 14, 1759, 1997.

[117] Subramanian, A., Ranganathan, P., and Diamond, S.L., Nuclear targeting peptide scaffolds for lipofection of nondividing mammalian cells, *Nat. Biotechnol.*, 17, 873, 1999.

[118] Boutorine, A.S. and Kostina, E.V., Reversible covalent attachment of cholesterol to oligodeoxyribo-nucleotides for studies of the mechanisms of their penetration into eucaryotic cells, *Biochimie*, 75, 35, 1993.

[119] Alahari, S.K. et al., Inhibition of expression of the multidrug resistance-associated P-glycoprotein of by phosphorothioate and 5′ cholesterol-conjugated phosphorothioate antisense oligonucleotides, *Mol. Pharmacol.*, 50, 808, 1996.

[120] Krieg, A.M. et al., Modification of antisense phosphodiester oligodeoxynucleotides by a 5′ cholesteryl moiety increases cellular association and improves efficacy, *Proc. Natl Acad. Sci. USA*, 90, 1048, 1993.

[121] Corrias, M.V., Guarnaccia, F., and Ponzoni, M., Bioavailability of antisense oligonucleotides in neuroblastoma cells: comparison of efficacy among different types of molecules, *J. Neurooncol.*, 31, 171, 1997.

[122] Shoji, Y. et al., Enhancement of anti-herpetic activity of antisense phosphorothioate oligonucleotides 5′ end modified with geraniol, *J. Drug Target*, 5, 261, 1998.

[123] Prasad, V. et al., Oligonucleotides tethered to a short polyguanylic acid stretch are targeted to macrophages: enhanced antiviral activity of a vesicular stomatitis virus-specific antisense oligonucleotide, *Antimicrob. Agents Chemother.*, 43, 2689, 1999.

[124] Sazani, P. et al., Systemically delivered antisense oligomers upregulate gene expression in mouse tissues, *Nat. Biotechnol.*, 20, 1228, 2002.

[125] Pooga, M. et al., Cellular translocation of proteins by transportan, *FASEB J.*, 15, 1451, 2001.

[126] Astriab-Fisher, A. et al., Conjugates of antisense oligonucleotides with the Tat and antennapedia cell-penetrating peptides: effects on cellular uptake, binding to target sequences, and biologic actions, *Pharm. Res.*, 19, 744, 2002.

[127] Probst, J.C., Antisense oligodeoxynucleotide and ribozyme design, *Methods*, 22, 271, 2000.

[128] Khan, A. et al., Site-specific administration of antisense oligonucleotides using biodegradable polymer microspheres provides sustained delivery and improved subcellular biodistribution in the neostriatum of the rat brain, *J. Drug Target*, 8, 319, 2000.

[129] Moulds, C. et al., Site and mechanism of antisense inhibition by C-5 propyne oligonucleotides, *Biochemistry*, 34, 5044, 1995.

[130] Jayaraman, A. et al., Rational selection and quantitative evaluation of antisense oligonucleotides, *Biochim. Biophys. Acta*, 1520, 105, 2001.

[131] Walton, S.P. et al., Prediction of antisense oligonucleotide binding affinity to a structured RNA target, *Biotechnol. Bioeng.*, 65, 1, 1999.

[132] Mathews, D.H. et al., Predicting oligonucleotide affinity to nucleic acid targets, *RNA*, 5, 1458, 1999.

[133] Freier, S.M. and Altmann, K.H., The ups and downs of nucleic acid duplex stability: structure-stability studies on chemically-modified DNA:RNA duplexes, *Nucleic Acids Res.*, 25, 4429, 1997.

[134] Agrawal, S. et al., Mixed-backbone oligonucleotides as second generation antisense oligonucleotides: *in vitro* and *in vivo* studies, *Proc. Natl Acad. Sci. USA*, 94, 2620, 1997.

[135] Gryaznov, S. and Chen, J.K., Oligodeoxyribonucleotide N3′-]P5′ phosphoramidates — synthesis and hybridization properties, *J. Am. Chem. Soc.*, 116, 3143, 1994.

[136] Michel, T. et al., Cationic phosphoramidate alpha-oligonucleotides efficiently target single-stranded DNA and RNA and inhibit hepatitis C virus IRES-mediated translation, *Nucleic Acids Res.*, 31, 5282, 2003.

[137] Jones, R.J. et al., Synthesis and binding-properties of pyrimidine oligodeoxynucleoside analogs containing neutral phosphodiester replacements — the formacetal and 3′-thioformacetal internucleoside linkages, *J. Org. Chem.*, 58, 2983, 1993.

[138] Peoc'h, D. et al., Synthesis of 2′-substituted MMI linked nucleosidic dimers: an optimization study in search of high affinity oligonucleotides for use in antisense constructs, *Nucleosides Nucleotides Nucleic Acids*, 23, 411, 2004.

[139] Weiler, J. et al., Hybridisation based DNA screening on peptide nucleic acid (PNA) oligomer arrays, *Nucleic Acids Res.*, 25, 2792, 1997.

[140] Igloi, G.L., Variability in the stability of DNA-peptide nucleic acid (PNA) single-base mismatched duplexes: real-time hybridization during affinity electrophoresis in PNA-containing gels, *Proc. Natl Acad. Sci. USA*, 95, 8562, 1998.

[141] Lesnik, E.A. and Freier, S.M., Relative thermodynamic stability of DNA, RNA, and DNA:RNA hybrid duplexes: relationship with base composition and structure, *Biochemistry*, 34, 10807, 1995.

[142] Sugimoto, N. et al., Thermodynamic parameters to predict stability of RNA/DNA hybrid duplexes, *Biochemistry*, 34, 11211, 1995.

[143] Yamana, K. et al., Incorporation of two anthraquinonylmethyl groups into the 2′-O-positions of oligonucleotides: increased affinity and sequence specificity of anthraquinone-modified oligonucleotides in hybrid formation with DNA and RNA, *Bioconjug. Chem.*, 7, 715, 1996.

[144] Herdewijn, P., Conformationally restricted carbohydrate-modified nucleic acids and antisense technology, *Biochim. Biophys. Acta*, 1489, 167, 1999.

[145] Petersen, M. and Wengel, J., LNA: a versatile tool for therapeutics and genomics, *Trends Biotechnol.*, 21, 74, 2003.

[146] Kvaerno, L. et al., Synthesis of abasic locked nucleic acid and two seco-LNA derivatives and evaluation of their hybridization properties compared with their more flexible DNA counterparts, *J. Org. Chem.*, 65, 5167, 2000.

[147] Petersen, M. et al., The conformations of locked nucleic acids (LNA), *J. Mol. Recognit.*, 13, 44, 2000.

[148] Christensen, U. et al., Stopped-flow kinetics of locked nucleic acid (LNA)–oligonucleotide duplex formation: studies of LNA–DNA and DNA–DNA interactions, *Biochem. J.*, 354, 481, 2001.

[149] Torigoe, H. et al., 2′-O,4′-C-methylene bridged nucleic acid modification promotes pyrimidine motif triplex DNA formation at physiological pH: thermodynamic and kinetic studies, *J. Biol. Chem.*, 276, 2354, 2001.

[150] Froehler, B.C. et al., Oligonucleotides derived from 5-(1-propynyl)-2′-O-allyl-uridine and 5-(1-propynyl)-2′-O-allyl-cytidine — synthesis and RNA duplex formation, *Tetrahedron Lett.*, 34, 1003, 1993.

[151] Wagner, R.W. et al., Antisense gene inhibition by oligonucleotides containing C-5 propyne pyrimidines, *Science*, 260, 1510, 1993.

[152] Tona, R., Bertolini, R., and Hunziker, J., Synthesis of aminoglycoside-modified oligonucleotides, *Org. Lett.*, 2, 1693, 2000.

[153] Zhu, T. et al., Oligonucleotide-poly-L-ornithine conjugates: binding to complementary DNA and RNA, *Antisense Res. Dev.*, 3, 265, 1993.

[154] Francois, J.C. and Helene, C., Recognition of hairpin-containing single-stranded DNA by oligonucleotides containing internal acridine derivatives, *Bioconjug. Chem.*, 10, 439, 1999.

[155] Christensen, U.B. and Pedersen, E.B., Intercalating nucleic acids containing insertions of 1-O-(1-pyrenylmethyl)glycerol: stabilisation of dsDNA and discrimination of DNA over RNA, *Nucleic Acids Res.*, 30, 4918, 2002.

[156] Ellington, A.D. and Szostak, J.W., In vitro selection of RNA molecules that bind specific ligands, *Nature*, 346, 818, 1990.

[157] Lorsch, J.R. and Szostak, J.W., *In vitro* selection of RNA aptamers specific for cyanocobalamin, *Biochemistry*, 33, 973, 1994.

[158] Tuerk, C. and Gold, L., Systematic evolution of ligands by exponential enrichment: RNA ligands to bacteriophage T4 DNA polymerase, *Science*, 249, 505, 1990.

[159] Bock, L.C. et al., Selection of single-stranded DNA molecules that bind and inhibit human thrombin, *Nature*, 355, 564, 1992.

[160] Padmanabhan, K. et al., The structure of alpha-thrombin inhibited by a 15-mer single-stranded DNA aptamer, *J. Biol. Chem.*, 268, 17651, 1993.

[161] Macaya, R.F. et al., Thrombin-binding DNA aptamer forms a unimolecular quadruplex structure in solution, *Proc. Natl Acad. Sci. USA*, 90, 3745, 1993.

[162] Smirnov, I. and Shafer, R.H., Effect of loop sequence and size on DNA aptamer stability, *Biochemistry*, 39, 1462, 2000.

[163] Latham, J.A., Johnson, R., and Toole, J.J., The application of a modified nucleotide in aptamer selection: novel thrombin aptamers containing 5-(1-pentynyl)-2'-deoxyuridine, *Nucleic Acids Res.*, 22, 2817, 1994.

[164] Akhtar, S. et al., Sequence and chemistry requirements for a novel aptameric oligonucleotide inhibitor of EGF receptor tyrosine kinase activity, *Biochem. Pharmacol.*, 63, 2187, 2002.

[165] Jellinek, D. et al., Potent 2'-amino-2'-deoxypyrimidine RNA inhibitors of basic fibroblast growth factor, *Biochemistry*, 34, 11363, 1995.

[166] Kujau, M.J. and Wolfl, S., Intramolecular derivatization of 2'-amino-pyrimidine modified RNA with functional groups that is compatible with re-amplification, *Nucleic Acids Res.*, 26, 1851, 1998.

[167] Dewey, T.M. et al., New uridine derivatives for systematic evolution of RNA ligands by exponential enrichment, *J. Am. Chem. Soc.*, 117, 8474, 1995.

[168] Ruckman, J. et al., 2'-fluoropyrimidine RNA-based aptamers to the 165-amino acid form of vascular endothelial growth factor (VEGF165). Inhibition of receptor binding and VEGF-induced vascular permeability through interactions requiring the exon 7-encoded domain, *J. Biol. Chem.*, 273, 20556, 1998.

[169] Willis, M.C. et al., Liposome-anchored vascular endothelial growth factor aptamers, *Bioconjug. Chem.*, 9, 573, 1998.

[170] Shi, H., Hoffman, B.E., and Lis, J.T., RNA aptamers as effective protein antagonists in a multicellular organism, *Proc. Natl Acad. Sci. USA*, 96, 10033, 1999.

[171] Wang, W. et al., Effects of S-dC28 on vascular smooth muscle cell adhesion and plasminogen activator production, *Antisense Nucleic Acid Drug Dev.*, 7, 101, 1997.

[172] Wang, W. et al., Sequence-independent inhibition of *in vitro* vascular smooth muscle cell proliferation, migration, and *in vivo* neointimal formation by phosphorothioate oligodeoxynucleotides, *J. Clin. Invest.*, 98, 443, 1996.

[173] Volk, D.E. et al., Solution structure and design of dithiophosphate backbone aptamers targeting transcription factor NF-kappaB, *Bioorg. Chem.*, 30, 396, 2002.

[174] Nolte, A. et al., Mirror-design of L-oligonucleotide ligands binding to L-arginine, *Nat. Biotechnol.*, 14, 1116, 1996.

[175] Milton, R.C., Milton, S.C., and Kent, S.B., Total chemical synthesis of a D-enzyme: the enantiomers of HIV-1 protease show reciprocal chiral substrate specificity [corrected], *Science*, 256, 1445, 1992.

[176] Leva, S. et al., GnRH binding RNA and DNA spiegelmers: a novel approach toward GnRH antagonism, *Chem. Biol.*, 9, 351, 2002.

[177] Wlotzka, B. et al.,*In vivo* properties of an anti-GnRH Spiegelmer: an example of an oligonucleotide-based therapeutic substance class, *Proc. Natl Acad. Sci. USA*, 99, 8898, 2002.

[178] Purschke, W.G. et al., A DNA spiegelmer to staphylococcal enterotoxin B, *Nucleic Acids Res.*, 31, 3027, 2003.

[179] Vater, A. et al., Short bioactive spiegelmers to migraine-associated calcitonin gene-related peptide rapidly identified by a novel approach: tailored-SELEX, *Nucleic Acids Res.*, 31, e130, 2003.

[180] Faulhammer, D. et al., Biostable aptamers with antagonistic properties to the neuropeptide nociceptin/orphanin FQ, *RNA*, 10, 516, 2004.

[181] Williams, K.P. et al., Bioactive and nuclease-resistant L-DNA ligand of vasopressin, *Proc. Natl Acad. Sci. USA*, 94, 11285, 1997.

[182] Boiziau, C. et al., DNA aptamers selected against the HIV-1 trans-activation-responsive RNA element form RNA-DNA kissing complexes, *J. Biol. Chem.*, 274, 12730, 1999.

[183] Duconge, F. and Toulme, J.J., *In vitro* selection identifies key determinants for loop–loop interactions: RNA aptamers selective for the TAR RNA element of HIV-1, *RNA*, 5, 1605, 1999.

[184] Collin, D. et al., NMR characterization of a kissing complex formed between the TAR RNA element of HIV-1 and a DNA aptamer, *Nucleic Acids Res.*, 28, 3386, 2000.

[185] Darfeuille, F. et al., 2'-O-methyl-RNA hairpins generate loop-loop complexes and selectively inhibit HIV-1 Tat-mediated transcription, *Biochemistry*, 41, 12186, 2002.

[186] Darfeuille, F. et al., Loop–loop interaction of HIV-1 TAR RNA with N3′–>P5′ deoxyphosphoramidate aptamers inhibits *in vitro* Tat-mediated transcription, *Proc. Natl Acad. Sci. USA*, 99, 9709, 2002.

[187] Beaurain, F. et al., Molecular dynamics reveals the stabilizing role of loop closing residues in kissing interactions: comparison between TAR–TAR* and TAR–aptamer, *Nucleic Acids Res.*, 31, 4275, 2003.

[188] Elbashir, S.M. et al., Duplexes of 21-nucleotide RNAs mediate RNA interference in cultured mammalian cells, *Nature*, 411, 494, 2001.

[189] Elbashir, S.M., Lendeckel, W., and Tuschl, T., RNA interference is mediated by 21- and 22-nucleotide RNAs, *Genes Dev.*, 15, 188, 2001.

[190] Elbashir, S.M. et al., Functional anatomy of siRNAs for mediating efficient RNAi in *Drosophila melanogaster* embryo lysate, *EMBO J.*, 20, 6877, 2001.

[191] *AG 105 Tuschl: siRNA*. http://www.rockefeller.edu/labheads/tuschl/sirna.html, 2004.

[192] Reynolds, A. et al., Rational siRNA design for RNA interference, *Nat. Biotechnol.*, 22, 326, 2004.

[193] Chiu, Y.L. and Rana, T.M., RNAi in human cells: basic structural and functional features of small interfering RNA, *Mol. Cell*, 10, 549, 2002.

[194] Nykanen, A., Haley, B., and Zamore, P.D., ATP requirements and small interfering RNA structure in the RNA interference pathway, *Cell*, 107, 309, 2001.

[195] Chiu, Y.L. and Rana, T.M., siRNA function in RNAi: a chemical modification analysis, *RNA*, 9, 1034, 2003.

[196] Smolke, C.D., Carrier, T.A., and Keasling, J.D., Coordinated, differential expression of two genes through directed mRNA cleavage and stabilization by secondary structures, *Appl. Environ. Microbiol.*, 66, 5399, 2000.

[197] McManus, M.T. et al., Gene silencing using micro-RNA designed hairpins, *RNA*, 8, 842, 2002.

[198] Czauderna, F. et al., Structural variations and stabilising modifications of synthetic siRNAs in mammalian cells, *Nucleic Acids Res.*, 31, 2705, 2003.

[199] Amarzguioui, M. et al., Tolerance for mutations and chemical modifications in a siRNA, *Nucleic Acids Res.*, 31, 589, 2003.

[200] Braasch, D.A. et al., RNA interference in mammalian cells by chemically-modified RNA, *Biochemistry*, 42, 7967, 2003.

[201] Layzer, J.M. et al., *In vivo* activity of nuclease-resistant siRNAs, *RNA*, 10, 766, 2004.

[202] Guvakova, M.A. et al., Phosphorothioate oligodeoxynucleotides bind to basic fibroblast growth factor, inhibit its binding to cell surface receptors, and remove it from low affinity binding sites on extracellular matrix, *J. Biol. Chem.*, 270, 2620, 1995.

[203] Khaled, Z. et al., Multiple mechanisms may contribute to the cellular anti-adhesive effects of phosphorothioate oligodeoxynucleotides, *Nucleic Acids Res.*, 24, 737, 1996.

[204] Akhtar, S. and Juliano, R.L., Cellular uptake and intracellular fate of antisense oligonucleotides, *Trends Cell. Biol.*, 2, 139, 1992.

[205] Reynolds, M.A. et al., Synthesis and thermodynamics of oligonucleotides containing chirally pure R(P) methylphosphonate linkages, *Nucleic Acids Res.*, 24, 4584, 1996.

[206] Nielsen, P.E. et al., Sequence-selective recognition of DNA by strand displacement with a thymine-substituted polyamide, *Science*, 254, 1497, 1991.

[207] Gray, G.D., Basu, S., and Wickstrom, E., Transformed and immortalized cellular uptake of oligodeoxynucleoside phosphorothioates, 3′-alkylamino oligodeoxynucleotides, 2′-O-methyl oligoribonucleotides, oligodeoxynucleoside methylphosphonates, and peptide nucleic acids, *Biochem. Pharmacol.*, 53, 1465, 1997.

18

Gene Therapy

Cindy Jung
Georgia Tech

Joseph M. Le Doux
Emory University

Gene therapy, the transfer of genes into cells for a therapeutic effect, is an experimental approach to the treatment of disease. The first clinically applicable system for efficiently delivering genes into mammalian cells was developed in the early 1980s and was based on a genetically engineered **retrovirus**, which, as part of its lifecycle, stably integrates its genome into the target cell's chromosomal DNA. Using **recombinant** DNA technology perfected in the mid-1970s, investigators replaced the viral genes with therapeutic genes and the resulting recombinant retrovirus shuttled these genes into the target cells. The potential applications of gene therapy are far reaching (Table 18.1) since there are over 4000 known human genetic diseases (many of which have no viable treatment) and virtually every human disease is profoundly influenced by genetic factors [1]. In addition to inherited diseases, other viable targets for gene therapy include more prevalent disorders that show a complex genetic dependence (i.e., cancer and heart disease) as well as infectious diseases (i.e., human immunodeficiency virus) and applications in tissue engineering [1,2].

18.1   Background

Gene therapy protocols conduct gene transfer in one of two settings; either *ex vivo* or *in vivo* [3]. For *ex vivo* gene therapy, target cells or tissue are removed from the patient, grown in culture, genetically modified, and then reinfused or retransplanted into the patient [4]. *Ex vivo* gene therapy is limited to those tissues which can be removed, cultured *in vitro* and returned to the patient and cannot be applied to many important target tissues and organs such as the lungs, brain, and heart. For *in vivo* gene therapy, the gene transfer agent is delivered directly to the target tissue or organ, and gene transfer occurs in the patient

TABLE 18.1   Target Diseases for Gene Therapy

Target disease	Target tissues	Corrective gene
Inherited		
ADA deficiency	Hematopoietic cells	ADA
α-1 antitrypsin deficiency	Fibroblasts	α-1 antitrypsin
	Hepatocytes	
	Lung epithelia cells	
	Peritoneal mesothelial cells	
Alzheimer's disease	Nervous system	nerve growth factor
Cystic fibrosis	Lung epithelial cells	CFTR
Diabetes	Fibroblasts	human insulin
	Hepatocytes	
Duchenne muscular dystrophy	Muscle cells	dystrophin
Familial hypercholesterolemia	Hepatocytes	LDL receptor
Gaucher disease	Hematopoietic cells	glucocerebrosidase
	Fibroblasts	
Growth hormone deficiency	Endothelial cells	human growth hormone
	Fibroblasts	
	Keratinocytes	
	Muscle cells	
Hemoglobinopathies	Hematopoietic cells	α- or β-globin
Hemophilia	Fibroblasts	factor VIII, IX
	Keratinocytes	
	Hepatocytes	
	Muscle cells	
Leukocyte adhesion deficiency	Hematopoietic cells	CD-18
Parkinson's Disease	Nervous system	tyrosine hydroxylase
Phenylketonuria	Hepatocytes	phenylalanine hydroxylase
Purine nucleoside phosphorylase deficiency	Fibroblasts	Purine nucleoside phosphorylase
Urea cycle disorders	Hepatocytes	Ornithine transcarbamylase or arginosuccinate synthetase
Acquired		
Cancer	Acute lymphoblastic leukemia	p53 HSV thymidine kinase
	Brain tumors	γ-interferon
	Carcinoma	tumor necrosis factor
	Melanoma	retinoblastoma gene
	Retinoblastoma	
Infectious diseases	HIV	dominant negative Rev
		TAR decoy
		RRE decoy
		diptheria toxin A
Cardiomyopathy	Muscle cells	(used reporter gene)
Emphysema	Lung epithelia cells	α-1 antitrypsin
Local thrombosis	Endothelial cells	anticlotting factors
Vaccines	Muscle cells	various

rather than in the tissue culture dish [3]. Both strategies have inherent advantages and disadvantages and current research is determining which approach can best meet the needs of a particular disease.

Gene delivery systems can be classified as either viral or nonviral [5]. For viral gene transfer, one of several different types of viruses is engineered to deliver genes. Typically, viral genes are removed to prevent self-replication of the virus and to provide room for the insertion of one or more therapeutic genes that the recombinant virus will carry. To further ensure the safety of the recombinant viruses, specialized packaging cell lines have been developed to produce the recombinant viruses and minimize the production of infectious wild-type viruses. Some viruses are able to integrate the therapeutic genes into the target cell's nuclear DNA (retroviruses, adeno-associated viruses [AAVs]), whereas others are not (adenoviruses) (Table 18.2).

TABLE 18.2 Physical Characteristics of Wild Type Virions

Characteristic	Retroviruses	Adenoviruses	AAV
Genome type	ssRNA (2 per virion)	dsDNA	ssDNA
Genome size (bases)	8300	36,000	4700
Genome MW (daltons)	3×10^6	$20{-}25 \times 10^6$	$1.2{-}1.8 \times 10^6$
Particle diameter (nm)	90–147	65–80	20–24
Particle mass (grams)	3.6×10^{-16}	2.9×10^{-16}	1.0×10^{-17}
Composition			
DNA/RNA (%)	2	13	26
Protein (%)	62	87	74
Lipid (%)	36	0	0
Density (g/cm^{3}CsCl)	1.15–1.16	1.33–1.35	1.39–1.42
Enveloped? (yes/no)	yes	no	no
Shape	spherical	icosahedral	icosahedral
Surface projections (yes/no)	yes	yes	no
Number	~60–200	12	
Length (nm)	5	25–30	
Max diameter (nm)	8	4	
Virus titer (pfu/ml)	$10^6{-}10^7$	$10^{10}{-}10^{12}$	$10^5{-}10^7$
Integration?	yes — random	no — episomal	yes — chromosome 19

TABLE 18.3 Features of the Various Gene Transfer Systems

Features	Retrovirus	AAV	Adenovirus	Nonviral
Maximum transgene size	8 kb	4.7 kb	36 kb	≫36 kb
Maximum concentration (vectors/ml)	~10^7	~10^{12}	~10^{12}	
Transfers genes to quiescent cells	No/Yes[a]	Yes	Yes	Yes
Integrates transgene into target cell genome	Yes	Yes	No	No
Persistance of gene expression	weeks–years	years	weeks–months	days–weeks
Immunological problems	Few	None known	Extensive	None
Preexisting host immunity	No	Yes	Yes	No
Stability of vector	Poor	Good	Good	Good
Ease of large-scale production	Difficult	Difficult	Easy	Easy
Safety concerns	Insertional mutagenesis	Inflammation toxicity	Inflammation toxicity	Toxicity

[a] Recombinant lentiviruses, such as human immunodeficiency virus, are capable of transducing quiescent cells.

Nonviral gene transfer systems are based on a variety of technologies that employ physical/chemical means to deliver genes [6]. These technologies include direct plasmid injection, bombardment with DNA coated microprojectiles, and DNA complexed with **liposomes** or polymers. Some nonviral transfection techniques are too inefficient (e.g., coprecipitation of DNA with calcium phosphate [7], DNA complexed with diethylaminoethyl (DEAE)-dextran [8], electroporation [9]), or laborious (e.g., microinjection of DNA [10]) for clinical use. Only those gene delivery systems (viral and nonviral) with potential for clinical application are discussed in this chapter. The main features of these technologies (Table 18.3) are described and specific examples of their applications highlighted.

18.2 Recombinant Retroviruses

Many of the approved clinical trials have utilized recombinant retroviruses for gene delivery. Retroviral particles contain two copies of identical RNA genomes that are wrapped in a protein coat and further encapsidated by a lipid bilayer membrane. The virus attaches to specific cell surface receptors via surface proteins that protrude from the viral membrane. The particle is then internalized and its genome is released into the cytoplasm, reverse transcribed from RNA to DNA, transported into the nucleus, and then integrated into the cell's chromosomal DNA. The integrated viral genome has LTRs (long terminal repeats) at both ends, which encode the regulatory sequences that drive the expression of the viral genome [11].

Retroviruses used for gene transfer are most frequently derived from wild-type murine retroviruses. The recombinant viral particles are structurally identical to the wild-type virus but carry a genetically engineered genome (retroviral **vector**) which encodes the therapeutic gene of interest. These recombinant viruses are incapable of self-replication but can infect and insert their genomes into a target cell's genome [12].

Recombinant retroviruses, like all other recombinant viruses, are produced by a two-part system composed of a **packaging cell line** and a recombinant vector (Figure 18.1) [1,13]. The packaging cell line has been engineered to express all the structural viral genes (*gag, pol,* and *env*) necessary for the formation of an infectious virus particle. The *gag* encodes the capsid proteins and is necessary for encapsidation of the vector. The *pol* encodes the enzymatic activities of the virus including reverse transcriptase and integrase. The *env* encodes the surface proteins on the virus particle, which are necessary for attachment to the target cell's receptors.

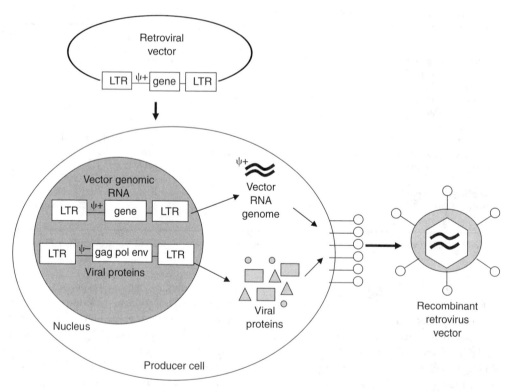

FIGURE 18.1 Packaging cell line for retrovirus. A simple retroviral vector composed of two LTR regions, which flank sequences encoding the packaging sequence (ψ) and a therapeutic gene. Packaging cell line is transfected with this vector. The packaging cell line expresses the three structural proteins necessary for formation of a virus particle (*gag, pol,* and *env*). These proteins recognize the packaging sequence on the vector and form an infectious virion around it. Infectious virions bud from the cell surface into the culture medium. The virus-laden culture medium is filtered to remove cell debris and is then either immediately used to transduce target cells or the virions are purified or concentrated and frozen for later use.

The retroviral vector is essentially the wild-type genome with all the viral genes removed. This vector encodes the transgene(s) and the regulatory sequences necessary for their expression as well as a special packaging sequence (ψ) that is required for encapsidation of the genome into an infectious viral particle [12]. To produce recombinant retrovirus particles, the retroviral vector is transfected into the packaging cell line. The structural proteins expressed by the packaging cell line recognize the packaging sequence on RNAs transcribed from the transfected vector and encapsidate them into an infectious virus particle that is subsequently exocytosed by the cell and released into the culture medium. This medium containing infectious recombinant viruses is harvested and used to **transduce** target cells.

As with all gene transfer technologies, there are advantages and disadvantages to the use of recombinant retroviruses. Retroviruses can only transduce dividing cells since integration requires passage of the target cells through mitosis, which limits their use for *in vivo* gene therapy since few normal cells are actively dividing [14]. Lentivirus vectors, derived from a family of complex retroviruses that are capable of infecting nondividing cells, have helped to overcome this limitation and have been used to transduce a number of different cell types *in vivo*, including neurons [15], hepatocytes [16], muscle cells [17], retinal cells [18], dendritic cells [19], and airway epithelial cells [20]. Lentivirus vectors appear unable to transduce some nonproliferative cell types, however, including hematopoietic stem cells in G_0 and nonactivated primary blood lymphocytes and monocytes [21–23].

Other drawbacks of retroviral vectors include (a) a limitation to the size of inserted genes (<8 kilobases) [24]; (b) the particles are unstable and lose activity at 37°C with a half-life of 5 to 7 h [25,26]; and (c) virus producer cell lines typically produce retrovirus in relatively low titers (10^5 to 10^7 infectious particles per milliliter) [27]. The viral titer is a function of several factors including the producer cell line, the type of transgene, and the vector construction. Moreover, purification and concentration of retroviruses without loss of infectivity is difficult [28]. Standard techniques such as centrifugation, column filtration, or ultrafiltration have, for the most part, failed [29,30]. Hollow fiber [27] and tangential flow filtration [25] have been used with some success. More commonly, retroviruses **pseudotyped** with VSV-G envelope proteins are used because they are not easily inactivated and can be readily concentrated by ultracentrifugation. More recently, complexation of retroviruses with charged polymers has been used to rapidly concentrate, purify, and deliver retroviruses to cells *ex vivo* without the need to pseudotype the viruses with VSV-G or any other specific envelope protein [31].

Though retroviruses have a low toxicity profile in the clinical setting, the use of recombinant retroviruses has raised two major safety concerns [24,32]. Replication competent virus was occasionally produced by some of the older packaging cell lines due to homologous recombination between the retroviral vector and the packaging cell line's retroviral sequences. New packaging cell lines have made the production of replication competent viruses essentially impossible [33]. Another safety concern is the possibility that the integration of a recombinant retrovirus can activate a proto-oncogene and cause cellular transformation. The probability of this event is very low and is typically outweighed by the potential therapeutic benefits [32,34]. Unfortunately, these events were manifested for the first time in a gene therapy clinical trial for the X-linked form of severe combined immune deficiency (SCID). Three of nine patients developed T-cell leukemia due to retrovirus-mediated insertional mutagenesis of *LMO2*, a gene involved in the onset of T-cell leukemia [35]. Although the FDA Biologics Response Modifier Advisory Committee (BRMAC) recommended that retroviral clinical trials continue, the incident highlighted the need for a more quantitative and systematic understanding of retrovirus-mediated gene transfer [36].

18.3   Recombinant Adenoviruses

Recombinant adenoviruses have a number of properties that make them a useful alternative to recombinant retroviruses for human gene transfer. Recombinant adenoviruses are well characterized, relatively easy to manipulate, can be grown and concentrated to very high titers (up to 10^{13} infectious particles/ml), are stable particles, and can transduce a wide variety of cell types [37,38]. Furthermore, genes transferred by recombinant adenoviruses do not integrate, eliminating the risk of insertional mutagenesis of the chromosomal DNA of the target cell [37]. Most important, recombinant adenoviruses efficiently transfer genes to nondividing, as well as dividing, cells which make possible the *in vivo* transduction of tissues composed of fully differentiated or slowly dividing cells such as the liver and lung [3].

Adenoviruses consist of a large double-stranded DNA genome (about 36 kilobase pairs long) packaged within a nonenveloped icosahedral capsid that is primarily composed of three virus-encoded proteins (hexon, penton base, and fiber proteins) [39]. The fiber proteins protrude from the surface of the virus and mediate its attachment to target cells via a high affinity interaction with the cellular receptor CAR (coxsackievirus and adenovirus receptor) [40]. The virus is then internalized into endosomal vesicles via specific interactions between the penton base proteins and α_v integrins [41]. Adenoviruses escape these vesicles by an acid-induced endosomolytic activity and are transported to the nucleus, into which they enter via pores in the nuclear membrane [42].

The wild-type adenovirus genome consists primarily of five early genes (E1 to E5), each of which is expressed from their own promoters [39]. There are also five late genes (L1 to L5), which are expressed from the major late promoter (MLP). The first generation of recombinant adenoviruses were based on a mutant adenovirus in which the E1 region (and in some cases the E3 region) was deleted. The E1 region is required for replication. Nevertheless, E1 minus mutants can be grown on specialized packaging cell lines (293 cells), which express the E1 gene and therefore provide the necessary functions for virus production [13]. To generate recombinant adenoviruses, a **plasmid** that contains the gene of interest, flanked by adenovirus inverted terminal repeat ITR sequences, is transfected into 293 cells in which adenoviruses that lack the E1 region are actively replicating (Figure 18.2). The virus stock is screened for

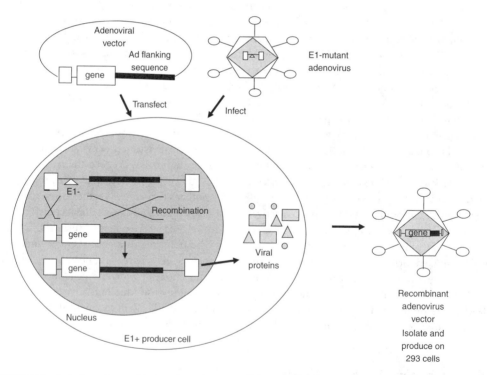

FIGURE 18.2 Isolation of recombinant adenovirus. A packaging cell line (293 cells) which expresses the E1 gene is infected with an E1 minus mutant adenovirus. The adenovirus is derived from a plasmid encoding the wild-type adenovirus genome. The E1 region of the adenovirus genome is replaced with the therapeutic gene, and the resultant plasmid (the adenovirus vector) is transfected into the 293 cell line, which is infected by the mutant adenovirus. Since the therapeutic gene is flanked by adenoviral sequences, the mutant adenovirus genome and the adenovirus vector will occasionally undergo homologous recombination and form an infectious recombinant adenovirus whose genome encodes the therapeutic gene. These rare recombinants are isolated and then grown on another 293 cell line.

the rare recombinants in which the gene of interest has correctly recombined with the E1 minus mutant by homologous recombination. These recombinant virions are purified and grown to high titer on 293 cells [43]. Second and third generation vectors, which removed the E2 or E4 regions or both, increased the packaging capacity and similarly required producer cells that additionally express E2 or E4 or both [44,45]. More recently, gutless vectors were developed that retain only the viral (ITR) and the packaging signal [46]. However these vectors require a helper virus that supplies the necessary viral proteins in *trans*.

Recombinant adenoviruses have been successfully used for *in vivo* gene transfer in a number of animal models and in several clinical protocols, including those which delivered a functional copy of the cystic fibrosis transmembrane conductance regulator (CFTR) gene into the nasal epithelium and lungs of cystic fibrosis patients [47–49]. Unfortunately, transgene expression was short-lived (5 to 10 days) [50] and led to acute, albeit transient, toxicity at higher doses ($\sim 2 \times 10^{11}$ particles/dose) [51]. The toxicity of these vectors has proven to be a significant problem, the urgency of which was underscored by the tragic death of a patient in a Phase I clinical trial [52,53]. The toxicity associated with adenoviral vectors involves both the innate and adaptive immune responses [54,55], is dose dependent and related to the route of administration [56,57], is dependent on tissue and cell type [58], and even varies between strains of the same species [59]. Numerous strategies have been pursued to reduce the immunogenicity and improve the safety of these vectors. One strategy has been to construct recombinant adenoviruses that encode fewer immunogenic adenoviral proteins, such as in the second and third generation and gutless or helper-dependent adenoviral vectors. Such vectors have the added benefit of being able to accommodate the cloning of much larger inserts of therapeutic DNA (to as much as 36 kilobases) than was possible with the first generation (E1 and E3 minus) of recombinant adenoviruses, which could accommodate only 7 kilobases of foreign DNA [46,60].

Another strategy has been to modulate the immune response to adenovirus proteins and transgenes. Immunomodulatory compounds (e.g., deoxyspergualin, interleukin [IL]-12, interferon [IFN]-γ) have been co-injected with recombinant adenoviruses to transiently suppress the immune system, eliminate the humoral response, and make possible repeat administration of the vector [38]. Similarly, immunosuppressive compounds that induce tolerance (e.g., CTLA4Ig) have been co-injected with the vectors or have been incorporated into their genomes and expressed by the vectors themselves (e.g., Ad5 E3 19-kDa protein or HSV ICP47) [61–63].

Adenovirus vectors that infect only the cell type of interest and no others (targeted adenoviruses) have also been developed as a means to increase their safety. In principle, the use of targeted adenoviruses should reduce the number of viruses needed to achieve the desired therapeutic effect, as well as reduce the number of infected "innocent bystander" cells. Genetic and nongenetic approaches have been used to develop targeted adenoviruses. Adenovirus fiber proteins have been replaced with fibers from different adenovirus serotypes to avoid problems with the preexisting neutralizing antibody response against the original serotype [64]. Fiber and capsid proteins have been modified to include ectopic peptides or targeting motifs designed to cause the adenovirus to bind to cell-specific receptors or proteins [65–67]. Bispecific molecules that bind to adenoviruses have been used to prevent the viruses from binding to their normal cellular receptors (CAR) while enabling them to bind to different cell-specific receptors [68]. Similarly, polyethylene glycol polymers functionalized with cell-targeting peptides have been used to chemically modify adenoviruses to increase the specificity and reduce the immunogenicity of infection [69].

In part because of their immunogenicity, adenovirus-mediated gene expression is relatively short-lived. Short-lived gene expressioin can be advantageous for applications where transient expression is preferred such as in the stimulation of angiogenesis by expression of vascular endothelial growth factor (VEGF) [2,70], or in the generation of immune responses against cancer or for vaccines [71]. Unfortunately, short-lived expression is a disadvantage for the treatment of genetic or chronic disorders because, in order to maintain the therapeutic effect of the transgene, recombinant adenoviruses would have to be administered to the patient repeatedly. Repeat administration has been effective in certain limited applications [72,73] but often fails due to the presence of neutralizing antibodies that form in response to the first administration of the recombinant adenoviruses [38]. Although short-lived gene expression could be the result of vector cytotoxicity, promoter shutoff, or loss of the transgene DNA, most investigators believe it is primarily due to the elimination of transduced cells by transgene or adenovirus-specific cytotoxic T-lymphocytes [74–77]. As a result, most efforts to increase the longevity of gene expression have focused on eliminating the immune rejection of cells transduced by recombinant adenoviruses.

As a result of these and similar efforts, the persistance of gene expression *in vivo* has been extended to as long as 12 months [78]. It remains to be determined, however, if these methods can eliminate the immune response against recombinant adenoviruses and their products, whether or not elimination of the immune response results in long-term gene expression, and if these methods will be effective in human gene therapy protocols.

18.4   Recombinant Adeno-Associated Viruses

Adeno-associated viruses are another virus-based gene transfer system that has significant potential for use in human gene therapy. AAVs are small, nonenveloped human parvoviruses that contain a single-stranded DNA genome (4.7 kilobases) and encodes two genes required for replication, *rep* and *cap* [79]. The primary receptor for AAV is heparan sulfate proteoglycan [80]. Fibroblast growth factor receptor 1 and $\alpha_v\beta_5$ integrin serve as co-receptors for AAV endocytosis [81,82]. AAVs are stable, have a broad host range, can transduce dividing and nondividing cells, and do not cause any known human disease [50]. AAVs require the presence of a helper virus (typically adenovirus) to replicate [83]. When no helper virus is present, AAVs do not replicate but instead tend to establish a latent infection in which they permanently integrate into the chromosomal DNA of the target cells [84]. Wild-type AAVs preferentially integrate into a specific site in chromosome 19 due to the interaction of the virus-encoded protein Rep with the host cell DNA [79]. Recombinant AAVs, however, are Rep-negative and as a result integrate randomly into the chromosomal DNA of the target cell.

To generate recombinant AAV, human 293 cells are transfected with the AAV vector, a plasmid that contains the therapeutic gene of interest flanked by the 145-bp AAV ITRs that are necessary for its encapsidation into a virus particle [85] (Figure 18.3). The cells are also transfected with a helper plasmid, a plasmid that encodes for the virus proteins necessary for particle formation and replication (i.e., AAV *rep* and *cap* genes). The transfected cells are infected with wild-type adenovirus, which supplies the helper functions required for amplification of the AAV vector [2] or transfected with a plasmid that contains the adenoviral helper functions but do not support the production of adenovirus proteins or viruses [86]. If present, contaminating adenovirus is removed or inactivated by density gradient centrifugation and heat inactivation or column chromatography [87]. Recombinant AAVs generated by this and similar methods have been successfully used to achieve long-term expression of therapeutic proteins in a number of cell types and tissues, including in the lung, muscle, liver, central nervous system, retina, and cardiac myocytes [88–93]. Therapeutic effects have been achieved in a number of model systems, including in a dog model of hemophilia and a mouse model for obesity and diabetes [92,94].

Despite these early successes, several technical issues must be addressed before recombinant AAVs can be used for human gene therapy on a routine basis. For example, little is known about the conditions or factors that control the efficiency with which recombinant AAVs integrate into the chromosomal DNA of target cells or why the efficiency of integration is so low (<1%). An additional concern is the immunogenicity of the vectors. Though activation of the immune system is substantially lower than that of adenoviral vectors, AAV vectors have been shown to activate cellular immunity [95–97] and also activate humoral immunity, which reduces the success of readministration through neutralizing antibodies [98,99]. The recent discovery of several new serotypes of AAVs should help to alleviate this problem [100,101]. Perhaps the most significant technical issue, however, is that the current methods for producing recombinant AAVs (see above) are tedious, labor intensive, and not well-suited for producing clinical grade virus.

Current methods are not adequate for producing clinical grade virus for several reasons. First, current methods do not produce enough virus particles to be useful for many gene therapies. For example, it has been estimated that 10^{14} recombinant viruses will be needed to achieve systemic production of therapeutic levels of proteins such as factor IX or erythropoietin [84]. With current production methods,

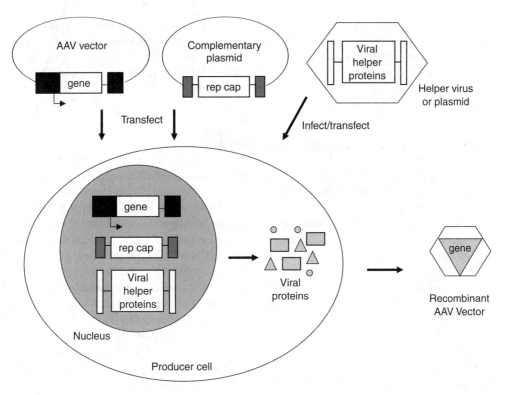

FIGURE 18.3   Production of a recombinant AAV. Human cells are transfected with a plasmid encoding the therapeutic gene, which is driven from a heterologous promoter (*crosshatched box*) and flanked with AAV terminal repeats (*stippled boxes*). The cells are also transfected with a complementing plasmid encoding the AAV *rep* and *cap* genes, which cannot be packaged because they are not flanked by AAV terminal repeats. The *rep* and *cap* genes, whose products are required for particle formation, are flanked by adenovirus 5 terminal fragments (*black boxes*), which enhance their expression. The transfected cells are infected or transfected with adenoviral helper functions required for amplification of the AAV vector. The virus stock may contain both AAV recombinant virus and adenovirus. The adenovirus is either separated by density gradient centrifugation or heat inactivated.

which yield 10^8 to 10^9 viruses per ml, about 100 to 1000 liters of virus would have to be produced for each treatment. Second, some current methods require the use of helper adenovirus, which is a significant disadvantage because their removal is tedious and labor intensive. In addition, there is the risk that residual contaminating adenovirus proteins will be present and stimulate the immune rejection of transduced cells [86]. Finally, the use of transient transfection is not amenable to scale-up and significantly increases the likelihood that replication competent AAVs will be generated by recombinogenic events [84].

To overcome these problems, investigators are working toward the development of stable packaging cell lines that produce recombinant AAVs Stable rep-cap cell lines have been made that can produce AAV particles from 293T cells but improvements in their stability and yield are needed [102]. In a different approach, a packaging cell line has been created that will produce AAV vectors without the use of plasmid transfection [103]. AAVs are created when the packaging cell line is infected with wild-type adenovirus and a hybrid recombinant adenovirus that contains a complete rAAV vector genome in the E1 region. Substantial increases in the yield of recombinant AAVs have been also achieved by increasing in the virus producer cell lines the number of copies of the AAV vector or of the helper plasmid. For example, one group developed an AAV packaging cell line which contained integrated helper and vector constructs that were linked to the simian virus 40 replication origin [84]. These packaging cells could be induced to express SV40 T antigen, which then amplified the helper and vector constructs by 4- to 10-fold, resulting in 5- to 20-fold increases in recombinant AAV production. Purification techniques have also been addressed to facilitate large-scale production of AAV vectors. Heparin affinity chromatography has been used to purify rAAVs with a titer of 10^{14} viruses per ml [87] and a two-step chromatography process recently developed for AAV purification has the additional advantage of easy scale-up [104]. In addition, investigators have begun to overcome the restricted packaging capacity of AAVs [105–108], and have begun to reduce the immunogenicity and increase the specificity of AAV vectors with techniques similar to those used with recombinant adenoviruses [109–114].

18.5   Direct Injection of Naked DNA

Direct injection of plasmid DNA intramuscularly, intraepidermally, and intravenously is a simple and direct technique for modifying cells *in vivo*. DNA injected intramuscularly or intraepidermally is internalized by cells proximal to the injection site [115,116]. DNA injected intravenously is rapidly degraded in the blood ($t_{1/2} < 10$ min) or retained in various organs in the body, preferentially in the nonparenchymal cells of the liver [117,118]. Gene expression after direct injection has been demonstrated in skeletal muscle cells of rodents and nonhuman primates, cardiac muscle cells of rodents, livers of cats and rats, and in thyroid follicular cells of rabbits [13,115,119,120].

The efficiency of gene transfer by direct injection is somewhat inefficient and variable [121]. As little as 60 to 100 myocardial cells have been reported to be modified per injection [122]. Higher efficiencies were observed when plasmids were injected into regenerating muscle cells [123] or co-injected with recombinant adenoviruses [124]. Injected DNA does not integrate, yet gene expression can persist for as long as two months [116]. Levels of gene expression are often low but can be increased by improvements in vector design [125]. Other factors shown to influence gene expression are cell death, increased cell cycling leading to loss of nonintegrated DNA, loss of DNA in the cytoplasm, promoter inactivation, and antigen-specific immune responses [126].

Despite the low efficiency of gene transfer and expression, direct injection of plasmid DNA has many promising applications in gene therapy, particularly when low levels of expression are sufficient to achieve the desired biological effect. For example, several patients suffering from critical limb ischemia were successfully treated by injection of DNA encoding human VEGF, a potent angiogenic factor [127–130]. Following injection of DNA into the ischemic limbs of ten patients, VEGF expression was detected in their serum, new blood vessels were formed in 7 of the 10 patients, and 3 patients were able to avoid scheduled below-the-knee amputations [131]. Similar results were obtained when fibroblast growth factor type 1 was injected intramuscularly to treat lower leg ischemia [132]. The study demonstrated safety and tolerance in addition to reducing pain and ulcer size and increasing transcutaneous oxygen pressure and ankle-brachial index.

Direct injection of DNA could also be used to vaccinate patients against pathogens as evidenced by the effects of direct injection of plasmid DNA encoding pathogen proteins or immunomodulatory cytokines [133,134]. Direct injection may also be an effective way to systemically deliver therapeutic proteins [135]. For example, the incidence of autoimmune diabetes in a mouse model of the disease was significantly reduced in mice that were injected intramuscularly with DNA encoding IL-10, an immunosuppressive cytokine [136].

In contrast to viral-based delivery systems, there is little restriction on the size of the transgene that can be delivered by direct DNA injection. As a result, direct DNA injection is particularly well suited for treating disorders that require the delivery of a large transgene. For example, Duchenne's muscular dystrophy, a genetic disease of the muscle caused by a defect in the gene for dystrophin (12 kilobases) can potentially be treated by direct DNA injection [137,138].

18.6   Particle-Mediated Gene Transfer

Particle-mediated gene transfer is an alternative method used to deliver plasmid DNA to cells. DNA-coated gold particles are loaded onto a macro-projectile, which is then accelerated through a vacuum chamber to high velocity by a burst of helium or a voltage discharge until it hits a stopping plate [139]. Upon impact, the DNA-coated microprojectiles are released through a hole in the stopping plate, penetrate the target tissue and cell and nuclear membranes, and the transferred gene is expressed [2,139]. Genes have been introduced and expressed in a number of cell types and tissues, including skin, liver, spleen, muscle, intestine, hematopoietic cells, brain, oral mucosa and epidermis, tumor explants, and cells of developing mouse embryos[2,140–144]. Similar to direct DNA injection, there are few constraints on the size of the DNA that can be delivered.

The efficiency of particle-mediated gene transfer varies with tissue type, but in general it is most efficient in the liver, pancreas, and epidermis of the skin, and least efficient in muscle, vascular, and cardiac tissues [145–147]. Because of the low level of penetration, particle-mediated gene transfer is being used to introduce antigens or cytokines primarily for vaccination and immunotherapy [148–150].

18.7 Liposome-Mediated Gene Delivery

Liposomes made from a mixture of neutral and cationic lipids have also been used to deliver plasmid DNA to cells. Liposomes are relatively easy to make, can be made with well-defined biophysical properties, and can accommodate virtually any size transgene [151,152]. Small unilamellar liposomes ranging from 20 to 100 nm in diameter are prepared by sonication of a mixture of cationic (e.g., DOTMA, N-{1-(2,3-dioleyloxy)propyl}-N, N, N-triethylammonium) and neutral (e.g., DOPE, dioleoylphosphatidylethanolamine) lipids, followed by extrusion through a porous polycarbonate filter (e.g., 100 nm pore size) [2,153]. DNA is added to the cationic liposomes, binds noncovalently to the positively charged cationic lipids, and induces a topological transition from liposomes to multilamellar structures composed of lipid bilayers alternating with DNA monolayers [153,154]. The size of the structures depends on their overall charge, with charged structures (negative or positive) being the smallest (about 100 nm in diameter) due to stabilization by electrostatic repulsion and neutral structures being the largest (>3000 nm in diameter) due to aggregation as a result of van der Waals attractive forces [153]. The relationship between structure and transfection efficiency is not well understood, although in general a slight excess of cationic lipid is needed for optimal gene transfer [151].

Gene transfer is accomplished by simply mixing or applying the lipid–DNA complexes to the target cells or tissue. Cationic liposome–DNA complexes have been used in a number of applications including transfer of genes to the arterial wall, lung, skin, and systemically by intravenous injection [2,155]. Genes delivered by cationic liposomes do not integrate so gene expression is transient and there is minimal risk of insertional mutagenesis. Liposomes do not carry any viral sequences or proteins, and are relatively nontoxic and nonimmunogenic [155,156].

Liposome-mediated gene transfer is somewhat inefficient, however, in part due to the failure of a large fraction of lipid-complexed DNA to escape degradation in cellular endosomes [157,158]. Several strategies have been taken to overcome this limitation, including use of acidotropic bases to reduce the rate of degradation by raising the pH of the endosomes, coupling of liposomes to endosomolytic or fusogenic virus proteins, and developing new liposome formulations that use pH-sensitive cationic lipids that become fusogenic in the acidic cellular endosomes [159–162]. Limitations due to inefficient transport of DNA to the nucleus have been addressed by increasing the mitotic activity of the cells [163], adding nuclear localization signals and targeting ligands [164,165], and through the use of cytoplasmic expression systems [166,167].

18.8 Other Gene Transfer Methods

Several other gene transfer technologies have been tested in clinical trials or are in various stages of development. These include recombinant viruses such as vaccinia virus [168], herpes simplex virus [169], canarypox virus [170], fowlpox [171], and Sendai virus [172], and nonviral vectors such as the use of magnetofection [173], DNA delivery with nanoparticles [174] or polymers [175,176], and DNA

TABLE 18.4   Current Clinical Experience Using Gene Transfer
(as of January 31, 2004)

Human gene transfer protocols	Number	Percentage
Gene marking studies	53	5.7
Nontherapeutic protocols	7	1
Therapeutic protocols	858	93
Infectious diseases	60	6.5
Inherited diseases	90	9.8
Cancer	608	66
Other diseases	100	11
Phases of gene delivery		
Phase I	589	64
Phase I/II	185	20
Phase II	120	13
Phase II/III	9	1
Phase III	15	1.6
Gene transfer technologies		
Permanent genetic modification		
Recombinant retroviruses	255	28
Recombinant adeno-associated virus	19	2.1
Temporary genetic modification		
Recombinant adenovirus	240	26
Cationic liposomes	85	9.3
Plasmid DNA	132	14
Particle mediated	5	0.5
Other[a]		
Viral vectors	122	13
Nonviral vector	60	6.5

[a]"Other" viral vectors refers to recombinant canarypox virus, vaccinia virus, fowlpox, and herpes simplex virus. "Other" nonviral vector refers to RNA transfer and antisense delivery.

conjugated to proteins that promote binding to specific cell-surface receptors, fusion, or localization to the nucleus [177]. Hybrid vectors between different types of viruses [178] and between viral and nonviral components [179,180] are also being developed. These methods are not discussed here in greater detail because even though they are capable of transferring genes to cells they have not yet been well developed or extensively tested in the clinic.

18.9   Summary and Conclusion

Several gene transfer systems have been developed that have successfully transferred genes to cells and elicited various biological effects. To date, nearly 900 clinical trials have been approved to test their safety and efficacy (Table 18.4) [181]. Each system has unique features, advantages, and disadvantages that determine if its use in a particular application is appropriate. One principal consideration is whether or not permanent or temporary genetic modification is desired. Other important considerations include what the setting of gene transfer will be (*ex vivo* or *in vivo*), what level of gene expression is needed, and whether or not the host has preexisting immunity against the vector. No single gene transfer system is ideal for any particular application and it is unlikely that such a universal gene transfer system will ever be developed. More likely, the current gene transfer systems will be further improved and modified, and new systems developed, that are optimal for the treatment of specific diseases.

Defining Terms

Ex vivo: Outside the living body, referring to a process or reaction occurring therein.

In vitro: In an artificial environment, referring to a process or reaction occurring therein, as in a test tube or culture dish.

In vivo: In the living body, referring to a process or reaction occurring therein.

Liposome: A spherical particle of lipid substance suspended in an aqueous medium.

Packaging cell line: Cells that express all the structural proteins required to form an infectious viral particle.

Plasmid: A small, circular extrachromosomal DNA molecule capable of independent replication in a host cell, typically a bacterial cell.

Pseudotype: A recombinant virus whose structural proteins are derived from two or more different viruses.

Recombinant: A virus or vector that has DNA sequences not originally (naturally) present in their DNA.

Retrovirus: A virus that possesses RNA-dependent DNA polymerase (reverse transcriptase), which reverse transcribes the virus' RNA genome into DNA, then integrates that DNA into the host cell's genome.

Transduce: To effect transfer and integration of genetic material to a cell by infection with a recombinant retrovirus.

Vector: A plasmid or viral DNA molecule into which a DNA sequence (typically encoding a therapeutic protein) is inserted.

References

 [1] Anderson, W.F., Human gene therapy, *Science*, 256, 808, 1992.
 [2] Morgan, J.R. and Yarmush, M.L., Gene therapy in tissue engineering. In *Frontiers in Tissue Engineering*. C.W. Patrick Jr., A.G. Mikos, and L.V. Mcintire (Eds). Oxford, Elsevier Science Ltd, p. 278, 1998.
 [3] Mulligan, R.C., The basic science of gene therapy, *Science*, 260, 926, 1993.
 [4] Ledley, F.D., Hepatic gene therapy: present and future, *Hepatology*, 18, 1263, 1993.
 [5] Friedmann, T., Progress toward human gene therapy, *Science*, 244, 1275, 1989.
 [6] Felgner, P.L. and Rhodes, G., Gene therapeutics, *Nature*, 349, 351, 1991.
 [7] Chen, C. and Okayama, H., High-efficiency transformation of mammalian cells by plasmid DNA, *Mol. Cell Biol.*, 7, 2745, 1987.
 [8] Pagano, J.S., McCutchan, J.H., and Vaheri, A., Factors influencing the enhancement of the infectivity of poliovirus ribonucleic acid by diethylaminoethyl-dextran, *J. Virol.*, 1, 891, 1967.
 [9] Neumann, E. et al., Gene transfer into mouse lyoma cells by electroporation in high electric fields, *EMBO J.*, 1, 841, 1982.
[10] Capecchi, M.R., High efficiency transformation by direct microinjection of DNA into cultured mammalian cells, *Cell*, 22, 479, 1980.
[11] Weiss, R. et al. *Molecular Biology of Tumor Viruses*. Cold Spring Harbor, Cold Spring Harbor Laboratory, 1982.
[12] Morgan, J.R., Tompkins, R.G., and Yarmush, M.L., Advances in recombinant retroviruses for gene delivery, *Adv. Drug Deliv. Rev.*, 12, 143, 1993.
[13] Levine, F. and Friedmann, T., Gene therapy, *Am. J. Dis. Child*, 147, 1167, 1993.
[14] Roe, T. et al., Integration of murine leukemia virus DNA depends on mitosis, *EMBO J.*, 12, 2099, 1993.
[15] Naldini, L. et al., *In vivo* gene delivery and stable transduction of nondividing cells by a lentiviral vector [see comments], *Science*, 272, 263, 1996.

[16] Follenzi, A. et al., Efficient gene delivery and targeted expression to hepatocytes *in vivo* by improved lentiviral vectors, *Hum. Gene Ther.*, 13, 243, 2002.

[17] Kafri, T. et al., Sustained expression of genes delivered directly into liver and muscle by lentiviral vectors, *Nat. Genet.*, 17, 314, 1997.

[18] Miyoshi, H. et al., Stable and efficient gene transfer into the retina using an HIV-based lentiviral vector, *Proc. Natl Acad. Sci. USA*, 94, 10319, 1997.

[19] Esslinger, C. et al., *In vivo* administration of a lentiviral vaccine targets DCs and induces efficient CD8(+) T cell responses, *J. Clin. Invest.*, 111, 1673, 2003.

[20] Johnson, L.G. et al., Pseudotyped human lentiviral vector-mediated gene transfer to airway epithelia *in vivo*, *Gene Ther.*, 7, 568, 2000.

[21] Sutton, R.E. et al., Transduction of human progenitor hematopoietic stem cells by human immunodeficiency virus type 1-based vectors is cell cycle dependent, *J. Virol.*, 73, 3649, 1999.

[22] Neil, S. et al., Postentry restriction to human immunodeficiency virus-based vector transduction in human monocytes, *J. Virol.*, 75, 5448, 2001.

[23] Korin, Y.D. and Zack, J.A., Progression to the G1b phase of the cell cycle is required for completion of human immunodeficiency virus type 1 reverse transcription in T cells, *J. Virol.*, 72, 3161, 1998.

[24] Roemer, K. and Friedmann, T., Concepts and strategies for human gene therapy, *Eur. J. Biochem.*, 208, 211, 1992.

[25] Kotani, H. et al., Improved methods of retroviral vector transduction and production for gene therapy, *Hum. Gene Ther.*, 5, 19, 1994.

[26] Le Doux, J.M. et al., Kinetics of retrovirus production and decay, *Biotech. Bioeng. Prog.*, 63, 654, 1999.

[27] Paul, R.W. et al., Increased viral titer through concentration of viral harvests from retroviral packaging lines, *Hum. Gene Ther.*, 4, 609, 1993.

[28] Andreadis, S.T. et al., Large scale processing of recombinant retroviruses for gene therapy, *Biotechnol. Prog.*, 15, 1, 1999.

[29] Le Doux, J.M., Morgan, J.R., and Yarmush, M.L., Removal of proteoglycans increases efficiency of retroviral gene transfer, *Biotechnol. Bioeng.*, 58, 23, 1998.

[30] McGrath, M. et al., Retrovirus purification: method that conserves envelope glycoprotein and maximizes infectivity, *J. Virol.*, 25, 923, 1978.

[31] Le Doux, J.M. et al., Complexation of retrovirus with cationic and anionic polymers increases the efficiency of gene transfer, *Hum. Gene Ther.*, 12, 1611, 2001.

[32] Temin, H.M., Safety considerations in somatic gene therapy of human disease with retrovirus vectors, *Hum. Gene Ther.*, 1, 111, 1990.

[33] Danos, O. and Mulligan, R.C., Safe and efficient generation of recombinant retroviruses with amphotropic and ecotropic host ranges, *Proc. Natl Acad. Sci. USA*, 85, 6460, 1988.

[34] Stocking, C. et al., Distinct classes of factor-independent mutants can be isolated after retroviral mutagenesis of a human myeloid stem cell line, *Growth Factors*, 8, 197, 1993.

[35] Hacein-Bey-Abina, S. et al., A serious adverse event after successful gene therapy for X-linked severe combined immunodeficiency, *N. Eng. J. Med.*, 348, 255, 2003.

[36] Andreadis, S. et al., Toward a more accurate quantitation of the activity of recombinant retroviruses: alternatives to titer and multiplicity of infection, *J. Virol.*, 74, 1258, 2000.

[37] Crystal, R.G., Transfer of genes to humans: early lessons and obstacles to success, *Science*, 270, 404, 1995.

[38] Hitt, M.M., Addison, C.L., and Graham, F.L., Human adenovirus vectors for gene transfer into mammalian cells, *Adv. Pharmacol.*, 40, 137, 1997.

[39] Horwitz, M.S., Adenoviridae and their replication. In *Fields Virology*. B.N. Fields, D.M. Knipe, R.M. Chanock et al. (Eds). New York, Raven Press, Vol. 2, p. 1679, 1990.

[40] Bergelson, J.M. et al., Isolation of a common receptor for Coxsackie B viruses and adenoviruses 2 and 5, *Science*, 275, 1320, 1997.

[41] Wickham, T.J. et al., Integrins alpha v beta 3 and alpha v beta 5 promote adenovirus internalization but not virus attachment, *Cell*, 73, 309, 1993.

[42] Greber, U.F. et al., Stepwise dismantling of adenovirus 2 during entry into cells, *Cell*, 75, 477, 1993.

[43] Morgan, J.R., Tompkins, R.G., and Yarmush, M.L., Genetic engineering and therapeutics. In *Implantation Biology: The Host Responses and Biomedical Devices*. R.S. Greco (Ed.). Boca Raton, FL, CRC Press. p. 387, 1994.

[44] Wang, Q. and Finer, M.H., Second-generation adenovirus vectors, *Nat. Med.*, 2, 714, 1996.

[45] Yeh, P. et al., Efficient dual transcomplementation of adenovirus E1 and E4 regions from a 293-derived cell line expressing a minimal E4 functional unit, *J. Virol.*, 70, 559, 1996.

[46] Parks, R.J. et al., A helper-dependent adenovirus vector system: removal of helper virus by Cre-mediated excision of the viral packaging signal, *Proc. Natl Acad. Sci. USA*, 93, 13565, 1996.

[47] Boucher, R.C. and Knowles, M.R., Gene therapy for cystic fibrosis using E1 deleted adenovirus: a phase I trial in the nasal cavity. Bethesda, MD, Office of Recombinant DNA Activity, NIH.

[48] Welsh, M.J., Adenovirus-mediated gene transfer of CFTR to the nasal epithelium and maxillary sinus of patients with cystic fibrosis. Bethesda, MD, Office of Recombinant DNA Activity, NIH.

[49] Wilmott, R.W. and Whitsett, J., A phase I study of gene therapy of cystic fibrosis utilizing a replication deficient recombinant adenovirus vector to deliver the human cystic fibrosis transmembrane conductance regulator cDNA to the airways. Bethesda, MD, Office of Recombinant DNA Activity, NIH.

[50] Verma, I.M. and Somia, N., Gene therapy — promises, problems and prospects [news], *Nature*, 389, 239, 1997.

[51] Zuckerman, J.B. et al., A phase I study of adenovirus-mediated transfer of the human cystic fibrosis transmembrane conductance regulator gene to a lung segment of individuals with cystic fibrosis, *Hum. Gene Ther.*, 10, 2973, 1999.

[52] Batshaw, M.L. et al., Recombinant adenovirus gene transfer in adults with partial ornithine transcarbamylase deficiency (OTCD), *Hum. Gene Ther.*, 10, 2419, 1999.

[53] Raper, S.E. et al., A pilot study of *in vivo* liver-directed gene transfer with an adenoviral vector in partial ornithine transcarbamylase deficiency, *Hum. Gene Ther.*, 13, 163, 2002.

[54] Zhang, Y., Chirmule, N., and Wilson, J.M., Acute cytokine responses to systemic adenovirus vector is mediated by dendritic cells and macrophages, *Mol. Ther.*, 3, 697, 2001.

[55] Kafri, T. et al., Cellular immune response to adenoviral vector infected cells does not require de novo viral gene expression: implications for gene therapy, *Proc. Natl Acad. Sci. USA*, 95, 11377, 1998.

[56] Thomas, C.E. et al., Acute direct adenoviral vector cytotoxicity and chronic, but not acute, inflammatory responses correlate with decreased vector-mediated transgene expression in the brain, *Mol. Ther.*, 3, 36, 2001.

[57] Harvey, B.G. et al., Variability of human systemic humoral immune responses to adenovirus gene transfer vectors administered to different organs, *J. Virol.*, 73, 6729, 1999.

[58] Lowenstein, P.R. and Castro, M.G., Inflammation and adaptive immune responses to adenoviral vectors injected into the brain: peculiarities, mechanisms, and consequences, *Gene Ther.*, 10, 946, 2003.

[59] Peng, Y., Falck-Pedersen, E., and Elkon, K.B., Variation in adenovirus transgene expression between BALB/c and C57BL/6 mice is associated with differences in interleukin-12 and gamma interferon production and NK cell activation, *J. Virol.*, 75, 4540, 2001.

[60] Morsy, M.A. et al., An adenoviral vector deleted for all viral coding sequences results in enhanced safety and extended expression of a leptin transgene, *Proc. Natl Acad. Sci. USA*, 95, 7866, 1998.

[61] Nakagawa, I. et al., Persistent and secondary adenovirus-mediated hepatic gene expression using adenovirus vector containing CTLA4IgG [In Process Citation], *Hum. Gene Ther.*, 9, 1739, 1998.

[62] Wold, W.S. and Gooding, L.R., Adenovirus region E3 proteins that prevent cytolysis by cytotoxic T cells and tumor necrosis factor, *Mol. Biol. Med.*, 6, 433, 1989.

[63] York, I.A. et al., A cytosolic herpes simplex virus protein inhibits antigen presentation to CD8+ T lymphocytes, *Cell*, 77, 525, 1994.

[64] Krasnykh, V.N. et al., Generation of recombinant adenovirus vectors with modified fibers for altering viral tropism, *J. Virol.*, 70, 6839, 1996.

[65] Micheal, S.I. et al., Addition of a short peptide ligand to the adenovirus fiber protein, *Gene Ther.*, 2, 660, 1995.

[66] Wickham, T.J. et al., Adenovirus targeted to heparan-containing receptors increases its gene delivery efficiency to multiple cell types, *Nat. Biotechnol.*, 14, 1570, 1996.

[67] Krasnykh, V.N. et al., Genetic targeting of an adenovirus vector via replacement of the fiber protein with phage T$ fibritin, *J. Virol.*, 75, 4176, 2001.

[68] Wickham, T.J. et al., Targeted adenovirus gene transfer to endothelial and smooth muscle cells by using bispecific antibodies, *J. Virol.*, 70, 6831, 1996.

[69] Fisher, K.D. et al., Polymer-coated adenovirus permits efficient retargeting and evades neutralising antibodies, *Gene Ther.*, 8, 341, 2001.

[70] Magovern, C.J. et al., Regional angiogenesis induced in nonischemic tissue by an adenoviral vector expressing vascular endothelial growth factor, *Hum. Gene Ther.*, 8, 215, 1997.

[71] Geutskens, S.B. et al., Recombinant adenoviral vectors have adjuvant activity and stimulate T cell responses against tumor cells, *Gene Ther.*, 7, 1410, 2000.

[72] Chen, P., Kovesdi, I., and Bruder, J.T., Effective repeat administration with adenovirus vectors to the muscle, *Gene Ther.*, 7, 587, 2000.

[73] Buller, R.E. et al., A phase I/II trial of rAd/p53 (SCH 58500) gene replacement in recurrent ovarian cancer, *Cancer Gene Ther.*, 9, 553, 2002.

[74] Dai, Y. et al., Cellular and humoral immune responses to adenoviral vectors containing factor IX gene: tolerization of factor IX and vector antigens allows for long-term expression, *Proc. Natl Acad. Sci. USA*, 92, 1401, 1995.

[75] Engelhardt, J.F. et al., Ablation of E2A in recombinant adenoviruses improves transgene persistence and decreases inflammatory response in mouse liver, *Proc. Natl Acad. Sci. USA*, 91, 6196, 1994.

[76] Scaria, A. et al., Adenovirus-mediated persistent cystic fibrosis transmembrane conductance regulator expression in mouse airway epithelium, *J. Virol.*, 72, 7302, 1998.

[77] Zsengeller, Z.K. et al., Persistence of replication-deficient adenovirus-mediated gene transfer in lungs of immune-deficient (nu/nu) mice, *Hum. Gene Ther.*, 6, 457, 1995.

[78] Morral, N. et al., Administration of helper-dependent adenoviral vectors and sequential delivery of different vector serotype for long-term liver-directed gene transfer in baboons, *Proc. Natl Acad. Sci. USA*, 96, 12816, 1999.

[79] McCarty, D.M. and Samulski, R.J., Adeno-associated viral vectors. In *Concepts in Gene Therapy*. M. Strauss and J.A. Barranger (Eds). Berlin, Walter de Gruyter & Co., p. 61, 1997.

[80] Summerford, C. and Samulski, R.J., Membrane-associated heparan sulfate proteoglycan is a receptor for adeno-associated virus type 2 virions, *J. Virol.*, 1438, 1998.

[81] Summerford, C., Bartlett, J.S., and Samulski, R.J., AlphaVbeta5 integrin: a co-receptor for adeno-associated virus type 2 infection, *Nat. Med.*, 5, 78, 1999.

[82] Qing, K. et al., Human fibroblast growth factor receptor 1 is a co-receptor for infection by adeno-associated virus 2, *Nat. Med.*, 5, 71, 1999.

[83] Muzyczka, N., Use of adeno-associated virus as a general transduction vector for mammalian cells, *Curr. Top. Microbiol. Immunol.*, 158, 97, 1992.

[84] Inoue, N. and Russell, D.W., Packaging cells based on inducible gene amplification for the production of adeno-associated virus vectors, *J. Virol.*, 72, 7024, 1998.

[85] Ferrari, F.K. et al., New developments in the generation of Ad-free, high-titer rAAVs gene therapy vectors, *Nat. Med.*, 3, 1295, 1997.

[86] Xiao, X., Li, J., and Samulski, R.J., Production of high-titer recombinant adeno-associated virus vectors in the absence of helper adenovirus, *J. Virol.*, 72, 2224, 1998.

[87] Zolotukhin, S. et al., Recombinant adeno-associated virus purification using novel methods improves infectious titer and yield, *Gene Ther.*, 6, 973, 1999.

[88] Bartlett, J.S., Samulski, R.J., and McCown, T.J., Selective and rapid uptake of adeno-associated virus type 2 in brain, *Hum. Gene Ther.*, 9, 1181, 1998.

[89] Flannery, J.G. et al., Efficient photoreceptor-targeted gene expression in vivo by recombinant adeno-associated virus, *Proc. Natl Acad. Sci. USA*, 94, 6916, 1997.

[90] Flotte, T.R. et al., Stable *in vivo* expression of the cystic fibrosis transmembrane conductance regulator with an adeno-associated virus vector, *Proc. Natl Acad. Sci. USA*, 90, 10613, 1993.

[91] Maeda, Y. et al., Efficient gene transfer into cardiac myocytes using adeno-associated virus (AAV) vectors [In Process Citation], *J. Mol. Cell Cardiol.*, 30, 1341, 1998.

[92] Monahan, P.E. et al., Direct intramuscular injection with recombinant AAV vectors results in sustained expression in a dog model of hemophilia, *Gene Ther.*, 5, 40, 1998.

[93] Xiao, W. et al., Adeno-associated virus as a vector for liver-directed gene therapy [In Process Citation], *J. Virol.*, 72, 10222, 1998.

[94] Murphy, J.E. et al., Long-term correction of obesity and diabetes in genetically obese mice by a single intramuscular injection of recombinant adeno-associated virus encoding mouse leptin, *Proc. Natl Acad. Sci. USA*, 94, 13921, 1997.

[95] Brockstedt, D.G. et al., Induction of immunity to antigens expressed by recombinant adeno-associated virus depends on the route of administration, *Clin. Immunol.*, 92, 67, 1999.

[96] Zhang, Y. et al., CD40 ligand-dependent activation of cytotoxic T lymphocytes by adeno-associated virus vectors *in vivo*: role of immature dendritic cells, *J. Virol.*, 74, 8003, 2000.

[97] Zaiss, A.K. et al., Differential activation of innate immune responses by adenovirus and adeno-associated virus vectors, *J. Virol.*, 76, 4580, 2002.

[98] Chirmule, N. et al., Humoral immunity to adeno-associated virus type 2 vectors following administration to murine and nonhuman primate muscle, *J. Virol.*, 74, 2420, 2000.

[99] Xiao, W. et al., Gene therapy vectors based on adeno-associated virus type 1, *J. Virol.*, 70, 8098, 1999.

[100] Gao, G.P. et al., Novel adeno-associated viruses from rhesus monkeys as vectors for human gene therapy, *Proc. Natl Acad. Sci. USA*, 99, 11854, 2002.

[101] Rabinowitz, J.E. et al., Cross-dressing the virion: the transcapsidation of adeno-associated virus serotypes functionally defines subgroups, *J. Virol.*, 78, 4421, 2004.

[102] Qiao, C. et al., A novel gene expression control system and its use in stable, high-titer 293 cell-based adeno-associated virus packaging cell lines, *J. Virol.*, 76, 13015, 2002.

[103] Liu, X.L., Clark, K.R., and Johnson, P.R., Production of recombinant adeno-associated virus vectors using a packaging cell line and a hybrid recombinant adenovirus, *Gene Ther.*, 6, 293, 1999.

[104] Brument, N. et al., A versatile and scalable two-step ion-exchange chromatography process for the purification of recombinant adeno-associated virus serotypes-2 and -5, *Mol. Ther.*, 6, 678, 2002.

[105] Duan, D., Yue, Y., and Engelhardt, J.F., A new dual-vector approach to enhance recombinant adeno-associated virus-mediated gene expression through intermolecular cis activation, *Nat. Med.*, 6, 595, 2001.

[106] Nakai, H., Storm, T.A., and Kay, M.A., Increasing the size of rAAV-mediated expression cassettes *in vivo* by intermolecular joining of two complementary vectors, *Nat. Biotechnol.*, 18, 527, 2000.

[107] Sun, L., Li, J., and Xiao, X., Overcoming adeno-associated virus vector size limitation through viral DNA heterodimerization, *Nat. Med.*, 6, 599, 2000.

[108] Yan, Z. et al., Recombinant AAV-mediated gene delivery using dual vector heterodimerization, *Meth. Enzymol.*, 346, 334, 2002.

[109] Cordier, L. et al., Muscle-specific promotors may be necessary for adeno-associated virus-mediated gene transfer in the treatment of muscular dystrophies, *Hum. Gene Ther.*, 12, 205, 2001.

[110] Sarukhan, A. et al., Successful interference with cellular immune responses to immunogenic proteins encoded by recombinant viral vectors, *J. Virol.*, 75, 269, 2001.

[111] Rabinowitz, J.E., Xiao, W., and Samulski, R.J., Insertional mutagenesis of AAV2 capsid and the production of recombinant virus, *Virology*, 265, 274, 1999.

[112] Auricchio, A. et al., Exchange of surface proteins impacts on viral vector cellular specificity and transduction characteristics: the retina as a model, *Hum. Mol. Genet.*, 10, 3075, 2001.

[113] Bartlett, J.S. et al., Targeted adeno-associated virus vector transduction of nonpermissive cells mediated by a bispecific F(ab'gamma)2 antibody, *Nat. Biotechnol.*, 17, 181, 1999.

[114] Wu, P., et al. Mutational analysis of the adeno-associated virus type 2 (AAV2) capsid gene and construction of AAV2 vectors with altered tropism, *J. Virol.*, 74, 8635, 2002.

[115] Hengge, U.R. et al., Cytokine gene expression in epidermis with biological effects following injection of naked DNA, *Nat. Genet.*, 10, 161, 1995.

[116] Wolff, J.A. et al., Direct gene transfer into mouse muscle *in vivo*, *Science*, 247, 1465, 1990.

[117] Kawabata, K., Takakura, Y., and Hashida, M., The fate of plasmid DNA after intravenous injection in mice: involvement of scavenger receptors in its hepatic uptake, *Pharm. Res.*, 12, 825, 1995.

[118] Lew, D. et al., Cancer gene therapy using plasmid DNA: pharmacokinetic study of DNA following injection in mice [see comments], *Hum. Gene Ther.*, 6, 553, 1995.

[119] Hickman, M.A. et al., Gene expression following direct injection of DNA into liver, *Hum. Gene Ther.*, 5, 1477, 1994.

[120] Sikes, M.L. et al., *In vivo* gene transfer into rabbit thyroid follicular cells by direct DNA injection, *Hum. Gene Ther.*, 5, 837, 1994.

[121] Doh, S.G. et al., Spatial–temporal patterns of gene expression in mouse skeletal muscle after injection of lacZ plasmid DNA, *Gene Ther.*, 4, 648, 1997.

[122] Acsadi, G. et al., Direct gene transfer and expression into rat heart *in vivo*, *New Biol.*, 3, 71, 1991.

[123] Wells, D.J., Improved gene transfer by direct plasmid injection associated with regeneration in mouse skeletal muscle, *FEBS Lett.*, 332, 179, 1993.

[124] Yoshimura, K. et al., Adenovirus-mediated augmentation of cell transfection with unmodified plasmid vectors, *J. Biol. Chem.*, 268, 2300, 1993.

[125] Hartikka, J. et al., An improved plasmid DNA expression vector for direct injection into skeletal muscle, *Hum. Gene Ther.*, 7, 1205, 1996.

[126] Herweijer, H. and Wolff, J.A., Progress and prospects: naked DNA gene transfer and therapy, *Gene Ther.*, 10, 453, 2003.

[127] Isner, J.M. et al., Clinical evidence of angiogenesis after arterial gene transfer of phVEGF165 in patient with ischaemic limb [see comments], *Lancet*, 348, 370, 1996.

[128] Isner, J.M. et al., Arterial gene transfer for therapeutic angiogenesis in patients with peripheral artery disease, *Hum. Gene Ther.*, 7, 959, 1996.

[129] Melillo, G. et al., Gene therapy for collateral vessel development, *Cardiovasc. Res.*, 35, 480, 1997.

[130] Tsurumi, Y. et al., Direct intramuscular gene transfer of naked DNA encoding vascular endothelial growth factor augments collateral development and tissue perfusion [see comments], *Circulation*, 94, 3281, 1996.

[131] Baumgartner, I. et al., Constitutive expression of phVEGF165 after intramuscular gene transfer promotes collateral vessel development in patients with critical limb ischemia [see comments], *Circulation*, 97, 1114, 1998.

[132] Comerota, A.J. et al., Naked plasmid DNA encoding fibroblast growth factor type 1 for the treatment of end-stage unreconstructible lower extremity ischemia: preliminary results of a phase I trial, *J. Vasc. Surg.*, 35, 930, 2002.

[133] Donnelly, J.J. et al., DNA vaccines, *Annu. Rev. Immunol.*, 15, 617, 1997.

[134] Sato, Y. et al., Immunostimulatory DNA sequences necessary for effective intradermal gene immunization, *Science*, 273, 352, 1996.

[135] Tripathy, S.K. et al., Long-term expression of erythropoietin in the systemic circulation of mice after intramuscular injection of a plasmid DNA vector, *Proc. Natl Acad. Sci. USA*, 93, 10876, 1996.

[136] Nitta, Y. et al., Systemic delivery of interleukin 10 by intramuscular injection of expression plasmid DNA prevents autoimmune diabetes in nonobese diabetic mice [In Process Citation], *Hum. Gene Ther.*, 9, 1701, 1998.

[137] van Deutekom, J.C. and van Ommen, G.J., Advances in Duchenne muscular dystrophy gene therapy, *Nat. Rev. Genet.*, 4, 774, 2003.

[138] Liang, K.W. et al., Restoration of dystrophin expression in mdx mice by intravascular injection of naked DNA containing full-length dystrophin cDNA, *Gene Ther.*, 11, 901, 2004.

[139] Yang, N.S., Sun, W.H., and McCabe, D., Developing particle-mediated gene-transfer technology for research into gene therapy of cancer, *Mol. Med. Today*, 2, 476, 1996.

[140] Jiao, S. et al., Particle bombardment-mediated gene transfer and expression in rat brain tissues, *Biotechnology (N Y)*, 11, 497, 1993.

[141] Keller, E.T. et al., *In vivo* particle-mediated cytokine gene transfer into canine oral mucosa and epidermis, *Cancer Gene Ther.*, 3, 186, 1996.

[142] Mahvi, D.M. et al., Particle-mediated gene transfer of granulocyte-macrophage colony-stimulating factor cDNA to tumor cells: implications for a clinically relevant tumor vaccine, *Hum. Gene Ther.*, 7, 1535, 1996.

[143] Verma, S. et al., Gene transfer into human umbilical cord blood-derived CD34+ cells by particle-mediated gene transfer [In Process Citation], *Gene Ther.*, 5, 692, 1998.

[144] Zelenin, A.V. et al., Transfer of foreign DNA into the cells of developing mouse embryos by microprojectile bombardment, *FEBS Lett.*, 315, 29, 1993.

[145] Rakhmilevich, A.L. and Yang, N.-S. (1997). Particle-mediated gene delivery system for cancer research. In *Concepts in Gene Therapy*. M. Strauss and J.A. Barranger (Eds). Berlin, Walter de Gruyter, p. 109.

[146] Williams, R.S. et al., Introduction of foreign genes into tissues of living mice by DNA-coated microprojectiles, *Proc. Natl Acad. Sci. USA*, 88, 2726, 1991.

[147] Yang, N.S. et al., *In vivo* and *in vitro* gene transfer to mammalian somatic cells by particle bombardment, *Proc. Natl Acad. Sci. USA*, 87, 9568, 1990.

[148] Lin, M.T. et al., The gene gun: current application in cutaneous gene therapy, *Int. J. Dermatol.*, 39, 161, 2000.

[149] Davidson, J.M., Krieg, T., and Eming, S.A., Particle-mediated gene therapy of wounds, *Wound Repair Regen.*, 8, 452, 2000.

[150] Muangmoonchai, R. et al., Transfection of liver *in vivo* by biolistic particle delivery: its use in the investigation of cytochrome P450 gene regulation, *Mol. Biotechnol.*, 20, 145, 2002.

[151] Kay, M.A., Liu, D., and Hoogerbrugge, P.M., Gene therapy, *Proc. Natl Acad. Sci. USA*, 94, 12744, 1997.

[152] Tomlinson, E. and Rolland, A.P., Controllable gene therapy pharmaceutics of non-viral gene delivery systems, *J. Control. Release*, 39, 357, 1996.

[153] Radler, J.O. et al., Structure of DNA-cationic liposome complexes: DNA intercalation in multilamellar membranes in distinct interhelical packing regimes [see comments], *Science*, 275, 810, 1997.

[154] Felgner, P.L. and Ringold, G.M., Cationic liposome-mediated transfection, *Nature*, 337, 387, 1989.

[155] Zhu, N. et al., Systemic gene expression after intravenous DNA delivery into adult mice, *Science*, 261, 209, 1993.

[156] Nabel, G.J. et al., Direct gene transfer with DNA-liposome complexes in melanoma: expression, biologic activity, and lack of toxicity in humans, *Proc. Natl Acad. Sci. USA*, 90, 11307, 1993.

[157] Xu, Y. and Szoka, F.C., Jr., Mechanism of DNA release from cationic liposome/DNA complexes used in cell transfection, *Biochemistry*, 35, 5616, 1996.

[158] Zabner, J. et al., Cellular and molecular barriers to gene transfer by a cationic lipid, *J. Biol. Chem.*, 270, 18997, 1995.

[159] Budker, V. et al., pH-sensitive, cationic liposomes: a new synthetic virus-like vector, *Nat. Biotechnol.*, 14, 760, 1996.

[160] Legendre, J.Y. and Szoka, F.C., Jr., Delivery of plasmid DNA into mammalian cell lines using pH-sensitive liposomes: comparison with cationic liposomes, *Pharm. Res.*, 9, 1235, 1992.

[161] Yonemitsu, Y. et al., HVJ (Sendai virus)-cationic liposomes: a novel and potentially effective liposome-mediated technique for gene transfer to the airway epithelium, *Gene Ther.*, 4, 631, 1997.

[162] Cheung, C.Y. et al., A pH-sensitive polymer that enhances cationic lipid-mediated gene transfer, *Bioconj. Chem.*, 12, 906, 2001.

[163] Escrion, V. et al., Critical assessment of the nuclear import of plasmid during cationic lipid-mediated gene transfer, *J. Gene Med.*, 3, 179, 2001.

[164] Zanta, M.A., Belguise-Valladier, P., and Behr, J.P., Gene delivery: a single nuclear localization signal peptide is sufficient to carry DNA to the cell nucleus, *Proc. Natl Acad. Sci. USA*, 96, 91, 1999.

[165] Fisher, K.D. et al., A versatile system for receptor-mediated gene delivery permits increased entry of DNA into target cells, enhanced delivery to the nucleus and elevated rates of transgene expression, *Gene Ther.*, 7, 1337, 2000.

[166] Brisson, M. et al., A novel T7 RNA polymerase autogene for efficient cytoplasmic expression of target genes, *Gene Ther.*, 6, 263, 1999.

[167] Chen, X. et al., A novel nonviral cytoplasmic gene expression system and its implications in cancer gene therapy, *Cancer Gene Ther.*, 2, 281, 1995.

[168] Qin, H. and Chatterjee, S.K., Cancer gene therapy using tumor cells infected with recombinant vaccinia virus expressing GM-CSF, *Hum. Gene Ther.*, 7, 1853, 1996.

[169] Glorioso, J.C. et al., Engineering herpes simplex virus vectors for human gene therapy, *Adv. Pharmacol.*, 40, 103, 1997.

[170] Kawakita, M. et al., Effect of canarypox virus (ALVAC)-mediated cytokine expression on murine prostate tumor growth [see comments], *J. Natl Cancer Inst.*, 89, 428, 1997.

[171] Wang, M. et al., Active immunotherapy of cancer with a nonreplicating recombinant fowlpox virus encoding a model tumor-associated antigen, *J. Immunol.*, 154, 4685, 1995.

[172] Bitzer, M. et al., Sendai virus vectors as an emerging negative-strand RNA viral vector system, *J. Gene Med.*, 5, 543, 2003.

[173] Scherer, F. et al., Megnetofection: enhancing and targeting gene delivery by magnetic force *in vitro* and *in vivo*, *Gene Ther.*, 9, 102, 2002.

[174] Lunsford, L. et al., Tissue distribution and persistence in mice of plasmid DNA encapsulated in a PLGA-based microsphere delivery vehicle, *J. Drug Target.*, 8, 39, 2000.

[175] Luo, D. and Saltzman, W.M., Synthetic DNA delivery systems, *Nat. Biotechnol.*, 18, 33, 2000.

[176] Koh, J.J. et al., Degradable polymeric carrier for the delivery of IL-10 plasmid DNA to prevent autoimmune insulitis of NOD mice, *Gene Ther.*, 7, 2099, 2000.

[177] Wu, G.Y. et al., Incorporation of adenovirus into a ligand-based DNA carrier system results in retention of original receptor specificity and enhances targeted gene expression, *J. Biol. Chem.*, 269, 11542, 1994.

[178] Recchia, A. et al., Site-specific integration mediated by a hybrid adenovirus/adeno-associated virus vector, *Proc. Natl Acad. Sci. USA*, 96, 2615, 1999.

[179] Curiel, D.T. et al., Adenovirus enhancement of transferrin-polylysine-mediated gene delivery, *Proc. Natl Acad. Sci. USA*, 88, 8850, 1991.

[180] Schuster, M.J. et al., Multicomponent DNA carrier with a vesicular stomatitis virus G-peptide greatly enhances liver-targeted gene expression in mice, *Bioconj. Chem.*, 10, 1075, 1999.

[181] Edelstein, M.L. et al., Gene therapy clinical trials worldwide 1989–2004 an overview, *J. Gene Med.*, 6, 597, 2004.

19

Bio-Nanorobotics: State of the Art and Future Challenges

Ajay Ummat
Gaurav Sharma
C. Mavroidis
Northeastern University

Atul Dubey
Northeastern University
Rutgers University

19.1　Introduction

Nanotechnology can best be defined as a description of activities at the level of atoms and molecules that have applications in the real world. A nanometer is a billionth of a meter, that is, about 1/80,000 of the diameter of a human hair, or 10 times the diameter of a hydrogen atom. The size-related challenge is the ability to measure, manipulate, and assemble matter with features on the scale of 1 to 100 nm. In order to achieve cost-effectiveness in nanotechnology it will be necessary to automate molecular manufacturing. The engineering of molecular products needs to be carried out by robotic devices, which have been termed as *nanorobots*. A nanorobot is essentially a controllable machine at the nanometer or molecular scale that is composed of nanoscale components. The field of nanorobotics studies the design, manufacturing, programming, and control of the nanoscale robots.

This review chapter focuses on the state of the art in the emerging field of nanorobotics, its applications and discusses in brief some of the essential properties and dynamical laws which make this field more challenging and unique than its macroscale counterpart. This chapter is only reviewing nanoscale robotic devices and does not include studies related to nanoprecision tasks with macrorobotic devices that are usually included in the field of nanorobotics.

Nanorobots would constitute any passive or active structure capable of actuation, sensing, signaling, information processing, intelligence, swarm behavior at the nano scale. These functionalities could be illustrated individually by a nanorobot or in combinations of nanorobots (swarm intelligence and cooperative behavior). Some of the abilities that are desirable for a nanorobot to function are:

1. *Swarm Intelligence* — decentralization and distributive intelligence
2. *Cooperative behavior* — emergent and evolutionary behavior
3. *Self-assembly and replication* — assemblage at nano scale and *"nanomaintenance"*
4. *Nanoinformation processing and programmability* — for programming and controlling nanorobots (autonomous nanorobots)
5. Nano to macroworld *interface architecture* — an architecture enabling instant access to the nanorobots and its control and maintenance

There are many differences between macro and nanoscale robots. These occur mainly in the basic laws that govern their dynamics. Macroscaled robots are essentially in the Newtonian mechanics domain whereas the laws governing nanorobots are in the molecular quantum mechanics domain. Furthermore, uncertainty plays a crucial role in nanorobotic systems. The fundamental barrier for dealing with uncertainty at the nano scale is imposed by the quantum and the statistical mechanics and thermal excitations. For a certain nanosystem at some particular temperature, there are positional uncertainties, which cannot be modified or further reduced [1].

The nanorobots are invisible to naked eye, which makes them hard to manipulate and work with. Techniques like scanning electron microscopy (SEM) and atomic force microscopy (AFM) are being employed to establish a visual and haptic interface to enable us to sense the molecular structure of these nanoscaled devices. Virtual reality (VR) techniques are currently being explored in nanoscience and biotechnology research as a way to enhance the operator's perception (vision and haptics) by approaching more or less a state of "full immersion" or "telepresence." The development of nanorobots or nanomachine components presents difficult fabrication and control challenges. Such devices will operate in microenvironments whose physical properties differ from those encountered by conventional parts. Since these nanoscale devices have not yet been fabricated, evaluating possible designs and control algorithms requires using theoretical estimates and virtual interfaces/environments. Such interfaces/simulations can operate at various levels of detail to trade-off physical accuracy, computational cost, number of components and the time over which the simulation follows the nanoobject behaviors. They can enable nanoscientists to extend their eyes and hands into the nanoworld and also enable new types of exploration and whole new classes of experiments in the biological and physical sciences. VR simulations can also be used to develop virtual assemblies of nano and bio-nanocomponents into mobile linkages and predict their performance.

Nanorobots with completely artificial components have not been realized yet. The active area of research in this field is focused more on molecular robots, which are thoroughly inspired by nature's way of doing things at nano scale. Mother Nature has her own set of molecular machines that have been working for centuries, and have been optimized for performance and design over the ages. As our knowledge and understanding of these numerous machines continues to increase, we now see a possibility of using the natural machines, or creating synthetic ones from scratch, using nature's components. This chapter focuses more on such molecular machines, called also *bio-nanorobots*, and explores various designs and research prevalent in this field. The main goal in the field of molecular machines is to use various biological elements — whose function at the cellular level creates motion, force or a signal — as machine components. These components perform their preprogrammed biological function in response to the specific physiochemical stimuli but in an artificial setting. In this way proteins and DNA could act as motors, mechanical joints, transmission elements, or sensors. If all these different components were assembled together in the proper proportion and orientation they would form nanodevices with multiple degrees of freedom, able to apply forces and manipulate objects in the nanoscale world. The advantage of using nature's machine components is that they are highly efficient and reliable.

Nanorobotics is a field, which calls for collaborative efforts between physicists, chemists, biologists, computer scientists, engineers, and other specialists to work towards this common objective. Figure 19.1 shows various fields, that are involved in the study of bio-nanorobotics (this is just a representative figure and not exhaustive in nature). Currently this field is still evolving, but several substantial steps have been

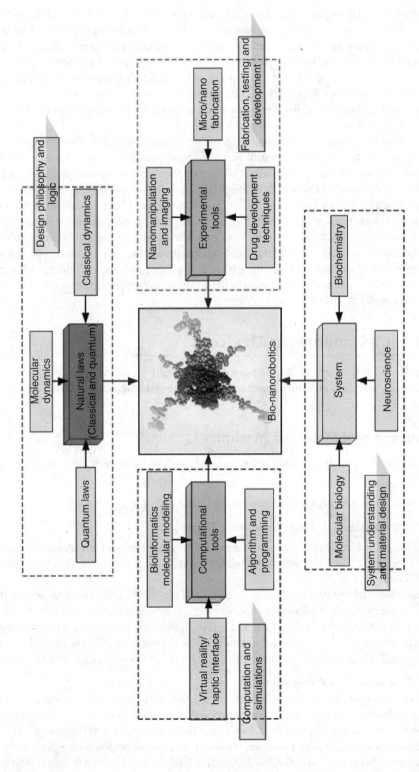

FIGURE 19.1 (See color insert following page **20**-14.) Bio-nanorobotics — a truly multidisciplinary field.

taken by great researchers all over the world and are contributing to this ever challenging and exciting field.

The ability to manipulate matter at the nano scale is one core application for which nanorobots could be the technological solution. A lot has been written in the literature about the significance and motivation behind constructing a nanorobot. The applications range from medical to environmental sensing to space and military applications. Molecular construction of complex devices could be possible by nanorobots of the future. From precise drug delivery to repairing cells and fighting tumor cells, nanorobots are expected to revolutionize the medical industry in the future. These applications come under the field of nanomedicine, which is a very active area of research in nanotechnology. These molecular machines hence form the basic enablers of future nanoscale applications.

In the next section, we shall try to understand the principles, theory, and utility of the known molecular machines and look into the design and control issues for their creation and modification. A majority of natural molecular machines are protein-based, while the DNA-based molecular machines are mostly synthetic. Nature deploys proteins to perform various cellular tasks — from moving cargo, to catalyzing reactions, while it has kept DNA as an information carrier. It is hence understandable that most of the natural machinery is built from proteins. With the powerful crystallographic techniques available in the modern world, the protein structures are clearer than ever. The ever-increasing computing power makes it possible to dynamically model protein folding processes and predict the conformations and structure of lesser known proteins. All this helps unravel the mysteries associated with the molecular machinery and paves the way for the production and application of these miniature machines in various fields including medicine, space exploration, electronics, and military.

19.2 Nature's Nanorobotic Devices

In this section we will detail some of the man-made and naturally occurring molecular machines. We divide the molecular machines into three broad categories — protein-based, DNA-based, and chemical molecular motors.

19.2.1 Protein-Based Molecular Machines

This section focuses on the study of the following main protein-based molecular machines:

1. ATP Synthase
2. The kinesin, myosin, dynein, and flagella molecular motors

19.2.1.1 ATP Synthase — A True Nanorotary Motor [2]

Synthesis of ATP is carried out by an enzyme, known as ATP Synthase. The inner mitochondrial membrane contains the ATP Synthase. The ATP Synthase is actually a combination of two motors functioning together as described in Figure 19.2 [3].

This enzyme consists of a proton-conducting F_0 unit and a catalytic F_1 unit. The figure also illustrates the subunits that constitutes the two motor components. F_1 constitutes of $\alpha_3\beta_3\gamma\delta\epsilon$ subunits. F_0 has three different protein molecules, namely, subunit a, b, and c. The γ subunit of F_1 is attached to the c subunit of F_0 and is hence rotated along with it. The $\alpha_3\beta_3$ subunits are fixed to the b subunit of F_0 and hence do not move. Further the b subunit is held inside the membrane by a subunit of F_0 (shown in Figure 19.2 by Walker [3]).

19.2.1.1.1 ATP Synthase "Nano" Properties

19.2.1.1.1.1 Reversibility of the ATP Synthase — There are two directions in ATP Synthase system and these two directions correspond to two different functionalities and behavior. This two-way behavior is because of the reversible nature of the ATP–ADP cycle and the structure of the ATP Synthase. Let us term the forward direction as when the F_0 drives the γ subunit (because of proton motive force) of F_1 and hence ATP synthesis takes place. And the backward direction is when hydrolysis of ATP counter-rotated the γ subunit and hence the F_0 motor and leads to pumping back the protons. Therefore, the forward direction

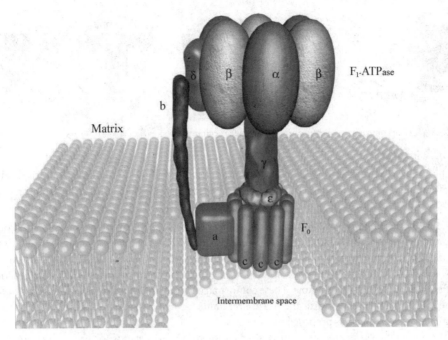

FIGURE 19.2 (See color insert.) The basic structure of the ATP Synthase. Shown is the flow of protons from the outer membrane toward the inner through the F_0 motor. This proton motive force is responsible for the synthesis of ATP in F_1.

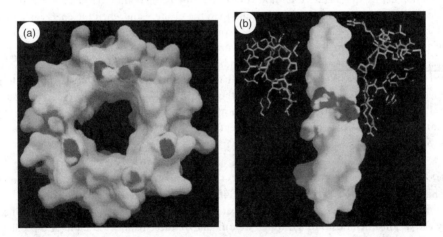

FIGURE 19.3 (See color insert.) The electrostatic surface potential on the $\alpha_3\beta_3$ and γ subunits.

is powered by the proton motive force and the backward direction is powered by the ATP hydrolysis. Which particular direction is being followed depends upon the situation and the environmental factors around the ATP Synthase.

19.2.1.1.1.2 Coupling of Proton Flow (F_0) and the ATP Synthesis and Hydrolysis (in F_1) — Boyer proposed a model which predicted that the F_0 and F_1 motors are connected through the γ subunit. Further he proposed that this connection was mechanical in nature. Figure 19.3 [4] illustrates the electrostatic surface potential on $\alpha_3\beta_3$ subunits. The red color represents a negatively charged surface and blue a positively charged surface. Shown in the Figure 19.3a, a predominately neutral hole in the $\alpha_3\beta_3$ subunit through

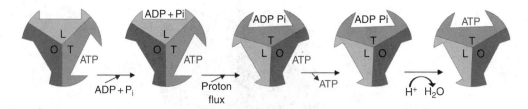

FIGURE 19.4   (See color insert.) Boyer's binding change mechanism.

which the γ subunit protrudes. Figure 19.3b shows a γ subunit with a significantly negatively charged region around half across its length. The γ subunit slides through the hole of the $\alpha_3\beta_3$ subunits.

19.2.1.1.1.3 Boyer's Binding Change Mechanism — Boyer isolated the F_1 part of the ATP Synthase complex. It was found that the α and β subunits alternate in this cylindrical part of the F_1 structure. As per this model each α and β pair forms a catalytic site. The rotation of the γ subunit induces structural conformation in the $\alpha_3\beta_3$ subunits. Although the three catalytic units are identical in their chemistry, they are functionally very different at any given point in time. These conformal changes induce a change in the binding affinities of all the three catalytic sites towards the ATPase reactants (ADP, P_i, ATP, etc.). Figure 19.4 [5] shows the binding change mechanism as proposed by Boyer.

The three catalytic sites could be in three distinct forms. O form stands for open which implies that it has got very low affinity for reactants; L form stands for loose, which implies that it would bind the reactants loosely but is still catalytically inactive; T form stands for tight, which binds the reactant tightly and is catalytically active.

The situation depicted in Figure 19.4 shows one of the sites being bound to ATP at T. The site for ADP and P_i would probably be L as it is more binding than the O site. Now when the energy is input to the system the sites are changed. T becomes O, O becomes L, and L becomes T. Due to these changes the ATP which was previously in T is now released. Further the ADP and P_i are now tightly bound due to the conversion of L site to the T site. This tight binding of ADP and P_i allows them to spontaneously get converted into ATP. Hence, this model proposed that the proton flow from the F_0 is coupled to the site inter conversions in the F_1 unit which triggers synthesis–hydrolysis of ATP. Boyer's theory was supported when Walker and his group solved the structure of the F_1-ATPase motor. The high-resolution structure thus obtained gave hints towards many experiments which proved the fact that the γ subunit indeed rotated against the α and β subunits.

19.2.1.1.1.4 F_1-ATPase a True Nanorotary Motor — Till today the exact mechanism of the molecular motor characterized by F_1-ATPase has not been fully determined. Research by Kinosita's lab is a step toward this goal and proposes some very conclusive models for the same. The results obtained show not only the various methods through which we can analyze these nanodevices, but also predicts many characteristics for these.

What is known till now is that the γ subunit rotates inside the α–β hexamer, but whether the rotation is continuous or random was not known. Kinosita's lab solved this problem by imaging the F_1-ATPase molecule. The objective of their experiment was to determine the uniqueness of the rotary motion and its characteristics. Figure 19.5 [2] depicts the experiment that was performed by this group. They attached a micrometer long actin filament to the γ subunit. This actin filament was fluorescently labeled, so that its fluorescence could be measured under a microscope. Hydrolysis of the ATP (when introduced in the experiment) led to the rotation of the γ subunit and in effect the rotation of the actin filament. As reported by the authors, not all the actin filaments were observed to have rotation. But some percentage of them did rotate and that too in a unique direction and without having much reversibility in the direction. This direct imaging proved that the structure solved by Walker and group was indeed correct and there exists rotary motion between γ subunit and the α and β hexamer.

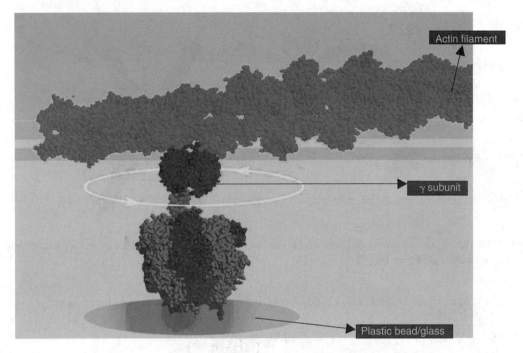

FIGURE 19.5   (See color insert.) Experiment performed for Imaging of F_1-ATPase. (From Kinosita, K., Jr., Yasuda, R., Noji, H., and Adachi, K. 2000. *Philos. Trans.: Biol. Sci.* 355 (1396): 473–489. With permission.)

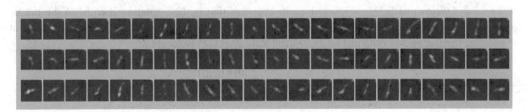

FIGURE 19.6   (See color insert.) Images of a rotating actin filament (sequential image at 33 msec intervals). (From Kinosita, K., Jr., Yasuda, R., Noji, H., and Adachi, K. 2000. *Philos. Trans.: Biol. Sci.* 355 (1396): 473–489. With permission.)

Figure 19.6 [2] shows the imaging of the actin filament that was obtained. The rotation is not restricted to some particular rotational angle but is continuously progressive in a particular direction. As the rotational motion is a continuous one, possibility of it being a twisting motion is ruled out. Hence, there should be no direct linkage between the γ subunit and the α–β hexamer in F_1-ATPase. It was further observed by the authors that the rotation of the actin filament was in certain steps. These step sizes were approximately equal to 120°.

19.2.1.1.2   *Other Observed Behaviors of the F_1-ATPase Motor [2]*

19.2.1.1.2.1   Rotational Rates [2] — Rotational rates were dependent upon the length of the actin filament. Rotational rates were found to be inversely proportional to the filament length. This could be attributed to the fact that the hydrodynamic friction is proportional to the cube of the length of the filament, therefore, longer length implied that the frictional forces were higher and rotational speeds in effect slower. As reported in the principle article, if the filament were to rotate at the speed of 6 rev/sec and the length of the actin filament were 1 μm, then as per the relation:

$$N = \omega\xi$$

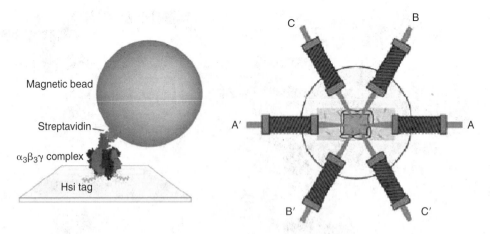

FIGURE 19.7   (See color insert.) Magnetic bead is attached to the γ subunit here (left figure) and the arrangement of the magnets (right figure) [6].

The torque required would be 40 pN nm. Here ξ is the drag coefficient given by the relation:

$$\xi = \frac{4\pi}{3}\eta L^3 \frac{1}{[\ln(L/r) - 0.447]}$$

where μ is the viscosity of the medium $= 10^{-3}$ N sec/m^2 and $r = 5$ nm, the radius of the filament.

19.2.1.1.2.2 Efficiency of F_1 [2] — Work done in one step, that is, 120° rotation is equal to the torque generated (i.e., 40 pN nm) times the angular displacement for that step (i.e., $2\pi/3$). This comes to about 80 pN nm. The free energy obtained by the hydrolysis of one ATP molecule is:

$$\Delta G = \Delta G_0 + k_B T \frac{\ln[\text{ADP}][\text{P}_i]}{[\text{ATP}]}$$

Here, the standard free energy change per ATP molecule is equal to -50 pN nm at pH 7. The thermal energy at room temperature is equal to 4.1 pN nm. At intracellular conditions, [ATP] and [P$_i$] is in the order of 10^{-3} M. Therefore, for [ADP] of 50 μM, ΔG is equal to -90.604 pN nm. Comparing this value of the free energy obtained by the hydrolysis of one molecule of ATP with the mechanical work done by the motor (i.e., 80 pN nm), we can deduce that the F_1-ATPase motor works on efficiency close to 100%!

19.2.1.1.2.3 Chemical Synthesis of ATP Powered by Mechanical Energy — In another study [6], evidence has been provided to justify the claim that the chemical synthesis of ATP occurs when propelled by mechanical energy. This basic nature of the F_1-ATPase was known for quite some time, but it is the first time that it is being experimentally verified. To prove this concept, the F_1 was bound to the glass surface through histidine residues attached at the end of the γ subunits. A magnetic bead coated with streptavidin was attached to the γ subunit (Figure 19.7 [6]).

Electric magnets were used to rotate this bead attached to the γ subunit. The rotation resulted in appearance of ATP in the medium (which was initially immersed in ADP). Thus, the connection between the syntheses of ATP as a result of the mechanical energy input is established.

The exact mechanism of the F_1-ATPase rotation is still an active area of research today and many groups are working towards finding it. The key to solving the mechanism is solving the *transient conformation* of the catalytic sites and the γ subunit when rotation is taking place. What is not clear is the correspondence between the chemical reactions at the catalytic sites and their influence on the rotation of the γ subunit. Which event triggers the rotation and which does not has still to be exactly determined? Many models have been predicted, but they all still elude the reality of the rotational mechanism.

19.2.1.2 The Kinesin, Myosin, Dynein, and Flagella Molecular Motors

With modern microscopic tools, we view a cell as a set of many different moving components powered by molecular machines rather than a static environment. Molecular motors that move unidirectionally along protein polymers (actin or microtubules) drive the motions of muscles as well as much smaller intracellular cargoes. In addition to the F_0–F_1-ATPase motors inside the cell, there are linear transport motors present as tiny vehicles known as motor proteins that transport molecular cargoes [7] that also require ATP for functioning. These minute cellular machines exist in three families — the kinesins, the myosins, and the dyneins [8]. The cargoes can be organelles, lipids, or proteins etc. They play an important role in cell division and motility. There are over 250 kinesin-like proteins, and they are involved in processes as diverse as the movement of chromosomes and the dynamics of cell membranes. The only part they have in common is the catalytic portion known as the motor domain. They have significant differences in their location within cells, their structural organization, and the movement they generate [9]. Muscle myosin, whose study dates back to 1864, has served as a model system for understanding motility for decades. Kinesin, however, was discovered rather recently using *in vitro* motility assays in 1985 [10]. Conventional kinesin is a highly processive motor that can take several hundred steps on a microtubule without detaching [11,12] whereas muscle myosin executes a single "stroke" and then dissociates [13]. A detailed analysis and modeling of these motors has been done [10,14].

Kinesin and myosin make up for an interesting comparison. Kinesin is microtubule-based; it binds to and carries cargoes along microtubules whereas myosin is actin-based. The motor domain of kinesin weighs one third the size of that of myosin and one tenth of that of dynein [15]. Before the advent of modern microscopic and analytic techniques, it was believed that these two have little in common. However, the crystal structures available today indicate that they probably originated from a common ancestor [16].

19.2.1.2.1 The Myosin Linear Motor

Myosin is a diverse superfamily of motor proteins [17]. Myosin-based molecular machines transport cargoes along actin filaments — the two stranded helical polymers of the protein actin, about 5 to 9 nm in diameter. They do this by hydrolyzing ATP and utilizing the energy released [18]. In addition to transport, they are also involved in the process of force generation during muscle contraction, wherein thin actin filaments and thick myosin filaments slide past each other. Not all members of the myosin superfamily have been characterized as of now. However, much is known about the structure and function. Myosin molecules were first sighted through electron microscope protruding out from thick filaments and interacting with the thin actin filaments in late 1950s [19–21]. Since then it was known that ATP plays a role in myosin related muscle movement along actin [22]. However, the exact mechanism was unknown, which was explained later in 1971 by Lymn and Taylor [23].

19.2.1.2.1.1 Structure of Myosin Molecular Motor — A myosin molecule binding to an actin polymer is shown in Figure 19.8a [24]. Myosin molecule has a size of about 520 kDa including two 220 kDa heavy chains and light chains of sizes between 15 and 22 kDa [25,26]. They can be visualized as two identical globular "motor heads," also known as motor domains, each comprising of a catalytic domain (actin, nucleotide as well as light chain binding sites) and about 8 nm long lever arms. The heads, also sometimes referred to as S1 regions (subfragment 1) are shown in blue, while the lever arms or the light chains, in yellow. Both these heads are connected via a coiled coil made of two α-helical coils (gray) to the thick base filament. The light chains have considerable sequence similarity with the protein "calmodulin" and troponin C, and are sometimes referred to as calmodulin-like chains. They act as links to the motor domains and do not play any role in their ATP binding activity [27] but for some exceptions [28,29]. The motor domain in itself is sufficient for moving actin filaments [30]. Three-dimensional (3D) structures of myosin head revealed that it is a pear-shaped domain, about 19 nm long and 5 nm in maximum diameter [30,31].

19.2.1.2.1.2 Function of Myosin Molecular Motor — A crossbridge-cycle model for the action of myosin on actin has been widely accepted since 1957 [19,32,33]. Since the atomic structures of actin monomer

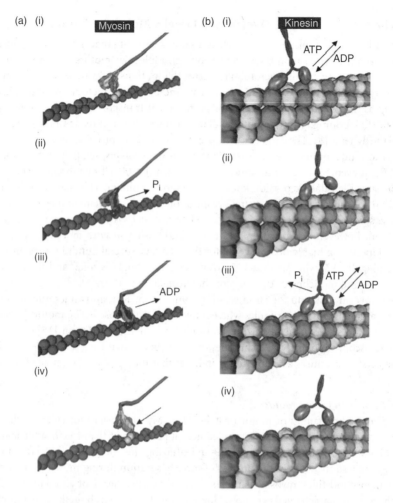

FIGURE 19.8 (See color insert.) The kinesin–myosin walks: (a) Myosin motor mechanism. (i) Motor head loosely docking to the actin binding site; (ii) The binding becomes tighter along with the release of P_i; (iii) Lever arm swings to the left with the release of ADP, and; (iv) replacement of the lost ADP with a fresh ATP molecule results in dissociation of the head; (b) Kinesin heads working in conjunction. (i) Both ADP-carrying heads come near the microtubule and one of them (black neck) binds; (ii) Loss of bound ADP and addition of fresh ATP in the bound head moves the other (red neck) to the right; (iii) The second head (red) binds to microtubule while losing its ADP, and replacing it with a new ATP molecule while the first head hydrolyses its ATP and loses P_i; (iv) The ADP-carrying black-neck will now be snapped forward, and the cycle will be repeated.

[34,35] and myosin [31] were resolved, this model has been refined into a "lever-arm model," which is now acceptable [36]. Only one motor head is able to connect to the actin filament at a time, the other head remains passive. Initially, the catalytic domain in the head has ADP and P_i bound to it and as a result, its binding with actin is weak. With the active motor head docking properly to the actin-binding site, the P_i has to be released. As soon as this happens, the lever arm swings counterclockwise [37] due to a conformational change [21,38–43]. This pushes the actin filament down by about 10 nm along its longitudinal axis [44]. The active motor head now releases its bound ADP and another ATP molecule by way of Brownian motion quickly replaces it, making the binding of the head to the actin filament weak again. The myosin motor then dissociates from the actin filament, and a new cycle starts. However, nanomanipulation of single S1 molecules (motor domains) show that myosin can take multiple steps per ATP molecule hydrolyzed, moving in 5.3 nm steps and resulting in displacements of 11 to 30 nm [45].

19.2.1.2.2 The Kinesin Linear Motor

Kinesin [15] and dynein family of proteins are involved in cellular cargo transport along microtubules as opposed to actin in the case of myosin [46]. Microtubules are 25 nm diameter tubes made of protein tubulin and are present in the cells in an organized manner. Microtubules have polarity; one end being the plus (fast growing) end while the other end is the minus (slow growing) end [47]. Kinesins move from minus end to plus end, while dyneins move from plus end to the minus end of the microtubules. Microtubule arrangement varies in different cell systems. In nerve axons, they are arranged longitudinally in such a manner that their plus ends point away from the cell body and into the axon. In epithelial cells, their plus end points toward the basement membrane. They deviate radially out of the cell center in fibroblasts and macrophages with the plus end protruding outwards [48]. Like myosin, kinesin is also an ATP-driven motor. One unique characteristic of kinesin family of proteins is their processivity — they bind to microtubules and literally "walk" on it for many enzymatic cycles before detaching [49,50]. Also, each of the globular heads/motor domains of kinesin is made of one single polypeptide unlike myosin (heavy and light chains and dynein heavy, intermediate, and light chains).

19.2.1.2.2.1 Structure of Kinesin Molecular Motor — A lot of structural information about kinesin is now available through the crystal structures [16,51,52]. The motor domain contains a folding motif similar to that of myosin and G proteins [8]. The two heads or the motor domains of kinesin are linked via "neck linkers" to a long coiled coil, which extends up to the cargo (Figure 19.8b). They interact with the α and β subunits of the tubulin hetrodimer along the microtubule protofilament. The heads have the nucleotide and the microtubule binding domains in them.

19.2.1.2.2.2 Function of Kinesin Molecular Motor — While Kinesin is also a two-headed linear motor, its modus operandi is different from myosin in the sense that *both* its head work together in a coordinated manner rather than one was being left out. Figure 19.8b shows the kinesin walk. Each of the motor heads is near the microtubule in the initial state with each motor head carrying an ADP molecule. When one of the heads loosely binds to the microtubule, it looses its ADP molecule to facilitate a stronger binding. Another ATP molecule replaces the ADP, which facilitates a conformational change such that the neck region of the bound head snaps forward and zips on to the head [9]. In the process it pulls the other ADP carrying motor head forward by about 16 nm so that it can bind to the next microtubule-binding site. This results in the net movement of the cargo by about 8 nm [53]. The second head now binds to the microtubule by losing its ADP, which is promptly replaced by another ATP molecule due to Brownian motion. The first head meanwhile hydrolyses the ATP and loses the resulting P_i. It is then snapped forward by the second head while it carries its ADP forward. Hence, coordinated hydrolysis of ATP in the two motor heads is the key to the kinesin processivity [54,55]. Kinesin is able to take about 100 steps before detaching from the microtubule [11,49,56] while moving at 1000 nm/sec and exerting forces of the order of 5 to 6 pN at stall [57,58].

19.2.1.2.3 The Dynein Motor

The Dynein superfamily of proteins was introduced in 1965 [59]. Dyneins exist in two isoforms, the cytoplasmic and the axonemal. Cytoplasmic dyneins are involved in cargo movement, while axonemal dyneins are involved in producing bending motions of cilia and flagella [60–70]. Figure 19.9 shows a typical cytoplasmic dynein molecule.

19.2.1.2.3.1 Structure of Dynein Molecular Motor — The structure consists of two heavy chains in the form of globular heads, three intermediate chains and four light intermediate chains [71,72]. Recent studies have exposed a linker domain connecting the "stem" region below the heads to the head itself [73]. Also from the top of the heads the microtubule binding domains (the stalk region, not visible in the figure) protrude out [74]. The ends of these stalks have smaller ATP sensitive globular domains, which bind to the microtubules. Cytoplasmic dynein is associated with a protein complex known as dynactin, which contains ten subunits [75]. Some of them are shown in the figure as p150, p135, actin-related protein 1 (Arp1), actin, dynamitin, capping protein, and p62 subunit. These play an important regulatory role in the

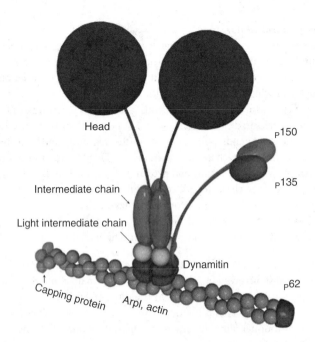

FIGURE 19.9   (See color insert.) A dynein molecule. Shown in blue are the globular heads (heavy chains) connected to the intermediate chains (red) and the light chains (light blue). Dynactin complex components p150, p135, dynamitin, p62, capping proteins, Arp1, actin is also shown.

binding ability of dynein to the microtubules. The heavy chains forming the two globular heads contain the ATPase and microtubule motor domains [76].

One striking difference that dynein exhibits compared to kinesins and myosins is that dynein has AAA (ATPases Associated with a variety of cellular Activities) modules [77–79], which indicate that its mode of working will be entirely different from kinesins and myosins. This puts dyneins into the AAA superfamily of mechanoenzymes. The dynein heavy chains contain six tandemly linked AAA modules [80,81] with the head having a ring-like domain organization, typical of AAA superfamily. Four of these are nucleotide binding motifs, named P1–P4, but only P1 (AAA1) is able to hydrolyze ATP.

19.2.1.2.3.2 Function of Dynein Molecular Motor — Because dynein is larger and more complex structure as compared to other motor proteins, its mode of operation is not as well known. However, very recently, Burgess et al. [73] have used electron microscopy and image processing to show the structure of a flagellar dynein at the start and end of its power stroke, giving some insight into its possible mode of force generation. When the dynein contains bound ADP and V_i (vandate), it is in the prepower stroke conformation. The state when it has lost the two, known as the apostate is the more compact postpower stroke state. There is a distinct conformational change involving the stem, linker, head, and the stalk that produces about 15 nm of translation onto the microtubule bound to the stalk [73].

19.2.1.2.4 The Flagella Motors

Unicellular organisms, such as, *Escherichia coli* have an interesting mode of motility (for reviews see [82–84]). They have a number of molecular motors, about 45 nm in diameter, that drive their "feet" or the flagella that help the cell to swim. Motility is critical for cells, as they often have to travel from a less favorable to a more favorable environment. The flagella are helical filaments that extend out of the cell into the medium and perform a function analogous to what the oars perform to a boat. The flagella and the motor assembly are called a flagellum. The flagella motors impart a rotary motion into the flagella [85,86]. In addition to a rotary mechanism, the flagella machines consist of components such as rate meters, particle counters, and gearboxes [87]. These are necessary to help the cell decide which way to go, depending on the change of concentration of nutrients in the surroundings. The rotary motion imparted to the flagella needs to be modulated to ensure the cell is moving in the proper direction as well as all flagella of the given cell are providing a concerted effort toward it [88]. When the motors rotate the flagella in a counterclockwise direction as viewed along the flagella filament from outside, the helical flagella create a wave away from the cell body. Adjacent flagella subsequently intertwine in a propulsive corkscrew manner and propel the bacteria. When the motors rotate clockwise, the flagella fly apart, causing the bacteria to tumble, or change its direction [89]. These reversals occur randomly, giving the bacterium a "random walk," unless of course, there is a preferential direction of motility due to reasons mentioned earlier. The flagella motors allow the bacteria to move at speeds of as much as 25 μm/sec with directional reversals occurring approximately 1 per sec [90]. A number of bacterial species in addition to *E. coli*, depend on flagella motors for motility. Some of these are *Salmonella enterica serovar Typhimurium* (Salmonella), *Streptococcus*, *Vibrio* spp., *Caulobacter*, *Leptospira*, *Aquaspirillum serpens*, and *Bacillus*. The rotation of flagella motors is stimulated by a flow of ions through them which is a result of a build-up of a transmembrane ion gradient. There is no direct ATP-involvement, however, the proton gradient needed for the functioning of flagella motors can be produced by ATPase.

19.2.1.2.4.1 Structure of the Flagella Motors — A complete part list of the flagella motors may not be available as of now. Continued efforts dating back to early 1970s have, however, revealed much of their structure, composition, genetics, and function. Newer models of the motor function are still being proposed with an aim to explain observed experimental phenomena [91,92]. That means that we do not fully understand the functioning of this motor [83]. A typical flagella motor from *E. coli* consists of about 20 different proteins [83], while there are yet more that are involved in the assembly and functioning. There are 14 Flg-type proteins named FlgA to FlgN; 5 Flh-type proteins called FlhA to FlhE; 19 Fli-type proteins named FliA to FliT; MotA and MotB making a total of 40 related proteins. The name groups Flg, Flh, Fli, and Flg originate from the names of the corresponding genes [93]. Out of these the main structural proteins are FliC or the filament; FliD (filament cap); FliF or the MS-ring; FliG; FliM, and FliN (C-ring); FlgB, FlgC, and FlgF (proximal rod); FlgG (distal rod); FlgH (L-ring); FlgI (P-ring); FlgK and FlgL (hook-filament junction); and MotA-MotB (torque generating units). Earlier it was believed that the M and S are two separate rings and M was named after membrane and S after supramembranous [94]. Now they are jointly called the MS-ring as it has been found that they are two domains of the same protein FliF [95,96]. The C-ring is named after cytoplasmic [97–99], while the names of the P- and L-rings come from "peptidoglycan" and "lipopolysaccharide," respectively. The FlhA, B, FliH, I, O, P, Q, R constitute the "transport apparatus."

The hook and filament part of the flagellum is located outside the cell body, while the motor portion is embedded in the cell membrane with parts (the C-ring and the transport apparatus) that are inside the inner membrane in the cytoplasmic region. MotA and MotB are arranged in a circular array embedded in the inner membrane, with the MS-ring at the center. Connected to the MS-ring is the proximal end of a shaft, to which the P-ring, which is embedded in the peptidoglycan layer, is attached. Moving further outwards, there is the L-ring embedded in the outer cell membrane followed by the distal shaft end that protrudes out of the cell. To this end there is an attachment of the hook and the filament, both of which are polymers of hook-protein and flagellin, respectively.

19.2.1.2.4.2 Function of the Flagella Motors — The flagellar motors in most cases are powered by protons flowing through the cell membrane (protonmotive force, defined earlier) barring exceptions such as certain marine bacteria, for example, the *Vibrio* spp., which are driven by Na^+ ions [100]. There are about 1200 protons required to rotate the motor by one rotation [101]. A complete explanation of how this proton flow is able to generate torque is not available as of today. From what is known, the stator units of MotA and MotB play an important role in torque generation. They form a MotA/MotB complex which when oriented properly binds to the peptidoglycan and opens proton channels through which protons can flow [102]. It is believed that there are eight such channels per motor [103]. The protonmotive force is a result of the difference of pH in the outside and the inside of the cell. The *E. coli* cells like to maintain a pH of 7.6–7.8 on their inside, hence depending on the pH of the surroundings, the protonmotive force will vary, and hence the speed of rotation of their motors. To test how the speed of rotation depends on the protonmotive force, the motors were powered by external voltage with markers acting as heavy loads attached to them [104]. It was found that the rotation indeed depends directly on the protonmotive force. According to the most widely accepted model, MotA/MotB complex interacts with the rotor via binding sites. The passage of protons through a MotA/MotB complex (stator or torque generator) moves it so that they bind to the next available binding site on the rotor, thereby stretching their linkage. When the linkage recoils, the rotor assembly has to rotate by one step. Hence, whichever complex receives protons from the flux will rotate the rotor, generating torque. The torque–speed dependence of the motor has been studied in detail [105,106] and indicates the torque range of about 2700 to 4600 pN nm.

19.2.2 DNA-Based Molecular Machines

As mentioned earlier, nature chose DNA mainly as an information carrier. There was no mechanical work assigned to it. Energy conversion, trafficking, sensing, etc., were the tasks assigned mainly to proteins. Probably for this reason, DNA turns out to be a simpler structure — with only four kinds of nucleotide bases adenosine, thiamine, guanine, and cytosine (A, T, G, and C) attached in a linear fashion that take a double helical conformation when paired with a complementary strand. Such structural simplicity vis-à-vis proteins — made of 20 odd amino acids with complex folding patterns — results in a simpler structure and predictable behavior. There are certain qualities that make DNA an attractive choice for the construction of artificial nanomachines. In recent years, DNA has found use in not only mechanochemical, but also in nanoelectronic systems as well [107–110]. A DNA double-helical molecule is about 2 nm in diameter and has 3.4–3.6 nm helical pitch no matter what its base composition is; a structural uniformity is not achievable with protein structures if one changes their sequence. Furthermore, double-stranded DNA (ds-DNA) has a respectable persistence length of about 50 nm [111] which provides it enough rigidity to be a candidate component of molecular machinery. Single stranded DNA (ss-DNA) is very flexible and cannot be used where rigidity is required, however, this flexibility allows its application in machine components like hinges or nanoactuators [112]. Its persistence length is about 1 nm nm covering up to three base pairs [113] at 1 M salt concentration.

Other than the above structural features there are two important and exclusive properties that make DNA suitable for molecular level constructions. These are molecular recognition and self-assembly. The nucleotide bases A and T on two different ss-DNA have affinity towards each other, so do G and C. Effective and stable ds-DNA structures are only formed if the base orders of the individual strands are complement-ary. Hence, if two complementary single strands of DNA are in a solution, they will eventually recognize each other and hybridize or zip-up forming a ds-DNA. This property of molecular recognition and self-assembly has been exploited in a number of ways to build complex molecular structures [114–121]. In the mechanical perspective, if the free energy released by hybridization of two complementary DNA strands is used to lift a hypothetical load, a force capacity of 15 pN can be achieved [122], comparable to that of other molecular machines like kinesin (5 pN) [123].

Dr. Nadrian Seeman and colleagues built the first artificial DNA-based structure in the form of a cube in 1991 [116,124]. They then went on to create more complex structures such as knots [125,126] and Borromean rings [127]. In addition to these individual constructs, 2D arrays [118,127,128] with the help of the double-crossover (DX) DNA molecule [129–131]. This DX molecule gave the structural rigidity required to create a dynamic molecular device, the B–Z switch [132]. DNA double helices can be of three types — the A, B, or the Z-DNA. The B-DNA is the natural, right-handed helical form of DNA, while the A-DNA is a shrunken, low-humidity form of the B-DNA. Z-DNA can be obtained from certain C–G base repeat sequences occurring in B-DNA that can take a left-handed double helical form [133]. The CG repeated base pair regions can be switched between the left and the right-handed conformations by changing ionic concentration [134]. The switch was designed in such a way that it had three cyclic strands of DNA, two of them wrapped around a central strand that had the CG-repeat region in the middle. On the two free ends of the side strands fluorescent dyes were attached in order to monitor the conformational change. With the change in ionic concentration the central CG-repeat sequence could alternate between the B and the Z modes bidirectionally which was observed through Förster resonance energy transfer (FRET) spectroscopy.

19.2.2.1 The DNA Tweezers

In 2000, Dr. Bernard Yurke and colleagues made an artificial DNA based molecular machine that also accepted DNA as a fuel [135]. The machine, called DNA tweezers, consisted of three strands of DNA labeled A, B, and C. Strands B and C are partially hybridized on to the central strand A with overhangs on both ends. This conformation of the machine is the open conformation. When an auxiliary fuel strand F is introduced, that is designed to hybridize with both overhang regions, the machine attains a closed conformation. The fuel strand is then removed from the system by the introduction of its exact complement, leaving the system to go back to its original open conformation. This way, a reversible motion is produced, which can be observed by attaching fluorescent tags to the two ends of the strand A. In this case the 5′ end was labeled with the dye TET (tetrachloro-fluorescein phosphoramidite) and the 3′ end was labeled with TAMRA (carboxy-tertamethylrhodamine). Aside from the creation of a completely new molecular machine, this showed a way of selective fueling of such machines. The fuel strands are sequence-specific, hence they will work on only those machines towards which they are directed, and not trigger other machines surrounding them. This machine was later improved to form a Three-State Device [136] which had two robust states and one flexible intermediate state. A variation of the tweezers came about as the DNA-scissors [137].

19.2.3 Inorganic (Chemical) Molecular Machines

In the past two decades, chemists have been able to create, modify, and control many different types of molecular machines. Many of these machines carry a striking resemblance with our everyday macroscale machines such as gears, propellers, shuttles, etc. Not only this, all of these machines are easy to synthesize artificially and are generally more robust than the natural molecular machines. Most of these machines are organic compounds of carbon, nitrogen, and hydrogen, with the presence of a metal ion being required occasionally. Electrostatic interactions, covalent and hydrogen bonding play essential role in the performance of these machines. Such artificial chemical machines are controllable in various ways — chemically, electrochemically, and photochemically (through irradiation by light). Some of them are even controllable by more than one way, rendering more flexibility and enhancing their utility. A scientist can have more freedom with respect to the design of chemical molecular machines depending on the performance requirements and conditions. Rotaxanes [138–140] and catenanes [141,142] make the basis of many of the molecular machines described in this section. These are families of interlocked organic molecular compounds with a distinctive shape and properties that guide their performance and control.

19.2.3.1 The Rotaxanes

The Rotaxane family of molecular machines is characterized by two parts — a dumbbell shaped compound with two heavy chemical groups at the ends and a light, cyclic component, called macrocycle, interlocked between the heads as shown in Figure 19.10. It has been shown [143] that a reversible switch can be made with a rotaxane setup. For this, one needs to have two chemically active recognition sites in the neck region of the dumbbell. In this particular example, the thread was made of polyether, marked by recognition sites hydroquinol units and terminated at the ends by large triisoproplylsilyl groups. A tetracationic bead was designed and self-assembled into the system that interacts with the recognition sites.

The macrocycle has a natural low energy state on the first recognition site, but can be switched among the two sites reversibly upon application of suitable stimuli. Depending on the type of rotaxane setup the stimuli can be chemical, electrochemical, or photochemical [144,145]. The stereo-electronic properties of the recognition sites can be altered by protonation or deprotonation, or by oxidation or reduction, thereby changing their affinity towards the macrocycle. In a recent example, light-induced acceleration of

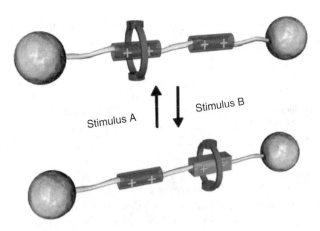

FIGURE 19.10 (See color insert.) A typical rotaxane shuttle set-up. The macrocycle encircles the thread-like portion of the dumbbell with heavy groups at its ends. The thread has two recognition sites which can be altered reversibly so as to make the macrocycle shuttle between the two sites (states 0 and 1).

rotaxane motion was achieved by photoisomerization [146], while similar controls through alternating current (oscillating electric fields) was shown before [147].

19.2.3.2 The Catenanes

The catenanes are also special type of interlocked structures that represent a growing family of molecular machines. They are synthesized by supramolecular assistance to molecular synthesis [148,149]. The general structure of a catenane is that of two interlocked ring-like components that are noncovalently linked via a mechanical bond, that is, they are held together without any valence forces. Both the macrocyclic components have recognition sites that are atoms of groups that are redox-active or photochemically reactive. It is possible to have both rings with similar recognition sites. In such a scenario, one of the rings may rotate inside the other with the conformations stabilized by noncovalent interactions, but the two states of the inner ring differing by 180° will be undistinguishable (degenerate) [150]. For better control and distinguishable molecular conformations, it is desirable to have different recognition sites within the macrocycles. Then they can be controlled independently through their own specific stimuli. The stereo-electronic property of one recognition site within a macrocycle can be varied such that at one point it has more affinity to the sites on the other ring. At this instant, the force balance will guide the rotating macrocycle for a stable conformation that requires that particular site to be inside the other macrocycle. Similarly, with other stimulus, this affinity can be turned off, or even reversed along with the affinity of the second recognition site on the rotating macrocycle increased towards those on the static one. There is a need for computational modeling, simulation, and analysis of such molecular machine motion [151]. Like rotaxanes, catenanes also can be designed for chemical, photochemical, or electrochemical control [152–156]. Figure 19.11 describes one such catenane molecular motor.

For both rotaxane and catenane-based molecular machines, it is desirable to have recognition sites such that they can be easily controlled externally. Hence, it is preferable to build sites that are either redox-active or photo-active [144]. Catenanes can also be self-assembled [157]. An example of catenane assembled molecular motors is the electronically controllable bistable switch [158]. An intuitive way of looking at catenanes is to think of them as molecular equivalents of ball and socket and universal joints [153,159,160].

Pseudorotaxanes are structures that contain a ring-like element and a thread-like element that can be "threaded" or "dethreaded" onto the ring upon application of various stimuli. Again, the stimuli can be chemical, photochemical, or electrochemical [161]. These contain a promise of forming molecular machine components analogous to switches and nuts and bolts from the macroscopic world.

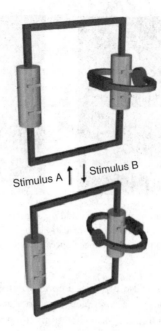

FIGURE 19.11 (See color insert.) A nondegenerate catenane. One of the rings (the moving ring) has two different recognition sites in it. Both sites can be turned "off" or "on" with different stimuli. When the green site is activated, the force and energy balance results in the first conformation, whereas when the red one is activated, the second conformation results. They can be named states 0 and 1 analogous to binary machine language.

19.2.3.3 Other Inorganic Molecular Machines

Many other molecular devices have been reported in the past four decades that bear a striking resemblance to macroscopic machinery. Chemical compounds behaving as bevel gears and propellers that were reported in the late 1960s and early 1970s are still being studied today [162–165]. A molecular propeller can be formed when two bulky rings such as the aryl rings [166] are connected to one central atom, often called the focal atom. Clockwise rotation of one such ring induces a counterclockwise rotation of the opposite ring about the bond connecting it to the central atom. It is possible to have a three-propeller system as well [167–169]. Triptycyl and amide ring systems have been shown to observe a coordinated gear-like rotation [170–174]. "Molecular Turnstiles" which are rotating plates inside a macrocycle, have been created [175,176]. Such rotations, however, were not controllable. A rotation of a molecular ring about a bond could be controlled by chemical stimuli, and this was shown by Kelly et al. [177] when they demonstrated a molecular brake. A propeller-like rotation of a 9-triptycyl ring system, which was used in gears, this time connected to a 2, 2'-bipyridine unit could be controlled by the addition and subsequent removal of a metal. Thus, free rotations along single bonds can be stopped and released at will.

Another type of molecular switch is the 1 "chiroptical molecular switch" [178]. Another large cyclic compound was found to be switchable between its two stable isomeric forms P and M' (right and left handed) stimulated by light. Depending on the frequency of light bombarded on it the *cis* and the *trans* conformations of the compound 4-[9'(2'-meth-oxythioxanthylidene)]-7-methyl-1,2,3,4-tetrahydrophenanthrene can be interconverted. Allowing a slight variation to this switch, a striking molecular motor driven by light or heat or both was introduced by Koumura et al. [179]. As opposed to the rotation around a single bond in the ratchet described above, the rotation was achieved around a carbon–carbon double bond in a helical alkene. Ultraviolet light or the change in temperature could trigger a rotation involving four isomerization steps in the compound (3R,3'R)-(P,P)-*trans*-1,1',2,2',3,3',4,4'-octahydro-3,3'-dimethyl-4,4',-biphenanthrylidene. A second generation motor along with eight other motors from the same material is now operational [180]. This redesigned motor has distinct upper and lower portions and it

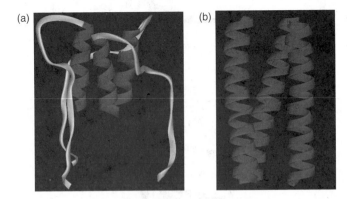

FIGURE 19.12   (See color insert.) VPL motor at (a) neutral and (b) acidic pH. (a) Front view of the partially α-helical triple stranded coiled coil. VPL motor is in the closed conformation. (b) VPL Motor in the open conformation. The random coil regions (white) are converted into well-defined helices and an extension occurs at lower pH.

operates at a higher speed. This motor also provides a good example of how controlled motion at the molecular level can be used to produce a macroscopic change in a system that is visible to the naked eye. The light-driven motors when inside liquid crystal (LC) films can produce a color change by inducing a reorganization of mesogenic molecules [181].

19.2.4   Other Protein-Based Motors Under Development

In this section we present two protein-based motors that are at initial developmental stages and yet possess some very original and interesting characteristics.

19.2.4.1   Viral Protein Linear Motors

The idea of Viral Protein Linear (VPL) motors [182] stems from the fact that families of retroviruses like the influenza virus [183] and the HIV-1 [184] has a typical mechanism of infecting a human cell. When such a virus comes near the cell it is believed that due to the environment surrounding the cell it experiences a drop in pH of its surroundings. This is a kind of a signal to the virus that its future host is near. The drop in pH changes the energetics of the outer (envelope glycoprotein) protein of the viral membrane in such a way that there is a distinct conformational change in a part of it [185,186]. A triple stranded coiled coil domain of the membrane protein changes conformation from a loose random structure to a distinctive α-helical conformation [187]. It is proposed to isolate this domain from the virus and trigger the conformational change by variation of pH *in vitro*. Once this is realized, attachments can be added to the N or C (or both) terminals of the peptide and a reversible linear motion can be achieved. Figure 19.12 shows a triple stranded coiled coil structure at a pH of 7.0; the inverted hairpin-like coils shown in the front view in Figure 19.12a and top view in Figure 19.12b change conformation into extended helical coils as seen in Figure 19.12b.

19.2.4.2   Synthetic Contractile Polymers

In a recent development, large plant proteins that can change conformation when stimulated by positively charged ions were separated from their natural environment and shown to exert forces in orthogonal directions [188,189]. Proteins from sieve elements of higher plants that are a part of the microfluidics system of the plant were chosen to build a new protein molecular machine element. These elements change conformations in the presence of Ca^{2+} ions and organize themselves inside the tubes so as to stop the fluid flow in case there is a rupture downstream. This is a natural defense mechanism seen in such plants. The change in conformation is akin to a balloon inflating and extending in its lateral as well as longitudinal directions. These elements, designated as "forisomes" adhered on to glass tubes were shown to reversibly swell in the presence of Ca^{2+} ions and shrink in their absence, hence performing a pulling/pushing action in both directions. Artificially prepared protein bodies like the forisomes could be a useful molecular machine component in a future molecular assembly, producing forces of the order of micronewtons [188]. Unlike the ATP-dependant motors discussed previously, these machine elements are more robust because they can perform in the absence of their natural environment as well.

19.3   Nanorobotics Design and Control

19.3.1   Design of Nanorobotic Systems

The design of nanorobotic systems requires the use of information from a vast variety of sciences ranging from quantum molecular dynamics to kinematic analysis. In this chapter we assume that the components of a nanorobot are made of biological components, such as, proteins and DNAs. So far, there does not exist any particular guideline or a prescribed manner, which details the methodology of designing a bio-nanorobot. There are many complexities, which are associated with using biocomponents (such as protein folding and presence of aqueous medium), but the advantages of using these are also quite considerable. These biocomponents offer immense variety and functionality at a scale where creating a man-made material with such capabilities would be extremely difficult. These biocomponents have been perfected by nature through millions of years of evolution and hence these are very accurate and efficient. As noted in the review section on molecular machines, F_1-ATPase is known to work at efficiencies which are close to 100%. Such efficiencies, variety, and form are not existent in any other form of material found today. Also, the other significant advantages in using protein-based bio-nanocomponents is the development and refinement over the last 30 years of tools and techniques that enable researchers to mutate proteins in almost any way imaginable. These mutations can consist of anything from simple amino acid side-chain swapping, to amino acid insertions or deletions, incorporation of nonnatural amino acids, and even the combination of unrelated peptide domains into whole new structures. An excellent example of this approach is the engineering of the F_1-ATPase, which is able to rotate a nanopropeller in the presence of ATP. A computational algorithm [190] was used to determine the mutations necessary to engineer an allosteric zinc-binding site into the F_1-ATPase using site-directed mutagenesis. The mutant F_1-ATPase was then shown to rotate an actin filament in the presence of ATP with average torque of 34 pN nm. This rotation could be stopped with the addition of zinc, and restored with the addition of a chelator to remove the zinc from the allosteric binding site [191]. This type of approach can be used for the improvement of other protein-based nanocomponents.

   Hence, these biocomponents seem to be a very logical choice for designing nanorobots. Some of the core applications of nanorobots are in the medical field and using biocomponents for these applications seems to be a good choice as they offer both efficiency and variety of functionality. This idea is clearly inspired by nature's construction of nanorobots, bacteria, and viruses which could be termed as *intelligent* organisms capable of movement, sensing, and organized control. Hence, our scope would be limited to the usage of these biocomponents in the construction of bio-nanorobotics. A roadmap is proposed which details the main steps towards the design and development of bio-nanorobots.

19.3.1.1   The Roadmap

The roadmap for the development of bio-nanorobotic systems for future applications (medical, space, and military) is shown in Figure 19.13. The roadmap progresses through the following main steps.

19.3.1.1.1   Step 1: Bio-Nanocomponents

Development of bio-nanocomponents from biological systems is the first step towards the design and development of an advanced bio-nanorobot, which could be used for future applications (see Figure 19.14). Since the planned systems and devices will be composed of these components, we must have a sound understanding of how these behave and how could they be controlled. From the simple elements such as structural links to more advanced concepts such as motors, each component must be carefully studied and possibly manipulated to understand the functional limits of each one of them. DNA and

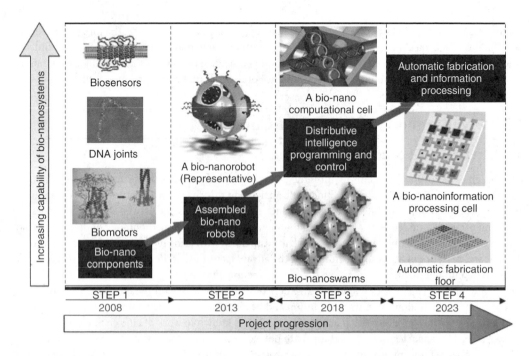

FIGURE 19.13   (See color insert.) The roadmap, illustrating the system capability targeted as the project progresses.

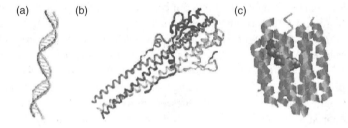

FIGURE 19.14   (See color insert.) (Step 1) 5 years from now — understanding of basic biological components and controlling their functions as robotic components. Examples are: (a) DNA which may be used in a variety of ways such as a structural element and a power source; (b) hemagglutinin virus may be used as a motor; (c) bacteriorhodopsin could be used as a sensor or a power source.

carbon nanotubes are being fabricated into various shapes, enabling possibilities of constructing newer and complex devices. These nanostructures are potential candidates for integrating and housing the bio-nanocomponents within them. Proteins such as *rhodopsin* and *bacteriorhodopsin* are a few examples of such bio-nanocomponents. Both these proteins are naturally found in biological systems as light sensors. They can essentially be used as solar collectors to gather abundant energy from the sun. This energy could either be harvested (in terms of proton motive force) for later use or could be consumed immediately by other components, such as the ATP Synthase nanorotary motor. The initial work is intended to be on the biosensors, such as, heat shock factor. These sensors will form an integral part of the proposed bio-nanoassemblies, where these will be integrated within a nanostructure and will get activated, as programmed, for gathering the required information at the nano scale. Tools and techniques from *molecular modeling* and *protein engineering* will be used to design these modular components.

19.3.1.1.2   Step 2: Assembled Bio-Nanorobots

The next step involves the assembly of functionally stable bio-nanocomponents into complex assemblies. Some examples of such complex assemblies or bio-nanorobots are shown in Figure 19.15. Figure 19.15a

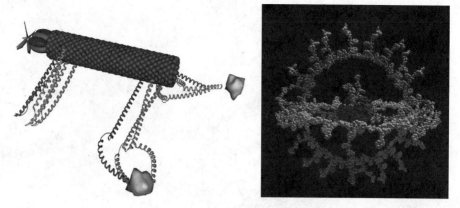

FIGURE 19.15   (See color insert.) (Step 2) (a) The bio-nanocomponents will be used to fabricate complex biorobotic systems. A vision of a nano-organism: carbon nanotubes form the main body; peptide limbs can be used for locomotion and object manipulation and the biomolecular motor located at the head can propel the device in various environments. (b) Modular organization concept for the bio-nanorobots. Spatial arrangements of the various modules of the robots are shown. A single bio-nanorobot will have actuation, sensory, and information processing capabilities.

shows a bio-nanorobot with its "*feet*" made of helical peptides and its body of carbon nano tubes, while the power unit is a biomolecular motor. Figure 19.15b shows a conceptual representation of *modular organization* of a bio-nanorobot. The modular organization defines the hierarchy rules and spatial arrangements of various modules of the bio-nanorobots such as: the inner core (the brain/energy source for the robot); the actuation unit; the sensory unit; and the signaling and information processing unit. By the beginning of this phase a "*library of bio-nanocomponents*" will be developed, which will include various categories such as, actuation, energy source, sensory, signaling, etc. Thereon, one will be able to design and develop such bio-nanosystems that will have enhanced mobile characteristics, and will be able to transport themselves as well as other objects to desired locations at nano scale. Furthermore, some bio-nanorobots will have the capability of assembling various biocomponents and nanostructures from *in situ* resources to house fabrication sites and storage areas, while others will just manipulate existing structures by repairing damaged walls or making other renovations. There will also be robots that not only perform physical labor, but also sense the environment and react accordingly. There will be systems that will sense an oxygen deprivation and stimulate other components to generate oxygen, creating an environment with stable homoeostasis.

19.3.1.1.3   Step 3: Distributive Intelligence Programming and Control
With the individual bio-nanorobots in full function, they will now need to collaborate with one another to further develop systems and "colonies" of similar and diverse nanorobots. This step will lay the foundation to the concept of *bio-nanoswarms* (distributive bio-nanorobots) (see Figure 19.16a). Here work has to be performed towards control and programming of bio-nanoswarms. This will evolve concepts like distributive intelligence in the context of bio-nanorobots. Designing swarms of bio-nanorobots capable of carrying out complex tasks and capable of computing and collaborating amongst the group will be the focus. Therefore, the basic computational architectures need to be developed and rules need to be evolved for the bio-nanorobots to make intelligent decisions at the nano scale.

To establish an interface with the macroworld, the computers and electronic hardware have to be designed as well. Figure 19.17 shows the overall electronic communication architecture. From a location, humans should be able to control and monitor the behavior and action of these swarms. Also, the basic computational capabilities required for functioning of the swarms will be developed. A representative computational bio-nanocell, which will be deployed within a bio-nanorobot, is shown in Figure 19.16b. This basic computational cell will initially be designed for data retrieval and storage at the nano scale. This capability will enable us to program (within certain degrees of freedom) the swarm behavior in the

(a)   (b)

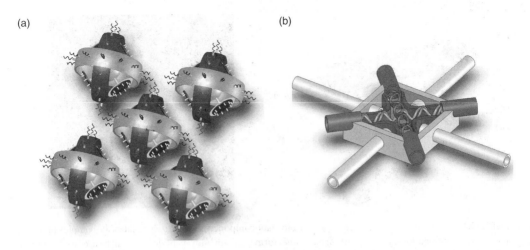

FIGURE 19.16   (See color insert.) (Step 3) (a) Basic bio-nanorobot forming a small swarm of five robots. The spatial arrangement of the individual bio-nanorobot will define the arrangement of the swarm. Also, these swarms could be re-programmed to form bindings with various other types of robots. The number of robots making a swarm will be dependent of the resulting capability required by the mission. Also the capability of attaching new robots at run time and replacing the nonfunctional robots will be added. (b) A basic bio-nanocomputational cell. This will be based on one of the properties of the biomolecules, which is "reversibility."

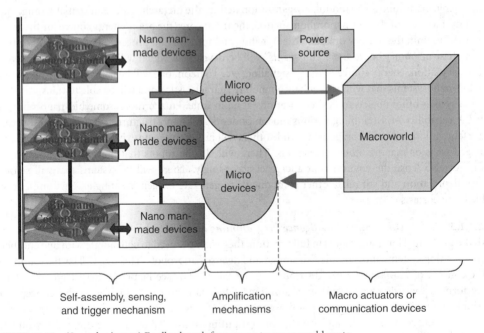

FIGURE 19.17   (See color insert.) Feedback path from nano to macroworld route.

bio-nanorobots. We will further be able to get their sensory data (from nanoworld) back to the macroworld through these storage devices. This programming capability would form the core essence of a bio-nanorobotics system and hence enables them with immense power.

19.3.1.1.4 Step 4: Automatic Fabrication and Information Processing Machines
For carrying out complex missions, such as sensing, signaling, and storing, colonies of these bio-nanorobotic swarms need to be created. The next step in nanorobotic designing would see the emergence

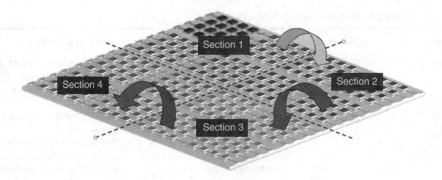

FIGURE 19.18 (See color insert.) (Step 4) 20–30 years — an automatic fabrication floor layout. Different color represents different functions in automatic fabrication mechanisms. The arrows indicate the flow of components on the floor layout. *Section 1* → Basic stimuli storage — control expression; *Section 2* → Biomolecular component manufacturing (actuator/sensor); *Section 3* → Linking of bio-nanocomponents; *Section 4* → Fabrication of bio-nanorobots (assemblage of linked bio-nanocomponents).

of automatic fabrication methodologies (see Figure 19.18) of such bio-nanorobots *in vivo* and *in vitro*. Capability of information processing, which will involve learning and decision making abilities, will be a key consideration of this step. This would enable bioswarms to have capability of *self-evolving* based on the environment they will be subjected to. These swarms could be programmed to search for *alternate* energy sources and would have an ability to adapt as per that resource. Energy management, self-repairing, and evolving will be some of the characteristics of these swarms.

19.3.1.2 Design Philosophy and Architecture for the Bio-Nanorobotic Systems

19.3.1.2.1 Modular Organization

Modular organization defines the fundamental rule and hierarchy for constructing a bio-nanorobotic system. Such construction is performed through *stable integration* of the individual "*bio-modules or components*," which constitute the bio-nanorobot. For example, if the entity ABCD, defines a bio-nanorobot having some *functional specificity* (as per the capability matrix defined in Table 19.1) then, A, B, C, and D are said to be the basic biomodules defining it. The basic construction will be based on the techniques of molecular modeling with emphasis on principles such as *Energy Minimization* on the hyper surfaces of the biomodules; *Hybrid Quantum-Mechanical and Molecular Mechanical* methods; *Empirical Force field* methods; and *Maximum Entropy Production* in least time.

Modular organization also enables the bio-nanorobots with capabilities such as, organizing into *swarms*, a feature, which is extremely desirable for various applications. Figure 19.19a,b shows the conceptual representation of modular organization. Figure 19.19c shows a more realistic scenario in which all the modules are defined in some particular spatial arrangements based on their functionality and structure. A particular module could consist of other group of modules, just like a fractal structure (defined as *fractal modularity*). The concept of *bio-nanocode* has been devised, which basically describes the unique functionality of a bio-nanocomponent in terms of alphabetic codes. Each bio-nanocode represents a particular module defining the structure of the bio-nanorobot. For instance, a code like E-M-S will describe a bio-nanorobot having capabilities of energy storage, mechanical actuation, and signaling at the nano scale. Such representations will help in general classifications and representative mathematics of bio-nanorobots and their swarms. Table 19.1 summarizes the proposed capabilities of the biomodules along with their targeted general applications. The bio-nanocode EIWR‖M‖S‖FG representing the bio-nanosystem shown in Figure 19.19b which could be decoded as shown in Figure 19.20. This depicts the "*Fractal modularity*" principle of the proposed concept.

19.3.1.2.2 The Universal Template — Bio-Nano-Stem System

The modular construction concept involves designing a universal template for bio-nanosystems, which could be "programmed and grown" into any possible bio-nanocoded system. This concept mimics the

TABLE 19.1   Defining the Capability Matrix for the Biomodules

Functionality	Bionanocode	Capabilities targeted	General applications
Energy storage and carrier	E	Ability to store energy from various sources such as, solar, chemical for future usage and for its own working	Required for the working of all the biochemical mechanisms of the proposed bio-nanorobotic systems
Mechanical	M	Ability to precisely move and orient other molecules or modules at nano scale. This includes ability to mechanically bind to various target objects, and carry them at desired location	Carry drugs and deliver it to the precise locations Move micro world objects with nanoprecision. For example, *Parallel platforms* for nanoorientation and displacements
Sensory	S	Sensing capabilities in various domains such as, chemical, mechanical, visual, auditory, electrical, and magnetic	Evaluation and discovery of target locations based on either chemical properties, temperature, or other characteristics
Signaling	G	Ability to amplify the sensory data and communicate with biosystems or with the microcontrollers. Capability to identify their locations through various trigger mechanisms such as fluorescence	Imaging for medical applications or for imaging changes in nanostructures
Information storage	F	Ability to store information collected by the sensory element Behave similar to a read–write mechanism in computer field	Store the sensory data for future signaling or usage Read the stored data to carry out programmed functions Backbone for the sensory bio-module Store nanoworld phenomenon currently not observed with ease
Swarm behavior	W	Exhibit binding capabilities with "similar" bio-nanorobots so as to perform distributive sensing, intelligence, and action (energy storage) functions	All the tasks to be performed by the bio-nanorobots will be planned and programmed keeping in mind the swarm behavior and capabilities
Bio-nanointelligence	I	Capability of making decisions and performing intelligent functions	Ability to make decision
Replication	R	Replicate themselves when required	Replicate at the target site Replication of a particular biomodule as per the demand of the situation

embryonic stem cells (bio-nanosystem would mimic this property and hence the name bio-nano-stem system) found in the human beings, that are a kind of primitive human cells which give rise to all other specialized tissues found in a human fetus, and ultimately to all the three trillion cells in an adult human body. Our bio-nano-stem system will act in a similar way. This universal growth template will be constituted of some basic bio-nanocodes, which will define the bio-nano-stem system. This stem system will be designed in a manner that could enable it to be programmed at run-time to any other required biomodule. Figure 19.21 shows one such variant of the bio-nano-stem system, having the bio-nanocode: EIWR∥M∥S∥FG and having enhanced sensory abilities.

19.3.1.3   Computational and Experimental Tools for Studying Bio-Nanorobotic Systems
19.3.1.3.1   *Computational Methods* [192–194]
Molecular modeling techniques in sync with extensive experimentations will form the basis for studying bio-nanorobotic systems. Some of the molecular modeling techniques that can be used are described below.

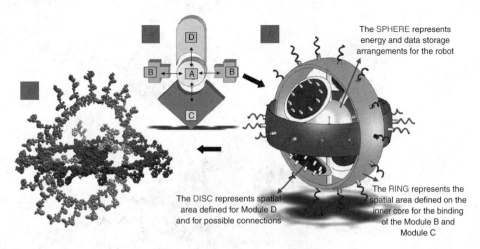

FIGURE 19.19 (See color insert.) (a) A bio-nanorobotic Entity "ABCD," where A, B, C, and D are the various biomodules constituting the bio-nanorobot. In our case these biomodules will be set of stable configurations of various proteins and DNAs. (b) A bio-nanorobot (representative), as a result of the concept of modular organization. All the modules will be integrated in such a way so as to preserve the basic behavior (of self-assembly, self-replication, and self-organization) of the biocomponents at all the hierarchies. The number of modules employed is not limited to four or any number. It is a function of the various capabilities required for a particular mission. (c) A molecular representation of the figure (b). It shows the red core and green and blue sensory and actuation biomodules.

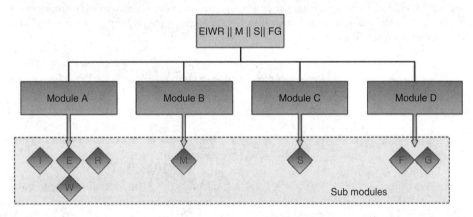

FIGURE 19.20 (See color insert.) The bio-nanocode and the fractal modularity principle. The letter symbols have the values specified in Table 19.1. The "‖" symbol integrates the various biomodules and collectively represents a higher order module or a bio-nanorobot.

19.3.1.3.1.1 Empirical Force Field Methods: (Molecular Mechanics) — In this method, the motion of the electrons is ignored and the energy of the system is calculated based on the position of the nucleus in a particular molecular configuration. There are several approximations which are used in this method with the very basic being the Born–Oppenheimer. The modeling of bio-nanocomponents or their assemblies could be done using one of the energy functions:

$$V(r^N) = \sum_{\text{bonds}} \frac{k_i}{2}(l_i - l_{i,0})^2 + \sum_{\text{angles}} \frac{k_i}{2}(\theta_i - \theta_{i,0})^2 + \sum_{\text{torsions}} \frac{v_n}{2}(1 + \cos(n\omega - \gamma))$$

$$+ \sum_{i=1}^{N} \sum_{j=i+1}^{N} \left(4\varepsilon_{ij} \left[\left(\frac{\sigma_{ij}}{r_{ij}}\right)^{12} - \left(\frac{\sigma_{ij}}{r_{ij}}\right)^{6} \right] + \frac{q_i q_j}{4\pi \varepsilon_0 r_{ij}} \right)$$

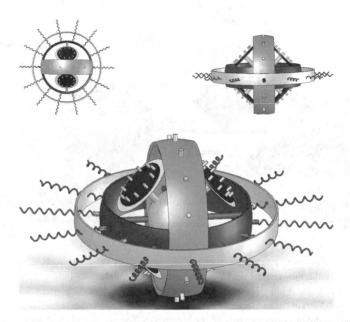

FIGURE 19.21   (See color insert.) A variant of the initial bio-nano-stem system, see Figure 19.19b, fabricated with enhanced bio-nanocode S, which defines it as a bio-nanorobot having enhanced sensory capabilities. The other features could be either suppressed or enhanced depending upon the requirement at hand. The main advantage of using bio-nano-stem system is that we could at run-time decide which particular type of bio-nanorobots we require for a given situation. The suppression ability of the bio-nano-stem systems is due to the property of "*Reversibility*" of the bio components found in living systems.

where $V(r^N)$ denotes the potential energy of N particles having position vector (**r**). The terms of the previous equation are:

$\sum\limits_{\text{bonds}} \frac{k_i}{2}(l_i - l_{i,0})^2$ Denotes the energy variations due to bond extension

$\sum\limits_{\text{angles}} \frac{k_i}{2}(\theta_i - \theta_{i,0})^2$ Denotes the energy variations due to bond angle bending

$\sum\limits_{\text{torsions}} \frac{v_n}{2}(1 + \cos(n\omega - \gamma))$ Denotes the energy variations due to bond torsion

$\sum\limits_{i=1}^{N}\sum\limits_{j=i+1}^{N}\left(4\varepsilon_{ij}\left[\left(\frac{\sigma_{ij}}{r_{ij}}\right)^{12} - \left(\frac{\sigma_{ij}}{r_{ij}}\right)^{6}\right] + \frac{q_i q_j}{4\pi\varepsilon_o r_{ij}}\right)$ Denotes the energy variation due to nonbonded terms, usually modeled using Coulomb's potential

19.3.1.3.1.2 Energy Minimization Methods — The potential energy depends upon the coordinates of the molecular configuration considered. In this method, points on the *hypersurface* (potential energy surface) are calculated for which the function has the minimum value. Such geometries, which correspond to the minimum energy, are the stable states of the molecular configuration considered. By this method we can also analyze the change in the configuration of the system from one minimum state to another. Methods such as the Newton–Raphson and Quasi-Newton are employed to calculate these minima. This method of finding minimum energy points in the molecule is used to prepare for other advanced calculations such as molecular dynamics or Monte-Carlo simulations. It is further used to predict various properties of the system under study.

19.3.1.3.1.3 Molecular Dynamics Simulation Methods — To begin predicting the dynamic performance (i.e., energy and force calculation) of a biocomponent (say a peptide) molecular dynamics (MD) is performed. This method utilizes Newton's Law of motion through the successive configuration of the system to determine its dynamics. Another variant of molecular dynamics employed in the industry is the Monte-Carlo simulation, which utilizes stochastic approaches to generate the required configuration of a system. Simulations are performed based on the calculation of the free energy that is released during the transition from one configuration state to the other (e.g., using the MD software CHARMM, Chemistry at Harvard Molecular Mechanics [195]). In MD, the feasibility of a particular conformation of a biomolecule is dictated by the energy constraints. Hence, a transition from one given state to another must be energetically favorable, unless there is an external impetus that helps the molecule overcome the energy barrier. When a macromolecule changes conformation, the interactions of its individual atoms with each other — as well as with the solvent — constitute a very complex force system. With one of the aspects of CHARMM, it is possible to model say, a peptide based on its amino acid sequence and allow a transition between two known states of the protein using targeted molecular dynamics (TMD) [196]. TMD is used for approximate modeling of processes spanning long time-scales and relatively large displacements.

19.3.1.3.1.4 Molecular Kinematic Simulations — They are also being used to study the geometric properties and conformational space of the biomolecules (peptides). The kinematic analysis is based on the development of direct and inverse kinematic models and their use towards the workspace analysis of the biomolecules. This computational study calculates all geometrically feasible conformations of the biomolecule, that is, all conformations that can be achieved without any atom interference. This analysis suggests the geometric paths that could be followed by a biomolecule during the transition from the initial to a final state, while molecular dynamics narrow downs the possibilities by identifying the only energetically feasible paths. The workspace analysis also characterizes the geometrically feasible workspace in terms of dexterity.

19.3.1.3.1.5 Modular Pattern Recognition and Clustering Function — The instantaneous value of the *property A* of a molecular system can be written as $A(p^n(t), r^n(t))$, where $p^n(t)$ and $r^n(t)$ represent the n momenta and positions of a molecular system at time t. This instantaneous value would vary with respect to the interactions between the particles. There are two parts to this function (termed as M function). One part (function A), evaluates and hence recognizes the equivalent modules (in term of properties) in the molecular system. The second part of the function (D) forms the cluster (like a bioisosteres, which are atom, molecules, or functional groups with similar physical and chemical properties) of various modular patterns according to the characteristic behaviors as identified by function A and also tracks their variations with rest to time.

$$M \equiv \{A(p^n(t), r^n(t), C^n[n]), D(A(p, r, C, t), f(x, y, \ldots), Bn(t))\}$$

where, A *is the first part* of the function; $p^n(t)$ and $r^n(t)$ represents the n momenta and positions of a molecular system at time t; and $C^n[n]$ is an n-dimensional matrix element for the individual components of the molecular system, which would store the categorized values of the modular patterns. D is the second part of the function, and it takes on function A recursively. It also maps these clusters based on a fitness function and stores the time-variant value in subfunction B. Figure 19.22 represents the conceptual version of the M-function.

This function is based on the hypothesis that in a complex molecular system, there are certain parts, which have similar properties and behavior as the system goes from one state to the other. By identifying these property patterns we can considerably reduce the simulation and computational

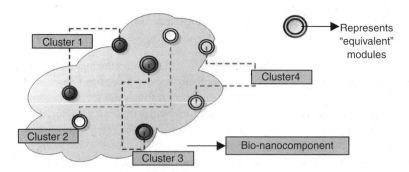

FIGURE 19.22 (See color insert.) Representing the modular pattern recognition and clustering function (the *M*-function.)

time frames and can have better predictability of the system. Having established the design for the bio-nanocomponents, computational studies would focus on determining the overall design and architecture of the bio-nanoassemblies. One of the methods used in the industry is of molecular docking.

19.3.1.3.1.6 Molecular Docking and Scoring Functions — The molecular docking method is very important for the design of nanorobotic systems. This method is utilized to fit two molecules together in 3D space [197]. The method of molecular docking could be used to computationally design the bio-nanoassemblies. The algorithms like DOCK, genetic algorithms and distance geometry are being specifically explored. Many drug-design companies are using depth-first systematic conformational search algorithms for docking, and therefore, is a primary candidate for current research. The docking algorithm generates a large number of solutions. Therefore, we require scoring functions to refine the results so produced. Scoring functions in use today approximate the "*binding free energy*" of the molecules. The free energy of binding can be written as an additive equation of various components reflecting the various contributions to binding. A typical equation would be:

$$\Delta G_{\text{bind}} = \Delta G_{\text{solvent}} + \Delta G_{\text{cont}} + \Delta G_{\text{int}} + \Delta G_{\text{rot}} + \Delta G_{t/r} + \Delta G_{\text{vib}}$$

where, $\Delta G_{\text{solvent}}$ is the solvent effects contribution, ΔG_{conf} is due to conformational changes in the bio-molecule, ΔG_{int} due to specific molecular interactions, ΔG_{rot} due to restrictive internal rotation of the binding bio-molecules, $\Delta G_{t/r}$ is due to loss in the translational and rotational free energies due to binding, and ΔG_{vib} is due to vibrational mode variations. Once the overall architecture to bind the bio-nanocomponents is carried out through molecular docking, we will need to combine the components into real assemblies. The molecular component binding is the next step in the design scheme.

19.3.1.3.1.7 Connecting Bio-Nanocomponents in a Binding Site — There are typically two approaches to design connectors for binding the bio-nanocomponents. One method searches the molecular database and selects a connector based on geometrical parameters. CAVEAT is a traditional routine, which employs this method. The other approach is to design a connector from scratch atom by atom. The geometrical parameters being known (as the configuration and the architecture was defined by molecular docking) these connectors are designed. A typical method employs designing molecular templates (which do not interfere with the basic geometry and design of the binding bio-nanocomponents) for defining a basic connector for binding the bio-nanocomponents. Feasibility of designing these connectors in real life is one challenge faced by molecular modelers. The minimum energy criterion is employed via the Metropolis Monte-Carlo simulation annealing method to select the basic structure of the final connector. Genetic algorithm approaches are also employed to generate such designs.

19.3.1.3.2 Experimental Methods

The step 1 in the roadmap requires that we have a library of biocomponents, which are characterized based on their potentials for using them for developing nanorobots. Various molecular techniques could be employed for assessing the usefulness of the biocomponents. For developing a nanorobot, we require the knowledge of the structure of the biocomponents used and the degree of conformational change that each element is capable of undergoing, and the environmental cues (e.g., T, pH) that induce these structural changes. Based on the computational methods detailed in the previous section, the following experimental techniques could be used to obtain this information.

19.3.1.3.2.1 Circular Dichroism Spectroscopy (CD) — CD spectroscopy can be utilized to gain insights into the secondary structure of each biomolecule such as peptides. In this technique, polarized far-UV light is used to probe the extent of secondary structure formation in solutions. This technique represents a proven method for estimating the structural composition of the nanorobotic elements during a change in environmental conditions. The effect of temperature on the structure of the nanorobotic elements can be evaluated by cooling the samples to $+1°C$ and then heating to $+85°C$, with a 5-min equilibration at each temperature interval. Intervals could be determined by first conducting CD scans with broad intervals, with subsequent narrowing as the location of the transition is identified. The effect of pH and ionic strength on the transitions could be monitored using separate, equilibrated preparations for each condition.

19.3.1.3.2.2 Förster Resonance Energy Transfer — Another method that can be used to rapidly assess the extent of conformational changes by the nanorobotic elements is FRET. In order to employ this method, the nanorobotic components have to be engineered to have cysteine residues at both ends. One end of the biocomponent then has to be labeled with a donor dye molecule (Alexa Fluor 488, Molecular Probes), and the other end labeled with an acceptor dye molecule (Alexa Fluor 594). The resulting FRET signal can be monitored with a laser (488 nm), whereby the signal changes would depend on the spatial separation of the ends of the bio component.

19.3.1.3.2.3 Nuclear Magnetic Resonance (NMR) — NMR is utilized to determine the exact 3D structure of the nanorobotic components. Although CD spectroscopy can be used to estimate the changes in the structural composition of the bio components, it does not provide the exact 3D configuration. This information can be obtained through the use NMR spectroscopy and the labeling of the biocomponent with NMR-active atoms. In addition to determining the endpoint structures of the components, NMR can also be used to follow the kinetics of the biomolecule conformational changes, in real time.

19.3.1.3.2.4 Laser-Based Optical Tweezers (LBOT) and Single-Molecule Fluorescence — LBOT and single-molecule fluorescence could be used to estimate the forces exerted by the nanorobotic elements, and the structural changes that occur during the genesis of these forces, after exposure to different stimuli. LBOT can provide force and displacement results with a resolution of sub-picoNewton and approximately one nanometer, respectively. Single-molecule fluorescence measurements, based on the previously described FRET method, can simultaneously provide information about the structural state of the molecule at each point of the force–displacement curve. To correlate force measurements with structural changes, combination of the LBOT method with FRET can be used [198]. The recent development of this technique has enabled the simultaneous assessment of nanoscale structural changes and their associated biomechanical forces.

19.3.1.4 Nanomanipulation — Virtual Reality-Based Design Techniques

For scanning and manipulating matter at the nanoscale, scanning tunneling microscopy (STM) [199], scanning electron microscopy (SEM), atomic force microscopy (AFM) [197] and scanned-probe microscope (SPM) [201] seem to be the common tools. Current work is mainly focused on using AFM nanoprobes for teleoperated physical interactions and manipulation at the nano scale. Precise manipulation could help scientists better understand the principles of nanorobots [202,203].

To achieve this it is essential to visualize the atom-to-atom interaction in real time and see the results in a fully immersive 3D environment. Also, to facilitate user input in nanorobotic systems it is essential to develop voice, gesture, and touch recognition features in addition to the conventional visualization and manipulation techniques. Virtual reality technology is applied here, which not only provides immersive visualization but also gives an added functionality of *navigation* and *interactive manipulation* of molecular graphical objects. VR technology comes to our aid by providing the experience of perception and interaction with the nanoworld through the use of sensors, effectors and interfaces in a simulated environment. These interfaces transform the signals occurring at nanoscale processes into signals at macrolevel and vice-versa. The requirement is that the communication with the nanoworld must be at high level and in real time, preferably in a natural, possibly intuitive "language." Considering the nanospecific problems related to task application, tools, and the interconnection technologies it leads to many flexible nanomanipulation concepts. They can range from pure master/slave teleoperation (through 3D visual/VR or haptic force feedback or both), over shared autonomy control (where, e.g., some degrees of freedom are teleoperated and other are operating autonomously) to fully autonomous operation.

In order to precisely control and manipulate biomolecules, we need tools that can interact with these objects at the nano scale in their native environments [204,205]. Existing bio-nanomanipulation techniques can be classified as noncontact manipulations including laser trapping [206,207] and electro-rotation [208], and contact manipulation referred to as mechanical stylus-, AFM-, or STM-based nanomanipulation [209]. The rapid expansion of AFM studies in biology/biotechnology results from the fact that AFM techniques offer several unique advantages: *first*, they require little sample preparation, with native biomolecules usually being imaged directly; *second*, they can provide a 3D reconstruction of the sample surface in real space at ultra-high resolution; *third*, they are less destructive than other techniques (e.g., electron microscopy) commonly employed in biology; and *fourth*, they can operate in several environments, including air, liquid, and vacuum. Rather than drying the sample, one can image quite successfully with AFM in fluid. The operation of AFM in aqueous solution offers an unprecedented opportunity for imaging biological molecules and cells in their physiological environments and for studying biologically important dynamic processes in real time [210].

Currently, these bio-nanomanipulations are conducted manually, however, long training, disappointingly low success rates from poor reproducibility in manual operations, and contamination call for the elimination of direct human involvement. Furthermore, there are many sources of spatial uncertainty in AFM manipulation, for example, tip effects, thermal drift, slow creeping motion, and hysteresis. To improve the bio-nanomanipulation techniques, automatic manipulation must be addressed. Visual tracking of patterns from multiple views is a promising approach, which is currently investigated in autonomous embryo pronuclei DNA injection [210]. Interactive nanomanipulation can be improved by imaging 3D viewpoint in a virtual environment. Construction of a VR space in an off-line operation mode for trajectory planning combined with a real-time operation mode for vision tracking of environmental change ensures a complete "immersed" visual display. Figure 19.23 shows an example of 3D bio-micro/nanomanipulation system with a 3D VR model of the environment including the biocell, and carrying out the user viewpoint change in the virtual space [211].

19.3.1.4.1 Molecular Dynamics Simulations in Virtual Environment

Molecular dynamics simulations of complex molecular systems require enormous computational power and produces large amount of data in each step. The resulting data includes number of atoms per unit volume, atomic positions, velocity of each atom, force applied on each atom, and the energy contents. These results of MD simulations need to be visualized to give the user a more intuitive feel of what is happening. Haptic interaction used in conjunction with VR visualization helps the scientist to control/monitor the simulation progress and to get feedback from the simulation process as well [212]. Figure 19.24 shows the virtual reality visualization of molecular dynamics simulation. Figure 19.25 shows a VR representation of MD simulations in CAVE virtual environment.

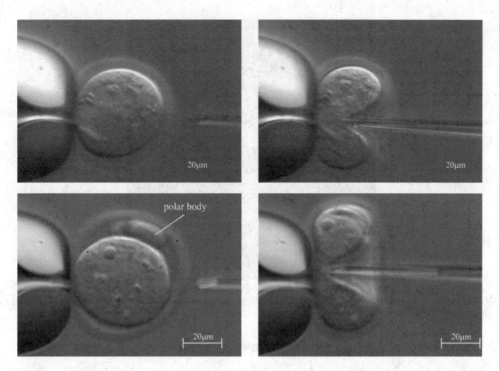

FIGURE 19.23 Haptic force measurement process on the Zona pellucida of mouse oocytes and embryos. (Courtesy of Dr. Brad Nelson, Swiss Federal Institute of Technology [ETH], Zurich and ©2003 IEEE.)

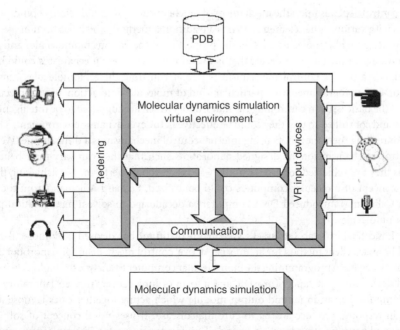

FIGURE 19.24 A block diagram showing virtual environment for molecular dynamics simulations (Reprinted from Z. Ai and T. Frohlich, *Molecular Dynamics Simulation in Virtual Environment*, Computer Graphics Forum, Volume 17, September 1998. With permission from Eurographics Association.)

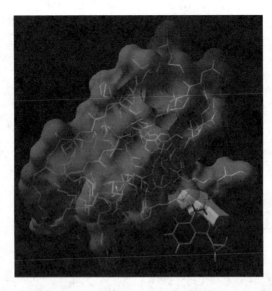

FIGURE 19.25   (See color insert.) Molecular dynamics simulation visualized in the CAVE. (Courtesy of Dr. Zhuming Ai, VRMedLab, University of Illinois at Chicago.)

19.3.2   Control of Nanorobotic Systems

The control of nanorobotic systems could be classified in two categories:

1. Internal control mechanisms
2. External control mechanisms

Another category could be a hybrid of internal and external control mechanisms.

19.3.2.1   Internal Control Mechanism — Active and Passive

This type of control depends upon the mechanism of biochemical sensing and selective binding of various biomolecules with various other elements. This is a traditional method, which has been in use since quite sometime for designing biomolecules. Using the properties of the various biomolecules and combining with the knowledge of the target molecule that is to be influenced, these mechanisms could be effective. But again, this is a passive control mechanism where at run time these biomolecules cannot change their behavior. Once programmed for a particular kind of molecular interaction, these molecules stick to that. Here lies the basic issue in controlling the nanorobots which are supposed to be intelligent and hence programmed and controlled so that they could be effective in the ever dynamic environment. The question of actively controlling the nanorobots using internal control mechanism is a difficult one. We require an "active" control mechanism for the designed nanorobots such that they can vary their behavior based on situations they are subjected to, similar to the way macrorobots perform. For achieving this internal control, the concept of molecular computers could be utilized. Leonard Adleman (from the University of Southern California) introduced DNA computers a decade ago to solve a mathematical problem by utilizing DNA molecules.

Professor Ehud Shapiro's lab (at Israel's Weizmann Institute) has devised a biomolecular computer which could be an excellent method for an internal 'active' control mechanism for nanorobots. They have recently been successful in programming the biomolecular computer to analyze the biological information, which could detect and treat cancer (prostate and a form of lung cancer) in their laboratory [213]. The molecular computer has an input and output module which acting together can diagnose a particular disease and in response produce a drug to cure that disease. It uses novel concept of software (made up of DNAs) and hardware (made up of enzymes) molecular elements. This molecular computer is in generalized form and can be used for any disease which produces a particular pattern of gene expression related to it [214].

19.3.2.2   External Control Mechanism

This type of control mechanism employs affecting the dynamics of the nanorobot in its work environment through the application of external potential fields. Researchers are actively looking at using MRI as an external control mechanism for guiding the nanoparticles. Professor Sylvain Martel's NanoRobotics Laboratory (at École Polytechnique de Montréal, Canada) is actively looking at using MRI system as a mean of propulsion for nanorobots. An MRI system is capable of generating variable magnetic field gradients, which can exert force on the nanorobot in the three dimensions and hence control its movement and orientation. Professor Martel's laboratory is exploring effect of such variable magnetic field on a ferromagnetic core that could probably be embedded into the nanorobots [215].

Other possibilities being explored are in the category of "hybrid" control mechanisms where the target is located and fixed by an external navigational system [216] but the behavior of the nanorobot is determined locally through an active internal control mechanism. The use of nanosensors and evolutionary agents to determine the nanorobots behavior is suggested by the mentioned reference.

19.4   Conclusions

Manipulating matter at molecular scale and influencing their behavior (dynamics and properties) is the biggest challenges for the nanorobotic systems. This field is still in very early stages of development and still a lot has to be figured out before any substantial outcome is produced.

The recent explosion of research in nanotechnology, combined with important discoveries in molecular biology have created a new interest in bio-nanorobotic systems. The preliminary goal in this field is to use various biological elements — whose function at the cellular level creates a motion, force, or a signal — as nanorobotic components that perform the same function in response to the same biological stimuli but in an artificial setting. In this way proteins and DNA could act as motors, mechanical joints, transmission elements, or sensors. If all these different components were assembled together they can form nanorobots and nanodevices with multiple degrees of freedom, with ability to apply forces and manipulate objects in the nanoscale world, transfer information from the nano- to the macroscale world and even travel in a nanoscale environment.

The ability to determine the structure, behavior, and properties of the nanocomponents is the first step which requires focused research thrust. Only when the preliminary results on these nanocomponents are achieved, steps toward actually building complex assemblies could be thought of. Still problems like protein (i.e., a basic bio-nanocomponent) folding and the precise mechanism behind the operation of the molecular motors like ATP Synthase have to be solved. The active control of nanorobots has to be further refined. Hybrid control mechanisms, wherein, a molecular computer and external (navigational) control system work in sync to produce the precise results seem very promising. Further, concepts like swarm behavior in context of nanorobotics is still to be worked out. As it would require colonies of such nanorobots for accomplishing a particular task, the concepts of cooperative behavior and distributed intelligence have to be evolved.

The future of bio-nanorobots (molecular robots) is bright. We are at the dawn of a new era in which many disciplines will merge including robotics, mechanical, chemical and biomedical engineering, chemistry, biology, physics, and mathematics so that fully functional systems will be developed. However, challenges towards such a goal abound. Developing a complete database of different biomolecular machine components and the ability to interface or assemble different machine components are some of the challenges to be faced in the near future.

References

[1] Drexler Eric K. 1992. *Nanosystems: Molecular Machinery, Manufacturing and Computation*, John Wiley & Sons.

[2] Kinosita K., Jr., Yasuda R., Noji H., and Adachi K. 2000. A rotary molecular motor that can work at near 100% efficiency. *Philos. Trans.: Biol. Sci.* 355: 473–489.

[3] Mavroidis C., Dubey A., and Yarmush M.L. 2004. Molecular machines. *Annu. Rev. Biomed. Eng.* 6: 10.1–10.33.

[4] Antony Crofts, Lecture 10, ATP Synthase. University of Illinois at Urbana-Champaign, http://www.life.uiuc.edu/crofts/bioph354/lect10.html

[5] Lubert S. 1995. *Biochemistry*, 4th ed., W.H. Freeman and Company.

[6] Itoh H., Takahashi A., Adachi K., Noji H., Yasuda R., Yoshida M., and Kinosita K., Jr. 2004. Mechanically driven ATP synthesis by F_1-ATPase. *Nature* 427: 465–468.

[7] Howard J. 1997. Molecular motors: structural adaptations to cellular functions. *Nature* 389: 561–567.

[8] Vale R. 1996. Switches, latches, and amplifiers: common themes of G proteins and molecular motors. *J. Cell Biol.* 135: 291–302.

[9] Farrell C.M., Mackey A.T., Klumpp L.M., and Gilbert S.P. 2002. The role of ATP hydrolysis for kinesin processivity. *J. Biol. Chem.* 277: 17079–17087.

[10] Vale R.D. and Milligan R.A. 2000. The way things move: looking under the hood of molecular motor proteins. *Science* 288: 88–95.

[11] Block S.M., Goldstein L.S., and Schnapp B.J. 1990. Bead movement by single kinesin molecules studied with optical tweezers. *Nature* 348: 348–352.

[12] Howard J., Hudspeth A.J., and Vale R.D. 1989. Movement of microtubules by single kinesin molecules. *Nature* 342: 154–158.

[13] Finer J.T., Simmons R.M., and Spudich J.A. 1994. Single myosin molecule mechanics: piconewton forces and nanometre steps. *Nature* 368: 113–119.

[14] Hackney D.D. 1996. The kinetic cycles of myosin, kinesin, and dynein. *Annu. Rev. Physiol.* 58: 731–750.

[15] Block S.M. 1998. Kinesin, what gives? *Cell* 93: 5–8.

[16] Kull F.J., Sablin E.P., Lau R., Fletterick R.J., and Vale R.D. 1996. Crystal structure of the kinesin motor domain reveals a structural similarity to myosin. *Nature* 380: 550–555.

[17] Sellers J.R. 2000. Myosins: a diverse superfamily. *Biochim. Biophys. Acta (BBA) — Mol. Cell Res.* 1496: 3–22.

[18] Howard J. 1994. Molecular motors. Clamping down on myosin. *Nature* 368: 98–99.

[19] Huxley H.E. 1957. The double array of filaments in cross-striated muscle. *J. Biophys. Biochem. Cytol.* 3: 631–648.

[20] Huxley H.E. 1953. Electron microscope studies of the organisation of the filaments in striated muscle. *Biochim. Biophys. Acta* 12: 387–394.

[21] Hanson J. and Huxley H.E. 1953. Structural basis of the cross-striations in muscle. *Nature* 153: 530–532.

[22] Huxley H.E. 1969. The mechanism of muscular contraction. *Science* 164: 1356–1365.

[23] Lymn R.W. and Taylor E.W. 1971. Mechanism of adenosine triphosphate hydrolysis by actomyosin. *Biochemistry* 10: 4617–4624.

[24] For videos of myosin and kinesin movement visit http://sciencemag.org/feature/data/1049155.shl

[25] Lowey S., Slayter H.S., Weeds A.G., and Baker H. 1969. Substructure of the myosin molecule. I. Subfragments of myosin by enzymic degradation. *J. Mol. Biol.* 42: 1–29.

[26] Weeds A.G. and Lowey S. 1971. Substructure of the myosin molecule. II. The light chains of myosin. *J. Mol. Biol.* 61: 701–725.

[27] Wagner P.D. and Giniger E. 1981. Hydrolysis of ATP and reversible binding to F-actin by myosin heavy chains free of all light chains. *Nature* 292: 560–562.

[28] Citi S. and Kendrick-Jones J. 1987. Regulation of non-muscle myosin structure and function. *Bioessays* 7: 155–159.

[29] Sellers J.R. 1991. Regulation of cytoplasmic and smooth muscle myosin. *Curr. Opin. Cell Biol.* 3: 98–104.

[30] Schroder R.R., Manstein D.J., Jahn W., Holden H., Rayment I. et al. 1993. Three-dimensional atomic model of F-actin decorated with Dictyostelium myosin S1. *Nature* 364: 171–174.

[31] Rayment I., Rypniewski W.R., Schmidt-Base K., Smith R., Tomchick D.R. et al. 1993. Three-dimensional structure of myosin subfragment-1: a molecular motor. *Science* 261: 50–58.

[32] Huxley A.F. 2000. Cross-bridge action: present views, prospects, and unknowns. *J. Biomech.* 33: 1189–1195.

[33] Huxley A.F. and Simmons R.M. 1971. Proposed mechanism of force generation in striated muscle. *Nature* 233: 533–538.

[34] Kabsch W., Mannherz H.G., Suck D., Pai E.F., and Holmes K.C. 1990. Atomic structure of the actin: DNase I complex. *Nature* 347: 37–44.

[35] Holmes K.C., Popp D., Gebhard W., and Kabsch W. 1990. Atomic model of the actin filament. *Nature* 347: 44–49.

[36] Spudich J.A. 1994. How molecular motors work. *Nature* 372: 515–518.

[37] Baker J.E., Brust-Mascher I., Ramachandran S., LaConte L.E., and Thomas D.D. 1998. A large and distinct rotation of the myosin light chain domain occurs upon muscle contraction. *Proc. Natl Acad. Sci. USA* 95: 2944–2949.

[38] Houdusse A., Kalabokis V.N., Himmel D., Szent-Gyorgyi A.G., and Cohen C. 1999. Atomic structure of scallop myosin subfragment S1 complexed with MgADP: a novel conformation of the myosin head. *Cell* 97: 459–470.

[39] Jontes J.D., Wilson-Kubalek E.M., and Milligan R.A. 1995. A 32 degree tail swing in brush border myosin I on ADP release. *Nature* 378: 751–753.

[40] Veigel C., Coluccio L.M., Jontes J.D., Sparrow J.C., Milligan R.A., and Molloy J.E. 1999. The motor protein myosin-I produces its working stroke in two steps. *Nature* 398: 530–533.

[41] Corrie J.E., Brandmeier B.D., Ferguson R.E., Trentham D.R., Kendrick-Jones J. et al. 1999. Dynamic measurement of myosin light-chain-domain tilt and twist in muscle contraction. *Nature* 400: 425–430.

[42] Irving M., St Claire Allen T., Sabido-David C., Craik J.S., Brandmeier B. et al. 1995. Tilting of the light-chain region of myosin during step length changes and active force generation in skeletal muscle. *Nature* 375: 688–691.

[43] Forkey J.N., Quinlan M.E., Shaw M.A., Corrie J.E., and Goldman Y.E. 2003. Three-dimensional structural dynamics of myosin V by single-molecule fluorescence polarization. *Nature* 422: 399–404.

[44] Vale R.D. and Milligan R.A. 2000. The way things move: looking under the hood of molecular motor proteins. *Science* 288: 88–95.

[45] Kitamura K., Tokunaga M., Iwane A.H., and Yanagida T. 1999. A single myosin head moves along an actin filament with regular steps of ~5.3 nm. *Nature* 397: 129–134.

[46] Howard J. 1996. The movement of kinesin along microtubules. *Annu. Rev. Physiol.* 58: 703–729.

[47] Howard J. and Hyman A.A. 2003. Dynamics and mechanics of the microtubule plus end. *Nature* 422: 753–758.

[48] Hirokawa N. 1998. Kinesin and dynein superfamily proteins and the mechanism of organelle transport. *Science* 279: 519–526.

[49] Vale R.D., Funatsu T., Pierce D.W., Romberg L., Harada Y., and Yanagida T. 1996. Direct observation of single kinesin molecules moving along microtubules. *Nature* 380: 451–453.

[50] Berliner E., Young E.C., Anderson K., Mahtani H.K., and Gelles J. 1995. Failure of a single-headed kinesin to track parallel to microtubule protofilaments. *Nature* 373: 718–721.

[51] Sablin E.P., Kull F.J., Cooke R., Vale R.D., and Fletterick R.J. 1996. Crystal structure of the motor domain of the kinesin-related motor ncd. *Nature* 380: 555–559.

[52] Sack S., Muller J., Marx A., Thormahlen M., Mandelkow E.M. et al. 1997. X-ray structure of motor and neck domains from rat brain kinesin. *Biochemistry* 36: 16155–16165.

[53] Schnitzer M.J. and Block S.M. 1997. Kinesin hydrolyses one ATP per 8-nm step. *Nature* 388: 386–390.

[54] Peskin C.S. and Oster G. 1995. Coordinated hydrolysis explains the mechanical behavior of kinesin. *Biophys. J.* 68: 202–211.

[55] Lohman T.M., Thorn K., and Vale R.D. 1998. Staying on track: common features of DNA helicases and microtubule motors. *Cell* 93: 9–12.

[56] Hackney D.D. 1995. Highly processive microtubule-stimulated ATP hydrolysis by dimeric kinesin head domains. *Nature* 377: 448–450.

[57] Hunt A.J., Gittes F., and Howard J. 1994. The force exerted by a single kinesin molecule against a viscous load. *Biophys. J.* 67: 766–781.

[58] Svoboda K. and Block S.M. 1994. Force and velocity measured for single kinesin molecules. *Cell* 77: 773–784.

[59] Gibbons I.R. and Rowe A.J. 1965. Dynein: a protein with adenosine triphosphate activity from cilia. *Science* 149: 424–426.

[60] Schroer T.A., Steuer E.R., and Sheetz M.P. 1989. Cytoplasmic dynein is a minus end-directed motor for membranous organelles. *Cell* 56: 937–946.

[61] Schnapp B.J. and Reese T.S. 1989. Dynein is the motor for retrograde axonal transport of organelles. *Proc. Natl Acad. Sci. USA* 86: 1548–1552.

[62] Lye R.J., Porter M.E., Scholey J.M., and McIntosh J.R. 1987. Identification of a microtubule-based cytoplasmic motor in the nematode *C. elegans*. *Cell* 51: 309–318.

[63] Paschal B.M., Shpetner H.S., and Vallee R.B. 1987. MAP 1C is a microtubule-activated ATPase which translocates microtubules in vitro and has dynein-like properties. *J. Cell Biol.* 105: 1273–1282.

[64] Hirokawa N., Sato-Yoshitake R., Yoshida T., and Kawashima T. 1990. Brain dynein (MAP1C) localizes on both anterogradely and retrogradely transported membranous organelles *in vivo*. *J. Cell Biol.* 111: 1027–1037.

[65] Waterman-Storer C.M., Karki S.B., Kuznetsov S.A., Tabb J.S., Weiss D.G. et al. 1997. The interaction between cytoplasmic dynein and dynactin is required for fast axonal transport. *Proc. Natl Acad. Sci. USA* 94: 12180–12185.

[66] Lin S.X. and Collins C.A. 1992. Immunolocalization of cytoplasmic dynein to lysosomes in cultured cells. *J. Cell. Sci.* 101 (Pt 1): 125–137.

[67] Corthesy-Theulaz I., Pauloin A., and Rfeffer S.R. 1992. Cytoplasmic dynein participates in the centrosomal localization of the Golgi complex. *J. Cell Biol.* 118: 1333–1345.

[68] Aniento F., Emans N., Griffiths G., and Gruenberg J. 1993. Cytoplasmic dynein-dependent vesicular transport from early to late endosomes. *J. Cell Biol.* 123: 1373–1387.

[69] Fath K.R., Trimbur G.M., and Burgess D.R. 1994. Molecular motors are differentially distributed on Golgi membranes from polarized epithelial cells. *J. Cell Biol.* 126: 661–675.

[70] Blocker A., Severin F.F., Burkhardt J.K., Bingham J.B., Yu H. et al. 1997. Molecular require-ments for bi-directional movement of phagosomes along microtubules. *J. Cell Biol.* 137: 113–129.

[71] King S.J., Bonilla M., Rodgers M.E., and Schroer T.A. 2002. Subunit organization in cytoplasmic dynein subcomplexes. *Protein Sci.* 11: 1239–1250.

[72] King S.M. 2000. The dynein microtubule motor. *Biochim. Biophys. Acta* 1496: 60–75.

[73] Burgess S., Walker M.L., Sakakibara H., Knight P.J., and Oiwa K. 2003. Dynein structure and power stroke. *Nature* 421: 715–718.

[74] Koonce M.P. 1997. Identification of a microtubule-binding domain in a cytoplasmic dynein heavy chain. *J. Biol. Chem.* 272: 19714–19718.

[75] Gill S., Schroer T., Szilak I., Steuer E., Sheetz M., and Cleveland D. 1991. Dynactin, a conserved, ubiquitously expressed component of an activator of vesicle motility mediated by cytoplasmic dynein. *J. Cell Biol.* 115: 1639–1650.

[76] Straube A., Enard W., Berner A., Wedlich-Soldner R., Kahmann R., and Steinberg G. 2001. A split motor domain in a cytoplasmic dynein. *EMBO J.* 20: 5091–5100.

[77] Vale R.D. 2000. AAA proteins: lords of the ring. *J. Cell Biol.* 150: 13F–20.

[78] Neuwald A.F., Aravind L., Spouge J.L., and Koonin E.V. 1999. AAA+: a class of chaperone-like ATPases associated with the assembly, operation, and disassembly of protein complexes. *Genom. Res.* 9: 27–43.

[79] Confalonieri F. and Duguet M. 1995. A 200-amino acid ATPase module in search of a basic function. *BioEssays* 17: 639–650.

[80] King S.M. 2000. AAA domains and organization of the dynein motor unit. *J. Cell Sci.* 113 (Pt 14): 2521–2526.

[81] Asai D.J. and Koonce M.P. 2001. The dynein heavy chain: structure, mechanics and evolution. *Trends Cell Biol.* 11: 196–202

[82] Berry R.M. and Armitage J.P. 1999. The bacterial flagella motor. *Adv. Microb. Physiol.* 41: 291–337.

[83] Berg H.C. 2003. The rotary motor of bacterial flagella. *Ann. Rev. Biochem.* 72: 19–54.

[84] Blair D.F. 1995. How bacteria sense and swim. *Annu. Rev. Microbiol.* 49: 489–522.

[85] Berg H.C. and Anderson R.A. 1973. Bacteria swim by rotating their flagellar filaments. *Nature* 245: 380–382.

[86] Fahrner K.A., Ryu W.S., and Berg H.C. 2003. Biomechanics: bacterial flagellar switching under load. *Nature* 423: 938.

[87] Berg H.C. 2000. Motile behavior of bacteria. *Phys. Today* 53: 24–29.

[88] Scharf B.E., Fahrner K.A., Turner L., and Berg H.C. 1998. Control of direction of flagellar rotation in bacterial chemotaxis. *Proc. Natl Acad. Sci. USA* 95: 201–206.

[89] Macnab R.M. 1977. Bacterial flagella rotating in bundles: a study in helical geometry. *Proc. Natl Acad. Sci. USA* 74: 221–225.

[90] Elston T.C. and Oster G. 1997. Protein turbines. I: the bacterial flagellar motor. *Biophys. J.* 73: 703–721.

[91] Walz D. and Caplan S.R. 2000. An electrostatic mechanism closely reproducing observed behavior in the bacterial flagellar motor. *Biophys. J.* 78: 626–651.

[92] Schmitt R. 2003. Helix rotation model of the flagellar rotary motor. *Biophys. J.* 85: 843–852.

[93] Iino T., Komeda Y., Kutsukake K., Macnab R.M., Matsumura P. et al. 1988. New unified nomenclature for the flagellar genes of *Escherichia coli* and *Salmonella typhimurium*. *Microbiol. Rev.* 52: 533–535.

[94] Berg H.C. 1974. Dynamic properties of bacterial flagellar motors. *Nature* 249: 77–79.

[95] Ueno T., Oosawa K., and Aizawa S. 1992. M ring, S ring and proximal rod of the flagellar basal body of *Salmonella typhimurium* are composed of subunits of a single protein, FliF. *J. Mol. Biol.* 227: 672–677.

[96] Ueno T., Oosawa K., and Aizawa S. 1994. Domain structures of the MS ring component protein (FliF) of the flagellar basal body of *Salmonella typhimurium*. *J. Mol. Biol.* 236: 546–555.

[97] Driks A. and DeRosier D.J. 1990. Additional structures associated with bacterial flagellar basal body. *J. Mol. Biol.* 211: 669–672.

[98] Khan I.H., Reese T.S., and Khan S. 1992. The cytoplasmic component of the bacterial flagellar motor. *Proc. Natl Acad. Sci. USA* 89: 5956–5960.

[99] Francis N.R., Sosinsky G.E., Thomas D., and DeRosier D.J. 1994. Isolation, characterization and structure of bacterial flagellar motors containing the switch complex. *J. Mol. Biol.* 235: 1261–1270.

[100] Yorimitsu T. and Homma M. 2001. Na+-driven flagellar motor of *Vibrio*. *Biochim. Biophys. Acta (BBA) — Bioenerg.* 1505: 82–93.

[101] Meister M., Lowe G., and Berg H.C. 1987. The proton flux through the bacterial flagellar motor. *Cell* 49: 643–650.

[102] Van Way S.M., Hosking E.R., Braun T.F., and Manson M.D. 2000. Mot protein assembly into the bacterial flagellum: a model based on mutational analysis of the motB gene. *J. Mol. Biol.* 297: 7–24.

[103] Blair D.F. and Berg H.C. 1988. Restoration of torque in defective flagellar motors. *Science* 242: 1678–1681.

[104] Fung D.C. and Berg H.C. 1995. Powering the flagellar motor of *Escherichia coli* with an external voltage source. *Nature* 375: 809–812.

[105] Berg H. and Turner L. 1993. Torque generated by the flagellar motor of *Escherichia coli*. *Biophys. J.* 65: 2201–2216.

[106] Chen X. and Berg H.C. 2000. Torque–speed relationship of the flagellar rotary motor of *Escherichia coli*. *Biophys. J.* 78: 1036–1041.

[107] Seeman N.C. 2003. DNA in a material world. *Nature* 421: 427–431.

[108] Dekker C.R. and M.A. 2001. Electronic properties of DNA. *Phys. World*, 29–33.

[109] Robinson B.H. and Seeman N.C. 1987. The design of a biochip: a self-assembling molecular-scale memory device. *Protein Eng.* 1: 295–300.

[110] Seeman N.C. and Belcher A.M. 2002. Emulating biology: building nanostructures from the bottom up. *PNAS* 99: 6451–6455.

[111] Smith S.B., Cui Y., and Bustamante C. 1996. Overstretching B-DNA: the elastic response of individual double-stranded and single-stranded DNA molecules. *Science* 271: 795–799.

[112] Simmel F.C. and Yurke B. 2001. Using DNA to construct and power a nanoactuator. *Phys. Rev. E Stat. Nonlin. Soft Matter Phys.* 63: 041913.

[113] Tinland B., Pluen A., Sturm J., and Weill G. 1997. Persistence length of single-stranded DNA. *Macromolecules* 30: 5763–5765.

[114] Seeman N.C. 1997. DNA Components for molecular architecture. *Acc. Chem. Res.* 30: 347–391.

[115] Niemeyer C.M. 1999. Progress in "engineering up" nanotechnology devices utilizing DNA as a construction material. *Appl. Phys. A: Mater. Sci. Process.* 68: 119–124.

[116] Chen J.H. and Seeman N.C. 1991. Synthesis from DNA of a molecule with the connectivity of a cube. *Nature* 350: 631–633.

[117] Zhang Y. and Seeman N.C. 1994. Construction of a DNA-truncated octahedron. *J. Am. Chem. Soc.* 116: 1661–1669.

[118] Winfree E., Liu F., Wenzler L.A., and Seeman N.C. 1998. Design and self-assembly of two-dimensional DNA crystals. *Nature* 394: 539–544.

[119] Yan H., Zhang X., Shen Z., and Seeman N.C. 2002. A robust DNA mechanical device controlled by hybridization topology. *Nature* 415: 62–65.

[120] Mao C., Sun W., and Seeman N.C. 1997. Assembly of Borromean rings from DNA. *Nature* 386: 137–138.

[121] Mao C., LaBean T.H., Relf J.H., and Seeman N.C. 2000. Logical computation using algorithmic self-assembly of DNA triple-crossover molecules. *Nature* 407: 493–496.

[122] Simmel F.C. and Yurke B., DNA-based Nanodevices. http://www2.nano.physik.uni-muenchen.de/publikationen/Preprints/index.html

[123] Coppin C.M., Pierce D.W., Hsu L., and Vale R.D. 1997. The load dependence of kinesin's mechanical cycle. *Proc. Natl Acad. Sci. USA* 94: 8539–8544.

[124] Seeman N.C. 1991. Construction of three-dimensional stick figures from branched DNA. *DNA Cell Biol.* 10: 475–486.

[125] Wang H., Du S.M., and Seeman N.C. 1993. Tight single-stranded DNA knots. *J. Biomol. Struct. Dyn.* 10: 853–863.

[126] Seeman N.C. 1998. Nucleic acid nanostructures and topology. *Ang. Chem. Int. Ed.* 37: 3220–3238.

[127] Mao C., Sun W., and Seeman N.C. 1999. Designed two-dimensional DNA Holliday junction arrays visualized by atomic force microscopy. *J. Am. Chem. Soc.* 121: 5437–5443.

[128] LaBean T.H., Yan H., Kopatsch J., Liu F., Winfree E., Reif J.H., and Seeman N.C. 2000. Construction, analysis, ligation, and self-assembly of DNA triple crossover complexes. *J. Am. Chem. Soc.* 122: 1848–1860.

[129] Fu T.J. and Seeman N.C. 1993. DNA double-crossover molecules. *Biochemistry* 32: 3211–3220.

[130] Zhang S., Fu T.J., and Seeman N.C. 1993. Symmetric immobile DNA branched junctions. *Biochemistry* 32: 8062–8067.

[131] Li X., Yang X., Jing Q., and Seeman N.C. 1996. Antiparallel DNA double crossover molecules as components for nanoconstruction. *J. Am. Chem. Soc.* 118: 6131–6140.

[132] Mao C., Sun W., Shen Z., and Seeman N.C. 1999. A nanomechanical device based on the B-Z transition of DNA. *Nature* 397: 144–146.

[133] Rich A., Nordheim A., and Wang A.H.-J. 1984. The chemistry and biology of left handed Z-DNA. *Ann. Rev. Biochem.* 53: 791–846.

[134] Pohl F.M. and Jovin T.M. 1972. Salt-induced co-operative conformational change of a synthetic DNA: equilibrium and kinetic studies with poly (dG-dC). *J. Mol. Biol.* 67: 375–396.

[135] Yurke B., Turberfield A.J., Mills A.P., Simmel F.C., and Neumann, J.L. 2000. A DNA-fuelled molecular machine made of DNA. *Nature* 415: 62–65.

[136] Simmel F.C. and Yurke B. 2002. A DNA-based molecular device switchable between three distinct mechanical states. *Appl. Phys. Lett.* 80: 883–885.

[137] Mitchell J.C. and Yurke B. 2002. DNA scissors. In *DNA Computing, Proceedings of the 7th International Meeting on DNA-Based Computers, DNA7*, S.N. Jonoska and N. Seeman (Eds.), Tampa, FL: Springer Verlag, Heidelberg.

[138] Schill G. 1971. *Catenanes Rotaxanes and Knots.* New York: Academic Press.

[139] Ashton P.R., Ballardini R., Balzani V., Belohradsky M., Gandolfi, M.T., Philp D., Prodi L., Raymo F.M., Reddington M.V., Spencer, N., Stoddart J.F., Venturi M., and Williams D.J. 1996. Self-assembly, spectroscopic, and electrochemical properties of [n]rotaxanes. *J. Am. Chem. Soc.* 118: 4931–4951.

[140] Amabilino D.B., Asakawa M., Ashton P.R., Ballardini R., Balzani, V., Belohradsky M., Credi A., Higuchi M., Raymo F.M., Shimizu T., Stoddart J.F., Venturi M., and Yase K. 1998. Aggregation of self-assembling branched [n]rotaxanes. *N. J. Chem.* 9: 959–972.

[141] Sauvage J.-P. and Dietrich-Buchecker C. 1999. *Molecular Catenanes, Rotaxanes and Knots.* Weinheim: Wiley-VCH.

[142] Harada A. 2001. Cyclodextrin-based molecular machines. *Acc. Chem. Res.* 34: 456–464.

[143] Anelli P.-L., Spencer N., and Stoddart J.F. 1991. A molecular shuttle. *J. Am. Chem. Soc.* 113: 5131–5133.

[144] Balzani V.V., Credi A., Raymo F.M., and Stoddart J.F. 2000. Artificial molecular machines. *Angew. Chem. Int. Ed. Engl.* 39: 3348–3391.

[145] Schalley C.A., Beizai K., and Vogtle F., 2001. On the way to rotaxane-based molecular motors: studies in molecular mobility and topological chirality. *Acc. Chem. Res.* 34: 465–476.

[146] Gatti F.G., Leon S., Wong J.K.Y., Bottari G., Altieri A. et al. 2003. Photoisomerization of a rotaxane hydrogen bonding template: light-induced acceleration of a large amplitude rotational motion. *PNAS* 100: 10–14.

[147] Bermudez V.V., Capron N., Gase T., Gatti F.G., Kajzar F. et al. 2000. Influencing intramolecular motion with an alternating electric field. *Nature* 406: 608–611.

[148] Fyfe M.C.T. and Stoddart J.F. 1997. Synthetic supramolecular chemistry. *Acc. Chem. Res.* 30: 393–401.

[149] Whitesides G.M., Mathias J.P., and Seto C.T. 1991. Molecular self-assembly and nanochemistry: a chemical strategy for the synthesis of nanostructures. *Science* 254: 1312–1319.

[150] Ashton P.R., Goodnow T.T., Kaifer A.W., Reddington M.V., Slawin A.M.Z., Spencer N., Stoddart J.F., Vicent C., and Williams D.J. 1989. A [2]catenane made to order. *Ang. Chem. Int. Ed. Eng.* 28: 1396–1399.

[151] Deleuze M.S. 2000. Can benzylic amide [2] catenane rings rotate on graphite? *J. Am. Chem. Soc.* 122: 1130–1143.

[152] Raymo F.M., Houk K.N., and Stoddart J.F. 1998. Origins of selectivity in molecular and supramolecular entities: solvent and electrostatic control of the translational isomerism in [2]catenanes. *J. Org. Chem.* 63: 6523–6528.

[153] Sauvage J.-P. 1998. Transition metal containing rotaxanes and catenanes in motion: toward molecular machines and motors. *Acc. Chem. Res.* 31: 611–619.

[154] Cambron J.-C. and Sauvage J.-P. 1998. Functional rotaxanes: from controlled molecular motions to electron transfer between chemically nonconnected chromophores. *Chem. A Euro. J.* 4: 1362–1366.

[155] Blanco M.J., Jimenez M.C., Chambron J.-C., Heitz V., Linke M., and Sauvage J.-P. 1999. Rotaxanes as new architectures for photoinduced electron transfer and molecular motions. *Chem. Soc. Rev.* 28: 293–305.

[156] Leigh D.A., Murphy A., Smart J.P., Deleuze M.S., and Zerbetto, F. 1998. Controlling the frequency of macrocyclic ring rotation in benzylic amide [2]catenanes. *J. Am. Chem. Soc.* 120: 6458–6467.

[157] Fujita M. 1999. Self-assembly OF [2]catenanes containing metals in their backbones. *Acc. Chem. Res.* 32: 53–61.

[158] Collier C.P., Mattersteig G., Wong E.W., Luo Y., Beverly K. et al. 2000. A [2]catenane-based solid state electronically reconfigurable switch. *Science* 289: 1172–1175.

[159] Balzani V.V., Gomez-Lopez M., and Stoddart J.F. 1998. Molecular machines. *Acc. Chem. Res.* 31: 405–414.

[160] Johnston M.R., Gunter M.J., and Warrener R.N. 1998. Templated formation of multi-porphyrin assemblies resembling a molecular universal joint. *Chem. Commun.* 28: 2739–2740.

[161] Amabilino D.B., Anelli P.-L., Ashton P.R., Brown G.R., Cordova E., Godinez L.A., Hayes W., Kaifer A.E., Philip D., Slawin A.M.Z., Spencer N., Stoddart J.F., Tolley M.S., and Williams D.J. 1995. Molecular meccano. 3. Constitutional and translational isomerism in [2]catenanes and [n]pseudorotaxanes. *J. Am. Chem. Soc.* 117: 11142–11170.

[162] Vacek J. and Michl J. 1997. A molecular "Tinkertoy" construction kit: computer simulation of molecular propellers. *N. J. Chem.* 21: 1259–1268.

[163] Michl J. and Magnera T.F. 2002. Supramolecular chemistry and self-assembly special feature: two-dimensional supramolecular chemistry with molecular Tinkertoys. *PNAS* 99: 4788–4792.

[164] Vacek J. and Michl J. 2001. Molecular dynamics of a grid-mounted molecular dipolar rotor in a rotating electric field. *PNAS* 98: 5481–5486.

[165] Gimzewski J.K., Joachim C., Schlittler R.R., Langlais V., Tang H., and Johannsen I. 1998. Rotation of a single molecule within a supramolecular bearing. *Science* 281: 531–533.

[166] Gust D. and Mislow K. 1973. Analysis of isomerization in compounds displaying restricted rotation of aryl groups. *J. Am. Chem. Soc.* 95: 1535–1547.

[167] Finocchiaro P., Gust D., and Mislow K. 1974. Correlated rotation in complex triarylmethanes. I. 32-isomer system and residual diastereoisomerism. *J. Am. Chem. Soc.* 96: 3198–3205.

[168] Finocchiaro P., Gust D., and Mislow K. 1974. Correlated rotation in complex triarylmethanes. II. 16- and 8-isomer systems and residual diastereotopicity. *J. Am. Chem. Soc.* 96: 3205–3213.

[169] Mislow K. 1976. Stereochemical consequences of correlated rotation in molecular propellers. *Acc. Chem. Res.* 9: 26–33.

[170] Clayden J. and Pink J.H. 1998. Concerted rotation in a tertiary aromatic amide: towards a simple molecular gear. *Ang. Chem. Int. Ed. Engl.* 37: 1937–1939.

[171] Hounshell W.D., Johnson C.A., Guenzi A., Cozzi F., and Mislow K. 1980. Stereochemical consequences of dynamic gearing in substituted bis (9-triptycyl) methanes and related molecules. *Proc. Natl Acad. Sci. USA* 77: 6961–6964.

[172] Cozzi F., Guenzi A., Johnson C.A., Mislow K., Hounshell W.D., and Blount J.F. 1981. Stereoisomerism and correlated rotation in molecular gear systems. Residual diastereomers of bis(2,3-dimethyl-9-triptycyl)methane. *J. Am. Chem. Soc.* 103: 957–958.

[173] Kawada Y.I.H. 1981. Bis(4-chloro-1-triptycyl) ether. Separation of a pair of phase isomers of labeled bevel gears. *J. Am. Chem. Soc.* 103: 958–960.

[174] Johnson C.A., Guenzi A., and Mislow K. 1981. Restricted gearing and residual stereoisomerism in bis(1,4-dimethyl-9-triptycyl)methane. *J. Am. Chem. Soc.* 103: 6240–6242.

[175] Bedard T.C.M.J.S. 1995. Design and synthesis of a "molecular turnstile." *J. Am. Chem. Soc.* 117: 10662–10671.

[176] Ugi I., Marquarding D., Klusacek H., Gillespie P., and Ramirez F. 1971. Berry pseudorotation and turnstile rotation. *Acc. Chem. Res.* 4: 288–296.

[177] Kelly T.R., Bowyer M.C., Bhaskar K.V., Bebbington D., Garcia A., Lang F., Kim M.H., and Jette M.P. 1994. A molecular brake. *J. Am. Chem. Soc.* 116: 3657–3658.

[178] Feringa B.L., Jager W.F., De Lange B., and Meijer E.W. 1991. Chiroptical molecular switch. *J. Am. Chem. Soc.* 113: 5468–5470.

[179] Koumura N., Zijlstra R.W., van Delden R.A, Harada N., and Feringa B.L. 1999. Light-driven monodirectional molecular rotor. *Nature* 401: 152–155.

[180] Koumura N., Geertsema E.M., van Gelder M.B., Meetsma A., and Feringa B.L. 2002. Second generation light-driven molecular motors. Unidirectional rotation controlled by a single stereogenic center with near-perfect photoequilibria and acceleration of the speed of rotation by structural modification. *J. Am. Chem. Soc.* 124: 5037–5051.

[181] van Delden R.A., Koumura N., Harada N., and Feringa B.L.. 2002. Unidirectional rotary motion in a liquid crystalline environment: color tuning by a molecular motor. *Proc. Natl Acad. Sci. USA* 99: 4945–4949.

[182] Dubey A., Thornton A., Nikitczuk K.P., Mavroidis C., and Yarmush M.L. 2003. Viral Protein Linear (VPL) Nano-Actuators. *Proceedings of the 2003 3rd IEEE Conference on Nanotechnology*, San Francisco, USA.

[183] Wilson I.A., Skehel J.J., and Wiley D.C. 1981. Structure of the haemagglutinin membrane glycoprotein of influenza virus at 3Å resolution. *Nature* 289: 366–373.

[184] Chan D.C., Fass D., Berger J.M., and Kim P.S. 1997. Core structure of gp41 from the HIV envelope glycoprotein. *Cell* 89: 263–273.

[185] Bentz J. 2000. Minimal aggregate size and minimal fusion unit for the first fusion pore of influenza hemagglutinin-mediated membrane fusion. *Biophys. J.* 78: 227–245.

[186] Bentz J. 2000. Membrane fusion mediated by coiled coils: a hypothesis. *Biophys. J.* 78: 886–900

[187] Carr C.M. and Kim P.S. 1993. A spring-loaded mechanism for the conformational change of influenza hemagglutinin. *Cell* 73: 823–832.

[188] Knoblauch M., Noll G.A., Muller T., Prufer D., Schneider-Huther I. et al. 2003. ATP-independent contractile proteins from plants. *Nat. Mater.* 2: 600–603.

[189] Mavroidis C. and Dubey A. 2003. Biomimetics: from pulses to motors. *Nat. Mater.* 2: 573–574.

[190] Hellinga H.W. and Richards F.M. 1991. Construction of new ligand binding sites in proteins of known structure. I. Computer-aided modeling of sites with pre-defined geometry. *J. Mol. Biol.* 222: 763–785.

[191] Liu H., Schmidt J.J., Bachand G.D., Rizk S.S., Looger L.L. et al. 2002. Control of a biomolecular motor-powered nanodevice with an engineered chemical switch. *Nat. Mater.* 1: 173–177.

[192] Leach Andrew R. 2001. *Molecular Modelling*, 2nd ed., Prentice Hall.

[193] Hinchliffe A. 2002. *Modelling Molecular Structures*, 2nd ed., John Wiley & Sons.

[194] Vinter J.G. and Gardner Mark. 1994. *Molecular Modelling and Drug Design*. CRC Press.

[195] Brooks R., Bruccoleri R.E., Olafson B.D, States D.J, Swaminathan S. et al. 1983. CHARMM: a program for macromolecular energy, minimization, and dynamics calculations. *J. Comput. Chem.* 4: 187–217.

[196] Schlitter J., Engels M., and Kruger P. 1994. Targeted molecular dynamics: a new approach for searching pathways of conformational transitions. *J. Mol. Graph.* 12: 84–89.

[197] Morris G.M. *Molecular Docking Web*, http://www.scripps.edu/pub/olson-web/people/gmm

[198] Lang M.J., Fordyce P.M., and Block S.M. 2003. Combined optical trapping and single-molecule fluorescence. *J. Biol.* 2: 6.

[199] Binnig G., Rohrer H., Gerber C., and Weibel E. 1986. Surface studies by scanning tunnelling microscopy, *Phys. Rev. Lett.*, 56: 930–933.

[200] Binnig G. 1982. Atomic force microscope, *Phys. Rev. Lett.*, 49: 57–61.

[201] Wickramasinghe H.K. 1989. Scanned-probe microscopes, *Sci. Am.*, 261: 89–105.

[202] Funatsu T., Harada Y., Higuchi H. et al. 1997. Imaging and nano-manipulation of single biomolecules, *Biophys. Chem.*, 68: 63–77.

[203] Svoboda K., Schmidt C., Schnapp B., and Block S. 1993. Direct observation of kinesin stepping by optical trapping interferometry, *Nature* 365: 721–727.

[204] Castelino K. 2002. Biological Object Nanomanipulation, *Review Report, University of California, Berkeley.*

[205] Fukuda T., Arai F., and Dong L. 2002. Nano Robotic World — From Micro to Nano, *Int'l Workshop on Nano- \ Micro-Robotics in Thailand.*

[206] Ashkin A. 1970. Acceleration and trapping of particles by radiation pressure, *Phys. Rev. Lett.,* 24: 156–156.

[207] Bruican T.N., Smyth M.J., Crissman H.A., Salzman G.C., Stewart C.C., and Martin J.C. 1987. Automated single-cell manipulation and sorting by light trapping, *Appl. Opt.,* 26: 5311–5316.

[208] Nishioka M., Katsura S., Hirano K., and Mizuno A. 1997. Evaluation of cell characteristics by step-wise orientational rotation using optoelectrostatic micromanipulation, *IEEE Trans. Ind. Appl.,* 33: 1381–1388.

[209] Riquicha A.A.G. et al. 2001. Manipulation of Nanoscale Components with the AFM: Principles and Applications, *IEEE Int. Conf. Nanotechnol.,* Maui, HI, October 28–30, 2001.

[210] Sun Y., Wan K.T., Roberts K.P., Bischof J.C., and Nelson B.J. 2003. Mechanical property characterization of the mouse zona pellucida, *IEEE Trans. NanoBioSci.,* 2.

[211] Arai F. and Fukuda T. 1998. 3D Bio Micromanipulation , *International Workshop on Microfactoryies IWMF'98,* December 7–9, pp. 143–148.

[212] Disz M., Papka M., Pellegrino Stevens R., and Taylor V. 1995. Virtual reality visualization of parallel molecular dynamics simulation, in *Proc. 1995 Simulation Multi-conference Symposium,* (Phoenix, Arizona), pp. 483 -487, Society for Computer Simulation (April 1995).

[213] Professor Shapiro: *Laboratory for Biomolecular Computers*: http://www.weizmann.ac.il/mathusers/lbn/index.html

[214] Benenson Y., Gil B., Ben-Dor U., Adar R., and Shapiro E. 2004. An autonomous molecular computer for logical control of gene expression. *Nature,* 429: 423–429.

[215] Mathieu J.-B., Martel S., Yahia L'H., Soulez G., and Beaudoin G. 2003. MRI systems as a mean of propulsion for a microdevice in blood vessels. *EMBC.*

[216] Cavalcanti A., Freitas Robert A. Jr., and Kretly Luiz C. Nanorobotics control design: a practical approach tutorial. *ASME 28th Biennial Mechanisms and Robotics Conference,* Salt Lake City Utah, USA, September 2004.

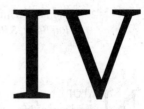

Bionanotechnology

David E. Reisner
Inframat® Corporation

N ATURE has been engaged in its own unfathomable and uncanny nanotechnology project since
the dawn of life, billions of years ago. It is only recently that humans have had their own tools
to watch nature as she assembles and manipulates structures so complex and purposeful so as
to defy their imagination. No one would argue that all molecular biology is based on nanotechnology;
after all, these structural building blocks comprising ordered elements are well within the 100 nanometer
scale that is generally agreed upon as the upper physical dimension with which nanotechnology processes
occur. It is no wonder that man is now attempting to mimic nature by building analogous structures from
the bottom up.

Now, a word about the chapter title. The temptation to consider "nanobiotechnology" as a subset of
biotechnology, fails to pay homage to the gargantuan impact of the burgeoning nanotechnology field, a
field which is in the throes of revolutionary growth. The phrase "nanobiotechnology" feels redundant and
trite. In distinction, the term "bionanotechnology" connotes a rapidly evolving sector of the nanotechnology field that deals strictly with biological processes and structures. Many refer to this synthesis, if you
will, as "convergence." As will be demonstrated in this new edition CRC Handbook chapter, the seeds of
bionanotechnology development have been planted. Commercial products will be on the marketplace well
before the next edition appears. Many nanotech soothsayers predict that as time goes on, this convergence
of biotechnology and nanotechnology will become a dominant focus area for technological innovation
worldwide and will impact all of our lives on a daily basis.

Of course, this is an engineering handbook. One need not stretch the imagination very far to appreciate
that nature has fundamentally engineered life as we know it, culminating in our own species. This fact
has not gone unnoticed on the part of nanotechnologists, who have begun in earnest to mimic nature's
fundamental engineering processes through invoking precise controls over her building blocks. Self-
assembly, a key construct of nanotechnology, forms the backbone of biological processes. For example,
exploiting DNA as scaffolding for the engineering of DNA-templated molecular electronic devices is an
inspiring example of our newfound ability to insinuate our own design skills at the nanoscale level in
living systems. Using this approach, it is possible to create self-assembling electronic circuits or devices
in solution. Directed evolution based on repeated mutagenesis experiments can be conducted at the
nanoscale level. Along these lines, the use of the solar energy conversion properties of bacteriorhodopsin
for making thin film memories, photovoltaic convertors, holographic processors, artificial memories, logic
gates, and protein–semiconductor hybrid devices is astounding.

Quantum dots are tiny light-emitting particles on the nanoscale. They have been developed as a new class
of biological fluorophore. Once rendered hydrophilic with appropriate functional groups, quantum dots
can act as biosensors that can detect biomolecular targets on a real-time or continuous basis. Different
colors of quantum dots could be combined into a larger structure to yield an optical barcode. Gold
nanoparticles can be functionalized to serve as biological tags.

Nanomedicine is a burgeoning area of development, encompassing drug delivery by nanoparticulates,
including fullerenes, as well as new enabling opportunities in medical diagnostics, labeling, and imaging.
Quantum dots will certainly play a large role in nanomedicine. Years from now, we will laugh at the archaic
approach to treating disease we presently take for granted, carried over from the 20th century, relying on
a single drug formulation to treat a specific disease in all people without acknowledging each individual's
unique genetic makeup. Nanocoatings also play an important near-term role in the lifetime of medical
devices, especially orthopedic prosthetics. Nanocrystalline hydroxyapatite is far less soluble in human
body fluid than conventional amorphous material, thereby anticipating great increases in calendar life.

It is not our intention to provide a comprehensive treatise on bionanotechnology, rather we hope to
provide representative reporting on a wide variety of activity in the field. We have attempted to assemble
papers that are relevant to looming product opportunities and instructional for those readers interested

in developing the bionanotechnology products of the future. To that end, we have felt it appropriate to conclude our discussion with an article that reviews the patent landscape for bionanotechnology, which is presently in a state of great flux. Now more than ever, intellectual property is relevant to both the academic and corporate sectors, and as such patents are being ascribed greater value and importance. Bionanotechnology commercialization will be driven by the increases in federal funding as well as the expiration of more traditional drug patents.

I would like to acknowledge the tireless efforts of both Raj Bawa, who acted as an informal editor during the tedious process of inviting authors to submit new articles for this new Handbook chapter, as well as Cindy McGovern who spent many a thankless hour chasing down authors all over the globe to deliver their manuscripts, organize and package them for the editors.

20

DNA as a Scaffold for Nano-Structure Assembly

Michael Connolly
Integrated Nano-Technologies

20.1 Introduction

Advances in technology have led to increasingly smaller levels of manipulation to achieve greater results. As this trend continues, we begin to approach the limits of conventional processes to the point where improvements go from small, to incremental, to significant. In microelectronics, the theoretical end of the silicon-based lithographic process is drawing near, while in material science the need to control characteristics beyond the macroscale is becoming necessary to continue innovating. There is an imminent need for controlled manipulation at the nanoscale, and until it is reliably achieved, progress in some arenas may plateau. Once it is achieved, however, a new chapter in technical innovation will be open.

Nanotechnology has been put forward as the approach to solve this fabrication problem. Nanoscale structures would be self-assembled from the "bottom-up." Over the past several years, new materials having unique properties have been identified. For example, carbon nanotubes have extraordinary strength and electrical properties [1–2], and numerous labs have demonstrated simple patterning of these materials. However, more complex structures require a material capable of directing multiple components to precise locations.

Molecular biotechnology is a promising point from which nanotechnology can evolve, because living systems are successful examples of atomic and molecular manipulation on the nanoscale. Although enzymes manipulate atoms and molecular fragments on the Angstrom scale, biological systems make their structural components on the nanometer scale, where weak intermolecular energies direct the self-assembly process. This latter approach is likely to be the simplest motif for building the first nanoscale devices whose synthesis and assembly are controlled, to a degree, with current technology. These objects can be used for scaffolding to orient and juxtapose other molecules to form devices, mechanisms, and structures [3].

Because the predominant examples of nanotechnology in nature derive from living systems, it is reasonable to look to those systems for the components of the first nanotechnological objects and devices. Because of this, nanotechnology, which can come from many routes, is likely to evolve in part from molecular biotechnology. The bottom-up approach entails making objects and devices on the nanoscale from molecular and macromolecular components. There is good reason to believe that this approach is practical to some extent, since living systems already exemplify its success: cells manipulate chemical structure on the Angstrom scale via their enzymatic proteins; in addition, they contain self-assembling structural components. Self-assembly is spontaneous. Manipulation that involves the breaking or formation of bonds requires the control of processes in which large amounts of energy can be liberated or consumed [3].

Although processes for manipulating, enhancing, and modifying biological entities exist, they are predominantly effective on a sample en masse, rather than on an individual cell or molecule. By applying chemical, electrical, mechanical, and biological processes, a volume of a sample can be affected. This is useful in a serial manner, but what about when a multistep process is required to achieve a result? Batch processes quickly become either too cumbersome or ineffective, rendering the desired result either too complicated or functionally impractical. If there were a way to direct manipulation at the nanoscale, whereby molecules would behave in a predictable and reliable fashion, the goal of nanoscale achievement could begin to be realized.

Nature has been doing nanotechnology for millennia, and one of the most powerful nanotechnology mechanisms is present in every living thing. That mechanism is called Watson–Crick base pairing of DNA. DNA can store and transfer information, perform computations, and build structures. These things already occur in nature without human interaction; however, manipulating them for a specific purpose and connecting the activity to a useful human interface is what lies between theory and practical application.

20.2   DNA as a Scaffold for Building Structures

Nature has designed DNA such that it is an ideal molecule for building nanoscale structures. Because of how the molecule is constructed, strands of DNA can be "programmed" to assemble themselves into complex arrangements in two and three dimensions. Self-assembly requires information to be carried on the substrates, therefore the greater the information carrying capacity, the greater the complexity of the structures that are produced. This specific programmability stems from the four nucleic acids that make up the rungs of the DNA double helix. These four acids (adenine, thymine, guanine, and cytosine) are represented by the letters A, T, G, and C, respectively. The characteristics of these acids (also referred to as nucleotides or bases) dictate specific pairings of A and T, and G and C. Each nucleic acid makes up one half of each rung in the twisted ladder structure of a complete DNA strand. Because each base will only match up with an appropriate complement, both naturally occurring and synthesized DNA is predictable and stable.

An important property of DNA is its double-stranded nature. Since every DNA sequence has a natural complement (i.e., if a sequence is ATTACGTCG, its complement is TAATGCAGC). These two strands will come together (or hybridize) to form double-stranded DNA, as shown in Figure 20.1.

By producing strands with the appropriate combinations of complementary bases, DNA can be designed to automatically create a nearly infinite number of self-assembling structures. These structures can be as simple as a naturally occurring double helix or a highly complex, three-dimensional shape.

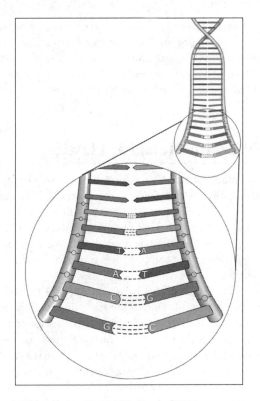

FIGURE 20.1 (See color insert following page 20-14.) Structure of DNA.

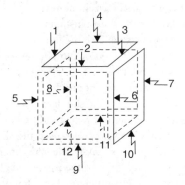

FIGURE 20.2 Seeman cube.

Nadrian C. Seeman, Professor of Chemistry at New York University, has published extensively on this subject and has put forth several models for using DNA to create simple, compound, and complex structures. Using a combination of ligation, restriction, and hybridization steps, Dr. Seeman has been able to create three-dimensional structures like the cube in Figure 20.2 [4].

A group of scientists at The Scripps Research Institute has designed, constructed, and imaged a single strand of DNA that spontaneously folds into a highly rigid, nanoscale octahedron [5].

Beyond the specificity and predictability of DNA, nature has provided a comprehensive tool box to manipulate DNA. In fact, nature provides virtually every tool an engineer would need to build. Restriction enzymes cut DNA at specific sequences of bases. Ligase fuses the ends of two molecules. More complex sets of enzymes can be used to make virtually unlimited copies of a DNA molecule. Polymerase chain reaction technology uses DNA polymerases to exponentially copy DNA molecules. Enzymes facilitate restriction (cutting), ligation (fusing), and polymerization (copying) of DNA strands. Numerous site-specific DNA-binding proteins can be used to mask specific locations on DNA. Other enzymes can edit mistakes, twist, or untwist DNA. Similar proteins also work with ribonucleic acid (RNA). When combined with the macro effects of temperature and Ph, these naturally occurring substances provide for a nearly infinite number of creation and assembly combinations.

20.3   Coating DNA with Metals or Plastics

As discussed earlier, DNA is uniquely suited for the formation of complex three dimensional structures. However, to produce electronic circuits and nanoscale structures, it is necessary to be able to alter the properties of the DNA molecules. Fortunately DNA reacts with a wide variety of materials. Charged molecules are attracted to the negatively charged phosphate backbone. Other reagents react with the active groups on the bases. Yet other compounds intercalate between the stacked bases of the single- or double-stranded molecules. Using these compounds it is possible to alter the electronic and physical properties of the DNA molecules.

Over the last decade, several research efforts have concluded that a strand of DNA can act as an electrical conductor or semiconductor [6]. During the same time period, an almost equal number of studies concluded just the opposite; that DNA is either a poor conductor or a resistor [7]. While it is true that under certain circumstances, DNA may appear to carry a current, no research has been able to put forth consistent circumstances under which DNA, in its natural form, is a reliable conductor.

In order to convert a DNA molecule into a highly conductive wire, researchers at the Technion (Israel Institute of Technology) began work on a process to coat DNA with metal. To instill electrical functionality, silver metal is deposited along the DNA molecule, as shown in Figure 20.3. The three-step chemical deposition process is based on selective localization of silver ions along the DNA through Ag^+/Na^+ ion-exchange 18 and formation of complexes between the silver and the DNA bases. The Ag^+/Na^+ ion-exchange process is monitored by following the almost instantaneous quenching of the fluorescence signal of the labeled DNA. The ion-exchange process, which is highly selective and restricted to the DNA template alone, is terminated when the fluorescence signal drops to 1 to 5% of its initial value (the quenching is much faster than normal bleaching of the fluorescent dye). The silver ion-exchanged DNA is then reduced to form nanometer-sized metallic silver aggregates bound to the DNA skeleton. These silver aggregates are subsequently further "developed," much as in the standard photographic procedure, using an acidic solution of hydroquinone and silver ions under low light conditions. Such solutions are metastable and spontaneous metal deposition is normally very slow. However, the silver aggregates on the DNA act as catalysts and significantly accelerate the process. Under the experimental conditions, metal deposition therefore occurs only along the DNA skeleton, leaving the passivated glass practically clean of silver. The silver deposition process is monitored *in situ* by differential interference contrast (DIC) microscopy and terminated when a trace of the metal wire is clearly observable under the microscope. The metal wire follows precisely the previous fluorescence image of the DNA skeleton. The structure, size, and conduction properties of the metal wire are reproducible and dictated by the "developing" conditions [8].

The coating process works equally well with compounds other than metal and has therefore been developed into a process for coating DNA for purposes beyond conductivity. The process in its most simplified form (as shown in Figure 20.4) is as follows:

1. Synthesized or naturally occurring DNA is isolated
2. Positively charged (primary) ions are introduced and are attracted to the negatively charged phosphates (along the DNA backbone) and the negatively charged NH_2 on the bases
3. Once the ions attach, the DNA is rinsed and the secondary substance is added. This substance develops (or grows) on the primary ions creating a continuum of material along the entirety of the DNA strand [9]

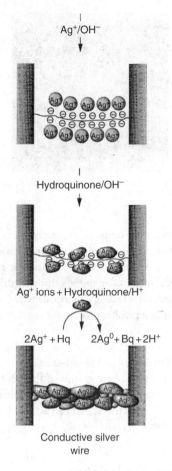

FIGURE 20.3   Silver DNA wire development. (Taken from Braun, E., Eichen, Y., Sivan, U., and Ben-Joseph, G., 1998, *Nature*, 391, 775. With permission.)

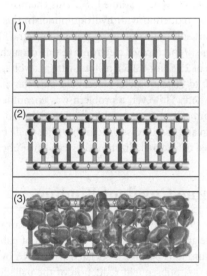

FIGURE 20.4   (See color insert.) DNA Coating (1) interdigitated wires DNA strand. (2) Oligo-nucleotide probes primary ions applied. (3) Hybridized target secondary material developed on the primary. (Taken from Keren, K., Berman, R., Buchstab, E., Sivan, U., and Braun, E., 2003, *Science*, 302, 1380–1382. With permission.)

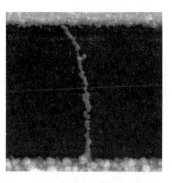

FIGURE 20.5   SEM of metal coated DNA.

The coated DNA can now possess a wide range of characteristics depending on the type of material used in the coating process. The coated strand can now bear electrical characteristics of a conductor, semiconductor, or a resistor as shown in Figure 20.5. Structurally it can be rigid, semirigid or with any level of flexibility. By running a wide range of materials through this process, DNA becomes an ideal foundation for both electrical and structural tasks. A nanoscale wire (or any other coated strand) by itself is not particularly useful; however, once a reliable process for coating DNA was established, a whole new world of possibility was opened.

Three DNA metallization chemistries have been used to convert DNA into a conducting wire [5,8–10]. These chemistries fall into two reaction categories (1) ion-exchange of a metal (silver) ion for the positive sodium counter ion associated with the phosphate groups of the DNA backbone and (2) formation of a covalent bond between a metal ion (palladium or platinum) and amine groups of the DNA bases. In both cases, the attached ions are reduced to form a metal that can act as a catalytic site for the deposition of an alternate metal on the surface of the DNA [11].

20.4   Sodium–Silver Ion Exchange

A silver-catalyzed gold chemistry has also been studied [8]. This chemistry also involves ion exchange of silver ions for sodium followed by reduction with hydroquinone. In this case, the particles of metallic silver are incubated in a three-part solution containing potassium tetrachloroaurate to develop gold on the surface of the DNA. Keren et al. [9] performed electronic testing on such metallized DNA and reported ohmic behavior with a resistance of 25 Ω for a 2.5 μm-long wire at a voltage of 0 to 2 mV. This chemistry has also been shown to form 60 to 70 nanometer-sized gold particles along the surface of DNA with no background deposition elsewhere. However, a problem was encountered with a precipitate of gold thiocyanate produced during synthesis of the tetrachloroaurate solution. This precipitate is formed as particles with diameters ≤ 0.8 μm and then redissolved into a phosphate buffer. If these particles are not completely redissolved or removed before metallization they can cause aberrant results.

20.5   Palladium–Amine Covalent Binding

Another metallization chemistry [9–11] involves the formation of a covalent bond between palladium and platinum ions and the amine groups of DNA bases. A solution of palladium acetate is mixed with a solution of DNA and the palladium ions become associated with DNA by forming covalent bonds with the amine groups of the DNA bases. Subsequent reduction of the palladium ions allows them to form autocatalytic sites for the deposition of a palladium metal coating on the surface of the DNA. Reduction of the palladium bonded to the DNA results in very small metal deposits of palladium. However, there may not be enough metal to form a continuous conducting wire after a single treatment with the palladium acetate solution. The initial palladium deposits can serve as catalytic sites for the further deposition of palladium. Subsequent rounds of treatment with palladium acetate and the reducing agent enhance these deposits with additional metallic palladium.

Richter et al. [12,13] electrically characterized wires formed by the palladium-catalyzed deposition of palladium on lambda DNA immobilized between gold electrodes with an inter-electrode gap of 5 to 10 μm. DNA was dried on the surface of a comb-shaped contact structure so that the DNA strands were perpendicular to the gold electrodes. Palladium metallization was then carried out on the microchips and voltages applied across the wires. Applied voltages in the range of tens of millivolts produced currents in the range of tens of microamps. Resistance measurements were reported for individual wires by comparing the system resistance before and after individual wires were broken. Resistance measurements were made for more than 100 wires and all showed ohmic behavior at room temperature. Data showed that a diameter of approximately 50 nm is sufficient to achieve continuous metallization of the DNA. Although the initial resistance of the wires was proportional to their length, none of the wires exhibited resistance less than 5 kΩ even when wire diameter was increased to 200 nm. These higher resistances were attributed to contact resistances between the palladium wire and the gold electrodes when electron-beam-induced carbon lines were written over the ends of the wires where contact was made with the gold electrodes. The resistance of individual wires was less than 1 kΩ. For example, a 16.5 μm wire with an average diameter of 50 nm had a resistance of 743 Ω. The two-terminal $I-V$ curve of this wire was recorded after cutting all other wires. Linear current–voltage dependence was observed for bias voltages down to 1 mV and no evidence of a nonconducting region or diode-like behavior was found at room temperature.

20.6 Patterning Materials on DNA

To fully take advantage of DNA as a substrate, one would like to direct coatings to specific regions of the DNA molecule. Reaching into nature's toolbox, it is possible to mask regions of the DNA molecule using sequence specific DNA binding proteins. During the synthesis of the DNA molecules, binding sites for masking proteins are engineered into the molecules. With the engineered molecules it is possible to mimic the lithography process on DNA to produce structures with more than one coating on a DNA molecule. Nanoscale electronic components are created through the multistep process outlined below [14]:

A specifically designed DNA strand is synthesized with single-stranded "tailed" ends. These ends will be used in the selfassembly/manipulation process once the component is created.

1. Blocking proteins are applied to specific locations along the strand, providing a mask from the coating process. Depending on the complexity of the component, several different proteins may be used
2. Once the proteins are applied, the first coating step is applied to the unblocked section of DNA
3. The masking proteins are removed with enzymes
4. The now exposed area is coated with the next coating material. Steps 4 and 5 may be repeated several times to achieve the desired characteristics
5. Once the internal areas are coated, the blocking proteins on the ends are removed and the nanoscale component is created (see Figure 20.6)

Proper design of the components is the key to assembly. The unique ends of each component will only bond to its intended counterpart. Designs can create circuits in two or three dimensions and can be independent (free floating) or be joined to a substrate like silicon for connection to more conventional circuitry. With complete circuits thousands of times smaller than their conventional counterparts, an entirely new (previously unthinkable) world of development is created.

In 2002, Keren et al. [9] demonstrated a detailed masking process for creating DNA-based electronic components. A region of DNA was coated with RecA protein. The DNA was then exposed to silver nitrate and then gold was deposited onto the regions of DNA unprotected by RecA. The RecA protein was then

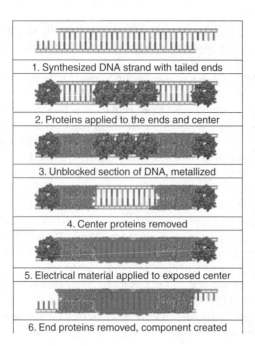

FIGURE 20.6   (See color insert.) DNA patterning process. (Taken from Thorstenson, Y.R., Hunicke-Smith, S.P., Oefner, P.J., and Davis, R.W., 1998, *Genome Res.*, 8, 848–855. With permission.)

removed to expose an uncoated region of the DNA molecule. This demonstration of sequence-specific lithography on a single molecule was an important step toward DNA-templated electronics.

In November 2003, the same group took the approach further with the creation of a DNA-templated field effect transistor (FET). The details of the FET creation are summarized here.

Assembly of a DNA-templated FET:

1. RecA monomers polymerize on a ssDNA molecule to form a nucleoprotein filament
2. Homologous recombination reaction leads to binding of the nucleoprotein filament at the desired address on an aldehydederivatized scaffold dsDNA molecule
3. The DNA-bound RecA is used to localize a streptavidin-functionalized single-walled nano tubules (SWNT), utilizing a primary antibody to RecA and a biotin-conjugated secondary antibody
4. Incubation in an $AgNO_3$ solution leads to the formation of silver clusters on the segments that are unprotected by RecA
5. Electroless gold deposition, using the silver clusters as nucleation centers, results in the formation of two DNA-templated gold wires contacting the SWNT bound at the gap (Figure 20.7) [9]

These DNA-based components can be synthesized in solution and then combined to make electronic circuits. As indicated above, single-stranded DNA ends can be protected using single-stranded DNA binding protein (SSB) to leave the ends available for binding with other components. The single stranded regions are designed to specifically bind to the end of another component. Using this approach it is possible to create selfassembling electronic circuits or devices in solution (see Figure 20.8).

20.7   Coated DNA Structures in Practice — A PCR Free, Biological Detection, and Identification Systems

A growing percentage of the things that threaten health, safety, economy, and national security are nearly invisible. From bacteria on a piece of uncooked chicken, to a stranger with a contagious cough,

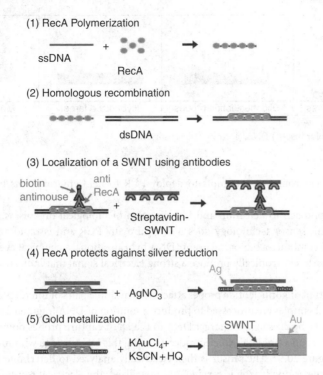

(1) RecA Polymerization

ssDNA + RecA →

(2) Homologous recombination

dsDNA →

(3) Localization of a SWNT using antibodies

biotin
antimouse   anti RecA
+ Streptavidin-SWNT →

(4) RecA protects against silver reduction

+ AgNO₃ → Ag

(5) Gold metallization

+ KAuCl₄+ KSCN+HQ → SWNT   Au

FIGURE 20.7 (See color insert.) Assembly of a DNA based field effect transistor. (Taken from Keren, K., Berman, R., Buchstab, E., Sivan, U., and Braun, E., 2003, *Science*, 302, 1380–1382. With permission.)

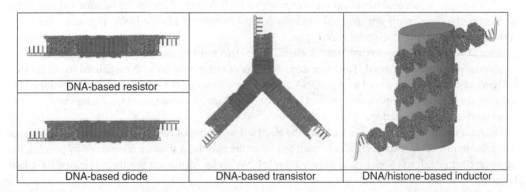

DNA-based resistor

DNA-based diode

DNA-based transistor

DNA/histone-based inductor

FIGURE 20.8 (See color insert.) DNA-based, nanoscale, electronic components. (Taken from Thorstenson, Y.R., Hunicke-Smith, S.P., Oefner, P.J., and Davis, R.W., 1998, *Genome Res.*, 8, 848–855. With permission.)

to the looming threat of bioterrorism, pathogens can cause disease ranging from a simple inconvenience to a catastrophic pandemic. Because of their size, detection and accurate identification of biological pathogens is difficult through traditional means. Current technology has proven moderately accurate, but often too slow to be effective in many situations.

A technology that could read the DNA from a sample and rapidly and accurately identify the organisms therein would address this problem. Using the mechanisms discussed heretofore in this chapter, a system has been developed with these capabilities. Currently, polymerase chain reaction (PCR) amplification followed by fluorescent analysis is the most common method of DNA identification. PCR is a well-understood and reliable laboratory process, but it is highly susceptible to contamination, is labor intensive, and requires a skilled operator and specialized equipment. It is best suited to use within a laboratory

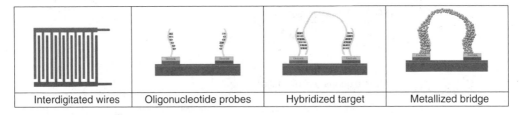

| Interdigitated wires | Oligonucleotide probes | Hybridized target | Metallized bridge |

FIGURE 20.9   (See color insert.) DNA/electronic biosensor process.

or other controlled environment. Attempts to deploy PCR to field environments have proven largely ineffective.

This electronic approach to detection and identification of biological organisms actually uses DNA to identify DNA. This sensor technology does not require any PCR and is rapid and highly accurate. The sensor uniquely combines a biological event (DNA hybridization), a chemical event (metal coating), and microelectronics, to electronically produce a strong electrical signal that indicates the presence of an organism [16].

The sensor consists of oligonucleotide probes attached to multiple pairs of interdigitated electrodes on a microchip. Biological samples are processed to produce a solution of DNA fragments that are passed over the sensor's surface. Hybridization of a target DNA to the DNA capture probes bound to the electrodes forms a DNA bridge connecting the two electrodes. Coating this DNA bridge with metal converts it to a conductive wire (Figure 20.9). The sensor is then electrically analyzed to determine if any bridges have formed. When as little as one bridge is formed and metallized, the electrical resistance of the sensor is reduced more than 1000 fold.

Once prepared, the DNA is introduced to the chip surface containing capture probes complementary to a DNA target sequence. Hybridization occurs with a high degree of specificity because (1) two complementary binding events are required (one to each electrode) and (2) the DNA fragment must be of sufficient length to span the interelectrode gap.

Since DNA by itself is not a reliable conductor [7], the DNA must be made conductive using the coating techniques previously discussed. The decreased resistance of test structures with metallized (coated) DNA bridges indicates the presence of a target DNA. Several metallization chemistries have been developed for use with the biosensor focusing on the ideal balance of rapid reaction time, minimal background, and no adverse effect on hybridization.

The final step in the process is to measure the electrical resistance of each of the test structures. Voltage is applied to one of the two electrodes in each test structure and the resistance is obtained by probing the opposite electrode. It has been observed that a single DNA bridge formation results in at least a 1000-fold reduction in resistance on the test structure.

Other groups have developed technologies that rely on electronic signals for the detection of modified DNA [17–19], but these systems are limited by a requirement for a high concentration of target DNA within the sample. Motorola used a gold electrode to form a complicated sandwich of target and reporter probes that contained ferrocene capable of donating electrons [19]. In the presence of a specific target DNA, ferrocene reporters donated electrons that were captured by the gold electrode. However, in this system, many molecules of target DNA were required to generate enough electrons to give a robust signal. Park et al. [10] reported an electronic DNA detection technology based on a gold sol hybridization technique. Gold sols were used to immobilize specific target DNAs from solution to gold surfaces in between two electrodes. Silver was then deposited on the gold sols to close the electrode gap and form a conductive bridge. This technique also required a high concentration of specific target DNA molecules to capture sufficient gold sols to produce an electrical signal.

The approach detailed above is not dependent on the presence of a high concentration of target DNA within the sample, and has a high signal to noise ratio. In this approach, prior amplification of the target DNA is unnecessary. The target DNA itself forms the connection between the two electrodes and

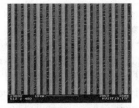

FIGURE 20.10 Thousands of DNA bridges on a sensor.

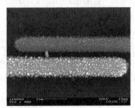

FIGURE 20.11 Single DNA bridge.

is converted to a conductive wire by direct metallization. Thus, in theory with this technology it might be possible to detect even a single hybridization event.

20.8 Components

The biosensor system is built around a two component design: a self-contained disposable test cartridge and an analyzer into which the cartridge is loaded for testing. Within each test cartridge, there is a simple silicon chip with multiple independently addressable test structures arrayed upon it. Current chip architecture supports 14 and 64 test structures, each of which may test for the same or multiple-target organisms simultaneously. Each independently addressable test structure measures about $400 \times 400 \ \mu$m. The next chip in development will have 250+ independently addressable test structures with embedded logic that will permit quantitation assays in addition to identification.

The SEMs of the sensors after metallization reveal the conductive nanowires formed between electrodes when a target biological is present. Figure 20.10 shows a test structure of target DNA hybridized to capture probes and Figure 20.11 shows a magnified view of a single wire (20 to 40 nm in diameter).

The system has successfully demonstrated electronic detection of gene targets from samples of genomic DNA from *Bacillus anthracis*. No amplification of the target sequences is performed before detection. Current research involves an expanding list of pathogens.

20.9 Sample Preparation

For a sample to be read by the electronic biosensor, preparation requires efficient release and isolation of DNA and breaking the DNA down to an appropriate size. Because the system does not require amplification of the target nucleic acid molecules, sample prep and processing requirements can be incorporated into a simple, automated procedure. Most inhibitors of the enzymes required for amplification will not have an effect on the process utilized. Additionally, detergents and organic solvents can be used to decrease nonspecific binding and inhibit degradation of target nucleic acid molecules, especially RNA targets.

There are several effective methods for releasing DNA from cells, including chemical lysis and sonication. Chemical lysis works well for human cells, common bacteria, and viruses. Sonication is more effective for disrupting bacterial spores. For most samples, chemical disruption is sufficient. After lysis, the sample is filtered to remove anything in the sample that could aberrantly short the sensors. Again, because the system does not use enzymes, it is not necessary to remove all chemical contaminants. Furthermore, the nucleic acid analog probes are not affected by salt concentrations.

The released DNA must be sheared to a length that works with the BioDetect sensor. Current DNA fragment size is between 1000 and 6000 base pairs in length. Future chip designs will lower the required target DNA length to several hundred base pairs. A mechanical shearing method provides fragments within the desired ranges [15,20]. This method involves pushing DNA through a small bore opening into a larger-bore vessel. The average length can be controlled by changes to flow rate and the size of the opening. The resulting fragments fall within a twofold size distribution.

The sheared DNA is then moved into the hybridization chamber where it can bind to the test sites on the sensor. The DNA is manipulated by mechanical mixing, electrical fields, and pulsing of the fluids. After hybridization, all unbound DNA is washed into a waste chamber.

In summary, the system requires minimal sample prep. The process which involves cell lysis, DNA shearing, and filtering can be accomplished in a single pass through cartridge which can be integrated with the detection sensor to produce a fully automated system (Figure 20.12).

20.10   Future Capabilities

The system can be highly multiplexed to test for numerous biological agents simultaneously, to provide confirmatory tests for different unique sequences from a target organism, and to provide highly accurate and quantitative results.

The new design under development will incorporate CMOS-based logic. This will allow the system to produce highly multiplexed results quickly and inexpensively using a combination of on-chip logic, statistics, and bioinformatics. The logic chips will have 256 separately addressable test sites. Future chips may have several thousands of test sites with each site possessing a unique set of probes. Additionally, each test site will be subdivided into thousands of subsensors, allowing for the collection of data for statistical and quantitative analysis. The data will be analyzed using algorithms which will weigh results from the various sensors and calculate the statistical level of certainty of a positive or negative result and provide quantitative results. Error recognition software will be utilized to recognize patterns from handling damage to electrical signals from debris, further increasing the reliability of the system.

Due to the ability to multiplex, the system can provide for more information regarding an agent than simply a yes or no identification. Through the proper design of probe sets, the chips can identify genetically altered organisms, determine drug resistances, and even provide a taxonomic analysis of an unknown organism.

This detection system provides a glimpse into the possibilities of DNA-based nanostructures. Using a simple nanowire based on a naturally occurring strand, the system provides a significant advance over current technologies, matching or exceeding the sensitivity and accuracy of PCR-based assays in the field while delivering the speed, portability, and ease-of-use of much simpler assays.

20.11   Conclusion

DNA-directed assembly is making the promise of selfassembling nanosized devices a reality. The ability to realize the dream of selfassembly allows for low-cost fabrication of simple devices which, to date, could not be produced. DNA based nanoelectronics and mechanisms will start appearing in products in the foreseeable future. Research and development in this arena holds the promise of great possibilities. Imagine: Materials that can communicate with the devices that they comprise, nanoscale machines that can accurately perform medical tasks currently dependent on high-risk surgery, high-efficiency hydrogen fuel cells, radio frequency identification (RFID) tags embedded into products at the material level, virtually eliminating time spent checking out in stores. These things and many more are not only possible, but

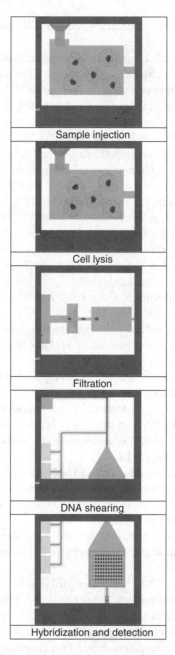

FIGURE 20.12 DNA sample prep for electronic detection.

likely in a world where DNA based nanoelectronics are used. The example of the DNA sensor system is only the beginning of the kinds of things that are possible as this exciting new arena begins to take shape.

References

[1] Dürkop, T., Brintlinger, T., and Fuhrer, M.S., 2002, Nanotubes are high mobility semiconductors, in *Structural and Electronic Properties of Molecular Nanostructures*, H. Kuzmany, J. Fink, M. Mehring, and S. Roth (Eds.) (API Conference Proceedings, New York, 2002), pp. 242–246.

[2] Tersoff, J. and Ruoff, R.S., 1994, Structural properties of a carbon-nanotube crystal, *Phys. Rev. Lett.*, 73, 676–679.

[3] Seeman, N.C., 1989, Nanoscale assembly and manipulation of branched DNA: a biological starting point for nanotechnology, NANOCON Proceedings, J. Lewis and J.L. Quel, NANOCON, Bellevue, WA, pp. 101–123; transcript of oral presentation, pp. 30–36.

[4] Seeman, N.C., 2003, DNA in a material world, *Nature*, 421, 427.

[5] Shih, W.M., Quispe, J.D., and Joyce, G.F., 2004, A 1.7-kilobase single-stranded DNA that folds into a nanoscale octahedron, *J. Nature Lett.*, 427, 618–621.

[6] Henderson, P.T., Jones, D., Hampikian, G., Kan, Y., and Schuster, G.B., 1999, Long-distance charge transport in duplex DNA: the phonon-assisted polaron-like hopping mechanism, *Proc. Natl Acad. Sci. USA*, 96, 8353–8358.

[7] Zhang, Y., Austin, R.H., Kraeft, J., Cox, E.C., and Ong, N.P., 2002, Insulating behavior of Lambda-DNA on the micron scale, *Phys. Rev. Lett.*, 89, 198–102.

[8] Braun, E., Eichen, Y., Sivan, U., and Ben-Joseph, G., 1998, DNA-templated assembly and electrode attachment of a conducting silver wire, *Nature*, 391, 775–778.

[9] Keren, K., Berman, R., Buchstab, E., Sivan, U., and Braun, E., 2003, DNA-templated carbon nanotube field-effect transistor, *Science*, 302, 1380–1382.

[10] Park, S.J., Taton, T.A., and Mirkin, C.A., 2002, Array-based electrical detection of DNA with nanoparticle probes, *Science*, 295, 1503–1506.

[11] Onoa, G.B. and Moreno, V., 2002, Study of the modifications caused by cisplatin, transplatin, and Pd(II) and Pt(II) mepirizole derivatives on pBR322 DNA by atomic force microscopy, *Int. J. Pharm.*, 245, 55–65.

[12] Richter, J., Seidel, R., Kirsch, R., Mertig, M., Pompe, W., Plaschke, J., and Schackert, K., 2000, Nanoscale palladium metallization of DNA, *Adv. Mater.*, 12, 507–510.

[13] Richter, J., Mertig, M., Pompe, W., Monch, I., and Schackert, H.K., 2001, Construction of highly conductive nanowires on a DNA template, *Appl. Phys. Lett.*, 78, 536–538.

[14] Connolly, D.M., Integrated Nano-Technologies, 2001, Method of Chemically Assembling Nano-Scale Devices, US Patent 6,248,529 B1.

[15] Thorstenson, Y.R., Hunicke-Smith, S.P., Oefner, P.J., and Davis, R.W., 1998, An automated hydrodynamic process for controlled, unbiased DNA shearing, *Genome Res.*, 8, 848–855.

[16] Connolly, D.M., Integrated Nano-Technologies, 2003, High Resolution DNA Detection Methods and Devices, US Patent 6,593,090.

[17] LaBean, T.H., Yan, H., Kopatsch, J., Liu, F., Winfree, E., Reif, J.H., and Seeman, N.C., 2000, The construction, analysis, ligation and self-assembly of DNA triple crossover molecules, *J. Am. Chem. Soc.*, 122, 1848–1860.

[18] Mao, C., Sun, W., and Seeman, N.C., 1999, Designed two-dimensional DNA holliday junction arrays visualized by atomic force microscopy, *J. Am. Chem. Soc.*, 121, 5437–5443.

[19] Umek, R.M., Lin, S.W., Vielmetter, J., Terbrueggen, R.H., Irvine, B., Yu, C.J., Kayyem, J.F., Yowanto, H., Blackburn, G.F., Farkas, D.H., and Chen, Y.P., 2001, Electronic detection of nucleic acids: versatile platform for molecular diagnostics, *J. Mol. Diagn.*, 3, 74–84.

[20] Oefner, P.J., Hunicke-Smith, S.P., Chiang, L., Dietrich, F., Mulligan, J., and Davis, R.W., 1996, Efficient random subcloning of DNA sheared in a recirculating point- sink flow system, *Nucleic Acids Res.*, 24, 3879–3886

[21] Winfree, E., Sun, W., and Seeman, N.C., 1998, Design and self-assembly of two-dimensional DNA crystals, *Nature*, 394, 539–544.

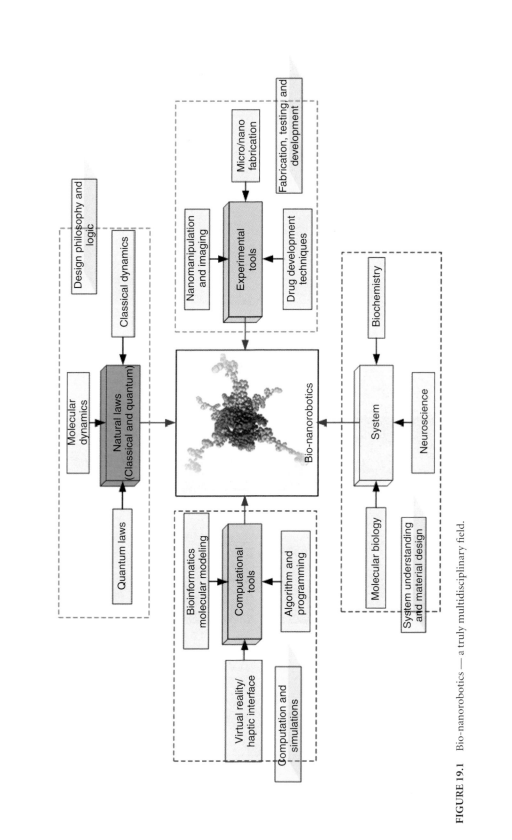

FIGURE 19.1 Bio-nanorobotics — a truly multidisciplinary field.

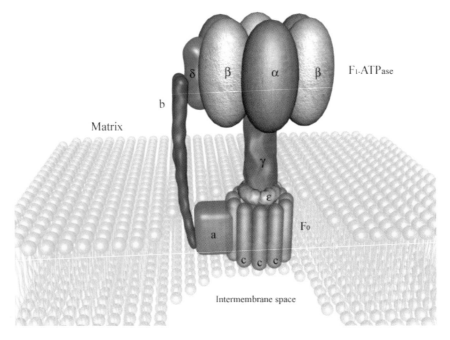

FIGURE 19.2 The basic structure of the ATP Synthase. Shown is the flow of protons from the outer membrane towards the inner through the F_0 motor. This proton motive force is responsible for the synthesis of ATP in F_1.

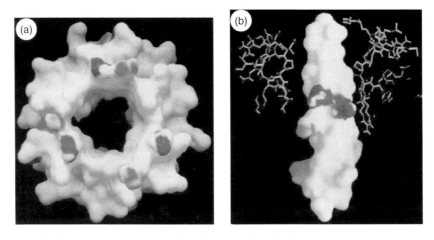

FIGURE 19.3 The electrostatic surface potential on the $\alpha_3\beta_3$ and γ subunits.

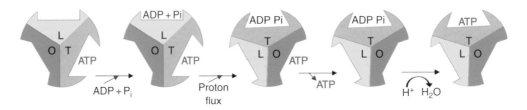

FIGURE 19.4 Boyer's binding change mechanism.

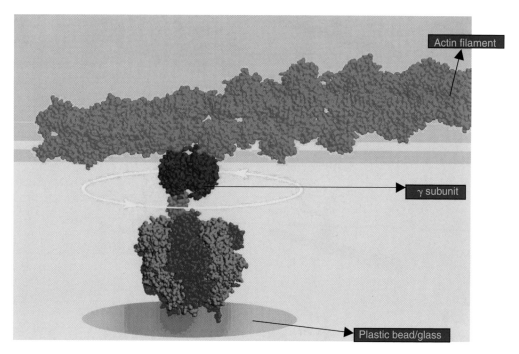

FIGURE 19.5 Experiment performed for Imaging of F_1-ATPase (Kinosita, K., Jr., Yasuda, R., Noji, H., and Adachi, K. 2000. *Philos. Trans.: Biol. Sci.* 355 (1396): 473–489. With permission).

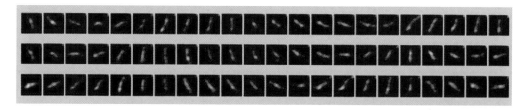

FIGURE 19.6 Images of a rotating actin filament (sequential image at 33 ms intervals)(Kinosita, K., Jr., Yasuda, R., Noji, H., and Adachi, K. 2000. *Philos. Trans.: Biol. Sci.* 355 (1396): 473–489. With permission).

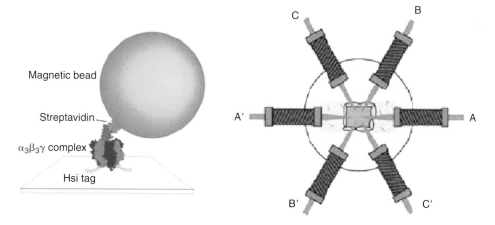

FIGURE 19.7 Magnetic bead is attached to the γ subunit here (left figure) and the arrangement of the magnets (right figure) [6].

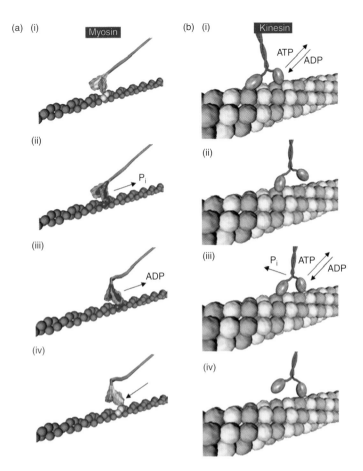

FIGURE 19.8 The kinesin–myosin walks: (a) Myosin motor mechanism. (i) Motor head loosely docking to the actin binding site; (ii) The binding becomes tighter along with the release of P_i; (iii) Lever arm swings to the left with the release of ADP, and; (iv) replacement of the lost ADP with a fresh ATP molecule results in dissociation of the head; (b) Kinesin heads working in conjunction. (i) Both ADP-carrying heads come near the microtubule and one of them (black neck) binds; (ii) Loss of bound ADP and addition of fresh ATP in the bound head moves the other (red neck) to the right; (iii) The second head (red) binds to microtubule while losing its ADP, and replacing it with a new ATP molecule while the first head hydrolyses its ATP and loses P_i; (iv) The ADP-carrying black-neck will now be snapped forward, and the cycle will be repeated.

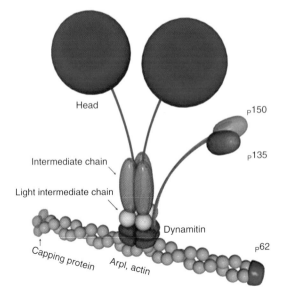

FIGURE 19.9 A dynein molecule. Shown in blue are the globular heads (heavy chains) connected to the intermediate chains (red) and the light chains (light blue). Dynactin complex components p150, p135, dynamitin, p62, capping proteins, Arp1, actin is also shown.

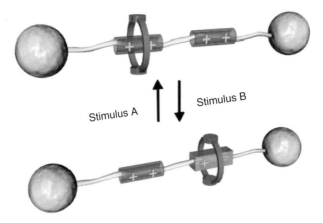

FIGURE 19.10 A typical rotaxane shuttle set-up. The macrocycle encircles the thread-like portion of the dumbbell with heavy groups at its ends. The thread has two recognition sites which can be altered reversibly so as to make the macrocycle shuttle between the two sites (state 0 and state 1).

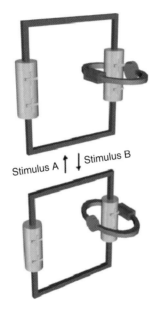

FIGURE 19.11 A nondegenerate catenane. One of the rings (the moving ring) has two different recognition sites in it. Both sites can be turned "off" or "on" with different stimuli. When the green site is activated, the force and energy balance results in the first conformation, whereas when the red one is activated, the second conformation results. They can be named states 0 and 1 analogous to binary machine language.

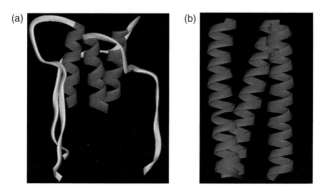

FIGURE 19.12 VPL motor at (a) neutral and (b) acidic pH. (a) Front view of the partially α-helical triple stranded coiled coil. VPL motor is in the closed conformation. (b) VPL Motor in the open conformation. The random coil regions (white) are converted into well-defined helices and an extension occurs at lower pH.

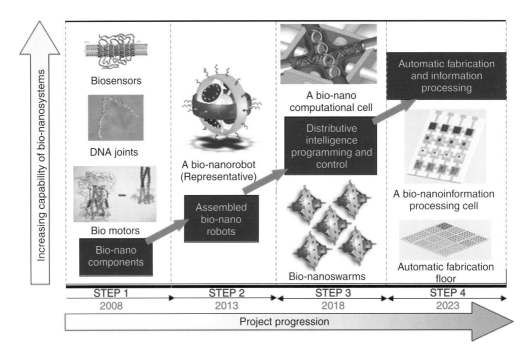

FIGURE 19.13   The roadmap, illustrating the system capability targeted as the project progresses.

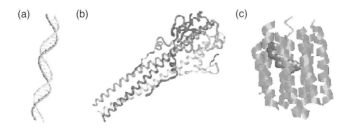

FIGURE 19.14   (Step 1) 5 years from now — understanding of basic biological components and controlling their functions as robotic components. Examples are: (a) DNA which may be used in a variety of ways such as a structural element and a power source; (b) hemagglutinin virus may be used as a motor; (c) bacteriorhodopsin could be used as a sensor or a power source.

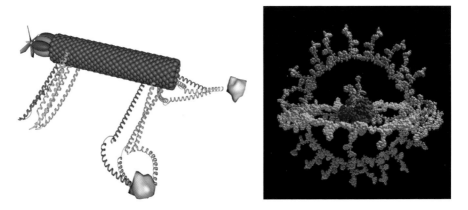

FIGURE 19.15   (Step 2) (a) The bio-nanocomponents will be used to fabricate complex biorobotic systems. A vision of a nano-organism: carbon nanotubes form the main body; peptide limbs can be used for locomotion and object manipulation and the biomolecular motor located at the head can propel the device in various environments. (b) Modular organization concept for the bio-nanorobots. Spatial arrangements of the various modules of the robots are shown. A single bio-nanorobot will have actuation, sensory, and information processing capabilities.

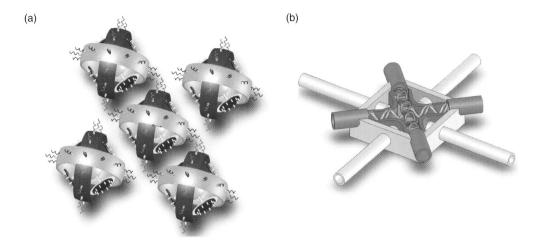

FIGURE 19.16 (Step 3) (a) Basic bio-nanorobot forming a small swarm of five robots. The spatial arrangement of the individual bio-nanorobot will define the arrangement of the swarm. Also, these swarms could be re-programmed to form bindings with various other types of robots. The number of robots making a swarm will be dependent of the resulting capability required by the mission. Also the capability of attaching new robots at run time and replacing the nonfunctional robots will be added. (b) A basic bio-nanocomputational cell. This will be based on one of the properties of the biomolecules, which is "reversibility."

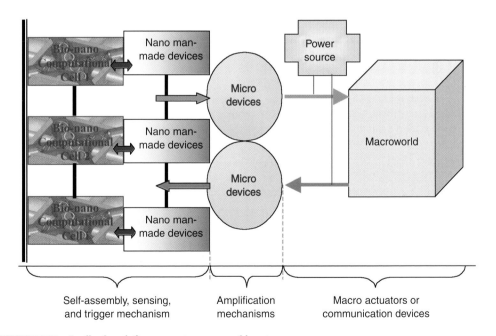

FIGURE 19.17 Feedback path from nano to macroworld route.

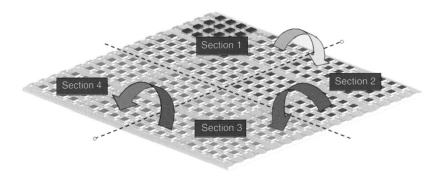

FIGURE 19.18 (Step 4): 20–30 years — an automatic fabrication floor layout. Different color represents different functions in automatic fabrication mechanisms. The arrows indicate the flow of components on the floor layout. *Section 1* → Basic stimuli storage — control expression; *Section 2* → Biomolecular component manufacturing (actuator/sensor); *Section 3* → Linking of bio-nanocomponents; *Section 4* → Fabrication of bio-nanorobots (assemblage of linked bio-nanocomponents).

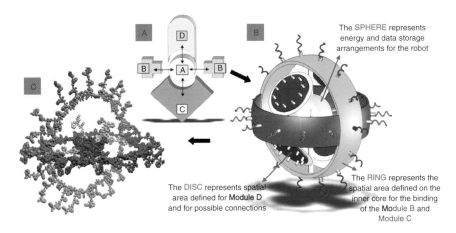

FIGURE 19.19 (a) A bio-nanorobotic Entity "ABCD," where A, B, C, and D are the various biomodules constituting the bio-nanorobot. In our case these biomodules will be set of stable configurations of various proteins and DNAs. (b) A bio-nanorobot (representative), as a result of the concept of modular organization. All the modules will be integrated in such a way so as to preserve the basic behavior (of self-assembly, self-replication, and self-organization) of the biocomponents at all the hierarchies. The number of modules employed is not limited to four or any number. It is a function of the various capabilities required for a particular mission. (c) A molecular representation of the figure (b). It shows the red core and green and blue sensory and actuation biomodules.

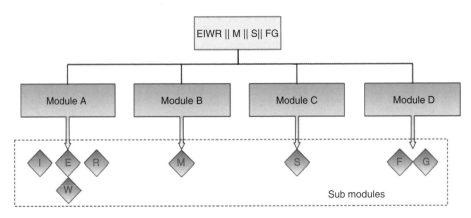

FIGURE 19.20 The bio-nanocode and the fractal modularity principle. The letter symbols have the values specified in Table 19.1. The "∥" symbol integrates the various biomodules and collectively represents a higher order module or a bio-nanorobot.

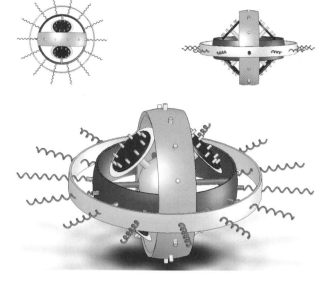

FIGURE 19.21 A variant of the initial bio-nanostem system (b), fabricated with enhanced bio-nanocode S, which defines it as a bio-nanorobot having enhanced sensory capabilities. The other features could be either suppressed or enhanced depending upon the requirement at hand. The main advantage of using bio-nanostem system is that we could at run-time decide which particular type of bio-nanorobots we require for a given situation. The suppression ability of the bio-nanostem systems is due to the property of "*Reversibility*" of the bio components found in living systems.

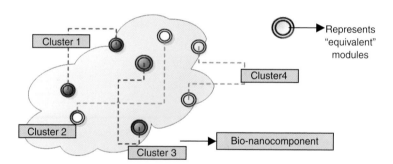

FIGURE 19.22 Representing the modular pattern recognition and clustering function (the *M*-function.)

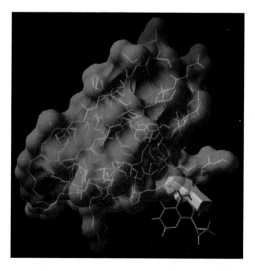

FIGURE 19.25 Molecular dynamics simulation visualized in the CAVE. (Courtesy of: Dr. Zhuming Ai, VRMedLab, University of Illinois at Chicago.)

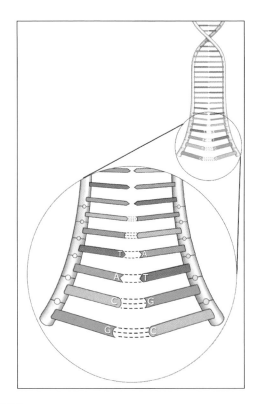

FIGURE 20.1 Structure of DNA.

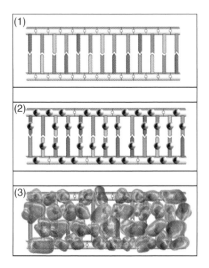

FIGURE 20.4 DNA Coating (1) interdigitated wires DNA strand. (2) Oligo-nucleotide probes primary ions applied. (3) Hybridized target secondary material developed on the primary. (Taken from Keren, K., Berman, R., Buchstab, E., Sivan, U., and Braun, E., 2003, *Science*, 302, 1380–1382. With permission.)

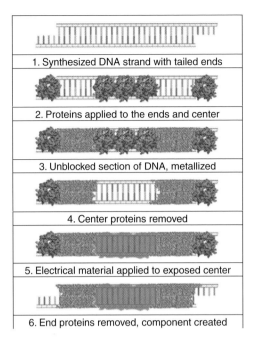

FIGURE 20.6 DNA patterning process. (Taken from Thorstenson, Y.R., Hunicke-Smith, S.P., Oefner, P.J., and Davis, R.W., 1998, *Genome Res.*, 8, 848–855. With permission.)

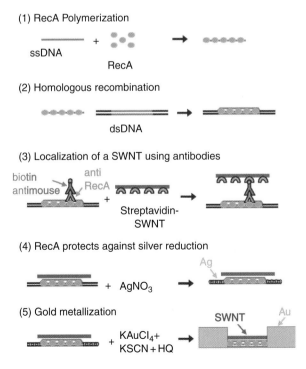

FIGURE 20.7 Assembly of a DNA based field effect transistor (Taken from Keren, K., Berman, R., Buchstab, E., Sivan, U., and Braun, E., 2003, *Science*, 302, 1380–1382. With permission.)

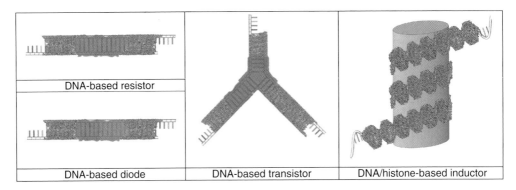

FIGURE 20.8 DNA-based, nanoscale, electronic components (Taken from Thorstenson, Y.R., Hunicke-Smith, S.P., Oefner, P.J., and Davis, R.W., 1998, *Genome Res.*, 8, 848–855. With permission.)

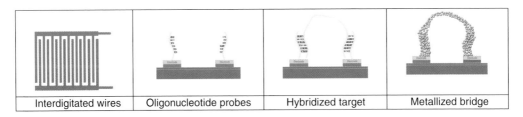

| Interdigitated wires | Oligonucleotide probes | Hybridized target | Metallized bridge |

FIGURE 20.9 DNA/electronic biosensor process.

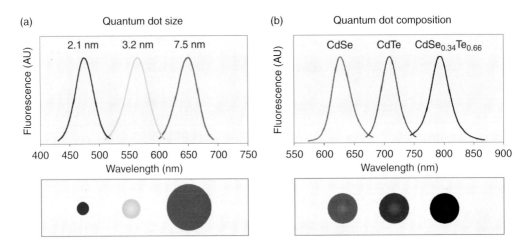

FIGURE 22.1 Size and composition tuning of optical emission for binary CdSe and ternary CdSeTe quantum dots. (a) CdSe QDs with various sizes (given as diameter) may be tuned to emit throughout the visible region by changing the nanoparticle size while keeping the composition constant. (b) The size of QDs may also be held constant, and the composition may be used to alter the emission wavelength. In the above example, 5 nm diameter quantum dots of the ternary alloy $CdSe_xTe_{1-x}$ may be tuned to emit at longer wavelengths than either of the binary compounds CdSe and CdTe due to a nonlinear relationship between the alloy bandgap energy and composition (Taken from, Bailey, R.E. and Nie, S.M. (2003). *J. Am. Chem. Soc.* 125, 7100–7106. With permission.)

Quantum dot water solubilization

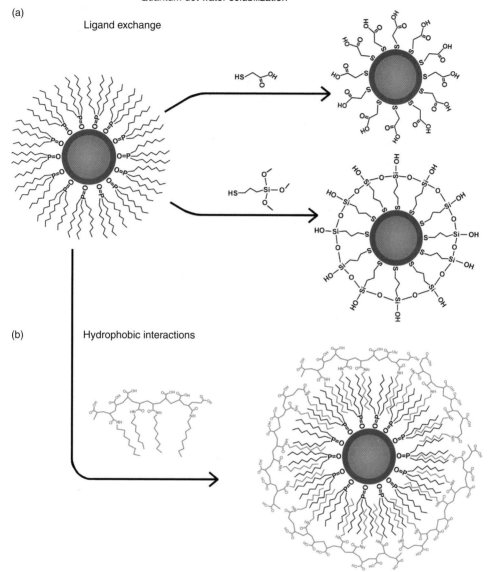

FIGURE 22.2 Diagram of two general strategies for phase transfer of TOPO-coated QDs into aqueous solution. Ligands are drawn disproportionately large for detail. (a) TOPO ligands may be exchanged for hetero-bifunctional ligands for dispersion in aqueous solution. This scheme can be used to generate a hydrophilic QD with carboxylic acids or a shell of silica on the QD surface. (b) The hydrophobic ligands may be retained on the QD surface and rendered water soluble through micelle-like interactions with an amphiphilic polymer like octylamine-modified polyacrylic acid.

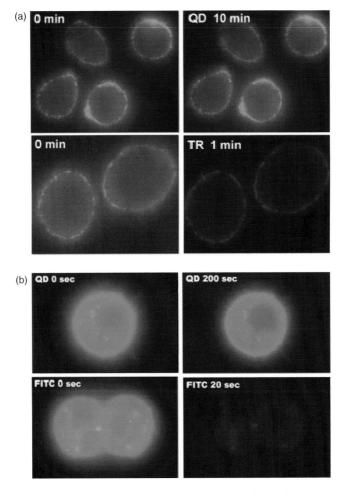

FIGURE 22.3 Immunofluorescent labeling of human breast tumor cells with antibody-conjugated quantum dots, and comparison of signal brightness and photostability with organic dyes. (a) Cancer cells labeled with antibody-conjugated QD or Texas Red (TR) targeting cell surface antigen uPAR. (b) Cancer cells labeled with antibody-conjugated QD or FITC targeting cell surface antigen Her-2/neu. Excitation from a 100 W mercury lamp caused negligible photobleaching of QDs, compared to the two organic fluorophores. (Courtesy of Dr. Xiaohu Gao, Emory University).

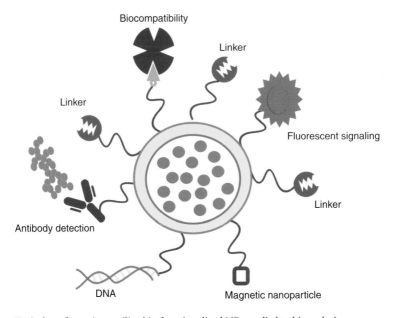

FIGURE 23.1 Typical configurations utilized in functionalized NPs applied to bioanalysis.

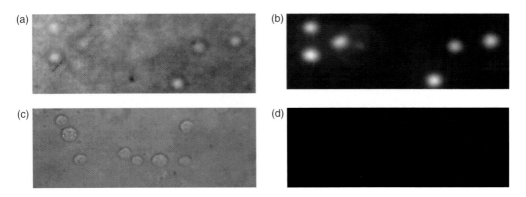

FIGURE 23.3 NPs as biomarkers for cell labeling. (a) Optical and (b) fluorescence images of leukemia cells incubated with antibody-immobilized RuBpy-doped NPs, (c) optical, and (d) fluorescence images of leukemia cells incubated with unmodified RuBpy-doped NPs as a control.

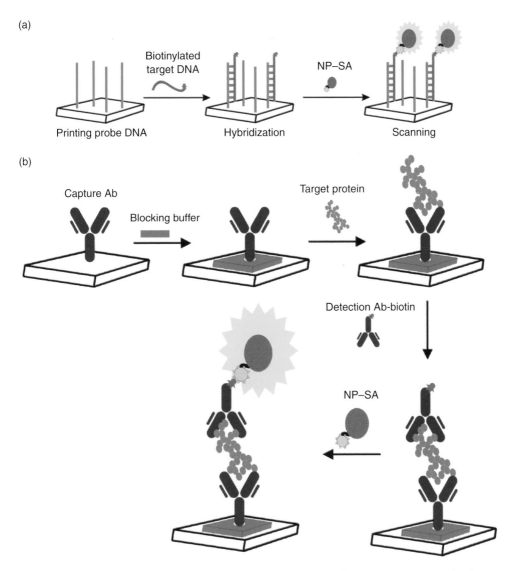

FIGURE 23.4 Strategies of NP-based labeling for (a) DNA microarray and (b) protein microarray technology.

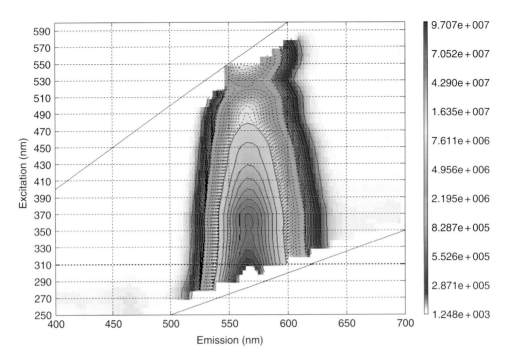

FIGURE 25.1   Semiconductor nanocrystals, also referred to as "quantum dots," are highly light absorbing, luminescent nanoparticles whose absorbance onset and emission maximum shift to higher energy with decreasing particle size due to quantum confinement effects. As seen in this typical excitation–emission plot for a type of quantum dot, strong emission is observed over a broad range of excitation wavelengths.

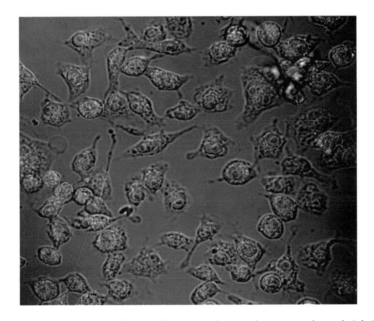

FIGURE 25.2   Quantum dots can be used for live cell imaging. They are advantageous due to their bright fluorescence over a broad range of excitation wavelengths, resistance to photobleaching, and stability. Surface modifications are required for biocompatibility.

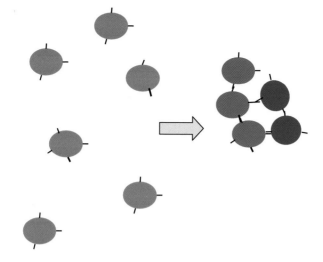

FIGURE 25.3 When gold nanoparticles come into close proximity, plasmon–plasmon interactions cause dramatic changes in optical properties. Using appropriately conjugated nanoparticles, this behavior can be exploited for DNA hybridization assays and immunoassays.

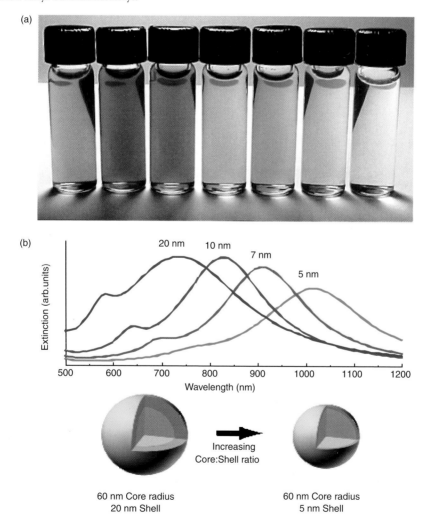

FIGURE 25.4 Gold nanoshells consist of a dielectric core nanoparticle surrounded by a thin metal shell. By varying the relative dimensions of the core and shell constituents, one can design particles to either absorb or scatter light over the visible and much of the infrared regions of the electromagnetic spectrum. A). These vials contain suspensions of either gold colloid (far left with its characteristic red color) or gold nanoshells with varying core:shell dimensions. B). The optical properties of nanoshells are predicted by Mie scattering theory. For a core of a given size, forming thinner shells pushes the optical resonance to longer wavelengths.

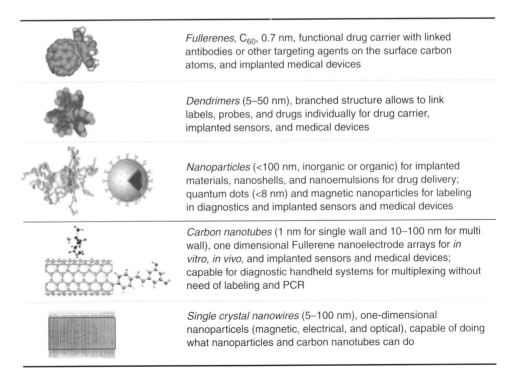

FIGURE 25.6 Breast carcinoma cells were exposed to either nanoshells (a), near infrared light (b), or the combination of nanoshells and near infrared light (c). As demonstrated by staining with the fluorescent viability marker calcein AM, the carcinoma cells in the circular region corresponding to the laser spot were completely destroyed, while neither the nanoshells nor the light treatment alone compromised viability.

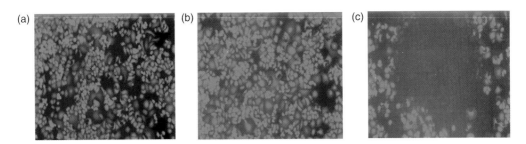

2000	1985	1972	Year
0.18 μm	1.5 μm	10 μm	Transistor size
42 million	275,000	3,500	Transistor number
1,500 MHz	33 MHz	0.2 MHz	Speed
Pentium4	80386	8008	Computer

Fullerene, nanotube, dendrimer, nanoparticle, nanowire

Silicon transistors, integrated circuit and computer

by Dr. Jie Han, 1992

FIGURE 27.1 Nano and microscale materials, devices, and systems.

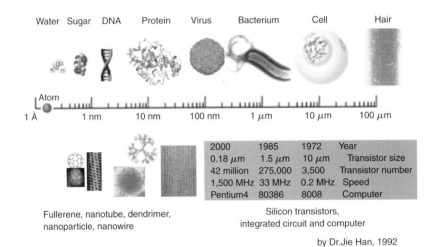

Fullerenes, C$_{60}$, 0.7 nm, functional drug carrier with linked antibodies or other targeting agents on the surface carbon atoms, and implanted medical devices

Dendrimers (5–50 nm), branched structure allows to link labels, probes, and drugs individually for drug carrier, implanted sensors, and medical devices

Nanoparticles (<100 nm, inorganic or organic) for implanted materials, nanoshells, and nanoemulsions for drug delivery; quantum dots (<8 nm) and magnetic nanoparticles for labeling in diagnostics and implanted sensors and medical devices

Carbon nanotubes (1 nm for single wall and 10–100 nm for multi wall), one dimensional Fullerene nanoelectrode arrays for *in vitro*, *in vivo*, and implanted sensors and medical devices; capable for diagnostic handheld systems for multiplexing without need of labeling and PCR

Single crystal nanowires (5–100 nm), one-dimensional nanoparticels (magnetic, electrical, and optical), capable of doing what nanoparticles and carbon nanotubes can do

FIGURE 27.2 Biologically functional nanomaterials and biomedical applications.

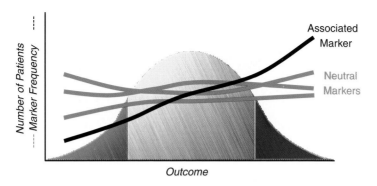

FIGURE 28.1 Physiogenomic analysis of gene marker frequency as a function of phenotype variability (association: a specific genomic marker is enriched selectively in the patients with a specific outcome).

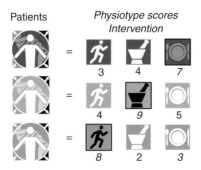

FIGURE 28.2 Physiotypes for personalized health.

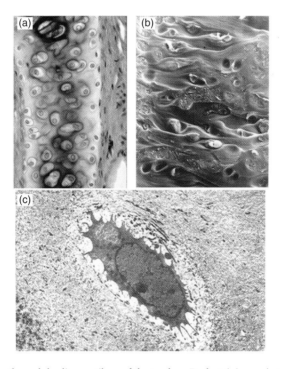

FIGURE 32.3 (a) Section through hyaline cartilage of the trachea. Dark staining regions surrounding cells (chondrocytes) are pericellular or "territorial" matrix and represent most recently-deposited cartilage matrix. (b) SEM of hyaline cartilage showing lacunae or "little lakes" in which chondrocytes reside. In this preparation some are occupied by cells and others are empty because the cells have fallen out during cutting of the cartilage. The fibrous nature of the matrix (due to the presence of type II collagen) is evident. (c) TEM of a chondrocyte within a lacuna. Collagen fibers can be seen in the cartilage matrix surrounding the lacunae. These fibers are not seen in light microscopic preparations such as those in panel a since they have the same refractive index as the collagen matrix material.

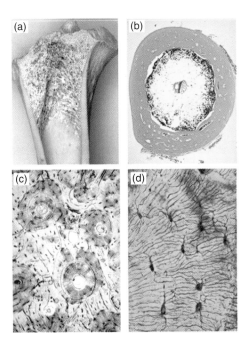

FIGURE 32.4 (a) Transverse cut through the metaphysis of a calf femur. The bone shaft is compact bone and spongy bone with bony trabeculae lining the interior. (b) Cross-section through a decalcified preparation of a fetal femur. Compact bone encloses the marrow cavity. (c) Preparation of compact bone. Concentric lamellae of Haversian systems surround blood vessels. Interstitial lamellae represent older Haversian systems replaced during bone remodeling. (d) High magnification image of a compact bone preparation. India ink fills lacunae in which embedded bone cells (osteocytes) are normally found. Channels connecting lacunae are called "canaliculi." These are occupied by cell processes and provide a means whereby osteocytes communicate with one another.

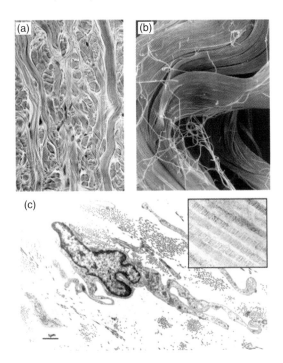

FIGURE 32.5 (a) Light micrograph of collagen fiber bundles in dense, irregular connective tissue such as the dermis of the skin. Nuclei of fibroblasts (cells that secrete procollagen which is processed and assembled into collagen extracellularly) can be seen closely associated with the fibers. (b) SEM of bands of type I collagen fiber bundles. Individual fibers can be seen independent of the fiber bundles. (c) TEM of a fibroblast in close association with bundles of collagen fibers sectioned transversely, obliquely and longitudinally. The inset shows individual collagen fibers exhibiting the characteristic periodic banding pattern.

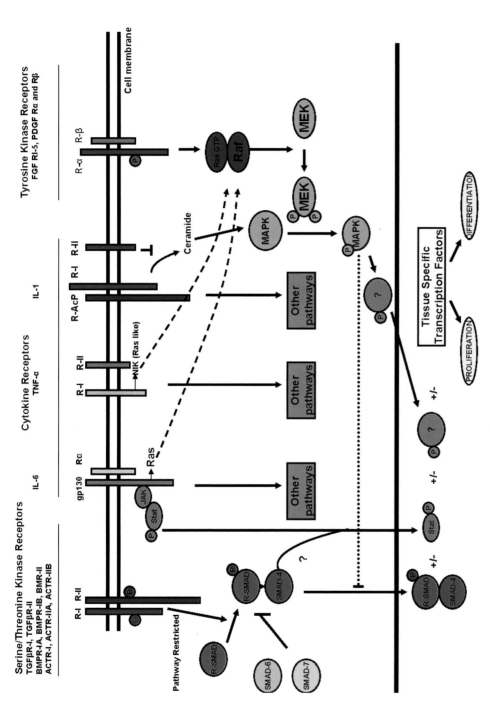

FIGURE 50.1 Major growth factors and cytokines involved in fracture repair. Reproduced from *J. Bone Miner. Res.* 1999, 14:1808 with permission of the American Society for Bone and Mineral Research.

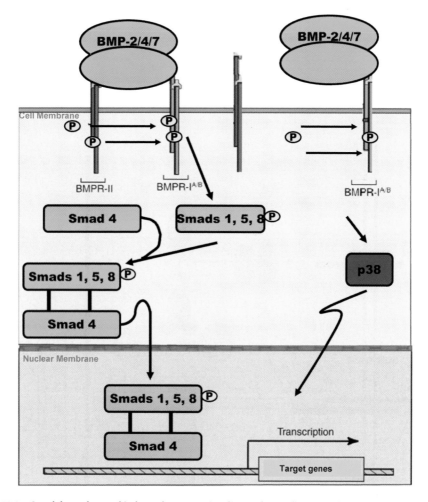

FIGURE 50.3 Smad dependent and independent BMP signaling pathways. "Reprinted from Schmitt J.M., Hwang K., Winn S.R., and Hollinger J.O. 1999. *J. Orthop. Res.* 17: 269–278. With permission from the Orthopedic Research Society."

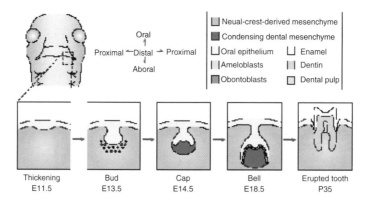

FIGURE 61.2 Stages of tooth development. A schematic frontal view of an embryo head at embryonic day (E)11.5 is shown with a dashed box to indicate the site where the lower (mandibular) molars will form. Below, the stages of tooth development are laid out from the first signs of thickening at E11.5 to eruption of the tooth at around 5 weeks after birth. The tooth germ is formed from the oral epithelium and neural-crest-derived mesenchyme. At the bell stage of development, the ameloblasts and odontoblasts form in adjacent layers at the site of interaction between the epithelium and mesenchyme. These layers produce the enamel and dentin of the fully formed tooth. (Reproduced from Tucker, A. and Sharpe, P. *Nat. Rev. Genet.* 5: 499–508, 2004. With permission.)

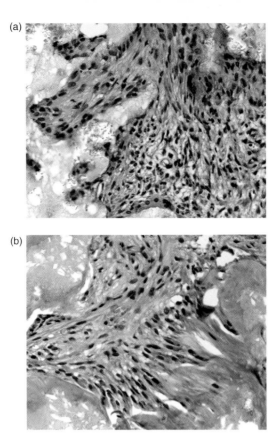

FIGURE 61.3 Hematoxylin and eosin staining of representative DPSC transplants. (a) After one week posttransplantation, DPSC transplants contain connective tissue (*CT*) around HA/TCP carrier (*HA*), without any sign of dentin formation. (b) After six week posttransplantation, DPSCs differentiate into odontoblasts (arrows) that are responsible for the dentin formation on the surface of HA/TCP (*HA*). Original magnification: 40X.

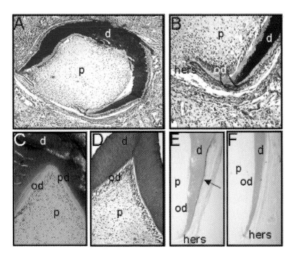

FIGURE 61.4 Histology and immunohistochemistry of a 20-week implant. (a) Von Kossa stain for calcified mineralization in bioengineered tooth crown (50× magnification). Dark brown stain is positive for mineralized tissues. (b) A high-magnification (400×) photomicrograph of the Hertwig's epithelial root sheath is shown, stained by the Von Kossa method to detect calcified mineralization. (c) High-magnification (200×) photomicrograph of cuspal region in bioengineered tooth crown. The tissue was stained by the Von Kossa method. (d) Hematoxylin and eosin (H&E) stain of a positive control porcine third molar cuspal region demonstrates morphology similar to that of the bioengineered tooth structure (200×). (e) BSP immunostain of 20-week bioengineered tooth crown (100×). Positive BSP expression is indicated by the arrow. (f) Negative preimmune control immunostain for BSP in bioengineered tooth crown (100×). Abbreviations: d, dentin; od, odontoblasts; p, pulp; pd, predentin, hers, Hertwig's epithelial root sheath.

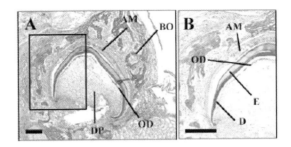

FIGURE 61.5 Recombinant explant between bone-marrow-derived cells and oral epithelium following 12 days of development in a renal capsule. All the tissues visible are donor-derived, since the host kidney makes no cellular contribution to the tissue. Where epithelium in the recombinations was from GFP mice, *in situ* hybridization of sections of these tissues confirmed that all mesenchyme-derived cells were of wildtype origin (not shown). BO, bone; Am, ameloblasts; DP, dental pulp; OD, odontoblasts, E, enamel; D, dentin. Scale bar: 80 μm. (Reproduced from Ohazama, et al. *J. Dent. Res.* 83: 518–522. With permission.)

21

Directed Evolution of Proteins for Device Applications

Jeremy F. Koscielecki
Jason R. Hillebrecht
Robert R. Birge
University of Connecticut

21.1 Protein-Based Devices

Protein-based photonic devices gain comparative advantage from the unique properties of proteins, and the fact that nature has optimized many proteins for the efficient conversion of light to structural changes. Additional advantages derive from the fact that many proteins produce a voltage, a current or change in polarizability in response to light absorption, and carry out this function with a high quantum efficiency and speed [1]. More recently, investigators are approaching the use of proteins in device applications from the perspective that nature has provided a template for optimization rather than a material with optimal properties. This view is made possible by significant advances in genetic engineering and the use of techniques such as directed evolution. The combination of *in vitro* genetic diversification with tunable selective pressures has enabled investigators to tailor biological macromolecules for electronic and photonic device applications [2–5].

The topic of this brief chapter is bacteriorhodopsin (BR) and the use of genetic engineering to optimize the protein for devices that are based on the long-lived Q state. BR is grown by the halophile archaeon *Halobacterium salinarum*, which uses the protein as a solar energy converter [6]. *H. salinarum* has survived on Earth for more than 3 billion years and has evolved a light-transducing protein that has intrinsic properties appropriate to device applications. These properties include high quantum efficiency, thermal stability, and photochemical cyclicity that combine to make the native protein useful for making thin film memories [7,8], photovoltaic converters [9], holographic processors [10], artificial retinas [11–13], associative memories [14], logic gates [15], and protein-semiconductor hybrid devices [16]. In all cases investigated, however, a genetically or chemically modified form of the protein outperforms the native protein when a systematic study is carried out to identify or create an optimized variant [17,18]. There are a number of techniques currently used to make modifications to the structure of proteins at different levels of variability. These techniques include site-directed, semirandom, and random mutagenesis. However, the most efficient technique in optimizing the structure or function of biological materials is known as directed evolution where repeated mutagenesis experiments of screening and selection yield a material with a particular characteristic [3]. In this chapter, the use of mutagenesis techniques are discussed as a method for the optimization of BR for the use in biomolecular devices.

21.2 Bacteriorhodopsin

Bacteriorhodopsin is a membrane-bound protein with seven transmembrane helices, 248 amino acid residues, and a chromophore (retinal) covalently bound via a protonated Schiff base linkage to Lys-216 near the center of the protein. BR is used by *H. Salinarum* as a photosynthetic protein and upon the absorption of light, this protein pumps protons across the cell membrane. The resulting pH gradient is used to convert ADP and inorganic phosphate into ATP [6]. The primary photochemical event involves the photoisomerization of the chromophore from all-*trans* to 13-*cis*, which forms the ground state species called K (Figure 21.1). The proton pumping process then takes place in the dark through a complex photocycle as shown in Figure 21.1. The figure also shows the branched photocycle involving the P and Q states [19]. The change in the absorption maximum of each intermediate is caused by three factors: the conformation and protonation state of the chromophore (indicated under the absorption max in Figure 21.1), protonation changes of amino acids near the chromophore, and other protein–chromophore interactions [20]. Note that the symbol bR is used to reference the light-adapted resting state of bacteriorhodopsin and the symbol BR is used to reference the protein or a protein variant in an undefined state.

The two states that are of primary interest for photonic applications are the blue-shifted M and Q states. In general, the M state is used for real-time holographic devices and memories [10,17,21,22] and the Q state, the long-lived state within the "branched photocycle," is used for both long-term holographic storage and three-dimensional memories [11,19]. The M state has significant advantages for holography because it is produced with high quantum efficiency (0.65) and generates a significant change in refractive index (Figure 21.2). A thin film of BR adjusted to have an absorptivity of 5 at 280 nm produces a film with a 6.4% holographic efficiency at 670 nm. The only disadvantage is that the holographic image is relatively short-lived (milliseconds to hours), and M-state holograms find primary application in real-time holographic processing [10,17,21,22]. A single mutation involving the replacement of Asp96 with Asn (D96N) has generated one of the most useful holographic materials known [17]. Long-term holography and data storage is carried out using the branched photocycle to form the Q state (Figure 21.1). The branching reaction from O to P is the gateway to the Q state and involves an all-*trans* to 9-*cis* photochemical event. The Q state is unique because the chromophore separates from the covalent bond to the protein to form an isolated 9-*cis* retinal chromophore, which remains caged in the binding site. The Q state

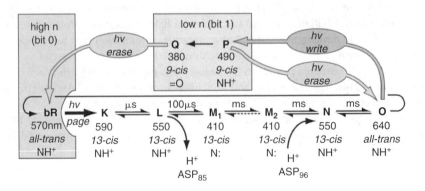

FIGURE 21.1   The main and branched photocycles of bacteriorhodopsin.

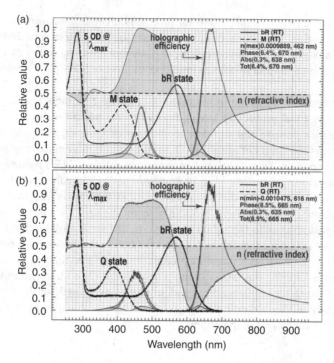

FIGURE 21.2 The diffractive and refractive properties of M-state (a) and Q-state (b) films of bR.

is a very long-lived blue shifted intermediate that has a lifetime of many years at ambient temperature (Figure 21.2). Because this state has a lower oscillator strength and is blue shifted relative to the M state, the holographic efficiency of comparable BR films based on Q-state formation have higher holographic efficiency (8.5%) than M-state films (see Figure 21.2). Furthermore, the Q state has additional uses as a binary storage component in three-dimensional memories. Space constraints prevent a detailed discussion of the three-dimensional memory, and the interested reader is directed to References 3 and 11 for details.

Holographic systems based on the M state and the D96N variant are near optimal for real-time holography [10,17,21,22]. But the native protein can also be used for real-time holography with adequate results. In contrast, competitive devices based on the Q state cannot be generated by using the native protein. Some form of chemical or genetic optimization of the protein is required to create a viable system [3,11]. The problem can be explained by reference to Figure 21.1. Note that the only method of generating Q is via a branching reaction involving photoconversion of the red-shifted O intermediate. In the native protein, the O-state concentration rarely exceeds 3 to 5% of the activated protein concentration and thus the O → P photoreaction is compromised by a lack of available O state. One of the first characteristics that needs to be optimized is the O-state concentration, and the remaining portion of this chapter will focus on methods to manipulate the formation and decay kinetics of this red-shifted intermediate. In addition, the quantum efficiency of the O → P all-*trans* to 9-*cis* photochemistry is also a problem, but one which can be addressed by using site-directed mutagenesis.

21.3 Protein Optimization via Mutagenesis

Genetic modifications can be created by using site-directed (SDM) or semirandom mutagenesis (SRM) to insert, delete, or more often, replace one or more residues. SDM is a method which carries out the substitution of a given residue with a specific replacement residue, normally involving a single site. Using a commercially available mutagenesis kit, protein variants are easily engineered once an expression system for protein production is in place. SDM requires mutation of the protein coding sequence, then expression of this gene in a host (*E. coli* or *H. salinarum*) for protein production. Because of the large number of mutations that are possible, SDM methods are not useful tools for protein optimization unless a good structure–function model of the protein is available to guide mutation. In most cases, theory is incapable of accurately predicting the impact of a given mutation, and hence SDM plays a minor role in protein optimization.

Semirandom mutagenesis or saturation mutagenesis allows each amino acid in a specified region to be mutated with an equal probability leaving the rest of the protein unchanged. SRM generates a large number of mutant proteins and therefore requires an effective screening method to analyze the photokinetic properties of a library of mutations. In some cases it is more efficient to generate mutations throughout the entire protein. Error-prone polymerase chain reaction (PCR) is one such technique and introduces mutations at a frequency from 1 to 20 mutations per 1 kb by enhancing the natural error rate of polymerase (usually *Taq*) by the modification of standard PCR methods [23]. In the case of BR, there is enough structural and prior mutagenesis work to preempt the need for a purely random search. For example, we know that residues in the region from 190 to 210 are involved in the exit channel of the protein. Thus, it is not surprising that the mutation of residues in this region has a profound impact on the lifetime of the O-state, which must transfer a proton from Asp85 into this region prior to reformation of the bR resting state. Carrying out random mutagenesis in this region has a much higher probability of generating long-lived O-state mutants than random mutations throughout the entire protein. As we explore in the next section, directed evolution may offer the best combination of efficiency and speed in finding an optimal mutation or set of mutations.

21.4 Directed Evolution

Biological systems have evolved over the past 3 billion years via an algorithm of mutation and natural selection [23]. Present day mutagenesis techniques and *in vitro* recombination methods are aimed to mimic the genetic diversification that occurs in natural ecosystems. The major advantage to the artificial creation of genetic diversity is its attenuated timescale, relative to natural mutation rates. Countless mutations can be inserted into the genetic code of nearly any biological macromolecule in a matter of hours. Combining this technology with a selection method that is specific to a parameter of interest is the fundamental essence of directed evolution.

While mutagenesis and *in vitro* recombination methods can be applied to any genetically amenable system, the limiting factor in most directed evolution investigations is the screening system used to select for optimized variants. The architectural design and stringency of the system must be tailored to the biochemical and biophysical parameters that are being optimized. Selection of optimized variants is followed by genetic and phenotypic characterization of the molecule. Select variants are then used as parental templates in subsequent rounds of directed evolution. The selective pressure in ensuing rounds of directed evolution is typically increased, in order to drive and direct the evolution of the macromolecule.

For BR to serve as a biomaterial in photochromic and optoelectronic device applications, the branched photochemistry of the protein must be optimized. Optimization of the O-state concentration and the quantum efficiency of the O $\rightarrow$ P transition are key to the architecture of BR-based optical memories. While traditional mutagenesis techniques (SDM and SRM) are useful for probing localized regions of a protein, global modifications account for more of the complicated and oftentimes distant molecular interactions that contribute to the photochemistry of a protein. Random mutagenesis, DNA shuffling, and *in vitro* recombination are just a few of the methods available for introducing global diversity into a biological macromolecule [23].

Photochemical selection of BR variants require a high throughput screening method for mutants with long O-state concentrations and efficient O $\rightarrow$ P transitions. Two types of selection methods currently exist for BR-based libraries. Type 1 selection involves the *in vitro* characterization of isolated purple membrane fragments, while type 2 involves screening the photochemistry of whole cell cultures. The photokinetic properties of each variant protein are directly measured in type 1 screening. The drawback to this method is the time and cost involved with isolating each variant protein from whole cell cultures. Type 2 screening probes the photocycle of whole cell cultures and indirectly selects for variants with optimized branched photochemistry (long Q-state concentrations). Selecting for variants with long Q-state concentrations is automated by using a modified, bioflow cell reactor. These apparatus sort out variants with undesirable photochemistry while cataloging the cells with high Q-state yields. Candidate mutants are then grown in large quantities and isolated for more detailed photochemical analysis. Mutants with favorable photochemistry are used as starting points for subsequent rounds of diversification and differential selection.

The ability to tailor a biomaterial to the demands of protein-based applications is a testament to the flexibility of directed evolution and its usefulness to the field of biomolecular electronics.

21.5 Conclusions

By using directed evolution and other mutagenesis techniques, we greatly increase the possibility for discovering a genetic variant of BR with optimal performance in a biomolecular device. Starting with a protein that nature has provided as a template will allow researchers to optimize proteins for device applications by achieving a high level of optimization in a short period of time. BR variants with altered photochemistry have already been produced that are functional and stable; directed evolution could enhance these properties even further.

References

[1] Xu, J. et al., Direct measurement of the photoelectric response time of bacteriorhodospin via electro-optic sampling. *Biophysic. J.*, 2003, **85**: 1128–1134.

[2] Arnold, F.H., Design by directed evolution. *Acc. Chem. Res.*, 1998, **31**: 125–131.

[3] Wise, K.J. et al., Optimization of bacteriorhodopsin for bioelectronic devices. *Trends Biotechnol.*, 2002, **20**: 387–394.

[4] Arnold, F. and J.C. Moore, Optimizing industrial enzymes by directed evolution. *Adv. Biochem. Eng.*, 1997, **58**: 1–14.

[5] Dalby, P.A., Optimising enzyme function by directed evolution. *Curr. Opin. Struct. Biol.*, 2003, **13**: 500–505.

[6] Oesterhelt, D. and W. Stoeckenius, Rhodopsin-like protein from the purple membrane of *Halobacterium halobium. Nature (London), New Biol.*, 1971, **233**: 149–152.

[7] Lawrence, A.F. and R.R. Birge, Communication with submicron structures. Perspectives in the application of biomolecules to computer technology. In *Nonlinear Electrodynamics in Biological Systems*, H.R. Adey and A.F. Lawrence, Eds. 1984, Plenum: New York, pp. 207–218.

[8] Schick, G.A., A.F. Lawrence, and R.R. Birge, Biotechnology and molecular computing. *Trends Biotechnol.*, 1988, **6**: 159–163.

[9] Marwan, W., P. Hegemann, and D. Oesterhelt, Single photon detection by an archaebacterium. *J. Mol. Biol.*, 1988, 663–664.

[10] Hampp, N. and T. Juchem, Fringemaker — the first technical system based on bacteriorhodopsin. In *Bioelectronic Applications of Photochromic Pigments*, 2000, IOS Press: Szeged, Hungary.

[11] Birge, R.R. et al., Biomolecular electronics: protein-based associative processors and volumetric memories. *J. Phys. Chem. B.*, 1999, **103**: 10746–10766.

[12] Miyasaka, T., K. Koyama, and I. Itoh, Quantum conversion and image detection by a bacteriorhodopsin-based artifical photoreceptor. *Science*, 1992, **255**: 342–344.

[13] Chen, Z. and R.R. Birge, Protein-based artificial retinas. *Trends Biotechnol.*, 1993, **11**: 292–300.

[14] Birge, R.R., Photophysics and molecular electronic applications of the rhodopsins. *Annu. Rev. Phys. Chem.*, 1990, **41**: 683–733.

[15] Mobarry, C. and A. Lewis, Implementations of neural networks using photoactivated biological molecules. *Proc. SPIE*, 1986, **700**: 304.

[16] Bhattacharya, P. et al., Monolithically integrated bacteriorhodopsin-GaAs field-effect transistor photoreceiver. *Opt. Lett.*, 2002, **27**: 839–841.

[17] Hampp, N., Bacteriorhodopsin: mutating a biomaterial into an optoelectronic material. *Appl. Microbiol. Biotechnol.*, 2000, **53**: 633–639.

[18] Wise, K.J. and R.R. Birge, Biomolecular photonics based on bacteriorhodopsin. In *CRC Organic Handbook of Photochemistry and Photobiology*, W. Horspool and F. Lenci, Eds. 2003, Boca Raton, FL, CRC Press, Chapter 135.

[19] Gillespie, N.B. et al., Characterization of the branched-photocycle intermediates P and Q of bacteriorhodopsin. *J. Phys. Chem. B*, 2002, **106**: 13352–13361.

[20] Ebrey, T.G., Light energy transduction in bacteriorhodopsin. In *Thermodynamics of Membrane Receptors and Channels*, M.B. Jackson, Ed. 1993, CRC Press: Boca Raton, FL, pp. 353–387.

[21] Juchem, T. and N. Hampp, Interferometric system for non-destructive testing based on large diameter bacteriorhodopsin films. *Optics Lasers Eng.*, 2000, **34**: 87–100.

[22] Oesterhelt, D., C. Bräuchle, and N. Hampp, Bacteriorhodopsin: a biological material for information processing. *Quart. Rev. Biophys.*, 1991, **24**: 425–478.

[23] Arnold, F.H. and G. Georgiou, Eds. Directed evolution library creation. *Meth. Mol. Biol.*, 2003, **231**: 3.

22

Semiconductor Quantum Dots for Molecular and Cellular Imaging

Andrew Michael Smith
Shuming Nie
Emory University
Georgia Institute of Technology

22.1 Introduction

Biological probes are indispensable tools for studying biological samples, cells in culture, and animal models. Exogenous probes are frequently multifunctional, having one component that can detect a biological molecule or event, and another component that reports the presence of the probe. A fundamental example of this functionality is a fluorescently labeled antibody: when administered to a monolayer of fixed cells, the antibody binds to its target molecule, and the fluorophore emits light to signal its presence. Of the many available reporters (e.g., radioactive isotopes, chromophores, and fluorophores), fluorescent molecules have been found to be invaluable due to their inherently high sensitivity of detection, low cost, ease of conjugation to biological molecules, and lack of ionizing radiation. Indeed, organic fluorophores and fluorescent proteins have been used in nearly all avenues of biological sensing, from *in vitro* assays, to living animal imaging. Recently quantum dots have been developed as a new class of biological fluorophore. With easily tunable properties and significant spectral advantages over conventional fluorophores, QDs have already been used for ultrasensitive biological detection.

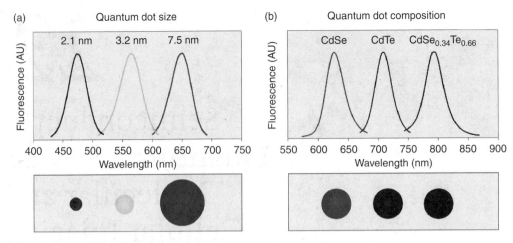

FIGURE 22.1 (See color insert following page **20**-14.) Size and composition tuning of optical emission for binary CdSe and ternary CdSeTe quantum dots. (a) CdSe QDs with various sizes (given as diameter) may be tuned to emit throughout the visible region by changing the nanoparticle size while keeping the composition constant. (b) The size of QDs may also be held constant, and the composition may be used to alter the emission wavelength. In the above example, 5 nm diameter quantum dots of the ternary alloy $CdSe_xTe_{1-x}$ may be tuned to emit at longer wavelengths than either of the binary compounds CdSe and CdTe due to a nonlinear relationship between the alloy bandgap energy and composition (Taken from Bailey, R.E. and Nie, S.M. (2003). *J. Am. Chem. Soc.* 125, 7100–7106. With permission.)

Semiconductor QDs have captivated scientists and engineers over the past two decades due to their fascinating optical and electronic properties that are neither available from isolated molecules nor from bulk solids. QDs are nanocrystals of inorganic semiconductors that are restricted in three dimensions to a somewhat spherical shape, typically with a diameter of 2 to 8 nm (on the order of 200 to 10,000 atoms). Bulk-phase semiconductors are characterized by valence electrons that can be excited to a higher-energy conduction band. The energy difference between the valence band and the conduction band is the bandgap energy of the semiconductor. The excited electron may then relax to its ground state through the emission of a photon with energy equal to that of the bandgap. When a semiconductor is of nanoscale dimensions, the bandgap is dependent on the size of the nanocrystal. As the size of a semiconductor nanocrystal decreases, the bandgap increases, resulting in shorter wavelengths of light emission. This quantum confinement effect is analogous to the quantum mechanical "particle in a box," in which the energy of the particle increases as the size of the box decreases. Cadmium selenide (CdSe) is the prototypical QD, and its size-tunable fluorescence throughout the visible light spectrum is depicted in Figure 22.1a. Other semiconductor materials display fluorescence in different spectral ranges, so that QDs can be synthesized to emit at wavelengths between 400 and 2000 nm by changing their composition and size [1–3]. An important consequence of this quantum confinement effect for biologists is that these size-tunable properties occur at the same size regime as biological macromolecules like proteins and nucleic acids.

22.2 Quantum Dots vs. Organic Fluorophores

Fluorescent dyes have been valuable in the study of biological phenomena due to their inherent high sensitivity of detection and ease of use. QDs may provide a new class of biological labels that could overcome the limitations of organic dyes and fluorescent proteins. With size-tunable fluorescence emission, QDs can be generated for any specific wavelength, from the UV through the near-infrared [4]. QD emission peaks are narrow (FWHM typically 25 to 35 nm) and symmetric compared to organic fluorophores, making them ideal for applications involving the simultaneous detection of multiple fluorophores [5].

In addition, the broad absorption spectra of QDs allow the excitation of multiple fluorophores with a single light source, at any wavelength shorter than the emission peak wavelength [5]. QDs are highly resistant to photobleaching, a commonly occurring problem for organic fluorophores, thus making them useful for continuous monitoring of fluorescence [6]. QDs have very large molar extinction coefficients and high quantum yields, resulting in bright fluorescent probes in aqueous solution [7]. Moreover, QDs have long fluorescence lifetimes on the order of 20 to 50 nsec, which may allow them to be distinguished from background and other fluorophores for increased sensitivity of detection [4].

It should be noted, however, that QDs are unlikely to replace organic dyes. Although QDs are commercially available, they are currently expensive compared to organic dyes, and changing an already established biological detection system from dyes to QDs will require time and optimization. Also QDs are an order of magnitude larger than organic dyes. Therefore, applications such as real-time monitoring of biomolecular interactions (in which steric hindrance is of concern) may require the use of organic dyes, as QDs smaller than 1 nm are inherently unstable. In addition, most organic dyes are of similar sizes, so that fluorophores of different emissions are similar sterically, compared to the large difference in QD size required to tune their wavelength. However, it has been shown that the emission wavelengths of alloy QDs may be tuned by altering the alloy composition, while keeping the size constant (Figure 22.1b) [1].

22.3 Synthesis and Bioconjugation

22.3.1 Synthesis and Capping

The prototypical QD is CdSe because colloidal syntheses for monodisperse nanocrystals of this semiconductor are well established. CdSe is most often synthesized through the combination of cadmium and selenium precursors in the presence of a QD-binding ligand that stabilizes the growing QD particles and prevents their aggregation into bulk semiconductor. Among various synthetic methods reported in the literature, high-temperature synthesis in coordinating solvents has yielded the best size monodispersity and fluorescence efficiencies. A coordinating solvent serves as a solvent and as a ligand, and is most commonly a mixture of trioctylphosphine (TOP), trioctylphosphine oxide (TOPO), and hexadecylamine (HDA). The basic functional groups of these ligands (phosphines, phosphine oxides, and amines) attach to the QD surface during synthesis, leaving the ligand alkyl chains directed away from the surface. The resulting QDs are highly hydrophobic, and only soluble in nonpolar solvents such as chloroform and hexane. The CdSe core is often capped with a thin layer of a higher bandgap material, such as ZnS or CdS, which removes surface defects, significantly improving fluorescence quantum yields.

22.3.2 Water Solubilization and Bioconjugation

For use in biological labeling, QDs must be rendered hydrophilic so that they are soluble in aqueous buffers. Two general strategies have been developed for phase transfer of QDs to aqueous solution (Figure 22.2). In the first approach, hydrophobic surface ligands are replaced with bifunctional ligands such as mercaptoacetic acid, which contains a thiol group that binds strongly to the QD surface as well as a carboxylic acid group that is hydrophilic [7]. Other functional groups may also be used; for example, silane groups can be polymerized into a silica shell around the QD after ligand exchange [4]. In the second method, coordinating ligands (e.g., TOPO) on the QD surface are used to interact with amphiphilic polymers or lipids [6,8], resulting in micelle-like encapsulation of the QD. This later method is more effective than ligand exchange at maintaining the QD optical properties and storage stability in aqueous buffer, but it increases the overall size of QD probes. Water-soluble QDs may be rendered biologically active through conjugation to biomolecules, such as nucleic acids, proteins, or small molecules. Attachment of these biomolecules has been demonstrated using a variety of intermolecular interactions, including covalent coupling [4,7], ionic attraction [9], and streptavidin–biotin bridging [6].

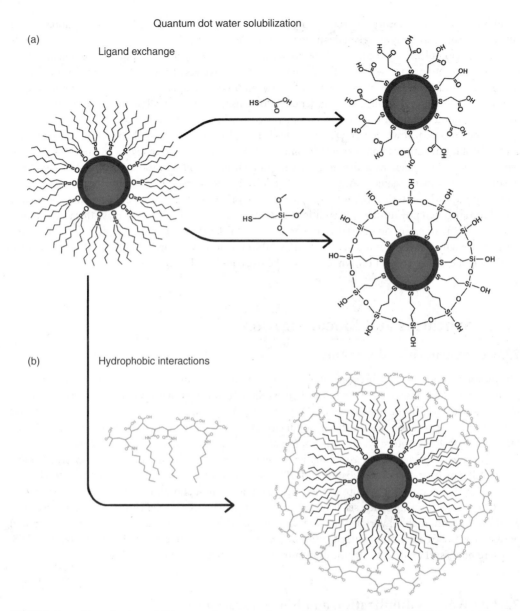

FIGURE 22.2 (See color insert.) Diagram of two general strategies for phase transfer of TOPO-coated QDs into aqueous solution. Ligands are drawn disproportionately large for detail. (a) TOPO ligands may be exchanged for hetero-bifunctional ligands for dispersion in aqueous solution. This scheme can be used to generate a hydrophilic QD with carboxylic acids or a shell of silica on the QD surface. (b) The hydrophobic ligands may be retained on the QD surface and rendered water soluble through micelle-like interactions with an amphiphilic polymer like octylamine-modified polyacrylic acid.

22.4   Biological Applications

Fluorescence is a sensitive and routine means for monitoring biological events using fluorescent dyes and fluorescent proteins. Since 1998, QDs have also been used as biological labels in a variety of bioassays, some of which would not have been possible with conventional fluorophores. *In vitro* bioanalytic assays were developed by using QD-tagged antibodies, FRET-QD biosensors, as well as by using QD-encoded microbeads. In addition to solution-based assays, the spectroscopic advantages of QDs have also allowed sensitive optical imaging in living cells and animal models. Many reports have concentrated on simply replacing organic dyes with QDs, without utilizing their unique properties. This analysis will focus on the publications that have exploited their resistance to photobleaching and potential for multiplexed detection.

22.4.1 Bioanalytic Assays

Organic fluorophores are commonly used as reporters in a large number of *in vitro* bioassays, such as quantitative immunoassays and fluorescence quenching assays for macromolecular interactions. High sensitivity has been realized with the use of organic dyes, but the spectral properties of QDs could lead to further improvements. Research in the application of QDs for *in vitro* bioanalysis has been advanced primarily by Mattoussi and his coworkers at the U.S. Naval Research Laboratory [9,10], and can be divided into two areas: immunoassays and biosensors.

Immunoassays typically involve the specific binding of a labeled antibody to an analyte, followed by physical removal of unbound antibody to allow the quantification of the bound label. QDs have been conjugated to antibodies for use in an assortment of these fluoroimmunoassays for detection of proteins and small molecules [10]. The results of these studies proved that QDs may be used as "generalized" reporters in immunoassays, but did not demonstrate an advantage over organic fluorophores, in that their sensitivity was comparable to that of commercial assays (protein concentrations down to 2 ng/ml, or 100 pM) [11]. The main advantages of QDs for immunoassays are their narrow, symmetric emission profiles and the excitability of many different QDs with a single light source, allowing the detection of multiple analytes simultaneously. Taking advantage of these spectral properties, Goldman et al. [10] simultaneously detected four toxins using four different QDs, emitting between 510 and 610, in a sandwich immunoassay configuration. Although there was spectral overlap of the emission peaks, deconvolution of the spectra revealed fluorescence contributions from all four toxins. This assay was far from quantitative, however, and it is apparent that fine-tuning of antibody cross-reactivity will be required to make multiplexed immunoassays useful.

Whereas immunoassays require the physical separation of unbound QD conjugates prior to analysis, biosensors can be developed to detect biomolecular targets on a real-time or continuous basis. QDs are ideal for biosensor applications due to their resistance to photobleaching, allowing for continuous monitoring of a signal. Fluorescence resonance energy transfer (FRET) has been the major proposed mechanism to render QDs switchable from a quenched "off" state to a fluorescent "on" state. FRET is the nonradiative energy transfer from an excited donor fluorophore to an acceptor. The acceptor can be any molecule (another nanoparticle, a nonemissive organic dye, or fluorophore) that absorbs radiation at the wavelength of donor emission. QDs are promising donors for FRET-based applications due to their continuously tunable emissions that can be matched to any desired acceptor, and their broadband absorption, allowing excitation at a short wavelength that does not directly excite the acceptor.

It has been confirmed that QDs can be FRET donors, quenchable with efficiencies up to 99%, using organic fluorophores, nonemissive dyes, gold nanoparticles, or other QDs as acceptors. Medintz et al. [9] used QDs conjugated to maltose binding proteins as an *in situ* biosensor for carbohydrate detection. Adding a maltose derivative covalently bound to a FRET acceptor dye caused QD quenching, and fluorescence was restored upon addition of native maltose, which displaced the sugar-dye compound. A key element of this work was that the physical orientation and stoichiometry of the maltose receptors on the QDs were controlled so that the restoration of QD fluorescence upon maltose addition could be directly related to maltose concentration. Although the FRET quenching efficiency was low, this work demonstrates the potential of QD-based *in situ* biosensing.

22.4.2 QD-Encoding

Rather than using single QDs for biological detection schemes, it has been proposed that different colors of QDs can be combined into a larger structure, such as a microbead, to yield an "optical barcode" [5].

With the combination of six QD emission colors and ten QD intensity levels for each color, one million different codes are theoretically possible. Biological molecules may be optically encoded by conjugation to these beads, opening the door to the multiplexed identification of many biomolecules for high-throughput screening of biological samples. Pioneering work was reported by Han et al. [5] in 2001, in which 1.2 μm polystyrene beads were encoded with three colors of QDs (red, green, and blue) and different intensity levels. The beads were then conjugated to DNA, resulting in different nucleic acids being distinguished by their spectrally distinct optical codes. These encoded probes were incubated with their complementary DNA sequences, which were also labeled with a fluorescent dye as a target signal. The hybridized DNA was detected through co-localization of the target signal and the probe optical code, via single-bead spectroscopy, using only one excitation source. The bead code identified the sequence, while the intensity of the target signal corresponded to the presence and abundance of the target DNA sequence.

The high-throughput potential of this seminal report was realized in 2003 with the use of a similar system to detect DNA sequences that differed by only one nucleotide (single nucleotide polymorphisms) [12]. In this work, 194 samples of 10 different DNA sequences from specific alleles of the human cytochrome P450 gene family were correctly identified by hybridization to encoded probes. High-throughput analysis was achieved by the use of flow cytometry to identify spectral codes, rather than single-bead spectroscopy. This identification would have been considerably more difficult with organic fluorophores due to the fact that their emission peaks overlap, obscuring the distinct codes, and the fact that multiple excitation sources would be required.

Once encoded libraries have been developed for identification of nucleic acid sequences and proteins, solution-based multiplexing of QD-encoded beads could quickly produce a vast amount of genomic and protein expression data. Another approach to gene multiplexing has been the use of planar chips, but bead-based multiplexing has advantages of greater statistical analysis, faster assaying time, and the flexibility to add additional probes at lower costs.

22.4.3 Imaging of Cells and Tissues

Fluorescent dyes are used routinely for determining the presence and location of biological molecules in cultured cells and tissue sections. Two original papers in 1998 demonstrated the feasibility of using QDs for cell labeling, displaying distinct advantages over organic dyes (Figure 22.3). Bruchez et al. [4] demonstrated dual-color labeling of fixed mouse fibroblasts, staining the nucleus with green QDs, and labeling the F-actin filaments in the cytoplasm with red QDs. Chan et al. [7] showed that QDs maintained their bright fluorescence in live cells, by imaging the uptake of transferrin-conjugated QDs by HeLa cells. These studies showed that QDs were brighter and more photostable than organic fluorophores, a claim that has been verified by independent reports [6].

In 2003, QDs were used for the first time to visualize cellular structures at high resolution, as Wu et al. [6] illustrated immunocytochemical stains of membrane, cytoplasmic, and nuclear antigens in fixed cells. Although imaging of fixed cells is useful and sufficient for many applications, live cell microscopy is ideal for visualizing cellular processes, but is considerably more difficult. It has been shown that many cell types naturally engulf QDs through a nonspecific uptake mechanism [13]. This mechanism was used to track the migration of breast tumor cells on a substrate coated with red QDs; the fluorescence inside the cells increased as the cells transversed and engulfed the QDs, leaving behind a dark path [13]. This and other studies demonstrated that QDs can be imaged inside living cells for long periods of time (over a week), a task that is not possible with organic fluorophores due to photobleaching. Indeed, QDs have opened up a new avenue for studying biomolecular processes inside living cells.

Two true marvels of real-time live cell imaging have recently been demonstrated using QDs. Dahan et al. [14] labeled glycine receptors on neuronal membranes with QDs. Imaging of the cells revealed the ability to observe the motion of single QDs, in real time (single, isolated QDs can be identified visually because they "blink"). This first example of single molecule detection using QDs in living cells produced remarkable movies of glycine receptor diffusion. In a second report, Lidke et al. [15] used QDs conjugated to epidermal growth factor (EGF) to monitor the interactions between EGF and the erbB/HER

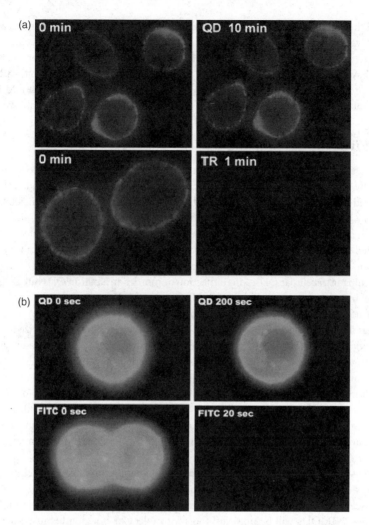

FIGURE 22.3   (See color insert.) Immunofluorescent labeling of human breast tumor cells with antibody-conjugated quantum dots, and comparison of signal brightness and photostability with organic dyes. (a) Cancer cells labeled with antibody-conjugated QD or Texas Red (TR) targeting cell surface antigen uPAR. (b) Cancer cells labeled with antibody-conjugated QD or FITC targeting cell surface antigen Her-2/neu. Excitation from a 100 W mercury lamp caused negligible photobleaching of QDs, compared to the two organic fluorophores. (Courtesy of Dr. Xiaohu Gao, Emory University.)

receptor on living cell membranes. Single molecules of EGF were visualized, in real time, as they bound to receptors and were endocytosed. This allowed the study of receptor interactions, and revealed a new cellular filopodial transport phenomenon.

Because the use of QDs as reporters in living cells may soon become conventional, the possibility of QD cytotoxicity is of interest and concern. Almost all of the reports of QDs in living cells have revealed little or no obvious cytotoxicity or changes in cellular differentiation [8,13]. Although QDs contain toxic elements, most importantly divalent cadmium, cytotoxicity issues may only become relevant for truly long-term (months to years) visualization of QDs in cells, a time period in which QD degradation could become significant.

QDs have been used as labels for studying single molecules that interact with the membranes of living cells. Performing the same task with intracellular targets will be much more difficult, but is essential for visualizing processes in living cells. Advanced delivery methods are needed to deliver QD probes into living cells, and the delivered probes must be available for binding to intracellular targets, and not trapped in endosomes, lysosomes, or other organelles. Until this becomes possible, intracellular processes can only be modeled by using isolated macromolecules under *in vitro* conditions. For example, QD-actin bioconjugates have been used to observe single molecule motorized motion of actin filaments sliding across myosin proteins in an ATP-driven reaction [16]. These model systems should be visualizable intracellularly once a protocol for translocation across the cellular membrane is established.

22.4.4 *In Vivo* Animal Imaging

The progression from optical microscopy of cells *in vitro* to optical imaging of entire organisms has mainly been inhibited by poor penetration of visible light through tissue. Due to this attenuation problem, QDs were initially used as optical imaging contrast agents only in simple model systems. In 2002, Akerman et al. [17] conjugated QDs to peptides for targeting endothelial cell receptors in specific tissues (lung, tumor blood vessels, or tumor lymphatic vessels). Intravenous injection of these bioconjugated nanoparticles into a mouse revealed accumulation of QDs in the targeted tissue, visualized histologically. Whole organism imaging was not performed in this work, but was achieved by Dubertret et al. [8] on small *Xenopus* embryos containing intracellular QDs. Microinjection of more than a billion QDs into single cells allowed cell lineage tracking and real-time imaging of stably fluorescent QDs.

To solve the attenuation problem for optical imaging in larger organisms and in deeper tissue, it has been shown that the far-red and near-infrared (NIR) spectral regions are characterized by less scattering and absorption by biological tissue. For sensitive detection, wavelengths must be chosen so that excitation light can penetrate tissue to the desired depth, and the emitted light must be able to travel back to a photodetector. Several semiconductor materials have been used to generate bright QDs that emit between 650 and 2000 nm [1,3]. There are no conventional dyes that that are bright and photostable that can emit fluorescence light beyond ~850 nm, which is why QDs are expected to provide substantial advantages for NIR optical imaging. NIR QDs with emission maxima between 750 and 860 nm were used to image coronary vasculature in a rat model [18], and to visualize sentinel lymph nodes in a pig, in 1-cm deep tissue [19].

Most imaging systems generate image contrast based on attenuation of radiation through tissue. Imaging with contrast based on molecular differences in tissue is called molecular imaging. Organic fluorescent dyes and fluorescent proteins have already been used as contrast agents for fluorescent molecular imaging in animal models. NIR QDs will be powerful tools for molecular imaging because they can be imaged in real time with multiplexed detection to monitor biomolecular phenomena *in vivo*. In our own lab we have recently been able to perform molecular imaging for the detection of subdermal tumors. Targeting of antibody-conjugated QDs to tumors has allowed generation of whole-body fluorescence imaging of mice with contrast based on biomolecular differences between normal and cancerous tissue [20].

22.5 Future Directions

Quantum dots have already fulfilled some of their promise as groundbreaking biological labels. The tremendous amount of interest in QDs is sure to quickly improve the previous applications and inspire new ones. Organic fluorophores may never be completely supplanted due to their inherently small size, but research in the past five years has shown that QDs offer remarkable advantages.

In the near future, the development of efficient QD biosensors may make QDs into powerful tools not just for *in vitro* biosensing, but also for living cell studies and *in vivo* imaging. Biosensors based on organic fluorophores have already shown promise *in vivo*, as tumors in mice were detected with "stealth" quenched probes, activatable upon exposure to proteases in the tumor microenvironment. The ability of a biochemical signal to switch a QD from an "off" to an "on" state would be an important and powerful tool for studying intracellular signaling. The development of a "quantum dot beacon" would be a monumental advance. For this to become a reality, however, biosensing QDs must be translocated across the cell membrane. Although microinjection and nonspecific uptake have been used, widespread applications must wait for a generalizable methodology for efficient delivery of QD probes into living cells. Recent research in our lab has shown that delivery peptides can be used for rapid intracellular QD translocation, and other groups have already demonstrated their efficacy for the delivery of other types of nanoparticles. The QD combination of real-time imaging, multiplexing capabilities, single molecule detection, and biological sensing on the nanoscale should allow scientists to address a broad array of analytical problems and biological questions.

A major goal in nanotechnology research is to develop smart multifunctional devices with nanometer dimensions. Although this is a lofty goal seemingly for the distant future, many multifunctional devices have already been created, and many tools have been developed for the assembly of QDs into complex, ordered structures. One proposed multifunctional device is a nanoscale contrast agent for multimodality imaging. QDs are fluorescent contrast agents, but can also be used as markers for electron microscopy due to their high electron density. Multimodal imaging has already been performed in cells to correlate fluorescence staining with electron micrographs using QDs [14]. As well, QDs may be combined with MRI contrast agents like Fe_2O_3 and FePt nanoparticles. By correlating the deep imaging capabilities of magnetic resonance imaging (MRI) with ultrasensitive optical fluorescence, a surgeon could visually identify tiny tumors or other small lesions during an operation and remove the diseased cells and tissue completely. Medical imaging modalities such as MRI and PET (positron emission tomography) can identify diseases noninvasively, but they do not provide a visual guide during surgery. The development of magnetic or radioactive QD probes could solve this problem.

Another desired multifunctional device would be the combination of a QD imaging agent with a therapeutic agent. Not only would this allow tracking of pharmacokinetics, but diseased tissue could be treated and monitored simultaneously and in real time. Surprisingly QDs may be innately multimodal in this fashion, as they have been shown to have potential activity as photodynamic therapy agents. These combinations are only a few possible achievements for the future. Practical applications of these multifunctional nanodevices will not come without careful research, but the multidisciplinary nature of nanotechnology may expedite these goals by combining the great minds of many different fields. The success seen so far with QDs points toward the success of QDs in biological systems, and also predicts the success of other avenues of bionanotechnology.

Acknowledgments

This work was supported by a grant from the National Institutes of Health (R01 GM60562), the Georgia Cancer Coalition (Distinguished Cancer Scholar Award to S.N.), and the Coulter Translational Research Program at Georgia Tech and Emory University. We are grateful to Dr. Xiaohu Gao for stimulating discussions and for providing Figure 22.3 for this article. A.M.S. acknowledges the Whitaker Foundation for generous fellowship support.

References

[1] R.E. Bailey and S.M. Nie (2003) Alloyed semiconductor quantum dots: tuning the optical properties without changing the particle size. *J. Am. Chem. Soc.* 125, 7100–7106.

[2] X.H. Zhong, Y.Y. Feng, W. Knoll, and M.Y. Han (2003) Alloyed $Zn_xCd_{1-x}S$ nanocrystals with highly narrow luminescence spectral width. *J. Am. Chem. Soc.* 125, 13559–13563.

[3] B.L. Wehrenberg, C.J. Wang, and P. Guyot-Sionnest (2002) Interband and intraband optical studies of PbSe colloidal quantum dots. *J. Phys. Chem. B* 106, 10634–10640.

[4] M. Bruchez, M. Moronne, P. Gin, S. Weiss, and A.P. Alivisatos (1998) Semiconductor nanocrystals as fluorescent biological labels. *Science* 281, 2013–2016.

[5] M.Y. Han, X.H. Gao, J.Z. Su, and S. Nie (2001) Quantum-dot-tagged microbeads for multiplexed optical coding of biomolecules. *Nat. Biotechnol.* 19, 631–635.

[6] X.Y. Wu, H.J. Liu, J.Q. Liu, K.N. Haley, J.A. Treadway, J.P. Larson, N.F. Ge, F. Peale, and M.P. Bruchez (2003) Immunofluorescent labeling of cancer marker Her2 and other cellular targets with semiconductor quantum dots. *Nat. Biotechnol.* 21, 41–46.

[7] W.C.W. Chan and S.M. Nie (1998) Quantum dot bioconjugates for ultrasensitive nonisotopic detection. *Science* 281, 2016–2018.

[8] B. Dubertret, P. Skourides, D.J. Norris, V. Noireaux, A.H. Brivanlou, and A. Libchaber (2002) *In vivo* imaging of quantum dots encapsulated in phospholipid micelles. *Science* 298, 1759–1762.

[9] I.L. Medintz, A.R. Clapp, H. Mattoussi, E.R. Goldman, B. Fisher, and J.M. Mauro (2003) Self-assembled nanoscale biosensors based on quantum dot FRET donors. *Nat. Mater.* 2, 630–638.

[10] E.R. Goldman, A.R. Clapp, G.P. Anderson, H.T. Uyeda, J.M. Mauro, I.L. Medintz, and H. Mattoussi (2004) Multiplexed toxin analysis using four colors of quantum dot fluororeagents. *Anal. Chem.* 76, 684–688.

[11] E.R. Goldman, G.P. Anderson, P.T. Tran, H. Mattoussi, P.T. Charles, and J.M. Mauro (2002) Conjugation of luminescent quantum dots with antibodies using an engineered adaptor protein to provide new reagents for fluoroimmunoassays. *Anal. Chem.* 74, 841–847.

[12] H.X. Xu, M.Y. Sha, E.Y. Wong, J. Uphoff, Y.H. Xu, J.A. Treadway, A. Truong, E. O'Brien, S. Asquith, M. Stubbins, N.K. Spurr, E.H. Lai, and W. Mahoney (2003) Multiplexed SNP genotyping using the Qbead (TM) system: a quantum dot-encoded microsphere-based assay. *Nucleic Acids Res.* 31, e43.

[13] W.J. Parak, R. Boudreau, M. Le Gros, D. Gerion, D. Zanchet, C.M. Micheel, S.C. Williams, A.P. Alivisatos, and C. Larabell (2002) Cell motility and metastatic potential studies based on quantum dot imaging of phagokinetic tracks. *Adv. Mater.* 14, 882–885.

[14] M. Dahan, S. Levi, C. Luccardini, P. Rostaing, B. Riveau, and A. Triller (2003) Diffusion dynamics of glycine receptors revealed by single-quantum dot tracking. *Science* 302, 442–445.

[15] D.S. Lidke, P. Nagy, R. Heintzmann, D.J. Arndt-Jovin, J.N. Post, H.E. Grecco, E.A. Jares-Erijman, and T.M. Jovin (2004) Quantum dot ligands provide new insights into erbB/HER receptor-mediated signal transduction. *Nat. Biotechnol.* 22, 198–203.

[16] A. Mansson, M. Sundberg, M. Balaz, R. Bunk, I.A. Nicholls, P. Omling, S. Tagerud, and L. Montelius (2004) *In vitro* sliding of actin filaments labelled with single quantum dots. *Biochem. Biophys. Res. Commun.* 314, 529–534.

[17] M.E. Akerman, W.C.W. Chan, P. Laakkonen, S.N. Bhatia, and E. Ruoslahti (2002) Nanocrystal targeting *in vivo*. *Proc. Natl Acad. Sci. USA* 99, 12617–12621.

[18] Y.T. Lim, S. Kim, A. Nakayama, N.E. Stott, M.G. Bawendi, and J.V. Frangioni (2003) Selection of quantum dot wavelengths for biomedical assays and imaging. *Mol. Imag.* 2, 50–64.

[19] S. Kim, Y.T. Lim, E.G. Soltesz, A.M. De Grand, J. Lee, A. Nakayama, J.A. Parker, T. Mihaljevic, R.G. Laurence, D.M. Dor, L.H. Cohn, M.G. Bawendi, and J.V. Frangioni (2004) Near-infrared fluorescent type II quantum dots for sentinel lymph node mapping. *Nat. Biotechnol.* 22, 93–97.

[20] X.H. Gao, Y.Y. Cui, R.M. Levenson, L.W.K. Chung, and S.M. Nie (2004) *In vivo* cancer targeting and imaging with semiconductor quantum dots. *Nat. Biotechnol.* 22, 969–976.

23

Bionanotechnology for Bioanalysis

Lin Wang
Weihong Tan
University of Florida

23.1 Overview

Bionanotechnology is defined by science's growing ability to work at the molecular level, atom by atom, combining biological materials and the rules of physics, chemistry, and genetics to create tiny synthetic structures. The end result of bionanotechnology is to create a highly functional system of biosensors, electronic circuits, nanosized microchips, molecular "switches," and even tissue analogs for growing skin, bones, muscle, and other organs of the body — all accomplished in ways that allow these structures to assemble themselves, molecule by molecule. On the other side, medical and biotechnological advances in the area of disease diagnosis and treatment are dependent on an in-depth understanding of biochemical processes. Diseases can be identified based on anomalies at the molecular level and treatments are designed based on activities in such low dimensions. Although a multitude of methods for disease identification as well as treatment already exists, it would be ideal to use research tools with dimensions close to the molecular level to better understand the mechanisms involved in the processes. These tools can be nanoparticles (NPs), nanoprobes, or other nanomaterials, all of which exist in ultrasmall dimensions and can be designed to interrogate a biochemical process of interest.

Nanomaterials are at the leading edge of the rapidly evolving field of nanotechnology. NPs usually form the core of nanobiomaterials [1]. The unique size-dependent physical and chemical properties of NPs make them superior and indispensable in many areas of human activity. Typical size dimensions of biomolecular components are in the range of 5 to 200 nm, which is comparable with the dimensions of man-made NPs. Using NPs as biomolecular probes allows us to probe biological processes without interfering with them [2].

The representative NP probes include semiconductor NPs (quantum dots), gold NPs, polystyrene latex NPs, magnetic NPs and dye-doped NPs. In our laboratory, dye-doped silica NPs have been developed, which possess unique properties of high signal amplification [3], excellent photostability, and easy surface modification.

23.2 Nanoparticle Surface Modification

To employ NPs as biological tags, a biological or molecular coating or layer acting as a bioinorganic interface should be attached to the NPs. The approaches used in constructing nano-biomaterials are schematically presented (Figure 23.1). To prepare such conjugates from NPs and biomolecules, the surface chemistry of the NPs must be such that the ligands are fixed to the NPs and possess terminal functional groups that are available for biochemical coupling reactions. A variety of surface modification and immobilization procedures have been utilized in our laboratory [4–8]. Recently we have developed new methods by cohydrolysis of organosilanes with TEOS (tetra ethyl orthosilicate) [9–13] for NP surface modification, which facilitates NP bioconjugation as well as NP dispersion.

Dye-doped silica NPs are first prepared using a water-in-oil microemulsion system. After a 24 h polymerization process, organosilanes with a range of terminal functional groups (Figure 23.2) are introduced into the microemulsion together with TEOS. Thiol groups (Figure 23.2a) are immobilized onto NPs by cohydrolysis of TEOS with MPTS (3-mercaptopropyltrimethoxy-silane). Amino groups can be introduced

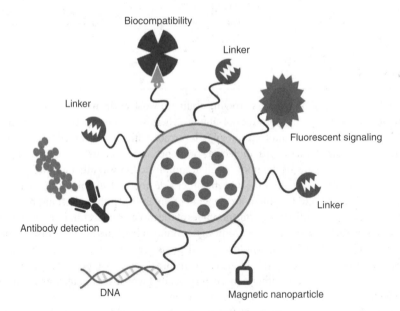

FIGURE 23.1 (See color insert following page **20**-14.) Typical configurations utilized in functionalized NPs applied to bioanalysis.

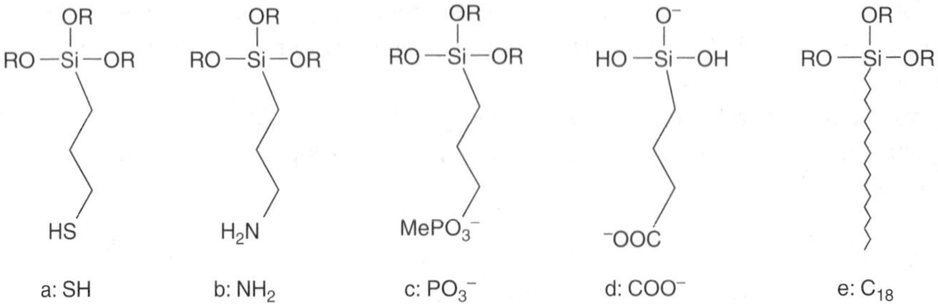

FIGURE 23.2 Structure of representative organosilanes for NP surface modification.

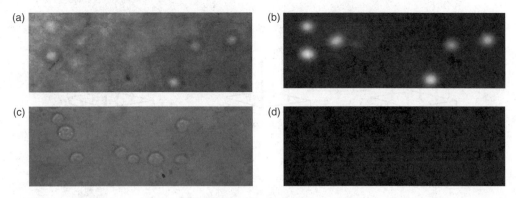

FIGURE 23.3 (See color insert.) NPs as biomarkers for cell labeling. (a) Optical and (b) fluorescence images of leukemia cells incubated with antibody-immobilized dye-doped NPs, (c) optical, and (d) fluorescence images of leukemia cells incubated with unmodified dye-doped NPs as a control.

onto NPs with the addition of APTS (3-aminopropyltriethoxysilane) (Figure 23.2b) and carboxyl groups modified NPs can be obtained by cohydrolyzing CTES (carboxyethylsilanetriol, sodium salt) (Figure 23.2d) with TEOS. To produce an overall negative surface charge, inert phosphonate groups (Figure 23.2c) can also be introduced onto NP surfaces.

Silica NPs are hydrophilic in nature and can be easily dispersed in water. For reactions in a nonpolar medium, it is essential to coat the NPs with hydrophobic alkyl groups. These hydrophobic silica NPs can be prepared during a postcoating process by cocondensation of alkyl functionalized triethoxy silane, such as octadecyl triethoxysilane (Figure 23.2e) and TEOS. The surface modified NPs thus act as a scaffold for the grafting of biological moieties (DNA oligonucleotides or aptamers, enzymes, proteins, etc.). To the functional groups by means of standard covalent bioconjugation schemes or electrostatic interactions between NPs and charged adapter molecules.

23.3   Nanoparticles for Cellular Imaging

For effective cellular labeling techniques, biomarkers need to have excellent specificity toward biomolecules of interest and also have optically stable signal transducers. Dye-doped silica NPs are ideal candidates for cellular membrane labeling and imaging. An example was demonstrated for the biomarking of leukemia cells. Mouse antihuman CD10 antibody was used as the cell recognition element and labeled with NPs pretreated with CNBr [7]. The mononuclear lymphoid cells were incubated with CD10 labeled NPs. After incubation, unbound NPs were washed away with phosphate buffered saline (PBS) buffer (pH 6.8). The cell suspension was then imaged with both optical and fluorescence microscopy. As shown in Figure 23.3, all of the cells in the field of view of the microscope were labeled, indicated by the bright emission of the dye-doped NPs. The optical image (Figure 23.3a) correlated well with the fluorescence image (Figure 23.3b). The control experiments with bare dye-doped NPs (no antibody attached) did not show labeling of the cells as shown in Figure 23.3c,d (optical image and fluorescence image). This clearly shows that the NPs conjugated with antibody are able to perform as a biomarker for cells via antibody–antigen recognition. With further development of this system, the NPs can serve as an efficient biomolecular analysis tool.

23.4   Nanoparticles for Microarray Technology

Dye-doped NPs have distinct advantages over conventional dye molecules in terms of their excellent photostability and extremely high signal amplification, which allow them to be favorably used as luminescent

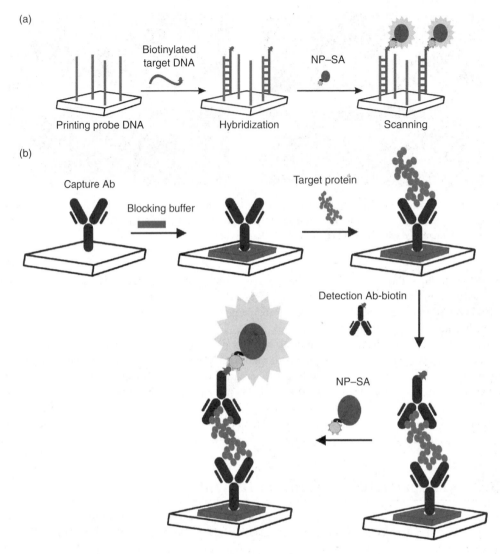

FIGURE 23.4 (See color insert.) Strategies of NP-based labeling for (a) DNA microarray and (b) protein microarray technology.

probes for bioassays. For every binding event, one NP provides thousands of dye molecules rather than only a few, resulting in an increased sensitivity for most bioanalytical applications such as ultrasensitive DNA detection.

Dye-doped NPs can be potentially applied as staining probes for DNA/protein microarray-based technology. Current imaging and detection of microarrays suffer from weak signal intensities and low photobleaching threshold of the staining probes. To overcome these problems, NP-based microarray detection has been proposed as an alternative for microarray technology. Metal NPs [14–16], magnetic NPs [17–18], and semiconductor nanocrystals [19] have been employed as labels for chip-based DNA detection. To further increase the sensitivity to lower molecular concentrations, dye-doped silica NPs can be employed as fluorescent labels for DNA and protein microarray detection. The strategies are shown in Figure 23.4a,b for DNA and protein microarray applications. Basically, streptavidin labeled NPs bind to biotinylated target DNA (DNA microarray) or biotinylated detection antibody (protein microarray). The highly fluorescent NPs provide amplified signal for trace amounts of samples, solve the major sensitivity limitation of microarray technology and push the boundaries of discovery. This advance is of significant importance when microarray analysis is applied in areas such as genetic screening, proteomics, safety assessment, and medical diagnosis.

23.5 Future Perspectives

Although NPs have been successfully utilized as biomolecular probes, they have not yet been exploited to their full potential. Some key advances include making NPs for drug delivery regimes and targeting biologically relevant diseases, using NPs for whole-cell labeling and cytoplasmic or nuclear target labeling, and developing NP detection probes for single molecule separation and detection techniques. All of these promising techniques, designed with nanometer dimensions, show that NPs will have a far-reaching impact on the ultrasensitive detection and monitoring of biological events.

Acknowledgments

This work is partially supported by NIH and NSF grants and by a Packard Foundation Science and Technology Award. We thank our colleagues at the University of Florida for their contributions.

References

[1] Feynman, R., There's plenty of room at the bottom. *Science*, 1991, 254, 1300–1301.

[2] Taton, T.A., Nanostructures as tailored biological probes. *Trends Biotechnol.*, 2002, 20, 277–279.

[3] Zhao, X., Bagwe, R.P., and Tan, W., Development of organic-dye-doped silica nanoparticles in a reverse microemulsion. *Adv. Mater.*, 2004, 16, 173–176.

[4] Qhobosheane, M., Santra, S., Zhang, P., and Tan, W., Biochemically functionalized silica nanoparticles. *Analyst*, 2001, 126, 1274–1278.

[5] Zhao, X., Tapec, R., and Tan, W., Ultrasensitive DNA detection using bioconjugated nanoparticles. *J. Am. Chem. Soc.*, 2003, 125, 11474–11475.

[6] Tapec, R., Zhao, X., and Tan, W., Development of organic dye-doped silica nanoparticle for bioanalysis and biosensors. *J. Nanosci. Nanotechnol.*, 2002, 2, 405–409.

[7] Hilliard, L., Zhao, X., and Tan, W., Immobilization of oligonucleotides onto silica nanoparticles for DNA hybridization studies. *Anal. Chim. Acta*, 2002, 470, 51–56.

[8] Santra, S., Zhang, P., Wang, K., Tapec, R., and Tan, W., Conjugation of biomolecules with luminophore-doped silica nanoparticles for photostable biomarkers. *Anal. Chem.*, 2001, 73, 4988–4993.

[9] Kriesel, J.W. and Tilley, T.D., Synthesis and chemical functionalization of high surface area dendrimer-based xerogels and their use as new catalyst supports. *Chem. Mater.*, 2000, 12, 1171–1179.

[10] Epinard, P., Mark, J.E., and Guyot, A., A novel technique for preparing organophilic silica by water-in-oil microemulsions. *Polym. Bull.*, 1990, 24, 173–179.

[11] Izutsu, H., Mizukami, F., Sashida, T., Maeda, K., Kiyozumi, Y., and Akiyama, Y., Effect of malic acid on structure of silicon alkoxide derived silica. *J. Non-Cryst. Solids*, 1997, 212, 40–48.

[12] van Blaaderen, A. and Vrij, A., In Bergna, H.E., Ed., *The Colloid Chemistry of Silica, American Chemical Society*, Washington, DC, 1994, p. 83.

[13] Markowitz, M.A., Schoen, P.E., Kust, P., and Gaber, B.P., Surface acidity and basicity of functionalized silica particles. *Colloids Surfaces A*, 1999, 150, 85–94.

[14] Fritzsche, W., Craki, A., and Moller, R., Nanoparticle-based optical detection of molecular interactions for DNA-chip technology. *Proc. SPIE*, 2002, 4626, 17–22.

[15] Caski, A., Maubach, G., Born, D., Reichert, J., and Fritzsche, W., DNA-based molecular nanotechnology. *Single Mol.*, 2002, 3, 275–280.

[16] Fritzsche, W. and Taton, T.A., Metal nanoparticles as labels for heterogeneous, chip-based DNA detection. *Nanotechnology*, 2003, 14, R63–R73.

[17] Schotter, J., Kamp, P.B., Beckere, A., Puhler, A., Reiss, G., and Bruckl, H., Comparison of a prototype magnetoresistive biosensor to standard fluorescent DNA detection. *Biosensors Bioelectron.*, 2004, 19, 1149–1156.

[18] Zhao, X., Tapec R., Wang, K., and Tan, W., Efficient collection of trace amounts of DNA/mRNA molecules using genomagnetic nano-capturers. *Anal. Chem.*, 2003, 75, 11474–11475.

[19] Gerion, D., Chen, F., Kannan, B., Fu, A., Parak, W.J., Chen, D.J., Majurndar, A., and Alivisatos, A.P., Room-temperature single-nucleotide polymorphism and multiallele DNA detection using fluorescent nanocrystals and microarrays. *Anal. Chem.*, 2003, 75, 4766–4772.

24

Nano-Hydroxyapatite for Biomedical Applications

Zongtao Zhang
Inframat Corporation

Yunzhi Yang
Joo L. Ong
University of Tennessee

24.1 Introduction

Pure crystalline hydroxyapatite (HA) has the composition of $Ca_{10}(PO_4)_6(OH)_2$ with the calcium to phosphor mole ratio Ca/P = 1.67. The main composition of the biological bone is nano-grained hydroxyapatite (HA) with the grain size of about 5 to 50 nm (see Figure 24.1). In a physiological environment, bone is a nonstoichemical HA of Ca/P mole ratio = 1.5 to 1.67, dependent on the age and bone site. Some ions such as HPO_4^{2-}, CO_3^{2-}, and F^{-1} replace partial PO_4^{3-} and OH^{-1}. Some other earth elements such as Mg^{2+} and Sr^{2+} can replace Ca^{2+}, too. The common formula should be $Ca_{10-x+y}(PO_4)_{6-x}(OH)_{2-x-2y}$, where $0 < x < 2$ and $0 < y < x/2$. For example, the bone composition can be represented by the formula of

$$Ca_{8.3}(PO_4)_{4.3}(HPO_4, CO_3)_{1.7}(OH, CO_3)_{0.3}$$

Bone is a living tissue and undergoes a constant change in composition by either dissolving or deposition of bone minerals through osteoclast and osteobalst cells, respectively. The nano-HA has a nano-crystalline feature similar to the bone, thus being sued as the bone substitute material [1–3].

Synthetic nano-HA has been introduced in medical application since the 1970s. The major products are coatings on metallic dental, hip, and spine implants for the acceleration of early stage healing and decreasing the pain. Other products such as nano-HA powders or porous blocks are used as bone fillers. From 1980s to 1990s, a calcium phosphate cement (Nano-HA formed after cementation) has been used

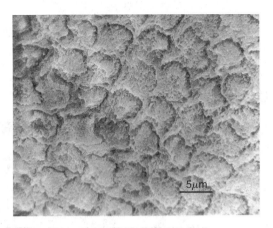

FIGURE 24.1   Biological HA from dental enamel etched by 30 sec with 35% phosphoric acid (Taken from Buddy D. Ratner, Allan S. Hoffman, Frederick J. Schosen, and Jack E. Lemons, *Biomaterials Science*, Academic Press, New York, 1996, p. 321. With permission.)

for cosmetic surgery and spine fusion. From 1990s to the present, nano-HA has been used for tissue engineering and drug delivery. In this chapter, we will briefly introduce the basic science of HA material, manufacturing process, application, and try to reflect on the latest progress of applications.

24.2   Basic Science of Nano-Hydroxyapatite

Nanostructured hydroxyapatite is defined as the HA material with the grain size of less than 100 nm. The nanostructured materials exhibited some unique properties that normal microstructured materials do not have, such as high hardness and low wear rate for engineering materials. For hydroxyapatite, the nanomaterial will have extremely high surface area. Since the atoms in the surface layer has un-saturated atomic bond, nano-HA exhibit a high bioactivity, which accelerates the early stage bone growth and tissue healing [3–10]. Supposing the 0.8 nm-thick surface layer (about one crystal lattice parameter, $a = 9.418$ Å, $c = 6.884$ Å) on the spherical ball, the volume fraction of surface bioactive atoms can be calculated to be $1 - (1 - 0.8/D)^3$, where D is the diameter of the particle. The calculated result is shown in Figure 24.2. For 10 nm grain size, the surfaced atoms account for about 22%, while the 50 nm grains have only 5% atoms on the surface. If the grain size is larger than 100 nm, the surface atoms account for less than 2.5%. The smaller the grain size, the higher the surface atoms, this results in quicker bone growth and faster dissolution rate. Experimental results of magnetic nano-$NiZnFe_2O_4$ particles have been demonstrated in Figure 24.2 model [11–13].

24.3   Nano-HA Chemistry

Hydroxyapatite is composed of CaO, P_2O_5, and H_2O, thus its stability is dependent on both the temperature and water vapor pressure. Figure 24.3 shows the phase diagram of CaO and P_2O_5 at 500 mm Hg partial pressure of water. At 500 mm Hg water vapor, HA is the stable phase below 1360°C, and decomposed into tetracalcium phosphate (C_4P or TTCP), ($Ca_4(PO_4)_2O$) and alfa-tricalcium phosphate (α-C_3P), $Ca_3(PO_4)_2$ at >1360°C. The complete decomposition occurs at 1550 to 1570°C and HA becomes the mixture of liquid, C_4P, and α-C_3P at >1570°C. Without water vapor, HA starts losing OH even as low as 900°C and the decomposition is significant at >1000°C in Air, N_2, or Ar. For sintering, the preferred temperature is at <1360°C under at least 500 mm Hg water vapor pressure. For plasma thermal spray at temperature >5000°C, the decomposition is inevitable. The final phase composition of HA coating contains crystalline HA, amorphous phase, C_4P, α-C_3P, β-C_3P, and CaO.

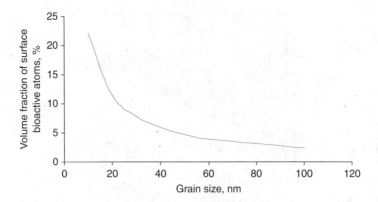

FIGURE 24.2 Surface atoms fraction as a function of grain size for a spherical particle, supposing the surface layer is 0.8 nm.

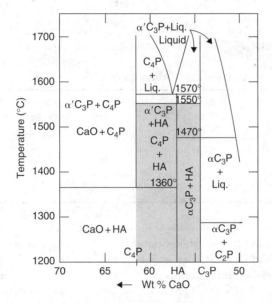

FIGURE 24.3 Phase diagram of $CaO-P_2O_5$. (Taken from Buddy D. Ratner, Allan S. Hoffman, Frederick J. Schosen, and Jack E. Lemons, *Biomaterials Science*, Academic Press, New York, 1996, p. 82. With permission.)

Hydroxyapatite stability in water is shown in Figure 24.4 [15]. HA has lowest calcium ion concentration and is the stable phase at the same pH when pH > 4.2, while all other calcium phosphate compounds such as $Ca_4(PO_4)_2O$ (TTCP), $CaHPO_4$ (DCPA), etc., transfer to HA through reaction with water. At pH < 4.2, $CaHPO_4 2H_2O$, is the stable compound and HA decomposes into $CaHPO_4 2H_2O$. Figure 24.4 is the base of calcium phosphate cement. For powder synthesis, the chemical precipitation process should be controlled at pH 8.5 to 9.5, where the Ca ion concentration in the solution is minimum. In body fluid system, the pH is 7.3 at 37°C, therefore any kind of calcium phosphate fillers or coatings will finally form HA, then the HA is gradually transformed into bone through balancing with the Ca^{2+} and PO_4^{3-} as well as other ions such as Mg^{2+}, F^- in body fluids.

24.4 Nano-HA Mechanics

The HA mechanical properties are listed in Table 24.1 for different forms of products as compared with bone. It is found that the sintered HA has the grain size >500 nm, which has the highest compressive

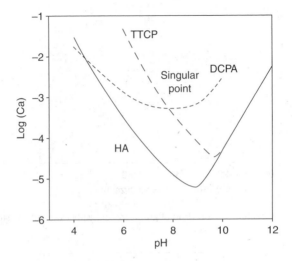

FIGURE 24.4   Phase diagram of $Ca(OH)_2$-H_3PO_4-H_2O at 25°C. (Taken from L.C. Chow and S. Takagi, *J. Res. Natl Inst. Standard Technol.* 2001; 106: 1029–1033. With permission.)

TABLE 24.1   Mechanical Properties of Hydroxyapatite

	Sintered HA (99% density)	Coralline HA	Cemented HA	Bone
Grain size, nm	>500	50–500	50–500	5–50
Tensile strength, MPa	80–180	2.8	2.1	3 (Cancellous) 151 (Cortical)
Compress strength, MPa	470	9.3	55	5.5 (Cancellous) 162 (Cortical)

and tensile strength. Researches have demonstrated that the mechanical properties are dominated by composition, porosity, and microstructure. For sintered HA bulk material, the compressive strength (σ_c) and tensile strength (σ_t) exponentially decrease with volume porosity (V_p), that is, $\sigma_c = 700 \exp(-5 V_p)$ and $\sigma_t = 220 \exp(-20 V_p)$ [1]. Using hot pressing or sintering in water vapor at 1150 to 1250°C, the HA relative density was reached 99%. The CO_3^{2-} or F^- replaced HA has the different values. The sintered HA is a hard and brittle material, too. Its Young's modulus is 110 GPa, Vicker's hardness 500 kg/mm^2 at 200 g load, and fracture toughness of about 1.0 to 1.2 MPa m$^{1/2}$ [16–19]. Since the sintered HA has very low Weibull factor ($n = 12$) in physiological solution, the bulk HA can not be used in load bearing applications [1]. Most applications of the bulk HA are under the nonload conditions such as middle ear.

The majority of HA products are powder blocks, cements, and coatings, with grain size about 50–100 nm and they are highly porous (30–80% pores). These pores make the HA have extremely low tensile strength of 2–3 MPa and compressive 9–60 MPa, which are similar to cancellous bone of 3 and 5.5 MPa, but far lower than the cortical bone. For nonload applications, the porous coralline and cemented HA has little foreign body reaction and finally merge and transform into physiological bone after surgery 3–5 years; this is the real advantage of HA materials [15,20].

24.5   Nano-HA Biology *In Vitro* and *In Vivo*

Since the biological apatite of bone mineral is a nanoapatite, the synthesized nano-HA is expected to be recognized as belonging to the body [21]. In other words, the synthesized nano-HA could be directly involved in the natural bone remodeling process, rather than being phagocytosized [21]. On the other hand, the biocompatibility of HA is being governed by a thin layer of apatitic mineral matrix as a result of the dissolution and reprecipitation of HA [22,23]. The biological responses to HA surfaces are known to be influenced by the size, morphology, and structure of HA particles [3,4,24,25]. For example, as-received HA with smaller crystal particles have been reported to stimulate greater inflammatory cytokine release as compared to well-sintered HA with bigger crystal particles [5]. In addition, well-sintered HA was observed to significantly enhance osteoblast differentiation as compared to as-received HA [6]. In contrast, nano-HA is expected to lead to different biological responses since nano-HA may have higher solubility.

In the *in vitro* study, human monocyte-derived macrophages and human osteoblast-like (HOB) cell models have been used to study the biocompatibility of nano-HA coatings [5]. The nano-HA coatings were prepared by means of electrospraying nano-HA particles onto glass substrates. The cells were seeded onto the nano-HA coatings and cultured for a week. The release of lactate dehydrogenase (LDH) and tumor necrosis factor alpha (TNF-α) from cells were used to evaluate the cytotoxicity and inflammatory responses, respectively. Although there was some evidence of LDH release from macrophages in the presence of high concentrations of nano-HA particles, there was no significant release of TNF-α. In addition, nano-HA was observed to support the attachment and the spread of HOB cells [5]. In another study using porous nano-HA scaffolds, periosteal-derived osteoblast (POB) was isolated from the periosteum of four-month human embryos aborting and seeded on porous nano-HA scaffolds. The attachment and the growth of POB on the scaffolds were evaluated by measuring the POB morphology, proliferative abilities, and osteogenic activity. POB could fully attach to and extend on HA scaffolds, and form extracellular matrix. Moreover the presence of nano-HA scaffolds in cell culture could promote cell proliferation as compared to tissue culture plate ($p < .05$) [7]. In another separate study, a porous nano-HA/collagen composite was produced in sheet form and convolved into a three-dimensional scaffold. Bone-derived mesenchymal cells from neonatal Wistar rats were seeded on the scaffolds and cultured up to 21 days. Spindle-shaped cells were found to continuously proliferate and migrate throughout the network of the coil. Eventually, three-dimensional polygonal cells and new bone matrix were observed within the composite scaffolds [8].

In a comparison study between nanosize HA filler and micronize HA filler using a rat calvarial defect model, histological analysis and mechanical evaluation showed a more advanced bone formation and a more rapid increase in stiffness in the defects with the nanosize HA augmented poly(propylene glycol-co-fumaric acid), suggesting an improved biological response to the nano-HA particles [9]. Other studies investigating the tissue response to a nano-HA/collagen composite implanted in the marrow cavity of New Zealand rabbit femur reported implant degradation and bone substitution during bone remodeling [10]. The process of implant degradation and bone substitution during bone remodeling suggested that the composite can be involved in bone metabolism. In addition to the process of degradation and bone substitution, the composite exhibited an isotropic mechanical behavior and similar microhardness when compared to the femur compacta [10].

24.6 HA Products and Their Applications

As indicated in HA biology, the HA as bone substitute has the ability of osteo-integration and osteo-conduction. The clinical applications are basically divided into two categories, nano-HA granular and calcium phosphate cement for bone repair and nano-HA coating for bone replacement. In research areas, nano-HA combined with polymer and bone growth factors (BMPs) have been used for drug delivery and tissue engineering. The details are described below.

24.6.1 Porous Nano-HA Granules or Blocks

Porous nano-HA can be prepared by two methods, sintering and hydrothermal reaction. The sintering method is first mixing naphthalene with HA particles, then compact the particles into a composite, and finally sintering. Naphthalene particles would sublime during the sintering, thus leaving a pore filled

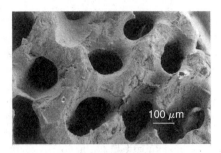

FIGURE 24.5 SEM of coralline HA. (Taken from B. Ben-Nissa, A. Milev, and R. Vago, *Biomaterials* 2004; 25: 4571–4975. With permission.)

structure. This method can make spherical porous HA particles, but pores are isolated. Hydrothermal reaction is using natural coral as raw material. This method was developed in 1971, marked as ProOsteon (interpore International, Irvine, CA, USA). The coral is first treated in boiling water with about 5% sodium hypochrorite (NaClO) to remove the organics and left calcium carbonate ($CaCO_3$) and pores. Then the $CaCO_3$ is reacted with ammonium monohydrogen phosphate ((NH_4)$_2HPO_4$) to form a coralline HA under temperature abound 250°C at 3.8 MPa for 24 h. The coralline HA has both needle-like grains with a length of 1–2 μm and a width of 100–200 nm. The most important is that the coralline HA has the micro-connective pores of 100–150 μm (Figure 24.5), which provide bone in growth channel. Fifty to eighty percent of the voids is filled within three months. When the fibro-osteous tissue ingrowth is complete, the implant consists of about 17% bone, 43% soft tissue, and 40% residual HA. Therefore, the coralline HA becomes as strong and tough as the cancellous bone [26–28].

24.6.2 Nano-HA Cement

Calcium phosphate cements are another kind of porous HA product which is used as a bone filler. Different from coral HA, the cements are paste-like slurries or gels that can be directly injected to the void site and molded to shape and set *in vivo*. This flow ability is unique and specially suitable for cosmetic surgery. There are two kinds of calcium cements. One is invented by Chow et al. and made by equal mole percent of $Ca_4(PO_4)_2O$ and $CaHPO_4$ mixed with water to form a paste [15]. This cement sets via isothermal reaction in 15 min and then fully hardens over 4 h. Another calcium cement uses $CaHPO_4H_2O$ and $CaCO_3$ as raw materials and H_3PO_4 as the liquid [26,27]. At 37°C, the cement has 2 min working time (mixing and injection while kept flowing ability) and sets in about 8 min. In all the calcium phosphate cements, the raw materials particle size, powder to liquid ratio, temperature, pH, seeding are all variables to influence the microstructure, working and setting times, and mechanical properties [31–37]. There are many manufacturers in the world to commercially supply these two types of cements. In the U.S. market, Bone Source, made by Leibinger, Dallas, TX, USA is a trade name of the first type of cement. Norrian SRS Cement is another commercial product for the second type of cement, which is made by Norian Corp., Cupertino, CA, USA [26,27].

All these products have similar mechanical properties as mentioned before. A porous needle-like structure $Ca_{10}(PO_4)_6(OH)_2$ crystals are their typical microstructure (Figure 24.6). These cements have been successfully used in sinus repair, cranioplasty, distal radial and calcaneal fracture. It has also been reported that the calcium phosphate cement has been used for percutanous Vertebroplasty [15,26–37].

24.6.3 Nano-HA Coating

Hydroxyapatite has been coated on metallic dental and orthopedic implants by high-temperature plasma thermal spray since the 1980s [24,25]. In this process, HA powders are fed into a plasma flame (temperature 5,000 to 15,000°C). The powders are quickly melted and quenched on the metallic implant substrate to

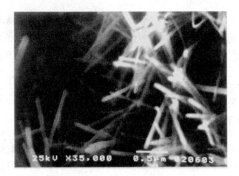

FIGURE 24.6   Nano-HA formed by calcium phosphate cementation. (Taken from L.C. Chow and S. Takagi, *J. Res. Natl Inst. Standard Technol.* 2001; 106: 1029–1033. With permission.)

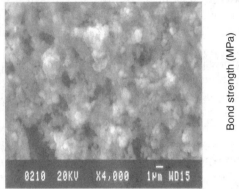 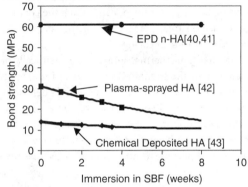

FIGURE 24.7   SEM picture (left) and tensile bond strength of electrophoresis deposited (EPD) nano-HA coating in SBF at 37°C, as compared to the commercial products [40–43].

form a thick film coating. Because the temperature is high, the coating contains melted and crystallized HA, unmelted HA, amorphous phase, and some decomposed phases such as $C_4P, \alpha\text{-}C_3P, \beta\text{-}C_3P$, and CaO as shown in Figure 24.2. Clinically, plasma thermal sprayed HA coating has been successfully used in dental implants and femoral stems for hip replacement, but the HA coating on cups has a high failure rate. The special advantage of plasma sprayed HA coating on the stems is the acceleration of cups early stage healing, no sigh-pain, and the enhancement of bone growth across a gap of 1 mm between the bone and the implants under stable and unstable mechanical conditions. Filling the gap is very important for the revision hips, where the patients had bone-loss during the primary hip replacement.

   However, the plasma thermal sprayed HA has the disadvantage of low bond strength at coating/implant interface, and the strength decreases over time in simulated fluid (SBF) (Figure 24.7). This is attributed to its low crystallinity (typically 70%) and microcracks formed due to high-temperature quenching, decomposition, and thermal expansion mismatch between the HA and metallic substrates ($\alpha_{HA} = 13 \times 10^{-6}/°C, \alpha_{Ti} = 9.8 \times 10^{-6}/°C, \alpha_{CoCr} = 16 \times 10^{-6}/°C$). There was a controversy about the amorphous HA. Theoretically, the amorphous HA is quickly dissolved *in vivo*, which generates high local Ca^{2+} and PO_4^{3-} ions concentration and form supersaturated conditions. Based on thermodynamics (Figure 24.4), the supersaturated Ca^{2+} and PO_4^{3-} will be deposited into the biological bone, thus proving beneficial to the early stage gap healing, about 30% amorphous phase is necessary [24,25,38,39]. Experimentally, the beneficial effect of the amorphous phase did not happen [40–44]. In a recent specific study, HA-coated titanium of 50% (low), 70% (medium), and 90% (high) crystallinity were inserted into the canine femur for 1, 4, 12, and 26 weeks. No significant differences could be found in the percentage of bone contact and interfacial attachment strength between the three types of HA-coated implants throughout the four implantation periods [44]. In another study, after three months of implantation, the high crystallinity (98%) coating showed the higher shear bond strength and integrated bone/coating interface, whereas the separation of the coating fragments was clearly observed in the coating that had low crystallinity (56%) [45].

In order to avoid the disadvantages of the plasma thermal spray, a chemical precipitation was introduced in the 1990s [46,47]. This method is a room-temperature process, depositing nano-HA thin film (grain size 60 to 100 nm and thickness $<5\ \mu$m) on porous beaded implants in the supersaturated Ca^{2+}, and PO_4^{3-} solution. This process has been successfully used for coating porous cups and porous stems too. Because the chemical precipitation is a liquid-based room-temperature process, the coating is uniform on the beads and in the inside of pores, which help the tissue and bone ingrowth in the pores. Therefore, this is the fixation of combined mechanical interlocking and osteo-integration. Some companies even only coat β-C_3P on the porous implant and let β-C_3P transform into HA *in vivo*. The basic function of the thin film nano-HA coating is stimulation of early bone growth into the macropores. Unfortunately, the chemical precipitated HA is only mechanically bonded on the implant surface with an extremely low bond strength, even one's finger can scratch the coating off. This requires a careful handling of the coated implants during surgery. Any chips of the coating might migrate in the articulating area and result in accelerated wear of the bearing surface.

Since both plasma thermal sprayed and chemically precipitated HA coatings have disadvantages in low bond strength or the strength decrease over time, many other processes have been used for coating HA, including sol-gel, dip coating, electrophoretic deposition, ion-implantation, chemical vapora deposition, and sputtering, etc. [48–55]. In all of these new processes, Inframat Corporation has developed an innovative electrophoretic deposition process to coat a special nano-HA coating. This nano-HA coating has the combined advantages of nano-grain structure, high crystallinity ($>90\%$), and the capability to coat the beaded porous surfaces. Figure 24.7 shows the typical surface microstructure and bond strength comparison [40,41].

In addition to the dental, hip, knee, and maxillofacial applications, nano-HA is also used for drug delivery and tissue engineering. These usually make a composite containing HA and other ingredients, such as anti-infection drugs, bone growth factors, and biodegradable polymers [56–65].

Acknowledgment

The authors gratefully acknowledge support from NIH SBIR programs under the grant Nos 1 R43 DE 015881-01 and 2-R44-AR047278-02A1.

References

[1] Buddy D. Ratner, Allan S. Hoffman, Frederick J. Schosen, and Jack E. Lemons. *Biomaterials Science* Academic Press, New York, 1996, pp. 82 and 321.

[2] Jill Dill Pasteris, Brigitte Wopenka, John J. Freeman, Keith Rogers, Eugenia Valsami-Jones, Jacqueline A.M. Van der Houwen, and Matthew J. Silva. Lack of OH in nanocrystalline apatite as a function of degree of atomic order: implications for bone and biomaterials. *Biomaterials* 2004; 2: 229–238.

[3] Sun J., Tsuang Y., Chang W.H., Li H., Liu H., and Lin F. Effect of hydroxyapatite particle size on myoblasts and fibroblasts. *Biomaterials* 1997; 18: 683–690.

[4] Ninomiya J.T., Struve J.A., Stelloh C.T., Toth J.M., and Crosby K.E. Effects of hydroxyapatite particulate debris on the production of cytokines and proteases in human fibroblasts. *J. Ortho. Res.* 2001; 19: 621–628.

[5] Ong J.L., Hoppe C.A., Cardenas H.L., Cavin R., Carnes D.L., Sogal A., and Raikar G.N. Osteoblast precursor cell activity on HA surfaces of different treatments. *J. Biomed. Mater. Res.* 1998; 39: 176–183.

[6] Huang J., Best S.M., Bonfield W., Brooks R.A., Rushton N., Jayasinghe S.N., and Edirisinghe M.J. *In vitro* assessment of the biological response to nano-sized hydroxyapatite. *J. Mater. Sci. Mater. Med.* 2004; 15: 441–445.

[7] Zhang Q., Zhao S., Guo Z., Dong Y., Lin P., and Pu Y. Research of biocompatibility of nano-bioceramics using human periosteum *in vitro. J. Southeast Univ. Natural Science Edition* 2004; 34: 219–223.

[8] Du C., Cui F.Z., Zhu X.D., and de Groot K. Three-dimensional nano-Hap/collagen matrix loading with osteogenic cells in organ culture. *J. Biomed. Mater. Res.* 1999; 44: 407–415.

[9] Doherty S.A., Hile D.D., Wise D.L., Ying J.Y., Sonis S.T., and Trantolo D.J. Nanoparticulate hydroxyapatite enhances the bioactivity of a resorbable bone graft. *Proc. Mater. Res. Soc. Symp.* 2003; 735: 75–79.

[10] Du C., Cui F.Z., Zhu X.D., and de Groot K. Tissue response to nano-hydroxyapatite/collagen composite implants in marrow cavity. *J. Biomed. Mater. Res.* 1998; 42: 540–548.

[11] Zongtao Zhang. Non-magnetic surface for magnetic nano-materials, a limit of exchange coupling. Inframat Corporation, Inner report, February 27, 2002.

[12] Yang, De-Ping, Lavoie, Lindsey K., Zhang, Yide, Zhang, Zongtao, Ge, Shihui. Mossbauer spectroscopic and x-ray diffraction studies of structural and magnetic properties of heat-treated $Ni0.5Zn0.5Fe_2O_4$ nanoparticles. *J. Appl. Phys.* 2003; 93: 7492–7494.

[13] Zongtao Zhang, Zhang, Y.D., Xiao, T.D., Shihui Ge, and Mingzhong Wu. Nanostructured $NiFe_2O_4$ ferrite. *Proc. Mater. Res. Soc. Symp. Nanophase Nanocomposite Mater. IV,* 2002; 703: 111–116.

[14] Hines W.A., Budnick J.I., Gromek J.M., Yacaman M.J., Troiani H.E., Chen Q.Z., Wong C.T., Lu W.W., Cheung K.M.C., Leong J.C.Y., and Luk K.D.K. Strengthening mechanisms of bone bonding to crystalline hydroxyapatite *in vivo. Biomaterials* 2004; 25: 4243–4254.

[15] Chow, L.C. and Takagi, S. A natural bone cement — a laboratory novelty led to the development of reutional new biomaterials. *J. Res. Natl Inst. Standard Technol.* 2001; 106: 1029–1033.

[16] Raynaud S., Champion E., and Bernache-Assollant D. Calcium phosphate apatites with variable Ca/P atomic ratio II. Calcination and sintering. *Biomaterials* 2002; 23: 1073–1080.

[17] Elena Landi, Anna Tampieri, Giancarlo Celotti, Lucia Vichi, and Monica Sandri. Influence of synthesis and sintering parameters on the characteristics of carbonate apatite. *Biomaterials* 2004; 23: 1763–1770.

[18] Raynaud S., Champion E., Lafon J., and Bernache-Assollant D. Calcium phosphate apatites with variable Ca/P atomic ratio III. Mechanical properties and degradation in solution of hot presses ceramics. *Biomaterials* 2002; 23: 1081–1089.

[19] Kārlis A. Gross and Kinnari A. Bhadang, Sintered hydroxyfluorapatite. Part II: sintering and resultant mechanical properties of sintered blends of hydroxyapatite and fluorapatite. *Biomaterials* 2004; 25: 1395.

[20] Hing K.A., Best S.M., Tanner K.E., and Bonfield W. Quantification of bone ingrowth within bone-derived porous hydroxyapatite implants of varying density. *J. Mater. Sci.* 1999; 10: 663–670.

[21] Driessens F.C.M., Boltong M.G., Khairoun I., De Maeyer E.A.P., Ginebra M.P., Wenz R., Planell J.A., and Verbeeck R.M.H. Applied aspects of calcium phosphate bone cement application. In Wise D.L., Trantolo D.J., Lewandrowski K.U., Gresser M.V., and Yaszemski M.J. (Eds). *Biomaterials Engineering and Devices. Human Applications.* Volume 2. Humana Press, New Jersey, Totowa. 2000, pp. 253–260.

[22] Hench L.L. Bioceramics: from concept to clinic. *J. Am. Ceram. Soc.* 1991; 74: 1487–1510.

[23] Kokubo T. Recent progress in glass based materials for biomedical applications. *J. Ceram. Soc. Japan* 1991; 99: 965–973.

[24] Yunzhi Yang, Kim K.-H., and Ong J.L. A review on calcium phosphate coatings produced using a sputtering process — an alternative to plasma spraying. *Biomaterials* 2005; 26: 327–337.

[25] Yang Y., Bessho K., and Ong J.L. Plasma-sprayed hydroxyapatite-coated and plasma-sprayed titanium-coated implants. In Yaszemski M.J., Trantolo D.J., Lewandrowski K.U., Hasirci V., Altobelli D.E., and Wise D.L. (Eds). *Biomaterials in Orthopedics.* Marcel Dekker, Inc., New York, 2004, pp. 401–423.

[26] Ben-Nissa B., Milev A., and Vago R. Morphology of sol–gel derived nano-coated Coralline hydroxyapatite. *Biomaterials* 2004; 25: 4571–4975.

[27] William R. Moore, Stephen E. Graves, and Gregory I. Bain. Synthetic bone graft substitutes. *ANZ J. Surg.* 2001; 71: 354–361.

[28] Lu W.W., Cheung K.M.C., Li Y.W., Luk D.K., Holmes A.D., Zhu Q.A., and Leong J.C.Y. Bioactive bone cement as a principal fixture for spinal fracture, An *in vitro* biomechanical and morphological study. *Spine* 2001; 26: 2684–2691.

[29] Tetsuya Yussa, Youji Miyamoto, Kunio Ishikawa, Masaaki Takechi, Yukihiro Momota, Seiko Tatehara, and Masaru Nagayama. Effects of apatite cements on proliferation and differentiation of human osteoblasts *in vitro. Biomaterials* 2004; 25: 1159–1166.

[30] Changsheng Liu, Wei Shen, and Jiangua Chen. Solution properties of calcium phosphate cement hardening body. *Mater. Chem. Phys.* 1999; 58: 78–83.

[31] Ginebra M., Driessens F.C.M., and Planell J.A. Effect of the particle size on the micro and nano-structural features of a calcium phosphate cement: a kinetic analysis. *Biomaterials* 2004; 25: 3453–3462.

[32] Changsheng Liu, Yue Huang, and Haiyan Zheng. Study of the hydration process of calcium phosphate cement by AC Impedance Spectroscopy. *J. Am. Ceram. Soc.* 1999; 82: 1052–1057.

[33] Changsheng Liu, Wei Gai, Songhua Pan, and Zisheng Liu. The exothermal behaviour in the hydration process of calcium phosphate cement. *Biomaterials* 2003; 24: 2995–3003.

[34] Bigi A., Bracci B., and Panzata S. Effect of added gelatin on the properties of calcium phosphate cement. *Biomaterials* 2004; 25: 2893–2999.

[35] Savarino L., Breschi L., Tedaldi M., Ciapetti G., Tarabusi C., Greco M., Giunti A., and Prati C. Ability of restorative and fluoride releasing materials to prevent marginal dentine demineralization. *Biomaterials* 2004; 25: 1011–1017.

[36] Changsheng Liu, Yue Huang, and Jianguo Chen. The physicochemical properties of the solidification of calcium phosphate cement. *J. Biomed. Mater. Res. Appl. Biomater.* 2004; 69: B:73–78.

[37] Apelt A., Theiss F., El-Warrak A.O., Zilinazky K., Bettschart-Wolfisberger R., Bohner M., Matter S., Auer J.A., and von Rechenberg B. *In vivo* behaviour of three injectable hydraulic calcium phosphate cements. *Biomaterials* 2004; 25: 1439–1451.

[38] Ricardo M. Souto, Maria M. Laz, and Rui L. Reis. Degradation characteristics of hydroxyapatite coatings on orthopedic TiAlV in simulated physiological media investigated by electrochemical impedance spectroscopy. *Biomaterials* 2003; 24: 4213–4221.

[39] Yu-Peng Lu, Mu-Sen Li, Shi-Tong Li, Zhi-Gang Wang, and Rui-Fu Zhu. Plasma-sprayed hydroxyapatite + titania composite bond coat for hydroxyapatite coating on titanium substrate. *Biomaterials* 2004; 25: 4393–4403.

[40] Zongtao Zhang, Xiao, and Tongsan D. Multi-layer coating useful for the coating of implants. U.S. Patent No. 2003099762 A1 2003.

[41] Zongtao Zhang, Matthew F. Dunn, Xiao, T.D., Antoni P. Tomsia, and Saiz, E. Nanostructured hydroxyapatite coatings for improved adhesion and corrosion resistance for medical implants. *Proc. Mater. Res. Soc. Symp. 703 Nanophase and Nanocomposite Mater. IV*, 2002, pp. 291–296.

[42] Yang C.Y., Wang B.C., Chang E., and Wu B.C. Bond degradation at the plasma-sprayed HA coating/Ti-6Al-4V alloy interface: an *in vitro* study. *J. Mater. Sci. Mater. Med.* 1995; 6: 258–265.

[43] Yong Han, Tao Fu, Jian Lu, and Kewei Xu. Characterization and stability of hydroxyapatite coatings prepared by an electrodeposition and alkaline-treated process. *J. Biomed. Mater. Res.* 2000; 54: 96–101.

[44] Chang Y.L., Lew D., Park J.B., and Keller J.C., Biomechanical and morphometric analysis of hydroxyapatite-coated implants with varying crystallinity. *J. Oral Maxillofac. Surg.* 1999; 579: 1096–1108.

[45] Xue W., Tao S., Liu X., Zheng X., and Ding C. *In vivo* evaluation of plasma sprayed hydroxyapatite coatings having different crystallinity. *Biomaterials* 2004; 253: 415–421.

[46] Leitao Eugenia Ribeiro de Sousa Fidalgo, Implant material. US patent No. 6,069,295, 2000.

[47] Florence Barrere, Margot M.E. Snel, Clemens A. Van Blitterswijk, Klass de Groot, and Pierre Layrolle. Nano-scale study of the nucleation and growth of calcium phosphate coating on titanium implants. *Biomaterials* 2004; 25: 2901–2910.

[48] Hao-Won kim, Young-Min Kong, Chang-Jun Bae, Yoon-Jung Noh, and Hyoun-Ee, kim. Sol–gel derived fluro-hydroxyapatite biocoatings on zircornia substrate. *Biomaterials* 2004; 25: 2919–2926.

[49] Hiroshi Kusakabe, Toyonori Sakamaki, Kotaro Nihei, Yasuo Oyama, Shigeru Yanagimoto, Masaru Ichimiya, Jun Kimura, and Yoshiaki Toyama, Osseointegration of a hydroxyapatite-coated multilayered mesh stem. 2004; 25: 2957–2969.

[50] Hao-Won kim, Hyoun-Ee, kim, and Jonathan C. Knowles. Fluro-hydroxyapatite sol–gel coating on titanium substrate for hardtissue implants. *Biomaterials* 2004; 25: 3351–3358.

[51] Michele Rocca, Milena Fini, Gianluca Giavaresi, Nicoló Nicoli Aldini, and Roberto Giardino. Osteointegration of hydroxyapatite-coated and uncoated titanium screw in long-term ovariec-tomized shee. *Biomaterials* 2002; 23: 1017–1023.

[52] Mark T. Fulmer, Ira C. Ison, Christine R. Hankermayer, Brent R. Constantz, and John Ross. Meas-urements of the solubilities and dissolution rates of several hydroxyapatites. *Biomaterials* 2004; 23: 751–755.

[53] Rößler S., Sewing A., Stölzel M., Born R., Scharnweber D., Dard M., and Worch H. Electrochemically assisted deposition of thin calcium phosphate coatings at near-physiological pH and temperature. *J. Biomed. Mater. Res.* 2002; 64A: 655–663.

[54] Leeuwenburgh S.C.G., Wolke J.G.C., Schoonman J., and Jansen J.A. Influence of precursor solution parameters on chemical properties of calcium phosphate coatings prepared using electrostatic spray deposition (ESD). *Biomaterials* 2004; 641–649.

[55] Nguyen H.Q., Deporter D.A., Pilliar R.M., Valiquette N., and Yakubovich R. The effect of sol–gel-formed calcium phosphate coatings on bone ingrowth and osteoconductivity of porous-surfaced Ti alloy implants. *Biomaterials* 2004; 25: 865–876.

[56] Paul W. and Sharma C.P. Development of porous spherical hydroxyapatite granules: application towards protein delivery. *J. Mater. Sci.* 1999; 10: 383–388.

[57] Rotter N., Aigner J., and Naumann A. Behaviour of tissue-engineered human cartilage after transplantation in nude mice. *J. Mater. Sci.* 1999; 10: 689–693.

[58] Qiaoling Hu, Baoqiang Li, Mang Wang, and Jiacong Shen. Preparation and characterization of biodegradable chitosan/hydroxyapatite nanocomposite rods via *in situ* hybridization: a potential material as internal fixation of bone fracture. *Biomaterials* 2004; 25: 779–785.

[59] Hassna R.R. Ramay and Zhang, M. Biophasic calcium phosphate nanocomposite porous scaffolds for load-bearing bone tissue engineering. *Biomaterials* 2004; 25: 5171–5180.

[60] Skrtic D., Antonucci J.M., Evance E.D., and Eidelman N. Dental composites based on hybrid and surface-modified amorphous calcium phosphates. *Biomaterials* 2004; 25: 1141–1150.

[61] Zigang Ge, Sophie Baguenard, Lee Yong Lim, Ailen Wee, and Eugene Khor. Hydroxyapatite-chitin materials as potential tissue engineered bone substitutes. *Biomaterials* 2004; 25: 1049–1058.

[62] Yoshio Ota, Tetsushi Iwashita, Toshihiro Kasuga, and Yoshihiro Abe. Process for producing hydroxyaptite fibers. US Patent No. 6,228,339 B1, 2001.

[63] Hockin H.K. Xu, Janet B. Quinn, Shozo Takagi, and Laurence C. Chow. Synergistic reinforcement of *in situ* hardening of calcium phosphate composite scaffold for bone tissue engineering. *Biomaterials* 2004; 25: 1029–1037.

[64] Eugenia Ribeiro de Sousa Fildago Leitao, Implant material and process for using it. US Patent No. 6,146,686, 2000.

[65] Gu Y.W., Khor K.A., Pan D., and Cheang P. Activity of plasma sprayed ytristablized zirconia rein-forced hydroxyl apatite/Ti–6Al–4V composite coatings in simulated body fluid. *Biomaterials* 2004; 25: 3177–3185.

25

Nanotechnology Provides New Tools for Biomedical Optics

Jennifer L. West
Rebekah A. Drezek
Naomi J. Halas
Rice University

25.1 Introduction

Continuing advances in nanotechnology are generating a variety of nanostructured materials with highly controlled and interesting properties — from exceptionally high strength to the ability to carry and target drugs to unique optical properties. By controlling structure at the nanoscale dimensions, one can control and tailor the properties of nanostructures, such as semiconductor nanoscrystals and metal nanoshells, in a very accurate manner to meet the needs of a specific application. These materials can provide new and unique capabilities for a variety of biomedical applications ranging from diagnosis of diseases to novel therapies. In particular, nanotechnology may greatly expand the impact of biophotonics by providing more robust contrast agents, fluorescent probes, and sensing substrates.

In addition, the size scale of nanomaterials is very interesting for many biomedical applications. Nanoparticles are similar in size scale to many common biomolecules, making them interesting for applications such as intracellular tagging and for bioconjugate applications such as antibody-targeting of imaging contrast agents. In many cases, one can make modifications to nanostructures to better suit their integration with biological systems; for example, modifying their surface layer for enhanced aqueous solubility, biocompatibility, or biorecognition. Nanostructures can also be embedded within other biocompatible materials to provide nanocomposites with unique properties.

Many of the biomedical applications of nanotechnology will involve bioconjugates. The idea of merging biological and nonbiological systems at the nanoscale has actually been investigated for many years.

The broad field of bioconjugate chemistry is based on combining the functionalities of biomolecules and nonbiologically derived molecular species for applications including markers for research in cellular and molecular biology, biosensing, and imaging [1]. Many current applications of nanotechnolgy, particularly in the area of biophotonics, are a natural evolution of this approach. In fact, several of the "breakthrough" applications recently demonstrated using nanostructure bioconjugates are in fact traditional applications originally addressed by standard molecular bioconjugate techniques that have been revisited with these newly designed nanostructure hybrids, often with far superior results. Typically, nanostructured materials possess optical properties far superior to the molecular species they replace — higher quantum efficiencies, greater scattering or absorbance cross sections, optical activity over more biocompatible wavelength regimes, and substantially greater chemical or photochemical stability. Additionally, some nanostructures provide optical properties that are highly dependent on particle size or dimension. The ability to systematically vary the optical properties via structure modification not only improves traditional applications but also may lead to applications well beyond the scope of conventional molecular bioconjugates. In this chapter, we introduce several successful examples of nanostructures that have been applied to relevant problems in biotechnology and medicine.

25.2 Quantum Dots as Fluorescent Biological Labels

Semiconductor nanocrystals, also referred to as "quantum dots," are highly light absorbing, luminescent nanoparticles whose absorbance onset and emission maximum shift to higher energy with decreasing particle size due to quantum confinement effects [2,3]. These nanocrystals are typically in the size range of 2 to 8 nm in diameter. Unlike molecular fluorophores, which typically have very narrow excitation spectra, semiconductor nanocrystals absorb light over a very broad spectral range (Figure 25.1). This makes

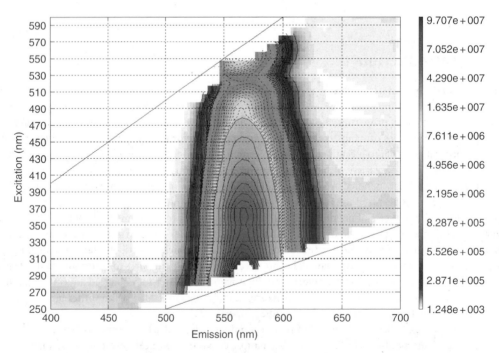

FIGURE 25.1 (See color insert following page 20-14.) Semiconductor nanocrystals, also referred to as "quantum dots," are highly light absorbing, luminescent nanoparticles whose absorbance onset and emission maximum shift to higher energy with decreasing particle size due to quantum confinement effects. As seen in this typical excitation–emission plot for a type of quantum dot, strong emission is observed over a broad range of excitation wavelengths.

it possible to optically excite a broad spectrum of quantum dot "colors" using a single excitation laser wavelength, which may enable one to simultaneously probe several markers in imaging, biosensing, and assay applications. Although the luminescence properties of semiconductor nanocrystals have historically been sensitive to their local environment and nanocrystal surface preparation, recent core-shell geometries where the nanocrystal is encased in a shell of a wider band gap semiconductor have resulted in increased fluorescence quantum efficiencies (>50%) and greatly improved photochemical stability. In the visible region, CdSe–CdS core-shell nanocrystals have been shown to span the visible region from approximately 550 nm (green) to 630 nm (red). Other material systems, such as InP and InAs, provide quantum dot fluorophores in the near infrared region of the optical spectrum, a region where transmission of light through tissues and blood is maximal [4]. Although neither II–VI nor III–V semiconductor nanocrystals are water soluble, let alone biocompatible, surface functionalization with molecular species such as mercaptoacetic acid or the growth of a thin silica layer on the nanoparticle surface facilitate aqueous solubility [5]. Both the silica layer and the covalent attachment of proteins to the mercaptoacetic acid coating permit the nanoparticles to be at least relatively biocompatible. Quantum dots have also been modified with dihydrolipoic acid to facilitate conjugation of avidin and subsequent binding of biotinylated targeting molecules [6]. Quantum dots can also be embedded within polymer nano- or microparticles to improve biocompatibility while maintaining the unique fluorescence.

Specific binding of quantum dots to cell surfaces, cellular uptake, and nuclear localization have all been demonstrated following conjugation of semiconductor nanocrystals to appropriate targeting proteins such as transferring, growth factors, peptides or antibodies [2,4,7,8]. This could be useful in a variety of microscopy and imaging applications (Figure 25.2). Several preliminary reports of *in vivo* imaging using quantum dots show considerable promise. For example, cancerous cells labeled with quantum dots *ex vivo* were injected intravenously to track extravasation and metastasis [9]. Five different populations of cells, each labeled with a different size of quantum dot, could be simultaneously tracked *in vivo* using multiphoton laser excitation. Another study evaluated *in vivo* imaging with quantum dots following direct injection [10]. A surface modification with polyethylene glycol of at least 5000 Da was required for sustained (>15 min) circulation of the particles in the bloodstream.

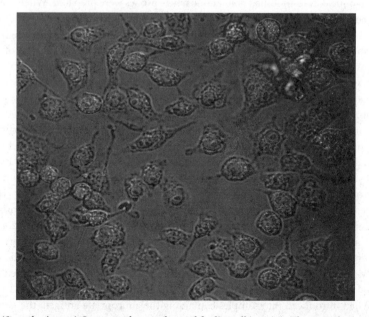

FIGURE 25.2   (See color insert.) Quantum dots can be used for live cell imaging. They are advantageous due to their bright fluorescence over a broad range of excitation wavelengths, resistance to photobleaching, and stability. Surface modifications are required for biocompatibility.

Quantum dots may also be useful in a variety of *in vitro* diagnostic applications, particularly since concerns about semiconductor nanocrystal biocompatibility can be neglected in such uses. One example is the development of a fluorescent immunoassay using antibody-conjugated quantum dots [6]; several protein toxins have been successfully detected using this system. In another example, quantum dots embedded in polymer microbeads have been used for DNA hybridization studies [11]. Encasing the nanocrystals in the polymer beads allows for simultaneous reading of a huge number of optical signals. The emission of different nanocrystal species can be tuned by varying the particle size. Microbeads can then be prepared with varying colors and intensities of quantum dots. Using 10 intensity levels and 6 colors, one could theoretically code 1 million optically differentiated signals to mark different nucleic acid or protein sequences for high throughput screening and diagnostics. Similarly, quantum dots bound to oligonucleotides have been used as probes for fluorescent *in situ* hybridization, or FISH [12]. This could enable more detailed analysis of gene expression profiles with localization within tissue than is currently possible with conventional molecular fluorophores.

25.3   Gold Nanoparticle Bioconjugate-Based Colorimetric Assays

The use of gold colloid in biological applications began in 1971 when Faulk and Taylor invented the immunogold staining procedure. Since that time, the labeling of targeting molecules, such as antibodies, with gold nanoparticles has revolutionized the visualization of cellular components by electron microscopy [13]. The optical and electron beam contrast properties of gold colloid have provided excellent detection capabilities for applications including immunoblotting, flow cytometry, and hybridization assays. Furthermore, conjugation protocols to attach proteins to gold nanoparticles are robust and simple [1], and gold nanoparticles were shown to have excellent biocompatibility [13].

Gold nanoparticle bioconjugates were recently applied to polynucleotide detection in a manner that exploited the change in optical properties resulting from plasmon–plasmon interactions between locally adjacent gold nanoparticles [14]. The characteristic red color of gold colloid has long been known to change to a bluish-purple color upon colloid aggregation due to this effect. In the case of polynucleotide detection, mercaptoalkyloligonucleotide-modified gold nanoparticle probes were prepared. When a single-stranded target oligonucleotide was introduced to the preparation, the nanoparticles aggregated due to the binding between the probe and target oligonucleotides, bringing the nanoparticles close enough to each other to induce a dramatic red-to-blue color change as depicted in Figure 25.3. Because of the extremely strong optical absorption of gold colloid, this colorimetric method can be used to detect ∼10 fmol of an oligonucleotide, which is ∼50 times more sensitive than the sandwich hybridization detection methods based on molecular fluorophores.

A similar approach has been used to develop a rapid immunoassay that can be performed in whole blood without sample preparation steps. This assay utilizes a relatively new type of gold nanoparticle called a gold nanoshell. Gold nanoshells are concentric sphere nanoparticles consisting of a dielectric core nanoparticle (typically gold sulfide or silica) surrounded by a thin gold shell [15]. By varying the relative dimensions of the core and shell layers, the plasmon-derived optical resonance of gold can be dramatically shifted in wavelength from the visible region into the mid infrared as depicted in Figure 25.4 [16]. By varying the absolute size of the gold nanoshells, they may be designed to either strongly absorb (for particles <∼75 nm) or scatter (for particles >∼150 nm) the incident light [16]. The gold shell layer is formed using the same chemical methods that are employed to form gold colloid; thus, the surface properties of gold nanoshells are virtually identical to gold colloid, providing the same ease of bioconjugation and excellent biocompatibility. To develop a whole blood immunoassay, gold nanoshells were designed and fabricated for near infrared resonance, and antibodies against target antigens were conjugated to the nanoshell surfaces [17]. When introduced into samples containing the appropriate antigen, the antibody–antigen linkages caused the gold nanoshells to aggregate, shifting the resonant wavelength further into the infrared. This assay system was shown to have sub-ng/ml sensitivity. More importantly, this assay can be performed in whole blood samples since the wavelengths utilized are in the near infrared, above the absorption of

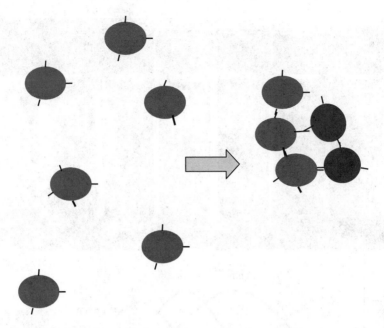

FIGURE 25.3   (See color insert.) When gold nanoparticles come into close proximity, plasmon–plasmon interactions cause dramatic changes in optical properties. Using appropriately conjugated nanoparticles, this behavior can be exploited for DNA hybridization assays and immunoassays.

hemoglobin yet below the water absorption band, where penetration of light through blood is relatively high [4]. Additionally, since gold nanoshells have highly tunable optical properties, it may be possible to probe for several antigens simultaneously using nanoshells with varying optical resonances. Nanoshells are also effective substrates for surface-enhanced Raman scattering [18], which may enable alternative methods for near infrared biosensing.

25.4 Photothermal Therapies

Gold nanoshells, described above, can be designed to strongly absorb light at desired wavelengths, in particular in the near infrared between 700 and 1100 nm where the tissue is relatively transparent [4]. Very few molecular chromophores are available in this region of the electromagnetic spectrum, let alone ones with low toxicity. When optically absorbing gold nanoshells are embedded in a matrix material, illuminating them at their resonance wavelength causes the nanoshells to transfer heat to their local environment. This photothermal effect can be used to optically modulate drug release from a nanoshell–polymer composite drug delivery system [19]. To accomplish photothermally modulated drug release, the matrix polymer material must be thermally responsive. Copolymers of N-isopropylacrylamide (NIPAAm) and acrylamide (AAm) exhibit a lower critical solution temperature (LCST) that is slightly above body temperature [20]. When the temperature of the copolymer exceeds its LCST, the resultant phase change in the polymer material causes the matrix to collapse, resulting in a burst release of any soluble material (i.e., drug) held within the polymer matrix [20]. As demonstrated in Figure 25.5, when gold nanoshells that were designed to strongly absorb near infrared light were embedded in NIPAAm-co-AAm hydrogels, pulsatile release of insulin and other proteins could be achieved in response to near infrared irradiation.

In another application, nanoshells are being used for photothermal tumor ablation [21,22]. When tumor cells are treated with nanoshells then exposed to near infrared light, cells are efficiently killed, while neither the nanoshells alone nor the near infrared light had any effect on cell viability, as shown in Figure 25.6 [21]. Furthermore, particles in the size range of 60 to 400 nm will extravasate and accumulate

(a)

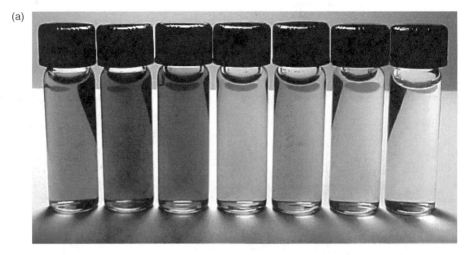

(b)

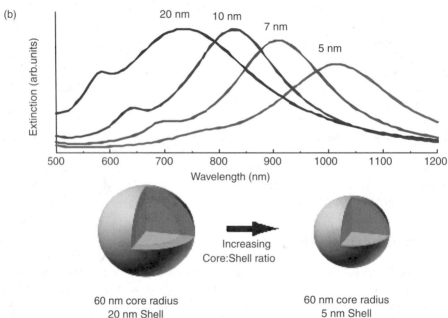

FIGURE 25.4   (See color insert.) Gold nanoshells consist of a dielectric core nanoparticle surrounded by a thin metal shell. By varying the relative dimensions of the core and shell constituents, one can design particles to either absorb or scatter light over the visible and much of the infrared regions of the electromagnetic spectrum. (a) These vials contain suspensions of either gold colloid (far left with its characteristic red color) or gold nanoshells with varying core:shell dimensions. (b) The optical properties of nanoshells are predicted by Mie scattering theory. For a core of a given size, forming thinner shells pushes the optical resonance to longer wavelengths.

in tumors due to the so-called enhanced permeability and retention effect that results from the leakiness of tumor vasculature [23]. Near infrared absorbing nanoshells are in the appropriate size range for this phenomenon. When polyethylene glycol-modified nanoshells were injected intravenously in tumor-bearing mice, the nanoshells accumulated in the tumor [22]. Subsequent exposure of the tissue region to near infrared light led to complete tumor regression and survival of the nanoshell-treated mice. The light alone had no effect. Nanoshells can be conjugated to antibodies against oncoproteins to potentially have cellular-level specificity of therapy [17,21].

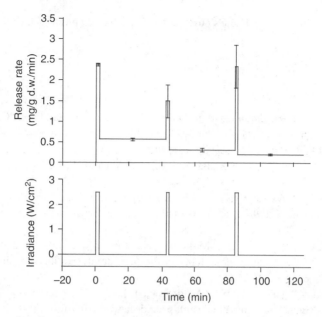

FIGURE 25.5 Release of insulin from NIPAAm-coAAm hydrogels with nanoshells embedded in their structure can be modulated by exposure to near infrared light (832 nm, 1.5 W/cm^2). The top panel is the release rate of insulin from the nanocomposite hydrogel materials vs. time, while the bottom panel indicates the pattern of laser illumination.

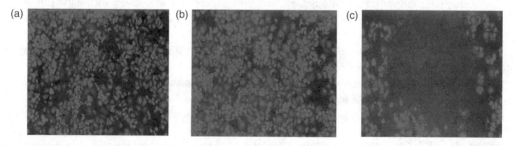

FIGURE 25.6 (See color insert.) Breast carcinoma cells were exposed to either nanoshells (a), near infrared light (b), or the combination of nanoshells and near infrared light (c). As demonstrated by staining with the fluorescent viability marker calcein AM, the carcinoma cells in the circular region corresponding to the laser spot were completely destroyed, while neither the nanoshells nor the light treatment alone compromised viability.

25.5 Silver Plasmon Resonant Particles for Bioassay Applications

Silver plasmon resonant particles have been used as reporter labels in microarray-based DNA hybridization studies [24] and sandwich immunoassays [25]. Silver plasmon resonant particles consist of a gold nanoparticle core onto which a silver shell is grown. Particles of this type in the size range of 40 to 100 nm scatter light very strongly, as many as 10^7 photons/sec to the detector [24], allowing them to act as diffraction-limited point sources that can be observed using a standard dark field microscope with white light illumination. In the bioassay applications that have been developed, bioconjugates are prepared with antibodies either against a target antigen for an immunoassay or against biotin for subsequent attachment of biotinylated DNA. In both the immunoassay and the hybridization assay, the results are determined by counting the number of particles bound to the substrate via microscopy. In the DNA hybridizationassay, the sensitivity obtained was approximately $60\times$ greater than what is typically achieved using conventional fluorescent labels.

References

[1] Hermanson, G.T. 1996. *Bioconjugate Techniques*. Academic Press, San Diego, CA.

[2] Bruchez, M., Moronne, M., Gin, P., Weiss, S., and Alivisatos, A.P. 1998. Semiconductor nanocrystals as fluorescent biological labels. *Science* 281: 2013–2016.

[3] Chan, W.C., Maxwell, D.J., Gao, X., Bailey, R.E., Han, M., and Nie, S. 2002. *Curr. Opin. Biotechnol.* 13: 40–46.

[4] Weissleder, R. 2001. A clearer vision for *in vivo* imaging. *Nat. Biotechnol.* 19: 316–317.

[5] Chan, W.C. and Nie, S. 1998. Quantum dot bioconjugates for ultrasensitive nonisotopic detection. *Science* 281: 2016–2018.

[6] Goldman, E.R., Balighian, E.D., Mattoussi, H., Kuno, M.L., Mauro, J.M., Tran, P.T., and Anderson, G.P. 2002. Avidin: a natural bridge for quantum dot-antibody conjugates. *J. Am. Chem. Soc.* 124: 6378–6382.

[7] Lidke, D.S., Nagy, P., Heintzmann, R., Arndt-Jovin, D.J., Post, J.N., Grecco, H.E., Jares-Erijman, E.A., and Jovin, T.M. 2004. Quantum dot ligands provide new insights into erbB/HER receptor-mediated signal transduction. *Nat. Biotechnol.* 22: 169–170.

[8] Lagerholm, B.C., Wang, M., Ernst, L.A., Ly, D.H., Liu, H., Bruchez, M.P., and Waggoner, A.S. 2004. Multicolor coding of cells with cationic peptide coated quantum dots. *NanoLetters* 10: 2019–2022.

[9] Voura, E.B., Jaiswal, J.K., Mattoussi, H., and Simon, S.M. 2004. Tracking metastatic tumor cell extravasation with quantum dot nanocrystals and fluorescence emission scanning microscopy. *Nat. Med.* 10: 993–998.

[10] Ballou, B., Lagerholm, B.C., Ernst, L.A., Bruchez, M.P., and Waggoner, A.S. Noninvasive imaging of quantum dots in mice. *Bioconjugate Chem.* 15: 79–86.

[11] Han, M., Gao, X., Su, J.Z., and Nie, S. 2001. Quantum-dot-tagged microbeads for multiplexed optical coding of biomolecules. *Nat. Biotechnol.* 19: 631–635.

[12] Pathak, S., Choi, S.K., Arnheim, N., and Thompson, M.E. 2001. Hydroxylated quantum dots as luminescent probes for *in situ* hybridization. *J. Am. Chem. Soc.* 123: 4103–4104.

[13] Hayat, M. 1989. *Colloidal Gold: Principles, Methods and Applications*. Academic Press, San Diego, CA.

[14] Elghanian, R., Storhoff, J.J., Mucic, R.C., Letsinger, R.L., and Mirkin, C.A. 1997. Selective colorimetric detection of polynucleotides based on the distance-dependent optical properties of gold nanoparticles. *Science* 277: 1078–1081.

[15] Averitt, R.D., Sarkar, D., and Halas, N.J. 1997. Plasmon resonance shifts of Au-coated Au_2S nanoshells: insight into multicomponent nanoparticle growth. *Phys. Rev. Lett.* 78: 4217–4220.

[16] Oldenburg, S.J., Averitt, R.D., Westcott, S.L., and Halas, N.J. 1998. Nanoengineering of optical resonances. *Chem. Phys. Lett.* 288: 243–247.

[17] Hirsch, L.R., Jackson, J.B., Lee, A., Halas, N.J., and West, J.L. 2003. A whole blood immunoassay using gold nanoshells. *Anal. Chem.* 75: 2377–2381.

[18] Jackson, J.B., Westcott, S.L., Hirsch, L.R., West, J.L., and Halas, N.J. 2003. Controlling the surface enhanced Raman effect via the nanoshell geometry. *Appl. Phys. Lett.* 82: 257–259.

[19] Sershen, S.R., Westcott, S.L., Halas, N.J., and West, J.L. 2000. Temperature-sensitive polymer-nanoshell composites for photothermally modulated drug delivery. *J. Biomed. Mater. Res.* 51: 293–298.

[20] Okano, T., Bae, Y.H., Jacobs, H., and Kim, S.W. 1990. Thermally on–off switching polymers for drug permeation and release. *J. Control. Release* 11: 255–265.

[21] Hirsch, L.R., Stafford, R.J., Bankson, J.A., Sershen, S.R., Rivera, B., Price, R.E., Hazle, J.D., Halas, N.J., and West, J.L. 2003. Nanoshell-mediated near infrared thermal therapy of tumors under magnetic resonance guidance. *Proc. Natl Acad. Sci. USA* 100: 13549–13554.

[22] O'Neal, D.P., Hirsch, L.R., Halas, N.J., Payne, J.D., and West, J.L. 2004. Photo-thermal tumor ablation in mice using near infrared-absorbing nanoparticles. *Cancer Lett.* 209: 171–176.

[23] Maeda, H. 2001. The enhanced permeability and retention (EPR) effect in tumor vasculature. *Adv. Enzyme Regul.* 41: 189–207.

[24] Oldenburg, S.J., Genick, C.C., Clark, K.A., and Schultz, D.A. 2002. Base pair mismatch recognition using plasmon resonant particle labels. *Anal. Biochem.* 309: 109–116.

[25] Schultz, S., Smith, D.R., Mock, J.J., and Schultz, D.A. 2000. Single-target molecule detection with nonbleaching multicolor optical immunolabels. *Proc. Natl Acad. Sci. USA* 97: 996–1001.

26

Nanomaterials Perspectives and Possibilities in Nanomedicine

Kimberly L. Douglas
Shawn D. Carrigan
Maryam Tabrizian
McGill University

Rapid advances in the field of nanotechnology have resulted in the development of methods to prepare, modify, and study materials and mechanisms at the molecular and atomic levels, providing tools to probe biological structures and processes on a scale not previously possible [1]. This greater understanding of biology has, in turn, fuelled nanotechnology by directing research in medical materials, devices, and treatments [2]. Divisible into complementary branches of biological discovery and biological mimicry, research in this field forms a nascent multifaceted domain requiring collaborative expertise from biologists, physicists, chemists, and engineers, that is collectively defined as nanobiotechnology [3]. Specific application of nanobiotechnology to nano- and molecular-scale design of devices for the prevention, treatment, and cure of illness and disease is called *nanomedicine* [1].

Nanotechnology, the parent research domain of nanobiotechnology, represents one of the few fields in which government funding has continued to increase. Between 1997 and 2003, government organizations globally increased funding in the nanotechnology sector from $432 million to almost $3 billion [3]. A report by the National Nanotechnology Initiative (NNI, USA) indicates that funding in nanobiotechnology accounts for less than 10% of this worldwide government support. In sharp contrast, over 50% of nanotechnology venture capital is invested in nanobiotechnology, an indicative of the potential benefit to be reaped from this burgeoning field [3].

Still in its infancy, nanomedicine has the potential to revolutionize the future practice of medicine. The majority of work in the area can be classified in one of the following three areas (1) therapeutic delivery systems with the potential to deliver genes and pharmaceuticals through specific cellular pathways, (2) novel biomaterials and tissue engineering for active tissue regeneration, and (3) biosensors, biochips, and novel imaging techniques for the purposes of diagnostic monitoring and imaging. In the sections that follow, each of these areas is discussed and supplemented by examples of current research.

26.1 Particle-Based Therapeutic Systems

Current pharmaceutical treatments for illnesses ranging from cystic fibrosis to cardiovascular intervention and the myriad of known cancers suffer a variety of drawbacks related to their methods of administration. Systemic delivery requires high concentrations, which can lead to adverse toxic side effects, unsustainable drug levels, and developed drug resistance. Additionally, oral medications are subject to individual patient compliance, further complicating the challenge of sustained therapeutic levels. Though illness-specific treatments each have unique associated detriments, the application of nanofabrication techniques promises to offer a range of delivery systems designed to remedy these obstacles by providing methods of controlled therapeutic delivery and release to specific tissues and tumors over a desired timeline.

Therapeutic delivery systems are designed to deliver a range of therapeutic agents, including poorly soluble drugs, proteins, vaccine adjuvants, and plasmid DNA (pDNA) for gene therapy, by exposing target cells to their payload. This requires the carrier to enter cells through endocytic or phagocytic pathways where, once internalized, the therapeutic agent is released through vehicle degradation and diffusion mechanisms. Accomplishing these tasks while addressing other issues, such as biocompatibility, biodegradability, and an ability to avoid capture and clearance by the reticuloendothelial system (RES), has proved challenging; systems excelling at certain aspects often fail to incorporate all required characteristics for *in vivo* application.

Current nanoscale delivery systems are divisible into two major categories: surface modification systems designed to prevent immune response or promote cell growth, and particle-based systems designed to deliver therapeutics to cells and tissues. The major research focus of surface modifications is antiproliferative drug eluting stent coatings designed to prevent restenosis, a reocclusion affecting 30 to 50% of angioplasty patients [4–7].

Alternatively, particle-based systems include viral carriers, organic and inorganic nanoparticles, and peptides. Current trends indicate that particle-based systems will likely replace surface modifications as treatments move towards less invasive interventions, as evidenced by recent research attempting to ameliorate the shortfalls in drugeluting stent coatings with nanoparticle systems [8–10].

Within the field of particle-based delivery, the major focus of research now lies in biocompatible polymers for gene therapy. While the efficient targeted delivery of therapeutic drugs remains a significant challenge with enormous potential benefit, the unfolding nature of proteomics has led more researchers to focus on the potential for gene therapy as the future of nanomedicine treatments. Accordingly, the majority of the studies discussed refer to gene transfection. However, the considerations necessary for efficient transfection are equally applicable to drug delivery systems.

Viruses, particularly retroviruses and adenoviruses, continue to be used for transfection, though their DNA carrying capacity is limited [11]. Despite their highly efficient transfection capabilities and the ability to achieve permanent insertion of the therapeutic gene into the cell genome, their immunogenic and mutagenic impacts have led research towards less hazardous vectors. The present design conundrum lies in developing vehicles that transfect as efficiently as viral vectors while avoiding the mutagenic and carcinogenic risks. Nonviral vectors include liposomes, and nanoparticles of peptides and synthetic and natural polymers, with vector selection governed by a myriad of factors including the therapeutic agent, desired pharmacokinetics, and the target cells.

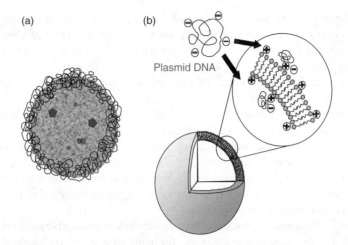

FIGURE 26.1 (a) The "conformational cloud" prevents opsonization of a PEG-coated polymeric nanoparticle loaded with a pharmaceutical. (b) Liposome section depicts how plasmid DNA is compacted by charge and encapsulated or adsorbed depending on fabrication method.

Liposomes are the primary choice for plasmid transfection, favorable for their ability to condense pDNA, protecting it against degradation by serum nucleases. Cationic lipids electrostatically compact DNA up to 2.3 Mb [12], forming complexes having a positive surface potential and diameter less than 200 nm; such particles are capable of being internalised through endocytic pathways. Complexes may consist of lipid cores with adsorbed plasmids [13] or lipid shells with internalized plasmids [14–16]. Due to the associated high surface charge, circulatory proteins are easily adsorbed and allow for rapid clearance of these vehicles from the circulatory system by the RES. This has led to the development of "stealth" coatings with hydrophilic polyethylene glycol (PEG) or longer chain polyethylene oxide (PEO), allowing circulation times in the range of hours rather than minutes [17]. Added through physical adsorption or as block copolymers, the flexible hydrophilic region of PEG chains form a "conformational cloud," preventing adhesion of opsonizing proteins [18] (Figure 26.1).

The incorporation of PEG is also commonplace for synthetic polymeric nanoparticles, generally used as block copolymers with the complementary polymer selected based on the properties of the drug to be delivered [19,20]. Cationic polymers commonly selected for their ability to condense negative plasmids demonstrate a positive surface charge, or zeta (ξ) potential, which permits binding of opsonizing proteins in the blood; as with liposomes, the integration of PEG in nanoparticles prevents opsonization. While the list of polymers employed is lengthy, the most common is FDA approved poly(D,L-lactide-co-glycolide) (PLGA) [5]. It should be noted that polyethyleneimine (PEI), whose proton sponge behavior is thought to cause endosome disruption, is generally the comparison standard for synthetic polymer transfection, though its cytotoxicity inhibits clinical application. In addition to plasmid transfection, synthetic polymers are also being developed for delivery of poorly soluble hydrophobic drugs such as cisplatin [21], clonazepam [22], and paclitaxel [9,18,23].

A common concern with synthetic polymers is the inability of cells to adequately metabolize the polymer vehicles and constituents that may be used in their fabrication, such as poly(vinyl alcohol) (PVA), which may comprise nearly 10% w/w of PLGA vehicles [5,24]. Though synthetic polymers provide better sustained release and gene expression profiles than their natural counterparts [5], recognition that *in vivo* safety is as important as therapeutic success has pushed research efforts toward natural biopolymers in the hopes of achieving true immune transparency [5].

Natural polymers such as chitosan and alginate have received recent attention due to their desirable biodegradability characteristics [25–27]. Research in this field, to date limited in contrast to liposomes and synthetic polymers, indicates that these natural vectors have inferior transfection capabilities when compared to viral and synthetic vectors. As nanoparticles are producible with similar size and surface charge, it remains to be ascertained where the breakdown in natural polymer transfection occurs. Though biopolymeric nanoparticles have yet to reach the transfection efficiency of commercial liposome formulations such as Lipofectaminea™, or that of synthetic polymers, their slow biodegradation, ensuring a burst-free release of therapeutic plasmid, and the promise of transfection without immune response continues to fuel research in this field.

In addition to natural biopolymers, recent attention has also focused on biocompatible peptides as delivery vectors. By condensing pDNA in a simple complexation fashion similar to polycations, protein transduction domain peptides demonstrate carrier uptake of 80 to 90% within 30 min, significantly more rapid than PEI or commercial liposomes [28]. These vectors are able to bypass traditional endocytic pathways to reach the nucleus within 1 h. Similarly, nuclear localization sequence (NLS) peptides allow superior transfection over synthetic polyplexes, and may be incorporated in traditional liposome complexes to assist in plasmid nuclear penetration [29,30].

It is evident that particle-based vectors have yet to reach their envisioned capabilities. Research focus has shifted from viral vectors, which continue to offer the highest transfection efficiency, through synthetic polymer and liposome systems, commercially available and suitable for *in vitro* transfection, to natural compounds in search of transfection using a biodegradable vector. The enhanced biocompatibility of peptides and natural biopolymers will certainly drive research as the quest for suitable *in vivo* vectors continues, though the balance between attaining biocompatibility while preserving transfection efficiency has yet to be found.

26.1.1 Practical Considerations for Nanoscale Vectors

Evident within the research to date is the superiority of certain vectors for particular aspects of the delivery process. The initial stage in the transfection process is endocytosis, which generally requires vectors to be less than 200 nm in diameter, though size limit is dependent on the target cells [24,28,31]. Size trials of a nonphagocytic cell line indicate that smaller particles are much more rapidly internalized, with 100 and 200 nm particles being internalized 3 to 4 and 8 to 10 times more slowly, respectively, than 50 nm particles [31]. Particle sizing methods must also be considered, as dynamic light scattering (DLS) frequently gives larger measurement than electron microscopy, and is particularly dependent on the presence of aggregate-inducing ions and proteins.

Cellular internalization is also strongly impacted by particle ξ potential. Though a positive ξ potential is required for binding to negative cell membranes, excessive surface charge leads to rapid systemic clearance and accumulation in the liver and spleen [27,32,33]. To control ξ potential, PEG and PEO are incorporated either as block copolymers for synthetic particles or as coatings for other vectors to produce a near neutral surface charge [17,21,34,35]. These elements also serve to prevent leeching of the therapeutic cargo by forming hydrogen bonds with the aqueous surroundings [20]. Unfortunately, the neutral ξ potential of these particles impairs the vector's ability to disrupt the lysosomal membrane for release to the cytosol, thought to occur upon a charge reversal as protons accumulate in nanoparticles within acidic lysosomes, limiting their transfection efficiency [5,33]. To exploit environmental pH change, polymers having degradable cross-linkers in acidic surroundings have been developed [36,37].

The increased circulation times provided by PEG coatings certainly increase the likelihood of vectors reaching the desired cells and do demonstrate enduring *in vivo* protein production following transfection [38,39]. To further improve delivery characteristics, a broad range of targeting moieties, including transferrin, folate, peptides, vitamins, and antibodies, have been incorporated into particle surfaces to actively target cells [10,33,40,41]. While transferrin and folate increase endocytosis in general, antibodies have the potential to target cell-specific membrane proteins. This enables targeting of particular cell types for specific therapies, such as localized delivery of costly and toxic chemotherapeutics to tumor growths. For example, antibody targeting of endothelial surface receptors results in a tenfold increase in cell binding and a doubling in transfection *in vitro* [10].

Vector targeting of specific tissues may also be achieved through magnetic, heat, and light-affected vehicles [17,19,36,42,43]. External fields retain magnetic vectors in the vasculature of a target region, giving cells greater contact time to endocytose the vector. Alternatively, heat-affected vectors can induce structural changes in polymeric vectors, leading to local pharmaceutical release in stimulated regions [17], while light stimulated vectors provide localized heating of metallic vectors. By active oncoprotein antibody targeting, or passive enhanced permeation and retention (EPR) targeting, which allows 50 to 100 nm vectors to extravasate from leaky tumor vasculature, gold nanoshells demonstrate tumor ablation when stimulated with near infrared lasers [43,44]. While such external targeting is effective, the biodegradability of the metallic and synthetic vectors remains an obstacle.

These noted considerations are further compounded by such factors as route of administration, target cells, vector stability, therapeutic cargo, and desired pharmacokinetics, as well as entrapment efficiency, loading rate, and release kinetics. Of primary importance is vector stability relative to the route of administration. Many synthetic polymer systems are rapidly cleared when injected intravenously as protein adsorption leads to agglomeration or RES removal, eliminating any potential therapeutic benefit. Similarly, a synergy is required between the target cell and the vector's pharmacokinetic characteristics. For example, slowly dividing cells require vectors capable of entering the nucleus or retarded system clearance and release profiles. Balance between the entrapment efficiency and the total mass loading of individual vectors must also be considered. Vectors with high encapsulation efficiency avoid waste of expensive therapeutic agents while vectors with high mass loading require fewer particles to be delivered to achieve therapeutic benefit. One study found that encapsulation efficiency was reduced by more than half when loading was increased from 1 to 3% w/w [18]. The vector must also be capable of releasing sufficient quantities with controllable kinetics. Finally, the dosage must ensure a continued presence of vector in the vicinity of the target cells while simultaneously assuring that overdosing does not lead to tumor development or toxic effects [5]. Ultimately, the current findings and the corollaries within indicate that suitable therapeutic delivery systems need to be developed for specific *in vivo* or *in vitro* applications.

26.1.2 Example Delivery Nanosystems

Vaccine adjuvants: Plasmid vaccines that can successfully elicit humoral and cellular immune response have the potential to provide safer alternatives than live viral or heat-killed bacterial vaccines. Therapeutically relevant immune response is attainable with adjuvants such as cholera toxin and lipid A delivered using cationic nanoparticles by topical and subcutaneous administration, respectively [45]. Additionally, protein-based vaccines may be encapsulated in pH sensitive polymers, where low pH in the phagosomes of antigen-presenting cells disrupt the vectors to release vaccines [37].

Drug delivery: Delivery of paclitaxel, a poorly soluble antitumoral, benefits from vector delivery by eliminating the hypersensitivity found in 25 to 30% of patients administered commercial Cremophor™ [23]. Relying on EPR, PEGcoated liposomes and synthetic particles such as polycaprolactone [46], polylactide [18], and PLGA [47] allow lower doses over prolonged periods. Similarly, hepatoma cells can be targeted through galactosylated ligands using 10 to 30 nm PEG–PLA (poly(lactic acid)) nanoparticles to deliver clonazepam [22], while cisplatin loaded PEG–polyglutamic acid block micelles demonstrate advanced tumor regression [21]. In an example of innovative drug delivery, temperature sensitive PEG-coated liposomes, whose drug diffusivity greatly increases in the 40 to 45°C range, demonstrate prolonged circulation and increased accumulation of a model drug in tumor tissue [17]. (See LaVan for a drug delivery review [36].)

Antimicrobial therapy: Bacterial detection using vancomycin-modified magnetic FePt particles demonstrates an ability to detect and entrap gram positive and gram negative strains, including highly lethal vancomycin-resistant *Enterococci* (VRE) [42]. Self-assembling peptides forming cylindrical nanotubes also display antimicrobial activity by penetrating bacterial cell membranes and increasing permeability, with demonstrated *in vivo* effectiveness against methicillin-resistant *S. aureus* (MRSA) [48].

Antisense therapy: Aimed at inhibiting the production of specific proteins, antisense oligonucleotides entrapped in PLGA nanospheres disrupt growth regulation of vascular smooth muscle cells and prevent restenosis following angioplasty [8]. Potential applications for this nascent field are innumerable and will become increasingly prominent as proteomics unfolds the nature of protein interactions and identifies the function of individual proteins.

Gene therapy: Contrary to antisense therapy, the ability to induce production of specific proteins identified by proteomics has similar potential for future clinical therapeutics. *In vitro* application is widespread, and researchers continue to develop new liposome [10,49], synthetic [33,34,50–52] and natural polymer [25,27], and peptide [28] vectors in pursuit of more efficient and compatible formulations. While human *in vivo* application of nonviral gene therapy remains limited, the wealth of research focused on developing suitable vectors cannot sufficiently emphasize the potential for successful application-specific transfection vehicles.

26.1.3 Summary

Given the range of therapeutic delivery systems presently available and the extent of continuing research, the above discussion is intended as a general background. Most evident in the majority of findings to date is the inability of individual vectors to simultaneously satisfy biocompatibility and delivery efficiency requirements. Further, results are nontransferable across applications, emphasising the necessity of developing systems for specific therapeutic agents, specific cells, and even specific cellular compartments [5]. Novel screening methods for transfection efficiency of new vectors will certainly accelerate advancement in this process [50]. Though delivery systems have yet to attain their promise, they are certainly well poised to revolutionize nanomedicine, therapeutic delivery, and most importantly, the range and acuteness of illnesses that are considered treatable.

26.2 Tissue Engineering

One of the main goals of biomedical engineering is the repair or replacement of defective or damaged organs and tissues [53]. To date, numerous methods have been used to fabricate constructs to repair tissues *in vitro* and *in vivo*, ranging from bone to blood vessels [54–56]. Recently, increasing awareness of the influence of molecular composition and nanoscale architecture on cellular responses to materials has focused nanobiotechnology research on controlling these fabrication parameters in the development of better materials for tissue engineering applications.

Present tissue engineering methods consist primarily of porous three-dimensional scaffolds of various materials designed to imitate and replace the extracellular matrix (ECM) that supports all cell growth in the body [57]. Ideal tissue engineering would result from full implant integration, followed by its gradual degradation and replacement by natural cell-produced ECM as new tissue is generated. For this to occur, scaffolds should promote cellular migration, adhesion, proliferation, and differentiation, while supporting natural cell processes [58]. Development of more suitable scaffolds requires materials that exhibit not only appropriate mechanical characteristics, but also that which elicit favorable cellular responses [59]. Fuelled by a greater understanding of surface topography and composition on cell–scaffold interaction, research continues to improve nanoscale control of scaffold architecture in the design of more compatible engineered materials [60].

The term "biocompatible," often used to describe ceramic, metal, and polymers utilized in biological applications, is rather imprecise given the broadness of its accepted definition: "the ability of a material to perform with an appropriate host response in a specific application." Such an indefinite description fails to suggest what type of host response should be desired or considered acceptable [61]. Despite the range of physical and chemical properties exhibited by biomaterials, the body reacts in a similar fashion after implantation; a layer of proteins is randomly adsorbed onto the surface immediately, followed by macrophage attack, and finally encapsulation of the device through the classic foreign body reaction (Figure 26.2) [62,63]. This encapsulation segregates the device from the body, impeding normal wound healing processes and preventing the device from functioning as intended.

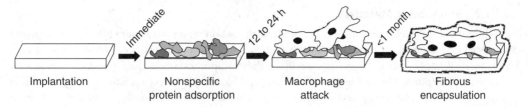

FIGURE 26.2 Implantation of a biomaterial ultimately leads to fibrous encapsulation of the device in the foreign body reaction, preventing natural tissue formation and device integration.

The need to develop biomaterials capable of eliciting specific responses was recognized as early as 1993 [58]. The resulting emerging class of engineered biomaterials aims to design bioactive materials that control the host response to promote full tissue–scaffold integration and natural wound healing while simultaneously preventing the foreign body reaction [62]. The main techniques presently investigated for tissue engineering endeavor to address one or more of the following objectives [58]:

1. Control of the chemical environment through surface biomolecule immobilization or self-assembled systems
2. Control of the nanostructure through surface modification or *de novo* fabrication
3. Control of the biological environment of the surface through cell patterning

Each of these seeks to reproduce an environment that successfully mimics *in vivo* conditions for successful tissue integration. It should be noted that very few examples of *in vivo* tissue replacement or repair have been reported. For this reason, promising *in vitro* results are discussed in the sections that follow, together with examples of preliminary tissue engineering applications.

26.2.1 Surface Molecular Engineering for Controlled Protein Interaction

It is hypothesized that nonordered protein adsorption on materials begins the cascade leading to the foreign body reaction, since all normal biological events operate on a system based on specific recognition of proteins and polysaccharides [62,63]. To control nonspecific adsorption, several surface modification approaches have been explored: "stealth" materials are designed to decrease nonspecific protein adsorption while others promote adsorption of specific proteins in an effort to direct biological processes [63,64].

26.2.1.1 Stealth Materials

There are three main methods used in the development of protein-resistant stealth materials, also referred to as nonfouling or noninteractive surfaces [65]:

1. Hydrophilic surfaces can be achieved through thin-film deposition of hydrogels, phospholipids, or other suitable materials, such as PEG and PEO.
2. Chemical surface modification leads to surface expression of specific functional groups known to inhibit protein adsorption. For example, surfaces rich in carboxylic acid groups support cell growth, whereas methyl, hydroxyl, and carboxymethyl ester groups generally do not. Interestingly, surfaces modified by random mixtures of organic functional groups can exhibit significant bioactivity and specificity [63].
3. Surface immobilization of biomolecules, including proteins, seeks to recreate the natural *in vivo* environment.

The first two approaches address the problem of nonspecific adsorption but fail to address the coexisting need to promote the favorable cell–surface interactions required to encourage natural healing and tissue repair processes. Alternatively, the last method represents a tactic that addresses both issues by creating materials that manage biological interactions while resisting nonspecific protein adsorption.

26.2.1.2 Biomimetic Materials

Immobilization of proteins to control tissue–surface interaction represents a more biomimetic approach to material development, in contrast to stealth materials that prevent interaction. Natural biomolecules have the dual capability of triggering specific cellular responses while their presence can prevent nonspecific adsorption. The techniques used to append biologically active moieties on surfaces can be grouped into three main categories: physical micro/nanofabrication, imprinting, and direct chemical immobilization.

Conventional microfabrication techniques used to pattern biomolecules on surfaces include photo-lithography, photochemistry, and microcontact printing [66]. Capable of immobilizing biomolecules on a variety of surfaces, the resolution of these techniques is generally limited to the micro scale. Though nanometrescale configurations are achievable through modifications of these techniques, including the application of lasers and finely focused ion beams (FFIB) to photolithography, they remain unable to meet the desired resolution [66,67].

Recently developed nanofabrication techniques include dip-pen nanolithography (DPN), which uses functionalized atomic force microscopy (AFM) tips to deposit biomolecules on surfaces with pattern features as small as 10 nm [68]. Used for the creation of protein nanoarrays and virus arrays, this technique can create patterns with multiple components [68,69]. Enzymes have also been selectively deposited for biochemical modification of self-assembled monolayers [70]. While nanofabrication techniques are effective for patterning two-dimensional surfaces, these methods are quite limited in terms of processing time and are not suitable for three-dimensional scaffolds.

Imprinting is an approach used to confer biological recognition to surfaces through the creation of templates in synthetic polymers. This process yields surfaces with imprint accuracy at the nanometrescale, resulting in binding cavities that possess the correct conformation and functionality to allow selective binding to the appropriate molecules [71]. Despite the promising results, this technique is also limited to two dimensions, and multicomponent systems would be difficult to achieve.

Chemical immobilization, a more facile method of introducing biomolecules on materials, exploits functional groups present at the surface as binding sites. Successful covalent and noncovalent immobilization of biomolecules on synthetic polymers has been reported extensively, resulting in modified bioactivity and specificity [63]. Polymers requiring functionalization are modified by blending, copolymerization, and chemical and physical treatments, among others [64]. While not amenable to specific patterning, multicomponent systems and three-dimensional surface modification is feasible. For example, the natural interaction between osteopontin and Type I collagen can be exploited to functionalize a surface with oriented protein binding, leading to increased endothelial cell adhesion and proliferation [72].

In many cases, it is preferential to chemically immobilize peptide segments rather than whole proteins, as they retain the activity of full proteins while being less likely to invoke immune responses and are more resistant to degradation. RGD (arginine–glycine–aspartic acid), perhaps the most studied peptide sequence for tissue engineering, is well documented as a stimulant for cell adhesion on synthetic surfaces and its ability to interact with multiple cell adhesion receptors (for a review see Reference 64). Several *in vivo* studies have investigated the fate of peptide covered surfaces in the body, including an RGD-functionalized hydrogel that demonstrates improved neural tissue adhesion, tissue regeneration, and host tissue infiltration when implanted into brain lesions, as compared to the nonmodified hydrogel [73]. A similar material also improves neurite repair and angiogenesis in spinal cord repair [74]. Bone tissue ingrowth and direct tissue-implant contact is also promoted on scaffolds with immobilized RGD-bearing peptides, whereas uncoated scaffolds become segregated by a fibrous tissue layer resulting from the foreign body reaction [75].

Control of protein–surface interaction is essential to the development of materials designed for bio-logical application. Reduction of nonspecific protein adsorption with stealth materials is a promising first step to avoiding the foreign body reaction. Surface immobilization of biological molecules is a more sophisticated approach, leading to materials exhibiting favorable cell interactions and having the potential to influence biological processes. Continued advancements in this area will require the development of additional nanoscale techniques to allow greater control over surface characteristics. Such advancements must be supported by microbiological research to elucidate the nature of interactions between proteins and surfaces, as well as the protein spatial arrangements and orientations necessary for the desired application-specific response.

26.2.2   Nanostructured Surfaces

In addition to the importance of recognition events, advances in microbiology provide a greater understanding of the effect of surface micro- and nanostructure on cell behavior. *In vivo*, all cells live within the structural support of a complex nanoscale topology of pores, ridges, and fibres provided by the ECM [53]. Interaction between the substrate and cells are thought to activate the cytoskeleton in a way that mediates attachment, migration, growth, and differentiation, in addition to affecting cytokine and growth factor production [60,76]. As noted by Miller et al. [77], it is surprising that the design of optimal tissue engineering structures has not focused more on nanostructure, given that ECM has been known for some time to be crucial to cell and tissue growth. However, advanced techniques allowing nanostructured construction have renewed research interest, with the majority of work to date related to blood vessel and bone tissue regeneration.

Several methods are used to create nanoscale architecture in polymers, including phase separation [53,57,59,78], electrospinning [79], rubbing [80], chemical etching [77,81], colloidal lithography [82], AFM-assisted nanolithography [83], and template patterning [76,84]. Phase separation is particularly useful since it is amenable to the production of three-dimensional scaffolds. In addition to polymers, hydroxyapatite (HAP) and collagen are generally the materials of choice for nanostructured bone regeneration scaffolds. Two novel ways of coating nanoscale HAP onto three-dimensional scaffolds include chemical vapor deposition and growth directly from aqueous solutions [85,86]. Regardless of the method or material used to produce nanostructures, cell adhesion and proliferation increase compared to smooth or microstructured surfaces, with cell morphology more closely resembling the native state [59,76,77,82,87,88]. Further, protein adsorption, a necessary precursor to cell adhesion, is improved on nanostructured surfaces [88]. Additionally, submicron sized grooves in surfaces can affect cell alignment for directed growth [87,89].

In addition to angiogenesis and osteogenesis, nanostructured materials demonstrate application for the growth of neurons and smooth muscle cells. Successful *in vitro* neurite growth is achievable with a biodegradable porous nanostructured PLA scaffold, where nanoscale topography promotes neuron adhesion and differentiation, including neurite outgrowth [53]. Similarly, bladder smooth muscle cell growth is improved on chemically-treated PLGA and polyurethane (PU) bearing nanostructures [81].

In a considerably different application, nanofabricated polyimide surfaces can be useful for the preparation of cell spheroids, roughly spherical masses composed of cells and associated ECM that demonstrate tissue-like morphological and physiological functions. Cell culture on nanostructured fluorinated polyimides results in fibroblast cell spheroids with a density comparable to tissue *in vivo*, fostering interest in their development for tissue engineering applications [90].

Research in this field demonstrates the importance of nanoscale architecture on cell adhesion, growth, differentiation, and phenotype expression. Furthermore, it promotes the development of techniques for producing nanostructured surfaces, which are certain to be an important component in the future of successful tissue engineering scaffolds.

26.2.3   Self-Assembled Systems

The techniques previously discussed represent approaches based on modifications to materials already employed in biomedical applications. Conversely, natural tissues consist of hierarchical organizations of molecules, giving rise to a multitude of nanostructures, microstructures, and macrostructures [91]. This has led researchers to explore the so-called "bottom-up" approach of self-assembling systems, using biological systems as a design base to create biomaterials with improved properties.

Biomimetic approaches to self-assembly are used to apply surface functionality onto materials to direct specific cell responses, while also displaying nanostructure resembling natural tissue ECM. Advantages of this approach include: ease with which functional groups can be incorporated; well-defined structures and intrinsic stability; and a lack of defects in the surfaces, which reduces nonspecific interactions [63,92]. The two main methods of self-assembly include the formation of self-assembled monolayers (SAMs) on surfaces and the formation of nano-, micro- and macroscopic structures from natural self-assembly. To date, the majority of research into SAMs uses molecularly flat surfaces as templates. Multicomponent SAMs with controllable nanoscale features are attainable with a variety of patterning techniques. (for a review see Reference 93). Though largely dependent on the functional groups of the surface on which they form and the nature of the molecules to be assembled [94], successful biomedical SAM application would require application to three-dimensional structures and to materials used for medical applications; such reports are limited [92].

In contrast to two-dimensional self-assembly, self-assembly of three-dimensional structures holds much promise and is of greater interest for tissue engineering. The challenge in this field remains the design of molecules that spontaneously self-organize into stable structures with desirable characteristics [95]. Peptides are particularly well suited as they are capable of self-assembly, are sufficiently robust, can confer biological activity to a surface, and degrade into nontoxic constituents. A particular advantage is that peptides may be designed to incorporate specific chains and functional groups to confer cell adhesive properties or cell differentiation signaling abilities to a surface. Several examples of synthetic and natural peptides demonstrate self-assembling abilities and form favorable structures, with amphiphilic peptides proving exceptionally useful in this domain [95].

In vitro, self-assembled peptide scaffolds facilitate cell attachment, migration, proliferation, and differentiation for a number of cell lines; cells are also found to produce components of natural ECM [95]. Primary rat neuronal cells project lengthy axons following the contours of a peptide nanofiber scaffold and form active and functional synapses. Chondrocytes encapsulated in the same scaffold produce components of natural ECM, including collagen and glycosaminoglycans. As well, liver progenitor cells differentiate and demonstrate natural enzyme activity. *In vivo*, these scaffolds promote repair of brain lesions [96]. In a separate application, an engineered amphiphilic self-assembling peptide forms collagen-like cylindrical structures that guide HAP crystal formation in orientations and sizes similar to natural bone [97]. Finally, an interesting combination of self-assembly and cell patterning techniques developed by Auger et al. employs a cohesive sheet of self-assembled human vascular cells as a template for fibroblast adhesion on the exterior surface. The interior surface then acts as a scaffold for endothelial cell growth, resulting in the formation of tissue-engineered blood vessels exhibiting appropriate structural characteristics and *in vitro* hemocompatibility [98,99].

26.2.4 Summary

It has long been recognized that the materials and constructs used to replace damaged tissues are vastly inferior to their natural counterparts. There is little doubt that an ability to induce healing processes to produce natural tissue would bestow an enormous wealth of medical treatment options. Expanded understanding of the processes involved in healing and tissue growth processes, provided by progress in nanobiotechnology and microbiology, has furthered insight into the interactions occurring between cells and substrates, leading to improved designs that demonstrate promising results for future *in vivo* tissue applications. Though nanomedicine has yet to benefit from the true promise held in tissue engineering, it is clear that further developments in this area, including fabrication processes amenable to three-dimensional constructs with modifiable bioactivity, possess the potential to provide achievable, application-specific, tissue engineering methods for medical treatments.

26.3 Diagnostic Imaging and Monitoring

The principles and methods employed in the nanoscale development of materials for therapeutic delivery systems and tissue engineering serve equally well in the design of imaging and monitoring diagnostics. Nanoparticles, primarily of inorganic materials such as silica, gold, and silver, serve as imaging aids for a range of *in vitro* and *in vivo* investigations, while tissue engineering methods of controlled biomolecule immobilization aid in the creation of biosensors to detect a range of proteins, DNA, and pathogenic compounds. Many of the techniques that now fall within the realm of nanomedicine were originally developed for other applications, such as the polymerase chain reaction (PCR) used to amplify DNA samples prior to diagnostic genetic screening [100]. The broad range of nanoscale manipulations used in diagnostic nanomedicine are highly cross-application tools, rendering difficult the categorization of such methods as biomolecule detection using nanoparticles for intracellular sensing [101]. The following division of imaging and diagnostic monitoring tools are intended to simplify these multidisciplinary applications, though the scope of current studies certainly exceeds these boundaries.

26.3.1 Biophotonics

Imaging techniques have benefited from progress in nanotechnology, with the main advances incorporating nanoparticles and quantum dots. Although not yet applicable for diagnostic purposes, new optical techniques are also being designed to improve nanoscale imaging.

26.3.1.1 Nanoparticles in Imaging

Advances in imaging have occurred in conjunction with the development of nanoparticles, which are used to enhance existing imaging techniques by serving as contrast agents or as markers in various optical techniques. The myriad of diagnostic imaging techniques currently used includes radiography (x-ray), magnetic resonance imaging (MRI), computed tomography (CT), positron emission tomography (PET), and ultrasound. Each of these methods represents an invaluable medical tool permitting diagnosis and monitoring of numerous conditions, however, each suffers from limitations due to one or more tissues that are difficult to image. Nanoparticles have been designed to overcome these limitations and to expand functionality of the techniques.

Radionuclide-encapsulating liposomes are used to prolong the lifetime of positron emitters in the body for improved diagnostic PET imaging. Liposomal radionuclides are designed to enhance blood pool imaging and specific tissue observation, with leaky tumor vasculature and subsequent accumulation making them particularly useful for diagnostic tumor imaging [102]. Radioisotope-carrying polymeric nanoparticles are similarly used to target bone and bone marrow [35]. As with drug delivery systems, these particles must be designed to avoid RES clearance and with appropriate molecular markers to allow accumulation in the target tissue.

Analogous strategies for improved radiography include the use of liposome-encapsulated contrast enhancers. In soluble form, these contrast enhancers are rapidly cleared from the body and pose some toxicity risks. In contrast, the nontoxic liposomal iohexol formulation increases residence time to 3 h, with applications in cardiac imaging and early tumor detection [103]. Similarly, improvements in MRI imaging result from the use of a gadolinium carrying polyamidoamine dendrimer as a contrast agent. This nanosized paramagnetic molecule allows noninvasive localization of sentinel lymph nodes and metastases in breast cancer patients, which is crucial for treatment design [104].

While nanoparticles provide improved imaging using existing techniques, image resolution remains limited by the system design. Therefore, nanoparticles are being designed to be used with systems capable of nanoscale resolution. New optical imaging techniques have emerged as supporting technology enables more precise imaging and labeling at the nano scale. Fluorescence-based imaging systems are by far the most popular and most studied systems for cell analysis. These systems, based on bioconjugation of an optical dye to biological molecules, offer the same resolution as optical microscopy systems, but allow for precise localization and sensitive quantification of individual biomolecules. However, fluorescent dyes suffer from limitations, including potential toxicity, reduced sensitivity compared to radioactivity, and interference from other molecules.

To improve upon the sensitivity of fluorescent imaging modalities, several methods of signal enhancement are employed in optical systems. Signal enhancement through fluorescence resonance energy transfer (FRET, also called fluorescence *in situ* hybridization, or FISH), which results when two fluorescent molecules are brought into close proximity leading to a change in fluorescence intensity, permits the intracellular detection of specific sequences in nucleic acids, including mRNA and DNA [105]. Signal enhancement is also achieved with plasmon–plasmon resonance interactions, which are similar to FRET. Gold and silver plasmon-resonant particles (PRPs), as well as superparticles consisting of colloidal gold nanoparticle shells around silica cores, strongly scatter optical light, making them easily visible using conventional microscopy or surface-enhanced Raman scattering (SERS) [44,106]. Two PRPs in close proximity produce changes in their plasmon optical resonance, allowing their distinct and bright signals to be quantified; a single PRP is as bright as $\sim 5 \times 10^6$ fluorescein molecules or 10^5 quantum dots [107]. These are used for highly sensitive detection of antibodies in whole blood, as well as investigations of intracellular transport pathways [44,106].

26.3.1.2 Nanosensor Probes

Nanoparticles are also used to enhance and exploit fluorescent signals in the form of optical nanosensors. These sensors, which generally consist of an encapsulated fluorescent detection system, are designed to take advantage of fluorescent systems while improving their sensing abilities and reducing toxicity [108]. Dendrimers, in particular, allow the colocalization of several chromophores, increasing the signal and sensitivity to levels provided by less-favorable radioactive tags [109]. Nanosensors are more complex than simple fluorescent tags, usually consisting of a fluorophore that is activated or quenched by a particular analyte.

Nanosensors incorporating several different molecules including fluorophores, enzymes, fluoriono-phores, and associated ionophores, are being designed for the detection of specific analytes, including intracellular pH, glucose, and potassium [108,110]. These show fast response time, reversible analyte detection, and high selectivity [111]. For example, quantitative glucose-sensing nanosensors, also called PEBBLEs, contain glucose oxidase and an oxygen sensitive fluorescent indicator to detect intracellular glucose levels (Figure 26.3) [112]. The versatility of nanosensors allows encapsulation of a variety of molecules, leading to "particle labs" that perform complex tests intracellularly through synergistic reactions. They can be targeted to specific organelles, though they do suffer some cell entry limitations. Physical cell delivery methods are also viable, including injection and gene gun delivery, though liposomal and ultrasound-based delivery leads to better cell survival [106,108]. Advances in delivery vehicle design will also benefit nanosensors, enabling improved cellular entry.

The development and use of nanoparticles for diagnostic imaging is a relatively new endeavor that is likely to increase, owing to the promising results obtained to date. It can be expected that the development and use of nanosensors and image enhancers for common diagnostic techniques will predominate in the coming years.

26.3.1.3 Quantum Dots in Imaging

Although these nanosized devices could technically be included with nanoparticles, their unique properties place quantum dots (Qdots) in their own category. Qdots are semiconductor nanocrystals (diameter 2 to 10 nm) that exhibit broad excitation spectra and narrow emission spectra in the visible range [44]. Originally designed for information technology purposes, their application to biophotonic imaging through conjugation with biomolecules was quickly realized. They demonstrate significant advantages over classic fluorescent dyes, including size-tuneable emission wavelength, photobleaching resistance, increased stability, reduced toxicity, and persistent residency in cells [113–115]; as well, simultaneous

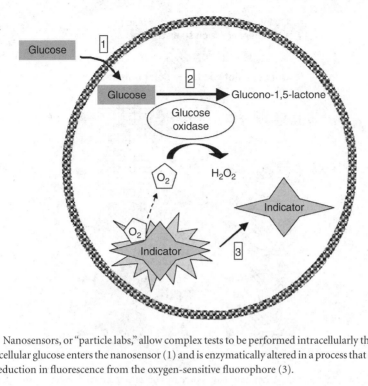

FIGURE 26.3 Nanosensors, or "particle labs," allow complex tests to be performed intracellularly through synergistic reactions. Intracellular glucose enters the nanosensor (1) and is enzymatically altered in a process that consumes oxygen (2), causing a reduction in fluorescence from the oxygen-sensitive fluorophore (3).

detection of multiple agents is possible due to their broad excitation and tuneable narrow emission spectra.

Qdots are used in a number of biological applications, including visualization of DNA hybridization [116], immunoassays [117], receptor-mediated endocytosis [118], and *in vivo* cellular imaging [113]. *In vitro* and *in vivo* intracellular labeling with Qdots does not interfere with cell viability, growth, or differentiation over extended periods of time [119], and no signs of systemic toxicity result from intravenous administration [120]. Their persistence in cells makes them amenable for following extended tissue development, including embryo development [116].

The versatility of Qdots is best demonstrated through the design of multicolour optical coding systems. Hundreds of thousands of unique Qdots can be created through the encapsulation of combinations of zinc sulphide-capped cadmium selenide nanocrystals of slightly different sizes in polymeric beads expressing various biomolecules at the surface (Figure 26.4) [121]. This ability makes them ideal for high-throughput parallel analysis of biological molecules, such as gene expression studies and medical diagnostics. The use of Qdots in analysis is expected to replace planar DNA chips due to reduced costs, faster binding kinetics, and greater flexibility in target selection [121].

Even greater promise for Qdots lies with *in vivo* application. As with all nanoparticles, these must be designed with surface coatings to reduce RES clearance and to promote cell-specific targeting; they must also demonstrate sufficient lifetimes to allow visualization. Amphiphilic poly(acrylic acid) surface coatings allow noninvasive whole body fluorescence imaging of targeted tissues up to 4 months postinjection [122]. Qdots are used for live imaging of tumors [123], capillaries, skin, and adipose tissue [120]. Further *in vivo* application will require Qdots with near infrared (NIR) emission spectra, since transmission of these wavelengths is possible through tissue [44,113,122]. They may also find application in tracking of viral particles, drug molecules, and migratory tumor cells *in vivo* [113]. Qdots may also play a role in the development of spectroscopic and spectral imaging techniques for molecular analysis of pathologic tissue, leading to the identification of "disease fingerprints" and subsequent diagnostic techniques [124]. As interest and research in Qdots increases, it is likely that the consequential development of new noninvasive imaging techniques will ensue.

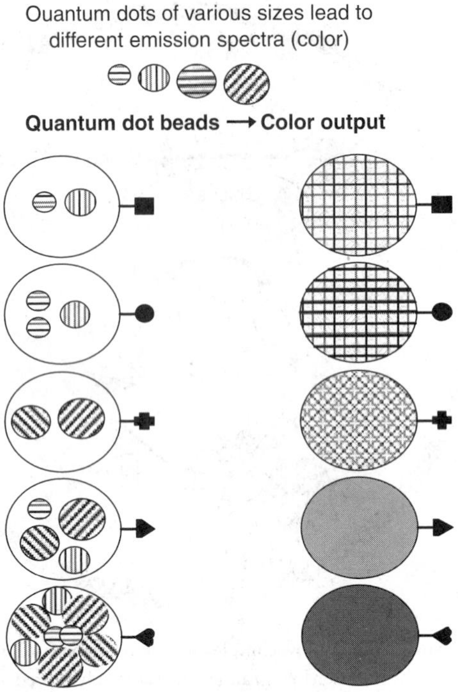

FIGURE 26.4 The versatility of quantum dots allows preparation of numerous distinctive tags using encapsulated combinations of uniquely colored dots.

26.3.2 Diagnostic Biosensors

Though the majority of biorecognition techniques incorporate nanoscale manipulations, the majority of these methods would more classically fall within the domains of analytical chemistry than applied nanomedicine. However, the increasing sensitivity of these techniques greatly improves their utility as diagnostic aids and broadens the scope of applied and investigative nanomedicine.

26.3.2.1 Molecular Biointerfaces for Gene and Protein Biorecognition

Biomolecule detectors incorporate a biorecognition device capable of selectively recognizing the analyte of interest in connection with a signal transducer and a suitable output device. Transduction methods include a variety of optical (surface plasmon resonance [SPR], fluorescence), electrochemical (voltammetry, impedance, field effect), mechanical (cantilever, surface probe microscopy), and mass-based systems (quartz crystal microgravimetry [QCM], mass spectrometry). Selection of the appropriate transduction system is partially determined by the nature of information sought (quantitative or qualitative), the analyte (concentration, molecular weight), the sample size, and assay timeline.

The study of genomics promises to unravel the link between specific gene sequences and phenotype. Consequently, the majority of present diagnostic research focuses on the recognition of specific oligo-nucleotide (ON) sequences, DNA mutations, and single nucleotide polymorphisms (SNP) in order to identify predisposition to genetic disorders or the presence of disease. Recognition using any of the above transduction methods requires the immobilization of biomolecules to a surface to form a biointerface in a manner similar to the design of tissue engineering scaffolds. However, biosensors not intended for *in vivo* implantation avoid biocompatibility requirements and can employ inorganic and metallic substrates.

Common DNA recognition protocols rely on thiolated ONs adhered to gold surfaces as recognition ligands. Following PCR amplification of DNA to increase assay sensitivity, samples are exposed to the biointerface with the immobilized ON. While label-free assays are possible [125], the majority of hybridization and mutation assays use labels to obtain additional sensitivity through transduction dependant signal amplification. For example, silver and gold nanoparticles (PRPs) act as reporters for hybridization monitoring of cystic fibrosis genes by Raman scattering detection of plasmon resonance [126], and in the quantitative detection of SNPs in breast cancer genes using optical microscopy [127]. Monitoring of plasmon effects has the added advantage of multiple labeling capacity, where particles may generate different colors to label different sequences.

Nanoparticles are also used for fluorescent transduction methods, with single base mutation detection using 2.5 nm gold particles as scaffolds for fluorescently labeled ONs [128], or 2 to 100 nm fluorophore-loaded silica nanoparticles conjugated to unlabeled ONs [129]. For nonoptical transduction, charged liposomes amplify DNA recognition in electrochemical methods [130]. Recent studies also demonstrate amplified recognition of DNA hybridization using gold nanoparticles with QCM, which act as secondary ligands to increase the mass of recognized sequences [131], and provide sub-layers to which the ligand ON is immobilized [132]. Continuing research has lowered the detection sensitivity of DNA hybridization events by three to four orders of magnitude in as many years, with current sensitivity in the subfemtomolar concentration range for fluorescence and QCM-based techniques [129,132]. For the more difficult task of identifying single base mutations, assays are approximately one order of magnitude less sensitive in terms of molar concentration [131].

The use of biosensors is not limited to genomic applications and DNA analysis. Proteomics, which seeks to identify and define the roles played by cellular proteins, has led to improved protein recognition sensors [133]. Traditional highly sensitive enzyme-linked immunosorbent assays (ELISA) are being replaced with microarray format protein assays similar to DNA analyses with the goal of increasing knowledge of associated disease biomarkers, protein functions, and drug target identification. Depending on the transduction method, detection relies on protein composition (mass spectroscopy), or on the immobilization of a monoclonal antibody to a biointerface for optical (SPR, fluorescence) [134,135] and mass (QCM)-based strategies [136,137]. Such methods require the oriented immobilization of a functional protein to allow correct binding with the target analyte.

To achieve proper antibody immobilization while preventing nonspecific protein adsorption, which is a particular necessity to maintain assay sensitivity and specificity for serum or unpurified samples, biointerfaces are designed using principles similar to those used in tissue engineering. The importance of such nanoscale design factors are clearly demonstrated by the tenfold increase in sensitivity obtained in one study upon a doubling of the distance at which the antibody was immobilized from the surface [138]. The sensitivity of immobilized ligands to their environment is an additional obstacle with protein arrays as individual antibodies require unique pH and ionic conditions to maintain functional conformation [139]. Despite the advances in this field, the sensitivity of specific protein biorecognition has yet to experience the enormous gain in sensitivity found with DNA assays, which benefit from the advantage of sample amplification.

The array formats popular for both protein and DNA detection are well adapted to genetic screening for a multitude of illnesses. By using automation to process large numbers of samples, databases generated from mass samplings are used to correlate genetic presence or susceptibility to illnesses such as breast cancer [140,141] and bacterial infection [142,143]. The genetic test for cystic fibrosis, which requires 25 genetic traits to be tested, highlights the utility of arrays for both exploratory and diagnostic studies [144]. Presently, the requirements of such broad analysis limit testing to optical methods. However, the prohibitive cost of specialized optical analysers, in conjunction with improvements in electrochemical and QCM sensors, may soon popularize alternative diagnostic techniques. Ideally, these technologies will soon permit nanomedicine diagnostics to attain current sensitivity limits in a point-of-care device that requires no sample preparation, amplification, or labeling.

26.3.2.2 Pathogen Recognition

In addition to providing identification of disease susceptibility, advances in DNA hybridization techniques have greatly enhanced pathogen detection. These improvements permit the diagnosis timeline for sepsis, a rapidly advancing systemic infection for which timely treatment is critical, to narrow from the 24 to 48 h required for culturing methods to 5 to 6 h using PCR amplification methods [145]. Specific pathogenic nucleotide sequences correlate with a variety of pathogens, allowing detection using biorecognition techniques: the 16S rRNA gene is detectable in a range of gram negative and positive bacteria [146], the mecA gene is specific for the detection of methicillin resistant staphylococci [147], and the 18S rRNA sequence is indicative of the fungus *Candida albicans* [148].

Viral genetic materials are also quantitatively detectable using PCR-amplified fluorescent techniques, the sensitivity of which is particularly important for measuring HIV loads in patients undergoing retroviral therapies that reduce viral loads to below the detection limit of commercial diagnostic methods [149]. Though the majority of pathogen detection relies on PCR amplification followed by electrophoretic or fluorescent identification, hybridization of viral DNA has recently been reported using alternate transduction methods. Thiolated ONs immobilized on gold nanoparticles provide a platform for optical Rayleigh scattering to detect hepatitis B and C viral DNA [150], while ester linkages to immobilize hepatitis B fragments allow for similar detection by voltammetry [151]. Silicon miniaturization technology also presents future possibilities for point-of-care viral detection using arrayed electrodes for amperometric techniques [152]. However, the true potential of bacterial and viral recognition techniques will not be achieved until assays are capable of detecting natural load levels, negating the necessity of PCR amplification, to provide more rapid and cost effective diagnosis.

26.3.3 Summary

Imaging and biorecognition systems used in diagnostic techniques rely predominantly on biophotonics, though alternate transduction methods are becoming more prevalent in biorecognition. Both domains mutually benefit from rapid technological advances, fueled by an enormous research focus in the application of nanoparticles for enhanced imaging and DNA recognition techniques. Nanoparticles have been developed to improve contrast and allow imaging of target tissues using conventional medical diagnostic equipment, such as PET, MRI, and x-ray. Fluorescence-based nanoparticle systems are also generating much interest, particularly as nanosensors demonstrate the capability for detecting and quantifying intracellular processes. Greater interest still stems from advances in quantum dots, which have already demonstrated superiority over conventional fluorescent tags, and demonstrate a capacity for *in vivo* live imaging. Such interest is paralleled in biorecognition techniques, where similar particle-based tagging and amplification strategies have vaulted hybridization sensitivity to subfemtomolar levels. These techniques expand medical diagnoses to include abilities to genetically screen for disease susceptibility using microarrays that simultaneously analyse thousands of genes, as well as to detect disease and pathogen presence through DNA fingerprints. Continued development of nanobiotechnology techniques will increase the ease with which such diagnostic routines are performed, ensuring that analytical nanomedicine will prevail in the future of medical diagnostics.

26.4   On the Horizons of Nanomedicine

While the methods discussed represent applied modalities that promise to be implemented within years, the scope of nanobiotechnology encompasses research which, though currently on the very frontiers of modern science, present innumerable possibilities for the future of nanomedicine. The prophesied ability of nanoscale machines, or nanobots, to provide molecular level construction and repair to exterminate disease and erase genetic defects represents the pinnacle of nanomedicine aspirations. Although the inherent difficulties in the design and manufacture of such devices raise questions as to their feasibility [153], research continues to explore nature's nanomachines and issues crucial to the development of nanobots. In cells, proteins are nanomachines that act as transporters, actuators, and motors, and are responsible for meticulous monitoring and repair processes [154,155].

Single molecule analysis can reveal the mechanistic details of protein function, with AFM and FRET imaging being the favored tools in such investigations. FRET imaging allows observation of biomolecular structure and intracellular motion [156,157] while AFM is used to explore molecular forces and energetics, and can be used to manipulate folding and structure [154]. A recently developed imaging technique, scanning near-field optical microscopy (SNOM), offers visual imaging with nanometre resolution, promising further developments in this field. Combining AFM and SNOM advances single molecule analysis by allowing simultaneous nanoscale topographic and fluorescence imaging, making nano-FRET analysis possible [158].

Through analysis of individual molecules, researchers aim to elucidate the principles of biomolecular machinery to understand the mechanisms governing gene activation, DNA repair, and motor proteins such as kinesin and myosin. These biological motors have the capability of precise molecular positioning in the construction of energetically unfavorable structures. Advances in this field could lead to the exploitation of nanomotors for molecular assembly; researchers have already begun to envisage the use of kinesin motors as molecular transporters in nanoscale syntheses [155]. Whether or not these discoveries ultimately contribute to the future development of nanorobots, the wealth of knowledge generated by single molecule analyses will undoubtedly expand the boundaries of treatment and diagnosis in nanomedicine.

26.5 Conclusions

The term "nanomedicine" presently incorporates a vast multitude of techniques that are roughly divisible into categories of therapeutic delivery systems, tissue engineering, and diagnostic imaging and biorecognition. As discoveries in various fields, such as nanofabrication, proteomics, and biophotonics continue, and given the enormous funding presently directed towards nanotechnology by government and private sector investors, this field will undoubtedly proliferate. Ultimately, nanomedicine treatments and diagnostics must bypass or control the host immune response to fulfill their function over a desired timeline. Though many of the treatments currently under development have yet to reach their envisioned performance at a research level, the potential clinical application of such interventions provide sufficient promise to ensure that nanomedicine does represent the future of medical care.

References

[1] National Institutes of Health 2004.
[2] NBTC 2004.
[3] DeFrancesco L. 2003. *Nat. Biotechnol.* 21: 1127.
[4] Kereiaks D.J., Choo J.K., and Young J.J. 2004. *Rev. Cardiovasc. Med.* 5: 9.
[5] Panyam J. and Labhasetwar V. 2003. *Adv. Drug Deliv. Rev.* 55: 329.
[6] Tanabe K., Regar E., Lee C.H. et al. 2004. *Curr. Pharm. Des.* 10: 357.
[7] Thierry B., Winnik F.M., Merhi Y. et al. 2003. *Biomacromolecules* 4: 1564.
[8] Cohen-Sacks H., Najajreh Y., Tchaikovski V. et al. 2002. *Gene Ther.* 9: 1607.
[9] Kolodgie F.D., John M., Khurana C. et al. 2002. *Circulation* 106: 1195.
[10] Tan P.H., Manunta M., Ardjomand N. et al. 2003. *J. Gene Med.* 5: 311.
[11] Baker A.H. 2004. *Prog. Biophys. Mol. Biol.* 84: 279.
[12] Vijayanathan V., Thomas T., and Thomas T.J. 2002. *Biochemistry* 41: 14085.
[13] Cui Z. and Mumper R.J. 2002. *Pharm. Res.* 19: 939.
[14] Ameller T., Marsaud V., Legrand P. et al. 2003. *Int. J. Cancer* 106: 446.
[15] Cui Z. and Mumper R.J. 2002. *Bioconjug. Chem.* 13: 1319.
[16] Dauty E., Behr J.P., and Remy J.S. 2002. *Gene Ther.* 9: 743.
[17] Lindner L.H., Eichhorn M.E., Eibl H. et al. 2004. *Clin. Cancer Res.* 10: 2168.
[18] Dong Y. and Feng S.S. 2004. *Biomaterials* 25: 2843.
[19] Kumar N., Ravikumar M.N., and Domb A.J. 2001. *Adv. Drug Deliv. Rev.* 53: 23.
[20] Rosler A., Vandermeulen G.W., and Klok H.A. 2001. *Adv. Drug Deliv. Rev.* 53: 95.
[21] Nishiyama N., Okazaki S., Cabral H. et al. 2003. *Cancer Res.* 63: 8977.

[22] Kim I.S. and Kim S.H. 2002. *Int. J. Pharm.* 245: 67.

[23] Ibrahim N.K., Desai N., Legha S. et al. 2002. *Clin. Cancer Res.* 8: 1038.

[24] Prabha S., Zhou W.Z., Panyam J. et al. 2002. *Int. J. Pharm.* 244: 105.

[25] Douglas K.D. and Tabrizian M. 2005. *J. Biomater. Sci. Polym. Ed.* 16: 43–56.

[26] Gonzalez F.M., Tillman L., Hardee G. et al. 2002. *Int. J. Pharm.* 239: 47.

[27] Kim T.H., Ihm J.E., Choi Y.J. et al. 2003. *J. Control Release* 93: 389.

[28] Park Y.J., Liang J.F., Ko K.S. et al. 2003. *J. Gene Med.* 5: 700.

[29] Bremner K.H., Seymour L.W., Logan A. et al. 2004. *Bioconjug. Chem.* 15: 152.

[30] Keller M., Harbottle R.P., Perouzel E. et al. 2003. *Chembiochem* 4: 286.

[31] Rejman J., Oberle V., Zuhorn I.S. et al. 2004. *J. Biochem.* 377: 159.

[32] Chesnoy S., Durand D., Doucet J. et al. 2001. *Pharm. Res.* 18: 1480.

[33] Merdan T., Callahan J., Petersen H. et al. 2003. *Bioconjug. Chem.* 14: 989.

[34] Itaka K., Yamauchi K., Harada A. et al. 2003. *Biomaterials* 24: 4495.

[35] Park Y.J., Nah S.H., Lee J.Y. et al. 2003. *J. Biomed. Mater. Res.* 67A: 751.

[36] LaVan D.A., McGuire T., and Langer R. 2003. *Nat. Biotechnol.* 21: 1184.

[37] Murthy N., Xu M., Schuck S. et al. 2003. *Proc. Natl Acad. Sci. USA* 100: 4995.

[38] Kim J.K., Choi S.H., Kim C.O. et al. 2003. *J. Pharm. Pharmacol.* 55: 453.

[39] Tang G.P., Zeng J.M., Gao S.J. et al. 2003. *Biomaterials* 24: 2351.

[40] Na K., Bum L.T., Park K.H. et al. 2003. *Eur. J. Pharm. Sci.* 18: 165.

[41] Quintana A., Raczka E., Piehler L. et al. 2002. *Pharm. Res.* 19: 1310.

[42] Gu H., Ho P.L., Tsang K.W. et al. 2003. *J. Am. Chem. Soc.* 125: 15702.

[43] O'Neal D.P., Hirsch L.R., Halas N.J. et al. 2004. *Cancer Lett.* 209: 171.

[44] West J.L. and Halas N.J. 2003. *Annu. Rev. Biomed. Eng.* 5: 285.

[45] Cui Z. and Mumper R.J. 2003. *Eur. J. Pharm. Biopharm.* 55: 11.

[46] Kim S.Y., Lee Y.M., Baik D.J. et al. 2003. *Biomaterials* 24: 55.

[47] Fonseca C., Simoes S., and Gaspar R. 2002. *J. Control Release* 83: 273.

[48] Fernandez-Lopez S., Kim H.S., Choi E.C. et al. 2001. *Nature* 412: 452.

[49] Lee M., Rentz J., Han S.O. et al. 2003. *Gene Ther.* 10: 585.

[50] Anderson D.G., Lynn D.M., and Langer R. 2003. *Angew. Chem. Int. Ed. Engl.* 42: 3153.

[51] Liu G., Li D., Pasumarthy M.K. et al. 2003. *J. Biol. Chem.* 278: 32578.

[52] Ziady A.G., Gedeon C.R., Miller T. et al. 2003. *Mol. Ther.* 8: 936.

[53] Yang F., Murugan R., Ramakrishna S. et al. 2004. *Biomaterials* 25: 1891.

[54] Matsuda T. 2004. *Artif. Organs* 28: 64.

[55] Ochi M., Adachi N., Nobuto H. et al. 2004. *Artif. Organs* 28: 28.

[56] Sharma B. and Elisseeff J.H. 2004. *Ann. Biomed. Eng.* 32: 148.

[57] Chen V.J. and Ma P.X. 2004. *Biomaterials* 25: 2065.

[58] Prokop A. 2001. *Ann. NY Acad. Sci.* 944: 472.

[59] Dalby M.J., Riehle M.O., Johnstone H.J. et al. 2003. *J. Biomed. Mater. Res.* 67A: 1025.

[60] Woo K.M., Chen V.J., and Ma P.X. 2003. *J. Biomed. Mater. Res.* 67A: 531.

[61] Ratner B.D. 2002. *J. Control Release* 78: 211.

[62] Garrison M.D., McDevitt T.C., Luginbuhl R. et al. 2000. *Ultramicroscopy* 82: 193.

[63] Ratner B.D. 1996. *J. Mol. Recognit.* 9: 617.

[64] Hersel U., Dahmen C., and Kessler H. 2003. *Biomaterials* 24: 4385.

[65] Martin S.M., Ganapathy R., Kim T.K. et al. 2003. *J. Biomed. Mater. Res.* 67A: 334.

[66] Lee K.B., Park S.J., Mirkin C.A. et al. 2002. *Science* 295: 1702.

[67] Blawas A.S. and Reichert W.M. 1998. *Biomaterials* 19: 595.

[68] Lee K.B., Lim J.H., and Mirkin C.A. 2003. *J. Am. Chem. Soc.* 125: 5588.

[69] Cheung C.L., Camarero J.A., Woods B.W. et al. 2003. *J. Am. Chem. Soc.* 125: 6848.

[70] Hyun J., Kim J., Craig S.L. et al. 2004. *J. Am. Chem. Soc.* 126: 4770.

[71] Shi H. and Ratner B.D. 2000. *J. Biomed. Mater. Res.* 49: 1.

[72] Martin S.M., Schwartz J.L., Giachelli C.M. et al. 2004. *J. Biomed. Mater. Res.* 70A: 10.

[73] Plant G.W., Woerly S., and Harvey A.R. 1997. *Exp. Neurol.* 143: 287.

[74] Woerly S., Pinet E., de Robertis L. et al. 2001. *Biomaterials* 22: 1095.

[75] Kantlehner M., Schaffner P., Finsinger D. et al. 2000. *Chembiochem* 1: 107.

[76] Goodman S.L., Sims P.A., and Albrecht R.M. 1996. *Biomaterials* 17: 2087.

[77] Miller D.C., Thapa A., Haberstroh K.M. et al. 2004. *Biomaterials* 25: 53.

[78] Ma P.X. and Zhang R. 1999. *J. Biomed. Mater. Res.* 46: 60.

[79] Boland E.D., Matthews J.A., Pawlowski K.J. et al. 2004. *Front Biosci.* 9: 1422.

[80] Nagaoka S., Ashiba K., and Kawakami H. 2002. *Artif. Organs* 26: 670.

[81] Thapa A., Miller D.C., Webster T.J. et al. 2003. *Biomaterials* 24: 2915.

[82] Dalby M.J., Berry C.C., Riehle M.O. et al. 2004. *Exp. Cell Res.* 295: 387.

[83] Lyuksyutov S.F., Vaia R.A., Paramonov P.B. et al. 2003. *Nat. Mater.* 2: 468.

[84] Guo C., Feng L., Zhai J. et al. 2004. *Chemphyschem* 5: 750.

[85] Price R.L., Haberstroh K.M., and Webster T.J. 2003. *Med. Biol. Eng. Comput.* 41: 372.

[86] Li P. 2003. *J. Biomed. Mater. Res.* 66A: 79.

[87] Flemming R.G., Murphy C.J., Abrams G.A. et al. 1999. *Biomaterials* 20: 573.

[88] Wei G. and Ma P.X. 2004. *Biomaterials* 25: 4749.

[89] Suzuki I., Sugio Y., Moriguchi H. et al. 2004. *J. Nanobiotechnol.* 2: 7.

[90] Nagaoka S., Ashiba K., Okuyama Y. et al. 2003. *Int. J. Artif. Organs* 26: 339.

[91] Sarikaya M., Tamerler C., Jen A.K. et al. 2003. *Nat. Mater.* 2: 577.

[92] Kwok C.S., Mourad P.D., Crum L.A. et al. 2000. *Biomacromolecules* 1: 139.

[93] Smith R.K., Lewis P.A., and Weiss P.S. 2004. *Prog. Surf. Sci.* 75: 1.

[94] Jang C.H., Stevens B.D., Carlier P.R. et al. 2002. *J. Am. Chem. Soc.* 124: 12114.

[95] Zhang S., Marini D.M., Hwang W. et al. 2002. *Curr. Opin. Chem. Biol.* 6: 865.

[96] Zhang S. 2003. *Nat. Biotechnol.* 21: 1171.

[97] Hartgerink J.D., Beniash E., and Stupp S.I. 2001. *Science* 294: 1684.

[98] L'Heureux N., Paquet S., Labbe R. et al. 1998. *FASEB J.* 12: 47.

[99] Remy-Zolghadri M., Laganiere J., Oligny J.F. et al. 2004. *J. Vasc. Surg.* 39: 613.

[100] Saiki R.K., Bugawan T.L., Horn G.T. et al. 1986. *Nature* 324: 163.

[101] Koo Y.E., Cao Y., Kopelman R. et al. 2004. *Anal. Chem.* 76: 2498.

[102] Oku N. 1999. *Adv. Drug Deliv. Rev.* 37: 53.

[103] Kao C.Y., Hoffman E.A., Beck K.C. et al. 2003. *Acad. Radiol.* 10: 475.

[104] Kobayashi H., Kawamoto S., Sakai Y. et al. 2004. *J. Natl Cancer Inst.* 96: 703.

[105] Tsuji A., Sato Y., Hirano M. et al. 2001. *Biophys. J.* 81: 501.

[106] Zhao Y., Sadtler B., Lin M. et al. 2004. *Chem. Commun. (Camb)* 7: 784–5.

[107] Schultz S., Smith D.R., Mock J.J. et al. 2000. *Proc. Natl Acad. Sci. USA* 97: 996.

[108] Aylott J.W. 2003. *Analyst* 128: 309.

[109] Abdalla M.A., Bayer J., Radler J. et al. 2003. *Nucleosides Nucleotides Nucl. Acids* 22: 1399.

[110] Brown J.Q. and McShane M.J. 2003. *IEEE Eng. Med. Biol. Mag.* 22: 118.

[111] Lu J., Rosenzweig Z., and Fresenius J. 2000. *Anal. Chem.* 366: 569.

[112] Xu H., Aylott J.W., and Kopelman R. 2002. *Analyst* 127: 1471.

[113] Chan W.C., Maxwell D.J., Gao X. et al. 2002. *Curr. Opin. Biotechnol.* 13: 40.

[114] Wu X., Liu H., Liu J. et al. 2003. *Nat. Biotechnol.* 21: 41.

[115] Kaul Z., Yaguchi T., Kaul S.C. et al. 2003. *Cell Res.* 13: 503.

[116] Dubertret B., Skourides P., Norris D.J. et al. 2002. *Science* 298: 1759.

[117] Sun B., Xie W., Yi G. et al. 2001. *J. Immunol. Meth.* 249: 85.

[118] Akerman M.E., Chan W.C., Laakkonen P. et al. 2002. *Proc. Natl Acad. Sci. USA* 99: 12617.

[119] Jaiswal J.K., Mattoussi H., Mauro J.M. et al. 2003. *Nat. Biotechnol.* 21: 47.

[120] Larson D.R., Zipfel W.R., Williams R.M. et al. 2003. *Science* 300: 1434.

[121] Han M., Gao X., Su J.Z. et al. 2001. *Nat. Biotechnol.* 19: 631.

[122] Ballou B., Lagerholm B.C., Ernst L.A. et al. 2004. *Bioconjug. Chem.* 15: 79.

[123] Weissleder R., Tung C.H., Mahmood U. et al. 1999. *Nat. Biotechnol.* 17: 375.

[124] Gao X. and Nie S. 2003. *Trends Biotechnol.* 21: 371.

[125] Uslu F., Ingebrandt S., Mayer D. et al. 2004. *Biosens. Bioelectron.* 19: 1723.

[126] Docherty F.T., Clark M., McNay G. et al. 2004. *Faraday Discuss.* 126: 281.

[127] Oldenburg S.J., Genick C.C., Clark K.A. et al. 2002. *Anal. Biochem.* 309: 109.

[128] Maxwell D.J., Taylor J.R., and Nie S. 2002. *J. Am. Chem. Soc.* 124: 9606.

[129] Zhao X., Tapec-Dytioco R., and Tan W. 2003. *J. Am. Chem. Soc.* 125: 11474.

[130] Patolsky F., Lichtenstein A., and Willner I. 2001. *J. Am. Chem. Soc.* 123: 5194.

[131] Liu T., Tang J., Han M. et al. 2003. *Biochem. Biophys. Res. Commun.* 304: 98.

[132] Liu T., Tang J., and Jiang L. 2004. *Biochem. Biophys. Res. Commun.* 313: 3.

[133] Walter G., Bussow K., Lueking A. et al. 2002. *Trends Mol. Med.* 8: 250.

[134] Brynda E., Houska M., Brandenburg A. et al. 2002. *Biosens. Bioelectron.* 17: 665.

[135] Deckert F. and Legay F. 2000. *J. Pharm. Biomed. Anal.* 23: 403.

[136] Liss M., Petersen B., Wolf H. et al. 2002. *Anal. Chem.* 74: 4488.

[137] Zhang J., Su X., and O'Shea S. 2002. *Biophys. Chem.* 99: 31.

[138] Grubor N.M., Shinar R., Jankowiak R. et al. 2004. *Biosens. Bioelectron.* 19: 547.

[139] Washburn M.P. 2003. *Nat. Biotechnol.* 21: 1156.

[140] Bertucci F., Viens P., Hingamp P. et al. 2003. *Int. J. Cancer* 103: 565.

[141] Hao X., Sun B., Hu L. et al. 2004. *Cancer* 100: 1110.

[142] Boldrick J.C., Alizadeh A.A., Diehn M. et al. 2002. *Proc. Natl Acad. Sci. USA* 99: 972.

[143] Nau G.J., Richmond J.F., Schlesinger A. et al. 2002. *Proc. Natl Acad. Sci. USA* 99: 1503.

[144] Grody W.W., Cutting G.R., Klinger K.W. et al. 2001. *Genet. Med.* 3: 149.

[145] Carrigan S.D., Scott G., and Tabrizian M. 2004. *Clin. Chem.* 50: 1301.

[146] Shang S., Chen Z., and Yu X. 2001. *Acta. Paediatr.* 90: 179.

[147] Tarkin I.S., Henry T.J., Fey P.I. et al. 2003. *Clin. Orthop.* 89.

[148] Tirodker U.H., Nataro J.P., Smith S. et al. 2003. *J. Perinatol.* 23: 117.

[149] Gibellini D., Vitone F., Schiavone P. et al. 2004. *J. Clin. Virol.* 29: 282.

[150] Wang Y.F., Pang D.W., Zhang Z.L. et al. 2003. *J. Med. Virol.* 70: 205.

[151] Ye Y.K., Zhao J.H., Yan F. et al. 2003. *Biosens. Bioelectron.* 18: 1501.

[152] Albers J., Grunwald T., Nebling E. et al. 2003. *Anal. Bioanal. Chem.* 377: 521.

[153] Smalley R.E. 2001. *Sci. Am.* 285: 76.

[154] Janicijevic A., Ristic D., and Wyman C. 2003. *J. Microsc.* 212: 264.

[155] Hess H., Bachand G.D., and Vogel V. 2004. *Chemistry* 10: 2110.

[156] Zhuang X. and Rief M. 2003. *Curr. Opin. Struct. Biol.* 13: 88.

[157] Murakoshi H., Iino R., Kobayashi T. et al. 2004. *Proc. Natl Acad. Sci. USA* 101: 7317.

[158] Yoshino T., Sugiyama S., Hagiwara S. et al. 2003. *Ultramicroscopy* 97: 81.

27

Biomedical Nanoengineering for Nanomedicine

Jie Han
NASA Ames Research Center

Nanomedicine is the medical application of nanotechnology in prevention, diagnostics and treatment of diseases. In this handbook, the term "Biomedical Nanoengineering" is used to address the engineering issues in the biomedical applications of nanomaterials and nanodevices. In October 2003, the NIH announced the NanoMedicine Initiative (NMI) [1]. The NMI envisions, for example, the biomedical nanodevices or nanosystems to search out and destroy the very first cancer cells of a tumor developing in the body, the biological nanomachines to remove and replace the cell's broken part, and the molecule-sized pumps to deliver life-saving medicines precisely where they are needed in the human body.

Nanomedicine was mentioned in many early publications. For example, in two books [2,3], the nanomachines were proposed to monitor and repair the damaged cells and the intracellular structures, the nanorobots equipped with wireless transmitters to circulate in the blood and lymph systems and send out warnings when chemical imbalances occur or worsen, and at the extreme, these nanosystems to replicate themselves or correct genetic deficiencies by altering or replacing DNA molecules.

These scenarios may have sounded unbelievable years ago and may sound so even now, but the rapid, tremendous progress in nanotechnology is promising the formation of the nanomedicine through development of the biomedical nanoengineering. For example, nanostructures such as functional nano-particles, dendrimers, fullerenes, carbon nanotubes, and semiconductor nanocrystals including quantum dots have been exploited for drug delivery, diagnostics, and treatment of diseases at molecular level; the assembled nanostructured fibrous scaffolds reminiscent of extracellular matrix have been used for mimic properties of bone; and protein nanotubes based on self-assembly of unique cyclic peptides for novel antibiotics. While most work is still in the laboratory research, some has found applications. For example, nanoparticles have been used in commercial products including drug delivery systems and point of care diagnostics.

Tremendous medical benefits for healthcare from nanotechnology have been repeatedly described in many publications and media reports. Continued nanotechnology research in biomedicine is bringing up as much challenge as opportunities if it is never the less. Nanomedicine is a multidisciplinary field that needs the integrated teamwork and mutual understanding from professionals and public in the areas of medicine, biology, chemistry, physics, materials science, engineering, healthcare, law, and government.

Biomedical nanoengineering is a very broad yet deep multidisciplinary field, and cannot be fully covered in this chapter. This chapter is only to offer a basic understanding of this emerging field for the professionals and public with different backgrounds. It will mainly discuss biologically functional nanomaterials such as dendrimers, single crystal nanoparticles and nanowires, and fullerenes and carbon nanotubes, and their biomedical applications mainly in the prevention, diagnostics, and treatment of diseases.

27.1   Nanomaterials and Nanodevices

The NIH defines nanotechnology as "the creation of functional materials, devices and systems through control of matters at the scale of 1 to 100 nanometers, and exploitation of novel properties and phenomena at the same scale." Nanomaterials can be simply defined to have three features: 1 to 100 nm in one dimension, functional in applications, and producible in manufacturing. They have to be biologically engineered for biomedical applications.

Living systems are built upon from molecular materials or nanostructures such as nucleic acids (DNA and RNA) and protein. They are 2 and 5 to 50 nm wide, respectively. They can be produced from the self-assembly or self-organization processes in the living system itself or by chemical synthesis. DNA or RNA and associated enzymes and proteins or lipids can be self-assembled into 75 to 100 nm wide viruses. They can be further assembled into bacteria. Bacteria are 1 to 10 μm in size, with thin, rubbery cell membrane surrounding the fluid (cytoplasm) and all genetic information needed to make copies of its own DNA. Viruses and bacteria cause many diseases. A white blood cell is about 10 μm big whereas all materials internalized by cells are smaller than 100 nm.

The size domain of nanomaterials is similar to that of the biological structures, as shown in Figure 27.1. For example, a single wall carbon nanotube is as wide as a double strand DNA; dendrimers and nanoparticles can be made similar to the sizes of proteins or viruses; and fullerene may present the smallest molecular nanostructures. These nanostructures have significantly different properties from bulk or microstructures and they are especially suitable for biomedical applications. For example,

- Nanoscale single crystal or ordered structures are stronger; lighter, less corrosive, yet cause less damage to cells or tissues
- High specific surface allows to load the recognition molecules and drugs, enter the cells, and seek out specific nucleic acids and proteins or other molecular marks
- Quantum confinement at nanoscale makes them more electrically conductive, superparamagnetic, and tunable optical emission for control of drug delivery and sensing at intra- and extracellular level through external light, magnetic or electric field
- Electricity or heat generated by external light, magnetic field, or electric field can destroy sick cells locally while leaving neighboring healthy cells intact, etc

The nanomaterials shown in Figure 27.1 are commercially available now. The biological functionalization to load drugs or recognition molecules chemically or physically is the critical step in their biomedical applications. A brief introduction to these nanomaterials and their properties and biomedical application is presented in Figure 27.2.

27.1.1   Fullerenes and Carbon Nanotubes

Fullerenes (C_{60} and C_{70}) were discovered in 1985 by Smalley, Curl, and Kroto, which won the 1997 Nobel Prize in Chemistry [4]. Fullerenes are roughly spherical in shape and approximately 1 nm big.

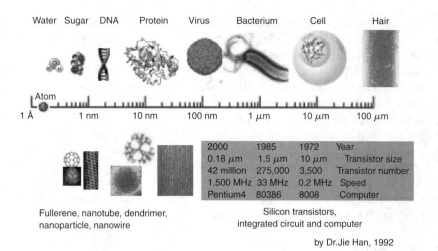

Water Sugar DNA Protein Virus Bacterium Cell Hair

Atom

1 Å   1 nm   10 nm   100 nm   1 μm   10 μm   100 μm

2000	1985	1972	Year
0.18 μm	1.5 μm	10 μm	Transistor size
42 million	275,000	3,500	Transistor number
1,500 MHz	33 MHz	0.2 MHz	Speed
Pentium4	80386	8008	Computer

Fullerene, nanotube, dendrimer,
nanoparticle, nanowire

Silicon transistors,
integrated circuit and computer

by Dr.Jie Han, 1992

FIGURE 27.1   (See color insert following page **20**-14.) Nano and microscale materials, devices, and systems.

Fullerenes, C_{60}, 0.7 nm, functional drug carrier with linked antibodies or other targeting agents on the surface carbon atoms, and implanted medical devices

Dendrimers (5–50 nm), branched structure allows to link labels, probes, and drugs individually for drug carrier, implanted sensors, and medical devices

Nanoparticles (<100 nm, inorganic or organic) for implanted materials, nanoshells, and nanoemulsions for drug delivery; quantum dots (<8 nm) and magnetic nanoparticles for labeling in diagnostics and implanted sensors and medical devices

Carbon nanotubes (1 nm for single wall and 10–100 nm for multi wall), one dimensional Fullerene nanoelectrode arrays for *in vitro*, *in vivo*, and implanted sensors and medical devices; capable for diagnostic handheld systems for multiplexing without need of labeling and PCR

Single crystal nanowires (5–100 nm), one-dimensional nanoparticels (magnetic, electrical, and optical), capable of doing what nanoparticles and carbon nanotubes can do

FIGURE 27.2   (See color insert.) Biologically functional nanomaterials and biomedical applications.

A carbon atom sits at each vertex of a buckyball, bonding with three of its neighbors. The strained sp2 configuration allows to be chemically or biologically modified with small or large molecules for the biomedical applications. Fullerenes are transparent over a wide spectral range extending from the mid-infrared throughout the visible. They possess a high thermal and oxidative stability compared to many other organic materials, and they are extremely resilient and relatively impervious to damage. They do not react with corrosive compounds and are capable of absorbing and releasing electrons without being harmed or without changing. Fullerenes are mainly used for drug delivery and implanted sensing and treatment devices. They allow active pharmacopheres to be grafted to its surface in three-dimensional orientations for precise control in matching biological targets, in entrapping atoms within the fullerene cage, and for attaching fullerene derivatives to targeting agents.

Carbon nanotubes (CNT) are one-dimensional fullerenes with a cylinder shape, discovered by Sumio Iijima in 1992 [4]. These cylinders can be closed or open in the ends, having single or multiple walls, can be metallic or semiconducting, tens of nanometers to tens of micrometers long. They are about 1 nm wide for single wall structures and 5 to 100 nm wide for multiwall structures. While retaining the properties of the fullerenes, the one-dimensional extension and the quantum confinement in the circumference make nanotubes intrinsically high electrical and thermal conductive, mechanically strong, but very gentle to biological structures. Therefore, carbon nanotubes can be made stand-alone functional devices such as probe tips for biological images and chemical force detection, and vertically aligned nanoelectrode arrays for diagnostics and implanted medical sensing and treatment devices. The chemical functionalization is relatively easier in the open end than in the sidewall or closed ends.

27.1.2 Dendrimer

Dendrimer, discovered by Don Tomalia in 1992 [5], is precisely constructed molecules built on the nanoscale in a multistep process through up to ten generations (5 to 50 nm). Each step doubles the complexity at the branching end. Drugs and recognition molecules can be attached to their ends or placed inside cavities within them. Dendrimers are versatile, with discrete numbers and high local densities of surface functionalities in one molecule, very attractive for biomedical applications, especially in cancer therapy. The dendritic multifunctional platform is ideal to combine various functions like imaging, targeting, and drug transfer into cell.

27.1.2.1 Nanoparticles and Nanowires

Nanoparticles might be the earliest nanomaterials [6,7]. Their research and applications started at least two decade ago. They can be made of almost all known materials whereas the biomedical applications have been mainly highlighted for organic and several types of inorganic nanoparticles.

- Polymer nanoparticles have been widely used for drug delivery and implantable materials. They can be made into nanoshells for drug encapsulation, and hydrophilic and hydrophobic for the expected biocompatibility. Their diameter ranges from 10 to 100 nm. The first nanoparticles were reported in 1976 with protein molecules entrapped inside 80 nm hydrophilic polymers.
- Magnetic nanoparticles can be made from most of the bulk magnetic materials such as cobalt, iron, and nickle, and their alloys, ferrite, nitride, or oxide, etc. The superparamagnetic properties of smaller nanoparticles (<10 nm) can provide control for drug delivery, implanted sensing, and heating treatment to destroy sick cells through external electromagnetic field.
- Quantum dot nanoparticles can be made of the semiconductors and metals when the particle size is less than 8 nm. They are capable of confining a single electron, or a few, and in which the electrons occupy discrete energy states just as they would in an atom (quantum dots have been called artificial atoms). These particles show optical gain and stimulated emission at room temperature. They are suitable for biological markers, drug delivery, and implanted sensing and heating devices through external lighting.

27.1.2.1.1 Single crystal nanowires

Single crystal nanowires (SNW) are one-dimensional single crystal nanoparticles like fullerenes vs. carbon nanotubes. While retaining the properties of nanoparticles, SNW have been made into functional devices such as transistors, nanoelectrode arrays, and probes for biological sensing. Depending on the materials type and diameter, SWN and devices can be made electrically, optically, or magnetically functional.

Nanomaterials and nanodevices can be fabricated basically using two approaches. Bottom-up approach builds up devices or systems from atoms or molecules through chemical synthesis, self-assembly, or self-organization processes. This has been a natural way in life science to build up viruses, bacteria, cells, and living systems from molecular materials such as DNA and proteins. Top-down approach works from bulky materials through machining, etching, and lithography processes. There has been a drive in semiconductor industry to make faster and more powerful computers by scaling down silicon transistor devices from 10 μm in 1972 to about 0.1 μm or 90 nm in 2004, as shown in Figure 27.1. In this chapter, we mainly discuss the bottom-up nanomaterials and nanodevices.

The scaling in top-down approaches is reaching the limit or so-called 100 nm barriers beyond which the previous working principle and optical lithography may no longer work or may work at an extremely high cost. On the other hand, the 100 nm is also a scale boundary in biotechnology and medicine between cellular or larger scale and molecular scale (DNA and protein level). Thus we can understand why nanotechnology defines the scale below 100 nm.

The impact of the semiconductor technology is felt far beyond laptop and desktop computers, account for personal electronics, telecommunications, medical devices, automotive, almost every aspect of our daily life, all reaping healthy benefits from the increasing power of semiconductor chips. It has enabled the Micro-Electrical-Mechanical-Systems (MEMS), microfluidics, DNA microarrays or gene chips, protein chips, and all kinds of micromedical devices. These technologies will be further brought down to nanoscale by using the bottom-up biologically functional nanomaterials.

Nanomaterials offer many unique, novel features in biomedical applications, which other scale materials and technologies may not reach. For example,

Intracellular delivery capability: The size of virus, bacterium, and cell is about approximately 100 nm, 1 and 10 μm or larger, respectively (which, interestingly, corresponds to the feature size of transistors in 2003, 1985, and 1972) as shown in Figure 27.1. The biologically functional nanostructures with the size of less than 100 nm can enter cells and the organelles inside them to interact with DNA and proteins or stick on the surface of specific cells or organelles. This enables earliest prevention and treatment of diseases. For example, detection of cancer at early stages is a critical step in improving cancer treatment. Currently, detection and diagnosis of cancer usually depend on changes in cells and tissues that are detected by a doctor's physical touch or imaging expertise. In many cases, it was too late to treat when it was diagnosed at microscale cellular or larger image scale level. The best way is to detect the earliest molecular changes, long before a physical exam or imaging technology is effective or even tumor is formed.

PCR- and label-free detection capability: Nanomaterials can readily be chemically attached with specific probes such as cDNA and antibody, which can seek out specific target DNA, RNA, or proteins for diagnostics and treatment. For example, a specific tag can be attached onto the nanotube ends to look for the specific mutations that are responsible for the diseases of interest. Nanoparticles or dendrimers can be attached with cDNA for gene expression analysis.Conventionally, gene expression analysis or mutation detection has to the carried out after or during the tedious sample amplification and optical labeling. However, the utilization of nanodevices as biosensor can get rid of these tedious laboratory steps for the sample preparations. For example, the carbon nanotube electrodes attached with DNA probes have been developed for label- and PCR-free detection for DNA samples.

Drug- and surgery-free intracellular treatment capability: The detection or diagnosis is carried out with optical, magnetic, and electrical response of the nanodevices to the interaction or binding. In addition, the treatment can also be carried out using the magnetic, optical, or electrical properties of nanostructures. For example, heat generated by the light absorbing, electrical thermal emission, and magnetic thermal generation can kill tumors cells while leaving neighboring cells intact.

In the following section, we will briefly introduce the biomedical applications associated with these unique features.

27.2 Biomedical Applications

Biomedical applications of nanotechnology or nanomedicine have been reviewed by the nanotechnology alliance in Canada [8] and classified into the following category, as summarized in Table 27.1. In this

TABLE 27.1   Nanomedicine Taxonomy

Biopharmaceutics
Drug delivery
    Drug encapsulation
    Functional drug carriers
Drug discovery

Implantable materials
Tissue repair and replacement
    Implant coatings
    Tissue regeneration scaffolds

Structural implant materials
Bone repair
Bioresorbable materials
Smart materials

Implantable devices
Assessment and treatment devices
    Implantable sensors
    Implantable medical devices
Sensory aids
    Retina implants
    Cochlear implants

Surgical aids
Operating tools
    Smart instruments
    Surgical robots

Diagnostic tools
Genetic testing
    Ultrasensitive labeling and detection technologies
    High throughput arrays and multiple analyses
Imaging
    Nanoparticle labels
    Imaging devices

chapter, we will only briefly introduce some of the applications listed in Table 27.1, which we believe will illustrate the unique features of nanomaterials and nanodevices in biomedical applications that conventional technologies may not reach. In addition, we will discuss these applications based on the prevention, diagnostics, and treatment of diseases. The nanomedicine and biomedical nanoengineering are only emerging, much information has been only appearing in the conferences, and not much from referred journals. Therefore, the references in this chapter are mainly from the Internet and Reference 8.

27.2.1 Prevention

The best health care or medicine is the preventive medicine. Common diseases to many people include diverticuiitis, kidney failure, dialysis, gallstones, diabetes, osteoporosis, hypertension, coronary artery disease, stroke, aging, and numerous cancers. Virtually all our major diseases are associated with the consumption of (1) smoke and pollutants through the respiratory system, (2) alcohol, colas, and caffeine, and (3) an abundance of fats, animal proteins, and sweets, and the neglect of exercise. In addition to air cleaning, exercise, and vegetarian program, nutritional approaches for personal care including skincare will be the best for multiple diseases prevention. Although it has not been greatly addressed in publications, the author believes that nanomaterials are promising the most effective preventive medicines. This is because of the intracellular delivery features of the nanomaterials.

Infection control is very important in the prevention of diseases. Conventional disinfectants for infection control have not been safe enough in applications. Nanoengineered delivery system technology is now offering a solution. For example, scientists at the University of Michigan and EnviroSystems, Inc. located in northern California have independently demonstrated safe and effective use of nanoemulsions as antimicrobial solutions. Nanoemulsions, which are suspensions of nanoparticles in water, have the emergent property of killing bacteria and inactivating enveloped viruses. EnviroSystems developed a nanoemulsion as a targeted delivery device for the biocide PCMX. This PCMX-loaded nanoemulsion has a broad spectrum of activity against bacteria including TB, both enveloped and nonenveloped viruses, and fungi. Because the nanoemulsion is targeted, it has no toxicity to higher animal cells. Other respective benefits of the new nanoemulsion disinfectants are contributions to institutional productivity. For example, because nanoemulsion disinfectants are not considered hazardous materials, they do not require any special compliance with the Occupational Safety and Health Administration (OSHA), the EPA, or local water systems. Many of the widely used disinfectants have been implicated in occupational dermatitis and respiratory illness. A reduction in the hazardous waste stream also contributes to a healthier local environment.

Another example of application in the marketplace is skincare products using nanoparticles [11]. Nanoparticles encapsulating different agents of cosmetic and pharmaceutical interest have been developed for novel skincare applications. The nanoparticles were found to show unique additional physical properties and offer new application possibilities that conventional technology cannot reach. The nanoparticles were also found to be very stable and have a high affinity to the stratum corneum. In addition, nanoparticle delivery systems have been developed to target the vesicles to hair and for that purpose they have dotted the nanoparticle shell with cationic molecules thus producing a positively charged surface.

Nanoparticles in skincare products include various types of delivery systems and can be subdivided on the basis of the encapsulating membrane structure into liposomes, nanoemulsions, nanosomes, and nanotopes. They can carry many actives to penetrate into skin quickly and into intracellular structures while conventional skincare products usually do not penetrate the skin and release the active by diffusion or by capsule destruction. Nanoparticles also bring up many other new applications. For example, skin whitening or lightening is a more recent application in which actives carried by nanoparticles penetrate beyond the skin barrier, and more active reaches the necessary site of action in the skin, resulting in improved performance.

In addition to novel drug delivery systems, biomedical nanoengineering also offers new approaches for the earlier detection of diseases or pathogens. This is also very important for the purpose of screening or diagnostics testing in the preventive medicine as well as treatment, as introduced below.

27.2.2 Diagnostics

Nanoparticles especially gold nanoparticles have been used for diagnostics applications. For example, Quantum Dot Corp. uses quantum dots to detect biological material [11]. Because their color can be tailored by changing the size of the dot, the potential for multiple colors increases the number of biological molecules that can be tracked simultaneously. In addition, quantum dots do not fade when exposed to ultraviolet light and the stability of their fluorescence allows longer periods of observation. These technologies are expected to be more sensitive than fluorescent dyes and could more effectively detect low abundance and low-level expressioning genes. They may also make use of smaller and less expensive equipment to light and detect the samples. Without the need for gene amplification, they can also provide results in less time.

In addition to optical detection approaches, new effort has been made in electrical detection. Chad Mirkin and Nanosphere Company [12] use gold nanoparticle probes coated with a string of nucleotides that complement one end of a target sequence in the sample. Another set of nucleotides, complementing the other end, is attached to a surface between two electrodes. If the target sequence is present, it anchors the nanoprobes to the surface like little balloons, and when treated with a silver solution, they create a bridge between the electrodes and produce a current. Nanotechnology group at NASA Ames Research Center has developed carbon nanotube electrodes with attached DNA probes for DNA diagnostics applications [13]. They claim their technology can detect 1000 DNA molecules and therefore does not need the sample amplification methods such as PCR. In addition, they use nanoelectrodes for guanine oxidation in the DNA sample and therefore do not need any sample labeling.

Nanomaterials also offer new biomedical imaging that provides high quality not possible with current technologies, along with new methods of treatment. Researchers at the University of Michigan [14] are developing magnetic nanoparticles attached to a cancer antibody and a dye that is highly visible on an MRI. When these nanoparticles latch onto cancer cells, the cancer cells will be detected on the MRI and then destroyed by laser or low dosage killing agents that attack only the diseased cells. Another group at Washington University [15] is using nanoparticles to attract to proteins emitted from newly forming capillaries that deliver blood to solid tumors. The nanoparticles circulate through the bloodstream and attach to blood vessels containing their complementary protein. Once attached, chemotherapy is released into the capillary membrane. The nanoparticles traveling in the bloodstream would be able to locate additional cancer sites that may have spread to other parts of the body.

Miniature wireless nanodevices are being developed for providing high quality images not possible with traditional devices. Given Imaging has developed a pill containing a miniature video system. When the pill is swallowed, it moves through the digestive system and takes pictures every few seconds. The entire digestive system can be assessed for tumors, bleeding, and diseases in areas not accessible with colonoscopies and endoscopies. A company, MediRad is trying to develop a miniature x-ray device that can be inserted into the body. They are attempting to make carbon nanotubes into a needle shaped cathode. The cathode would generate electron emissions to create extremely small x-ray doses directly at a target area without damaging surrounding normal tissue.

Implantable or wearable nanosensors are being developed for providing continuous and extremely accurate medical information, incorporated with complementary microprocessors to diagnose disease, transmit information, and administer treatment automatically if required. For examples, researchers at Texas A&M and Penn State use polyethylene glycol beads coated with fluorescent molecules to monitor diabetes blood sugar levels. The beads are injected under the skin and stay in the interstitial fluid. When glucose in the interstitial fluid drops to dangerous levels, glucose displaces the fluorescent molecules and creates a glow. This glow is seen on a tattoo placed on the arm.

Researchers at the University of Michigan [16] are using dendrimers attached with fluorescent tags to sense premalignant and cancerous changes inside living cells. The dendrimers are administered trans-dermally and pass through membranes into white blood cells to detect early signs of biochemical changes from radiation or infection. Radiation changes the flow of calcium ions within the white blood cells and eventually triggers apoptosis, or programmed cell death (PCD) due to the radiation or infection. The fluorescent tags attached to the dendrimers will glow in the presence of the death cells when passed through a retinal scanning device using a laser capable of detecting the fluorescence.

27.2.3 Treatment

Biomedical nanoengineering is showing great potentials in drug delivery nanosystems and biomedical nanodevices for safe and effective treatment.

For example, Advectus Life Sciences is developing a nanoparticle-based drug delivery system for the treatment of brain tumors. The antitumor drug doxorubicin is adhered to a Poly ButylCyano Acrylate (PBCA) nanoparticle and coated with polysorbate 80. The drug is injected intravenously and circulates through the blood stream. The polysorbate 80 attracts plasma apolipoproteins and is used by the blood stream to carry lipids. This is to create a camouflage effect similar to LDL cholesterol, allowing the drug to pass the blood–brain barrier. Neurotech company is developing a nanoencapsulated cell therapy to treat eye diseases. It uses a semipermeable membrane to encapsulate cells, which also permits therapeutic agents produced by the cells to diffuse through the membrane. The membrane isolates the cells from the local environment and minimizes immune rejection. The encapsulated cells are administered by a device implanted in the eye to permit the continuous release of therapeutic molecules from living cells. This avoids direct injections into the eye, which may not be practical for regular administrations.

C Sixty [17] is developing fullerene-based drug delivery platforms, which link fullerenes with antibodies and other targeting agents. Their drug delivery systems include fullerene-decorated chemotherapeutic constructs, fullerene-radiopharmaceuticals, and fullerene-based liposome systems for the delivery of single drug loads or multiple drug cocktails. Employing rational drug design, C Sixty has produced several drug candidates using its fullerene platform technology in the areas of HIV/AIDS, neuro-degenerative disorders, and cancer. Nanospectra Company is developing an interesting drug delivery nanosystem in which a gold exterior layer covers interior layers of silica and drugs. This nanoshell structure can be made to absorb light energy and then convert it to heat. As a result, when nanoshells are placed next to a target area such as tumor cell, they can release tumor-specific antibodies when infrared light is administered.

Perhaps the most exciting biomedical nanoengineering research is implantable nanodevices that can integrate sensing, monitoring, and treatment functionalities together. For example, researchers at Aalborg University in Denmark are applying nanostructures to the electrode surfaces to improve biocompatibility and acceptance in the neural/muscle tissue. When placed within a cell membrane, the nanostructures form a bioelectric interface with the neuron or muscle cell that enables the intracellular potential of the cell to be observed and manipulated. They are further using nanostructures to activate denervated muscles caused by injuries to the lower motor neurons located in the spinal cord. This can result from traumatic spinal cord injury, strokes in the spinal cord, repeated vertebral subluxation, brachial plexus injuries, and peripheral myopathies such as polio, which destroys the nerve cells controlling muscle (i.e., denervated muscle). Similar nanodevices can be also used to restore lost vision and hearing functions. The devices collect and transform data into precise electrical signals that are delivered directly to the human nervous system. Degenerative diseases of the retina, such as retinitis pigmentosa or age related macular degeneration, decrease night vision and can progress to diminishing peripheral vision and blindness. These retinal diseases may lead to blindness due to a progressive loss of photoreceptors (rods and cones), the light sensitive cells of the eye.

Retinal implants are being developed to restore vision by electrically stimulating functional neurons in the retina. One approach being developed by various groups including a project at Argonne National Laboratory is an artificial retina implanted in the back of the retina. The artificial retina uses a miniature video camera attached to a blind person's eyeglasses to capture visual signals. The signals are processed by a microcomputer worn on the belt and transmitted to an array of electrodes placed in the eye. The array stimulates optical nerves, which then carry a signal to the brain. Optobionics Company makes use of a subretinal implant designed to replace photoreceptors in the retina. The visual system is activated when the membrane potential of overlying neurons is altered by current generated by the implant in response to light stimulation. The implant makes use of a microelectrode array powered by as many as 3500 microscopic solar cells.

A new generation of smaller and more powerful cochlear implants is intended to be more precise and offer greater sound quality. An implanted transducer is pressure-fitted onto the incus bone in the inner ear. The transducer causes the bones to vibrate and move the fluid in the inner ear, which stimulates the auditory nerve. An array at the tip of the device makes use of up to 128 electrodes, which is five times higher than current devices. The higher number of electrodes provides more precision about where and how nerve fibers are stimulated. This can simulate a fuller range of sounds. The implant is connected to a small microprocessor and a microphone, which are built into a wearable device that clips behind the ear. This captures and translates sounds into electric pulses which are sent down a connecting wire through a tiny hole made in the middle ear. Implant electrodes are continuously decreasing in size and in time could enter the nanoscale. The nanotechnology group at NASA Ames Research Center is developing the carbon nanotube electrode arrays for this purpose [13].

27.3 Conclusion

Biomedical nanoengineering is an offshoot of biomedical engineering at nanoscale. It will be further defined, as the engineering issues at nanoscale in a biological system are being addressed during the application, research, and practice of nanotechnology to biomedicine. This chapter is intended for researchers to pay attention to many engineering issues in nanomedicine research.

For example, many engineering issues have not been addressed. They include fluid mechanics, diffusions, interactions, and self-assembling of nanomaterials and nanodevices in inter- and intracellular structures. Others to be studied include the characterization for the exact quantities and variations, location, timescales, interactions, affinities, force generation, flexibility, and internal motion of the nanomaterials and nanodevices. These engineering studies will help identify and define the design principles and operational parameters of nanodevices.

Biocomaptibility is another important issue to be addressed. The electrically, magnetically functional carbon nanotubes, inorganic nanoparticles and nanowires present the most existing nanomaterials, but may suffer from the poor biocompatibility. If so, can these materials be modified while retaining the expected properties or new nanomaterials be developed to be used *in vivo*?

It surely takes great effort and time to answer these and many other questions for nanomedicine practice. NIH Roadmap's Nanomedicine initiative anticipates Nanomedicine will yield medical benefits as early as 10 years from now.

References

[1] "NIH Nanomedicine Overview," http://nihroadmap.nih.gov/nanomedicine/index.asp

[2] "*Unbounding the Future — Nanotechnology Revolution*," Drexler and Peterson, William Morrow and Company, 1991.

[3] "*Nanomedicine*," Freitas Jr., Landes Bioscience, 1999.

[4] "*The Science of Fullerenes and Carbon Nanotubes*," M.S. Dresselhaus, G. Dresselhaus, and P. Eklund (Eds.), Academic (1996).

[5] "*Dendrimers III: Design, Dimension, Function Series : Topics in Current Chemistry*," Vol. 212, Vögtle, Fritz (Ed.), 2001.

[6] "*Nanoparticles: from Theory to Practice*" Gunter Smidt, John Wiley & Sons, 2004.

[7] "*Nanowires and Nanobelts: Materials, Properties and Devices*," Zhong-lin Wang (Ed.), Springer, 2004.

[8] "*Nanomedicine Taxonomy*," http://www.regenerativemedicine.ca/nanomed/Nanomedicine%20Taxonomy%20(Feb%202003).PDF

[9] "*Nanotechnology Enters Infection Control*," http://www.infectioncontroltoday.com/articles/391feat3.html

[10] "*Preparation & Properties of Small Nanoparticles for Skin and Hair Care*," F. Zuelli and F. Suter of Mibelle AG — Biochemistry (*SOEFW J.* 123, 1997, 880–885).

[11] Quantum Dots, http://www.qdots.com/new/corporate/team.html

[12] Chad Mirkin Northwestern, http://www.chem.nwu.edu/~mkngrp/pictmenu.html

[13] NASA Ames Center for Nanotechnology, http://www.ipt.arc.nasa.gov

[14] Martin Philbert U Michigan, http://www.sph.umich.edu/faculty/philbert.html

[15] Buddy Ratner U Washington, http://www.avs.org/dls/ratner.html

[16] James Baker U Michigan, http://nano.med.umich.edu/Personnel.html#Baker

[17] Uri Sagman C Sixty, http://www.asapsites.com/asap/db/tss/home.nsf/pages/s14-sagman

28

Physiogenomics: Integrating Systems Engineering and Nanotechnology for Personalized Medicine

Gualberto Ruaño
Andreas Windemuth
Genomas, Inc.

Theodore R. Holford
Yale University School of Medicine

28.1 Physiogenomics and Nanotechnology

28.1.1 Introduction

A revolution in our understanding of human health and disease has been launched by the sequencing of a prototypical human genome. To a large degree, this achievement represents the pinnacle of reductionist scientific thought, as having all genes dissected one could in principle allow reconstitution of the organism. In contrast, the classical discipline of physiology has been dealing with systems from its very outset. Although clinically extraordinarily relevant, physiology remained an engineering embodiment of scientific thought distant from the molecular basis of function. Physiogenomics bridges the gap between the systems approach and the reductionist approach by using human variability in physiological process, either in health or disease, to drive their understanding at the genome level. Physiogenomics is particularly relevant to the phenotypes of complex diseases and the clustering of phenotypes into domains according to measurement technique, ranging from functional imaging and clinical scales to protein serology and gene expression.

Nanotechnology probes can serve as ultrasensitive reporters of dynamic cellular phenomena and protein interactions, allowing precise physiological phenotypes to be coupled to genomics, the new discipline of physiogenomics. Nanotechnologies allow delivery of nutrients, supplements, and growth factors in localized and compartmentalized cellular environments. Nanotechnology allows veering into cellular function with materials and constructs of the same scale as biological organelles and even macromolecules. With the level of specificity and individualization achievable with nanotechnology, the emerging paradigm is "genomically guided nanotechnology." The coupling of physiogenomics and nanotechnology provides key underpinnings to personalized health preservation as well as disease management and treatment [Ruano, 2004].

Although single gene effects are the basis of "genetic diseases," partial penetrance is the rule in common clinical care. The pathways of physiology in personalized medicine are multigenetic, as they rely on networks of genes and not on single receptors and enzymes. With the advent of gene nanotechnology-based arrays, parallel processing of gene variability is practically possible at the level of physiological systems.

The concept of "average response" and "deviation from the mean" are ingrained in biomedical science. Learning from variability in response, and translating that into predictive diagnostics for personalized medicine is the challenge confronting physiogenomics and nanotechnology. Positioning each individual along a continuum of response to environmental inputs is the goal of array technology. There is a major need to couple the engineering advances in highly parallel genomic screens with statistical tools to derive valid information from pattern recognizing algorithms. The practical consequence is that by learning from variability, and not depending on means and standard deviations, we can expect reduced sample sizes in clinical studies, and most importantly the ability to discover the markers and implement them in practice for prototyping and clinical validation. In this chapter, we introduce physiogenomics theory and application through nanotechnology capabilities for the understanding of disease etiology and treatment and for the advancement of personalized medicine.

28.1.2 Fundamentals of Physiogenomics

Physiogenomics utilizes an integrated approach composed of genotypes and phenotypes and a population approach deriving signals from functional variability among individuals. In physiogenomics, genotype markers of gene variation or "alleles" (single nucleotide polymorphisms [SNPs], haplotypes, insertions/deletions) are analyzed to discover statistical associations to physiological characteristics (phenotypes). The phenotypes are measured in populations of individuals either at baseline or after they have been similarly exposed or challenged to environmental triggers. These environmental interactions span the gamut from exercise and diet to drugs and toxins, and from extremes of temperature, pressure, and altitude to radiation. In the case of complex diseases we are likely to find both baseline characteristics and response phenotypes to as yet undetermined environmental triggers. Variability in a genomic marker among individuals that tracks with the variability in physiological characteristics establishes associations and mechanistic links with specific genes (Figure 28.1).

Physiogenomics integrates the engineering systems approach with molecular probes stemming from genomic markers available from nanotechnologies that have altered the face of life sciences research. Physiogenomics is a biomedical application of sensitivity analysis, an engineering discipline concerned with how variation in the input of a system leads to changes in output quantities [Saltelli et al., 2000]. Physiogenomics marks the entry of genomics into systems biology, and requires novel analytical platforms to integrate the data and derive the most robust associations. Once physiological systems are under scrutiny, the industrial tools of high-throughput genomics do not suffice, as fundamental

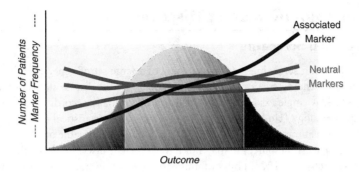

FIGURE 28.1 (See color insert following page 20-14.) Physiogenomic analysis of gene marker frequency as a function of phenotype variability. An associated gene marker is one whose frequency in the cohort tracks with the variability in physiological responses. A neutral marker is one whose frequency is unchanged along the spectrum of response in the cohort.

processes such as signal amplification, functional reserve, and feedback loops of homeostasis must be incorporated. Physiogenomics comprises marker discovery and model building. We will describe each of these interrelated components in a generalized fashion.

28.1.3 Physiotype Models

We term the diagnostic models derived from physiogenomic diagnostics as "physiotypes." Physiotypes have several unique features. Physiotypes are predictive models incorporating genotypes from various genes and any covariates (e.g., baseline levels). Physiotypes are thus multigenetic in nature, and also include clinical information routinely gathered in medical care. Physiotypes harness the combined power of genotypes ("nature") and phenotypes ("nurture") to predict drug responses and the responses to other environmental challenges. Physiotypes are multimodular, and each individual module is derived from whether a significant association is found by univariate testing of the respective end point. The overall operational features of physiotypes are specificity and sensitivity each of 80% or more. While each component has individual characteristics, physiotypes reflect combined features of the various modules. Physiotypes provide answers to clinical management questions with high reliability and impact and can be used to address issues such as the risk of side effects from a medication.

Various specific genetic features of physiotypes are attractive for studying environmental interactions in prevention and treatment of disease. The genotype component does not change and is not confounded with environment. Some genotypes associated with a phenotype can become a surrogate marker for the actual measurement of the phenotype. This capability may be particularly useful when measurement of the phenotype is difficult, expensive, or confounded by environmental conditions. Most importantly, genotyping technologies are rapidly decreasing in cost and are becoming increasingly automated. To this end, multiple genotypes from different genes coding for proteins in interacting pathways allow sampling the genetic variability in entire physiological networks quite economically.

Physiogenomics requires the highly multiplexed parallel processing capabilities available from nanotechnology. At Genomas we have employed automated, high-throughput genotype analysis with state-of-the-art fiber optic systems [Gunderson et al., 2004]. The genotyping analysis has an initial capacity of 300,000 SNPs per day and a multiplexing capability of 1,500 SNPs from each genomic DNA sample. Our approach is to analyze each gene for variation at the SNP and haplotype level [Stephens et al., 2001]. SNPs are available in the public domain from the National Center for Biotechnology Information (http://www.ncbi.nlm.nih.gov/SNP), and most have been confirmed for physical location in the chromosome locus of the gene, and validated as highly heterozygous in various populations by the International Haplotype Map Consortium [2003]. Genomas also has access to Illumina's "SNP Knowledge Resource," a large, rapidly expanding SNP database of currently more than 1,000,000 high-confidence, mapped, and annotated SNP markers.

28.2 Physiogenomic Marker Discovery

28.2.1 Association Screening

The purpose in association screening is to identify any of a large set of genetic markers (SNPs, haplo-types) and physiological characteristics that have an influence on the disease status of the patient, or the progression to disease. A single association test will proceed initially according to accepted multivariate methods in epidemiology [Holford, 2002]. The objective of the statistical analysis is to find a set of physiogenomic factors that together provide a way of predicting the outcome of interest. The association of an individual factor with the outcome may not have sufficient discrimination ability to provide the necessary sensitivity and specificity, but by combining the effect of several such factors this objective may be achieved.

The purpose of the analysis at first is to identify significant covariates among demographic data and the other phenotypes and delineate correlated phenotypes by principal component analysis. Covariates are determined by generating a covariance matrix for all markers and selecting each significantly correlated markers for use as a covariate in the association test of each marker. Serological markers and baseline outcomes are tested using linear regression.

Next in the analysis is performing unadjusted association tests between genotypes and linear regression for serum levels and baselines. Tests will be performed on each marker, and markers that clear a significance threshold of $p < .05$ are selected for permutation testing.

28.2.2 Physiogenomic Control and Negative Results

Each gene not associated with a particular outcome effectively serves as a negative control, and demonstrates neutral segregation of nonrelated markers. The negative controls altogether constitute a "genomic control" for the positive associations where segregation of alleles tracks segregation of outcomes by requiring the representation of the least common allele for each gene to be at least 5% of the population, one can ascertain associations clearly driven by statistical outliers. Negative results are particularly useful in physiogenomics since one can still gain mechanistic understanding of complex systems from those, especially for sorting out the influences of the various candidate genes among the various phenotypes.

28.3 Physiogenomic Modeling

28.3.1 Model Building

Once the associated markers have been determined, a model is built for the dependence of response on the markers. In phase I, linear regression models will be used of the following form:

$$R = R_0 + \sum_i \alpha_i M_i + \sum_j \beta_j D_j + \varepsilon$$

where R is the respective phenotype variable, M_i are the marker variables, D_j are demographic covariates, and ε is the residual unexplained variation. The model parameters that are to be estimated from the data are R_0, α_i, and β_j.

The association between each physiogenomic factor and the outcome is calculated using a regression model, controlling for the other factors that have been found to be relevant. The magnitude of these associations is measured with the odds ratio and statistical significance of these associations will be determined by constructing 95% confidence intervals. Multivariate analyses include all factors that have been found to be important based on univariate analyses.

28.3.2 Overall Rationale

The objective of these analyses is to search for genetic markers that modify the effect produced by a particular type of intervention, which epidemiologists refer to as an effect modifier. These markers are parameterized in our models as gene-intervention interactions. For example, if M_i is a 0 or 1 indicator of the presence of at least one recessive allele of gene i, and X_j represents the level of intervention, then the entire contribution to the outcome is given by the contribution of not only the gene and intervention main effects, but their interaction, as well, that is, $M_i\alpha_i + X_j\beta_j + M_iX_j(\alpha\beta)_{ij}$. Under this model, when the allele is absent ($M_i = 0$), the effect of a unit change in the intervention is described by the slope, β_j, but when the allele is present ($M_i = 1$), the effect of a unit change in the intervention is $\beta_j + (\alpha\beta)_{ij}$. Thus, the gene-intervention interaction parameter, $(\alpha\beta)_{ij}$, represents the difference in the effect of the intervention seen when the allele is present.

In the usual modeling framework, the response is assumed to be a continuous variable in which the error distribution is normal with mean 0 and a constant variance. However, it is not uncommon for the outcomes to have an alternative distribution that may be skewed, such as the gamma, or it may even be categorical. In these circumstances, we will make use of a generalized linear model, which includes a component of the model that is linear, referred to as the linear predictor, thus enabling us to still consider the concept of a gene-intervention interaction, as described earlier. The advantage of this broader framework is that it allows for considerable flexibility in formulating the model through the specification of the link function that describes the relationship between the mean and the linear predictor, and it also provides considerable flexibility in the specification of the error distribution, as well [McCullagh and Nelder, 1989]. The S-Plus statistical software provides functions that calculate the maximum likelihood estimates of the model parameters.

To this point, we have described an analysis in which the effect of the intervention is assumed to be linear, but in practice the effect may not take place until a threshold is past, or it may even change directions. Thus, an important component of our exploration of the intervention effect on a particular response will involve the form for the relationship. In this case we will make use of generalized additive models (GAMs) [Hastie and Tibshirani, 1986]. In GAMs the contribution of the marker and intervention is given by $M_i\alpha_i + \beta(X_j) + M_i\beta_\alpha(X_j)$. In this case, the effect when the allele is absent ($M_i = 0$) is $\beta(X_j)$ which is an unspecified function of the level of the intervention. In subject in which the allele is present ($M_i = 1$), the effect is given by the function $\beta(X_j) + M_i\beta_\alpha(X_j)$. In practice, we can estimate these functions through the use of cubic regression splines [Durlemann and Simon, 1989].

Predictive models may be sought by starting out with a hypothesis (which may be the null model of no marker dependence) and then adding each one out of a specified set of markers to the model in turn. The marker which most improves the p-value of the model is kept, and the process is repeated with the remaining set of markers until the model can no longer be improved by adding a marker. The p-value of a model is defined as the probability of observing a data set as consistent with the model as the actual data when in fact the null-model holds. The resulting model is then checked for any markers with coefficients that are not significantly (at $p < .05$) different from zero. Such markers are removed from the model.

28.3.3 Model Parameterization

The models built in the previous steps can be parameterized based on physiogenomic data. The maximum likelihood method is used, which is a well-established method for obtaining optimal estimates of parameters. S-plus provides very good support for algorithms that provide these estimates for the initial linear regression models, as well as other generalized linear models that we may use when the error in distribution is not normal.

In addition to optimizing the parameters, model refinement is performed by analyzing a set of simplified models and eliminating each variable in turn followed by reoptimizing the likelihood function. The ratio between the two maximum likelihoods of the original vs. the simplified model then provides a significance measure for the contribution of each variable to the model. In a probabilistic network model, the approach is exactly the same, except that instead of removing variables, dependency links are removed.

28.3.4 Model Validation

A cross-validation approach is used to evaluate the performance of models by separating the data used for parameterization (training set) from the data used for testing (test set). A model to be evaluated is reparameterized using all data except for one patient. The likelihood of the outcome for this patient is calculated using the outcome distribution from the model. The procedure is repeated for each patient, and the product of all likelihoods is computed. The resulting likelihood is compared with the likelihood of the data under the null model (no markers, predicted distribution equal to general distribution). If the likelihood ratio is less than the critical value for $p = .05$, the model will be evaluated as providing a significant improvement of the null model. If this threshold is not reached, the model is not sufficiently supported by the data, which could mean either that there is not enough data, or that the model does not reflect actual dependencies between the variables.

28.3.5 Multiple Comparison Corrections

Since the number of possible comparisons is very large in physiogenomics we routinely include in our analysis a random permutation test for the null hypothesis of no effect for two to five combinations of genes. The permutation test is accomplished by randomly assigning the outcome to each individual in the study, which is implied by the null distribution of no genetic effect, and estimating the test statistic that corresponds to the null hypothesis of the gene combination effect. Repeating this process provides an empirical estimate of the distribution for the test statistic, and hence a p-value that takes into account the process that gave rise to the multiple comparisons.

For permutation testing, 1000 permuted data sets are generated, and each candidate marker will be retested on each of those 1000 sets. A p-value is assigned according to the ranking of the original test result within the 1000 control results. A marker is selected for model building when the original test ranks within the top 50 of the 1000 ($p < .05$).

The purpose of multiple comparison corrections is to generate a nonparametric and marker complexity adjusted p-value by permutation testing. This procedure is important because the p-value is used for identifying a few significant markers out of the large number of candidates. Model-based p-values are unsuitable for such selection, because the multiple testing of every potential serological marker and every genetic marker will be likely to yield some results that appear to be statistically significant even though they occurred by chance alone. If not corrected, such differences will lead to spurious markers being picked as the most significant. The correction is made by permutation testing, that is, the same tests are performed on a large number of data sets that differ from the original by having the response variable permuted at random with respect to the marker, thereby providing a nonparametric estimate of the null distribution of the test statistics. The ranking of the unpermuted test result in the distribution of permuted test results provides a nonparametric and statistically rigorous estimate of the false positive rate for this marker. We also consider hierarchical regression analysis to generate estimates incorporating prior information about the biological activity of the gene variants. In this type of analysis, multiple genotypes and other risk factors can be considered simultaneously as a set, and estimates are adjusted based on prior information and the observed covariance, theoretically improving the accuracy and precision of effect estimates [Steenland et al., 2000].

28.3.6 Summary of Association Results

The basis of the physiogenomics informatics platform is a parallel search for associations between multiple phenotypes and genetic markers for several candidate genes. The summary in Table 28.1 depicts the data set gathered from a hypothetical application of physiogenomics to a complex environmental exposure such as exercise or diet. In the top panel, each column represents a single phenotype measurement.

TABLE 28.1 Example of Physiogenomics Data Analysis and Screening for Gene Marker/Phenotype Associations

	Biochemical						Physiological			
A	B	C	D	E	F	G	H	I	J	Genotypes
SNP Hits										
4	0	3	23	2	5	1	27	30	0	G1
4	3	1	5	3	16	17	25	23	3	G2
0	3	4	6	0	27	0	7	3	11	G3
0	0	3	0	3	2	4	1	5	16	G4
21	32	21	0	1	2	11	2	3	6	G5
9	5	0	0	23	5	3	9	12	11	G6
Genomic controls										
4	6	5	2	1	1	0	3	1	2	G7
1	2	0	1	5	8	9	1	0	0	G8
2	2	3	4	6	0	4	0	2	2	G9

Among the ten phenotypes in this example, various biochemical markers (denoted A–G) and physiological parameters (denoted H–J) are shown. Each row represents alleles for a given gene, and quantitatively render associations of specific alleles to the variability in the phenotype.

The various numbers in Table 28.1 refer to the negative logarithms of p-value times 10. These p-values are adjusted for multiple comparisons using the nonparametric permutation test described earlier. For example, 30 refers to a p-value of less than 10^{-3}, or $p < .001$. The interface currently under development will also include the capability of interacting with cell in the table to generate a further detailed analysis. As already noted, the p-value displayed in a cell is generated under the assumption of a linear trend for the effect of an intervention. The interface will be constructed to also generate a nonparametric estimate of the dose response relationship for the different alleles using cubic splines [Durrleman and Simon, 1989], as well as other summary statistics such as the distribution of different alleles.

The interface allows visual recognition of highly significant association domains to both biochemical and physiological responses. Note the phenotype associations of Gene 1 to both biochemical and physiological values. The biochemical and physiological outputs are associated by their relationship to the same gene. Noteworthy also are high ranking associations of Gene 2 to biochemical markers F–G and physiological phenotypes H and I. A summary table could list in order of significance the "hits" of positive association between genes and phenotypes.

There are also clearly negative fields. The same gene is associated to some phenotypes but not to others. Similarly, a given phenotype may have associations to some genes, but not others. Each negative result lends power to the positive associations. Some genes (G7 to G9) denoted as "genomic controls" have no association to any phenotype. Had a phenotype arisen from unsuspected population founder effects, most genes would have had specific founderallele frequencies reflected in the overall analysis. Such population stratification would give rise to a disproportionate number of genes associated to the phenotype.

The physiogenomics analysis includes the number of individuals with and without the associated allele. The individuals' counts among various phenotypes may be different depending on genotype sampling during a study. Physiogenomics can derive information from both well represented distributions among the "in" and "out" groups and also those potentially driven by outliers. Thus, an association given an "in" group of 33% is interesting in most analytical platforms, whereas another with an "in" group of only 6% is potentially tractable only with physiogenomics with well-represented genomic controls. If the phenotype represents an undesirable outcome, the power of physiogenomics to detect trends among a small group of outliers is particularly valuable. In the case of side effects, the outliers may actually represent the susceptible population associated with a lower frequency predictive marker.

28.4   Future Research and Prospects

28.4.1   Future Research

In the near future, more sophisticated models can be built using probabilistic networks. A probabilistic network is a factorization of the joint probability function over all the considered variables (markers, interventions, and outcomes) based on knowledge about the dependencies and independencies between the variables. Such knowledge is naturally provided by the hits coming out of the association screen, where each association can be interpreted as a dependency, and the absence of an association as an independency between variables. The model can then be parameterized by fitting to the data, similarly to the linear and logistic regression models, which are in fact special cases of probabilistic network models.

We also envision the informatics analysis to incorporate systems modules that could attribute various weights to each gene according to their relevance to the physiological mechanisms and predictive power statistically. The interface will include a framework for the expert physiologist to query the data set for mechanistic hypothesis, including feedback inhibition and signal amplification.

We know a priori that any list of candidate genes will miss some known key genes, and will certainly lack those genes not discovered so far or not identified yet as relevant. Physiogenomics posits the gene representation question in the following logic: representative genes are selected based on various functional criteria, and the associated genes are assembled into a predictive model. Through clinical research the predictive power of the model is ascertained. The hypothesis is that the genes in the panel together will explain a useful fraction of the variability in response among individuals. If the answer is affirmative, then the hypothesis is accepted, and the model is used. If the answer is inconclusive, the roster of genes will be modified until the multigene model's predictive level is clinically useful. Failure to establish predictive models with genes selected by either gene expression or pathway analysis can be circumvented with a supplementary analysis with other gene candidates.

An alternative physiogenomics strategy is genome-wide association study. The ultimate goal of The International Haplotype Map Consortium [2003] is to render such an approach feasible, and the high multiplexing capacity of the various nanotechnology array platforms would be perfectly suited for such analysis. Such a strategy has been successful in family study of genetic traits but remains unproven for population studies.

28.4.2   Prospects and Conclusions

The wealth of interesting associations, some certainly unexpected, points to the power of physiogenomics. The above-described analytical tools permit the extension of physiogenomics to several thousand additional genes with the modern array nanotechnologies. Phenotypes could be added as well, for example, inflammatory and neuroendocrine markers are an area of intense interest in clinical medicine. The ability to measure changes in these markers for disease prevention strategies provides us a unique opportunity to examine genes determining a path to personalized health. The research can now utilize saved blood plasma and DNA for each patient to measure the appropriate genotypes and biochemical markers in blood thus opening the possibility of retrospective analysis from archived clinical samples.

We conclude describing a prophetic embodiment of physiogenomics relevant to disease prevention. Figure 28.2 provides an example of personalized healthcare by customizing treatment intervention for the metabolic syndrome of obesity [Ford et al., 2002]. In the table, the choices are to recommend a given kind of exercise, drug, or diet regimen. If one of the options is high scoring, it can be used on its own. Thus in the example, diet is high scoring in the first patient, a drug in the second, and exercise in the third. If the options are midrange, they can be used in combination, if for example, exercise and diet each have a positive effect but are unlikely to be sufficient independently. If none of the options is high or at least midscoring, the physiotype analysis suggests that the patient requires another option not yet in the menu.

As more environmental responses are characterized through physiogenomics, the chance that all patients will be served at increased precision of intervention and with optimal outcome will be greater. That we may even contemplate this scenario is a testament to the combined power of physiogenomics

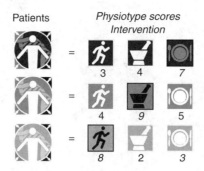

Patients   Physiotype scores
                Intervention

FIGURE 28.2   (See color insert.) Physiotypes for personalized health.

and nanotechnology. The highly parallel genome probing possible with nanotechnology and the systems engineering approach underlying physiogenomics in a real sense allow us to reconstitute the organism and its environmental response from the individual components. The specificity and individualization afforded by nanotechnology and physiogenomics are ushering medicine into the era of personalized health.

References

Durrleman, S. and Simon, R. Flexible regression models with cubic splines. *Stat. Med.* 1989; 8: 551–561.

Ford, E.S., Giles, W.H., and Dietz, W.H. Prevalence of the metabolic syndrome among US adults: findings from the third National Health and Nutrition Examination Survey. *JAMA* 2002; 287: 356–359.

Gunderson, K.L., Semyon, K., Graige, M.S. et al. Decoding randomly ordered DNA arrays. *Genome Res.* 2004; 14: 870–877.

Hastie, T. and Tibshirani, R. Generalized additive models. *Stat. Sci.* 1986; 1: 297–318.

Holford, T.R. *Multivariate Methods in Epidemiology.* New York: Oxford University Press, 2002.

International Haplotype Map Consortium. *Nature* 2003; 426: 789–796.

McCullagh, P. and Nelder, J.A. *Generalized Linear Models.* London: Chapman and Hall, 1989.

Saltelli, A., Chan, K., and Scott, E.M. *Sensitivity Analysis.* Chichester: John Wiley and Sons, 2000.

Ruano, G. Personalized Medicine Quo Vadis, *Personalized Medicine,* 2004 (in press).

Steenland, K., Bray, I., Greenland, S., and Boffetta, P. Empirical Bayes adjustments for multiple results in hypothesis-generating or surveillance studies. *Cancer Epidemiol. Biomarkers Prev.* 2000; 9: 895–903.

Stephens, J.C., Schneider, J.A., and Tanguay, D.A. Haplotype variation and linkage disequilibrium in 313 human genes. *Science* 2001; 293: 1048.

29

Bionanotechnology Patenting: Challenges and Opportunities

Raj Bawa
Bawa Biotechnology Consulting LLC
Rensselaer Polytechnic Institute, NVCC

S.R. Bawa
Bawa Biotechnology Consulting LLC

Stephen B. Maebius
Foley & Lardner

Chid Iyer
Sughrue Mion PLLC

Innovations at the intersection of engineering, biotechnology, medicine, physical sciences, and information technology are spurring new directions in research, education, commercialization, and technology transfer. The future of nanotechnology is likely to continue in this interdisciplinary manner. Perhaps the greatest impact of nanotechnology will take place in the context of biology, biotechnology, and medicine. For the sake of simplicity, in this chapter, we refer to this arena of nanotechnology as bionanotechnology.

The U.S. National Nanotechnology Initiative (NNI) defines nanotechnology as involving research and development at the atomic, molecular, or macromolecular levels in the sub-100 nm range to create and use structures, devices, and systems that have novel functional properties because of this size.[1] By manipulating atoms, scientists can create stronger, lighter more efficient materials ("nanomaterials") with tailored properties. In addition to the numerous advantages provided by this scale of miniaturization (over their conventional "bulk" counterparts), quantum physics effects at this scale provide additional

---

[1] A nanometer is one billionth of a meter, or 1/75,000th the size of a human hair. An atom is about one third of a nanometer in width. National Nanotechnology Initiative, *What is Nanotechnology?* at http://www.nano.gov/html/facts/whatIsNano.html

novel properties.[2] However, some experts have cautioned against such an overly rigid or restrictive definition of nanotechnology based on a size range, emphasizing instead the continuum of scale from the nano- to the microscale.[3] In fact, a definition based on physical limits tends to be an unorthodox way of defining a technology field, especially because other technologies tend to be defined by a key technology or breakthrough.[4] Genetic engineering technology, for example, is based upon recombinant DNA. It is well known that the Internet is a collection of "bulletin boards" networked in a World Wide Web. The broadness in scope and definition of nanotechnology presents difficulties for understanding the scientific, legal, environmental, regulatory, and ethical implications because nanotechnology may represent a cluster of technologies, each of which may have different characteristics and applications.

Although the definition of nanotechnology is at best arbitrary, industry is clearly beginning to envision its potential. For example, novel nanomaterials are used in materials applications, pharmaceutical applications, electronics, and elsewhere. According to the National Science Foundation (NSF), by 2015 the annual global market for nano-related goods and services will top 1 trillion U.S. dollars, making it one of the fastest growing industries in history. Although the process of converting basic research in nanoscience into commercially viable products will be long and difficult, governments across the globe are impressed by nanotechnology's potential and are staking their claims by doling out billions of dollars, euros, and yen for research. Political alliances and battle lines are starting to form. The passage of the 21st Century Nanotechnology Research and Development Act (Pub. L. No. 108-153), which authorized $3.7 billion in federal funding from 2005 through 2008 for the support of nanotechnology R&D, has further fueled the fervor over nanotechnology.[5] In the United States, nanotechnology is poised to become the largest government science initiative since the space race. A recent report from Lux Research [1] states: "sales of products incorporating emerging nanotechnology will rise from <0.1% of global manufacturing output today to 15% in 2014, totaling $2.6 trillion. This value will approach the size of the information technology and telecom industries combined and will be 10 times larger than biotechnology revenues. However, sales of basic nanomaterials like carbon nanotubes and quantum dots will total only $13 billion in 2014: nanotechnology's economic impact will arise from how these fundamental building blocks are used, not from sales of the materials themselves." This report projects that by 2014, 16% of goods in healthcare and life sciences (by revenue) will incorporate emerging nanotechnology. The report refutes the popular notion that nanotechnology is an industry or a sector, considering it to represent a set of tools and processes for manipulating matter that can be applied to virtually any manufactured goods. Similarly,

---

[2]Merging research from many disciplines, some near-term nanotechnology applications involve scratchproof glass, antifouling coatings, novel drug-delivery systems, while a future application could be a sugar cube-sized computer capable of storing the entire information content of the Library of Congress.

[3]NIH, *NHLBI Programs of Excellence in Nanotechnology*, at http://grants.nih.gov/grants/guide/rfa-files/RFA-HL-04-020.html

[4]There is confusion and disagreement among experts on the definition of nanotechnology. This is because nanotechnology is an umbrella term used to define the products and processes at the nano/microscale that have resulted from the convergence of the physical, chemical, and life sciences. The NNI defines it as "anything involving structures less than 100 nm in size." However, this rigid definition excludes numerous devices and materials of micron dimensions, a scale that is included within the definition of nanotechnology by many nanoscientists. Therefore, some have suggested the phrase "small technologies" to encompass both nanotechnology and microtechnology. A more appropriate definition may be "the design, characterization, production and application of structures, devices, and systems by controlled manipulation of size and shape at the nanometer scale (atomic, molecular and macromolecular scale) that produces structures, devices and systems with at least one novel/superior characteristic or property [2]." Also, note that this sub-100 nm size limitation is rarely critical to a drug company from a formulation, pharmacokinetic or efficacy perspective since the desire property (improved bioavailability reduced toxicity, enhanced solubility, etc.) may be achieved outside of this sub-100 nm size range.

[5]This legislation emphasizes the creation of R&D Centers in academia and government. At present, there are over 50 institutes and centers dedicated to nanotechnology R&D. For example, the NSF has established the National Nanotechnology Infrastructure Network — composed of 13 university sites that will form an integrated, nationwide system of user facilities to support research and education in nanoscale science, engineering, and technology. Similarly, there are currently 15 government agencies with R&D budgets dedicated to nanotechnology.

many experts caution against envisioning a "nanotechnology market" per se, recommending instead that industry and policy makers focus on how nanotechnology is being exploited across industry value chains, from basic materials to intermediate products to final goods.

29.1   Defining Bionanotechnology R&D

Nanotechnology promises to transform most industries and will have a particularly profound impact on healthcare and medicine. A significant sector within nanotechnology is bionanotechnology. Bionanotechnology (sometimes referred to as nanobiotechnology or nanomedicine) is in a broad sense the application of nanoscale technologies to the practice of medicine, namely, for diagnosis, prevention, and treatment of disease and to gain an increased understanding of complex disease mechanisms. The creation of nanodevices such as "nanobots" capable of performing real-time therapeutic functions *in vivo* is one eventual goal within this emerging interdisciplinary field of research. On the path to that goal, significant technological advances across multiple scientific disciplines will continue to be proposed, validated, patented, and commercialized. Advances in delivering therapies, miniaturization of analytical tools, improved computational and memory capabilities, and developments in remote communications will be integrated.

The scale of man-made components involved in nanotechnology is similar to that of biological structures. For example, quantum dot nanoparticles are similar in size to peptides (<10 nm) while drug-delivery nanoparticles are the same size as some viruses (<100 nm). Because of this similarity in scale and certain characteristics, nanotechnology is a natural progression of many areas of biomedical research. Bionanotechnology has many applications in drug development, drug delivery, detection, sensing, imaging, and devices and, again, depending on the definition used, many applications already exist. Bionanotechnology is poised to deliver [2]:

- Inexpensive and higher throughput DNA sequencers that can reduce the time for drug discovery and diagnostics
- Nanofluidic systems that transport fluids more efficiently because fluids move through micro- and nanoscale pipes with laminar flow, thereby avoiding turbulence and mixing
- More efficient and site-specific/targeted drug-delivery systems, such as close-looped sensing and drug-administration devices where sensors (to monitor biomolecules) and drug reservoirs (for precise delivery) are located on the same chip
- Nanomaterials that can solve unique biological issues not currently possible, such as detection of electrical changes from biological molecules via inorganic molecules, followed by a reaction of the two in a manner that detects or treats a disease
- Microsurgical devices or nanobots that are capable of navigating throughout the body, repairing injuries, destroying tumors or viruses, and even performing gene therapy

It is expected that significant research will be undertaken at least in the following areas in the coming years generating both evolutionary and revolutionary products: synthesis and use of novel nanomaterials and nanostructures (e.g., less antigenic); biomimetic nanostructures (synthetic products developed from an understanding of biological systems); biological nanostructures; electronic biological interfaces; devices and nanosensors for early detection of diseases and pathogens (e.g., PCR-coupled nano/micro fluidic devices); instruments for studying individual molecules; nanotechnology for tissue engineering (nanostructures scaffolds) and regenerative medicine. In the diagnostic area, much of the research has been focused on biochips, which are devices that contain many biological sensors. Nanotechnology has been proposed to increase the density of sensors on the biochips and to provide alternative detection mechanisms. In the area of therapeutics, some potential near term applications may involve dendrimers, nanoliposomes, and nanoparticles as vehicles for efficient gene or drug-delivery.

Bionanotechnology also aims to learn from nature — to understand the structure and function of biological devices and to utilize nature's solutions to advance science and engineering. Evolution has produced an overwhelming number and variety of biological devices, compounds, and processes that function at the nanometer or molecular level and that provide performance that is unsurpassed by manmade technologies. When nanotechnology is combined with molecular biology, the possible applications are widespread and may sound like the stuff of science fiction. In this regard, bionanotechnology can be characterized as a primitive technology that takes advantage of the properties of highly evolved natural products like nucleic acids and proteins by attempting to harness them to achieve new and useful functionalities on the nanoscale. The construction principles used in this field often originate in biology and the goals are often biomimetic or aimed at the solution of long-standing research problems. At the heart of the approaches in this field is the concept of self-assembly. Self-assembly of ordered elements is a defining property of living things. Bionanotechnology attempts to exploit both self-assembly and the ordered proximity of nanoscale structures found in biology.

29.2   Significance of Patents to Bionanotechnology Commercialization

As we can see, the time for bionanotechnology has come and a classic technological revolution is unfolding. According to *the Nanotech Report 2003*, venture funds are preferentially going to bionanotechnology, with 52% of the $900 million in venture capital funding for nanotechnology in the past four years going to bionanotechnology start-ups.[6] The market for bionanotechnology has existed only for a few years but it is expected to rapidly reach over US $3 billion by 2008, reflecting an annual growth at a rate of 28%.[7]

Commercial bionanotechnology, however, is at a nascent stage. Large-scale production challenges, high production cost, the public's general reluctance to embrace innovative technology without real safety data or products, scarcity of venture money, big pharma's reluctance to embrace bionanotechnology and a well-established micron-scale industry are just a few of the bottlenecks facing early-stage bionanotechnology commercialization. However, some major factors that will drive commercialization in bionanotechnology in the near future will be greater federal funding, an expiration of block buster drug patents an aging population's desire for novel drugs and therapies and an ever-increasing understanding of the molecular basis of disease.[8] Bionanotechnology will almost certainly develop as biotechnology has, through intensive research that produces novel products and processes. Similar to their importance to the development of the biotechnology and information technology industries, patents will also play a critical role in the success of the global bionanotechnology revolution. In fact, patents are already shaping the nascent and rapidly evolving field of nanoscience generally and bionanotechnology in particular [4]. As companies develop products and processes and begin to seek commercial applications for their inventions, securing valid and defensible patent protection will be vital to their long-term survival. In the future, bionanotechnology will mimic what the biotechnology start-ups of the early 1980s faced — namely, corporate partnerships, licensing, and venture opportunities. Patents are central to all these activities. As we enter the "golden era" of bionanotechnology in the next decade, with the field maturing and the promised breakthroughs accruing, patents will generate licensing revenue, provide leverage in deals and mergers, and reduce the likelihood of infringement. Because development of bionanotechnology-related products is one of the most research-intensive industries in existence, without the market exclusivity offered by a U.S. patent, development of these products and their introduction into the marketplace will be significantly hampered. Since this technology is multidisciplinary in nature, patenting here poses unique opportunities as well as challenges. As a result, the inventor needs to follow certain key patent strategies to succeed in this bourgeoning field (See Section 29.4).

---

[6]Lux Capital Releases Key Findings from *The Nanotech Report* 2003, at http://nanotech- now.com/Lux-Capital-release-06232003.htm

[7]Nanobiotechnology, opportunities and technical analysis. Front Line Strategic Consulting, Inc., San Mateo, California (2003).

[8]According to Merrill Lynch, 23 of the top global pharmaceutical patents will expire by 2008, accounting for an annual revenue loss of over $46 billion [3].

There is ample evidence that companies, start-ups, and research universities of all sizes are ascribing greater value and importance to patents. In general, they are willing to risk a larger part of their budgets to acquire, exercise, and defend patents. While patents are being sought more actively and enforced more vigorously, the entire patent system is under greater scrutiny and strain. The PTO has often struggled in the light of new technologies such as biotechnology and software patents. This disturbing trend continues with bionanotechnology patenting, as this 200-year-old federal agency continues to grapple with evaluating bionanotechnology-related patent applications [5].

For more than a decade, all the major patent offices of the world have faced an onslaught of nanopatent applications. This is likely to get worse as more applications are filed and the backlog of unexamined patent applications (pendency) skyrocket. Due to the potential market value of bionanotechnology-related products, researchers, executives, and patent lawyers are all on a quest to obtain broad protection for new nanoscale polymers and materials that have applications in bionanotechnology Researchers around the world are steadily filing patents in hopes of creating "toll booths" for future product development. Hence, a sort of "patent land grab" is in full swing by patent prospectors as startups and corporations compete to lock up broad bionanotechnology-related patents in these critical early days [4]. This land grab mentality has not only produced overlapping patents but the race to hurriedly patent anything "nano" has produced a pile of "unduly broad" patents, a proliferation that will ultimately produce a dense web of overlapping "patent thickets" requiring patent litigation to sort out, especially if sectors of bionanotechnology become financially lucrative. Given such a landscape, expensive litigation is inevitable. In most of the patent battles, the larger entity with the deeper pockets will rule the day, even if the brightest innovators were on the other side. It is very likely that the future bionanotechnology start-ups will be attractive takeover targets for larger companies since takeover is generally a more cost-effective alternative to litigation. Since there has been an explosion of overlapping and broad patent filing on nanomaterials, it is very likely that companies that want to use these building blocks in products will be forced to license patents from many different sources in order to practice their inventions. Therefore, business planners and patent practitioners should steer company researchers away from such potential patent entanglements. They may also need to analyze the patent landscape to gauge the "white space" opportunities (no overlapping patents) prior to R&D efforts, patent filing or commercialization activities. Most experts agree that the stage is set for a wave of cross-licensing agreements and bundles of intellectual property for specific bionanotechnology applications licensed by groups of large corporations.

The table below lists some of the possible technologies and techniques pertaining to bionanotechnology that can be protected via a U.S. patent:[9]

Biopharmaceutics
Drug delivery
   Drug encapsulation
   Functional drug carriers
Drug discovery

Implantable materials
Tissue repair and replacment
   Implant coatings
   Tissue regeneration scaffolds
Structural implant materials
   Bone repair
   Bioresorbable materials
   Smart materials

Continued

---

[9]Courtesy of Mr. Neil Gordon and Dr. Uri Sagman, Canadian NanoBusiness Alliance, Montréal, Canada.

Continues

Implantable devices
Assessment and treatment devices
    Implantable sensors
    Implantable medical devices
Sensory aids
    Retina implants
    Cochlear implants

Surgical aids
Operating tools
    Smart instruments
    Surgical robots

Diagnostic tools
Genetic testing
    Ultrasensitive labeling and
      detection technologies
    High throughput arrays and
      multiple analyses
Imaging
    Nanoparticle labels
    Imaging devices
Understanding basic life processes

29.3   The U.S. Patent System and the Criteria for Patenting

A patent is not a "hunting license"; it is merely a "no trespassing signpost" that clearly marks the boundaries of an invention.[10] Modern intellectual property consists of patents, trademarks, copyrights, and trade secrets.[11] Globally, industries that produce and manage "knowledge" and "creativity" have replaced capital, colonies, and raw materials as the new wealth of nations. Property, which has always been the essence of capitalism, is changing from tangible to intangible. Intangible assets as a portion of corporate market capital are steadily rising. Patent protection is the incentive for industry to invest in research and development programs that produce innovation. Clearly, without such protection, many companies would avoid costly R&D and society would be deprived of the many benefits thereof. Patents are the most complex, tightly regulated, and expensive forms of intellectual property. However, they offer protection for the broad design concept behind an invention in addition to the tangible form of the invention itself.

A U.S. patent is a legal document granted by the federal government whereby the recipient (or "patentee") is conferred the temporary right to exclude others from making, using, selling, offering for sale, or importing the patented invention into the United States for up to 20 years from the filing date. Similarly, if the invention is a process, then the products made by that process cannot be imported

---

[10] *Brenner v. Manson*, 383 U.S. 519, 536 (1966).

[11] In the case of nanotechnology, mask works may be added to this list. If chip layout information is novel in design, it can be protected to prevent unauthorized copying. The PTO issues three types of patents: (a) utility patents for "any new and useful process, machine, manufacture, or composition of matter, or any new and useful improvement thereof; (b) plant patents for "any distinct and new variety of plant"; and (c) design patents for "any new, original and ornamental design for an article of manufacture." Note that this chapter focuses solely on U.S. utility patents.

into the United States. A U.S. patent provides protection only in the United States, its territories, and its possessions for the term of the patent.

The rationale behind patent law is simple. An inventor is encouraged to apply for a patent by a promise from the U.S. government of a limited legal monopoly for the invention. This promise of limited monopoly rights justifies development costs and assures a reasonable return on profit. In exchange, the inventor publicly discloses the new technology that might have otherwise remained secret (the "immediate benefit" to the public) and allows the public to freely use, make, sell, or import the invention once the patent expires (the "delayed benefit"). Hence, the new technology that is brought to light encourages further innovation. In this way, society obtains a *quid pro quo* from inventors in exchange for the temporary grant of exclusive rights. Such an advantageous exchange spurs American industry and stimulates commerce (the "long-term benefit"). Although obtaining a patent does not ensure commercial success, economists view patenting as an indicator of scientific activity. They argue that this in turn is the basis for providing a nation with a competitive advantage, fueling its economy.[12] The Founding Fathers incorporated the concept of patents into the Constitution under Article 1, Section 8, Clause 8, whereby Congress has the authority "[t]o promote the progress of science and the useful arts, by securing for limited times to authors and inventors the exclusive right to their respective writings and discoveries." President Washington signed the first U.S. Patent Act on April 10, 1790. Title 35 of the *United States Code* codified the Patent Act of 1952, the Act currently in use. Since the granting of the first U.S. patent in 1790, more than 6.6 million patents have been issued by the PTO a bureau of the U.S. Department of Commerce.[13] In 1790, the PTO issued only three patents. For the past few years, the agency has received over 350,000 patent applications annually. The number of patent applications filed has been increasing, on average, by over 10% per year since 1996. The PTO issued almost 200,000 patents in fiscal year 2004.

Traditionally, patents and inventions of commercial interest have been viewed as the domain of industry while basic science and research have been viewed as the concern of academia. This separation has now blurred. In fact, there has been an upsurge of patents granted to U.S. universities. This has contributed to an increase in the number of university-related start-ups as well as an increase in income generated via patent licensing. An interesting trend is emerging with respect to Asian nanotechnology companies: they are funding U.S. research and striking deals for patents from U.S. universities.

As defined by the Constitution, U.S. patents are granted to chemical compositions, machines, industrial or chemical processes, manufactured articles, ornamental designs of an article of manufacture, and asexually reproduced nontuber plant varieties. Patentable inventions need not be pioneering breakthroughs. Improvements of existing inventions or unique combinations/arrangements of old formulations or components may also be patented.[14] In fact, the majority of inventions are improvements on existing

---

[12]See, e.g., Roger W. Ferguson, Jr., *Patent Policy in a Broader Context,* Remarks at 2003 Financial Markets Conference of the Federal Reserve Bank of Atlanta (April 5, 2003), at http://www.federalreserve.gov/boarddocs/speeches/2003/20030407/default.html

[13]Nearly 90% of the world's patents are issued through the three main Patent Offices: the United States, Europe, and Japan. According to PTO data (http://www.uspto.gov/web/offices/com/annual/2003/060406_table6.html), each fiscal year (October 1–September 30), the U.S. Patent Office grants more patents (excluding design, plant or reissue patents) than the European Patent Office or the Japanese Patent Office. In 2004, close to 44% of the total U.S. patents issued were to foreign residents. Note that because many patent applications remain under review at the PTO for more than one fiscal year, these annual patent figures do not represent a valid comparison. The United States has been the major foreign patenting system employed by foreign inventors. The primary reason for this is that the U.S. economy is particularly attractive to foreign innovators due to its large size and advanced nature. One highly controversial but important statistic worth mentioning is the PTO grant rate, that is, the patent application acceptance or allowance rate. The PTO grant rate may range from 70% to 97% (taking into account continuing patent applications), see, for example, Ebert, L.B. Things are not always what they seem to be. *Intellectual Property Today* 12(10): 20–22. Since the acceptance rates for the European, German, and Japanese Patent Offices are lower than the PTO, some patent experts argue that this indicates a less rigorous examination at the PTO, resulting in patents of poor quality.

[14]Works of art and writings, however, may be copyrighted. Various symbols may be trademarked.

technologies. However, not every innovation is patentable. For example, abstract ideas, laws of nature, works of art, mathematical algorithms, and unique symbols and writings cannot be patented.

To be patentable, an invention (or more accurately, the patent specification) must meet *all* of the following criteria:

- It must be novel (i.e., sufficiently new and unlike anything that has been previously patented, marketed, practiced, publicized, or published).
- It must be nonobvious to a person with knowledge in the field related to the invention, meaning that the person would not automatically arrive at the present invention from a review of existing ones (i.e., trivial variations that are readily apparent to a person with knowledge in the field related to the invention cannot be patented).
- It must have utility (i.e., the invention has some use and it actually works or accomplishes a useful task).[15]
- It must be adequately described to the public in order to demonstrate "possession" of the invention at the time of filing.
- It must enable a person with knowledge in the field related to the invention to make or carry out the invention without "undue experimentation" (i.e., to make the claimed product or carry out the claimed process).
- It must enable a person with knowledge in the field related to the invention to use the invention.
- It must be described in clear, unambiguous, and definite terms.
- It must set forth the best mode of making and using the invention contemplated by the inventor at the time of filing of the patent application.

29.4   Key Considerations and Strategies for Inventors

Millions of dollars may be lost if a company fails to take the necessary steps to protect its patent assets. Securing valid defensible patent protection is vital to the long-term viability of virtually any pharmaceutical or biotechnology company, whether nanotechnology is the platform technology involved or not. Often, loss of these critical assets is a result of the researcher's excitement with his work and ignorance about intellectual property. Hence, it is essential that managers and patent practitioners implement certain proactive measures to "box out" the competition. In other words, taking the correct preventive steps is critical to realizing the full commercial potential of a bionanotechnology invention.

Because bionanotechnology interfaces with fields such as biology, physics, chemistry, engineering, medicine, and computer science, filing a patent application (or conducting a patent search) in bionanotechnology may require expertise in these diverse disciplines. The quality and value of the issued bionanotechnology patent will largely determine its potential for commercialization, licensing opportunities, investor interest, and enforceability. Hence, employing qualified patent counsel (a patent agent, patent attorney, or a multidisciplinary team of lawyers) who understand the legal and technical complexities of bionanotechnology is a critical step in obtaining quality patents. In short, issued bionanotechnology-related patents should be carefully evaluated and effective patent-drafting strategies devised accordingly. Additionally, many complex marketing factors may also need to be carefully evaluated ("Inventor's Reality Checklist"):

- Does the invention offer a unique solution to a real problem?
- Does it offer a measurable improvement over previous attempts to solve the problem?
- Is it a stand-alone product or part of an existing product?

---

[15]Perpetual motion machines, time machines, and a random configuration of gears lack utility, and therefore, are unpatentable. Note that inventions that may be perceived as being immoral or illegal also fall under this clause. A hypothetical example is a drug aerosol formulation comprising toxic nanoparticles (e.g., anti-bound quantum dots) and lacking any known beneficial use. Although patent statutes are technology neutral, emerging areas such as biotechnology and nanotechnology may face PTO scrutiny in particular with respect to utility.

- Can it be easily manufactured or integrated into an existing product or system?
- How big is the potential market?
- Is the market growing or shrinking?
- Is the market global? Can the invention be expanded into new markets as they evolve?
- Will the invention become passé before a prototype is designed?
- Who are the prospective investors, partners, or licensing agents in the field?
- What price will consumers put on its value?
- What are the estimates for commercialization and marking?
- What are the incentives for the consumer to buy the product?
- Is federal regulatory approval required?
- How long will it take to bring the product to market?

Some key considerations for the bionanotechnology inventor and his/her company to adequately protect the invention prior to filing for a patent are discussed below [6]:

1. *Avoid early publication or any public disclosure*: The inventor must refrain from publishing a description of, publicly presenting, submitting grant proposals for, or offering the invention for sale prior[16] to filing a patent application. All of these activities create prior art against the inventor. Note that one of the criteria for patentability in the United States is that the invention must be "novel"[17] and not in the public domain in the form of "prior art."[18] According to current U.S. patent law, the applicant has one year to file for an application from the date that invention is known of, used by others, or offered for sale (meaning that any public disclosure triggers a one-year deadline to file a patent application in the United States). On the other hand, because this one-year grace period is not offered by foreign patent offices, any publication or public disclosure will prevent the inventor from obtaining a foreign patent altogether, or prevent the inventor from realizing the full range of potential applications of the bionanotechnology for which a patent is being sought overseas. In summary, a patent application should be drafted and filed as soon as possible after the completion date of the invention to realize its full commercial potential.

2. *Consider obtaining a foreign patent*: Filing a bionanotechnology patent in a foreign country should be carefully considered and should largely depend upon commercial considerations. If there is an interest in expanding into foreign markets, then obtaining patents abroad should be seriously considered. In fact, even if the inventor does not plan to establish a market for the particular bionanotechnology in a foreign country, obtaining a patent there could be critical in securing licensing deals (and discouraging unlicensed copying or use by foreign competitors). The danger of steering clear of foreign patent filing is that a competitor could commercialize the invention in a foreign country and capture a valuable market share there. For example, an inventor who patents new nanoparticles for drug delivery only in the United States is essentially giving away the entire technology to other countries because the patent may also disclose the best method of producing these novel nanoparticles.

   Most U.S. inventors seeking foreign bionanotechnology patents first file a U.S. patent application (known as the "national stage" application) and follow it with a patent application under the Patent Cooperation Treaty (PCT).[19] Inventors have a year after filing the national stage patent application

---

[16]Often a company releases information on a new product, or discusses details during negotiations prior to filing a patent application. This may also trigger a one-year "on-sale bar."

[17]Defined previously in Section 29.3.

[18]The phrase "prior art" generally refers to the state of knowledge existing or publicly available prior to the date of the invention. Prior art is often in the form of a printed document (any publication, prior patent, etc.) that contains a disclosure or description that is relevant to an invention for which a patent is being sought or enforced. Typically, prior art is submitted by the inventor during prosecution of his/her patent application.

[19]The PCT is a multilateral treaty, established in 1978, among more than 125 nations that allows reciprocal patent rights among its signatory nations. In other words, it simplifies the patenting process when an inventor seeks to patent the same invention in more than one country. It should be emphasized that there is no "world patent."

to file in the foreign country under the PCT. Under PCT rules, inventors can specify particular foreign countries where they intend to seek patent protection for their bionanotechnology invention and may take 30 months (or more) from their original national stage application filing date in their home country to complete all foreign application requirements. This delay may provide the inventors with time to determine whether their bionanotechnology invention is commercially viable and merits patenting in several countries, thereby sparing them substantial effort and expense should they decide not to file overseas.

3. *Beware of pre-grant publication of U.S. patent applications*: Today, as part of the application process, all U.S. patent applications are published eighteen months after filing (up to that point they are confidential), unless the applicant opts out and foregoes foreign patent filing.[20] This implies that a bionanotechnology application will generally appear in the public domain and be available to competitors, whether it is patented or not.

4. *Maintain proper laboratory notebooks*: Often, laboratory notebooks contain valuable and critical information not apparent to a company or R&D facility. It is critical that laboratory notebooks be maintained properly. This is especially important, when working in research teams. Here, proper laboratory notes documenting the creative effort, maintaining confidentiality and securing communication among the teams, and filing for a patent promptly are essential so that some members of one group do not inadvertently disclose the invention of another group prematurely. Laboratory notebooks are also useful to patent practitioners to establish the date of an invention, especially in light of a competitor challenge in court.

5. *Conduct a prior art search and/or a "freedom-to-operate" search*: It is wise to conduct a proper prior art search before filing a patent application in order to assess the competition. This may also assist the inventor to design around potential prior art. Moreover, because the patent owner does not automatically have the right to practice his invention, it may be wise to conduct a "freedom-to-operate search" of the issued patent prior to investing and commercializing the patented bionanotechnology. Note that filing a patent application (or conducting a prior art or freedom-to-operate search) on novel bionanotechnology such as a nanoparticle or delivery system may require expertise in diverse disciplines like biotechnology, physics, medicine, chemistry, engineering, and computer science. The quality and value of the issued patent will largely determine its potential for commercialization, licensing opportunities, investor interest, and enforceability. Hence, employing qualified patent counsel who understands the legal and technical complexities of the technology is a critical step to obtaining quality patents.

6. *Educate employees and researchers*: Educate scientists to spot potential inventions during research, since this may not always be apparent to them. Implement policies involving incentives where scientists are rewarded for reporting or submitting an invention disclosure. This may be especially critical in a university setting where scientists are generally promoted in terms of the research grants they receive. Often, scientists overlook their inventions that can be patented. In fact, "patent awareness" during the research process may enable a researcher to pursue a research path that leads to a patentable invention.

7. *Require strong employment agreements*: Require all company employees to sign agreements that clearly specify that all company inventions, intellectual property, and proprietary information is company property and cannot be disclosed or exploited by any employee. This could become critical if a former employee joins a competitor company or research laboratory. Similar agreements should be required of consultants and visiting scholars where all rights are assigned to the company or university. Furthermore, confidential materials should be properly labeled and safeguarded; otherwise, value associated with specific information or invention may be lost or reduced.

---

[20]Traditionally, applications filed at the PTO were kept secret until they matured into a patent. However, because of the American Inventors Protection Act (AIPA) of 1999, an application filed on or after November 29, 1999 loses its secret status when it is published.

8. *Use standard language while drafting patent applications*: The fact remains that bionanotechnology is an inherently difficult topic for discussion, in part due to the confusion surrounding its definition.[21] Although it is well recognized in patent law that a patent applicant can be his/her own lexicographer, it is recommended that an applicant should employ language in bionanotechnology patent applications whose meaning is well recognized in the pharmaceutical, biomedical, or biotechnology fields. Furthermore, the language should be precise and the use of terms consistent throughout the claims and specification (avoid synonyms and be repetitive in the use of phrases when appropriate). This will prevent confusion and possible prosecution delay at the PTO.

   Note that it is possible that the patent will be the subject of litigation such as an infringement suit initiated by the patentee against a competitor or a suit for declaratory relief initiated by an accused competitor (infringer). The success of the litigation may hinge on how the patent was drafted.[22] A poorly drafted patent will give an advantage to the competitor, causing significant aggravation and resulting in substantial litigation fees for the inventor. In conclusion, while drafting patent applications, the drafter should anticipate that the patent might have to be defended in court.

9. *Note the ease in obtaining "Broad" patents in bionanotechnology*: Broad patents continue to be issued by the PTO in bionanotechnology. The overburdened PTO faces new challenges and problems as it attempts to handle the enormous backlog in bionanotechnology applications filed and the torrent of improperly reviewed patents granted.[23] In this "patent proliferation climate" it is inevitable that in the near future there will be an increase in litigation in bionanotechnology as well. While new laws in the past 20 years have made it easier to secure broad patents, these laws have also tilted the table in favor of patent holders, no matter how broad or tenuous their claims.[24] At present, all these factors favor obtaining broad patents in bionanotechnology.

29.5   The Bionanotechnology Start-Up and Patents

Patents are of great importance to start-ups and smaller bionanotechnology companies because they may protect them from infringement by larger corporations. In fact, patents may also protect the clients of a patent owner because they may prevent a competitor from infringing or replicating the client's products made under license from the patentee. Moreover, patents offer credibility to any nanotechnology inventor with its backers, shareholders, and venture capitalists — groups that may not fully understand the science behind the technology. As start-ups evolve and grow in size, protecting trade secrets[25] in this information age may be difficult. Few venture capitalists are likely to support a start-up that relies on trade secrets instead of patents. For a start-up, patents are a means of validating the company's foundational technology in order to attract investment. Most experts agree that a start-up should focus on obtaining a broad intellectual property portfolio that includes both patents and trade secrets that cover clusters of an emerging sector in bionanotechnology. Alternatively, the start-up may seek dominant (or pioneering) patent protection as a means of gaining an advantage.[26] The start-up (or any skilled inventor) should

---

[21] See *supra* note 4.

[22] Often large competitors employ frivolous suits to pressure a company whose patent stands in their way, or which they wish to acquire. Frequently, the cost in executive time and corporate money for the smaller company or startup becomes so onerous that it caves into a licensing agreement. One viable strategy to avoid being taken over is to license the patent to the large competitor, in whose interest it then becomes to protect its position by protecting and defending the patent.

[23] Refer to Section 29.2.

[24] Some have charged that this has converted the patent system from a stimulator of innovation to a creator of litigation and uncertainty [7].

[25] A trade secret consists of any formula, pattern, device, method, idea, or any information that provides a company with a competitive advantage if kept secret from the public or competitors.

[26] Dominating patents are those that are generally the first ones to issue and detail a novel technology.

consider filing patents on their concepts to protect them from predatory inventors,[27] and later file on the details of these early concepts when they are worked out. A nanotechnology start-up should also consider patenting peripheral technology in addition to the base technology. This strategy may sustain it during times of economic downturn or provide it with additional revenue through licensing or sale to other companies that are better positioned to take advantage of the technology. Either of these intellectual property strategies provides a market advantage to the start-up. Even after the dissolution of a poorly performing nanotechnology start-up, patents on its vital technologies can be sold to another company, thereby providing some return for investors.

29.6 Searching Bionanotechnology-Related Patents

Because bionanotechnology by definition covers a broad class of materials and systems, searching for bionanotechnology-related patents and publications is complicated relative to other technology areas. At present, global patent classification systems are neither sufficiently defined nor descriptive enough to accommodate many of the unique properties that bionanotechnology inventions exhibit. Until recently, there was no formal classification scheme for U.S. bionanotechnology patents.[28] However, the PTO's flawed definition of nanotechnology (which is copied from the NNI) has resulted in a skewed classification system.

Additionally, the PTO lacks effective automation tools for bionanotechnology "prior art" searching. The fundamental nature of bionanotechnology is part of the challenge for effectively mapping the patent landscape. Many patent applications may result from a single bionanotechnology invention; hence, a single patent may generate many products or markets. Published patents that are truly bionanotechnological in nature may not use any specific nano-related terminology. Often patents are written "not to be found" in order to keep potential competitors at a "knowledge" disadvantage. Conversely, there are business savvy inventors and assignees who might use key words incorporating a nano prefix for the sake of marketing their invention or concept. Therefore, part of the challenge in finding truly bionanotechnology related patents is the judicious use of key terms and class codes while searching the patent databases. This searching, along with the additional filter of subject area expertise (which can be used to review patents for the problem being solved and the technology applied) is the most reliable way to find nanotechnology patents at the present time. A subject area expert can ultimately provide the judgment in determining whether a patent pertains to bionanotechnology.

Although the full potential of bionanotechnology has yet to be realized, patents granted in this field and applications containing the terms "nano" or "quantum" have shown an upward trend in the past five years. In fact, the number of bionanotechnology-related patents has been on the rise for more than a decade, with IBM leading all nanopatent recipients.[29] Because the patent landscape is getting crowded, commercialization of a bionanotechnology product should not be attempted without reviewing the patent literature. Although there has been a dramatic rise in bionanotechnology patent activity, most of the prior art exists in the form of journal publications and book articles. Web sites and pre-grant patent publications provide an additional resource. Various data sources and software tools can make a patent search more efficient and effective.[30]

---

[27] Predatory inventors are individuals who patent every possible application around a novel, early technology. This approach could become common in certain sectors of bionanotechnology.

[28] Refer to Section 29.7 (2).

[29] Judging from the explosion of U.S. nanopatents, it is clear that the PTO views a scale-down in physical dimensions patentable. In fact, current case law supports the proposition that a change in size can result in patentable subject matter because unique technical problems arise when physical dimensions are reduced.

[30] Some of the key data sources available for patent search and analysis include: Thomson Derwent (World Patents Index, Patents Citation Index); Thomson Delphion; various issuing authorities' websites (PTO, European Patent Office, Japanese Patent Office, etc.); IFI CLAIMS (U.S. Patents/Citations, Current Patent Legal Status); assignee websites; INPADOC (family and legal status); Dialog (e.g., Dialindex); JAPIO (patent abstracts of Japan); engineering, technology, and scientific databases (INSPEC, EiCompendex, SCISEARCH, CAS); and markets and business databases (Factiva or PROMT). Some key software tools useful for patent analysis include Internet-based or enabled systems

29.7   Challenges Facing the U.S. Patent and Trademark Office

As stated previously, patent offices around the world are struggling to evaluate and prosecute bionanotechnology patent applications. As the U.S. patent system expands to accommodate bionanotechnology-related inventions, the PTO has yet to implement a plan to handle the soaring number of patent applications being filed. The rise of nanotechnology is presenting new challenges and problems to this overburdened agency as it attempts to handle the enormous growth in applications filed and patents granted in a wide range of disciplines encompassing "nanoscience" or "nanotechnology."

Some shortcomings at the agency regarding examining bionanotechnology applications requiring urgent attention are discussed below:

1. *Lack of a technology center*: The various divisions, or technology centers (TCs) of the PTO are focused on reviewing patents in a specific technology sector or field. For example, TC 1600 reviews patents pertaining to biotechnology and organic chemistry while TC 1700 examines patent applications pertaining to chemical and materials engineering. At present, the agency lacks a dedicated TC to handle applications on nanotechnology. Because nanotechnology is interdisciplinary in nature, patent applications that are searched, examined, and prosecuted in one center could and should be examined more effectively by a coordinated review of more than one center. Experts have criticized this, especially because there is traditionally little collaboration or communication among the various TCs. However, the PTO has no plans to form a new technology center, primarily due to the interdisciplinary nature of nanotechnology. The authors consider the formation of a separate technology center premature, and instead suggest creating a working group/committee within each TC that identifies nanotechnology patent applications as they are filed, formulates examination guidelines, undertakes training of selected examiners, and periodically meets with its counterparts from other technology centers. A progress report should be periodically presented to PTO customers at nanotechnology partnership meetings.

2. *Lack of a thorough classification system*: There is no thorough classification scheme for U.S. nanotechnology patents. Additionally, the PTO lacks effective automation tools for nanotechnology "prior art" searching. This could render examination unfocused and inefficient, resulting in the issuance of unduly broad patents. Some patent practitioners argue that a separation of the search from the examination of a patent application, as proposed by the 21st *Century Strategic Plan of the PTO*, could further undermine the examination of small tech applications. Recently the PTO proposed to outsource PCT searches. In November 2004, the PTO formally created a new digest (Class 977/DIG 1)[31] for nanotechnology-related patents.[32]

   However, this rudimentary classification is not sufficient to address the interdisciplinary range of technologies encompassed by bionanotechnology. It seems to be more of a public relations move on the part of the PTO to satisfy its critics.

3. *High attrition rates*: The PTO continues to be under-staffed in numerous examining areas and it is plagued by high attrition rates.[33] Some experts believe that these attrition rates are likely to be

---

(Delphion, Derwent, MicroPatent, Government sites, Google, Dogpile, Vivisimo, Teleport Pro); text mining tools (ClearForest, VantagePoint); and Microsoft Office (Pivot tables, charting, and organizing data).

[31] The PTO's definition requires that at least one dimension of an invention be in the sub-100 nm range. However, scale alone is not enough: to qualify as nanotechnology the nanoscale element of the product or process must be essential to whatever properties make it novel. In other words, an inventor gets a nanotechnology patent only if its utility is made unique by its nanoscale size, see also Section 29.6.

[32] In an e-mail dated November 2004 to Dr. Bawa, the PTO defined a digest as follows: "A digest is a collection of cross-reference patent disclosures based on a concept that relates to the concepts of a class but not to any particular subclass of that class. Digests are listed in numeric sequence at the end of each class schedule. As necessary, Patent Examiners create digests to simplify searches within their assigned arts. A digest cannot be designated as the OR [original] classification of a patent. In most instances, digests are not defined and are not available in the [PTO] Public Search Room."

[33] The agency's inability to retain a talented pool of patent examiners is highlighted by the cumulative loss of examiners from its biotechnology group (TC 1600) since fiscal year 2001. Couple this to the average growth rate

further exacerbated by poorly designed quality initiatives and a flawed electronic file and search software.

4. *Funding problems*: PTO's funding problems are compounded by Congress's long-standing practice of "diverting" user fees collected from patent applicants to the general budget.[34] Naturally, many of the PTO's problems would be solved by ending this practice of diverting user fees to other agencies. In fact, the pending legislation encompassing the 21st *Century Strategic Plan of the PTO* promises to end this diversion.

5. *High patent pendency*: The backlog in patent applications continues to build. This slows the ability of businesses to bring innovative new products to market. Since there is a backlog of almost 700,000 patent applications (as of this writing), presently the average time to process an application (i.e., patent pendency) is over 2 years.[35] However, given the current trend, the agency expects this backlog of unexamined patent applications to skyrocket to more than 1 million by 2008 (it was 70,000 in the mid-1980s). This implies an average pendency of 3 to 5 years (or longer) for patent approvals.[36] Since small tech patent applications are spread throughout the agency, it may be virtually impossible even to gauge the precise backlog in this case.

6. *Limited industry–PTO interaction*: Only a handful of experts from industry or academia have lectured on nanotechnology at the PTO. In fact, the first-ever Nanotechnology Customer Partnership Meeting was held at the PTO on September 11, 2003. The meeting was designed and developed to be a forum to share ideas, experiences, and insights between individual users and the PTO. However, the agency does not intend to use the meeting to arrive at any consensus.

7. *Little examiner training or guidelines*: to date, no training modules or examination guidelines have been developed to educate patent examiners in the complexities and subtleties of nanotechnology. No written guidelines for the practitioner have been published in the *Official Gazette of the PTO*. According to a report, the PTO began training its examiners in nanotechnology concepts and terminology in November 2004. However, that has not been enough to head off confusion in a realm where the same invention might be called a carbon nanotube, an elongated cylinder made of carbon, or a carbonaceous cylinder in three separate patent applications. Because such problems with terminology have resulted in examination errors, a number of overlapping patents have already been issued. In fact, most experts agree that protracted legal battles resulting from such "patent thickets" could freeze nanotechnology development in its tracks, posing the biggest threat to commercialization.

The results of the shortcomings cited earlier could result in:

- An improper rejection of a nanotechnology patent application due to an examiner's erroneous conclusion that the subject matter is not novel
- Issuance of an "overly broad" nanotechnology patent that infringes on previously issued patents and gives far too much control over a particular swath of nanotechnology, allowing the patentees to unfairly exclude competition[37]

(i.e., new application filings per period) of greater than 10% for the past five years, and the pendency figures become more serious [8].

[34] Since 1990, the agency has been totally funded by user fees (not taxpayer money) collected from inventors, businesses, universities and corporations. The President's recent proposal to allow the PTO to keep all of its patent fees it collects each year is being praised. The proposal will allow the PTO to hire hundreds of new examiners to attack the enormous patent application backlog. It is yet to be seen if Congress will uphold this directive, or if the damaging drain on the agency's resources will continue.

[35] Latest patent pendency statistics are available on the PTO website (www.uspto.gov).

[36] The Director of the PTO described his agency as being in a state of "crisis" while discussing this issue [9]. In fact, the PTO plans to hire 1000 examiner's each year through 2011, in an effort to address the patent pendency problem.

[37] Issuance of overly broad patents may stifle future development of nanotechnology by allowing inventors and corporations control of basic technologies; this violates the primary directive of the patent system to stimulate innovation and commerce.

- Issuance of a nanotechnology patent in spite of existing prior art that was overlooked during patent examination

Any of the above results is unacceptable. Issuance of patents of poor quality[38] (or too many "invalid" patents on early-stage research) is likely to cause enormous damage to global commercialization efforts by causing one or more of the following:

- Suppressing market growth and innovation
- Causing a loss of revenues, resources, and time
- Discouraging industry from conducting R&D and inducing unnecessary licensing
- Resulting in a flood of appeals and infringement lawsuits[39]
- Distorting away from high-quality inventions (introducing noise into investment, valuation, and contracting decisions) and undermining the purpose of the patent system (to promote progress)
- Eroding public trust vis-à-vis nanotechnology

As industry and trade groups continue to highlight these concerns to the PTO, the agency appears to have finally taken notice. However, critics charge that the PTO has failed to take any concrete steps to address the numerous concerns of the nanotechnology community. They point to the fact that the PTO has not taken any proactive steps to train its patent examiners in nanotechnology or undertaken any serious classification projects setting out the sub- and cross disciplines in the field, generally first steps in organizing new technologies.[40]

For now, it appears that the PTO will continue to struggle with nanopatent applications. How many invalid or overly broad patents have been issued so far by the agency? At this point, it is anyone's guess. However, if its track record on gene-therapy, genomics, and "business method" patents is any indication, the current agency practice presents the frightening prospect of mismanagement of the patent application and prosecution process for nanobusiness. It is hoped that the agency will not take the same lax approach that has resulted in the present serious backlog of patent applications. If the shortcomings described above are not addressed promptly and effectively, U.S. patents of poor quality could stifle research and impede nanotechnology from realizing its true potential, undermining the future of this promising technology. Furthermore, it is likely to create legal wrangles sufficient to stifle innovation, causing a serious negative impact on business ventures, venture capital, and entrepreneurs — all vital contributors to the development, exploitation, and promotion of the nanotechnology revolution.

As a result, companies bringing new products to the market will certainly face considerable uncertainty regarding the validity of broad and potentially overlapping patents held by others [11,12]. The ongoing land grab will definitely worsen the problem for companies striving to develop commercially viable

---

[38] Many, including the Federal Trade Commission (http://ftc.gov), believe that the PTO is often issuing patents of poor quality. *See* Federal Trade Commission, *To Promote Innovation: The Proper Balance of Competition and Patent Law and Policy*, October 2003. In fact, more than ever before, many experts are suggesting removing the presumption of validity associated with issued patents. Some of the factors contributing to poor examination at the PTO are the increasing number of patent applications filed each year and the agency's inability to attract and retain a talented pool of patent examiners. Moreover, even today with all the quality initiatives underway at the agency, examiners are still largely rewarded on the quantity of their work, not quality. Although flawless patent examination is impossible, cooperation between the Patent Office Professional Association (the labor union representing the examiners), the U.S. Department of Commerce and Congress is urgently needed to address this critical issue.

[39] Costly litigation, generally a last resort for most companies, is an untested area with respect to most sectors of nanotechnology. Few patent infringement cases actually result in trial. Figures from past years have been below 5%. Unlike biotechnology, mechanical and chemical patent practice, patent practitioners in nanotechnology do not yet have a fully established body of patent law specific to nanotechnology. Some experts have proposed providing a means to invalidate a patent short of litigation (similar to the current European "patent opposition"). Such a process would be beyond the present limited reexamination procedure. In fact, this simple "postgrant review" of patents would provide an inexpensive option compared to litigation as it would allow for withdrawal of a patent when it fails to fulfill the criteria for patentability, thereby encouraging licensing and commercialization activity [10].

[40] In fact, the PTO has dismantled its classification center and sent its classification experts to the TCs.

products. Therefore, it is critical that reforms be undertaken at the PTO in order to ensure a better balance between innovation and competition, particularly in the bionanotechnology space. Otherwise, cursory patent examination at the PTO and resultant issuance of invalid patents will certainly generate a crowded, entangled patent landscape with few open space opportunities for commercialization [11,12]. If such a dismal patent climate persists, investors are unlikely to invest in risky commercialization efforts. For them, competing in this high-stakes patent game may prove to be costly. In fact, this patent thicket problem may prove to be *the* major bottleneck to viable commercialization, negatively affecting the whole bionanotechnology enterprise.

References

[1] *Sizing Nanotechnology's Value Chain*, Lux Research, New York (2004).

[2] Raj Bawa, S.R. Bawa, S.B. Maebius, T. Flynn, and C. Wei. Protecting new ideas and inventions in nanomedicine with patents. *Nanomedicine* 1(2): 150–158 (2005).

[3] D. Risinger, J. Boris, B. Li, and J. Calone, US major pharmaceutical model and pipeline book, 4th Quarter issue, Merrill Lynch, New York (2003).

[4] Raj Bawa, Nanotechnology Patents and the U.S. Patent Office, 4 Small Times IP8 (2004).

[5] Raj Bawa, Nanotechnology Patenting in the U.S. *Nanotechnoogy Law and Business* 1(1): 31–50 (2004).

[6] Drew Harris, John Miller, Raj Bawa, Janell T. Cleveland, and Sean O'Neill, Strategies for resolving patent disputes over nanoparticle drug delivery systems. *Nanotechnology Law and Business* 1(4): 101–118 (2004).

[7] Adam Jaffe and Josh Lerner, Innovation and Its Discontents, Princeton University Press (2004).

[8] Kathleen Madden Williams, Current State of the Art at the U.S. Patent & Trademark Office, Genetic Eng News, June 1, 2003, p. 6.

[9] Eriq Gardner, Patent pending, Corporate Counsel, October 2003, pp. 104–107.

[10] Wesley M. Cohen and Stephen A. Merrill (Eds.) Patents in the Knowledge-Based Economy 120-141 (2003).

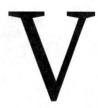

Tissue Engineering

John P. Fisher and Antonios G. Mikos
University of Maryland and Rice University

T ISSUE-ENGINEERING STUDIES are quickly becoming pervasive in not only biomedical engineering, but also cellular, and molecular biology. As evidenced in both the scientific and popular
   press, there exists considerable excitement surrounding the strategy of regenerative medicine.
Popular news magazines, including *Time, Barron's,* and *The Economist,* have recently reported on the
clinical possibilities as well as financial promise of tissue-engineered devices. Furthermore, a quick investigation of the National Library of Medicine database of scientific literature shows that tissue engineering
is a young field, with just over 4100 articles referencing the term and all references occurring since 1984.
Nevertheless, it is a field that has experienced an explosive growth, *with a remarkable 88% of these articles
published since the year 2000.* Qualitatively similar results are found in other databases, including the ISI
Web of Science.

In an effort to put the numerous advances in the field into a broad context, this section of the Biomedical Engineering Handbook is devoted to the dissemination of current thoughts on the development
of engineered tissues. To this end, the section has been divided into three parts: Fundamentals of Tissue
Engineering, Enabling Technologies, and Tissue-Engineering Applications. The Fundamentals of Tissue
Engineering subsection examines the properties of stem cells, primary cells, growth factors, and extracellular matrix as well as their impact on the development of tissue-engineered devices. The Enabling
Technologies subsection focuses upon those strategies typically incorporated into tissue-engineered
devices or utilized in their development, including scaffolds, nanocomposites, bioreactors, drug delivery
systems, and gene therapy techniques. Finally, the Tissue-Engineering Applications subsection presents
synthetic tissues and organs that are currently under development for regenerative medicine applications.

The contributing authors are a diverse group with backgrounds in academia, clinical medicine, and
industry. Furthermore, the section includes contributions from Europe, Asia, and North America, helping
to broaden the views on the development and application of tissue-engineered devices.

The format of this section is derived from the Advances in Tissue Engineering short course, which has
been held at Rice University since 1993. This short course has educated researchers, students, clinicians,
and engineers on both the fundamentals of tissue engineering and recent advances in many of the most

prominent tissue-engineering laboratories around the world. For many of the contributors, the chapter included in this section presents findings that have been recently discussed at the Advances in Tissue-Engineering short course.

The target audience for this section includes not only researchers, but also advanced students and industrial investigators. This section should be a useful reference for courses devoted to tissue engineering fundamentals and those laboratories developing tissue-engineered devices for regenerative medicine therapy.

30

Fundamentals of Stem Cell Tissue Engineering

Arnold I. Caplan
Case Western Reserve University

30.1 Introduction

In adults, stem cells are fundamental cell units within every tissue that function as a renewal source of highly specialized, terminally differentiated cells. The cell renewal serves to compensate for the normal cell turnover (cell death) or serves to provide reparative cells for the repair of minor defects. The stem cells can be thought of as the rejuvenation potential of the organism (high during the young or growth phase). Unfortunately, this renewal capacity decreases with age; even amphibians that are able to perfectly regenerate an entire limb lose this capacity with age [1]. Thus, one of the long-term goals of Tissue Engineering is to learn how to control and regulate this natural regeneration potential, so that tissue performance can be enhanced or massive defects can be repaired via an intrinsic regenerative pathway.

As a scientific discipline, Tissue Engineering is very young, and thus, is quite distant from its long-term goal. To approach this goal, a series of sequential technological advancements must be made. Our earliest achievements, material-assisted repair of various tissues, have been accomplished in a variety of preclinical models and, in the case of skin, with clinical success in humans [2–5]. In all these cases, scaffolds, cells and growth factors/cytokines, or a combination of these have been surgically implanted. Like the first crude cardiac pacemakers, their initial successful implantation served as a catalyst for their improvement and perfection, a process that is ongoing.

THE MESENGENIC PROCESS

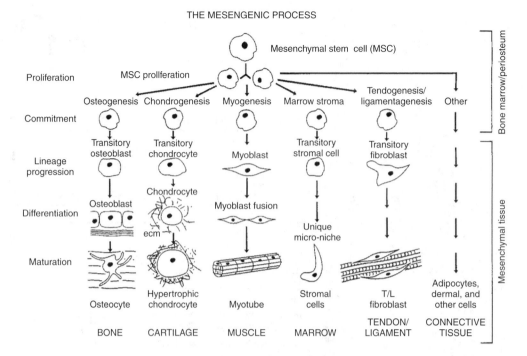

FIGURE 30.1   The mesengenic process involves the replication of MSCs and their entrances along multistep lineage pathways to produce differentiated cells that fabricate specific tissues such as bone, cartilage, and so on. We know most about the lineages on the left and least about those on the right of the diagram.

It follows that if we are to learn how to manage the various intrinsic organ stem cells to reconstruct or repair specific tissues, we must first obtain a deep understanding of these unique stem cells; we must understand what makes these cells divide, differentiate, grow old, and expire. We must learn how to position these stem cells in defects, how to coordinate the integration of blood vessels and nerves, and how to integrate the host tissue with the *neo*-tissue. Lastly, as Tissue Engineers, we must recognize that each individual has a genetically controlled variation, even between close family members, that will affect the fine-tuning of every repair logic.

It would be impossible to review the fundamental characteristics of every stem cell/organ system in the body in this chapter. Thus, I will focus on only one stem cell system, the mesenchymal stem cells (MSCs), that has already proven to be a versatile source of reparative cells for Tissue Engineering applications.

30.2   Mesenchymal Stem Cells

I suggested long ago that bone marrow contained a stem cell capable of differentiating into a number of mesenchymal tissues; I call this cell a mesenchymal stem cell (MSC) and the lineage sequences Mesengenesis, as pictured in Figure 30.1 [6–11]. This suggestion was based on my familiarity with embryonic mesenchymal progenitors [12–14] and partially on the early studies of Freidenstein [15] and, in particular, of Owen. Indeed, it was Owen [16] who drew me into the adult MSC realm by her scholarly treatise. In the late 1980s, Stephen Haynesworth and I [10,17,18] embarked in the task of isolating these rare MSCs from human bone marrow; the key to our success was a selected batch of fetal bovine serum that worked quite well with embryonic chick limb bud mesenchymal progenitor cells [19]. Subsequently, my collaborators have shown that marrow-derived MSCs are capable of differentiating into cartilage [20,21], bone [22,23], muscle [24,25], bone marrow stroma (hematopoietic support tissue) [26–28], fat [29], tendon [30,31], and other connective tissues. Other laboratories have provided evidence that MSCs can differentiate into neural cells [32,33], cardiac myocytes [34,35], vascular support cells (pericytes, smooth muscle cells) [36,37], and perhaps other tissues [38,39]. The multipotential of culture expanded MSCs provides the stimulus to consider them as candidates for various Tissue Engineering strategies. Such strategies, by necessity, require both scaffolds and various growth factors/cytokines to manage the proliferation and differentiation of MSCs to form specific tissues *in vivo*. In some cases, the tissue defect, itself, and its microenvironment provide instructional support; in other cases, pretreatment of the cells or placing the cells within unique scaffolds provides the instructional cues [40]. The details of these experiments provide the experimental basis for improving these early Tissue Engineering logics in preparation for their clinical use.

30.3 Fundamental Principles

When in doubt of how to manage the multiple parameters of tissue repair/regeneration, Mother Nature should be asked to reveal her secrets as a guide. Philosophically, we believe that many of the fundamental principles of Tissue Engineering involve the recapitulation of specific aspects of embryonic tissue formation [41,42]. For example, the embryonic mesenchyme that will form the cartilage anlagen of long bones has a high ratio of undifferentiated progenitor cells to extracellular matrix (ECM). This embryonic mesenchymal ECM is composed of type I collagen, hyaluronan, fibronectin, and water. In experiments with chick limb bud mesenchymal progenitor cells in culture, we showed that the molecular weight of hyaluronan is instructive to these progenitor cells, in that high molecular weight chondro-inductive or chondro-permissive [43,44]. Others have shown that high molecular weight hyaluronan is antiangiogenic. Indeed, the exclusion of blood vessels is also chondrogenic. Thus, a scaffold of hyaluronan coated with type I collagen or fibronectin to bind the MSCs would be expected to be chondrogenic; indeed, we have shown it to be just that [45]. The scaffold must be quite porous to allow the newly differentiated chondrocytes to fabricate their unique and voluminous ECM that controls the cushioning properties of the cartilaginous tissue. By mimicking the cell density and ECM of embryonic progenitor mesenchyme, cartilaginous tissue forms in large, full thickness defects in adult rabbit knees [41].

In the absence of hyaluronan, the key physical characteristic of prechondrocytes is their close proximity to their neighbors and maintenance of the cells in a rounded shape [20,21]. One way to achieve this condition is to place adult MSCs in a type I collagen lattice. The cells will bind to the lattice fibrils and rapidly contract the lattice to bring the cells into a high density configuration [46]. In culture, in the presence of TGF-β [20,21] or *in vivo* by the contracted network excluding blood vessels, the MSCs will form cartilage tissue. Thus, mimicking the embryonic microenvironment both chemically and physically can result in the specific differentiation of MSCs.

In contrast, the rules for bone formation are quite different from those governing cartilage formation [13,47,48]. In this case, we again studied embryonic chick limb development and observed that vasculature is the driver for bone formation. In the context of Tissue Engineering scaffolds, bone formation requires rapid invasion of blood vessels into the pores of the scaffold. For example, porous calcium phosphate ceramics coated with fibronectin to bind MSCs provide an inductive microenvironment for bone formation in subcutaneous or orthotopic sites [52]; it may be that the calcium phosphate, itself, is informational, but more likely it binds osteogenic growth factors that stimulate the MSCs. The MSCs bind to the walls of the pores in the ceramic where they divide and, as vasculature invades from the host tissue at the implantation site, the cells differentiate into sheets of osteoblasts and fabricate the lamellae of bone [49]. The vasculature does not go to the walls of dead-ends of the ceramic and in this location, the MSCs divide and pile-up on one another and form compact areas of cartilage. Thus, in the two different microenvironments (vascular and avascular), the MSCs form two very different tissues (bone and cartilage). This bone/cartilage forming capacity has been quantified and has become our gold standard for judging the quality of MSC preparations [19,50].

Again, for emphasis, mimicking Mother Nature, especially her very efficient embryological events, is, for us, a fundamental rule of engineering tissue repair or regeneration in adults.

30.3.1 *In Vitro* Assays for the Osteogenic and Chondrogenic Lineages

We have established an *in vitro* assay for the differentiation of human and animal MSCs into bone and cartilage phenotypes [20–23]. For osteogenesis, the inclusion of dexamethasone (*dex*), ascorbate, and eventually β-glycerophosphate (a phosphate donor) causes the MSCs to enter the osteogenic lineage, upregulate alkaline phosphatase activity (two- to ten-fold), secrete various bone proteins, and eventually, organize calcium apatite deposition within type I collagen fibrils comparable to that observed in *in vivo* osteoid.

Likewise, we have established the *in vitro* conditions for causing MSCs to differentiate into chondrocytes [21,22]. Simply, MSCs are pelleted to the bottom of 15-ml conical plastic tubes, and the medium is changed to a chemically defined medium containing TGF-β at a concentration of 2–10 ng/ml. The pelleted cells come off the bottom of the tube and form a sphere of cells that differentiate into chondrocytes that fabricate type II collagen- and aggrecan-rich ECM. Both of these *in vitro* assays and the porous ceramic assay *in vivo* have been tested by diluting the human or rat marrow-derived MSCs with dermal fibroblasts. In these experiments, the human dermal fibroblasts were shown to *not* differentiate into bone or cartilage phenotypes. The results of these assays are that MSC preparations can have 25–50% non-MSCs without experiencing a major loss of osteo- or chondrogenic tissue formation [51]. In the context of Tissue Engineering logics, these observations could mean that the implanted MSCs could be "contaminated" by host-derived fibroblasts, but would still retain their capacity to regenerate osteochondral tissue.

30.4 MSCs and Hematopoietic Support

The marrow stroma is a highly specialized connective tissue that provides different microenvironmental niches for the different lineage pathways of hematopoiesis. Each of the different lineage pathways of hematopoiesis requires a different combination of cytokines and growth factors. The marrow stromacytes not only fabricate these unique physical niches of connective tissue, but they secrete specific bioactive molecules for the initiation and control of these lineage pathways. The MSC differentiation sequence into these different hematopoietic lineage support phenotypes has yet to be described. However, just as complex multicellular Dexter cultures are able to support *in vitro* hematopoiesis, so can homogeneous populations of MSCs incubated in Dexter medium provide support for hematopoiesis. Because of these very specific hematopoietic-support functions, the term "marrow stromal cells" should be reserved for these highly differentiated marrow connective tissue cells that facilitate hematopoietic differentiation.

It is important to stress that the differentiation of MSCs into marrow stroma or osteoblasts involves a time-dependent sequence of differentiation steps (the lineage) with each step involving the up- and down-regulation of many genes. For example, we have compared the cytokine secretion into the medium in 24 h by human MSCs cultured in growth medium, in osteogenic medium (*dex*, ascorbate), and in stroma-generating medium (Dexter conditions or in the presence of IL-1α). The cytokine quantity is very different for these three culture conditions [28]. Also of considerable importance was the realization that the constitutive levels of these cytokines are different for each donor batch of cells under standard growth or differentiation conditions. These measured differences emphasize the influence of the genotype on the observed differentiation/lineage pathways and multigenic expression profiles of each MSC donor or recipient or both.

30.4.1 Muscle, Tendon, and Fat

Both *in vitro* and *in vivo*, microenvironments control the differentiation and expressional profile of the MSCs and their differentiated descendants. Without going into all of the details, MSCs have been shown to differentiate into skeletal muscle, into Achilles or patella tendon tissue, and into adipocytes as reviewed earlier in this chapter. The cell culture conditions or *in vivo* tissue sites were different for each of the phenotypes observed. Importantly, the introduction of MSCs into specific tissue locations was followed by using markers or molecular probes [53,54]. For example, normal rodent marrow-derived MSCs form

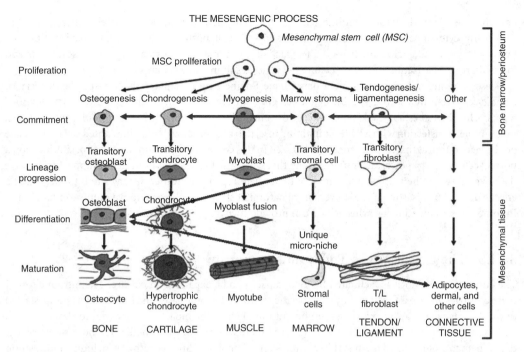

FIGURE 30.2   The mesengenic process in which transdifferentiation is depicted by horizontal arrows. For example, adipocytes can transdifferentiate into osteoblasts.

dystrophin-positive skeletal muscle in the limbs of *mdx* mice that are dystrophin-negative [25]. Likewise, reparative *neo*-tissue formed in rabbit tendon defects when autologous MSCs were introduced in suitable scaffolds [30,31].

The isolation of MSCs from fat provides an intriguing question of the origin of these progenitor cells [34,55]: Are these MSCs an intrinsic occupant of fat, are they associated with the blood vessels, or are they dedifferentiated adipocytes? Both marrow- and fat-derived MSCs differentiate into adipocytes and the other phenotypes of the Mesengenic Lineage (Figure 30.1). These observations raise the question of phenotypic *plasticity* and whether differentiated cells dedifferentiate into a stem cell and then rediffer-entiate into an alternate phenotype or whether the differentiated cells *transdifferentiate* directly into a different mesenchymal phenotype (as pictured in Figure 30.2). The current data indicate that cells can transdifferentiate along certain permissible routes without backing up to the stem cell status.

30.4.2   A New Fundamental Role for MSCs

Previously, all of the preclinical models used MSCs to provide the cells that fabricate the specialized, differentiated tissues. I propose that MSCs could be used in a different clinical context: that MSCs could provide a trophic influence to structure a reparative microenvironment. The precedent for cells secreting cytokines/growth factors that have regulator effects is well established in regenerative biology. For example, Singer long ago established the trophic effect of nerves on amphibian limb regeneration [56]. He showed that a certain quantum of nerves in the limb stump is required for successful limb regeneration; the nerves delivered neural trophic factors and the electrical or neural transmitter release was not associated with this trophic effect as evidenced by switching the ratios of different nerves into the limb stump.

In this regard, the bone marrow stroma derived from MSCs provides very specific instructional niches for various lineage pathways of hematopoiesis as discussed earlier. The question arises, "Can MSCs structure reparative microenvironments *without* differentiating into specific differentiated cells or tissue?" The answer appears to be "yes!" In the cases of cardiac infarct (ischemia) and stroke (brain ischemia), bone marrow-derived MSCs when injected into the ischemic zones do not massively differentiate into cardiac myocytes or neural cells. Rather, the MSCs appear to establish a trophic influence that is antifibrotic (antiscar tissue) and angiogenic [57–60]. The lack of the formation of extensive fibrotic, scar tissue and the rapid revascularization of the affected tissue zones result in clinically improved tissues.

These new findings suggest to me a new Tissue Engineering paradigm: the site-specific delivery of trophic cells (cells that secrete specific cytokines/growth factors) that structure reparative microenvironments. Already well established is the concept of genetically engineering the insertion of a specific gene, for example, transfection with a BMP-containing insert, to be synthesized by an implanted cell to stimulate bone regeneration at that implantation site [61,62]. In this context, why not implant to a specific location a normal cell that has a powerful trophic activity that will cause the implantation site to support restorative therapy? Likewise, the trophic effect may not stimulate repair, but rather, it may inhibit a debilitating effect, such as fibrosis, so that the slower, more natural host-mediated regenerative events can take place. In some cases, as mentioned earlier, MSCs can provide such a trophic effect.

30.4.3   The Use of MSCs Today and Tomorrow

The current use of MSCs is facilitated by their capacity to be expanded in culture. The introduction of these cells back *in vivo* is facilitated by site-specific scaffolds. In some cases, the MSCs can be jump-started down a lineage pathway by exposing them in culture to a specific bioactive agent (*dex* for bone [23,49], TGF-β for cartilage [20,21], etc.). In the long-term, there will be a way to mobilize the body's own MSCs, direct them to a site, expand them at the site, and signal them into a lineage pathway including modulation of the phenotypic expression of the cells to produce the appropriate tissues for that repair site (articular cartilage at the knee and auricular cartilage in the ear). There are at least two unknowns in this process. First, we do not know what mobilizes MSCs from marrow or other depots, although there are data that suggest such mobilization takes place following injury [34,35,63]. Second, we do not know how such mobilized MSCs dock into specific tissues. Consistent with this lack of knowledge is our inability to obtain high engraftment percentages for systemically administered, culture-expanded (marked) MSCs [64]. At best, only 2 to 3% of systemically administered MSCs home back to bone marrow with most of the infused cells lodging in the lung (probably a size issue) and liver (probably a fibronectin issue).

30.5   Cell Targeting

To systematically learn more about control of engraftment of systemically or locally introduced reparative cells, we have developed protocols which facilitate the targeting of cells to specific molecular docking sites. The approach is to insert specific targeting molecules into the cell membranes. The first approach involved palmitoylating protein G and painting this "primer" coat on cells, since the hydrophobic fatty acid tail of palmitic acid will quantitatively insert into the cell's plasma membrane lipid bilayer core. This positions the protein to orient out of the cell's surface. Protein G binds strongly to the Fc region of antibodies. Thus, we can put different paints (antibodies) on the primer coat on the cell's surface. Moreover, if we had specific addressing or docking peptides, we could construct a fusion protein with such addresses in series with the Fc-region of antibodies in a molecularly reconstructed fusion protein as pictured in Figure 30.3.

In a proof of this technology concept, Dennis et al. [65] have created a deep cartilage defect in the condyle of rabbits. A library of antibodies exists against various epitopes in the ECM of deep articular cartilage as opposed to the surface of the condylar cartilage. With these antibodies, cultured rabbit or human chondrocytes were shown to home to the defect and subsequently fabricate cartilage ECM in an organ culture test system. The painting moieties were shown to not affect the viability or replication of the painted cells nor the differentiation capacity of painted MSCs. The long-term goal is the injection of painted chondrogenic cells into the synovial space to direct their docking to cartilage defects and, then, to facilitate the repair/regeneration of the cartilage.

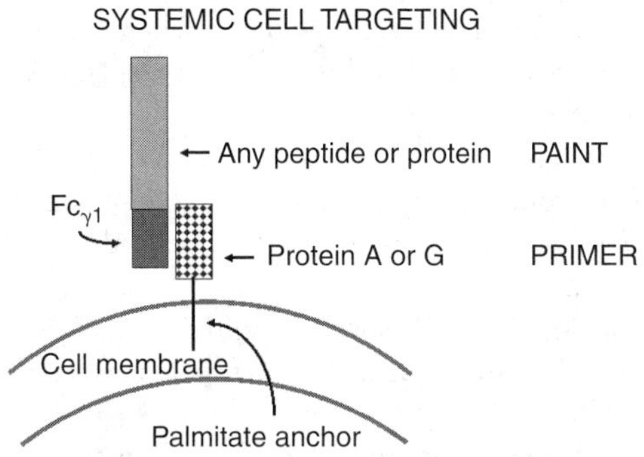

SYSTEMIC CELL TARGETING

FIGURE 30.3 Cell targeting technology involves palmitic acid that is derivatized with Protein A or G (PRIMER). The fatty acid hydrophobic tail quantitatively inserts into the lipid bilayer of the cell membrane. An antibody or fusion protein with the Fc domain at one end is referred to as the Paint.

I could imagine using the painting technology to insert tissue-specific address or targeting molecules to implanted scaffold docking sites as a basis for various systemically or locally supplied reparative cells, for example, stem cells for a variety of tissues. The docking of these cells could improve tissue performance or repair localized defects. Enhanced engraftment of stem cells, either by mobilizing intrinsic populations or by injecting extrinsically expanded cells, should provide useful Tissue Engineering strategies for tomorrow. Clearly, a lot of work needs to be done before this long-term goal will be realized.

Acknowledgments

The research was supported by grants from NIH, DOE, and the State of Ohio. I thank my colleagues at Case Western Reserve University and elsewhere for providing the experimental basis for this chapter.

References

[1] Nye, H.L. et al., Regeneration of the urodele limb: a review, *Dev. Dyn.*, 226, 280–294, 2003.

[2] Bell, E., Living tissue formed *in vitro* and accepted as skin-equivalent tissue of full thickness, *Science*, 211, 1052–1054, 1981.

[3] Boyce, S.T., Cultured skin for wound closure, in *Skin Substitute Production by Tissue Engineering: Clinical and Fundamental Applications*, chap. 4, Rouabhila, M. (Ed.), Landes Bioscience, Austin, 1997.

[4] Hardin-Young, J. et al., Approaches to transplanting engineered cells and tissues, in *Principles of Tissue Engineering*, chap. 23, Guilak, F., Butler, D.L., Goldstein, S.A., and Mooney, D.J. (Eds.), 2nd ed. Academic Press, 2000.

[5] Brisco, D.M. et al., The allogeneic response to cultured human skin equivalent in the hu-PBL-SCID mouse model of skin rejection, *Transplantation*, 67, 1590–1599, 1999.

[6] Caplan, A.I., Biomaterials and bone repair, *BIOMAT*, 87, 15–24, 1988.

[7] Caplan, A.I., Cell delivery and tissue regeneration, *J. Control. Release*, 11, 157–165, 1989.

[8] Caplan, A.I., Mesenchymal stem cells, *J. Orthop. Res.*, 9, 641–650, 1991.

[9] Caplan, A.I. et al., Cell-based technologies for cartilage repair, in *Biology and Biomechanics of the Traumatized Synovial Joint: The Knee as a Model*, Finerman, G.A.M. and Noyes, F.R. (Eds.), American Academy of Orthopaedic Surgeons, Rosemont, pp. 111–122, 1992.

[10] Haynesworth, S.E., Baber, M.A., and Caplan, A.I., Cell surface antigens on human marrow-derived mesenchymal cells are detected by monoclonal antibodies, *Bone*, 13, 69–80, 1992.

[11] Caplan, A.I., The mesengenic process, *Clin. Plast. Surg.*, 21, 429–435, 1994.

[12] Jargiello, D.M. and Caplan, A.I., The fluid flow dynamics in the developing chick wing, in *Limb Development and Regeneration, Part A*, Fallon, J.F. and Caplan, A.I. (Eds.), Alan R. Liss, Inc., New York, pp. 143–154, 1983.

[13] Caplan, A.I., Cartilage, *Sci. Am.*, 251, 84–94, 1984.

[14] Caplan, A.I., The molecular control of muscle and cartilage development, in *39th Annual Symposium of the Society for Developmental Biology*, Subtelney, S. and Abbott, U. (Eds.), Alan R. Liss, Inc., New York, pp. 37–68, 1981.

[15] Friedenstein, A.J., Petrakova, K.V., Kurolesova, A.I., and Frolova, G.P., Heterotopic of bone marrow. Analysis of precursor cells for osteogenic and hematopoietic tissues, *Transplantation*, 6, 230–247, 1968.

[16] Owen, M., Lineage of osteogenic cells and their relationship to the stromal system, in *Bone and Mineral Research,* chap. 1, Peck, W.A. (Ed.), Elsevier Science, Oxford, 1985.

[17] Haynesworth, S.E. et al., Characterization of cells with osteogenic potential from human marrow, *Bone*, 13, 81–88, 1992.

[18] Haynesworth, S.E., Goldberg, V.M., and Caplan, A.I., Diminution of the number of mesenchymal stem cells as a cause for skeletal aging, in *Musculoskeletal Soft-Tissue Aging: Impact on Mobility, Section 1,* chap. 7, Buckwalter, J.A., Goldberg, V.M., and Woo, S.L.-Y. (Eds.), American Academy of Orthopaedic Surgeons, Publishers, pp. 79–87, 1994.

[19] Lennon D.L. et al., Human and animal mesenchymal progenitor cells from bone marrow: identification of serum for optimal selection and proliferation, *In Vitro Cell Dev. Biol.*, 32, 602–611, 1996.

[20] Johnstone, B. et al., *In vitro* chondrogenesis of bone marrow-derived mesenchymal progenitor cells, *Exp. Cell Res.*, 238, 265–272, 1998.

[21] Yoo, J.U. et al., The chondrogenic potential of human bone-marrow-derived mesenchymal progenitor cells, *J. Bone Joint Surg.*, 80, 1745–1757, 1998.

[22] Dennis, J.E. and Caplan, A.I., Differentiation potential of conditionally immortalized mesenchymal progenitor cells from adult marrow of a H-2Kb-tsA58 transgenic mouse, *J. Cell. Physiol.*, 167, 523–538, 1996.

[23] Jaiswal, N., Haynesworth, S.E., Caplan, A.I., and Bruder, S.P., Osteogenic differentiation of purified, culture-expanded human mesenchymal stem cells *in vitro*, *J. Cell Biochem.*, 64, 295–312, 1997.

[24] Wakitani, S., Saito, T., and Caplan, A.I., Myogenic cells derived from rat bone marrow mesenchymal stem cells exposed to 5-azacytidine, *Muscle Nerve*, 18, 1417–1426, 1995.

[25] Saito, T. et al., Myogenic expression of mesenchymal stem cells within myotubes of mdx mice *in vitro* and *in vivo*, *Tissue Eng.*, 1, 327–344, 1996.

[26] Majumdar, M. et al., Human marrow-derived mesenchymal stem cells (MSCs) express hematopoietic cytokines and support long-term hematopoiesis when differentiated toward stromal and osteogenic lineages. *J. Hematother. Stem Cell Res.*, 9, 841–848, 2001.

[27] Dennis, J.E., Carbillet, J.-P., Caplan, A.I., and Charbord, P., The STRO-1+ marrow cell population is multi-potential, *Cells Tissues Organs*, 170, 73–82, 2002.

[28] Haynesworth, S.E., Baber, M.A., and Caplan, A.I., Cytokine expression by human marrow-derived mesenchymal progenitor cells *in vitro*: effects of dexamethasone and IL-1α, *J. Cell Physiol.*, 166, 585–592, 1996.

[29] Dennis, J.E. et al., A quadripotential mesenchymal progenitor cell isolated from the marrow of an adult mouse, *J. Bone Mineral. Res.*, 14, 1–10, 1999.

[30] Young, R.G. et al., The use of mesenchymal stem cells in Achilles tendon repair, *J. Orthop. Res.*, 16, 406–413, 1998.

[31] Awad, H. et al., Autologous mesenchymal stem cell-mediated repair of tendon, *Tissue Eng.*, 5, 267–277, 1999.

[32] Weimann, J.M. et al., Contribution of transplanted bone marrow cells to Purkinje neurons in human adult brains, *Proc. Natl Acad. Sci. USA*, 100, 2088–2093, 2003.

[33] Prockop, D.J., Marrow stromal cells as stem cells for nonhematopoetic tissues, *Science*, 276, 71–74, 1997.

[34] Laflamme, M.A., Myerson, D., Saffitz, J.E., and Murry, C.E., Evidence for cardiomyocyte repopulation by extracardiac progenitors in transplanted human hearts, *Circ. Res.*, 90, 634–640, 2002.

[35] Orlic, D. et al., Mobilized bone marrow cells repair the infracted heart, improving function and survival, *Proc. Natl Acad. Sci. USA*, 98, 10344–10349, 2001.

[36] Jackson, K.A. et al., Regeneration of ischemic cardiac muscle and vascular endothelium by adult stem cells, *J. Clin. Invest.*, 107, 1395–1402, 2001.

[37] Shi, S. and Gronthos, S., Pervascular niche of postnatal mesenchymal stem cells in human bone marrow dental pulp, *J. Bone Mineral Res.*, 18, 696–704, 2003.

[38] Jiang, Y. et al., Pluripotency of mesenchymal stem cells derived from adult marrow, *Nature*, 418, 41–49, 2002.

[39] Reyes, M. et al., Purification and *ex vivo* expansion of postnatal human marrow mesodermal progenitor cells, *Blood*, 98, 2615–2625, 2001.

[40] Caplan, A.I., Tissue engineering strategies for the use of mesenchymal stem cells to regenerate skeletal tissues, in *Functional Tissue Engineering*, chap. 10, Guilak F., Butler, D.L., Goldstein, S.A., and Mooney, D.J. (Eds.), Springer-verlag, New York, 2003.

[41] Caplan, A.I. et al., The principles of cartilage repair/regeneration, *Clin. Orthop. Relat. Res.*, 342, 254–269, 1997.

[42] Caplan, A.I., Embryonic development and the principles of tissue engineering, in *Novartis Foundation: Tissue Engineering of Cartilage and Bone*, John Wiley & Sons, London, pp. 17–33, 2003.

[43] Kujawa, M.J. and Caplan, A.I., Hyaluronic acid bonded to cell culture surfaces stimulates chondrogenesis in stage 24 limb mesenchyme cell cultures, *Dev. Biol.*, 114, 504–518, 1986.

[44] Kujawa, M.J., Carrino, D.A., and Caplan, A.I., Substrate-bonded hyaluronic acid exhibits a size-dependent stimulation of chondrogenic differentiation of stage 24 limb mesenchymal cells in culture, *Dev. Biol.*, 114, 519–528, 1986.

[45] Caplan, A.I., Tissue engineering designs for the future: new logics, old molecules, *Tissue Eng.*, 6, 1–8, 2000.

[46] Ponticiello, M.S. et al., Gelatin-based resorbable sponge as a carrier matrix for human mesenchymal stem cells in cartilage regeneration therapy, in *Osiris Therapeutics*, John Wiley & Sons, 2000.

[47] Caplan, A.I. and Pechak, D.G., The cellular and molecular embryology of bone formation, in *Bone and Mineral Research*, Vol. 5, Peck, W.A. (Ed.), Elsevier, New York, pp. 117–184, 1987.

[48] Caplan, A.I., Bone development, in *Cell and Molecular Biology of Vertebrate Hard Tissues*, CIBA Foundation Symposium 136, Wiley, Chichester, pp. 3–21, 1988.

[49] Ohgushi, H. and Caplan, A.I., Stem cell technology and bioceramics: from cell to gene engineering, *J. Biomed. Mater. Res.*, 48, 1–15, 1999.

[50] Dennis, J.E., Konstantakos, E.K., Arm, D., and Caplan, A.I., *In vivo* osteogenesis assay: a rapid method for quantitative analysis, *Biomaterials*, 19, 1323–1328, 1998.

[51] Lennon, D.P. et al., Dilution of human mesenchymal stem cells with dermal fibroblasts and the effects on *in vitro* and *in vivo* osteogenesis, *Dev. Dynam.*, 219, 50–62, 2000.

[52] Goshima, J., Goldberg, V.M., and Caplan, A.I., The osteogenic potential of culture-expanded rat marrow mesenchymal cells assayed *in vivo* in calcium phosphate ceramic blocks, *Clin. Orthop. Relat. Res.*, 262, 298–311, 1991.

[53] Allay, J.A. et al., LacZ and IL-3 expression *in vivo* after retroviral transduction of marrow-derived human osteogenic mesenchymal progenitors, *Hum. Gene Ther.*, 8, 1417–1427, 1997.

[54] Gimble, J.M. et al., The function of adipocytes in the bone marrow stroma: an update, *Bone*, 19, 421–428, 1996.

[55] Dragoo, J.L. et al., Tissue-engineered cartilage and bone using stem cells from human infrapatellar fat pads, *J. Bone Joint Surg.*, 85, 740–747, 2003.

[56] Singer, M., Neurothophic control of limb regeneration in the newt, *Ann. NY Acad. Sci.*, 228, 308–322, 1974.

[57] Stamm, C. et al., Autologous bone-marrow stem-cell transplantation for myocardial regeneration, *Lancet*, 361, 45–46, 2003.

[58] Shake, J.G. et al., *In-vivo* mesenchymal stem cell grafting in a swine myocardial infarct model: molecular and physiologic consequences, *Ann. Thorac. Surg.*, 73, 1919–1926, 2002.

[59] Chen, J. et al., Therapeutic benefit of intracerebral transplantation of bone marrow stromal cells after cerebral ischemia in rats, *J. Neurol. Sci.*, 189, 49–57, 2001.

[60] Chen, J. et al., Intravenous bone marrow stromal cell therapy reduces apoptosis and promotes endogenous cell proliferation after stroke in female rat, *J. Neurosci. Res.*, 73, 778–786, 2003.

[61] Lieberman, J.R. et al., The effect of regional gene therapy with bone morphogenetic protein-2 producing bone-marrow cells on the repair of segmental femoral defects in rats, *J. Bone Joint Surg. Am.*, 81, 905–917, 1999.

[62] Evans, C.H. and Robbins, P.D., Possible orthopaedic applications of gene therapy, *J. Bone Joint Surg. Am.*, 77, 1103–1114, 1995.

[63] Mahmood, A. et al., Treatment of traumatic brain injury in adult rats with intravenous administration of human bone marrow stromal cells, *Neurosurgery*, 53, 697–703, 2003.

[64] Gao, J. et al., The dynamic *in vivo* distribution of bone marrow-derived mesenchymal stem cells after infusion, *Cells Tissues Organs*, 169, 12–20, 2001.

[65] Dennis, J.E., Cohen, N., Goldberg, V.M., and Caplan, A.I., Targeted delivery of progenitor cells for cartilage repair, *J. Orthop. Res.*, 22, 735–741, 2004.

31

Growth Factors and Morphogens: Signals for Tissue Engineering

A. Hari Reddi
University of California

31.1 Introduction

Tissue engineering is the exciting discipline of design and construction of spare parts for the human body to restore function based on biology and biomedical engineering. The basis of tissue engineering is the triad of signals for tissue induction, responding stem cells, and the scaffolding of extracellular matrix. Among the many tissues in the human body bone has the highest power of regeneration and therefore is a prototype model for tissue engineering based on morphogenesis. Morphogenesis is the developmental cascade of pattern formation, body plan establishment, and culmination of the adult body form. The cascade of bone morphogenesis in the embryo is recapitulated by demineralized bone matrix-induced bone formation. The inductive signals for bone morphogenesis, the bone morphogenetic proteins (BMPs) were isolated from demineralized bone matrix. BMPs and related cartilage-derived morphogenetic proteins (CDMPs) initiate cartilage and bone formation. The promotion and maintenance of the initiated skeleton is regulated by several growth factors. Tissue engineering is the symbiosis of signals (growth factors and morphogens), stem cells, and scaffolds (extracellular matrix). The rules of architecture for tissue engineering are a true imitation of principles of developmental biology and morphogenesis.

31.2 Tissue Engineering and Morphogenesis

An understanding of the molecular principles of development and morphogenesis, is a prerequisite for tissue engineering. We define tissue engineering as the science of design and manufacture of new tissues for functional restoration of the impaired organs and replacement of lost parts due to disease, trauma, and tumors [1]. Tissue engineering is based on principles of developmental biology and morphogenesis, biomedical engineering, and biomechanics.

Morphogenesis is initiated by morphogens. The promotion and maintenance of morphogenesis is achieved by a variety of growth factors. Generally, morphogens are first identified in fly and frog embryos by genetic approaches, differential displays, and subtractive hybridization expression cloning. An alternate biochemical approach of "grind and find" from adult mammalian bone led to the isolation of BMPs, the premier signals for bone morphogenesis. We now discuss the identification, isolation, and molecular cloning of BMPs from a natural biomaterial, the demineralized bone matrix.

31.3   The Bone Morphogenetic Proteins

Bone grafts have been used to aid the healing of recalcitrant fractures. Demineralized bone matrix induced new bone formation. Bone induction by demineralized bone matrix is a sequential cascade [2–4]. The key steps in this cascade are chemotaxis of progenitor cells, proliferation of progenitor cells, and finally differentiation first into cartilage and then bone. The demineralized bone matrix is devoid of any living cells and is a biomaterial that elicits new bone formation. The insoluble collagenous bone matrix binds plasma fibronectin [3] and promotes the proliferation of cells. Proliferation was maximal on day 3, chondroblast differentiation was evident on day 5, and chondrocytes were abundant on day 7. The cartilage hypotrophied on day 9 with concominant vascular invasion and osteogenesis. On days 10 to 12 maximal alkaline phosphatase activity, a marker of bone formation, was observed. Hematopoietic differentiation was observed in the ossicle on day 21. The sequential bone development cascade is reminiscent of bone morphogenesis in limb.

A systematic study of the biochemical basis of bone induction was initiated. A bioassay for bone induction was established *in vivo* in rats. The insoluble demineralized bone matrix was extracted in 4 M guanidine hydrochloride, a dissociative extractant. About 3% of the proteins were solubilized and the rest was the insoluble residue. The extract and the residue alone were unable to induce bone formation. However, reconstitution of the extract to residue yielded new bone morphogenesis. Thus there is collaboration between soluble signals and the insoluble matrix scaffold to yield new bone formation [5,6]. This key experiment predates the term tissue engineering and demonstrates the collaboration of soluble signals and insoluble scaffolding as a critical concept in practical tissue engineering. Collagen appear to be an optimal scaffold [7]. The bone induction is dependent on the hormonal status including vitamin D [8,9]. Irradiation of the recipient blocked the cellular cascade of osteogenesis [10].

This bioassay was a critical development in the quest for the purification of the bioactive bone morphogens, the bone morphogenetic proteins [11–15]. There are nearly 15 members of BMPs in the human genome (Table 31.1). BMPs are dimeric molecules with a single disulfide bond. The mature monomer consists of seven canonical cysteines contributing to three interchain disulfides and one interchain disulfide bond.

BMPs stimulate chondrogenesis in limb bud mesodermal cells [16]. BMP 2 stimulates osteoblast maturation [17]. BMPs are chemotactic for human monocytes [18]. In addition to initiating chondrogenesis BMPs maintain proteoglycan biosynthesis in bovine articular cartilage explants [19,20]. Recombinant human growth/differentiation factors (GDF-5) stimulate chondrogenesis during limb development [21].

BMPs interact with BMP receptors I and II on the cell surface/membrane [1,22]. BMP receptors are serine/threonine kinases. The intracellular substrates for these kinases called Smads function as relays to activate the transcriptional machinery [23]. The three functional classes are (1) receptor-regulated Smads, namely, Smads 1, 5, and 8, (2) the common partner Smad — 4, and (3) the inhibitory Smads 6 and 7. There are Smad-dependent and independent pathways for activation of BMP signaling including new bone formation.

TABLE 31.1   The BMP Family in Mammals[a]

BMP subfamily	Generic name	BMP designation
BMP 2/4	BMP-2A	BMP-2
	BMP-2B	BMP-4
BMP-3	Osteogenin	BMP-3
	Growth/differentiation factor-10 (GDF-10)	BMP-3B
OP-1/ BMP-7	BMP-5	BMP-5
	Vegetal related-1 (Vgr-1)	BMP-6
	Osteogenic protein-1 (OP-1)	BMP-7
	Osteogenic protein-1 (OP-2)	BMP-8
	Osteogenic protein-1 (OP-3)	BMP-8B
	Growth/differentiation factor-2 (GDF-2)	BMP-9
	BMP-10	BMP-10
	Growth/differentiation factor-11 (GDF-11)	BMP-11
GDF-5,6,7	Growth/differentiation factor-7 (GDF-7) or cartilage-derived morphogenetic protein-3 (CDMP-3)	BMP-12
	Growth/differentiation factor-6 (GDF-6) or cartilage-derived morphogenetic protein-2 (CDMP-2)	BMP-13
	Growth/differentiation factor-5 (GDF-5) or cartilage-derived morphogenetic protein-1 (CDMP-1)	BMP-14
	BMP-15	BMP-15

[a] BMP-1 is not a BMP family member with seven canonical cysteines. It is a procollagen-C proteinase related to *Drosophila* Tolloid.

31.4   Growth Factors

Growth factors are proteins with profound influence on proliferation and growth of cells. Growth factors stimulate the differentiation of progenitor/stem cells. The growth factors include many subgroups and such as Insulin like growth factors (IGFs), fibroblast growth factors (FGFs), and platelet-derived growth factors (PDGFs).

Insulin like growth factors are polypeptides related to Insulin. There are two members, IGF-I and IGF-II. Liver is the predominant site of IGF-I synthesis, and is stimulated by pituitary growth hormone. IGF biological activity is modulated by IGF-binding proteins (IGFBP). There are six different IGFBPs. IGFs promote extracellular matrix biosynthesis by osteoblasts.

Fibroblast growth factors (FGFs) are proteins with multiple members. FGFs are mitogens for endothelial cells. Along with Vascular Endothelial Growth Factors (VEGFs), FGFs are critical for bone formation. It is well known that vascular invasion is a prerequisite for endochodral bone formation.

Platelet-derived growth factors come in three isoforms, namely, AA, AB, and BB. They are primarily produced by platelets in blood. Various isoforms stimulate bone formation.

31.5   BMPs Bind to Extracellular Matrix

The critical role of extracellular matrix in morphogenesis of many tissues during development is well known. The extracellular matrix is a supramolecular assembly of collagens, proteoglycans, and glycoproteins. The collagens are tissue specific and the proteoglycans include chondroitin sulfate, dermatan sulfate, heparan sulfate/heparin, and keratan sufate. Recombinant BMP 4 and BMP 7 bind to heparan sulfate/heparin, collagen IV of the basement membrane [24]. The binding of a soluble morphogen to insoluble extracellular matrix renders the morphogen to act locally and protects it from proteolytic degradation and therefore extends its biological half-life. Thus, extracellular matrix scaffolding is an efficient delivery system for tissue engineering. Growth factors such as FGFs bind to heparan sulfate. An emerging concept for tissue engineering is the tethering of signals to scaffolds to restrict their diffusion.

31.6   Clinical Applications

Recombinant BMP 2 has been approved by the Food and Drug administration for spine fusion and open fractures of tibia due to orthopaedic trauma. There have been several clinical applications of BMPs in orthopaedic surgery [25–29]. The developing experience of BMPs will be of immense utility to the nascent field of tissue engineering, the science of design-based manufacture of spare parts for human skeleton based on signals, stem cells, and scaffolding [1,30] in medicine and dentistry. A prototype paradigm has validated the proof of principle for tissue engineering based on tissue transformation by BMPs and scaffolding [31].

31.7   Challenges and Opportunities

Despite the exciting advances in clinical applications of BMPs there remain many challenges. Foremost among them is the need for developing synthetic scaffolds to deliver recombinant BMPs for skeletal tissue engineering. The development of synthetic scaffolds with an ability to respond to biomechanical influences that are known to be critical for musculoskeletal structures will lead to a quantum improvement of current tissue engineering approaches to bone, cartilage, and meniscus. The remaining challenges make the field of morphogen-based tissue engineering an exciting frontier with unlimited opportunities.

Acknowledgments

The research in the Center for Tissue Regeneration is supported by the Lawrence Ellison Chair in Musculoskeletal Molecular Biology and grants from NIH and DOD. I thank Danielle Neff for the outstanding help in completion of this article.

References

[1] Reddi, A.H., Role of morphogenetic proteins in skeletal tissue engineering and regeneration, *Nat. Biotechnol.*, 16, 247, 1998.

[2] Reddi, A.H. and Anderson, W.A., Collagenous bone matrix-induced endochondral ossification hemopoiesis, *J. Cell Biol.*, 69, 557, 1976.

[3] Weiss, R.E. and Reddi, A.H., Synthesis and localization of fibronectin during collagenous matrix-mesenchymal cell interaction and differentiation of cartilage and bone *in vivo*, *Proc. Natl Acad. Sci. USA*, 77, 2074, 1980.

[4] Reddi, A.H., Cell biology and biochemistry of endochondral bone development, *Coll. Relat. Res.*, 1, 209, 1981.

[5] Sampath, T.K. and Reddi, A.H., Dissociative extraction and reconstitution of extracellular matrix components involved in local bone differentiation, *Proc. Natl Acad. Sci. USA*, 78, 7599, 1981.

[6] Sampath, T.K. and Reddi, A.H., Homology of bone-inductive proteins from human, monkey, bovine, and rat extracellular matrix, *Proc. Natl Acad. Sci. USA*, 80, 6591, 1983.

[7] Ma, S., Chen, G., and Reddi, A.H., Collaboration between collagenous matrix and osteogenin is required for bone induction, *Ann. NY Acad. Sci.*, 580, 524, 1990.

[8] Reddi, A.H., Extracellular matrix and development, in *Extracellular Matrix Biochemistry*, Piez, K.A. and Reddi, A.H. Eds., Elsevier, New York, 1984, p. 247.

[9] Sampath, T.K., Wientroub, S., and Reddi, A.H., Extracellular matrix proteins involved in bone induction are vitamin D dependent, *Biochem. Biophys. Res. Commun.*, 124, 829, 1984.

[10] Wientroub, S. and Reddi, A.H., Influence of irradiation on the osteoinductive potential of demineralized bone matrix, *Calcif. Tissue Int.*, 42, 255, 1988.

[11] Wozney, J.M. et al., Novel regulators of bone formation: molecular clones and activities, *Science*, 242, 1528, 1988.

[12] Luyten, F.P. et al., Purification and partial amino acid sequence of osteogenin, a protein initiating bone differentiation, *J. Biol. Chem.*, 264, 13377, 1989.

[13] Celeste A.J. et al., Identification of transforming growth factor beta family members present in bone-inductive protein purified from bovine bone, *Proc. Natl Acad. Sci. USA*, 87, 9843, 1990.

[14] Ozkaynak, E. et al., OP-1 cDNA encodes an osteogenic protein in the TGF-beta family, *EMBO J.*, 9, 2085, 1990.

[15] Wang, E.A. et al., Recombinant human bone morphogenetic protein induces bone formation, *Proc. Natl Acad. Sci. USA*, 87, 2220, 1990.

[16] Chen, P. et al., Stimulation of chondrogenesis in limb bud mesoderm cells by recombinant human bone morphogenetic protein 2B (BMP-2B) and modulation by transforming growth factor beta 1 and beta 2, *Exp. Cell Res.*, 195, 509, 1991.

[17] Yamaguchi, A. et al., Recombinant human bone morphogenetic protein-2 stimulates osteoblastic maturation and inhibits myogenic differentiation *in vitro*, *J. Cell Biol.*, 113, 681, 1991.

[18] Cunningham, N.S., Paralkar, V., and Reddi, A.H., Osteogenin and recombinant bone morphogenetic protein 2B are chemotactic for human monocytes and stimulate transforming growth factor beta 1 mRNA expression, *Proc. Natl Acad. Sci. USA*, 89, 11740, 1992.

[19] Luyten, F.P. et al., Natural bovine osteogenin and recombinant human bone morphogenetic protein-2B are equipotent in the maintenance of proteoglycans in bovine articular cartilage explant cultures, *J. Biol. Chem.*, 267, 3691, 1992.

[20] Lietman, S.A. et al., Stimulation of proteoglycan synthesis in explants of porcine articular cartilage by recombinant osteogenic protein-1 (bone morphogenetic protein-7), *J. Bone Joint Surg. Am.*, 79, 1132, 1997.

[21] Khouri, R.K., Koudsi, B., and Reddi, A.H. M Tissue transformation into bone *invivo* a potential practical application, *JAMA*, 266, 1953, 1991.

[22] ten Dijke, P. et al., Identification of type I receptors for osteogenic protein-1 and bone morphogenetic protein-4, *J. Biol. Chem.*, 269, 16985, 1994.

[23] Imamura T. et al., Smad6 inhibits signalling by the TGF-beta superfamily (see comments), *Nature*, 389, 622, 1997.

[24] Paralkar, V.M. et al., Interaction of osteogenin, a heparin binding bone morphogenetic protein, with type IV collagen, *J. Biol. Chem.*, 265, 17281, 1990.

[25] Einhorn, T.A., Clinical applications of recombinant BMPs: early experience and future development, *J. Bone Joint Surg.*, 85A, 82, 2003.

[26] Li, R.H. and Wozney, J.M. Delivering on the promise of bone morphogenetic proteins, *Trends Biotechnol.*, 19, 255, 2001.

[27] Ripamonti, U., Ma, S., and Reddi A.H. The critical role of geometry of porous hydroxyapatite delivery system in induction of bone by osteogenin, a bone morphogenetic protein, *Matrix*, 12, 202, 1992.

[28] Geesink, R.G., Hoefnagels, N.H., and Bulstra, S.K. Osteogenic activity of OP1, bone morphogenetic protein 7 (BMP 7) in a human fibular defect, *J. Bone Joint Surg.*, 81, 710, 1999.

[29] Friedlaender, G.E. et al., Osteogenic protein 1 (bone morphogenic protein 7) in the treatment of tibial non-unions, *J. Bone Joint Surg. Am.*, 83A, S151, 2001.

[30] Govender et al., Recombinant human bone morphogenetic protein 2 for treatment of open tibiol fractures: a prospective, controlled, randomized study of four hundred and fifty patients. *J. Bone Joint Surg. Am.*, 84A, 2123, 2002.

[31] Nakashima, M. and Reddi, A.H. The application of bone morphogenetic protein to dental tissue engineering, *Nat. Biotechnol.*, 21, 1025, 2003.

[32] Khouri, R.K., Koudsi, B., and Reddi, A.H. Tissue transformation into bone *in vivo*: a potential practical application. *JAMA*, 266, 1953, 1991.

32

Extracellular Matrix: Structure, Function, and Applications to Tissue Engineering

Mary C. Farach-Carson
Roger C. Wagner
Kristi L. Kiick
University of Delaware

32.1   Introduction

A major goal of tissue engineering is to employ the principles of rational design to recreate appropriate signals to cells that promote biological processes leading to production of new tissues or repair of damaged ones. A key modulator of cell behavior is the ECM that provides individual cells with architectural cues of time and space, modulates bioavailability of soluble growth and differentiation factors, and organizes multicellular tissue development. This chapter will focus on key ECM components and their functions, emphasizing relationships between natural matrices present in both hard and soft tissues and cell function. The concept of "mining" the natural matrix for active motifs that are useful in tissue engineering applications also is introduced. Finally, the utility of translating knowledge gained from study of native ECM to controlled delivery of growth factors and deliberate modulation of cell and tissue phenotype for engineering purposes is discussed.

32.2 ECM and Functional Integration of Implanted Materials

Cells sense and respond to a variety of signals that include those that are soluble such as growth factors, differentiation factors, cytokines, and ion gradients. In addition, cell behavior and phenotype is governed by responses to other types of signals that include mechanical forces, electrical stimuli, and various physical cues. Immobilized protein matrices that generally are fixed in space also regulate cell function. The general term that has come to denote the complex mixture of proteins on the outside of cells that governs their behavior is ECM. Evolution has provided cells with surface receptors to ECM components that enable them to recognize and decipher the signals that they encounter from the ECM and which influence cell growth, division, and differentiation [1].

For descriptive purposes, cell adhesion is classified into categories of cell–substratum and cell–cell attachment. Cell–cell interactions may occur between like cells (homotypic events) or between dissimilar cells (heterotypic). Homotypic interactions stabilize epithelia, which typically lie upon a sheet of specialized ECM called the basement membrane, discussed in Section 32.2. Heterotypic interactions govern many normal cellular phenomena including embryo–uterine implantation, immune surveillance, cell migration during embryogenesis, and neurotransmission. They also characterize the pathological states of cancer metastasis, rejection of transplanted tissues and organs, and inflammation [2,3]. In the context of tissue engineering, both types of cellular interactions must be understood, and thus hopefully manipulated, to ensure successful integration of transplanted materials.

There exists in tissues an exquisite balance between the anabolic process of ECM production and the catabolic process of ECM turnover. Introduction of foreign materials inevitably disrupts this natural homeostasis. A goal of tissue engineering is to successfully introduce replacement tissues that will, through stimulation of anabolic processes, lead to ECM production and acceptance of engineered materials rather than their immediate or eventual destruction via activation of catabolic pathways. To facilitate biointegration, both degradable and nondegradable foreign materials can be modified with native ECM or motifs derived from proteins in the ECM. Achievement of this goal requires a thorough understanding of the structural relationships among molecules in the ECM, their molecular interactions directing cell adhesion events, their biosynthesis and turnover, and their natural functions.

32.3 Basement Membranes and Focal Adhesions

Basement membranes, also called basal lamina, are sheets of highly organized ECM that are associated with the basal membrane of epithelial cells, around muscle cells, below endothelial cells in blood vessels, supporting fat cells, and associated with Schwann cells surrounding peripheral nerve axons [4,5]. In addition to physically separating the cell layers comprising epithelia and stroma, they provide a diversity of functions including structural support, selective filtration, and serve as barriers to invasion. They also establish cell polarity, influence cell metabolism, induce cell differentiation, direct cell migration, and organize membrane receptors. Figure 32.1 depicts scanning and transmission (SEM and TEM, respectively) electron micrographs of natural basement membranes illustrating their typical functions and structural roles in separating cells in tissues. Note that cells contact the basement membrane on a single face that establishes cell polarity and creates the basal surface of attaching cell. The basement membrane exists as a complex meshwork comprised of the proteins collagen IV, laminin, proteoglycans including perlecan, agrin, and collagens XV and XVIII, fibulin, BM-40 (SPARC), and nidogen/entactin [4]. The spatial relationships among these molecules were examined using atomic force microscopy where thin, threadlike strands of heparan sulfate attached to certain proteoglycans were seen to protrude from the core meshwork and proposed to function as an "entropic brush" that could filter proteins by their constant thermal

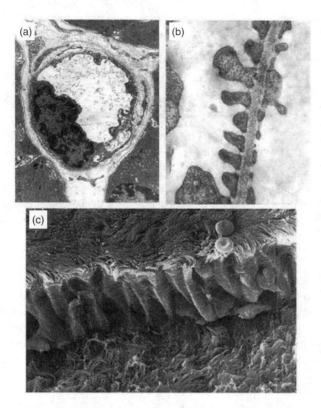

FIGURE 32.1   (a) Transmission electron micrograph of a transverse section through a blood capillary consisting of a single endothelial cell wrapped around to join upon itself to create a lumen. The endothelial cell is (as are all epithelia) bordered by a basement membrane on its external aspect. The basement membrane is shared by pericapillary cells called "pericytes" that are represented by the small bits of seemingly isolated cell material at the capillary periphery. (b) High magnification TEM of the glomerular basement membrane separating the capillaries of the kidney glomerulus and the "podocytes" on their surface. The capillary endothelium (on the right) contains apparent gaps which in three dimensions represent "fenestrae" or "little windows" in the capillary wall. The podocyte "pedicles" on the left actually are part of larger cell processes out of the plane of section. This panel highlights the function of the basement membrane as part of a filtration barrier which sieves large molecules and those with cationic charges. (c) A SEM of the ciliated respiratory epithelium of the trachea. Part of the epithelium has been denuded during preparation (bottom) to reveal meshwork collagen IV fibers of the underlying basement membrane and connective tissue underneath it.

motion within the basement membrane [5]. Collagen IV and laminin within the basement membrane form two overlapping polymeric networks [6,7] with which the other components interact in a highly organized fashion. The basement membrane provides an anchor for cells, which adhere to it using specific surface receptors called integrins [1]. Focal adhesions are the sites of cell–ECM attachment that were first identified ultrastructurally as cell surface electron dense regions near sites of cell attachment to substrata and then recognized as interfaces with the cytoskeleton [8]. Focal adhesions belong to the contractile class of matrix contacts, distinct from protrusive contacts or those that provide mechanical support [9]. Figure 32.2 diagrams a cartoon of a focal adhesion consisting of both integrin and nonintegrin receptors in the plasma membrane attached to ECM in the basement membrane. The processes of anchoring and spreading of cells on substrata occur as multistep processes that involve, among other things, clustering of surface receptors at sites of focal adhesions. Protein complexes link the cytoplasmic tails of surface receptors to the cytoskeleton, facilitating cell adhesion and transmitting signals through the intracellular network that ultimately signal to the nucleus to inform the cell that it has attached. This form of signaling has come to be called "outside in" signaling and is a key component of engineering functional interfaces between materials and living cells. It is important to note that cells seldom rely on one adhesion system

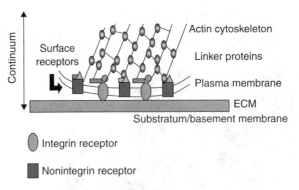

FIGURE 32.2   Focal adhesion schematic. The diagram illustrates the components of the focal adhesion attaching an adherent cell to an ECM substratum. Note the continuum of functional connections between the ECM and the cytoskeleton, bridged by both integrin and nonintegrin transmembrane receptors.

to support cell attachment, a concept thought to confer some degree of protection to cells against single mutations that would completely abolish adhesion-competence. Nonetheless, mutations in key adhesion molecules found in focal adhesions frequently have extreme and adverse consequences on tissue and organ development [10]. Guided tissue regeneration with artificial two-dimensional matrices such as GORE-TEX® (expanded polytetrafluoroethylene or ePTFE) that resemble basement membranes has been widely used for treatment of periodontal and bone defects and relies upon the membrane for physical separation of cell layers during healing [11].

32.4   Focal Adhesions as Signaling Complexes

Attachment of cells to substrata provides signals for spreading, migration, survival, and proliferation. As mentioned above, cell surface receptors recognize ECM components in a manner that is both specific and reversible. The initial attraction and attachment often involves nonintegrin adhesion events that may be related solely to charge or hydrophobic interactions between surfaces [12,13]. Examples include recognition of polyanionic polymers such as those presented by the heparan sulfate or chondroitin sulfate glycosaminoglycans (GAGS) attached to surface proteoglycans. Depending on the nature of the molecules involved, these adhesive events may or may not be dependent on the presence of divalent cations such as Ca^{2+} [14–16]. In any case, these early events tend to rely on multiple, low affinity interactions similar to the way that Velcro® functions as a two-sided hook and loop fastener. Once cells adhere, higher affinity interactions such as those involving integrin receptors are stabilized during the spreading phase of adhesion. A very interesting feature of integrin interactions with ECM proteins is that they display a wide range of ligand affinities ranging from 10^{-6} to 10^{-9} l/M under different conditions [17]. It is this quality that ensures reversibility of integrin-mediated cell adhesion and allows cells to *both* attach and detach from biological substrata at sites of focal adhesions. In general, cells attach to differentiate and carry out specialized cell functions such as secretion, absorption, or signal transmission. They detach in order to migrate and proliferate. Interestingly, many epithelia undergo a form of programmed cell death known as anoikis if forcibly detached from their substrata [18]. Elegant studies of migrating cells have shown simultaneous formation of focal adhesions with substrata on the leading edge of the cell, and dissolution of attachment sites on the trailing end [19].

Receptor clustering during adhesion triggers cascades of events involving protein phosphorylation and dephosphorylation that carry intracellular signals through the cell from surface to nucleus, ultimately leading to changes in gene transcription. Frequently, changes in cell shape mediated by the cytoskeleton accompany and promote these signals. An emerging paradigm for signal transduction involves the formation of protein complexes or "signalosomes" held together by specific interactions of regulatory molecules with scaffolding proteins that, like the electron transport chain of the mitochondrion, reduce diffusion and speed up signal transmission. The interested reader is referred to one of several recent reviews on this exciting subject [20–22].

Once activated, feedback loops within cells act quickly to attenuate signals, preventing desensitization to extracellular signals and in some cases preserving cell viability. For example, prolonged Ca^{2+} signals are associated with activation of apoptotic pathways and cell death [23]. These loops also allow cells to return to a responsive state in which they can respond to subsequent signals that they may encounter from the ECM. Changes that occur within cells and that feed back to modulate the activity of surface receptors have come to be called "inside out" signals and modulate activity of both integrin and nonintegrin receptors in focal adhesions.

32.5 ECM and Skeletal Tissues

The ECM in cartilage is frequently described as part of a pericellular or "territorial" matrix that is both avascular and noninnervated. Figure 32.3 depicts several views illustrating the architecture of cartilage at the cellular level. Note that, unlike cells interacting with basement membranes, cells in mesenchyme are surrounded on all sides by the territorial matrix. This is particularly evident in Figure 32.3c showing a single chondrocyte in its lacunae. The chondrocyte has a very unique relationship with its microenvironment that has been well described [24]. The cartilage matrix consists of type II collagen and various noncollagenous

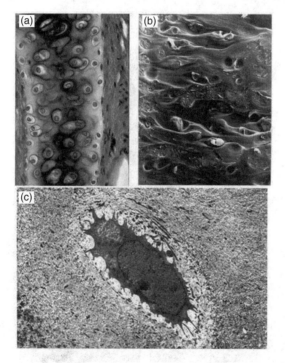

FIGURE 32.3 (See color insert following page **20**-14.) (a) Section through hyaline cartilage of the trachea. Dark staining regions surrounding cells (chondrocytes) are pericellular or "territorial" matrix and represent most recently-deposited cartilage matrix. (b) SEM of hyaline cartilage showing lacunae or "little lakes" in which chondrocytes reside. In this preparation some are occupied by cells and others are empty because the cells have fallen out during cutting of the cartilage. The fibrous nature of the matrix (due to the presence of type II collagen) is evident. (c) TEM of a chondrocyte within a lacuna. Collagen fibers can be seen in the cartilage matrix surrounding the lacunae. These fibers are not seen in light microscopic preparations such as those in panel a since they have the same refractive index as the collagen matrix material.

ECM molecules that differ depending on the type and differentiated state of cartilage. In articular cartilage, type II, IX, and XI collagens form a meshwork that provides form and tensile stiffness and strength [25]. Type VI collagen is present in the matrix surrounding the chondrocyte; aggrecan provides resilience to compressive forces, and small proteoglycans such as fibromodulin help to stabilize the matrix. Other noncollagenous proteins that are present include cartilage oligomeric matrix protein (COMP), perlecan, anchorin II, and tenascin. It has been proposed that the presence of tenascin-C in the articular cartilage matrix, a protein which is absent from growth plate cartilage, may help articular chondrocytes avoid endochondral ossification [26]. The role of the cartilage ECM in tissue engineering was reviewed recently [27]. In the growth plate, a progressive series of events occur to produce a cartilaginous matrix that gives way to bone matrix [28–30]. Early stages are marked by high rates of cell proliferation and ECM production. The final stage of development of growth plate cartilage is hypertrophy, marked by turnover of matrix, mineralization, invasion of marrow vasculature, and chondrocyte apoptosis. Type X collagen is the classical marker for hypertrophic cartilage ECM, and is absent from articular cartilage [31].

The ECM of bone is distinct from that of cartilage. Bone tissue (Figure 32.4a) is greater than 95% type I collagen based and includes noncollagenous proteins such as the acidic calcium binding proteins osteocalcin, bone sialoprotein, osteopontin, and osteonectin/SPARC. Of these, osteocalcin and bone sialoprotein can be considered specific to bone. It has been proposed that compact lamellar bone and woven trabecular bone have distinct matrix protein compositions and ratios [32]. The marrow compartment (Figure 32.4b) can be considered as structurally distinct from proper bone, although it houses cellular precursors for bone cells. As shown in Figure 32.4c,d, osteocytes, like chondrocytes, are surrounded by and embedded in matrix, but in this case the matrix normally remains fully mineralized. The processes of

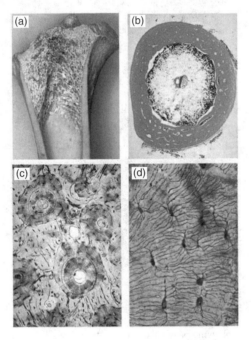

FIGURE 32.4   (See color insert.) (a) Transverse cut through the metaphysis of a calf femur. The bone shaft is compact bone and spongy bone with bony trabeculae lining the interior. (b) Cross-section through a decalcified preparation of a fetal femur. Compact bone encloses the marrow cavity. (c) Preparation of compact bone. Concentric lamellae of Haversian systems surround blood vessels. Interstitial lamellae represent older Haversian systems replaced during bone remodeling. (d) High magnification image of a compact bone preparation. India ink fills lacunae in which embedded bone cells (osteocytes) are normally found. Channels connecting lacunae are called "canaliculi." These are occupied by cell processes and provide a means whereby osteocytes communicate with one another.

bone remodeling that maintain structural integrity of bone and include a finely tuned balance between osteoclastic bone resorption and osteoblastic bone formation have been reviewed recently [33]. ECM is one of many influences on bone cell function that also include growth factors, physical stimuli, metabolic demands, and structural responsibilities [34].

32.6   Sources of ECM for Tissue Engineering Applications

It is critical to choose an ECM that will support cell adhesion, and also ensure survival, growth, and appropriate cell differentiation following adhesion. A number of alternatives exist for the tissue engineer including commercial mixed matrices based upon the composition of basement membranes (collagen IV, laminin, perlecan, nidogen/entactin). One example of such a commercial matrix is Matrigel™ that is available in both growth factor replete and depleted forms. This matrix is extracted from Engelbreth–Holm–Swam (EHS) mouse sarcoma and provides a material similar to the mammalian basement membrane. Available from the global nonprofit ATCC (http://www.atcc.org/) is an ECM solution also representing a solubilized basement membrane solution (30-2501) similar to Matrigel. This preparation contains tissue plasminogen activator as well as a number of growth factors including transforming growth factor β, epidermal growth factor, insulin-like growth factor 1, fibroblast growth factor 2, and platelet derived growth factor. Both these products form a gel at room temperature that will support growth and differentiation of cells grown on (or in) it as a two- or three-dimensional matrix.

Serum also provides a variety of adhesion factors including fibronectin and vitronectin, along with a rich selection of soluble, circulating growth factors. The response of cells to serum components is highly variable, as is the composition of serum itself. Because of the uncertainty in knowing the exact composition of serum for use in tissue engineering applications, batch testing of serum for long-term applications is encouraged when its use is necessitated. Purified ECM molecules provide a more reliable and predictable source for engineering applications. Smaller molecules can be expressed as recombinant proteins in either bacteria, insect, or mammalian cells in bioreactors [35–37]. Each of these expression systems provides a set of advantages and disadvantages that have been reviewed [38]. For ECM molecules of large size or complexity (collagens, many proteoglycans, noncollagenous glycoproteins), problems can occur related to size, microheterogeneity, yield, and scalability. For most of the molecules in this class, function requires posttranslational modifications that can only be acquired when expressed by mammalian cells. In this case, some luck has been achieved by expressing recombinant constructs in cell lines such as the HEK-293 cell line or even in tissue systems [37,39]. For very large matrix molecules, such as perlecan, that are too large to be expressed as full length recombinant proteins, it has been possible to create smaller expression constructs that retain functions of individual protein domains [37]. Of interest, there appears to be considerable cell type diversity in the manner and extent of posttranslational modification affecting the fine structure of the carbohydrate chains. For example, domain I of perlecan that contains consensus sites for both heparan and chondroitin sulfate chain addition can be produced in both active and inactive forms depending on the cells producing it [40].

An alternative to the use of recombinant ECM proteins is the use of synthetic peptides or proteolytic fragments of native molecules that retain selected functional properties of their parent molecules. Many ECM molecules contain a consensus sequence recognized by integrin receptors that consists of the triplet peptide, arginine–glycine–aspartate (RGD) sequence. The context in which this peptide is presented by the ECM molecule containing it determines the strength and the specificity of the interaction. Examples of common ECM molecules containing the RGD sequence include fibronectin, osteopontin, laminin, vitronectin, some collagens, and tenascin. Current effort is focused on identifying other active motifs present within ECM molecules that are small enough to be prepared as synthetic proteins. One promising example of this is the laminin-derived cell binding YIGSR sequence that has been proposed for derivatization of scaffolds for breast and soft tissue reconstruction [41]. Another is the tetrapeptide sequence REDV which simulates an active motif in the CS5 domain of fibronectin [42]. This subject is discussed further in Section 32.7 devoted to mining of the ECM.

32.7 Properties of ECM

Extracellular matrix in all tissues possesses certain properties that allow it to support tissue cohesion and provide microstructure. The most salient of these properties is that of *self-assembly* [43]. Protein and carbohydrate components of secreted ECM will self-associate in a highly ordered and predictable fashion that is tissue and cell type specific. Associations are based upon the presence of highly conserved motifs and independently folded domains whose structures are increasingly appreciated [44]. Interactions occur based upon complementary secondary and tertiary structural features including charge properties, ion and metal bridging, hydrophobic domains, redox interactions, and covalent bonding. The structures that form may produce either two-dimensional networks such as the meshwork of the basement membrane, or three-dimensional structures in space such as that of the territorial matrix. While most of the assembly is thought to occur extracellularly, there is evidence that some degree of assembly may be initiated during biosynthesis and take place within intracellular secretory vesicles creating a sort of "pre-fabricated" scaffold to promote rapid assembly once secretion into the extracellular compartment occurs [45]. In the sea urchin model system, it has been proposed that distinct intracellular vesicles form and are directionally released during exocytosis; these have been termed "basal laminar vesicles" and "apical vesicles" [46].

32.8 Mining the ECM for Functional Motifs

In the new age of the fruition of the genome projects, it is exciting to consider the possibility that bioinformatic approaches can be used to identify structure–function relationships in natural ECM molecules for use in translational biology including tissue engineering. This process, which has come to be termed "data mining," can identify motifs in larger molecules that can be used to manipulate behavior of cells and tissues *in vitro* and *in vivo*. Motifs can be included in small synthetic peptides, recombinant domains expressed in viral, bacterial, or mammalian expression systems, or rationally designed chemically synthesized mimics. The latter, in particular, frame the enormous potential of rational drug design when combined with computer modeling of protein interactions. The following sections will briefly describe the properties of some individual ECM molecules which provide the raw material for mining the ECM for functional motifs. In each case, the Swiss-Protein (http://au.expasy.org/sprot/) ID number for the *human* protein is provided as a link to the electronic database for that protein. The complete domain structure of each molecule may be accessed using Pfam (http://www.sanger.ac.uk/Software/Pfam/) and typing in the accession number in Protein Search.

32.8.1 Collagen

Members of the collagen family are diverse; they make up some one-third of all the protein in the body and model the framework of connective tissues [47,48]. Collagens form what can be thought of as "functional aggregates" with noncollagenous molecules to form macrostructures including fibrils, basement membranes, filaments, canals, and sheets. Fibril forming collagens are synthesized in precursor forms that are sequentially processed during or following secretion into the ECM [45]. Collagens and proteins with collagen-like domains now number at least 27 types with 42 distinct polypeptide chains; there are 20 additional proteins with collagen-like domains and 20 isoenzymes that modify collagen structure [49]. Examples of fibrillar collagens include type I collagen [collagen I α1 (PO2452), α2 (P08123)] found in connective tissues, and type II collagen [collagen II α1 (PO2458)] found in cartilage. Each of these assembles as a triple helix that once incorporated into rod-like fibrils can also assemble with other collagenous and noncollagenous proteins [48]. Figure 32.5 shows several views of collagen type I fibrils. Figure 32.5c depicts the structural relationship of a fibroblast and its ECM, including collagen fibrils seen in cross-section. The dimensional comparison between the cell and the collagen is also evident in this photograph (bar in the figure is 1 μm). The inset clearly shows the banding pattern characteristic of collagen type I when viewed by transmission electron microscope (TEM). Fibril associated collagens with interrupted triple helices (FACIT) collagens associate with surfaces of collagen fibrils in many tissues including skin,

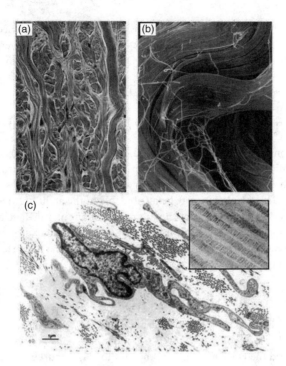

FIGURE 32.5 (See color insert.) (a) Light micrograph of collagen fiber bundles in dense, irregular connective tissue such as the dermis of the skin. Nuclei of fibroblasts (cells that secrete procollagen which is processed and assembled into collagen extracellularly) can be seen closely associated with the fibers. (b) SEM of bands of type I collagen fiber bundles. Individual fibers can be seen independent of the fiber bundles. (c) TEM of a fibroblast in close association with bundles of collagen fibers sectioned transversely, obliquely and longitudinally. The inset shows individual collagen fibers exhibiting the characteristic periodic banding pattern.

tendon, and cartilage. Meshwork or basement membrane collagens include basement membrane-localized collagen IV [α1 (PO2462) and α2 (P08572)], hypertrophic cartilage-specific collagen X [α1 (Q03692)] and endothelial collagen VIII [α1 (P27658)]. Collagen VII [α1 (Q99715)] is also a member of this family and forms anchoring fibrils that connect skin and mucosa to underlying tissue.

32.8.2 Fibronectin

Fibronectin (PO2751) is a glycoprotein found in soluble form in plasma and in insoluble form in loose connective tissue and basement membranes. Fibronectin binds cell surfaces as well as various other ECM molecules including collagen, heparan sulfate proteoglycans, and fibrin. Fibronectins are involved in diverse functions including cell migration, wound healing, cell proliferation, blood coagulation, and maintenance of cell cytoskeleton. Fibronectin is a multidomain protein that contains three types of domains (FN1, 2, 3) that are repeated multiple times depending on the isoform. Fibronectin was the first noncollagenous component of the ECM that was thoroughly studied as a ligand for its integrin receptor, now termed $\alpha_5\beta_1$, but originally studied as the "fibronectin receptor" [50]. Fibronectin served as the prototype for the development of the RGD-peptides now widely used in modification of biomaterials for the purpose of tissue engineering [51,52].

32.8.3 Laminin

Laminin is a common ECM component found in basement membranes and used as a substratum for cell migration by many cell types. It has a clear role in cell migration and tissue morphogenesis during embryonic development [4]. The classical laminin-1 is a cruciform shaped molecule composed of three chains [α1 (P25391), β1 (PO7942), and γ1 (P11047)]. There are at least 15 heterotrimers that can form using various α, β, and γ chains [see α2 (P24043), α3 (Q16787), α4 (Q16363), α5 (O15230), β2 (P55268), and β3 (Q13751), γ2 (Q13753)]. Laminin self-assembles into polygonal lattices *in vitro* [53]. It is a favorite ECM-based substrate for cells in the neural system [54].

32.8.4   Tenascin, Thrombospondin, and Osteonectin/SPARC/BM-40

Tenascin (P24821), thrombospondin-1 (P07996) and osteonectin/SPARC (P09486) are all modulators of cell adhesion, migration, and growth. Expression changes in these molecules are associated with neoplastic transformation and acquisition of migratory metastatic states such as those that occur during wound healing [55–57]. This regulation may be attributable to the ability of these molecules to trigger "de-adhesion," a process that has been speculated to represent an intermediate adaptive condition that facilitates expression of specific genes that are involved in repair and adaptation of cells and tissues [58]. In this regard, these molecules and motifs therein might be of particular importance in processes related to tissue engineering, although this has not yet been exploited.

32.8.5   Proteoglycans and Glycosaminoglycans

Perlecan (P98160), glypican (1-P35052) and syndecan (1-P18827, 2-P34741, 3-O75056, 4-P31431) are heparan sulfate proteoglycans (HSPGs) involved in diverse functions and essential to embryogenesis. Both the core proteins and the HS side chains are thought to play important functional roles. HS chains consist of a repeating disaccharide structure (glycosaminoglycan or GAG) that is regionally modified by enzymes that produce epimerization, vary sulfation patterns, and alter chain length [59]. The GAG chains create polycationic binding sites for attachment of proteins, primarily heparin-binding growth factors (HBGFs). Perlecan is secreted entirely into the matrix [60], syndecan possesses a transmembrane domain and remains as an integral component of the plasma membrane [61], and glypican is lipid-linked [62].

  Chondroitin sulfate proteoglycans (CSPGs) such as the large cartilage matrix protein aggrecan (P16112) have very large hydration spheres. Aggrecan is secreted into the pericellular matrix of cartilage where it self-assembles into a superstructure that can have as many as 50 monomers bound to a central filament composed of hyaluronic acid [63]. This structure is often described as resembling a "bottle brush." Aggrecan provides the osmotic resistance that cartilage needs to resist large compressive loads; its destruction during aging and in pathologic states contributes to skeletal erosion. The enzymes responsible for this destruction are matrix metalloproteinases (MMPs) called "aggrecanases" that are members of the ADAMTS (A Disintegrin And Metalloproteinase with Thrombospondin Motifs) gene family [64].

32.8.6   Osteopontin

Osteopontin (P10451) is a secreted matrix molecule that regulates cell responses through several integrin receptors and also is recognized by the CD44 receptor, through which it acts as a chemoattractant [65]. Osteopontin is thus a multifunctional molecule able to support both adhesion and migration, distinct properties that may be dependent on the degree and sites of phosphorylation [66]. The cell attachment site in osteopontin was mined and used to generate peptides for incorporation into peptide modified hydrogels that recently were used for modifying the function of marrow stromal osteoblasts [52].

32.9   Summary of Functions of ECM Molecules

The properties of ECM molecules make them ideal for cell and tissue engineering. ECM-derived molecules can be used to coat implants, modify surfaces, direct cell growth and differentiation, and engineer cell phenotype and behavior. Their multifunctional nature makes them ideal for promotion of cell specific adhesion via integrins and other surface receptors. Conversely, they can be used to release cells from adhesion ("counteradhesion") and thus migrate, for example, to cover a scaffold. They serve as efficient co-receptors for sequestration and delivery of growth factors, establishing morphogenic gradients recognized by cellular receptors during development, wound healing, and tissue repair [67,68]. For each of these functional roles, the context of the presentation of the ECM motif is critical in determination of outcome. For example, RGD peptides when presented to integrin-bearing cells *inhibit* adhesion and may lead to anoikis, but when immobilized these same motifs *support* adhesion, focal adhesion formation, and activate survival and proliferation pathways. These properties, if well understood, allow the ECM to serve as a rich source for mining and future development of novel tissue engineering applications.

32.10 Polymeric Materials and their Surface Modification

The rich biochemical and mechanical properties of the ECM have long been used as a model for tissue engineering constructs for the production of tissues such as cartilage, bone, nerve, and skin, as well as for the continued efforts toward the production of more complicated organs. Historically, the materials used for tissue engineering applications have relied primarily on readily available polymeric materials, both naturally derived and chemically synthesized. Polymers for specific applications are chosen on the basis of their aggregate mechanical properties, ease of processing, degradation profiles, and biochemical activity, with the latter becoming more prominent in the recent design of tissue engineering materials that elicit a specific and desired biological response. Among the most commonly utilized materials are natural ECM-based polymers such as collagen, fibrin glues, hyaluronic acid, and alginate. Although the biological activities and biocompatibility of these materials are useful, the lack of control over desired mechanical, degradation, and processing properties has motivated the use of synthetic polymers such as poly(glycolic acid), poly(lactic acid), poly(glycolic-*co*-lactic acid), poly(ethylene glycol) hydrogels, poly(*N*-isopropylacrylamide), poly(hydroxyethylmethacrylate), poly(anhydrides), and poly(*ortho*-esters). There are many good reviews on these and other polymeric systems and their use in tissue engineering [69–73], and descriptions of these materials are not included here.

Recent research effort in tissue engineering has focused on the incorporation of biologically active motifs derived from ECM proteins into matrices to integrate essential molecular elements of the ECM into the biomaterial and to promote a desired biological response. The choice of biologically active motifs incorporated into engineered matrices depend upon the ultimate end use of the matrix, but rely heavily on the coating of scaffolds with ECM-derived proteins, peptides, and glycosaminoglycans. Among the most straightforward of strategies is the simple coating of polymeric scaffolds (fibers, meshes, sponges, foams) with solutions of ECM protein(s) of interest based on adsorption via noncovalent interactions. While this method has demonstrated improvements in cell adhesion, proliferation, and secretion of ECM for a variety of cell types, it requires the adsorption of a high density of protein, since the protein can denature on the surface or adsorb in a suboptimal orientation, which significantly reduces affinity for given cell types. Alternatively, ECM proteins can be modified and then immobilized onto surfaces. In one recent example, fibronectin modified with Pluronic™ F108 could be easily attached to both poly(styrene) surfaces and poly(propylene) filaments with demonstrated improvements in neuronal cell attachment and neurite outgrowth [74].

Short, bioactive peptides from ECM proteins and growth factors, such as the RGD, YIGSR, IKVAV, REDV, heparin binding, and other sequences, also have been attached via straightforward chemical methods. The attachment of peptides (vs. proteins) is advantageous because the surface density and orientation of the peptide can be more easily controlled, allowing more quantitative understanding and manipulation of the surface modification process. Further, select peptides or combinations of peptides can yield materials that better mimic desirable signals present in the ECM. For example, the peptide REDV can be immobilized on surfaces instead of RGD to mediate the selective adhesion of endothelial cells over smooth muscle cells, fibroblasts, and platelets. Additionally, the combination of both the RGD and the heparin-binding motifs from bone sialoprotein (FHRRIKA) can synergistically improve cell adhesion and mineralization in osteoblast culture [75], and RGD modified polymers can impart desirable osteoblast adhesion and mineralization on titanium implants [76]. Peptides also can be incorporated into materials to reduce biodegradation, for example, the peptide aprotinin, which inhibits several serine proteases, has been used to derivatize the commercially available Tissucol® fibrin gels so that they maintain their bioactivity while exhibiting a reduced degradation rate (Immuno AG, Vienna, Austria). Numerous experiments have been conducted with surfaces and tissue engineering matrices covalently modified with ECM-derived peptides, and they have confirmed the bioactivity of these peptides and their utility in many tissue engineering applications. The most widely used methods for peptide immobilization, with just a few relevant examples, are summarized.

A very commonly employed strategy for peptide immobilization is the reaction of the thiol-terminated peptide with surfaces and polymers that are functionalized with maleimide, thiol, and vinyl sulfone groups. The reaction of thiol groups with vinyl sulfone modified polymers and surfaces has been employed in many recent investigations owing to its high selectivity over reactions with amines and its high reaction efficiency at physiological temperature and near physiological pH [77–79]. Reactions of amine-terminated side chains and carboxylic acid side chains also can be used for certain amino acid sequences in which these side chains are not required for biological activity. A variety of chemical reaction strategies can be used [80], one of the most common being the carbodiimide-activated coupling of amines with carboxylic acids. The advantage of the latter reactions is that they are generally applicable to a variety of proteins, synthetic polymers, and plasma-treated surfaces. The overall surface density of the peptides also can be controlled easily via these chemical modification strategies, which can have a large impact on cell proliferation and differentiation, particularly when coupled with manipulation of the chemical composition of the matrix material [81,82].

Another strategy for the incorporation of biologically active peptide motifs onto tissue engineering scaffolds involves the covalent coupling of the peptide into the matrix during matrix formation. Acrylated peptides such as RGD and plasmin substrate sequences have been incorporated into a variety of poly(ethylene glycol) (PEG) hydrogel materials in this manner and have imparted desirable cell adhesion and cell-mediated degradation [83,84]. Essentially, any peptide can be incorporated into hydrogels via these strategies, and recently, GRGDS or an osteopontin derived peptide (ODP), DVDVPDGRGDSLAYG, were incorporated in oligo(poly(ethylene glycol) fumarate) hydrogels to determine the impact on osteoblast migration. Osteoblasts migrate both faster and for longer distances on the ODP-modified hydrogels vs. the RGD modified hydrogels [52].

Enzymatic attachment of a peptide that carries both a cell attachment or signaling sequence and a domain that is a substrate for enzymatic coupling by Factor XIIIa (-NQEQVSP-) also has been used to covalently incorporate ECM-derived peptide sequences into tissue engineering materials. This strategy has been recently developed for the incorporation of a variety of cell adhesion peptides (derived from fibronectin, laminin, and N-cadherin), heparin-binding peptides, and growth factors into fibrin matrices, via the action of Factor XIIIa, to demonstrate improvements in cell adhesion, neurite outgrowth, and axonal regeneration [85–87].

Strategies that involve assembly and adsorption also have been useful for mediating the presentation of peptides at surfaces. For example, a very general strategy for surface modification of both polymeric and inorganic matrices involves the incorporation of mussel-adhesive-protein-derived dihydroxylphenylalanine (DOPA) residues at the termini of polymers [88]. Interaction of the DOPA residues with surfaces results in attachment, and although this method has currently been applied to the modification of surfaces with ethylene glycol oligomers, it should be equally applicable to the simple attachment of bioactive peptides to a variety of surfaces. Strategies for presenting labile ligands at an interface via the use of RGD-modified nanoparticles also have been developed as a strategy to improve cell migration on biomaterials surfaces [89]. Another emerging strategy is the use of peptide-modified self-assembling materials for the multivalent presentation of biologically active peptides. Peptide–amphiphiles, decorated with either phosphate-functionalized amino acids or sequences such as IKVAV, assemble into stable fibrous hydrogel materials and demonstrate promising activities such as mineralization and selective differentiation of neural progenitor cells *in vitro* [90,91].

A more experimentally complicated, but useful, method for the incorporation of biologically active peptide motifs is the inclusion of these peptide sequences directly in the backbone of recombinant artificial proteins and in protein/polymer conjugates. Cell adhesion sequences from fibronectin (RGD and REDV) have been incorporated into silk-like, collagen-like, and elastin-like artificial proteins. The mechanical properties of the silk, collagen, or elastin provide excellent adhesion and elasticity, and the ECM-derived proteins mimic some essential features of the ECM. The fibronectin-derived cell-binding sequences result in marked improvements in cell adhesion to films of these proteins [92–95]. The silk-fibronectin proteins form autoclave-stable coatings on polystyrene culture plates and are sold commercially as the Pronectins®, originally by Protein Polymer Technologies, Inc. The mechanical properties of the elastin-like protein polymers can be engineered via chemical cross-linking strategies to closely match those of native elastin [96,97], which aid in compliance matching of small-diameter vascular graft replacement materials with host tissues.

Investigations to engineer biologically active domains of other proteins also have been initiated. Given the prominent developmental and physiological functions of collagen, and its widespread use as a tissue engineering material, collagen proteins have received significant attention. Individual domains of collagen II have been isolated to determine their biological activity, and the amino acid region 704-938 in collagen II was identified in these studies as critical for the spreading of chondrocytes [98]. These studies may direct the production of repetitive proteins containing that amino acid sequence for improved chondrocyte adhesion and spreading. Chimeric proteins of collagen III and EGF also have been produced, and retain the fibril-forming properties of the collagen domain and the activity of EGF; these materials may find application in cell culture, wound healing, and tissue engineering applications [99]. Similarly, biologically active motifs can be genetically engineered and then conjugated to synthetic polymers to produce biologically active protein–polymer block copolymers. Specifically, an artificial protein equipped with an RGD sequence and two plasmin degradation sites from fibrinogen, and an ATIII-derived heparin binding site, was grafted to PEG-acrylates and incorporated into hydrogels. These hydrogels supported three-dimensional outgrowth of human fibroblasts mediated by adhesion to the RGD sequences [100].

32.11 Formation of Gradient Structures

While the coating of tissue engineering matrix surfaces with bioactive molecules has improved cell adhesion and biological properties of matrices, the native temporal and spatial presentation of molecules in the ECM also has been increasingly mimicked as a strategy to control materials response. The establishment of functional morphogen gradients and patterns in materials controls cell signaling and proliferation, and can be achieved by a variety of methods, including temporally controlled deposition, microfluidic approaches, photoinitiated polymerizations, photolithography, soft lithography, block copolymer assembly, and printing strategies. One area in which the deposition of functional gradients of ECM-derived proteins has had large impact is in the generation of materials for guiding neurite outgrowth. For example, the formation of simple concentration gradients via controlled photopolymerization of nerve growth factor (NGF) in poly(2-hydroxyethyl methacrylate) microporous gels has guided the growth of PC12 cell neurites up the concentration gradient [101]. Microfluidic methods also have been used to control deposition of proteins in channels; in one example, the deposition of laminin was controlled, and the growth of hippocampal neurons toward the regions of highest laminin deposition was observed [102]. Protein gradients also have been produced on surfaces via the temporally controlled deposition of protein-coated gold nanoparticles onto poly(lysine) derivatized surfaces [103]. Proteins immobilized in this manner retain their bioactivity, and the presence of the particles is not detrimental to the growth of hippocampal neurons. Furthermore, this method is generally applicable to the production of protein gradients on the surfaces of a variety of two-dimensional and three-dimensional scaffolds.

In addition to the production of concentration gradients in hydrogel materials and on surfaces, there has been increasing interest in controlling cell placement for studying and manipulating cellular responses to materials. Lithographic methods have emerged as a viable strategy for achieving this patterning. Photolithographic strategies permit the production of patterns of proteins on the micron length scale, via selective activation of photosensitive groups on a surface followed by coupling to a protein of interest. These methods have been used to create many patterned surfaces including those for controlling neuronal patterning [104,105]. Perhaps the most popular lithographic method for patterning surfaces is the soft lithographic approach of microcontact printing, in which an elastomeric stamp is used to directly "print" chemically or biologically active peptides and proteins onto surfaces of both hard and soft materials [106–108]. The methods have been used to print laminin, collagen, and a variety of other ECM-derived proteins and peptides, and provide a useful means to control cell adsorption and response to materials [109–112]. These methods have been used to pattern surfaces primarily at the micron length scale, but can also be used to pattern proteins at surfaces at length scales smaller than 1 μm.

Direct printing of ECM proteins and peptides also has been demonstrated. Ink jet printing can modify and fabricate scaffolds for tissue engineering applications, including the printing of active proteins [113], and the fabrication and surface modification of three-dimensional scaffolds [114]. In one recent example, automated ink jet printing was used to produce 350 μm features of collagen in lines, circles, arrays of dots, and gradients. Smooth muscle cells and dorsal root ganglia neurons adhere to these patterned regions and achieve confluency in the shape of the pattern in as few as 4 h [115]. Dip-pen nanolithography (DPN), in which an atomic force microscope (AFM) tip is "inked" with a solution of interest and then is used to deposit a pattern, also has been applied to produce protein patterns with feature sizes below 200 nm. Dots and lines of antibodies and ECM-derived proteins have been printed [116–118]. Collagen has been printed to feature sizes of 30 to 50 nm [116], and Retronectin, a recombinant fragment of fibronectin comprising the central cell-binding domain, the heparin binding domain II, and the CS1 site, was printed onto gold surfaces via DPN at feature sizes of approximately 200 nm [117]. Fibroblasts adhere selectively to the areas printed with Retronectin, but with morphologies different than those on unpatterned surfaces modified with Retronectin. The use of these methods may therefore permit the study and manipulation of cell adhesion and signaling phenomena via patterning at lengthscales relevant to individual receptors on cell surfaces.

The directed assembly of polymeric materials also can be used to pattern bioactive elements on the nanometer length scale. For example, the spatial distribution of RGD-containing peptides has been controlled by the presentation of the peptide on star-shaped polymers. By controlling the number of peptides per star polymer, as well as by controlling the density of peptide-functionalized star polymers on a surface, these methods have been useful for clustering peptides and increasing fibroblast adhesion strength and actin stress fiber formation [119]. The clustering of the ligands also has altered fibroblast adhesion behavior under centrifugal detachment forces, with clustered ligands increasing adhesion with increasing detachment force for forces from 70 to 150 pN/cell [120].

32.12 Delivery of Growth Factors

The development of polymeric controlled release systems has facilitated the development of tissue engineering scaffolds capable of the controlled release of growth factors, and has enabled the control of cellular processes for prolonged periods of times via a sustained release of appropriate growth factors directly into the cell microenvironment (for a recent review see Reference 121). Simple injection of growth factors has not reached its potential therapeutically owing to the very short half-lives of the growth factor *in vivo* (a few minutes), which has necessitated studies of their controlled release. Growth factors have been both noncovalently and covalently incorporated into a wide variety of materials over the past decade, which has resulted in numerous reports of their benefit in bone, cartilage, and nerve tissue engineering investigations. Growth factors can be simply encapsulated into matrices comprised of collagen, alginate, hyaluronic acid, or other synthetic hydrogels. In many cases the half-life of the growth factor is significantly increased vs. that of the free growth factor in solution. For example, in alginate matrices, electrostatic interactions stabilize the growth factor in the matrix and control its slow release [122]. Interest in extending the release time of the growth factors, improving their bioactivity, and allowing for delivery of multiple growth factors have led to additional strategies for incorporating growth factors into materials and onto surfaces [123,124]. There have been a myriad of studies on the passive encapsulation of growth factors into particles, fibers, and hydrogels; the discussion below focuses on recently described methods involving immobilization of growth factors via interaction with heparinized materials or via covalent attachment.

Heparin has been widely applied to surfaces and encapsulated into hydrogels as a strategy for immobilization of growth factors. The interaction of heparin and growth factors permits immobilization and stabilization of the growth factor via sequence-specific electrostatic interactions with heparin, which mimic the natural mechanisms by which growth factors are protected in the ECM via interactions with heparan sulfate. Accordingly, hydrogels in which growth factor and heparin are co-encapsulated show improvements in growth factor delivery and half-life. Heparin has been covalently attached to polymers to reduce heparin diffusion from the matrix and further increase retention and half-life of growth factors. For example, when bFGF is immobilized in a heparinized collagen matrix, bFGF retains its bioactivity and promotes endothelial cell growth [125]. A variety of other materials have been covalently modified with heparin using other chemical strategies to enable growth factor binding, and these achieve desirable cellular responses [126–128]. In a recent example with a slightly different approach, PEG star polymers were modified with heparin-binding peptides (hbp) and then cross-linked via noncovalent interactions with high molecular weight heparin. The mechanical properties and delivery rates of the hydrogels can be mediated by the affinity and kinetics of the heparin–hbp interactions [78]. Likewise, hydrogels have also been assembled via noncovalent interactions between PEG–hbp star copolymers and PEG star polymers modified with low molecular weight heparin. These networks have demonstrated release profiles for bFGF that correlate with erosion of the noncovalent network [129]. It is envisioned that growth factors noncovalently bound to the heparin will be released at rates that correlate with the heparin–hbp affinities and that can be tuned for a desired tissue engineering or drug delivery application.

Another recently developed approach for growth factor delivery is the development of fibrin matrices in which hbp have been covalently incorporated into fibrin via the action of Factor XIIIa [86]. Both heparin and growth factors are then incorporated into these matrices, and the passive release of the heparin-associated growth factor is minimized via the binding between the heparin and the covalently bound hbp. Prudent choice of the ratio of growth factor: heparin:hbp permits growth factor release to be controlled by cell-mediated degradation of the fibrin matrix, rather than by passive diffusion. When bFGF was delivered from this growth factor delivery system *in vitro*, the results demonstrated a nearly 100% enhancement in neurite extension over an unmodified fibrin control [86]. Additionally, NGF has been immobilized in similar matrices. Despite the fact that NGF does not bind heparin with high affinity, the electrostatic interactions between basic regions of the NGF and heparin immobilize NGF in the fibrin matrices. These materials also enhance neurite extension from chick dorsal root ganglia by up to 100% relative to unmodified fibrin at 48 h [130], and more recent investigations demonstrate that these materials perform similarly to isografts when tested in 13-mm rat sciatic nerve defects [131]. Another recently employed strategy for growth factory delivery takes advantage of the native heparan sulfate chains of the ECM protein, perlecan, which binds HBGFS including TGFB, BMP, and bFGF. A recombinant domain of perlecan was used to sequester and release bFGF from native collagen matrices [124].

While the rates of release of bioactive growth factors from hydrogels of all the above kinds can be controlled via control of matrix pore size and heparin loading, the release mechanism is passive. There have been several strategies developed for the localized delivery of growth factors, and the covalent attachment of bioactive growth factors, such as EGF and TGF-β1, to different surfaces is a useful strategy for producing bioactive biomaterials [132,133]. Although the growth factors are immobilized by chemical methods, the bioactivity of both EGF and TGF-β1 are well preserved in these systems. The EGF, immobilized to a glass surface using a PEG linker, retained its activity as assessed by mitogenic and morphological assays of primary rat hepatocytes, while physisorbed EGF demonstrated no bioactivity [132]. The incorporation of TGF-β1 into PEG hydrogels increases ECM production by smooth muscle cells grown in these gels [133]. The incorporation of collagenase or elastase sensitive amino acid sequences in cross-linking regions of the gels also permits the migration of the cells into the matrix during remodeling [134]. The combination of the increased ECM production stimulated by TGF-β1 and the cell-mediated degradation of the matrix may provide materials that can provide sufficient mechanical stability throughout all stages of cell remodeling of the implant material.

Growth factors such as VEGF and β-NGF also have been covalently incorporated into fibrin matrices via the enzymatic action of Factor XIIIa [87,135,136]. In these examples, the growth factors were genetically engineered to carry both a Factor XIIIa substrate domain (for cross-linking) as well as an MMP substrate domain, so that they could be covalently incorporated into fibrin gels, and liberated upon cell migration into the gel via enzymatic cleavage of the MMP substrate domain. The β-NGF containing fibrin matrices enhanced neurite extension from embryonic chick dorsal root ganglia by 50% relative to soluble β-NGF and by 350% relative to a negative control without β-NGF [87]. Subcutaneous implantation of the VEGF-containing fibrin materials (5.4 mm diameter, 2 mm thickness) in rats demonstrated that these tissue engineering materials, after 2 weeks, were completely remodeled into native, vascularized tissue [136]. These results suggest the promise of such approaches to the development of useful tissue engineering materials that are responsive to cellular demand.

32.13   Summary and Conclusions

This chapter has summarized the present status of the science of tissue engineering using the ECM as a rich source of biologically relevant motifs. No doubt the next decade will provide a wealth of knowledge both about the native ECM and its components and the application of this knowledge to engineering purposes. The deliberate modulation of cell behavior using rational design and ECM-based biomaterials will serve as a major growth area in future biotechnology.

Acknowledgments

The authors thank the editors for the opportunity to compile the information in this chapter. We gratefully acknowledge the contributions to Figure 32.1a,c, Figure 32.2b,c, and Figure 32.3b,c by Dr. Fred Hossler, Department of Anatomy and Cell Biology at East Tennessee State University, J.H. Quillen College of Medicine. The work in the authors laboratories is supported by NIH R01 DE13542 (DDC and MCFC) and NIH R01 EB003172 (to KLK).

References

[1] Danen, E.H. and Sonnenberg, A., Integrins in regulation of tissue development and function, *J. Pathol.* 201, 632–41, 2003.

[2] Mareel, M. and Leroy, A., Clinical, cellular, and molecular aspects of cancer invasion, *Physiol. Rev.* 83, 337–76, 2003.

[3] Mekori, Y.A. and Baram, D., Heterotypic adhesion-induced mast cell activation: biologic relevance in the inflammatory context, *Mol. Immunol.* 38, 1363–7, 2002.

[4] Sasaki, T., Fassler, R., and Hohenester, E., Laminin: the crux of basement membrane assembly, *J. Cell Biol.* 164, 959–63, 2004.

[5] Chen, C.H. and Hansma, H.G., Basement membrane macromolecules: insights from atomic force microscopy, *J. Struct. Biol.* 131, 44–55, 2000.

[6] Yurchenco, P.D., Cheng, Y.S., and Colognato, H., Laminin forms an independent network in basement membranes, *J. Cell Biol.* 117, 1119–33, 1992.

[7] Timpl, R. and Brown, J.C., Supramolecular assembly of basement membranes, *Bioessays* 18, 123–32, 1996.

[8] Otey, C.A. and Burridge, K., Patterning of the membrane cytoskeleton by the extracellular matrix, *Semin. Cell Biol.* 1, 391–9, 1990.

[9] Adams, J.C., Regulation of protrusive and contractile cell-matrix contacts, *J. Cell Sci.* 115, 257–65, 2002.

[10] Klinghoffer, R.A. et al., Src family kinases are required for integrin but not PDGFR signal transduction, *EMBO J.* 18, 2459–71, 1999.

[11] Murphy, K.G. and Gunsolley, J.C., Guided tissue regeneration for the treatment of periodontal intrabony and furcation defects. A systematic review, *Ann. Periodontol.* 8, 266–302, 2003.

[12] Krasteva, N. et al., The role of surface wettability on hepatocyte adhesive interactions and function, *J. Biomater. Sci. Polym. Ed.* 12, 613–27, 2001.

[13] Siczkowski, M., Clarke, D., and Gordon, M.Y., Binding of primitive hematopoietic progenitor cells to marrow stromal cells involves heparan sulfate, *Blood* 80, 912–9, 1992.

[14] Kan, M. et al., Divalent cations and heparin/heparan sulfate cooperate to control assembly and activity of the fibroblast growth factor receptor complex, *J. Biol. Chem.* 271, 26143–8, 1996.

[15] Dais, P., Peng, Q.J., and Perlin, A.S., A relationship between 13C-chemical-shift displacements and counterion-condensation theory, in the binding of calcium ion by heparin, *Carbohydr. Res.* 168, 163–79, 1987.

[16] Kirchhofer, D., Grzesiak, J., and Pierschbacher, M.D., Calcium as a potential physiological regulator of integrin-mediated cell adhesion, *J. Biol. Chem.* 266, 4471–7, 1991.

[17] Buck, C.A. and Horwitz, A.F., Cell surface receptors for extracellular matrix molecules, *Annu. Rev. Cell Biol.* 3, 179–205, 1987.

[18] Frisch, S.M. and Screaton, R.A., Anoikis mechanisms, *Curr. Opin. Cell Biol.* 13, 555–62, 2001.

[19] Wehrle-Haller, B. and Imhof, B.A., Actin, microtubules and focal adhesion dynamics during cell migration, *Int. J. Biochem. Cell Biol.* 35, 39–50, 2003.

[20] Farach-Carson, M.C. and Davis, P.J., Steroid hormone interactions with target cells: cross talk between membrane and nuclear pathways, *J. Pharmacol. Exp. Ther.* 307, 839–45, 2003.

[21] Werlen, G. and Palmer, E., The T-cell receptor signalosome: a dynamic structure with expanding complexity, *Curr. Opin. Immunol.* 14, 299–305, 2002.

[22] Elion, E.A., The Ste5p scaffold, *J. Cell Sci.* 114, 3967–78, 2001.

[23] Fawthrop, D.J., Boobis, A.R., and Davies, D.S., Mechanisms of cell death, *Arch. Toxicol.* 65, 437–44, 1991.

[24] Archer, C.W. and Francis-West, P., The chondrocyte, *Int. J. Biochem. Cell Biol.* 35, 401–4, 2003.

[25] Buckwalter, J.A. and Mankin, H.J., Articular cartilage: tissue design and chondrocyte matrix interactions, *Instr. Course Lect.* 47, 477–86, 1998.

[26] Pacifici, M., Tenascin-C and the development of articular cartilage, *Matrix Biol.* 14, 689–98, 1995.

[27] Goessler, U.R., Hormann, K., and Riedel, F., Tissue engineering with chondrocytes and function of the extracellular matrix (review), *Int. J. Mol. Med.* 13, 505–13, 2004.

[28] de Crombrugghe, B. et al., Transcriptional mechanisms of chondrocyte differentiation, *Matrix Biol.* 19, 389–94, 2000.

[29] van der Eerden, B.C., Karperien, M., and Wit, J.M., Systemic and local regulation of the growth plate, *Endocr. Rev.* 24, 782–801, 2003.

[30] Kronenberg, H.M., Developmental regulation of the growth plate, *Nature* 423, 332–6, 2003.

[31] Linsenmayer, T.F., Eavey, R.D., and Schmid, T.M., Type X collagen: a hypertrophic cartilage-specific molecule, *Pathol. Immunopathol. Res.* 7, 14–19, 1988.

[32] Gorski, J.P., Is all bone the same? Distinctive distributions and properties of non-collagenous matrix proteins in lamellar vs. woven bone imply the existence of different underlying osteogenic mechanisms, *Crit. Rev. Oral Biol. Med.* 9, 201–23, 1998.

[33] Jilka, R.L., Biology of the basic multicellular unit and the pathophysiology of osteoporosis, *Med. Pediatr. Oncol.* 41, 182–5, 2003.

[34] Sommerfeldt, D.W. and Rubin, C.T., Biology of bone and how it orchestrates the form and function of the skeleton, *Eur. Spine J.* 10, S86–95, 2001.

[35] Panda, A.K., Bioprocessing of therapeutic proteins from the inclusion bodies of *Escherichia coli*, *Adv. Biochem. Eng. Biotechnol.* 85, 43–93, 2003.

[36] Ikonomou, L., Schneider, Y.J., and Agathos, S.N., Insect cell culture for industrial production of recombinant proteins, *Appl. Microbiol. Biotechnol.* 62, 1–20, 2003.

[37] French, M.M. et al., Chondrogenic activity of the heparan sulfate proteoglycan perlecan maps to the N-terminal domain I, *J. Bone Miner. Res.* 17, 48–55, 2002.

[38] Sodoyer, R., Expression systems for the production of recombinant pharmaceuticals, *BioDrugs* 18, 51–62, 2004.

[39] Bulleid, N.J., John, D.C., and Kadler, K.E., Recombinant expression systems for the production of collagen, *Biochem. Soc. Trans.* 28, 350–3, 2000.

[40] Knox, S., Melrose, J., and Whitelock, J., Electrophoretic, biosensor, and bioactivity analyses of perlecans of different cellular origins, *Proteomics* 1, 1534–41, 2001.

[41] Patrick, C.W., Jr., Adipose tissue engineering: the future of breast and soft tissue reconstruction following tumor resection, *Semin. Surg. Oncol.* 19, 302–11, 2000.

[42] Heilshorn, S.C. et al., Endothelial cell adhesion to the fibronectin CS5 domain in artificial extracellular matrix proteins, *Biomaterials* 24, 4245–52, 2003.

[43] Yurchenco, P.D., Smirnov, S., and Mathus, T., Analysis of basement membrane self-assembly and cellular interactions with native and recombinant glycoproteins, *Meth. Cell Biol.* 69, 111–44, 2002.

[44] Hohenester, E. and Engel, J., Domain structure and organisation in extracellular matrix proteins, *Matrix Biol.* 21, 115–28, 2002.

[45] Hulmes, D.J., Building collagen molecules, fibrils, and suprafibrillar structures, *J. Struct. Biol.* 137, 2–10, 2002.

[46] Matese, J.C., Black, S., and McClay, D.R., Regulated exocytosis and sequential construction of the extracellular matrix surrounding the sea urchin zygote, *Dev. Biol.* 186, 16–26, 1997.

[47] Ottani, V. et al., Hierarchical structures in fibrillar collagens, *Micron* 33, 587–96, 2002.

[48] Gelse, K., Poschl, E., and Aigner, T., Collagens — structure, function, and biosynthesis, *Adv. Drug Deliv. Rev.* 55, 1531–46, 2003.

[49] Myllyharju, J. and Kivirikko, K.I., Collagens, modifying enzymes and their mutations in humans, flies and worms, *Trends Genet.* 20, 33–43, 2004.

[50] Brown, P.J. and Juliano, R.L., Expression and function of a putative cell surface receptor for fibronectin in hamster and human cell lines, *J. Cell Biol.* 103, 1595–603, 1986.

[51] Hersel, U., Dahmen, C., and Kessler, H., RGD modified polymers: biomaterials for stimulated cell adhesion and beyond, *Biomaterials* 24, 4385–415, 2003.

[52] Shin, H. et al., Attachment, proliferation, and migration of marrow stromal osteoblasts cultured in biomimetic hydrogels modified with an osteopontin-derived peptide, *Biomaterials* 25, 895–906, 2004.

[53] Colognato, H., Winkelmann, D.A., and Yurchenco, P.D., Laminin polymerization induces a receptor-cytoskeleton network, *J. Cell Biol.* 145, 619–31, 1999.

[54] Grimpe, B. and Silver, J., The extracellular matrix in axon regeneration, *Prog. Brain Res.* 137, 333–49, 2002.

[55] Mukaratirwa, S. and Nederbragt, H., Tenascin and proteoglycans: the role of tenascin and proteoglycans in canine tumours, *Res. Vet. Sci.* 73, 1–8, 2002.

[56] Sage, E.H., Regulation of interactions between cells and extracellular matrix: a command performance on several stages, *J. Clin. Invest.* 107, 781–3, 2001.

[57] Sid, B. et al., Thrombospondin 1: a multifunctional protein implicated in the regulation of tumor growth, *Crit. Rev. Oncol. Hematol.* 49, 245–58, 2004.

[58] Murphy-Ullrich, J.E., The de-adhesive activity of matricellular proteins: is intermediate cell adhesion an adaptive state? *J. Clin. Invest.* 107, 785–90, 2001.

[59] Esko, J.D. and Selleck, S.B., Order out of chaos: assembly of ligand binding sites in heparan sulfate, *Annu. Rev. Biochem.* 71, 435–71, 2002.

[60] Iozzo, R.V., Perlecan: a gem of a proteoglycan, *Matrix Biol.* 14, 203–8, 1994.

[61] Bernfield, M. et al., Biology of the syndecans: a family of transmembrane heparan sulfate proteoglycans, *Annu. Rev. Cell Biol.* 8, 365–93, 1992.

[62] Fransson, L.A., Glypicans, *Int. J. Biochem. Cell Biol.* 35, 125–9, 2003.

[63] Knudson, C.B. and Knudson, W., Cartilage proteoglycans, *Semin. Cell Dev. Biol.* 12, 69–78, 2001.

[64] Roberts, S. et al., Matrix metalloproteinases and aggrecanase: their role in disorders of the human intervertebral disc, *Spine* 25, 3005–13, 2000.

[65] Sodek, J. et al., Novel functions of the matricellular proteins osteopontin and osteonectin/SPARC, *Connect. Tissue Res.* 43, 308–19, 2002.

[66] Denhardt, D.T., The third international conference on osteopontin and related proteins, San Antonio, Texas, May 10–12, 2002, *Calcif. Tissue Int.* 74, 213–19, 2004.

[67] Gritli-Linde, A. et al., The whereabouts of a morphogen: direct evidence for short- and graded long-range activity of hedgehog signaling peptides, *Dev. Biol.* 236, 364–86, 2001.

[68] Cadigan, K.M., Regulating morphogen gradients in the *Drosophila* wing, *Semin. Cell Dev. Biol.* 13, 83–90, 2002.

[69] Hirano, Y. and Mooney, D.J., Peptide and protein presenting materials for tissue engineering, *Adv. Mater.* 16, 17–25, 2004.

[70] Drury, J.L. and Mooney, D.J., Hydrogels for tissue engineering: scaffold design variables and applications, *Biomaterials* 24, 4337–51, 2003.

[71] Shin, H., Jo, S., and Mikos, A.G., Biomimetic materials for tissue engineeering, *Biomaterials* 24, 4353–64, 2003.

[72] Sakiyama-Elbert, S.E. and Hubbell, J.A., Functional biomaterials: design of novel biomaterials, *Ann. Rev. Mater. Res.* 31, 183–201, 2001.

[73] Seal, B.L., Otero, T.C., and Panitch, A., Polymeric biomaterials for tissue and organ regeneration, *Mat. Sci. Eng. Res. Rep.* 34, 147–230, 2001.

[74] Biran, R. et al., Surfactant-immobilized fibronectin enhances bioactivty and regulates sensory neurite outgrowth, *J. Biomed. Mater. Res.* 55, 1–12, 2001.

[75] Healy, K.E., Rezania, A., and Stile, R.A., Designing biomaterials to direct biological responses, *Ann. NY Acad. Sci.* 875, 24–35, 1999.

[76] Barber, T.A. et al., Peptide-modified p(AAm-co-EG/AAc)IPNs grafted to bulk titanium modulate osteoblast behavior *in vitro*, *J. Biomed. Mater. Res. A.* 64A, 38–47, 2003.

[77] Lutolf, M.P. and Hubbell, J.A., Synthesis and physicochemical characterization of end-linked poly(ethylene glycol)-co-peptide hydrogels formed by Michael-type addition, *Biomacromolecules* 4, 713–2, 2003.

[78] Seal, B.L. and Panitch, A., Physical polymer matrices based on affinity interactions between peptides and polysaccharides, *Biomacromolecules* 4, 1572–82, 2003.

[79] Heggli, M. et al., Michael-type addition as a tool for surface functionalization, *Bioconj. Chem.* 14, 967–73, 2003.

[80] Hermanson, G.T., *Bioconjugate Techniques.* Academic Press, New York, 1996.

[81] Rezania, A. and Healy, K.E., The effect of peptide surface density on mineralization of a matrix deposited by osteogenic cells, *J. Biomed. Mater. Res.* 52, 595–600, 2000.

[82] Rowley, J.A. and Mooney, D.J., Alginate type and RGD density control myoblast phenotype, *J. Biomed. Mater. Res.* 60, 217–23, 2002.

[83] Hern, D.L. and Hubbell, J.A., Incorporation of adhesion peptides into nonadhesive hydrogels useful for tissue resurfacing, *J. Biomed. Mater. Res.* 39, 266–76, 1998.

[84] West, J.L. and Hubbell, J.A., Polymeric biomaterials with degradation sites for proteases involved in cell migration, *Macromolecules* 32, 241–4, 1999.

[85] Schense, J.C. et al., Enzymatic incorporation of bioactive peptides into fibrin matrices enhances neurite extension, *Nat. Biotechnol.* 18, 415–9, 2000.

[86] Sakiyama-Elbert, S.E. and Hubbell, J.A., Development of fibrin derivatives for controlled release of heparin-binding growth factors, *J. Control. Release* 65, 389–402, 2000a.

[87] Sakiyama-Elbert, S.E., Panitch, A., and Hubbell, J.A., Development of growth factor fusion proteins for cell-triggered delivery, *FASEB J.* 15, 1300–2, 2001.

[88] Dalsin, J.L. et al., Mussel adhesive protein mimetic polymers for the preparation of nonfouling surfaces, *J. Am. Chem. Soc.* 125, 4253–8, 2003.

[89] Tjia, J.S. and Moghe, P.V., "Cell-internalizable" ligand microinterfaces on biomaterials, in *Biomimetic Materials and Design*, Dillow, A.K. and Lowman, A.M. (Eds.), Marcel Dekker, Inc., New York, 2002, pp. 335–73.

[90] Hartgerink, J.D., Beniash, E., and Stupp, S.I., Self-assembly and mineralization of peptide-amphiphile nanofibers, *Science* 294, 1684–8, 2001.

[91] Silva, G.A. et al., Selective differentiation of neural progenitor cells by high-epitope density nanofibers, *Science* 303, 1352–5, 2004.

[92] Ferrari, F.A. and Cappello, J., Biosynthesis of protein polymers, in *Protein-Based Materials*, McGrath, K. and Kaplan, D. (Eds.), Birkhauser, Boston, 1997, pp. 37–60.

[93] Urry, D.W. et al., Transductional elastic and plastic protein-based polymers as potential medical devices, in *Drug Targeting and Delivery, Handbook of Biodegradable Polymers*, Domb, A.J., Kost, J., and Wiseman, D.M. (Eds.), Harwood Academic Publ., Amsterdam, 1997, pp. 367–86.

[94] Panitch, A. et al., Design and biosynthesis of elastin-like extracellular matrix proteins containing periodically spaced fibronectin CS5 domains, *Macromolecules* 32, 1701–3, 1999.

[95] Liu, J.C., Heilshorn, S.C., and Tirrell, D.A., Comparative cell response to artificial extracellular matrix proteins containing the RGD and CS5 cell-binding domains, *Biomacromolecules* 5, 497–504, 2004.

[96] Welsh, E.R. and Tirrell, D.A., Engineering the extracellular matrix: a novel approach to polymeric biomaterials. I. Control of the physical properties of artificial protein matrices designed to support adhesion of vascular endothelial cells, *Biomacromolecules* 1, 23–30, 2000.

[97] Di Zio, K. and Tirrell, D.A., Mechanical properties of artificial protein matrices engineered for control of cell and tissue behavior, *Macromolecules* 36, 1553–8, 2003.

[98] Fertala, A., Han, W.B., and Ko, F.K., Mapping critical sites in collagen II for rational design of gene-engineered proteins for cell-supporting materials, *J. Biomed. Mater. Res.* 57, 48–58, 2001.

[99] Hayashi, M., Tomita, M., and Yoshizato, K., Production of EGF-collagen chimeric protein which shows the mitogenic activity, *Biochim. Biophys. Acta* 1528, 187–95, 2001.

[100] Halstenberg, S. et al., Biologically engineered protein-graft-poly(ethylene glycol) hydrogels: a cell adhesive and plasmin-degradable biosynthetic material for tissue repair, *Biomacromolecules* 3, 710–23, 2002.

[101] Kapur, T.A. and Shoichet, M.S., Immobilized concentration gradients of nerve growth factor guide neurite outgrowth, *J. Biomed. Mater. Res. A* 68A, 235–43, 2004.

[102] Dertinger, S.K.W. et al., Gradients of substrate-bound laminin orient axonal specification of neurons, *Proc. Natl Acad. Sci. USA* 99, 12542–7, 2002.

[103] Kramer, S. et al., Preparation of protein gradients through the controlled deposition of protein-nanoparticle conjugates onto functionalized surfaces, *J. Am. Chem. Soc.* 126, 5388–95, 2004.

[104] Ravenscroft, M.S. et al., Developmental neurobiology implications from fabrication and analysis of hippocampal neuronal networks on patterned silane-modified surfaces, *J. Am. Chem. Soc.* 120, 12169–77, 1998.

[105] Chang, J.C., Brewer, G.J., and Wheller, B.C., Modulation of neural network activity by patterning, *Biosensors Bioelectron.* 16, 527–33, 2001.

[106] Mrksich, M. et al., Controlling cell attachment on contoured surfaces with self-assembled monolayers of alkanethiolates on gold, *Proc. Natl Acad. Sci. USA* 93, 10775–8, 1996.

[107] Kane, R.S. et al., Patterning proteins and cells using soft lithography, *Biomaterials* 20, 2363–76, 1999.

[108] Bernard, A. et al., Microcontact printing of proteins, *Adv. Mater.* 12, 1067–70, 2000.

[109] Patel, N. et al., Printing patterns of biospecifically adsorbed protein, *J. Biomater. Sci. Polym. Ed.* 11, 319–31, 2000.

[110] McDevitt, T.C. et al., Spatially organized layers of cardiomyocytes on biodegradable polyurethane films for myocardial repair, *J. Biomed. Mater. Res. A* 66A, 586–95, 2003.

[111] Lee, K.B. et al., Pattern generation of biological ligands on a biodegradable poly(glycolic acid) film, *Langmuir* 20, 2531–5, 2004.

[112] Schmalenberg, K.E., Buettner, H.M., and Uhrich, K.E., Microcontact printing of proteins on oxygen plasma-activated poly(methyl methacrylate), *Biomaterials* 25, 1851–7, 2004.

[113] Roda, A. et al., Protein microdeposition using a conventional ink-jet printer, *Biotechniques* 28, 492–6, 2000.

[114] Park, A., Wu, B., and Griffith, L.G., Integration of surface modification and 3D fabrication techniques to prepare patterned poly(L-lactide) substrates allowing regionally selective cell adhesion, *J. Biomater. Sci. Polym. Ed.* 9, 89–110, 1998.

[115] Roth, E.A. et al., Inkjet printing for high-throughput cell patterning, *Biomaterials* 25, 3707–15, 2004.

[116] Wilson, D.L. et al., Surface organization and nanopatterning of collagen by dip-pen nanolithography, *Proc. Natl Acad. Sci. USA* 98, 13660–4, 2001.

[117] Lee, K.B. et al., Protein nanoarrays generated by dip-pen nanolithography, *Science* 295, 1702–5, 2002.

[118] Lee, K.B., Lim, J.H., and Mirkin, C.A., Protein nanostructures formed via direct-write dip-pen nanolithography, *J. Am. Chem. Soc.* 125, 5588–9, 2003.

[119] Maheshwari, G. et al., Cell adhesion and motility depend on nanoscale RGD clustering, *J. Cell Sci.* 113, 1677–86, 2000.

[120] Koo, L.Y. et al., Co-regulation of cell adhesion by nanoscale RGD organization and mechanical stimulus, *J. Cell Sci.* 115, 1423–1433, 2002.

[121] Lee, K.Y. and Mooney, D.J., Controlled growth factor delivery for tissue engineering, in *Advances in Controlled Drug Delivery: Science, Technology, and Products*, American Chemical Society, New York, 2003, pp. 73–83.

[122] Peters, M.C. et al., Release from alginate enhances the biological activity of vascular endothelial growth factor, *J. Biomater. Sci. Polym. Ed.* 9, 1267–78, 1998.

[123] Richardson, T.P. et al., Polymeric system for dual growth factor delivery, *Nat. Biotechnol.* 19, 1029–34, 2001.

[124] Yang, W.D. et al., Perlecan domain I promotes FGF-2 delivery in collagen I fibril scaffolds, *Tissue Eng.*, 11, 76–89, 2005.

[125] Wissink, M.J.B. et al., Improved endothelialization of vascular grafts by local release of growth factor from heparinized collagen matrices, *J. Control. Release* 64, 103–14, 2000.

[126] Liu, L.S. et al., Hyaluronate-heparin conjugate gels for the delivery of basic fibroblast growth factor (FGF-2), *J. Biomed. Mater. Res.* 62, 128–35, 2002.

[127] Matsuda, T. and Magoshi, T., Preparation of vinylated polysaccharides and photofabrication of tubular scaffolds for potential use in tissue engineering, *Biomacromolecules* 3, 942–50, 2002.

[128] Chinen, N. et al., Action of microparticles of heparin and alginate crosslinked gel when used as injectable artificial matrices to stablilize basic fibroblast growth factor and induce angiogenesis by controlling its release, *J. Biomed. Mater. Res. A* 67A, 61–8, 2003.

[129] Yamaguchi, N. and Kiick, K.L., Polysaccharide-poly(ethylene glycol) star copolymers as scaffolds for the production of bioactive hydrogels, *Biomacromolecules* 6, 1921–30, 2005.

[130] Sakiyama-Elbert, S.E. and Hubbell, J.A., Controlled release of nerve growth factor from a heparin-containing fibrin-based cell ingrowth matrix, *J. Control. Release* 69, 149–58, 2000b.

[131] Lee, A.C. et al., Controlled release of nerve growth factor enhances sciatic nerve regeneration, *Exp. Neurol.* 184, 295–303, 2003.

[132] Kuhl, P.R. and Griffith-Cima, L.G., Tethered epidermal growth factor as a paradigm for growth factor-induced stimulation from the solid phase, *Nat. Med.* 2, 1022–7, 1996.

[133] Mann, B.K., Schmedlen, R.H., and West, J.L., Tethered-TGF-beta increases extracellular matrix production of vascular smooth muscle cells, *Biomaterials* 22, 439–44, 2001a.

[134] Mann, B.K. et al., Smooth muscle cell growth in photopolymerized hydrogels with cell adhesive and proteolytically degradable domains: synthetic ECM analogs for tissue engineering, *Biomaterials* 22, 3045–51, 2001b.

[135] Zisch, A.H. et al., Covalently conjugated VEGF-fibrin matrices for endothelialization, *J. Control. Release* 72, 101–13, 2001.

[136] Zisch, A.H. et al., Cell-demanded release of VEGF from synthetic, biointeractive cell-ingrowth matrices for vascularized tissue growth, *FASEB J.* 17, 2260–2, 2003.

33

Mechanical Forces on Cells

Yan-Ting Shiu
University of Utah

33.1 Introduction

All cells in the body are subjected to mechanical forces that are either self-generated or originate from the environment. Depending on their location within the body, cells may be selectively exposed to various forces such as pressure, fluid shear stress, stretch, and compression. These externally applied mechanical forces play a significant role in normal tissue homeostasis and remodeling. For example, gravitational compressive forces control bone deposition, mechanical loads on skeletal muscle determine muscle mass, and blood flow-associated mechanical forces regulate the homeostasis of vascular walls [1–3]. All external forces that impinge on cells are imposed on a dynamic backdrop of various internally generated forces necessary for carrying out fundamental cellular events (e.g., cell division and migration). When cells sense a change in their net external loading, they actively alter their internal forces to counteract external forces. There is growing recognition that the balance between internally generated forces and externally applied forces is a key determinant of cell fate [1,4].

The importance of mechanical forces in tissue engineering applications is clear. The main goal of tissue engineering is the fabrication of artificial tissues for replacing damaged body structures. To produce functional tissues outside the body, it is necessary to create an *in vitro* culture environment that embodies the basic parameters of a physiological setting. Enormous strides have been made to understand the biochemical aspects of the *in vivo* microenvironment. However, the same level of understanding does not exist for the mechanical contributions. The mechanical environment of mammalian cells in the body is defined by an intricate balance between external loading and intracellular tension. The goal of this chapter is to examine the characteristics of each component within the mechanical microenvironment and highlight their implications in tissue engineering applications. The discussion will focus on anchorage-dependent, nonsensory cells.

33.2   The Role of Cytoskeletal Tension in Anchorage-Dependent Cells

For anchorage-dependent cells, the ability to apply cytoskeletal forces against the extracellular matrix (ECM) through integrin receptors is essential for cell survival and proliferation [4–6]. When a cell resides on an ECM scaffold, its contractile bundles of actin and myosin filaments (i.e., stress fibers) pull on an array of well-established connections between the cell and ECM known as focal adhesions (FAs). FAs consist of clustered integrins that span the plasma membrane, interacting with specific ECM ligands on the outside and with bundles of actin filaments via cytoskeletal-associated proteins (e.g., paxillin, α-actinin, and vinculin) on the inside [7–9]. In this way, cytoskeletal forces are transmitted via integrins to the underlying ECM, which acts as an external support for anchoring the cell and balancing the forces that maintain cell shape (Figure 33.1a) [7,8]. Thus, the adherent cell is under tension due to the ECM's resistance to deformation. The tension residing in the cytoskeleton of a resting adherent cell (often referred to as initial tension, resting tension, or prestress) is a major determinant of cell shape and functions such as proliferation, differentiation, deformability, migration, signal transduction, and ECM remodeling (see References 1,6, and 10–12 for review). Cytoskeletal tension is dynamic and can change without external stimuli during specific fundamental cellular events such as cell division and migration. Cytoskeletal tension also changes when the cell receives and responds to externally applied mechanical stimuli. Importantly, cellular responses to an external load may differ depending on the level of the initial tension (or, the "mechanical tone") in the cell [4,10–12].

The amount of the initial tension in an adherent cell is collectively controlled by its own actomyosin contractile machinery and its interaction with the ECM. Actomyosin contraction is driven by the motor protein myosin II and is triggered by the phosphorylation of the myosin light chain (MLC) in nonmuscle and smooth muscle cells [13]. The Rho GTPase (a member of the Rho family of GTP binding proteins) and its effector Rho kinase (ROCK) are important regulators of myosin activity. Blocking cell contractility by inactivating Rho or ROCK inhibits the formation of tension-dependent structures such as stress fibers and FAs [14–17]. The intracellular contractile force exerted on the ECM (also called the traction force) is essential for the assembly of fibronectin fibrils [18]. When the cell is cultured on a silicone rubber membrane, traction forces distort the substrate, forming wrinkles that can be visualized using phase-contrast microscopy [19].

Several techniques have been developed to characterize traction forces by measuring the deformation of elastic substrates (see References 13, and 20–22 for review). These methods can be combined with fluorescence imaging of FA proteins in living cells (e.g., green fluorescent protein [GFP]-tagged vinculin) to examine the relationship between the size/shape of FAs and the forces transmitted through them over time. Many studies have demonstrated conclusively that FAs transmit cytoskeletal forces in the range of several nanonewtons per square micrometers to the underlying substrate [13]. In addition, it was found that in stationary fibroblasts expressing GFP-tagged vinculin, the size of FAs is proportional to the local transmitted force (Figure 33.1b) and the orientation of FAs is parallel to the direction of the force applied at each FA (Figure 33.1c); the relaxation of the forces (induced by contractility inhibitors) and the disassembly of FAs occurred simultaneously [23]. It is important to note that the traction force is directly related, but not identical, to the intracellular contractile force, part of which could be dissipated

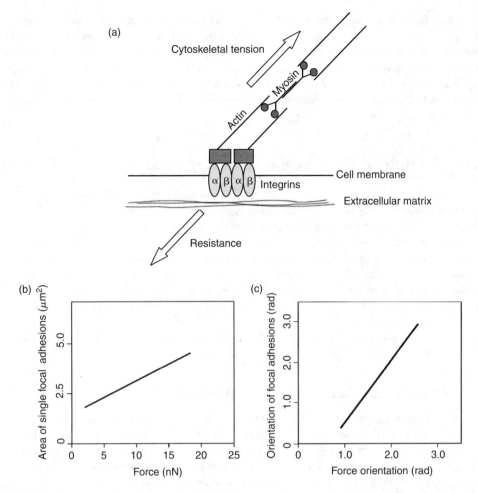

FIGURE 33.1 Forces on focal adhesions (FAs). (a) FAs are specialized sites of adhesion that form between cultured cells and a substrate. They contain clustered integrin receptors (heterodimeric transmembrane glycoproteins) whose extracellular domain binds to specific ECM ligands and intracellular domain interacts with bundles of actin filaments via cytoskeletal-associated proteins (the boxes between integrins and actin filaments). Myosin II-driven contractile forces applied to a cluster of integrins can lead to the development of tension if the underlying ECM is sufficiently rigid. (Adapted from Burridge, K. and Chrzanowska-Wodnika, M., *Annu. Rev. Cell Dev. Biol.*, 12, 463, 1996; Geiger, B. and Bershadsky, A., *Cell*, 110, 139, 2002. With permission.) (b) and (c) Fibroblasts expressing GFP-tagged vinculin were cultured on silicone elastomers imprinted with micropatterns of dots. The traction force applied by the cell on the substrate was calculated to the precision of a single adhesion site based on the displacements of dots (markers) and the locations of the FAs. In stationary fibroblasts, mature FAs were elongated structures; the size of vinculin-containing FAs was proportional to the local transmitted force (b) and the main axis of this elongation is parallel to the direction of the force applied at each FA (c). (Adapted from Balaban, N.Q., et al., *Nat. Cell Biol.*, 3, 466, 2001. With permission.)

due to cell deformation or other cellular processes [23,24]. Furthermore, the magnitude and direction of traction forces vary among different regions of a cell [13,23,25,26]. Experimental evidence shows that the average traction force magnitude over the entire cell area correlates with the state of cell contraction. Therefore, quantification of traction forces provides insightful information on the state of cellular tension.

Finally, in addition to the ECM, other structures exist that may provide mechanical support for the tensed actin network in the cytoplasm. Candidates include microtubules and cell–cell contacts. Several studies have reported that microtubules are under compression in living cells, and that compressive loads could be transferred from microtubules to the ECM based on the observation of an increase in traction forces upon the disruption of microtubules [27–30]. Cells can also transmit forces to their neighbors through cell–cell junctions. Cells in a confluent monolayer generally form fewer and smaller FAs with the ECM than subconfluent cells [31,32], suggesting a decreased tension at the interface between the ECM and a cell monolayer. The interactions between groups of cells and the ECM define "the resting stress field" within a tissue and are essential for guiding tissue development, remodeling, repair, and maintaining tissue homeostasis [6,33].

33.3   The Role of ECM Scaffolds in Regulating Cellular Tension

The effect of ECM molecules on cells is primarily mediated through integrins. It is well recognized that the chemical composition of the ECM influences integrin-mediated signaling pathways. However, a number of observations have shown that adhesion to the ECM (i.e., ligand occupation) alone is not sufficient to elicit a complete integrin-mediated response unless the matrix proteins are immobilized and can physically resist tension [34,35]. *In vitro* studies have demonstrated that although many integrin signaling events can be induced in suspended cells by allowing the cells to bind to ECM-coated microbeads, these cells never enter S phase and may even undergo apoptosis [36–38]. The tension-dependent control of cell growth is attributed to ensure that only anchored cells can grow. Loss of this control (i.e., anchorage independence) is a hallmark of cancerous cells [37].

While the chemical composition of the ECM determines whether a cell can bind to it or not, once ligation is established, the development of tension is influenced by the physicality of the ECM.

33.3.1   Effects of the Compliance of ECM Scaffolds

Because the mechanical properties of the ECM determine its deformation under compressive loads, they affect the level of tension that a cell can develop; a rigid surface can resist higher tension than a softer surface and thus allow cells to carry more tension in the cytoskeleton [1,37]. Experimental observations have confirmed this notion. Wang et al. [39,40] have developed ECM-coated polyacrylamide substrates that allow the compliance to be varied while maintaining a constant chemical environment. When compared with rigid substrates, fibroblasts grown on soft substrates exert smaller traction forces, indicating a decrease in their intracellular tension (Figure 33.2a). This response to a soft substrate is accompanied by a decrease in the cell spreading area, a decrease in the rate of DNA synthesis, and an increase in the rate of apoptosis [40]. Similar phenomena have also been observed in three-dimensional cell cultures using stabilized and freely floating collagen gels (i.e., stressed vs. relaxed gels). Fibroblasts grown in stabilized collagen gels generate isometric stresses within the gels while those cultured on freely floating gels do not [41]. The implication of these results for tissue engineering applications is clear; the compliance of the scaffolds for cells is an important regulator of cell behavior through its influence on cell tension.

It is worth noting that when cells are grown on a substrate containing a stiffness gradient, cells move preferentially toward the rigid side (a phenomenon known as durotaxis) [42]. This finding indicates that cells not only respond to but also actively probe substrate flexibility, most likely by applying contractile forces to the substrate via adhesion sites and then responding to the feedback (i.e., counter-forces from the substrate) via the same sites [39,40]. Hence, cell-substrate adhesion sites may act as mechanoprobing devices, translating "external" mechanical input into intracellular signals [39,40]. Several lines of experimental evidence strongly support a pivotal role for integrin-mediated adhesions in the mechanosensing process (see References 5,8,9,13,43, and 44 for review). FAs are multimolecular complexes consisting of more than 50 different proteins that link ECM-attached integrins to the actin cytoskeleton [7,8]. Enrichment of signaling and structural proteins at FAs could facilitate intracellular signaling by bringing enzymes and their substrates into close proximity, thereby enhancing rate and opportunity of the reaction [45]. It is hypothesized that external forces received by integrins may physically change the structure of specific FA molecules and rearrange the relative positions of FA components, thereby affecting the function of

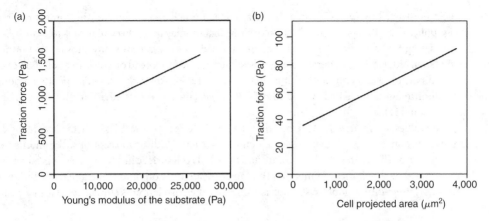

FIGURE 33.2 Effects of the physicality of ECM substrates on traction forces. Cells were cultured on polyacrylamide gels embedded with 0.2 μm-diameter fluorescent beads. Cellular traction forces were estimated based on the displacements of the beads (which reflected the deformation of the gel). The average traction force magnitude over the entire cell area was reported here. (a) Fibroblasts were cultured on collagen-coated polyacrylamide gels with different stiffness. Cells exerted larger traction forces on stiffer than softer gels. (Adapted from Wang, H.B., Dembo, M., and Wang,Y.L., *Am. J. Physiol. Cell Physiol.*, 279, C1345, 2000. With permission.) (b) Human airway smooth muscle cells were cultured on various micro-sized adhesive islands on the surface of polyacrylamide gels. The Young's modulus of the gels was $\approx$1,300 Pa. Promoting cell spreading resulted in increased traction forces. (Adapted from Wang, N. et al., *Cell Motil. Cytoskeleton*, 52, 97, 2002. With permission.)

associated signaling molecules and triggering a cascade of signaling events [8,13]. Alternatively, forces distributed along noncovalent bonds in a multimolecular FA complex may alter bond formation and dissociation kinetics, thereby altering signal transduction events [3,46].

33.3.2 Effects of the Spatial Distribution of ECM Ligands

An apparent effect of the ECM distribution on a cell is the cell shape (or projected area in a planar culture). It is well recognized that there is a close relationship between cell area and cell growth. Cells that are forced to spread over a large surface area survive better and proliferate faster than cells that are more confined [38,47]. Cell area may also affect the amount of cytoskeletal tension; a larger area underneath the cell body may resist greater levels of traction, thereby increasing isometric tension inside the cell [26,37,48]. A common and simple way to control cell area is to control the density of the ECM molecules coated on otherwise nonadhesive cell culture dishes. A higher ECM coating density allows cells to spread better and form more FAs than a lower coating density. However, because ECM coating density also affects integrin activation, it remained controversial whether the effect of increased cell area was due to the ECM density or was separate from it. This issue has been recently resolved by advances in micropatterning techniques, which allow the synthesis of surfaces on which different micron-sized islands are coated with the same ECM density and surrounded by nonadhesive regions to constrain cell spreading. When ECM islands are created on elastic substrates, traction forces can be estimated based on substrate deformation [26]. It was found that cultured cells spread to take the size and shape of the islands, and that traction forces increased as cell spreading was promoted (Figure 33.2b) [26]. These results indicate that larger cells carry greater cytoskeletal tension, and demonstrate that it is the extent of cell spreading, rather than ECM density, that influences cell tension. Furthermore, blocking the generation of actomyosin-based tension in well-spread cells (with an inhibitor that does not alter cell shape) was found to inhibit cell growth; thus, cytoskeletal tension is required for shape-dependent growth control [49].

It has been shown that myosin II-driven tension promotes cell spreading, and cell spreading stimulates MLC phosphorylation, thereby further increasing cytoskeletal tension generation [26,50]. Hence, there is an intimate crosstalk between the generation of cytoskeletal tension and the extent of cell distortion, the latter being restricted by the ECM area that is available for cell attachment. In the context of tissue engineering applications, the spatial distribution of ECM ligands may be a powerful means for controlling cell behavior. Using the micropatterned substrate mentioned above, a recent study showed that human mesenchymal stem cells (MSCs) undergo osteogenesis when allowed to spread out (cell area $\approx 10,000\ \mu m^2$) but become adipocytes when confined with a small area ($\approx 1,000\ \mu m^2$); this shape-dependent control of lineage commitment is mediated by the Rho GTPase, specifically via its effect on ROCK-mediated cytoskeletal tension [51].

Finally, the studies summarized above address the spatial effect of the ECM on the extent of cell distortion and tension in a two-dimensional cell culture system. With few exceptions, the mechanical interaction between a cell and the ECM occurs around the whole cell surface in a true physiological setting. While there is not yet a direct measurement method to correlate tractions and the spatial distribution of ECM ligands in a three-dimensional system, it is likely that the correlation is similar to that in a planar culture system.

33.3.3 Physicality of ECM Scaffolds in Tissue Engineering

The control of cell function by the ECM is a subject under vigorous investigation in the field of cell biology and has great potential in tissue engineering applications. While most studies have previously focused on the chemical composition of the ECM, it is becoming clear that the physicality of the ECM scaffold is equally important as it has a profound impact on the cellular tension. Thus, design of future artificial ECMs for tissue engineering applications should take into consideration both the chemical and physical properties of ECM scaffolds. It is important to note that the mechanical influence between cells and ECM scaffolds is mutual. Cells exert strong traction forces that deform and rearrange their surrounding matrix proteins [18,41]. Hence, traction forces may affect the structure of the scaffolds (e.g., porosity, pore size, etc.), and changes in material properties will feedback to affect cell functions. Finally, as discussed below, cells in the body exist in a dynamic mechanical environment. Cell-scaffold constructs that are formed *in situ* will inevitably experience mechanical loading. Therefore, it is important to understand how the material properties of the scaffold will be affected by mechanical forces, and how cells embedded within the scaffold will sense and respond to these physiologic loads transmitted through the scaffold.

33.4   The Role of Externally Applied Mechanical Forces in Cell Function

Throughout their lifetime, cells are exposed to various kinds of mechanical forces generated during common physiological processes. The ability to sense these external forces is not a unique property of cells in specialized sensory organs, but instead is shared by most, if not all, cell types. Furthermore, many nonsensory cells rely on appropriate mechanical inputs for regulating cell growth, function, and remodeling. For example, gravitational compressive forces control the deposition of bone, and mechanical load on skeletal muscle determines muscle mass; under conditions of diminished mechanical loading, such as prolonged bed rest or microgravity, bone and muscle mass is quickly lost [1–3]. From an engineering perspective, under normal conditions cells appear to convert "increases in the net external force acting on a tissue" into "internal tension" by increasing tissue mass or other responses [33,52]. Such a response is not always beneficial and may contribute to pathological states such as cardiac and vascular hypertrophy that is caused by chronic high blood pressure. It is generally agreed that forces beyond the physiological range, both over- and underloading, could lead to adverse consequences [11,45,52].

In order to influence cell growth and function, mechanical forces may trigger the same signaling pathways that are activated by conventional chemical stimuli (e.g., growth factors and hormones). A vast amount of data has shown that many of the biochemical events generated by cells in response to forces are similar to those that occur following recognition of chemical stimuli (see References 3,33,45, and 52–56

TABLE 33.1   A Summary of Devices Used for Mechanical Stimulation of Cells *In Vitro*

Name of device/method of developing forces	Primary force	Fluid flow in and out of device	Comments
Cone-and-plate	Shear stress	No	Possible presence of secondary flows
Parallel-plate flow chamber	Shear stress	Yes	Possible presence of not fully developed laminar flow where fluid enters device Pressure varies linearly as a function of position, though this variation is often ignored as it is very small
Uniaxial stretch	Tensional stress	No	May also generate shear stress due to motion of cells relative to fluid
Biaxial stretch	Tensional stress	No	May also generate shear stress due to motion of cells relative to fluid
Compression of gas phase by addition of an inert gas	Pressure	No	Change in concentration of dissolved gas due to nonideal behavior
Direct compression of liquid phase	Pressure	No	No gas phase present

Source: Adapted from Gooch, K.J. and Tennant, C.J., *Mechanical Forces: Their Effects on Cells and Tissues*, Springer-Verlag, New York, 1997. With permission.

for review). The exact mechanisms by which cells transduce mechanical stimuli into biochemical signaling events (mechanochemical transduction) are not yet clear and are an active area of research.

33.4.1   Devices and Methodology Used for Mechanical Stimulation of Cells *In Vitro*

In complex *in vivo* environments, it is difficult to clarify the exact effect of a specific force or to delineate the role of a specific signaling pathway in mechanotransduction processes due to the interference of myriad chemical factors and the presence of other mechanical forces. Therefore, investigations on cellular responses to mechanical stimulation have relied heavily on the use of *in vitro* systems. Table 33.1 summarizes devices that are commonly used to subject cultured cells to flow, stretch, and pressure [52]. These devices expose a large number of cells to well-defined mechanical stimuli that replicate physiological loading. Techniques for applying localized forces to individual cells have been developed. The reader is referred to other resources on the subject [2].

33.4.1.1   Shear Stress

It is possible that most cell types are exposed to fluid shearing due to interstitial flow. However, the effects of shear stress on cell behavior have been studied most extensively in vascular endothelial cells (ECs), as they are constantly exposed to blood flow. Two common flow systems used for *in vitro* studies of shear effects on cells are the cone-and-plate viscometer and the parallel-plate flow chamber. In a cone-and-plate device (Figure 33.3a), cells are placed on a plate that remains stationary. Medium is filled in the space between the plate and cone and fluid flow is achieved by rotating the cone. In a parallel-plate flow chamber (Figure 33.3b), cells are usually cultured on a glass slide that forms the floor of a rectangular flow channel. Flow is driven to pass over the cell surface by an imposed pressure gradient. Both devices generate macroscopically uniform shear stress acting on the surface of cells. The derivations for describing the velocity profile and shear stress for these two devices from hydrodynamic theory are described elsewhere [57,58]. Note that the estimated shear stress is usually nominal because only macro (or bulk) fluid dynamics is considered. At a subcellular length scale, the magnitude and gradient of shear stresses may vary significantly with the local cell surface topography [59–65]. In addition, the fluid is usually assumed to be an incompressible Newtonian fluid. The assumption of incompressibility is valid if

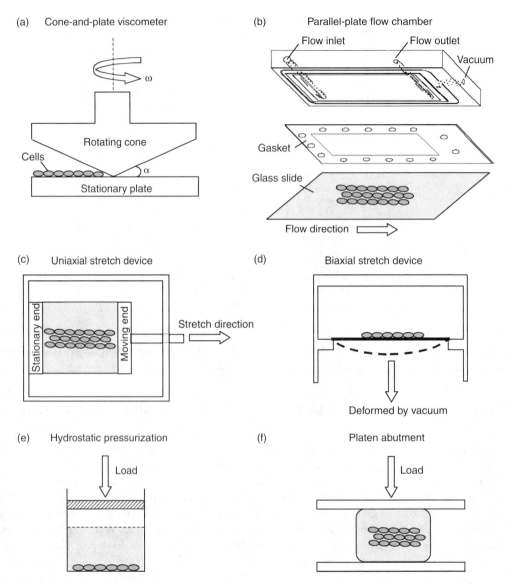

FIGURE 33.3 Schematic diagrams of devices used for mechanical stimulation of cells *in vitro*. (a) *The cone-and-plate viscometer*: cells are placed on the stationary plate and fluid flow is achieved by rotating the cone. For small cone angles ($\alpha \ll 1$) and small rotational rates ω, shear stress is uniform throughout the fluid phase between the cone and the plate. Although outside the scope of this chapter, it is important to note that this device is often used for studying the effect of bulk shear stress on suspended cells such as platelets and leukocytes. (Adapted from Tran-Son-Tay, R., *Physical Forces and the Mammalian Cell.*, Frangos, J.A. (Ed.) Academic Press, San Diego, 1993; Konstantopoulos, K., Kukreti,S., and McIntire, L.V., *Adv. Drug. Deliv. Rev.*, 33, 141, 1998. With permission.) (b) *The parallel-plate flow chamber*: the flow channel is formed by a cutout in a silicon gasket. The top plate of the flow channel is the surface of a polycarbonate base with flow inlet and outlet. The bottom plate is a glass slide where cells are cultured. The apparatus is held together by vacuum (shown here), clamps, or torqued screws. (c) *The uniaxial device*: cells are cultured on an elastic membrane, which is subjected to elongational stretch along one axis of the membrane in plane. (d) *The biaxial device*: cells are cultured on an elastic membrane, which is deformed by an applied vacuum. Solid and dashed lines are the positions of the membrane before and under deformation, respectively. (e, f) Devices for compressive loading. (Adapted from Brown, T.D., *J. Biomech.*, 33, 3, 2000. With permission.) See text for details.

water is the dominant component of the biological fluid under investigation. Other biological fluids such as blood, however, are non-Newtonian, and thereby limit the accuracy of the predictions [52,66].

33.4.1.2 Stretch

Many different cell types are constantly exposed to stretch during normal physiological processes. For example, cells on the compliant aortic wall are subjected to cyclic stretch due to pulsatile blood flow, and cells in the musculoskeletal system are subjected to cyclic stretch due to movement or gravity or both. A common method for *in vitro* studies of stretch effects on cells involves culturing cells on a flexible substrate, such as a silicone membrane, and then stretching the membrane with a controlled strain magnitude, frequency, and duration. Cells can be exposed to uniaxial or biaxial stretch (Figure 33.3c,d). This type of cell deformation device has several inherent problems. One problem is that the load delivered to cells is dependent on the state of adhesion between the cells and their substrate. Cells not fully adhered to the substrate do not experience the same amount of stretching as those fully adhered, and the subsequent data could be misleading [52]. Another problem is that fluid shear stress is often present concurrently with the imposed substrate deformation, due to coupled motion of the nutrient media [52,67]. Therefore, experimental design and data interpretation need to account for the relative contribution of stretch and shear stress.

33.4.1.3 Pressure/Compression

Hydrostatic pressurization is commonly used for investigating the effect of elevated pressure on cell functions (Figure 33.3e) [67]. This approach is simple and can deliver static and cyclic loading. However, the ensuing increase in the concentration of dissolved gases due to elevated pressure of the gas phase may affect cell functions, making it difficult to determine whether the effects observed in this system result from the pressure or from the change in gas concentration [52]. Two methods have been developed to circumvent this problem. One is to directly compress the fluid in the absence of a gas phase, and the other is to increase pressure by the addition of an inert gas (e.g., helium) while maintaining the partial pressure of biologically active gases (e.g., oxygen and carbon dioxide) [52,67].

An alternative approach to achieving compressive stress is to use direct platen abutment (Figure 33.3f) [67]. In this approach, a three-dimensional specimen (e.g., cells that are seeded in a matrix) is placed between two flat plates; the bottom plate remains stationary, whereas the top plate is pushed downward to deliver unconfined uniaxial compression (shown in Figure 33.3f; no peripheral support of the specimen so that it can freely expand laterally) or confined compression. This device can deliver static and cyclic compressive stresses. Direct platen abutment has an inherent problem that is similar to stretch devices: the loading delivered to cells is strongly dependent on the cell–matrix adhesion. Additionally, several variables arise concurrently with the compressive strain (e.g., flow, tensile strains, changes in specimen volume, etc.) [45,67]. When using them for experiments, it is important to include proper controls so that the effect due to compression can be distinguished from those due to other variables.

Finally, it should be noted that in all of the apparatuses mentioned earlier, cells usually are abruptly exposed to an imposed mechanical stimuli from static conditions. The sudden onset of mechanical inputs has been found to have a profound effect on some force-induced cell responses [68–72]. Detailed numerical analysis of the stress in the device may provide information for characterizing the time history of the mechanical stress under investigation, as well as for describing its spatial distribution and identifying the presence of unwanted inputs [52,67].

33.4.2 Responses of Cells to Mechanical Stimulation *In Vitro*

There is a rapidly growing list of reports detailing force-induced cellular responses by various experimental models as described earlier. Several excellent reviews have addressed the effects of particular forces on specific cell types *in vitro* [33,45,52–56,73–80]. The intention here is to avoid repetition with other papers and to address the general features of cellular responses to mechanical stimulation. The following discussion uses the force-induced responses of vascular ECs, vascular smooth muscle cells (SMCs), osteoblasts, and articular chondrocytes to illustrate the main points. These cell types are chosen because of the large body of data that are available.

Generally speaking, the responses of cells to a change in their external mechanical loads can be separated into rapid responses that occur within seconds to minutes and delayed responses that develop over many hours [45,75]. The rapid responses are due to the activation of a variety of intracellular signaling events, including potassium channel activation, elevated intracellular free calcium concentration, inositol trisphosphate generation, adelylate cyclase activation, G protein activation, phosphorylation of protein kinases, and, eventually activation of transcription factors [45,56,73,75]. Delayed responses usually require the modulation of gene expression [45,56,75]. Advances in the DNA microarray technology have allowed wide-scale screening of the genes affected by mechanical stimulation of cells, providing significant insights into the mechanical regulation of cell functions and homeostasis. For example, it was found that several genes related to inflammation and EC proliferation were downregulated after exposure of ECs to an arterial level of laminar shear stress (12 dyn/cm^2) for 24 h [81]. This finding suggests that long-term exposure to laminar flow may keep ECs in a relatively noninflammatory and nonproliferate state, which is consistent with the clinical observation that ECs at the straight part of arteries are mostly in a quiescent state and are relatively protected from the development of atherosclerotic plaques [81–85]. Reports concerning the genomic programming of other cell types in response to mechanical stimulation are available [86–89].

It is interesting to note that although force-induced delayed responses (and adaptive changes) vary at the cellular level among cell types, different mechanical stimuli induce several similar biochemical events in a variety of cells during rapid responses. For example, shear stress increases the concentration of intracellular free calcium and enhances the production of nitric oxide and at least one type of prostaglandin in osteoblasts, chondrocytes, SMCs, and ECs; in ECs, the above biochemical events can be induced by either shear stress or stretch [66,90–109]. The similarity of force-induced early biochemical events suggests that the way cells perceive different forces may be similar [52,73]. A cell may sense an imposed external force by detecting a deformation or resistance to deformation under stress. Different forces cause different kinds of cell deformation, thereby differentially inducing the common biochemical events and subsequently leading to diverse long-term changes. Indeed, it has been hypothesized that similar mechanisms might have evolved for cell recognition and response to external forces, since many cell types are subjected to external forces in the body, and even those thought not to be subjected to large forces *in vivo* respond to mechanical forces *in vitro* [45,52]. However, cell type-specific mechanosensing processes and the intrinsic heterogeneity among different cells cannot be excluded, but they are beyond the scope of this chapter.

33.4.3 Mechanosensing of Cultured Cells to Externally Applied Mechanical Forces

33.4.3.1 Direct Mechanosensing

Although intracellular signaling events triggered by external forces have been elucidated in many cell types, the primary mechanosensor for transducing mechanical input into biochemical signals remains elusive. It is hypothesized that forces may physically alter the molecular structure or displace the position of a sensor, thereby altering/triggering chemical signal transduction events. In conjunction, mechanosensors should be located at a site where the force acts directly or can be transmitted to efficiently [52,56,80]. Since most forces first act directly on the plasma membrane, the majority of the mechanotransensors that have been proposed are structures on the plasma membrane. Membrane structures that have been implicated in the role of mechanosensors in several cell types include ion channels, G protein-linked receptors, tyrosine kinase receptors, and integrins. Alternatively, because forces applied to the plasma membrane are transferred to the cytoskeleton, it too could act as a mechanosensor. Any reader interested in further details regarding the structures and signaling pathways associated with the proposed mechanosensors is referred to other resources [5,45,52–56,73,75,79,110–116].

Of the proposed mechanosensors, cytoskeleton and integrins have been the most extensively studied. Evidence suggests that they regulate mechanotransduction via mechanical and chemical mechanisms. The chemical nature of their functions is referred to the publications listed above. The mechanical nature of their actions is briefly considered here. As discussed in Section 33.2, an anchorage-dependent cell exists in a state of tension that is maintained by its cytoskeleton and balanced by the surrounding matrix via integrin-mediated adhesion sites (i.e., FAs). When an external force is loaded on the cell, the internal cellular tension changes to equalize the external force by actively rearranging its cytoskeleton and adhesion sites. The resulting change in cytoskeletal tension may convey a regulatory signal to the cell and subsequently alter its functional state. Dynamic changes in cytoskeleton organization, integrin-ECM binding, FAs, and traction forces may thus play a critical role in regulating mechanotransduction. These changes have been observed in EC responses to shear stress [117–121].

Finally, although each of the candidates mentioned above has been proposed to be a primary mechanosensor, it should be noted that they have a high degree of association with one another [3,56,75,80]. Considering the vast array of signaling pathways induced by forces, it is likely that several mechanosensors are induced simultaneously. Hence, forces may be transduced to biological signals through interactions of activated mechanoreceptors (Figure 33.4). Such a "decentralized model" was first proposed by Davies to describe EC responses to mechanical stresses but is applicable to mechanically induced responses in other cell types [56,80,122]. In this model, forces acting on one region of the cell surface are also transmitted by the cytoskeleton to other locations where signaling can occur, such as FAs at the cell–ECM interface, cell–cell junctions, the nuclear membrane, and, in case of two-dimensional culture, membrane proteins at the apical surface; the cytoskeleton itself is also a mechanosensor. This model predicts mechanotransduction as an integrated response of multiple signaling networks that are spatially organized in the cell. There is an increasing amount of data supporting the decentralization model (see References 13,56,75, and 122–124 for review).

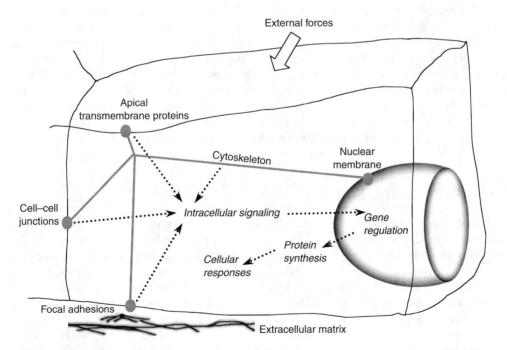

FIGURE 33.4 Model of initiation of signal transduction in cells in response to shear stress, stretch, and pressure. Forces may directly activate individual mechanosensors or may be transmitted by the cytoskeleton to intracellular locations where signaling can occur. In either case, cascades of intracellular signaling events are initiated, leading to altered gene expression and cell behavior. (Adapted from Davies, P.F., *Physiol. Rev.*, 75, 519, 1995. With permission.) See text for details.

33.4.3.2 Indirect Mechanosensing

It is important to note that mechanical forces may be accompanied by modifications of the chemical environment. For example, fluid flow influences the transport of agonists and other compounds to and from the cell surface (or, the local concentration of chemicals at the cell surface). If these agonists are degraded at the cell surface rapidly (as ATP is), flow will cause an increase in their concentration at the cell surface, and consequently modulate the cellular response [52,56,122]. Therefore, flow-induced responses may be mediated by increases in agonist concentrations (i.e., "indirect" mechanosensing), rather than physical alterations of mechanosensors (i.e., "direct" mechanosensing) by shear stress. There is *in vitro* experimental evidence that supports this mass transport hypothesis [125–132]. Indirect and direct mechanosensing are not mutually exclusive. It is likely that mechanical forces are incorporated into the biological signaling network by both physical alterations of mechanosensors and modifications of local chemical environments.

33.4.4 Applications of Externally Applied Mechanical Forces in Tissue Engineering

Conventional cell culture techniques grow cells under static conditions; in large-scale bioreactors (e.g., fluidized bed reactors, spinner flasks, rotating vessels, and perfused vessels), flow and mixing patterns are introduced merely to enhance spatially uniform cell distributions on three-dimensional scaffolds and provide efficient mass transfer to the growing tissues. As the significance of externally applied mechanical forces in maintaining appropriate cell physiology has come into the light, tissue engineers have incorporated mechanical stresses into bioreactor design and found that physiological loading has positive effects on growing cells/tissues *in vitro*. For example, increasing fluid shear forces significantly increases the mineral deposition by rat marrow stromal osteoblasts in a three-dimensional titanium fiber mesh scaffold [133,134], and the application of cyclic stretch to vascular SMCs cultured in collagen gels can help maintain the contractile phenotype of SMCs, align them in the correct physiological orientation, and improve the mechanical properties of cell–gel composites [135–137]. In the context of tissue-engineered cartilage, researchers have found that artificial cartilage grown under cyclic compressive loading has superior biochemical compositions and material properties than those grown statically [138–140]. Furthermore, cyclic compression can promote the chondrogenesis of rabbit bone-marrow MSCs by inducing the synthesis of transforming growth factor (TGF-β1), which then stimulates the MSCs to differentiate into chondrocytes [141]. These results show that appropriate mechanical stimulation may be a determining factor of tissue development *in vitro* and may improve the performance of engineered tissues in the body.

33.5 Concluding Remarks

This chapter has discussed three critical elements that define the mechanical microenvironment of a cell: self-generated forces, counter forces from the ECM, and externally applied forces in the body. Extensive work still needs to be done to create a coherent theory of mechanotransduction processes. At the cellular level, the nature of the primary mechanosensor(s) remains to be a central question. In this regard, investigations are limited by techniques that allow us to observe the force-induced changes in potential mechanosensors at a subcellular length scale and in a miniature time-frame. At the tissue level, tissue-scale responses to forces result from a dynamic and orchestrated interaction between different cell types in a three-dimensional matrix environment. In most of the *in vitro* studies described here, mechanical stimuli are imposed on monolayer cell cultures made of a single cell type. Although cultured cells sense and respond to mechanical stimulation in this setting, it is not yet clear whether the same responses or sensing mechanisms occur *in vivo*, but the wealth of *in vitro* data can guide *in vivo* experiments. Finally, in the context of tissue engineering, it is important to understand how the physicality of scaffolds affects cells, how the structure, composition, and mechanical properties of scaffolds may change as a result of traction forces from the cells and the external forces from the body, and how scaffolds affect cells to sense the external forces. These are just a few of the challenges for the future.

Acknowledgments

This work was supported by a Biomedical Engineering Research Grant from the Whitaker Foundation (RG-02-0133). The author thanks Matthew Iwamoto, Cole Quam, In Suk Joung, and Deepa Mishra for their help in manuscript preparation.

References

[1] Zhu, C., Bao, G., and Wang, N., Cell mechanics: mechanical responses, cell adhesion, and molecular deformation, *Annu. Rev. Biomed. Eng.*, 2, 189, 2000.

[2] Chen, C.S., Tan, J.L., and Tien, J., Mechanotransduction at cell–matrix and cell–cell contacts, *Annu. Rev. Biomed. Eng.*, 6, 3.1, 2004.

[3] Asthagiri, A.R. and Lauffenburger, D.A., Bioengineering models of cell signaling, *Annu. Rev. Biomed. Eng.*, 2, 31, 2000.

[4] Chicurel, M.E., Chen, C.S., and Ingber, D.E., Cellular control lies in the balance of forces, *Curr. Opin. Cell Biol.*, 10, 232, 1998.

[5] Katsumi, A. et al., Integrins in mechanotransduction, *J. Biol. Chem.*, 279, 12001, 2004.

[6] Galbraith, C.G. and Sheetz, M.P., Forces on adhesive contacts affect cell function, *Curr. Opin. Cell Biol.*, 10, 566, 1998.

[7] Burridge, K. and Chrzanowska-Wodnicka, M., Focal adhesions, contractility, and signaling, *Annu. Rev. Cell Dev. Biol.*, 12, 463, 1996.

[8] Geiger, B. and Bershadsky, A., Exploring the neighborhood: adhesion-coupled cell mechano-sensors, *Cell*, 110, 139, 2002.

[9] Geiger, B. and Bershadsky, A., Assembly and mechanosensory function of focal contacts, *Curr. Opin. Cell Biol.*, 13, 584, 2001.

[10] Ingber, D.E., Tensegrity I. Cell structure and hierarchical systems biology, *J. Cell Sci.*, 116, 1157, 2003.

[11] Ingber, D.E., Mechanobiology and diseases of mechanotransduction, *Ann. Med.*, 35, 564, 2003.

[12] Ingber, D.E., Tensegrity II. How structural networks influence cellular information processing networks, *J. Cell Sci.*, 116, 1397, 2003.

[13] Bershadsky, A.D., Balaban, N.Q., and Geiger, B., Adhesion-dependent cell mechanosensitivity, *Annu. Rev. Cell Dev. Biol.*, 19, 677, 2003.

[14] Narumiya, S., Ishizaki, T., and Watanabe, N., Rho effectors and reorganization of actin cytoskeleton, *FEBS Lett.*, 410, 68, 1997.

[15] Amano, M. et al., Phosphorylation and activation of myosin by Rho-associated kinase (Rho-kinase), *J. Biol. Chem.*, 271, 20246, 1996.

[16] Chrzanowska-Wodnicka, M. and Burridge, K., Rho-stimulated contractility drives the formation of stress fibers and focal adhesions, *J. Cell Biol.*, 133, 1403, 1996.

[17] Ridley, A.J. and Hall, A., The small GTP-binding protein rho regulates the assembly of focal adhesions and actin stress fibers in response to growth factors, *Cell*, 70, 389, 1992.

[18] Zhong, C. et al., Rho-mediated contractility exposes a cryptic site in fibronectin and induces fibronectin matrix assembly, *J. Cell Biol.*, 141, 539, 1998.

[19] Harris, A.K., Wild, P., and Stopak, D., Silicone rubber substrata: a new wrinkle in the study of cell locomotion, *Science*, 208, 177, 1980.

[20] Beningo, K.A., Lo, C.M., and Wang, Y.L., Flexible polyacrylamide substrata for the analysis of mechanical interactions at cell–substratum adhesions, *Meth. Cell Biol.*, 69, 325, 2002.

[21] Beningo, K.A. and Wang, Y.L., Flexible substrata for the detection of cellular traction forces, *Trends Cell Biol.*, 12, 79, 2002.

[22] Marganski, W.A., Dembo, M., and Wang, Y.L., Measurements of cell-generated deformations on flexible substrata using correlation-based optical flow, *Meth. Enzymol.*, 361, 197, 2003.

[23] Balaban, N.Q. et al., Force and focal adhesion assembly: a close relationship studied using elastic micropatterned substrates, *Nat. Cell Biol.*, 3, 466, 2001.

[24] Lauffenburger, D.A. and Horwitz, A.F., Cell migration: a physically integrated molecular process, *Cell*, 84, 359, 1996.

[25] Beningo, K.A. et al., Nascent focal adhesions are responsible for the generation of strong propulsive forces in migrating fibroblasts, *J. Cell Biol.*, 153, 881, 2001.

[26] Wang, N. et al., Micropatterning tractional forces in living cells, *Cell Motil. Cytoskeleton*, 52, 97, 2002.

[27] Wang, N. et al., Mechanical behavior in living cells consistent with the tensegrity model, *Proc. Natl Acad. Sci. USA*, 98, 7765, 2001.

[28] Stamenovic, D. et al., Effect of the cytoskeletal prestress on the mechanical impedance of cultured airway smooth muscle cells, *J. Appl. Physiol.*, 92, 1443, 2002.

[29] Brown, R.A. et al., Balanced mechanical forces and microtubule contribution to fibroblast contraction, *J. Cell Physiol.*, 169, 439, 1996.

[30] Dennerll, T.J. et al., Tension and compression in the cytoskeleton of PC-12 neurites. II: quantitative measurements, *J. Cell Biol.*, 107, 665, 1988.

[31] Ryan, P.L. et al., Tissue spreading on implantable substrates is a competitive outcome of cell–cell vs. cell–substratum adhesivity, *Proc. Natl Acad. Sci. USA*, 98, 4323, 2001.

[32] Nelson, C.M. et al., Vascular endothelial-cadherin regulates cytoskeletal tension, cell spreading, and focal adhesions by stimulating RhoA, *Mol. Biol. Cell*, 15, 2943, 2004.

[33] Silver, F.H. and Siperko, L.M., Mechanosensing and mechanochemical transduction: how is mechanical energy sensed and converted into chemical energy in an extracellular matrix? *Crit. Rev. Biomed. Eng.*, 31, 255, 2003.

[34] Miyamoto, S. et al., Integrin function: molecular hierarchies of cytoskeletal and signaling molecules, *J. Cell Biol.*, 131, 791, 1995.

[35] Miyamoto, S., Akiyama, S.K., and Yamada, K.M., Synergistic roles for receptor occupancy and aggregation in integrin transmembrane function, *Science*, 267, 883, 1995.

[36] Ingber, D.E., Fibronectin controls capillary endothelial cell growth by modulating cell shape, *Proc. Natl Acad. Sci. USA*, 87, 3579, 1990.

[37] Huang, S. and Ingber, D.E., The structural and mechanical complexity of cell-growth control, *Nat. Cell Biol.*, 1, E131, 1999.

[38] Chen, C.S. et al., Geometric control of cell life and death, *Science*, 276, 1425, 1997.

[39] Pelham, R.J., Jr. and Wang, Y., Cell locomotion and focal adhesions are regulated by substrate flexibility, *Proc. Natl Acad. Sci. USA*, 94, 13661, 1997.

[40] Wang, H.B., Dembo, M., and Wang, Y.L., Substrate flexibility regulates growth and apoptosis of normal but not transformed cells, *Am. J. Physiol. Cell Physiol.*, 279, C1345, 2000.

[41] Halliday, N.L. and Tomasek, J.J., Mechanical properties of the extracellular matrix influence fibronectin fibril assembly *in vitro*, *Exp. Cell Res.*, 217, 109, 1995.

[42] Lo, C.M. et al., Cell movement is guided by the rigidity of the substrate, *Biophys. J.*, 79, 144, 2000.

[43] Ingber, D.E., Mechanical signaling and the cellular response to extracellular matrix in angiogenesis and cardiovascular physiology, *Circ. Res.*, 91, 877, 2002.

[44] Geiger, B. et al., Transmembrane crosstalk between the extracellular matrix — cytoskeleton crosstalk, *Nat. Rev. Mol. Cell Biol.*, 2, 793, 2001.

[45] Millward-Sadler, S.J. and Salter, D.M., Integrin-dependent signal cascades in chondrocyte mechanotransduction, *Ann. Biomed. Eng.*, 32, 435, 2004.

[46] Bell, G.I., Models for the specific adhesion of cells to cells, *Science*, 200, 618, 1978.

[47] Ingber, D.E. and Folkman, J., Mechanochemical switching between growth and differentiation during fibroblast growth factor-stimulated angiogenesis *in vitro*: role of extracellular matrix, *J. Cell Biol.*, 109, 317, 1989.

[48] Huang, S. and Ingber, D.E., Shape-dependent control of cell growth, differentiation, and apoptosis: switching between attractors in cell regulatory networks, *Exp. Cell Res.*, 261, 91, 2000.

[49] Huang, S., Chen, C.S., and Ingber, D.E., Control of cyclin D1, p27(Kip1), and cell cycle progression in human capillary endothelial cells by cell shape and cytoskeletal tension, *Mol. Biol. Cell*, 9, 3179, 1998.

[50] Polte, T.R. et al., Extracellular matrix controls myosin light chain phosphorylation and cell contractility through modulation of cell shape and cytoskeletal prestress, *Am. J. Physiol. Cell Physiol.*, 286, C518, 2004.

[51] McBeath, R. et al., Cell shape, cytoskeletal tension, and RhoA regulate stem cell lineage commitment, *Dev. Cell*, 6, 483, 2004.

[52] Gooch, K.J. and Tennant, C.J., *Mechanical Forces: Their Effects on Cells and Tissues*, Springer-Verlag, New York, 1997.

[53] Hamill, O.P. and Martinac, B., Molecular basis of mechanotransduction in living cells, *Physiol. Rev.*, 81, 685, 2001.

[54] Apodaca, G., Modulation of membrane traffic by mechanical stimuli, *Am. J. Physiol. Renal Physiol.*, 282, F179, 2002.

[55] Shieh, A.C. and Athanasiou, K.A., Principles of cell mechanics for cartilage tissue engineering, *Ann. Biomed. Eng.*, 31, 1, 2003.

[56] Davies, P.F., Flow-mediated endothelial mechanotransduction, *Physiol. Rev.*, 75, 519, 1995.

[57] Bird, R.B., Stewart, W.E., and Lightfoot, E.N., *Transport Phenomena*, John Wiley & Sons, New York, 1960.

[58] Schlichting, H., *Boundary Layer Theory*, McGraw-Hill, New York, 1979.

[59] Liu, S.Q., Yen, M., and Fung, Y.C., On measuring the third dimension of cultured endothelial cells in shear flow, *Proc. Natl Acad. Sci. USA*, 91, 8782, 1994.

[60] Barbee, K.A., Davies, P.F., and Lal, R., Shear stress-induced reorganization of the surface topography of living endothelial cells imaged by atomic force microscopy, *Circ. Res.*, 74, 163, 1994.

[61] Barbee, K.A. et al., Subcellular distribution of shear stress at the surface of flow-aligned and nonaligned endothelial monolayers, *Am. J. Physiol.*, 268, H1765, 1995.

[62] Dewey, C.F., Jr. and DePaola, N. Exploring flow-cell interactions using computational fluid dynamics, in *Tissue Engineering*, Woo, S.-L.Y. and Seguchi, Y. (Eds.), ASME, New York, 1989.

[63] Satcher, R.L., Jr. et al., The distribution of fluid forces on model arterial endothelium using computational fluid dynamics, *J. Biomech. Eng.*, 114, 309, 1992.

[64] Sakurai, A. et al., A computational fluid mechanical study of flow over cultured endothelial cells, *Adv. Bioeng.*, 20, 299, 1991.

[65] Yamaguchi, T.H. et al., Shear stress distribution over confluently cultured endothelial cells studied by computational fluid dynamics, *Adv. Bioeng.*, 20, 167, 1993.

[66] Papadaki, M. and McIntire, L.V. Quantitative measurement of shear-stress effects on endothelial cells, in *Methods in Molecular Medicine, Vol. 18: Tissue Engineering Methods and Protocols.*, Morgan, J.R. and Yarmush, M.L. (Eds.), Humana Press, Totowa, NJ, 1998.

[67] Brown, T.D., Techniques for mechanical stimulation of cells *in vitro*: a review, *J. Biomech.*, 33, 3, 2000.

[68] Haidekker, M.A., White, C.R., and Frangos, J.A., Analysis of temporal shear stress gradients during the onset phase of flow over a backward-facing step, *J. Biomech. Eng.*, 123, 455, 2001.

[69] Frangos, J.A., Huang, T.Y., and Clark, C.B., Steady shear and step changes in shear stimulate endothelium via independent mechanisms — superposition of transient and sustained nitric oxide production, *Biochem. Biophys. Res. Commun.*, 224, 660, 1996.

[70] McKnight, N.L. and Frangos, J.A., Strain rate mechanotransduction in aligned human vascular smooth muscle cells, *Ann. Biomed. Eng.*, 31, 239, 2003.

[71] Clark, C.B., McKnight, N.L., and Frangos, J.A., Strain and strain rate activation of G proteins in human endothelial cells, *Biochem. Biophys. Res. Commun.*, 299, 258, 2002.

[72] Gudi, S.R. et al., Equibiaxial strain and strain rate stimulate early activation of G proteins in cardiac fibroblasts, *Am. J. Physiol.*, 274, C1424, 1998.

[73] Duncan, R.L. and Turner, C.H., Mechanotransduction and the functional response of bone to mechanical strain, *Calcif. Tissue Int.*, 57, 344, 1995.

[74] McIntire, L.V., 1992 ALZA Distinguished lecture: bioengineering and vascular biology, *Ann. Biomed. Eng.*, 22, 2, 1994.

[75] Papadaki, M. and Eskin, S.G., Effects of fluid shear stress on gene regulation of vascular cells, *Biotechnol. Prog.*, 13, 209, 1997.

[76] Patrick, C.W., Jr. and McIntire, L.V., Shear stress and cyclic strain modulation of gene expression in vascular endothelial cells, *Blood Purif.*, 13, 112, 1995.

[77] Skalak, T.C. and Price, R.J., The role of mechanical stresses in microvascular remodeling, *Microcirculation*, 3, 143, 1996.

[78] Liu, S.Q., Biomechanical basis of vascular tissue engineering, *Crit. Rev. Biomed. Eng.*, 27, 75, 1999.

[79] Chien, S., Li, S., and Shyy, Y.J., Effects of mechanical forces on signal transduction and gene expression in endothelial cells, *Hypertension*, 31, 162, 1998.

[80] Davies, P.F. and Tripathi, S.C., Mechanical stress mechanisms and the cell. An endothelial paradigm, *Circ. Res.*, 72, 239, 1993.

[81] Chen, B.P. et al., DNA microarray analysis of gene expression in endothelial cells in response to 24-h shear stress, *Physiol. Genom.*, 7, 55, 2001.

[82] Davies, P.F. et al., The convergence of haemodynamics, genomics, and endothelial structure in studies of the focal origin of atherosclerosis, *Biorheology*, 39, 299, 2002.

[83] Garcia-Cardena, G. et al., Biomechanical activation of vascular endothelium as a determinant of its functional phenotype, *Proc. Natl Acad. Sci. USA*, 98, 4478, 2001.

[84] McCormick, S.M. et al., DNA microarray reveals changes in gene expression of shear stressed human umbilical vein endothelial cells, *Proc. Natl Acad. Sci. USA*, 98, 8955, 2001.

[85] McCormick, S.M. et al., Microarray analysis of shear stressed endothelial cells, *Biorheology*, 40, 5, 2003.

[86] Segev, O. et al., CMF608-a novel mechanical strain-induced bone-specific protein expressed in early osteochondroprogenitor cells, *Bone*, 34, 246, 2004.

[87] Lee, R.T. et al., Mechanical strain induces specific changes in the synthesis and organization of proteoglycans by vascular smooth muscle cells, *J. Biol. Chem.*, 276, 13847, 2001.

[88] Karjalainen, H.M. et al., Gene expression profiles in chondrosarcoma cells subjected to cyclic stretching and hydrostatic pressure. A cDNA array study, *Biorheology*, 40, 93, 2003.

[89] Carinci, F. et al., Titanium–cell interaction: analysis of gene expression profiling, *J. Biomed. Mater. Res.*, 66B, 341, 2003.

[90] Schwarz, G. et al., Shear stress-induced calcium transients in endothelial cells from human umbilical cord veins, *J. Physiol.*, 458, 527, 1992.

[91] Segurola, R.J., Jr. et al., Cyclic strain is a weak inducer of prostacyclin synthase expression in bovine aortic endothelial cells, *J. Surg. Res.*, 69, 135, 1997.

[92] Rosales, O.R. et al., Exposure of endothelial cells to cyclic strain induces elevations of cytosolic Ca^{2+} concentration through mobilization of intracellular and extracellular pools, *Biochem. J.*, 326, 385, 1997.

[93] Reich, K.M. and Frangos, J.A., Effect of flow on prostaglandin E2 and inositol trisphosphate levels in osteoblasts, *Am. J. Physiol.*, 261, C428, 1991.

[94] Geiger, R.V. et al., Flow-induced calcium transients in single endothelial cells: spatial and temporal analysis, *Am. J. Physiol.*, 262, C1411, 1992.

[95] Shen, J. et al., Regulation of adenine nucleotide concentration at endothelium–fluid interface by viscous shear flow, *Biophys. J.*, 64, 1323, 1993.

[96] Kuchan, M.J. and Frangos, J.A., Role of calcium and calmodulin in flow-induced nitric oxide production in endothelial cells, *Am. J. Physiol.*, 266, C628, 1994.

[97] Frangos, J.A. et al., Flow effects on prostacyclin production by cultured human endothelial cells, *Science*, 227, 1477, 1985.

[98] Donahue, S.W., Donahue, H.J., and Jacobs, C.R., Osteoblastic cells have refractory periods for fluid-flow-induced intracellular calcium oscillations for short bouts of flow and display multiple low-magnitude oscillations during long-term flow, *J. Biomech.*, 36, 35, 2003.

[99] Hung, C.T. et al., Real-time calcium response of cultured bone cells to fluid flow, *Clin. Orthop.*, 256, 1995.

[100] Lee, M.S. et al., Effects of shear stress on nitric oxide and matrix protein gene expression in human osteoarthritic chondrocytes *in vitro*, *J. Orthop. Res.*, 20, 556, 2002.

[101] Osanai, T. et al., Cross talk between prostacyclin and nitric oxide under shear in smooth muscle cell: role in monocyte adhesion, *Am. J. Physiol. Heart Circ. Physiol.*, 281, H177, 2001.

[102] Sharma, R. et al., Intracellular calcium changes in rat aortic smooth muscle cells in response to fluid flow, *Ann. Biomed. Eng.*, 30, 371, 2002.

[103] Yellowley, C.E. et al., Effects of fluid flow on intracellular calcium in bovine articular chondrocytes, *Am. J. Physiol.*, 273, C30, 1997.

[104] Smalt, R. et al., Induction of NO and prostaglandin E2 in osteoblasts by wall-shear stress but not mechanical strain, *Am. J. Physiol.*, 273, E751, 1997.

[105] Smalt, R. et al., Mechanotransduction in bone cells: induction of nitric oxide and prostaglandin synthesis by fluid shear stress, but not by mechanical strain, *Adv. Exp. Med. Biol.*, 433, 311, 1997.

[106] McAllister, T.N. and Frangos, J.A., Steady and transient fluid shear stress stimulate NO release in osteoblasts through distinct biochemical pathways, *J. Bone Miner. Res.*, 14, 930, 1999.

[107] Johnson, D.L., McAllister, T.N., and Frangos, J.A., Fluid flow stimulates rapid and continuous release of nitric oxide in osteoblasts, *Am. J. Physiol.*, 271, E205, 1996.

[108] Abulencia, J.P. et al., Shear-induced cyclooxygenase-2 via a JNK2/c-Jun-dependent pathway regulates prostaglandin receptor expression in chondrocytic cells, *J. Biol. Chem.*, 278, 28388, 2003.

[109] Alshihabi, S.N. et al., Shear stress-induced release of PGE2 and PGI2 by vascular smooth muscle cells, *Biochem. Biophys. Res. Commun.*, 224, 808, 1996.

[110] Williams, B., Mechanical influences on vascular smooth muscle cell function, *J. Hypertens.*, 16, 1921, 1998.

[111] Lee, T. and Sumpio, B.E., Cell signalling in vascular cells exposed to cyclic strain: the emerging role of protein phosphatases, *Biotechnol. Appl. Biochem.*, 39, 129, 2004.

[112] Shyy, J.Y. and Chien, S., Role of integrins in cellular responses to mechanical stress and adhesion, *Curr. Opin. Cell Biol.*, 9, 707, 1997.

[113] Shyy, J.Y. and Chien, S., Role of integrins in endothelial mechanosensing of shear stress, *Circ. Res.*, 91, 769, 2002.

[114] Davidson, R.M., Membrane stretch activates a high-conductance K+ channel in G292 osteoblastic-like cells, *J. Membr. Biol.*, 131, 81, 1993.

[115] Berk, B.C. et al., Protein kinases as mediators of fluid shear stress stimulated signal transduction in endothelial cells: a hypothesis for calcium-dependent and calcium-independent events activated by flow, *J. Biomech.*, 28, 1439, 1995.

[116] Berk, B.C. et al., Atheroprotective mechanisms activated by fluid shear stress in endothelial cells, *Drug News Perspect.*, 15, 133, 2002.

[117] Helmke, B.P. et al., Spatiotemporal analysis of flow-induced intermediate filament displacement in living endothelial cells, *Biophys. J.*, 80, 184, 2001.

[118] Jalali, S. et al., Integrin-mediated mechanotransduction requires its dynamic interaction with specific extracellular matrix (ECM) ligands, *Proc. Natl Acad. Sci. USA*, 98, 1042, 2001.

[119] Li, S. et al., The role of the dynamics of focal adhesion kinase in the mechanotaxis of endothelial cells, *Proc. Natl Acad. Sci. USA*, 99, 3546, 2002.

[120] Shiu, Y.T. et al., Rho mediates the shear-enhancement of endothelial cell migration and traction force generation, *Biophys. J.*, 86, 2558, 2004.

[121] Stamatas, G.N. and McIntire, L.V., Rapid flow-induced responses in endothelial cells, *Biotechnol. Prog.*, 17, 383, 2001.

[122] Davies, P.F., Zilberberg, J., and Helmke, B.P., Spatial microstimuli in endothelial mechanosignaling, *Circ. Res.*, 92, 359, 2003.

[123] Helmke, B.P. and Davies, P.F., The cytoskeleton under external fluid mechanical forces: hemodynamic forces acting on the endothelium, *Ann. Biomed. Eng.*, 30, 284, 2002.

[124] Davies, P.F. et al., Spatial relationships in early signaling events of flow-mediated endothelial mechanotransduction, *Annu. Rev. Physiol.*, 59, 527, 1997.

[125] Ando, J. et al., Wall shear stress rather than shear rate regulates cytoplasmic Ca^{++} responses to flow in vascular endothelial cells, *Biochem. Biophys. Res. Commun.*, 190, 716, 1993.

[126] Ando, J. et al., Flow-induced calcium transients and release of endothelium-derived relaxing factor in cultured vascular endothelial cells, *Front. Med. Biol. Eng.*, 5, 17, 1993.

[127] Koller, A., Sun, D., and Kaley, G., Role of shear stress and endothelial prostaglandins in flow- and viscosity-induced dilation of arterioles *in vitro*, *Circ. Res.*, 72, 1276, 1993.

[128] Ando, J., Komatsuda, T., and Kamiya, A., Cytoplasmic calcium response to fluid shear stress in cultured vascular endothelial cells, *In Vitro Cell Dev. Biol.*, 24, 871, 1988.

[129] Dull, R.O. and Davies, P.F., Flow modulation of agonist (ATP)-response (Ca^2+) coupling in vascular endothelial cells, *Am. J. Physiol.*, 261, H149, 1991.

[130] Dull, R.O., Tarbell, J.M., and Davies, P.F., Mechanisms of flow-mediated signal transduction in endothelial cells: kinetics of ATP surface concentrations, *J. Vasc. Res.*, 29, 410, 1992.

[131] Mo, M., Eskin, S.G., and Schilling, W.P., Flow-induced changes in Ca^2+ signaling of vascular endothelial cells: effect of shear stress and ATP, *Am. J. Physiol.*, 260, H1698, 1991.

[132] Nollert, M.U. and McIntire, L.V., Convective mass transfer effects on the intracellular calcium response of endothelial cells, *J. Biomech. Eng.*, 114, 321, 1992.

[133] Bancroft, G.N. et al., Fluid flow increases mineralized matrix deposition in 3D perfusion culture of marrow stromal osteoblasts in a dose-dependent manner, *Proc. Natl Acad. Sci. USA*, 99, 12600, 2002.

[134] Sikavitsas, V.I. et al., Mineralized matrix deposition by marrow stromal osteoblasts in 3D perfusion culture increases with increasing fluid shear forces, *Proc. Natl Acad. Sci. USA*, 100, 14683, 2003.

[135] Nerem, R.M., Role of mechanics in vascular tissue engineering, *Biorheology*, 40, 281, 2003.

[136] Kanda, K. and Matsuda, T., Mechanical stress-induced orientation and ultrastructural change of smooth muscle cells cultured in three-dimensional collagen lattices, *Cell Transplant.*, 3, 481, 1994.

[137] Seliktar, D., Nerem, R.M., and Galis, Z.S., Mechanical strain-stimulated remodeling of tissue-engineered blood vessel constructs, *Tissue Eng.*, 9, 657, 2003.

[138] Davisson, T. et al., Static and dynamic compression modulate matrix metabolism in tissue engineered cartilage, *J. Orthop. Res.*, 20, 842, 2002.

[139] Park, S., Hung, C.T., and Ateshian, G.A., Mechanical response of bovine articular cartilage under dynamic unconfined compression loading at physiological stress levels, *Osteoarthr. Cartil.*, 12, 65, 2004.

[140] Hung, C.T. et al., A paradigm for functional tissue engineering of articular cartilage via applied physiologic deformational loading, *Ann. Biomed. Eng.*, 32, 35, 2004.

[141] Huang, C.Y. et al., Effects of cyclic compressive loading on chondrogenesis of rabbit bone-marrow derived mesenchymal stem cells, *Stem Cells*, 22, 313, 2004.

[142] Tran-Son-Tay, R. Techniques for studying the effects of physical forces on mammalian cells and measuring cell mechanical properties, in *Physical Forces and the Mammalian Cell*, Frangos, J.A. (Ed.), Academic Press, San Diego, 1993.

[143] Konstantopoulos, K., Kukreti, S., and McIntire, L.V., Biomechanics of cell interactions in shear fields, *Adv. Drug Deliv. Rev.*, 33, 141, 1998.

34

Cell Adhesion

Aaron S. Goldstein
Virginia Polytechnic Institute and State University

34.1 Introduction

Adhesion plays a critical role in the normal function of mammalian cells by regulating proliferation, differentiation, and phenotypic behavior. Although the molecular mechanism of adhesion involves several families of transmembrane receptors as well as numerous structural and regulatory proteins, they can be divided phenomenologically into two groups: those that mediate adhesive contacts to neighboring cells, and those that mediate adhesive contacts with structural extracellular matrix (ECM) proteins. In development, specific adhesive interactions between adjacent cells lead to the assembly of three-dimensional tissue structures, while cell adhesion to ECM proteins (e.g., collagens, elastin, and laminin) establishes cellular orientation and spatial organization of cells into tissues and organs. Consequently, both types are necessary for proper function of mammalian cells and tissues.

Initial efforts to design biomaterials — either to replace damaged tissues, or as a temporary scaffolds for the manufacture of engineered tissues and organs — have focused on achieving robust mechanical interactions between the biomaterial and adjacent cells (i.e., integration). However, evidence is emerging that cell/biomaterial interactions can affect cell/cell interactions, and consequently impact tissue development and function. Therefore, successful outcomes of tissue engineering efforts may require the development of advanced materials that can facilitate both cell/cell and cell/biomaterial adhesion.

This chapter discusses the phenomenon of cell adhesion both from a tissue perspective and from a biomaterial perspective. Section 34.2 describes the cell biology of adhesion receptors and their relevance to particular tissue functions. Section 34.3 addresses cell adhesion to biomaterials with specific focus on how the chemistry, biochemistry, and topography of biomaterial interfaces affect cell adhesion. Section 34.4 describes quantitative techniques to measure cell adhesion to biomaterials. Finally, Section 34.5 describes how cell spreading, proliferation, and migration depend on cell adhesion to biomaterials.

34.2 Adhesion Receptors in Tissue Structures

Mammalian cells establish and maintain adhesive contacts with extracellular structures and adjacent cells through several types of adhesion receptors that are displayed on the cell surface. The three main families of these receptors are integrins, cadherins, and members of the immunoglobulin superfamily [1–3]. Although they are involved in different adhesion-related tasks, they share several common features. First, when associated with extracellular ligands (e.g., ECM proteins, receptors on adjacent cells) they frequently assemble into clusters. Second, these transmembrane receptors are often linked to cytoskeletal structures (e.g., actin filaments, microtubules), and thus both anchor the cellular skeleton to extracellular structures and mediate the transmission of mechanical forces. Third, regulatory proteins (e.g., protein kinases) are associated with receptor clusters, and are responsible for controlling cluster stability and initiating signaling events that regulate cell proliferation and function.

34.2.1 Integrins

Integrins are a family of receptors that mediate cell adhesion to ECM proteins. They are found as heterodimers, consisting of α and β subunits, and to date at least 8 β and 18 α subunits and at least 24 different dimer combinations have been reported [4]. A short list of known integrin heterodimers and their respective ligands (Table 34.1) reveals that individual integrins can have multiple ligands (e.g., $\alpha_3\beta_1$ binds collagen, fibronectin, and laminin) and multiple integrins may bind the same ligand (e.g., laminin

TABLE 34.1   Integrin Dimers and Their Known Ligands

β subunit	α subunit	Ligand/counterreceptor	Binding site
β_1	α_1	LM (COL)	
	α_2	COL (LM)	DGEA (in COL I)
	α_3	FN, LM, COL	RGD?
	α_4	V-CAM (FN-alt)	REDV(in FN-alt)
	α_5	FN	RGD + PHSRN
	α_6	LM	RGD
	α_7	LM	
	α_8	?	
	α_V	FN	RGD
β_2	α_L	ICAM-1,2	
	α_M	FB, C3bi	
	α_X	FB, C3bi	GPRP
β_3	α_{IIb}	FB, FN, VN, VWF	RGD (+PHSRN in FN)
	α_V	VN, FB, VWF, TSP	RGD
β_5	α_V	VN, FN	RGD
β_6	α_V	FN	RGD

Adapted from Albelda, S.M. and Buck, C.A., *FASEB J.* 4, 2868, 1990. With permission and Hynes, R.O. and Lander, A.D., *Cell* 68, 303, 1992. With permission. LM laminin, COL collagens, FN fibronectin, VN vitronectin, FB fibrinogen, VWF von Willebrand Factor, TSP thrombospondin, C3bi breakdown product of third component of complement, FN-alt alternatively spliced fibronectin. DGEA, RGD, REDV, PHSRN, and GPRP are amino acid sequences.

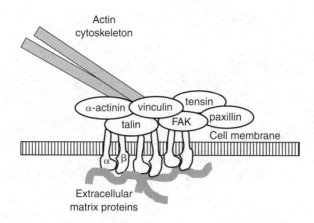

FIGURE 34.1 Illustration of a focal adhesion complex. A cluster of transmembrane integrin receptor heterodimers is shown interacting with extracellular matrix proteins and cytoplasmic proteins vinculin, α-actinin, talin, and focal adhesion kinase (FAK). This complex interacts with the actin cytoskeleton. Adapted from Petit, V. and Thiery, J.-P., *Biol. Cell.* 92, 477, 2000. With permission; Yamada, K.M. and Miyamoto, S., *Curr. Opin. Cell Biol.* 7, 681, 1995. With permission.

binds integrins $\alpha_1\beta_1$, $\alpha_2\beta_1$, $\alpha_3\beta_1$, $\alpha_6\beta_1$, $\alpha_7\beta_1$) [1,5]. In addition, most cell types express multiple integrin subunits. For example, the pluripotent mesenchymal progenitor bone marrow stromal cells have been shown to express integrin subunits α_1, α_5, α_6, and β_1 [6], while aortic smooth muscle cells express α_2, α_5, α_v, β_1, and β_5 [7]. It should be noted that integrins do not exclusively mediate cell/ECM adhesion: $\alpha_4\beta_1$ and $\alpha_M\beta_2$, presented on activated leukocytes and neutrophils mediate cell/cell adhesion by binding adhesion receptors of the immunoglobulin superfamily (e.g., vascular cell adhesion molecules [VCAM], intracellular adhesion molecules [ICAMs]) on activated endothelial cells [1,8].

Binding of integrin receptors to their extracellular ligands initiates a process of receptor clustering and the assembly of focal adhesion complexes [4,9–11] (Figure 34.1). Conserved sequences in the cytoplasmic tail of β subunit are responsible for recruiting integrins into clusters (except with β_4 and β_5 which do not aggregate), while the cytoplasmic tail of the α subunit plays a regulatory role to ensure aggregation of only ligand-bound receptors. The cytoplasmic proteins that associate with integrins in focal adhesion complexes can be divided into the categories of structural and regulatory proteins. The structural proteins — which include talin, α-actinin, filamin, and vinculin — stabilize the receptor aggregates and mechanically link the integrins to actin filaments, thus anchoring the cell cytoskeleton to extracellular structures. In particular, talin and α-actinin possess binding domains for β integrins, while vinculin has bonding domains for talin and actin. Regulatory proteins include paxillin, focal adhesion kinase (FAK), Src, and members of the Rho and Ras families [4]. FAK and Src are kinases that regulate focal adhesion complex assembly by phosphorylating structural proteins. In contrast, Rho and Ras are GTPases involved in initiating intracellular signaling. Rho is thought to act through a number of secondary messengers to stimulate focal adhesion assembly, actin stress fiber formation, and contraction, while Ras is thought to regulate integrin activation [12]. In addition, there is evidence that Ras activates mitogen-activated protein (MAP) kinase signaling cascades that are involved in regulating cell proliferation, apoptosis, migration, and development [10].

In addition to initiating signaling cascades, integrins also can stimulate signaling events initiated by cytokine receptors and growth factor receptors [12]. For example, interleukin (IL)-1 activation of MAP kinases requires integrin-mediated cell adhesion [13]. In addition, insulin and platelet-derived growth factor (PDGF) receptors — when bound to their respective ligands — physically interact with the $\alpha_v\beta_3$ integrin, and this association enhances MAP kinase signaling and cell proliferation [14]. Integrin binding also can modulate effects of other adhesion receptors. For example, the association of $\alpha_4\beta_1$ integrins with fibronectin has been shown to block the upregulation of metalloproteinase by $\alpha_5\beta_1$ binding to fibronectin

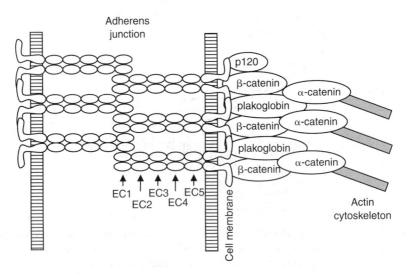

FIGURE 34.2 Illustration of cadherin receptors associated with actin cytoskeleton. Cadherin dimers are shown in a linear zipper structure with antiparallel binding of the EC1 domains. Cytoplasmic tails of cadherins interact with actin filaments through structural proteins β-catenin, p120^{cas} catenin, plakoglobin, and α-catenin.

[15]. Similarly, integrin-meditated adhesion to the ECM downregulates cadherin-mediated intercellular adhesion and cell clustering [16]. This last example illustrates a competition between integrin-mediated adhesion to the ECM and cadherin-mediated intercellular adhesion [17].

34.2.2 Cadherins

Cadherins are a family of calcium-dependent transmembrane glycoproteins that mediate cell/cell adhesion. Classical cadherins (e.g., E-, N-, P-, and VE-cad) possess five extracellular (EC) cadherin repeats, assemble into dimers, and mediate primarily homotypic binding between adjacent cells (Figure 34.2) [18–20]. Although the outermost repeat (EC1) is thought to be responsible for intercellular binding, it has been shown that cadherins can interact in at least three antiparallel alignments [21]. In addition, crystallography has revealed that cadherins may assemble into a linear zipper structure [22]. The cytoplasmic tails of classical cadherins interact with structural proteins β-catenin, p120^{cas} catenin, plakoglobin, and through them α-catenin and the actin cytoskeleton. The cytoplasmic tail of endothelial cell-specific receptor VE-cad also can interact vimentin intermediate filaments [18,20]. The protein p120^{cas} — a target of the Src kinase — is thought to be involved in regulating lateral clustering of cadherins, which has been shown to increase adhesive strength [23]. Thus, Src may be involved in regulating robust cadherin contacts.

Although cadherins do not exclusively cluster, the formation of adherens junctions is important for several tissue functions [18]. In epithelial tissues cadherins mediate zonula adherens junctions, which partition the cell membrane into apical and basolateral surfaces. In neuronal cells they mechanically stabilize synaptic junctions by mediating adhesion between the presynaptic and postsynaptic cells. In cardiac myocytes they establish intercalated discs, which both stabilize gap junctional coupling and transmit contractile forces.

In addition to classical cadherins, several other cadherin types have been identified [18,20]. Among these, desmocollins and desmogleins are expressed in cells that experience mechanical stress (e.g., epidermis, myocardium) and are the transmembrane proteins present in desmosomes [18,20]. Like classical cadherins, they have five extracellular cadherin repeats (except desmoglein 1, which has four repeats), but they form desmoglein/desmocollin heterodimers and are thought to mediate intercellular adhesion through heterotypic desmoglein/desmocollin interactions between adjacent cells. The cytoplasmic tails of these receptors interact, through structural proteins desmoglobin and desmoplakin, with the keratin intermediate filaments. To date three desmocollins and desmogleins have been identified. Desmoglein 2 and desmocollin 2 are expressed in all epithelial tissues that form desmosomes, while desmocollin 1 and desmoglein 1 are expressed predominantly in epidermal tissue.

In addition to regulating organized tissue functions, E-, N-, and VE-cadherin-mediated intercellular contacts have been shown to suppress cell proliferation [24–26]. This phenomenon is thought to be a consequence of cadherin-induced alterations in the cytoskeleton structure [27], and to contribute to the abrogation of cell proliferation of confluent tissue cultures.

34.2.3 Immunoglobulins

Members of the diverse immunoglobulin superfamily are characterized by the immunoglobulin (Ig) fold motif, a 70–110 amino acid structure consisting of two sheets of antiparallel β-strands stabilized by a disulfide bridge and numerous hydrophobic side chains [28,29]. Because the amine and carboxy termini extend from opposite ends of this structure, members of the immunoglobulin family frequently possess strings of Ig folds. Immunoglobulin proteins are most noted for their role in antigen presentation and recognition functions of the immune system, but at least ten members of the superfamily are involved in cell/cell adhesion. ICAM-1, ICAM-2, and VCAM, for example, are presented on the surface of activated endothelial cells and mediate heterotypic binding to integrins on activated leukocytes and neutrophils (Table 34.1) [8]. Neural cell adhesion molecules (NCAMs) and L1 — present in neurons and glia — primarily mediated homotypic binding and are involved in axon guidance, neuronal migration, neurite outgrowth, synapse formation, and maintenance of the integrity of myelinated fibers [29,30]. Finally, junctional adhesion molecules (JAMs) stabilize tight junctions, which regulate paracellular ion transport across epithelial and endothelial layers [31].

34.3 Cell Adhesion to Biomaterials

The efficacy of biomaterials — either as replacements for damaged tissues, or as a temporary scaffolds for the manufacture of engineered tissues and organs — relies on the ability of the material surface to regulate cell adhesion, and strategies to engineer this cell/biomaterial interaction have evolved over the past few decades through three basic generations [32]. The first generation is exemplified by bulk materials such as titanium, Dacron, and ultrahigh molecular weight polyethylene, which are durable and exhibit good mechanical properties, but are nondegradable and essentially bioinert (i.e., they elicit minimal effects *in vivo*). Second generation biomaterials are those that — when brought into contact with bodily fluids and cells — are modified chemically or biochemically to achieve more favorable biologic properties. Biochemical modifications include the adsorption of ECM proteins to the biomaterial surface in conformations that enhance cell and tissue behavior (e.g., adhesion [33], phenotype [34]), while examples of chemical modifications include the ion-exchange reactions of bioactive glasses, dissolution and reorganization of amorphous calcium phosphate, and hydrolytic degradation of polyurethanes and polyesters. Finally, third generation biomaterials are those that incorporate biomimetic moieties (e.g., peptides sequences) that are designed to interact with target proteins (e.g., adhesion receptors, growth factor receptors, matrix metalloproteinases) and elicit specific cell responses. Thus, third generation biomaterials are often referred to as bioactive materials because they act on cells and tissues.

Cell adhesion to biomaterials may be characterized in terms of specific and nonspecific interactions. Specific interactions entail cell receptor recognition and binding to proteins or biomimetic moieties on the biomaterial surface, whereas nonspecific interactions encompass noncovalent attractive forces (e.g., electrostatic interactions, hydrogen bonds, van der Waals forces) between the cell and biomaterial that are not associated with a specific receptor. In general, both specific and nonspecific interactions contribute to cell adhesion to biomaterials, and can be regulated through design of substratum chemistry and biochemistry. The following subsections address (a) the role of substratum chemistry on nonspecific adhesion, the roles of (b) proteins and (c) biomimetic moieties on specific adhesion, and (d) the effect of substratum topography on cell adhesion.

34.3.1   The Role of Interfacial Chemistry in Cell Adhesion

Although cells express receptors for ECM proteins and adjacent cells, they have been shown to adhere through nonspecific interactions to a variety of biomaterials. For example, a comprehensive study by Schakenraad et al. [35] demonstrated cell adhesion and spreading on 13 commercially available polymers. In particular, this study showed that cell spreading was markedly greater on materials with surface free energies greater than 50 erg/sec (hydrophilic surfaces) relative to low energy (hydrophobic) surfaces [35]. With the development of self-assembling methods (e.g., alkanethiolates on gold and alkylsilanes on glass), chemically well-defined model surfaces have been constructed and used to characterize cell adhesion [36–41]. These model studies indicate that terminal amine (NH_2) and carboxylic acid (COOH) groups produce superior adhesion relative to hydrophobic methyl-(CH_3)-terminated surfaces [36,38–40]. In contrast, surfaces presenting poly(ethylene glycol) subunits have been shown to inhibit cell adhesion [42]. In addition to organic polymers, alloys [43], and ceramics [44] have also been studied for their capacity to support cell adhesion. These materials have proven more difficult to characterize as the chemistries are complex, and the grain size appears to play an important role [44,45]. Nevertheless, a consistent theme that emerges from these studies is that cell adhesion increases with the material's capacity to promote adsorption of ECM proteins [33,38,40,45].

34.3.2   The Role of Interfacial Biochemistry in Cell Adhesion

A simple method to enhance cell adhesion to first and second generation biomaterials is to adsorb ECM proteins to the biomaterial surface from protein solutions (e.g., collagens [46], fibronectin [46–48]), serum, or serum-containing culture medium. Although albumin is the predominant protein in serum, vitronectin and fibronectin have been shown to deposit readily from serum onto both organic [49] and ceramic [50] biomaterial surfaces. The choice of ECM protein can be important to regulating cell behavior; cell adhesion and function have been shown to vary with the adhesive protein [46,49]. In addition, the chemistry of the biomaterial surface — to which the ECM proteins are adsorbed — can also affect cell adhesion and function [33,34,51] by altering protein orientation and inducing conformational changes (i.e., denaturation) [51–56] that undermine receptor binding. Conformational changes have been inferred from an increase in the ratio of β-turn to β-sheet structures, and indicate a higher degree of protein denaturation on hydrophobic methyl-terminated surfaces than on more hydrophilic carboxyl-terminated surfaces [54]. In addition, protein denaturation is inversely related to the rate of protein adsorption [57], and decreases as the protein concentration in solution is increased.

34.3.3   Biomimetic Approaches to Regulate Cell Adhesion

An attractive alternative to immobilization of entire ECM proteins at biomaterial interfaces is the use of short peptide sequences that are specifically recognized by integrin adhesion receptors [58–60]. Usually these peptides are immobilized in a random, spatially uniform manner across the biomaterial surface using bioconjugate techniques [61]. However, enhanced cell adhesion and migration has been reported when peptides are immobilized to surfaces in clusters that permit integrin clustering [62]. Particular peptide sequences that have been studied include argenine–glysine–aspartic acid (RGD), tyrosine–isoleucine–glycine–serine–aspartic acid (YIGSR), isoleucine–lysine–valine–alanine–valine (IKVAV), and arginine-glutamic acid–aspartic acid–valine (REDV). The RGD sequence — found in collagens, fibronectin, vitronectin, fibrinogen, von Willebrand factor, osteopontin, and bone sialoprotein [63–65] — is recognized by a large number of integrin receptors (Table 34.1), and consequently has been exploited extensively to promote integrin-mediated adhesion to biomaterials. Interestingly, the sequence proline–histidine–serine–arginine–asparagine (PHSRN) on fibronectin has been shown to act synergistically with RGD to enhance integrin-mediated adhesion and cell signaling via integrins $\alpha_5\beta_1$ and $\alpha_{11b}\beta_3$

[66,67]. REDV is an integrin binding sequence found in the alternatively spliced type III connecting segment region of fibronectin and is recognized by $\alpha_4\beta_1$ integrin (Table 34.1) [68]. It has been studied for its ability to support endothelial cell adhesion for development of engineered blood vessels [69–71]. Lastly, YIGSR [72] and IKVAV [73] are integrin binding sequences found in laminin. Because laminin is found in peripheral nerve tissue and the basal lamina of endothelial tissues, these peptide sequences hold promise for mediating adhesion and orientation of engineered epithelial [74] and neural tissues [75,76].

34.3.4 The Role of Interfacial Topography in Cell Adhesion

Cell adhesion to biomaterials is also influenced by topographical features, which restrict sites for cell adhesion. Studies performed nearly a century ago using spiderwebs revealed that adherent cells would spread with an orientation that could be dictated by the substratum topography [77]. This phenomenon, referred to as contact guidance, holds promise as a means to enhance engineered tissue function by inducing cell alignment [78,79]. Using microfabrication techniques (e.g., micromachining, photolithography) model substrates have been constructed to characterize the effect of topographical surface features on cell adhesion and function. For example, surfaces textured with parallel grooves can restrict focal adhesions to the raised edges of the substrate [80], while cytoskeletal elements — including microtubules, vimentin intermediate filaments, and actin filaments — are oriented parallel to the grooves [81]. Further, these effects are limited to feature sizes of 0.3 [81] to 2 μm [80]. When spacing between parallel grooves becomes too large, cells are able to attach to the depressed regions of the substratum and orientation is lost. Substrates exhibiting random topographies (e.g., acid-etched, sand blasted) also affect the behavior of adherent cells. Such substrates have been shown to enhance cell adhesion [82], synthesis of ECM proteins [82,83], and phenotypic behavior [83]. However, the effect of roughness on cell proliferation remains ambiguous: increasing roughness has been shown to decrease proliferation of osteoblasts [83], but may increase proliferation of endothelial and smooth muscle cells [84,85].

34.4 Measurement of Cell Adhesion to Biomaterials

Over the past two decades several devices have been developed to measure and characterize the adhesive interaction of cells with biomaterials, particles, and other cells. These devices share the common experimental strategy that nonadherent spherical cells are allowed to establish adhesive contacts to the test material under quiescent conditions and then are subjected to a well-defined distractive force. From the examination of large numbers of cells over a range of distractive forces, a probability distribution for cell adhesion as a function of distractive force can be constructed (Figure 34.3). From this distribution, an adhesion characteristic (e.g., τ_{50}, the shear stress necessary to detach 50% of the cells [47,86–88] may be determined. The primary differences between the various devices for measuring cell adhesion is the type of distractive force that is applied (e.g., membrane tension, buoyancy, and hydrodynamic shear stress) and the direction of the force relative to the plane of cell/surface contacts.

34.4.1 Micropipette Aspiration

Micropipette aspiration is a sensitive technique capable of measuring the strength of individual receptor/ligand adhesion complexes [89,90]. The advantage of this technique is its ability to probe cell contacts and adhesive structures with a range of forces (10^{-3} to 10^2 pN) that are capable of deforming the cell membrane (<0.1 pN) and extracting lipid-anchored receptors (~20 pN), but not breaking actin filaments (>100 pN) [90].

In this approach a cell is held at the end of micropipette by a small amount of suction. The cell is then brought into contact with a test surface, adhesive contacts are allowed to form, and then suction is applied to break this contact (Figure 34.4). The underlying principle is that suction, ΔP, used to draw a spherical cell of radius R_0 into the end of micropipette tip of radius R_p creates a membrane tension, T_m, at the

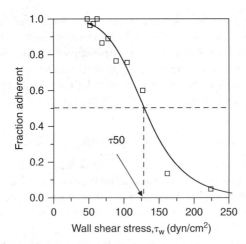

FIGURE 34.3   Probability distribution for cell adhesion. NIH 3T3 fibroblasts were detached from glass using a radial-flow chamber. Squares correspond to the fraction of cells that resisted detachment as a function of the applied shear stress. The curve is a best fit of the integral of a normal distribution function to the data. The characteristic measure of cell adhesion, τ_{50}, is 129 dyn/cm^2 for this test.

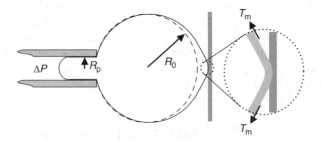

FIGURE 34.4   Micropipet aspiration. As suction, ΔP, is applied the cell is drawn into the pipet and membrane tension, T_m, is exerted at the point of cell/material contact. Adapted from Evans, E., Berk, D., and Leung, A., *Biophys. J.* 59, 838, 1991. With permission.

receptor/ligand contact [89]

$$T_m \approx \Delta P R_p / 2[1 - R_p/R_0] \tag{34.1}$$

The tension disrupts adhesive contacts in a manner that may be modeled as either a peeling process [91] or the failure of discrete cross-bridges [92], and can be used to predict receptor/ligand dissociation kinetics under mechanical strains [93].

34.4.2 Centrifugation

The centrifugation approach exploits the difference in density between cells, $\rho_c = 1.07$ [62], and culture medium, $\rho_m = 1.00$, to exert a supergravitational body force,

$$f = (\rho_c - \rho_m) V_c a \tag{34.2}$$

on the cell. Here V_c and a are the volume of the cell and the acceleration generated by the centrifuge, respectively. Distractive vectors both tangential [94] and normal [95,96] to the adhesive substrate have been used experimentally, although computational modeling predicts that tangential forces can be 20 to 56 times more disruptive to cell adhesion [97].

The experimental approach of Chu et al. [95] involves seeding cells onto substrates within 96 well plates, placing the plates into the 96 well-plate buckets of a table top centrifuge, and then applying accelerations of $a = 50, 100, 200$, or 300 g. Images are then collected to calculate the percent of cells that remain attached as a function of applied force, f. In contrast, the approach of Thoumine et al. [94] involves seeding cells onto plastic slides that are then fit into centrifuge tubes and placed in a swinging bucket centrifuge. Cells are then exposed to accelerations of 9,000 to 70,000 g for 5 to 60 min. Thoumine et al. also showed that the distractive force can be increased further by allowing the cells to phagocytose 1.5 μm gelatin-coated glass beads. As with Chu et al., images are analyzed to determine the percent of adherent cells as a function of time and distractive force.

34.4.3 Laminar Flow Chambers

Laminar flow devices are commonly used to characterize cell adhesion, and include rotating disc, parallel-plate (and variants), and radial-flow devices. These devices all employ tangential fluid flow to exert hydrodynamic drag and torque on adherent cells [98]. Among the different devices, the parallel-plate flow chamber (Figure 34.5a) is described most extensively, and has been used primarily to characterize cell and tissue phenomena under a well-defined hydrodynamic shear stress, τ. Here, τ can be predicted from fluid mechanics,

$$\tau = \frac{6\mu Q}{wh^2} \tag{34.3}$$

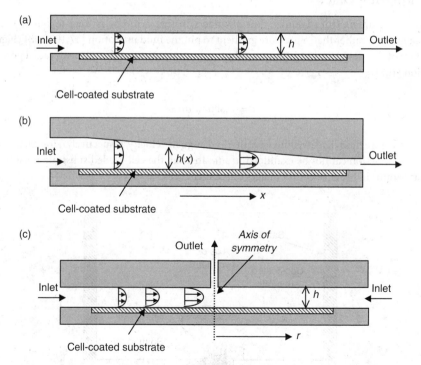

FIGURE 34.5 Various laminar flow chambers geometries. (a) Parallel-plate flow chamber uses linear laminar flow through a rectangular conduit with constant width, b, and height, h, where $b \gg h$. (b) Variable height laminar flow chamber uses flow through a tapered conduit, $h(x)$, of constant width to produce a flow profile that depends on position, x. (c) Radial-flow chamber uses cylindrical geometry to produce a flow profile that depends on position, r.

where Q is volumetric flow rate, h and w are the height and width of the flow path, respectively, and μ is the fluid viscosity [99]. The advantage of this device is that it permits nondestructive *in situ* visualization of cell attachment [100], detachment [101], and rolling processes [102]. However, because a single shear stress is generated across the cell-seeded substrate, multiple substrates must be tested at different shear stresses in order to construct shear-dependent patterns of cell adhesion [100,101].

Minor modifications have been made to the parallel-plate flow chamber geometry in order to produce a spatially dependent range of shear stresses across a single substrate. For example, a variable gap height device has been constructed in which h is a linear function of the distance from the inlet, x (Figure 34.5b) [103]. In another device the width of the flow path varies inversely with distance from the inlet, $w \propto 1/x$, to produce a Hele–Shaw flow pattern and a hydrodynamic shear stress that increases linearly with distance, $\tau \propto x$ [104,105].

An alternative device, the radial-flow chamber uses axisymmetric flow between parallel surfaces to generate a spatially dependent range of hydrodynamic shear stresses [65,106] (Figure 34.5c). Here, the magnitude of the shear stress is predicted by the equation

$$\tau = \left| \frac{3\mu Q}{\pi h^2 r} - \frac{3\rho Q^2}{70\pi^2 h r^3} \right| \tag{34.4}$$

where r is radial distance from the axis of symmetry, and ρ is fluid density. The first term of this equation is the creeping flow solution (analogous to Equation 34.3) and the second term is a first-order correction to account for inertial effects at high Reynolds numbers or low radial positions. It is interesting to note that the contribution of the second term depends on the direction of flow (i.e., the sign of Q) [106].

34.4.4 Rotating Disc

The rotating disc differs from laminar flow chambers in that a motor is used to put the cell-seeded substrate in motion, rather than a pressure gradient to put the fluid in motion [47,107,108] (Figure 34.6). An advantage of this device is that generates a shear stress, τ, that varies linearly with radial position, r, by the equation [107]

$$\tau = 0.800 r \sqrt{\rho \mu \omega^3} \tag{34.5}$$

Here, ρ, μ, and ω are fluid density, fluid viscosity, and angular velocity, respectively. However, a disadvantage is that cell adhesion cannot be examined *in situ*. Instead, the cell-seeded substrate must be removed from the apparatus in order to collect images of adherent cells.

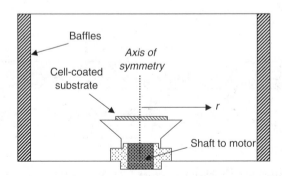

FIGURE 34.6 Rotating disc apparatus. The rapid rotation of the cell-seeded substrate generates a hydrodynamic shear that is proportional to radial position, r. Adapted from García, A.J., Huber, F., and Boettiger, D., *J. Biol. Chem.* 273, 10988, 1998. With permission.

34.4.5 Interpretation of Adhesion Data

Proper interpretation of adhesion data remains a technical challenge because quantitative measures are sensitive to cell history. As spherical, nonadherent cells are brought into contact with biomaterial interfaces, receptor-mediated contact initiates, followed by the clustering of receptors, cell spreading, and reorganization of the actin cytoskeleton. This dynamic process involves changes in the number and organization of adhesive contacts, cell shape, and the viscoelastic properties of the cell body — all of which influence the measured strength of adhesion. For example, quantitative measurements have demonstrated a linear dependence of the strength of cell adhesion on the density of adhesive ligands in the absence of cooperative binding [47] that is consistent with kinetic theory [109], but the strength of adhesion is increased by receptor activation [107] and modulated by receptor clustering [62]. In addition, cell adhesion has been shown to increase with the duration of cell/surface incubation [101], but it is difficult to deconvolve the individual effects of cell/surface contact area, focal adhesion organization, and filamentous actin content. Further, detachment assays that use hydrodynamic shear are sensitive to the hydrodynamic profile of the cell [110] and its deformability [111]. Consequently cells that are more spread or deform rapidly at the onset of shearing flow are more likely to resist detachment [48].

34.5 Effect of Biomaterial on Physiological Behavior

Establishment of adhesive cellular contacts with a biomaterial surface is critical for anchorage-dependent cell functions, such as spreading, proliferation, and migration. Studies of cell spreading indicate systematic increases in the rate and the extent of spreading with increasing density of adhesive ligands [112] or peptides [113]. In addition, microtubule and filamentous actin content increase during the initial spreading process [112]. Cell shape is also affected by the extent of cell spreading. For example, the aspect ratio of fibroblastic cells — which typically exhibit a spindle-shaped morphology — is maximal at an intermediate projected cell area [113]. Cell viability and proliferation also depend on projected cell area. Using microcontact printing to restrict the extent of cell spreading, Chen et al. [114] showed that when cells are able to adhere but not spread, apoptosis (programmed cell death) is significant. However, as the area for cell spreading is increased apoptosis declines and cell proliferation occurs.

Migration is another adhesion-dependent phenomenon, and requires polarized cells to execute coordinated steps that include pseudopodal extension, firm adhesion, contraction, and uropodal release [115]. Because both the pseudopodal attachment and uropodal release are adhesive processes, the capacity of the substratum to mediate cell adhesion directly affects the speed of cell migration. Manipulation of the strength of cell adhesion by changing the density, and type of ECM proteins has been shown to affect migration, with maximal speed occurring at an intermediate substratum adhesiveness [46]. In addition, migration rate can be modulated by depositing adhesive moieties as clusters [116] or by introducing topographical features [117].

34.6 Summary

In mammalian tissues and organs cell/cell and cell/ECM interactions are mediated through several families of adhesion receptors, which include integrins, cadherins, and members of the immunoglobulin superfamily. Biological studies have revealed that these adhesive contacts mechanically link the cell cytoskeleton to extracellular structures, initiate intercellular signaling cascades, and regulate cell viability, proliferation, organization of tissue structures, and cell function. Existing biomaterials — intended to replace tissue function or to serve as temporary scaffolds for engineered tissues — are capable of supporting cell adhesion, viability, and proliferation through a combination of nonspecific and integrin-mediated interactions. The current challenge is to develop bioactive materials that can act through different types of cell receptors to regulate cell and tissue behavior.

References

 [1] Albelda, S.M. and Buck, C.A., Integrins and other cell adhesion molecules, *FASEB J.* 4, 2868, 1990.

 [2] Hynes, R.O. and Lander, A.D., Contact and adhesive specificities in the associations, migrations, and targeting of cells and axons, *Cell* 68, 303, 1992.

 [3] Juliano, R.L., Signal transduction by cell adhesion receptors and the cytoskeleton: functions of integrins, cadherins, selectins, and immunoglobulin-superfamily members, *Ann. Rev. Pharmacol. Toxicol.* 42, 283, 2002.

 [4] Petit, V. and Thiery, J.-P., Focal adhesions: structure and dynamics, *Biol. Cell.* 92, 477, 2000.

 [5] Hynes, R.O., Integrins: versatility, modulation, and signaling in cell adhesion, *Cell* 69, 11, 1992.

 [6] ter Brugge, P.T., Torensma, R., de Ruijter, J.E. et al., Modulation of integrin expression on rat bone marrow cells by substrates with different characteristics, *Tissue Eng.* 8, 615, 2002.

 [7] Nikolovski, J. and Mooney, D.J., Smooth muscle cell adhesion to tissue engineering scaffolds, *Biomaterials* 21, 2025, 2000.

 [8] Springer, T.A., Adhesion receptors of the immune system, *Nature* 346, 425, 1990.

 [9] Sastry, S.K. and Burridge, K., Focal adhesions: a nexus for intercellular signalling and cytoskeletal dynamics, *Exp. Cell Res.* 261, 25, 2000.

 [10] Giancotti, F.G. and Ruoslahti, E., Integrin signaling, *Science* 285, 1028, 1999.

 [11] Yamada, K.M. and Miyamoto, S., Integrin transmembrane signaling and cytoskeletal control, *Curr. Opin. Cell Biol.* 7, 681, 1995.

 [12] Howe, A., Alpin, A.E., Alahari, S.K. et al., Integrin signaling and cell growth control, *Curr. Opin. Cell Biol.* 10, 220, 1998.

 [13] Lo, Y.Y.C., Luo, L., McCulloch, C.A. et al., Requirements of focal adhesions and calcium fluxes for interleukin-1-induced Erk kinase activation and c-fos expression in fibroblasts, *J. Biol. Chem.* 273, 7059, 1998.

 [14] Schneller, M., Vuori, K., and Ruoslahti, E., $\alpha v \beta 3$ integrin associates with activated insulin and PDGFβ receptors and potentiates the biological activity of PDGF, *EMBO J.* 16, 5600, 1997.

 [15] Huhtala, P., Humphries, M.J., McCarthy, J.B. et al., Cooperative signaling by $\alpha_5 \beta_1$ and $\alpha_4 \beta_1$ integrins regulates metalloproteinase gene expression in fibroblasts adhering to fibronectin, *J. Cell Biol.* 129, 867, 1995.

 [16] Monier-Gavelle, F. and Duband, J.L., Cross talk between adhesion molecules: control of N-cadherin activity by intercellular signals elicited by beta1 and beta3 integrins in migrating neural crest cells, *J. Cell Biol.* 137, 1663, 1997.

 [17] Lauffenburger, D.A. and Griffith, L.G., Who's got pull around here? Cell organization in development and tissue engineering, *Proc. Natl. Acad. Sci. USA* 98, 4282, 2001.

 [18] Wheelock, M.J. and Johnson, K.R., Cadherins as modulators of cellular phenotype, *Ann. Rev. Cell Dev. Biol.* 19, 207, 2003.

 [19] Yap, A.S., Brieher, W.M., and Gumbiner, B.M., Molecular and functional analysis of cadherin-based adherins junctions, *Ann. Rev. Cell Dev. Biol.* 13, 119, 1997.

 [20] Angst, B.D., Marcozzi, C., and Magee, A.I., The cadherin superfamily: diversity in form and function, *J. Cell Sci.* 114, 629, 2001.

 [21] Zhu, B., Chappuis-Flament, S., Wong, E. et al., Functional analysis of the structural basis of homophilic cadherin adhesion, *Biophys. J.* 84, 4033, 2003.

 [22] Shapiro, L., Fannon, A.M., Kwong, P.D. et al., Structural basis of cell–cell adhesion by cadherins, *Nature* 374, 327, 1995.

 [23] Yap, A.S., Brieher, W.M., Pruschy, M. et al., Lateral clustering of the adhesive ectodomain: a fundamental determinant of cadherin function, *Curr. Biol.* 7, 308, 1997.

 [24] St Croix, B., Sheehan, C., Rak, J.W. et al., E-cadherin-dependent growth suppression is mediated by the cyclin-dependent kinase inhibitor p27(KIP1), *J. Cell Biol.* 142, 557, 1998.

 [25] Levenberg, S., Yarden, A., Kam, Z. et al., p27 is involved in N-cadherin-mediated contact inhibition of cell growth and S-phase entry, *Oncogene* 18, 869, 1999.

[26] Caveda, L., Martin-Padura, I., Navarro, P. et al., Inhibition of cultured cell growth by vascular endothelial cadherin (cadherin-5/VE-cadherin), *J. Clin. Invest.* 98, 886, 1996.

[27] Nelson, C.M. and Chen, C.S., VE-cadherin simultaneously stimulates and inhibits cell proliferation by altering cytoskeletal structure and tension, *J. Cell Sci.* 116, 3571, 2003.

[28] Stryer, L., *Biochemistry*, 3rd ed., W.H. Freeman and Company, New York, 1988, p. 901.

[29] Walsh, F.S. and Doherty, P., Neural cell adhesion molecules of the immunoglobulin superfamily: role in axon growth and guidance, *Ann. Rev. Cell Dev. Biol.* 13, 425, 1997.

[30] Panicker, A.K., Buhusi, M., Thelen, K. et al., Cellular signalling mechanism of neural cell adhesion molecules, *Front. Biosci.* 8, 900, 2003.

[31] González-Mariscal, L., Betanzos, A., Nava, P. et al., Tight junction proteins, *Prog. Biophys. Mol. Biol.* 81, 1, 2003.

[32] Hench, L.L. and Polak, J.M., Third-generation biomedical materials, *Science* 295, 1014, 2002.

[33] García A.J., Ducheyne, P., and Boettiger, D., Effect of surface reaction stage on fibronectin-mediated adhesion of ostoblast-like cells to bioactive glass, *J. Biomed. Mater. Res.* 40, 48, 1998.

[34] Stephansson, S.N., Byers, B.A., and García A.J., Enhanced expression of the osteoblastic phenotype on substrates that modulate fibronectin conformation and integrin receptor binding, *Biomaterials* 23, 2527, 2002.

[35] Schakenraad, J.M., Busscher, H.J., Wildevuur, C.R.H. et al., The influence of substratum free energy on growth and spreading of human fibroblasts in the presence and absence of serum proteins, *J. Biomed. Mater. Res.* 20, 773, 1986.

[36] Tidwell, C.D., Ertel, S.I., Ratner, B.D. et al., Endothelial cell growth and protein adsorption on terminally functionalized, self-assembled monolayers of alkanethiolates on gold, *Langmuir* 13, 3404, 1997.

[37] Tegoulia, V.A. and Cooper, S.L., Leukocyte adhesion on model surfaces under flow: effects of surface chemistry, protein adsorption, and shear rate, *J. Biomed. Mater. Res.* 50, 291, 2000.

[38] McClary, K.B., Ugarova, T., and Grainger, D.W., Modulating fibroblast adhesion, spreading, and proliferation using self-assembled monolayer films of alkylthiolates on gold, *J. Biomed. Mater. Res.* 50, 428, 2000.

[39] Scotchford, C.A., Cooper, E., Leggett, G.J. et al., Growth of human osteoblast-like cells on alkane-thiol on gold self-assembled monolayers: the effect of surface chemistry, *J. Biomed. Mater. Res.* 41, 431, 1998.

[40] Faucheux, N., Schweiss, R., Lützow K. et al., Self-assembled monolaers with different terminating groups as model substrates for cell adhesion studies, *Biomaterials* 25, 2721, 2004.

[41] Webb, K., Hlady, V., and Tresco, P.A., Relationships among cell attachment, spreading, cytoskeletal organization, and migration rate for anchorage-dependent cells on model surfaces, *J. Biomed. Mater. Res.* 49, 362, 2000.

[42] López G.P., Albers, M.W., Schreiber, S.L. et al., Convenient methods for patterning the adhesion of mammalian cells to surfaces using self-assembled monolayers of alkanethiolates on gold, *J. Am. Chem. Soc.* 115, 5877, 1993.

[43] Puleo, D.A., Holleran, L.A., Doremus, R.H. et al., Osteoblast responses to orthopedic implant materials *in vitro, J. Biomed. Mater. Res.* 25, 711, 1991.

[44] Webster, T.J., Siegel, R.W., and Bizios, R., Osteoblast adhesion on nanophase ceramics, *Biomaterials* 20, 1221, 1999.

[45] Webster, T.J., Schadler, L.S., Siegel, R.W. et al., Mechanisms of enhanced osteoblast adhesion on nanophase alumina involve vitronectin, *Tissue Eng.* 7, 291, 2001.

[46] DiMilla, P.A., Stone, J.A., Quinn, J.A. et al., Maximal migration of human smooth muscle cells on fibronectin and type IV collagen occurs at an intermediate attachment strength, *J. Cell Biol.* 122, 729, 1993.

[47] García A.J., Ducheyne, P., and Boettiger, D., Cell adhesion strength increases linearly with adsorbed fibronectin surface density, *Tissue Eng.* 3, 197, 1997.

[48] Goldstein, A.S. and DiMilla, P.A., Effect of adsorbed fibronectin concentration on cell adhesion and deformation under shear on hydrophobic surfaces, *J. Biomed. Mater. Res.* 59, 665, 2001.

[49] Thomas, C.H., McFarland, C.D., Jenkins, M.L. et al., The role of vitronectin in the attachment and spatial distribution of bone-derived cells on materials with patterned surface chemistry, *J. Biomed. Mater. Res.* 37, 81, 1997.

[50] Kilpadi, K.L., Chang, P.L., and Bellis, S.L., Hydroxylapatite binds more serum proteins, purified integrins, and osteoblast precursor cells than titanium or steel, *J. Biomed. Mater. Res.* 57, 258, 2001.

[51] Iuliano, D.J., Saavedra, S.S., and Truskey, G.A., Effect of the conformation and orientation of adsorbed fibronectin on endothelial cell spreading and the strength of adhesion, *J. Biomed. Mater. Res.* 27, 1103, 1993.

[52] Yu, J.-L., Johansson, S., and Ljungh, Å., Fibronectin exposes different domains after adsorption to a heparinized and an unheparinized poly(vinyl chloride) surface, *Biomaterials* 18, 421, 1997.

[53] Giroux, T.A. and Cooper, S.L., FTIR/ATR studies of human fibronectin adsorption onto plasma derivatized polystyrene, *J. Colloid Interface Sci.* 139, 352, 1990.

[54] Cheng, S.-S., Chittur, K.K., Sukenik, C.N. et al., The conformation of fibronectin on self-assembled monolayers with different surface composition: an FTIR/ATR study, *J. Colloid Interface Sci.* 162, 135, 1994.

[55] Narasimhan, C. and Lai, C.-S., Conformational changes of plasma fibronectin detected upon adsorption to solid substrates, *Biochemistry* 28, 5041, 1989.

[56] Lhoest, J.-B., Detrait, E., van den Bosch de Aguilar, P. et al., Fibronectin adsorption, conformation, and orientation on polystyrene substrates studied by radiolabeling, XPS, and ToF SIMS, *J. Biomed. Mater. Res.* 41, 95, 1998.

[57] Wertz, C.F. and Santore, M.M., Effect of surface hydrophobicity on adsorption and relaxation kinetics of albumin and fibrinogen: single-species and competitive behavior, *Langmuir* 17, 3006, 2001.

[58] Mann, B.K., Gobin, A.S., Tsai, A.T. et al., Smooth muscle cell growth in photopolymerized hydrogels with cell adhesive and proteolytically degradable domains: synthetic ECM analogs for tissue engineering, *Biomaterials* 22, 3045, 2001.

[59] Massia, S.P. and Stark, J., Immobilized RGD peptides on surface-grafted dextran promote biospecific cell attachment, *J. Biomed. Mater. Res.* 56, 390, 2001.

[60] Alsberg, E., Anderson, K.W., Albeiruti, A. et al., Cell-interactive alginate hydrogels for bone tissue engineering, *J. Dental Res.* 80, 2025, 2001.

[61] Hermanson, G.T., Ed., *Bioconjugate Techniques*, Academic Press, San Diego, 1996,

[62] Koo, L.Y., Irvine, D.J., Mayes, A.M. et al., Co-regulation of cell adhesion by nanoscale RGD organization and mechanical stimulus, *J. Cell Sci.* 115, 1423, 2002.

[63] Pierschbacher, M.D. and Ruoslahti, E., Cell attachment activity of fibronectin can be duplicated by small synthetic fragments of the molecule, *Nature* 309, 30, 1984.

[64] Ruoslahti, E. and Pierschbacher, M.D., New perspectives in cell adhesion: RGD and integrins, *Science* 238, 491, 1987.

[65] Rezania, A., Thomas, C.H., Branger, A.B. et al., The detachment strength and morphology of bone cells contacting materials modified with a peptide sequence found within bone sialoprotein, *J. Biomed. Mater. Res.* 37, 9, 1997.

[66] Bowditch, R.D., Hariharan, M., Tominna, E.F. et al., Identification of a novel integrin binding site in fibronectin: differential utilization by β3 integrins, *J. Biol. Chem.* 269, 10856, 1994.

[67] Aota, S., Nomizu, M., and Yamada, K.M., The short amino acid sequence Pro–His–Ser–Arg–Asn in human fibronectin enhances cell-adhesive function, *J. Biol. Chem.* 269, 24756, 1994.

[68] Mould, A.P., Komoriya, A., Yamada, K.M. et al., The CS5 peptide is a second site in the IIICS region of fibronectin recognized by the integrin alpha 4 beta 1. Inhibition of alpha 4 beta 1 function by RGD peptide homologues, *J. Biol. Chem.* 266, 3579, 1991.

[69] Hodde, J., Record, R., Tullius, R. et al., Fibronectin peptides mediate HMEC adhesion to porcine-derived extracellular matrix, *Biomaterials* 23, 1841, 2002.

[70] Heilshorn, S.C., DiZio, K.A., Welsh, E.R. et al., Endothelial cell adhesion to the fibronectin CS5 domain in artificial extracellular matrix proteins, *Biomaterials* 24, 4245, 2003.

[71] Massia, S.P. and Hubbell, J.A., Vascular endothelial cell adhesion and spreading promoted by the peptide REDV of the IIICS region of plasma fibronectin is mediated by integrin a4b1, *J. Biol. Chem.* 267, 14019, 1992.

[72] Iwamoto, Y., Robey, F.A., Graf, J. et al., YIGSR, a synthetic laminin pentapeptide, inhibits experimental metastasis formation, *Science* 238, 1132, 1987.

[73] Tashiro, K., Sephel, G.C., Weeks, B. et al., A synthetic peptide containing the IKVAV sequence from the A chain of laminin mediates cell attachment, migration, and neurite outgrowth, *J. Biol. Chem.* 264, 16174, 1989.

[74] Li, F., Carlsson, D., Lohmann, C. et al., Cellular and nerve regeneration within a biosynthetic extracellular matrix for corneal transplantation, *Proc. Natl. Acad. Sci. USA* 100, 15346, 2003.

[75] Massia, S.P., Holecko, M.M., and Ehteshami, G.R., *In vitro* assessment of bioactive coatings for neural implant applications, *J. Biomed. Mater. Res.* 68A, 177, 2004.

[76] Shaw, D. and Shoichet, M.S., Toward spinal cord injury repair strategies: peptide surface modification of expanded poly(tetrafluoroethylene) fibers for guided neurite outgrowth *in vitro*, *J. Craniofac. Surg.* 14, 308, 2003.

[77] Harrison, R.G., The cultivation of tissues in extraneous media as a method of morphogenetic study, *Anat. Rec.* 6, 181, 1912.

[78] Singhvi, R., Stephanopoulos, G., and Wang, D.I.C., Review: effects of substratum morphology on cell physiology, *Biotechnol. Bioeng.* 43, 764, 1994.

[79] Flemming, R.G., Murphy, C.J., Abrams, G.A. et al., Effects of synthetic micro- and nano-structured surfaces on cell behavior, *Biomaterials* 20, 573, 1999.

[80] den Braber, E.T., Jansen, H.V., de Boer, H.J. et al., Scanning electron microscopic, transmission electron microscopic, and confocal laser scanning microscopic observation of fibroblasts cultured on microgrooved surfaces of bulk titanium substrata, *J. Biomed. Mater. Res.* 40, 425, 1998.

[81] Manwaring, M.E., Walsh, J.F., and Tresco, P.A., Contact guidance induced orientation of extracellular matrix, *Biomaterials* 25, 3631, 2004.

[82] Lampin, M., Warocquier-Clérout R., Legris, C. et al., Correlation between substratum roughness and wettability, cell adhesion, and cell migration, *J. Biomed. Mater. Res.* 36, 99, 1997.

[83] Martin, J.Y., Schwartz, Z., Hummert, T.W. et al., Effect of titatium surface roughness on proliferation, differentiation, and protein synthesis of human osteoblast-like cells (MG63), *J. Biomed. Mater. Res.* 29, 389, 1995.

[84] Miller, D.C., Thapa, A., Haberstroh, K.M. et al., Endothelial and vascular smooth muscle cell function on poly(lactic-co-glycolic acid) with nano-structured surface features, *Biomaterials* 25, 53, 2004.

[85] Chung, T.W., Liu, D.Z., Wang, S.Y. et al., Enhancement of the growth of human endothelial cells by surface roughness at nanometer scale, *Biomaterials* 24, 4655, 2003.

[86] Goldstein, A.S. and DiMilla, P.A., Application of fluid mechanic and kinetic models to characterize mammalian cell detachment in a radial-flow chamber, *Biotechnol. Bioeng.* 55, 616, 1997.

[87] Cozens-Roberts, C., Quinn, J.A., and Lauffenburger, D.A., Receptor-mediated adhesion phenomena: model studies with the radial-flow detachment assay, *Biophys. J.* 58, 107, 1990.

[88] Truskey, G.A. and Proulx, T.L., Relationship between 3T3 cell spreading and the strength of adhesion on glass and silane surfaces, *Biomaterials* 14, 243, 1993.

[89] Evans, E., Berk, D., and Leung, A., Detachment of agglutinin-bonded red blood cells, I. Forces to rupture molecular-point attachments, *Biophys. J.* 59, 838, 1991.

[90] Evans, E., Ritchie, K., and Merkel, R., Sensitive force technique to probe molecular adhesion and structural linkages at biological interfaces, *Biophys. J.* 68, 2580, 1995.

[91] Evans, E., Detailed mechanics of membrane–membrane adhesion and separation. I. Continuum of molecular cross-bridges, *Biophys. J.* 48, 175, 1985.

[92] Evans, E., Detailed mechanics of membrane-membrane adhesion and separation. II. Discrete, kinetically trapped molecular cross-bridges, *Biophys. J.* 48, 185, 1985.

[93] Chelsa, S.E., Selvaraj, P., and Zhu, C., Measuring two-dimensional receptor–ligand binding kinetics by micropipette, *Biophys. J.* 75, 1553, 1998.

[94] Thoumine, O., Ott, A., and Louvard, D., Critical centrifugal forces induce adhesion rupture or structural reorganization in cultured cells, *Cell Motil. Cytoskeleton* 33, 276, 1996.

[95] Chu, L., Tempelman, L.A., Miller, C. et al., Centrifugation assay of IgE-mediated rat basophilic leukemia cell adhesion to antigen-coated polyacrilimide gels, *AIChE J.* 40, 692, 1994.

[96] Piper, J.W., Swerlick, R.A., and Zhu, C., Determining force dependence of two-dimensional receptor-ligand binding affinity by centrifugation, *Biophys. J.* 74, 492, 1998.

[97] Chang, K.-C. and Hammer, D., Influence of direction and type of applied force on the detachment of macromolecularly-bound particles from surfaces, *Langmuir* 12, 2271, 1996.

[98] Hammer, D.A. and Lauffenburger, D.A., A dynamical model for receptor-mediated cell adhesion to surfaces, *Biophys. J.* 52, 475, 1987.

[99] Frangos, J.A., McIntire, L.V., and Eskin, S.G., Shear stress induced stimulation of mammalian cell metabolism, *Biotechnol. Bioeng.* 32, 1053, 1988.

[100] Tempelman, L.A. and Hammer, D.A., Receptor-mediated binding of IgE-sensitized rat basophilic leukemia cells to antigen-coated substrates under hydrodynamic flow, *Biophys. J.* 66, 1231, 1994.

[101] Truskey, G.A. and Pirone, J.S., The effect of fluid shear sress upon cell adhesion to fibronectin-treated surfaces, *J. Biomed. Mater. Res.* 24, 1333, 1990.

[102] Rinker, K.D., Prabhakar, V., and Truskey, G.A., Effect of contact time and force on monocyte adhesion to vascular endothelium, *Biophys. J.* 80, 1722, 2001.

[103] Xiao, Y. and Truskey, G.A., Effect of receptor–ligand affinity on the strength of endothelial cell adhesion, *Biophys. J.* 71, 2869, 1996.

[104] Usami, S., Chen, H.-H., Zhao, Y. et al., Design and construction of a linear shear stress flow chamber, *Ann. Biomed. Eng.* 21, 77, 1993.

[105] Powers, M.J., Rodriguez, R.E., and Griffith, L.G., Cell–substratum adhesive strength as a determinant of hepatocyte aggregate morphology, *Biotechnol. Bioeng.* 53, 415, 1997.

[106] Goldstein, A.S. and DiMilla, P.A., Comparison of converging and diverging radial flow for measuring cell adhesion, *AIChE J.* 44, 465, 1998.

[107] García, A.J., Huber, F., and Boettiger, D., Force required to break $\alpha_5\beta_1$ integrin–fibronectin bonds in intact adherent cells is sensitive to integrin activation state, *J. Biol. Chem.* 273, 10988, 1998.

[108] Reutelingsperger, C.P.M., van Gool, R.J.G., Heinjen, V. et al., The rotating disc as a device to study the adhesive properties of endothelial cells under differential shear stresses, *J. Mater. Sci., Mater. Med.* 5, 361, 1994.

[109] Cozens-Roberts, C., Lauffenburger, D.A., and Quinn, J.A., Receptor-mediated cell attachment and detachment kinetics: I. Probabilistic model and analysis, *Biophys. J.* 59, 841, 1990.

[110] Olivier, L.A. and Truskey, G.A., A numerical analysis of forces exerted by laminar flow on spreading cells in a parallel plate flow chamber assay, *Biotechnol. Bioeng.* 42, 963, 1993.

[111] Dong, C., Struble, E.J., and Lipowsky, H.H., Mechanics of leukocyte deformation and adhesion to the endothelium in shear flow, *Ann. Biomed. Eng.* 27, 298, 1999.

[112] Mooney, D.J., Langer, R., and Ingber, D.E., Cytoskeletal filament assembly and the control of cell spreading and function by extracellular matrix, *J. Cell Sci.* 108, 2311, 1995.

[113] Neff, J.A., Tresco, P.A., and Caldwell, K.D., Surface modification for controlled studies of cell–ligand interactions, *Biomaterials* 20, 2377, 1999.

[114] Chen, C.S., Mrksich, M., Huang, S. et al., Geometric control of cell life and death, *Science* 276, 1425, 1997.

[115] Lauffenburger, D.A. and Horwitz, A.F., Cell migration: a physically integrated molecular process, *Cell* 84, 359, 1996.

[116] Maheshwari, G., Brown, G., Lauffenburger, D.A. et al., Cell adhesion and motility depend on nanoscale RGD clustering, *J. Cell Sci.* 113, 1677, 2000.

[117] Tan, J., Shen, H., and Saltzman, W.M., Micron-scale positioning of features influences the rate of polymorphonuclear leukocyte migration, *Biophys. J.* 81, 2569, 2001.

35

Cell Migration

Gang Cheng
Kyriacos Zygourakis
Rice University

35.1 Introduction

Cell migration is an essential component of normal development, inflammation, tissue repair, angiogenesis, and tumor invasion. After conception, selected cells of the developing mammalian zygote invade the uterine wall to establish the placenta, while the intricately programmed migration of other cells within the embryo shapes the complex form of the emerging organism [1,2]. The nervous system is another example of large-scale cell migration during fetal development. The growth of axons and dendrites is preceded by a phase of cell migration in which immature neurons (or neuroblasts) move from their birthplace to settle in some other location in order to make the right connections [3]. Certain kinds of white blood cells are able to migrate through the walls of blood vessels and into the surrounding tissues, actively seeking and engulfing sources of decay [4]. Migrating fibroblastic and epithelial cells heal wounds, and osteoclasts and osteoblasts are in constant movement as they remodel bone [5–7]. Tumor cell motility is also required for invasion and metastasis. The crawling malignant tumor cells that invade and disrupt tissue architecture account as much or more for the lethality of cancer as does uncontrolled growth [8].

Cell migration also plays a key role in determining the structure and growth rate of bioartificial tissues built on scaffolds made from suitable biomaterials [9]. In recent years, a lot of attention has been focused on the development of *biomimetic* materials capable of promoting cell functions, including migration, by biomolecular recognition [10]. Such recognition can be achieved by surface or bulk modification of the material with bioactive molecules such as extracellular matrix (ECM) proteins or short peptide sequences that can induce specific interactions with cell receptors. In order to design biomimetic scaffolds with optimal properties for each application, however, we must thoroughly understand not only the mechanism of cell migration, but also the many factors that modulate this important process. We must also develop assays to accurately characterize cell movement on various biomaterials and, ultimately, build theoretical models that can quantitatively predict the effect of system parameters (scaffold properties, nutrient or growth factor concentrations, pH, etc.) on tissue development. Because tissues are highly *heterogeneous systems* exhibiting complicated cell population dynamics, such theoretical models must be able to accurately describe cell–cell and cell–substrate interactions.

This review attempts to address some of these issues for anchorage-dependent mammalian cells. After a brief description of the mechanism of cell movement, we outline the role that growth factors, substrate-adhesion molecules, and other environmental factors play in modulating cell migration. Since accurate measurements are essential for elucidating the effect of a specific stimulus on cell migration, we discuss the application of several assays that may be used to characterize cell motility. Finally, the use of theoretical models for analyzing cell population dynamics and predicting tissue growth rates is discussed.

35.2 Characteristics of Mammalian Cell Migration

35.2.1 Cell Movement Cycle

The movement of a mammalian cell on a substrate is an intricate process requiring at least three structural elements: an ECM ligand on the substrate, its cell surface receptor, and the intracellular cytoskeleton [6]. The receptors that play key roles for cell movement belong to a large family of transmembrane proteins called *integrins* [11]. Migration can be considered as a continual cycle consisting of four essential steps [4] (1) extension of the cell's leading margin over the substratum to form a lamellipod (i.e., a thin piece of membrane and cytoplasm at the front of the cell); (2) attachment to the substrate; (3) pulling or contraction using the newly formed points of adhesion as anchorage; and (4) release or detachment of adhesions at the rear of the cell. These four steps are orchestrated by the interaction of various extracellular and intracellular molecules. Extension of the leading margin of the cell is caused by the polymerization of actin filaments at the lamellipodia and crucial factors involved in this process are the Arp2/3 complex, gelsolin, and capping protein [4,12,13]. At the base of the cortical actin meshwork, cofilin promotes the disassembly of filaments [4,14]. Integrins anchor the cell to its substratum by binding both to ECM molecules on the outside of the cell and to the actin cytoskeleton on the inside. Cortical contractions due to myosin molecules pull structures toward the center of the cell, causing the uropod (lamellipod's counterpart at the rear of the cell) to retract and unattached structures on the dorsal surface to move backward [15–17]. The cycle is completed by a forward movement of actin and other constituents through the cytoplasm to the leading margin of the cell [4].

35.2.2 Persistent Random Walk

Migration of individual mammalian cells in isotropic environments can be described as a persistent random walk [18,19]. Over short time periods, cells follow a relatively straight path, showing persistence of movement (see Figure 35.1a). If long time intervals are used to observe the cell position, however, cell movement appears similar to Brownian motion with frequent direction changes (Figure 35.1b). At least two parameters are needed to describe persistent random walk [20]. The first one is the *speed S* that is intuitively defined as the displacement of the cell centroid per unit time. The second one is the *persistence time* (usually denoted by P) that is a measure of the average time between "significant" direction changes. The magnitude of P and S depend both on the type of the cell and on its microenvironment. Reported values of migration speed and persistence time range from 0.5 μm/min and 4 to 5 h, respectively for human microvessel endothelial cells and smooth muscle cells [20,21] to 20 μm/min and 4 min for rabbit neutrophils [22]. Lauffenburger and coworkers [23] pointed out that there exists a rough inverse relationship between S and P and that this could be understood by considering the product of these two parameters as the cell's analog to a "mean free-path length." Rigorous definition of P and S necessary for mathematical modeling and the assays to measure them will be described in Section 35.4.

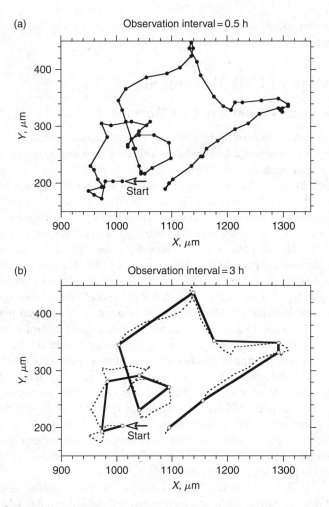

FIGURE 35.1 Typical trajectory of a bovine pulmonary artery endothelial cell migrating in a uniform environment. Symbols represent the position of the centroid of the same cell recorded at 30 min intervals (top panel) and 3 h intervals (bottom panel). When the observation interval is short (top panel), the cell clearly exhibits persistence in movement direction. If a long observation interval (bottom panel) is chosen, however, the movement of the same cell appears to be a random walk with frequent direction changes. (Adapted from Lee, Y., Mcintire, L.V., and Zygourakis, K., *Biochem. Cell Biol.*, 1995, **73**: 461–472. With permission.)

35.2.3 Cell–Cell Contacts

In a population of migrating cells, the persistent random walk of individual cells can be interrupted by contacts with other cells. Since cells usually stop and change the direction of their movement after such contacts, this phenomenon is often called *contact inhibition of locomotion* [6]. When two fibroblasts collide with each other, for example, ruffling of the membrane near the contact point stops to form a quiescent region, while ruffling continues at other regions of the membrane. After about 25 min, the cells break the adhesion and move away in new directions [6]. Cell–cell contacts have an even more profound effect on the migration of epithelial cells. Following a collision, the leading lamellae of the epithelial cells are gradually lost and an adhesion is formed between two cells. Sequential collisions with other cells result in the formation of small colonies and eventually a sheet of contiguous cells [6,4]. This process is essential for the coverage of the wounded area in wound healing [24,25]. It should be noted that cell–cell contacts also affect cell division and the effect is also often referred to as "contact inhibition," which actually means *contact inhibition of division.* As is shown later, the mechanisms of these two contact inhibitions are different, even though they are related in a rather complicated way.

35.3 Regulation of Cell Movement

35.3.1 Soluble Factors Modulate Cell Movement

Many polypeptide growth factors can upregulate cell motility. Sato and Rifkin [26] found that when a confluent monolayer of bovine aortic endothelial cells (BAECs) was wounded with a razor blade, cells at the edge of the wound released basic fibroblast growth factor (bFGF), which stimulated the rapid movement of nearby cells into the denuded area. Addition of anti-bFGF IgG slowed down considerably the cell movement and this inhibition was dose dependent. Sato and Rifkin also found that bFGF regulated the basal level of synthesis of the protease plasminogen activator (PA) and the basal level of DNA synthesis. These findings are consistent with earlier work demonstrating that plasmin contributed to cell migration [27,28]. Sato and Rifkin [26] also offer the alternative explanation that bFGF acts as a motility factor via its adhesive interactions described by Baird and coworkers [29]. Platelet-derived growth factor-BB (PDGF-BB) has been found to be the major motility enhancing factor in human serum for human dermal fibroblasts migrating on type I collagen, even though it is not needed for the initiation of cell movement [30]. Transforming growth factor-α (TGF-α) enhances locomotion of cultured human keratinocytes [31]. Stimulation of MTLn3 cells (a metastatic carcinoma cell line) with epidermal growth factor (EGF) causes rapid and transient lamellipod protrusion along with an increase in actin polymerization at the leading edge [32]. EGF was also found to greatly enhance random dispersion of fibroblasts by increasing the frequency of direction changes and at the same time slightly increasing the path length [33]. When multiple types of growth factors are present, they may affect cell motility synergistically with certain extent of specificity. For example, TGF-β1 has been found to synergistically enhance EGF-stimulated hepatocyte motility responses on collagen-containing extracellular matrices. However, the same effect was not achieved when TGF-β1 was added together with hepatocyte growth factor (HGF) [34]. Placental growth factor (PlGF) can augment the migration of endothelial cell in response to vascular endothelial growth factor (VEGF) in pathological angiogenesis [35].

Recent studies have revealed additional soluble motility-stimulating proteins, which include (a) The scatter factor or SF (also known as HGF), a mesenchymal cell-derived protein, which causes contiguous sheets of epithelium to separate into individual cells and stimulates the migration of epithelial as well as vascular endothelial cells [36–38]; (b) the autocrine motility factor (AMF), a tumor cell-derived protein, which stimulates migration of the producer cells [39–41]; and (c) the migration-stimulating factor (MSF), a protein produced by fetal and cancer patient fibroblasts, which stimulates penetration of three-dimensional collagen gels by nonproducing adult fibroblasts [42–44].

The direction of cell movement can be affected by the concentration gradient of certain growth factors, a response called *chemotaxis*. Chemotaxis is very important for processes such as normal development, inflammation, angiogenesis, and wound healing in which directed migration of specific cell types is essential. It has been found that when a wound is caused in the human body, large amounts of PDGF, EGF, and TGF-β are secreted at different times by cells around the wound to coordinate the influx of neutrophils, macrophages, fibroblasts, smooth muscle cells, and endothelial cells for fast and complete healing of the wound [45–48]. Lack of these chemotactic growth factors may impair the healing process, while overproduction can cause excessive repair or scarring [49]. A chemotactic response is typically a function of both the absolute concentration of the attractant and the steepness of its concentration gradient. Directional orientation bias increases with concentration gradient steepness, asymptotically approaching a maximal level as steepness increases. The dependence on attractant concentration is biphasic, increasing at low concentration to reach a maximum, then decreasing as concentration increases further [50–52].

Several hypotheses have been proposed to explain the underlying mechanisms of these phenomena. Lackie [6] suggested that cells decide their movement direction by receptor-mediated comparison of the spatial difference in attractant concentration across the cell dimension. This explains the biphasic dependence of directional orientation bias on attractant concentration for constant concentration gradient. At low-attractant concentrations, very few receptors are bound and, thus, only a small orientation bias results. At high-attractant concentrations almost all receptors are bound and, again, only a small bias is observed. Maximum bias is found for an intermediate attractant concentration, where the number of bound receptors is significant and most sensitive to differences in local attractant concentration. It should be noted that during the course of directed cell movement in chemotaxis, there are periods during which the cell may randomly stray toward the lower concentration or any other direction. Mechanistic models aimed at simulating chemotaxis must account for these random fluctuations in the cell's orientation even at the presence of the concentration gradient of a chemoattractant. Tranquillo and coworkers [53,54] hypothesized that this is caused primarily by the probabilistic kinetics of receptor/attractant binding. Their model divides a cell into two compartments along its polarization axis and assumes that the instantaneous numbers of receptor/attractant complexes at the compartment surfaces are governed by a stochastic differential equation with both a deterministic and a probabilistic part, which accounts for the random fluctuations in the binding process. The numbers of receptor/attractant complexes are then used to calculate the concentration of motile effectors in each intracellular compartment. Finally, the model postulates that the cell changes direction with an angular rate proportional to the imbalance between the levels of motile effectors in the two compartments. Model results were shown to provide good prediction for the chemotaxis of neutrophil leukocytes [55]. A recent extension of this model [56] relaxes several simplifying assumptions regarding receptor dynamics in the original model using newly obtained knowledge on transient G-protein signaling, cytoskeletal association, and receptor internalization and recycling, including statistical fluctuations in the numbers of receptors among the various states.

35.3.2 ECM Proteins and Cell–Substrate Interactions Regulate Cell Movement

As described earlier, each of the four phases in cell-movement cycle involves the interaction of cell-surface receptors with the ECM components on substratum surface. The ECM is a molecular complex whose components include collagens, glycoproteins, hyaluronic acid, proteoglycans, glycosaminoglycans, and elastins [57,58]. In addition, ECM harbors molecules such as growth factors, cytokines, matrix-degrading enzymes, and their inhibitors [57]. The distribution of these molecules varies from tissue to tissue and changes with time during tissue development, making the ECM a highly dynamic system [59,60]. The binding of ECM molecules to the extracellular domains of integrins triggers the receptor/ligand binding, trafficking and signaling cascade, activation of transcription factor and expression of target genes, and eventually results in the regulation of specific cell functions, which may include adhesion, migration, proliferation, and differentiation.

Integrin receptors are heterodimeric proteins composed of α and β subunits [11]. At least 15 α and β subunits have been identified so far and they pair with each other in a variety of combinations, giving rise to specific recognition on the ECM molecules with different selectivity. These combinations include the $\alpha_5\beta_1$ fibronectin receptor, $\alpha_2\beta_1$, $\alpha_3\beta_1$, and the vitronectin receptor $\alpha_v\beta_3$ [61–63]. While the $\alpha_5\beta_1$ integrin binds exclusively to fibronectin, $\alpha_1\beta_1$ can bind either to laminin or to collagen-IV and the $\alpha_v\beta_3$ receptor recognizes fibrinogen, vitronectin, and probably fibronectin. The $\alpha_4\beta_1$ integrin has also been found to mediate cell motility on fibronectin and vascular adhesion molecule-1 (VCAM-1) independently of the $\alpha_5\beta_1$ [64].

The ability of integrin receptors to recognize and bind the short peptide sequences corresponding to the adhesive domains of ECM proteins stimulated a lot of interest in developing *biomimetic* materials. Several studies by Hubbell and coworkers [65–71] have shown that covalent immobilization of adhesive peptides like RGD or YIGSR (which are the adhesive domains of fibronectin and laminin respectively) on the surface of glass or polymeric substrates can promote adhesion of endothelial cells. Kouvroukoglou and coworkers [72] found that such surface modifications significantly enhanced the migration of endothelial cells, a fact that might lead to higher endothelization rates of the surfaces of implantable biomaterials. Yang and coworkers [73] found that surface modification of poly(lactic acid) (PLA) films and poly(lactic-co-/glycolic acid) (PLGA) porous structures with RGD peptides or fibronectin greatly promoted human osteoprogenitor adhesion, migration, growth, and differentiation. Shin and coworkers [74] found that bulk modification of oligo(poly[ethylene glycol] fumarate) (OPF) hydrogel with a rat osteopontin-derived peptide (ODP) or a RGD peptide could increase the motility of marrow stromal osteoblasts and accelerate the expansion of megacolonies of these cells on the surface of the hydrogel.

The sudden introduction of a migratory ECM ligand into the environment of a cell may provide a key signal for the initiation of cell migration [75]. Similarly, the biosynthetic induction of such a migration protein or of its receptors might also promote migration [64,75–79]. The driving mechanism for migration appears to be provided by the physical interactions between specific sequences in adhesion proteins and their receptors [75], and by intracellular contractile proteins [4,17]. The signals involved in the termination of cell migration include the reacquisition of cell–cell adhesion molecules (e.g., N-cadherin), often accompanied by differentiation into the final tissue type [75].

The speed of cell movement on ECM proteins is regulated not only by the type of receptor/ligand interactions, but also by the ligand density on the substrate and the ligand affinity for cell adhesion receptors [80–83]. The complexity of these interactions leads to a *biphasic dependence* of cell speed on substrate adhesiveness. Goodman and coworkers [84] found that the migration speed of murine myoblasts on substrates covered with laminin or laminin fragment E8 depended in a biphasic fashion on the density of surface ligand. Maximum cell speeds were observed for ligand densities ranging from one third to one tenth of those required for strongest cell attachment. Low cell speeds were measured when the cells adhered very strongly or very weakly to the surface. A slow, monotonic increase of cell speed was observed, however, when the density of fibronectin ligands was increased. DiMilla and coworkers [22] measured the speed of human smooth muscle cells on fibronectin and collagen-IV. They found that cell speed varied in a biphasic fashion with increasing cell adhesion strengths for both ligands. Similar results are seen by varying the number of receptors on the cell surface. Keely and coworkers [85] found that the strength of adhesion of human breast carcinoma T47D cells to collagen I and IV decreased with decreasing levels of expression of the $\alpha_2\beta_1$ integrin (a collagen and laminin receptor). T47D clones that exhibited intermediate levels of adhesion to collagen had the highest motility across collagen-coated filters, suggesting that an intermediate density of cell-surface $\alpha_2\beta_1$ integrin optimally supports cell motility.

The reasons for this contrasting behavior were revealed by an elegant mathematical analysis of the cell-migration cycle by Lauffenburger [86] and DiMilla and coworkers [87]. The first key system parameter for explaining the experimental data is the *substratum adhesiveness* that is proportional to the surface ligand density and inversely proportional to the receptor/ligand equilibrium dissociation constant. Substrate adhesiveness, however, may not only depend on the strength of receptor/ligand association. A later analysis of Ward and Hammer [88] showed that the formation of focal contacts (which were modeled as cytoplasmic nucleation centers binding adhesion receptors) and the elastic rigidity of cytoskeletal connections may significantly affect cellular adhesive strength. The second parameter describes the *asymmetry in bond affinity* as the ratio of the dissociation rate constants between the front and the rear of the migrating cell. The model correctly predicted a biphasic dependence of cell speed on substrate adhesiveness, with cell locomotion occurring over an intermediate and (in many cases) limited range of adhesiveness. The size of this range was primarily governed by the asymmetry in adhesiveness between the front and the rear of the cell. Several mechanisms can provide a front-to-rear asymmetry in cell/substrate adhesiveness including dynamic integrin/cytoskeletal interactions [89] and polarized distributions of integrins maintained by receptor trafficking mechanisms [90].

The substratum adhesiveness can also affect the direction of cell movement, a response called *haptotaxis*. For example, cells cultured on a surface will move onto tracks of artificial adhesive material, such as polylysine or silicon oxide [4]. When fibroblasts are plated on a surface coated with a uniformly increasing gradient of a charged substance, they turn and move in the direction of increasing adhesiveness [91]. Dickinson and Tranquillo [92] have developed a stochastic mathematical model based on receptor/ligand binding and trafficking mechanism to provide a mechanistic understanding of how the magnitude and distribution of adhesion ligands in the substratum influence cell movement. Additional sources for directionality in movement may be simple population pressure, tissue or physical barriers [4,93], or the three-dimensional structure of the matrix. In a process known as *contact guidance*, matrix fibers can be spatially arranged as to facilitate cell movement in a preferred direction [94]. Micromachined grooves cut into the substratum have similar effect [95].

While properties of the substratum can greatly influence cell movement, cells can also direct their own migration by modifying the physical properties of the substratum. For example, pioneering cells within a population of migrating neural crest cells may be laying down extracellular cues that trailing cells recognize [96]. When a suspension of human keratinocytes is plated on a fibrin matrix, single cells invade the matrix and progress through it by dissolving the fibrin and thereby creating tunnels [97].

35.3.3 Electrical Fields Direct Cell Movement

The migration of many mammalian cells is affected by the presence of electric fields, a phenomenon called *galvanotaxis*. Nerve cells can detect electric field as weak as 10 mV/mm and turn their growth cones to move in the direction of the negative pole [4]. Fibroblasts and cells from the neural crest also move toward the negative pole in a steady electric field [98,99]. During wound healing in vertebrates, a steady lateral electric field of 40 to 200 mV/mm is generated in the disrupted epithelia layers to coordinate the directed migration of epithelial cells from the nearby regions [100]. Some experiments indicate that when the electric field is removed, the wound healing rate is 25% slower, while nearly every clinical trial using electric fields to stimulate healing in mammalian wounds reports a significant increase in the rate of healing from 13 to 50% [101].

Cell's response to electrical fields typically requires Ca^{2+} influx [102], the presence of specific growth factors [100] and intracellular kinase activity. Protein kinase C is required by neural crest cells [103] and cAMP-dependent protein kinase is used in keratinocytes [104], while mitogen-activated protein kinase is required by corneal epithelial cells [105]. Specifically, Zhao and coworkers [100] discovered that corneal epithelial cells cultured in serum-free medium showed no reorientation in an electric field until 250 mV/mm and addition of EGF, bFGF, or TGF-β 1 singly or in combination significantly restored the cathodal reorientation response at low field strengths. Interestingly, however, the directed migration of two fibroblastic cells, NIH 3T3 and SV101, was found to be calcium independent and was, instead, related to the lateral redistribution of plasma membrane glycoproteins involved in cell–substratum adhesion [98].

35.4 Cell Migration Assays

35.4.1 Cell-Population Assays

The methods used to assess the locomotory capabilities and characteristics of cells fall into two major categories. The first category includes techniques that monitor large populations of migrating cells and analyze the number density profiles of the population after a given time period of migration. The Boyden chamber is the most popular assay in this category [106–111]. According to this technique, cells are placed on the upper surface of a micropore filter installed in the chamber and incubated for a sufficient period of time to allow the cells to migrate to the lower surface of the filter. Cell motility is then quantified either by counting the number of cells that have migrated through the filter or by measuring the distance traveled into the filter by several of the fastest moving cells. A comparison of the number of cells that passed through the filter or of the migration distance measured for various experimental conditions reveal if, for example, a test substance is chemotactic for the cells under study. With appropriate modifications, the Boyden chamber can also be used to study cell migration under flow conditions or temporal chemotactic gradients [112,113].

Another cell-population assay measures the migration distance of endothelial cells or osteoblasts released from growth arrest using a silicon or steel template compartmentalization technique [74,114].

This assay system employs tissue culture dishes that are subdivided (using, for example, stainless steel annular rings) into two separate compartments: an inner circular core and an annular outer ring. Cells are seeded into the inner compartment and grown to confluence. The inner ring is then removed, and cells (released from growth arrest) start migrating from a sharp starting line. Cell motility is quantified by measuring the distance of the migrating front from the starting line. By using a growth-arrested mono-layer as a starting cell population for the quantification of migration, this assay system produces few or no wounded cells at the migration front. It also allows us to evaluate the migratory response to other cell types by coculturing them with the test cells after having seeded the effector cells into the outer compartment of the assay system. Since migration of endothelial cells is one of the critical features of wound repair, several researchers have also studied the movement of cells from a wound edge into a denuded area formed by scraping a confluent monolayer with a razor blade [26,115,116]. Migration is then quantified by counting the number of cells in successive 125-μm sections from the wound edge.

A third popular technique is the under-agarose assay where cells are allowed to migrate under a layer of agarose gel deposited on a glass or plastic surface [117–120]. For random motility experiments, a migration stimulus is incorporated at uniform concentration into the gel and the cell well medium. For chemotaxis experiments, the migration stimulus is placed in a separate well from which it forms a concentration gradient by diffusing through the gel. Typically measured quantities are again the location of the leading front or the total number of cells migrating away from the well.

However, intrinsic cell locomotory properties are not the only factors influencing the measurements obtained by cell-population assays. Parameters like the assay chamber geometry and size, initial cell num-ber, or attractant diffusivity can significantly affect the population dispersal and complicate comparison of different sets of experimental data. To alleviate these problems, a phenomenological model has been proposed by Keller and Segel [121] and reformulated by Rivero and coworkers [122]. This mathematical model takes the form of a *partial differential equation* describing the temporal evolution of the cell number density profile and having two key parameters (a) the random motility coefficient μ and (b) a chemotaxis coefficient χ. By comparing model predictions for cell number density profiles to experimental profiles measured with the linear under-agarose assay [123] or the filter assay [124], the random motility μ and the chemotaxis coefficient χ can be determined. A different approach was recently followed by Cheng and coworkers [125] to analyze the differential effect of cell migration and proliferation on the expan-sion of megacolonies of marrow stromal cells cultured on biomimetic hydrogels modified with RGD or osteopontin-derived peptides [74]. This study used a *discrete model* based on the Markov chain approach to simulate the cell-population dynamics of expanding megacolonies. A comparison of model predictions to experimental data showed that surface modifications enhance the expansion rates of cell megacolonies by upregulating the speeds of cell migration.

35.4.2 Individual-Cell Assays

Cell-population assays cannot provide detailed information on how cells move. They cannot directly quantify important locomotory parameters (like cell speed, persistence, turn angles, etc.) or evaluate the effects of external stimuli on these parameters. An accurate characterization of cell locomotion can only be obtained by continuously monitoring a sufficiently large population of migrating cells using a video microscopy system with digital or analog time-lapse capabilities. In most applications, cells migrate on two-dimensional surfaces beneath liquid culture media or agarose gels [21,72,126–129]. Procedures allowing tracking in three-dimensional collagen matrices have also been reported [50,130–136].

By analyzing a sequence of images obtained at fixed time intervals, the actual cell positions at the corresponding times can be identified to reconstruct the individual cell trajectories (see Figure 35.1a). The mean square *displacement* $\langle D^2 \rangle$ of the cells from their original positions can then be calculated and plotted vs. time. If cell movement were a random walk, the mean square *displacement* $\langle D^2 \rangle$ would vary with time according to

$$\langle D^2 \rangle = 2n\mu t \tag{35.1}$$

where μ is the *random motility coefficient* (formally equivalent to a *diffusion coefficient*) and n is a constant depending on the dimensionality of the random walk. For two-dimensional walks $n = 2$, while for three-dimensional walks $n = 3$ [18,137,138]. Equation 35.1 implies that the average distance traveled by a cell is proportional to the square root of the elapsed time.

As we mentioned in Section 35.2.2, however, mammalian cells migrating in isotropic environments execute *persistent random walks*. Dunn [19] and Othmer and coworkers [139] developed the following mathematical model to describe persistent random walks:

$$\langle D^2 \rangle = nS^2[Pt - P^2(1 - e^{-t/P})] \tag{35.2}$$

where $\langle D^2 \rangle$ is the *mean square displacement* of the tracked cells, S is the *root-mean-square cell speed*, P is the *persistence time*, and n is the constant that gives the dimensionality of the persistent random walk (n is 2 or 3 for 2D or 3D walks, respectively). This model assumes that S and P are time invariant. The root-mean-square cell speed S and persistence time P can be computed by fitting the experimental $\langle D^2 \rangle$ vs. time data with the persistent random walk model of Equation 35.2. Nonlinear parameter estimation algorithms [123] must be used, since graphical techniques [19] lead to results dependent on the size of the time interval. Note that for long times ($t \gg P$), Equation 35.2 reduces to the much simpler expression:

$$\langle D^2 \rangle = nS^2 Pt \tag{35.3}$$

Equation 35.3 implies *random walk* behavior and allows us to compute the *random motility coefficient* μ as follows:

$$\mu = \frac{1}{2} S^2 P \tag{35.4}$$

Many investigators have successfully used the persistent random walk model to quantify cell migration [72,140–144]. The chemotactic motion of cells in response to a chemical concentration gradient can also be modeled by adding a directional bias to the persistent random walk process [21]. The magnitude of the directional bias is characterized by the *chemotactic responsiveness* κ. By using experimentally measured values of S, P, and κ, Stokes and Lauffenburger generated computer simulations of theoretical individual cell paths, which were useful in elucidating the role of cell migration in physiological processes [21].

Although the persistent random walk model has been very successful in assaying and comparing the motility of cells under various conditions, it cannot provide all the parameters that may be necessary for an accurate quantification of the cell-migration process. Experimental observations with endothelial cells [127] have revealed that cells slow down or even stop migrating when they divide or when they collide with other cells. Migrating cells may also stop for a while before changing their direction of movement [127]. A detailed description of cell movement (suitable, e.g., for the computer implementation of migration-proliferation models of tissue growth [145]) requires the following information (1) the speed of cell locomotion (swimming speed); (2) the expected duration of cell movement in any given direction; (3) the probability distribution of turn angles that will decide the next direction of cell movement; (4) the frequency of cell stops; and (5) the duration of cell stops. The ultimate direction of cell movement should also be obtained to check for *spatial heterogeneities* or *chemotactic phenomena*.

When such a detailed description of the migration process is desired, models based on *Markov chain* concepts must be used to analyze the cell trajectory data [146–148]. At any time t, a migrating cell can exist in either a *directional state* (if it moves in a certain direction) or the *stationary state* (if it has stopped moving). Clearly, there is a *change of state* every time the migrating cell changes direction and when it starts or stops moving. The central assumption here is that state changes are random and do not depend either on the past history of the cell or on the length of time the cell spent in its current state. Under these assumptions, the sequence of states is a stochastic *Markov sequence*. Details for this analysis may be found in the monograph of Noble and Levine [147]. One usually allows only a finite number of *directional states* by partitioning the set of all possible directions of movement. Four or eight directional states are typically considered for two-dimensional walks (in addition to the stationary state) [147]. The reconstructed cell trajectories can then be modeled as Markov chains [146,149–151] and the following cell locomotory parameters can be extracted from the cell trajectory data using the well-known Markov chain theory [152] (a) *transition-state probabilities* that quantify the frequency with which the cells (individually or collectively) move from one state to another and, thus, characterize the turning and stopping behavior of the cells; (b) *waiting times* or the average time cells spend in a certain state (i.e., moving in a certain direction); and (c) *steady-state probabilities* that provide a measure of the directionality of cell movement (*chemotaxis*). The average speed of locomotion can also be estimated from the reconstructed cell trajectories using the formula:

$$v = \sum_{i=1}^{N} d_i / N \cdot \Delta t \tag{35.5}$$

where d_i is the displacement of the centroid of a cell between two successive observations, and N is the numbers of observations made at a fixed time interval Δt.

The Markov chain model can be used to analyze *chemotaxis* experiments. If there is a preferred direction for cell movement, its steady-state probability will be significantly higher than the steady-state probabilities of the other directions. The Markov chain approach can also provide a more detailed description of cell migration since it accounts for stops in cell movement and uses more than one descriptor (e.g., transition state probabilities and average waiting times) to define persistence [148].

A detailed comparison of the random walk and the Markov chain models using experimental data for migrating endothelial cells has shown [148] that all five locomotory parameters defined above affect the speed S and persistence time P estimated by the persistent random walk model. The persistent random walk model can provide a measure of the speed of locomotion S, appropriately weighted to account for the frequency and duration of cell stops (or slow-downs). The persistence time P, however, is a composite measure of all five locomotory parameters mentioned above. Hence, it may not be always possible to extract all the information necessary to describe cell locomotion from the two parameters of the persistent random walk model. The Markov chain approach, however, also has its drawbacks. Perhaps the most serious drawback is that the values of cell speeds computed according to Equation 35.5 depend on the time interval Δt between cell observations. Accurate estimations of locomotion speeds with Equation 35.5 are possible only when (a) cell trajectories are not very tortuous and (b) the cell positions are observed at short time intervals Δt. This time interval must be carefully chosen using Richardson plots to minimize errors in the computation of cell speed [148].

35.5 Mathematical Models for Cell Migration and Tissue Growth

Cell migration influences both the structure and the growth rate of bioartificial tissues built on biomimetic scaffolds. As we have seen in the previous sections, however, cell migration is a process modulated by a multitude of system parameters that include the local scaffold properties and nutrient or growth factor concentrations. Despite the complexity of this process, however, a purely empirical approach is still used to design scaffolds and select bioreactors appropriate for each application. Noting the limitations of this approach, Ratcliffe and Niklason [153] proposed an interdisciplinary effort to improve our fundamental understanding of the dynamic processes characterizing tissue growth and bioreactor operation. This goal can be achieved with the help of comprehensive computer models that allow for systematic analysis of tissue regeneration processes. Simulations can shorten the development stage by allowing tissue engineers to rapidly screen many alternatives on the computer and choose the most promising ones for laboratory experimentation.

The key challenge here involves the development of computationally efficient algorithms to describe the dynamics of large cell populations that evolve in a continuously changing environment. Early studies

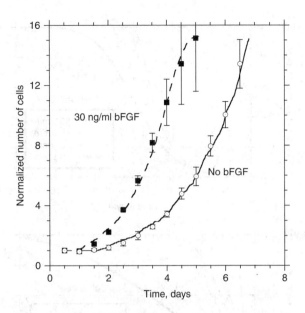

FIGURE 35.2 Normalized cell counts from experiments (symbols) and simulations (lines) for bovine pulmonary artery endothelial (BPAE) cells seeded uniformly on tissue culture plates and cultures without and with 30 ng/ml of bFGF. Standard errors are used as error bars. (Adapted from Lee, Y., Mcintire, L.V., and Zygourakis, K., *Biochem. Cell Biol.*, 1995, **69**: 1284–1298. With permission.)

utilized either discrete [154–156] or continuous models [157–161] to treat tissue growth problems. Using an approach that combined (a) modeling based on cellular automata, (b) computer simulations, and (c) experimentation (migration and proliferation assays), our group initially focused on the growth of two-dimensional tissues like vascular endothelium or keratinocyte colonies [145,155,156]. Using experimental data obtained from long-term tracking and analysis of cell locomotion [162], we developed a class of discrete models that described the population dynamics of cells migrating and proliferating on the surface of biomaterials. These models simulated persistent random walks on 2-D square lattices and accurately accounted for cell–cell collisions. Figure 35.2 shows that model predictions agreed well with experimentally measured proliferation rates of bovine pulmonary artery endothelial (BPAE) cells cultured with and without bFGF, a growth factor that upregulates cell motility. Results also showed that the seeding cell density, the population-average speed of locomotion, and the spatial distribution of the seed cells are crucial parameters in determining the temporal evolution of cell proliferation rates. More recently, models were developed to solve 2-D problems involving the aggregation and self-organization of the cellular slime mold *Dictyostelium discoideum* [163–166] and to study the interactions between extracellular matrix and fibroblasts [167]. To account for the effect of transport limitations that restrict our ability to grow bioartificial tissues [168,169], our group has also developed a *hybrid multi-scale model* that combines (a) partial differential equations modeling the simultaneous reaction–convection–diffusion problems for nutrients and growth factors, (b) discrete models describing the cell-population dynamics, and (c) single-cell models describing intracellular processes modulating cell function.

To demonstrate the potential of computational models for tissue engineering, we will briefly discuss the application of a 3-D model we have developed [170] to study a problem in *biomimetics*. Our objective was to evaluate the effectiveness of surface modifications in enhancing tissue-growth rates through increased cell-migration speeds. Such modifications may involve, for example, the immobilization of signaling or adhesive peptides on the surface of biomaterials [171–173]. To isolate the effect of population dynamics on tissue growth, simulations on 3-D scaffolds were performed by assuming that nutrient and growth factor concentrations remained constant throughout the tissue regeneration process. We considered cell-migration speeds varying across the entire range of observed values (from 0 to 50 μm/h) and used two different cell *seeding modes*. In the first mode, cells were seeded uniformly and randomly throughout the

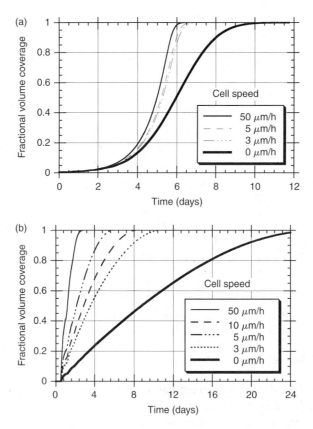

FIGURE 35.3 Effect of cell-migration speed on tissue-growth rates for two different cell-seeding modes. All simulations were carried out on a cubic domain with side equal to 1.9 mm ($128 \times 128 \times 128$ computational sites). (a) Cells were seeded uniformly and randomly with initial density equal to 0.5%. (b) Seeding simulated wound healing. The "wound" was a cylinder 0.95 mm in diameter and 1.9 mm in height. (Adapted from Belgacem, B.Y., Markenscoff, P., and Zygourakis, K. *Proceedings of the 3rd Chemical Engineering Symposium*, Athens, Greece, Vol. 2, pp. 1133–1136, 2001. With permission.)

scaffold. The second seeding mode was designed to simulate a "wound-healing" process. We assumed that a cylindrical wound was created in the center of a 3-D tissue. The wound was then filled with a biomaterial that allowed cells from the surrounding tissue to move into the wound and proliferate to heal it [170].

For uniform cell seeding, Figure 35.3a shows that increasing migration speeds initially enhanced tissue-growth rates. As cell speeds increased above 5 μm/h, however, this beneficial effect diminished and disappeared completely for large-migration speeds. For the wound-healing model, however, the simulations predicted significant enhancements of tissue-growth rates with increasing cell-migration speeds (Figure 35.3b). A careful analysis of the simulation results for these two cases revealed that the uniform cell seeding resulted in many more cell–cell collisions that slowed down the migration of cells. These results point out that the *cell-population dynamics*, the *geometry* of the problem, and the *initial conditions* can have a profound effect on tissue regeneration rates. The simulations also provide us with invaluable guidance for the design of experiments [174] that can test the efficacy of surface modifications designed to enhance cell-migration speeds.

References

[1] Le Douarin, N.M., Cell migrations in embryos. *Cell*, 1984, **38**: 353–360.
[2] Trinkaus, J.P., *Cells into Organs. The forces that Shape the Embryo*. Englewood Cliffs, NJ: Prentice-Hall, 1984.

[3] Condeelis, J., Life at the leading edge: the formation of cell protrusions. *Annu. Rev. Cell Biol.*, 1993, **9**: 411–444.

[4] Bray, D., *Cell Movements.* 2nd ed. New York: Garland Publishing, Inc., 2001.

[5] Devreotes, P.N. and Zigmond, S.H., Chemotaxis in eukaryotic cells: a focus on leukocytes and Dictyostelium. *Annu. Rev. Cell Biol.*, 1988, **4**: 649–686.

[6] Lackie, J.M., *Cell Movement and Cell Behaviour.* London: Allen and Unwin, 1986, pp. 253–275.

[7] Singer, S.J. and Kupfer, A., The directed migration of eukaryotic cells. *Annu. Rev. Cell Biol.*, 1986, **2**: 337–365.

[8] Liotta, L.A., Stracke, M.L., Aznavoorian, S.A., Beckner, M.E., and Schiffmann, E., Tumor cell motility. *Semin. Cancer Biol.*, 1991, **2**: 111–114.

[9] Langer, R. and Vacanti, J.P., Tissue engineering. *Science*, 1993, **260**: 920–926.

[10] Shin, H., Jo, S., and Mikos, A.G., Biomimetic materials for tissue engineering. *Biomaterials*, 2003, **24**: 4353–4364.

[11] Hynes, R.O., Integrins: a family of cell surface receptors. *Cell*, 1987, **48**: 549–554.

[12] Egelhoff, T.T. and Spudich, J.A., Molecular genetics of cell migration: dictyostelium as a model system. *Trends Genet.*, 1991, **7**: 161–166.

[13] Schafer, D.A., Welch, M.D., Machesky, L.M., Bridgman, P.C., Meyer, S.M. et al., Visualization and molecular analysis of actin assembly in living cells. *J. Cell Biol.*, 1998, **143**: 1919–1930.

[14] Carlier, M.F. and Pantaloni, D., Control of actin dynamics in cell motility. *J. Mol. Biol.*, 1997, **269**: 459–467.

[15] Novak, K.D. and Titus, M.A., Myosin I overexpression impairs cell migration. *J. Cell Biol.*, 1997, **136**: 633–647.

[16] Pollard, T.D. and Ostap, E.M., The chemical mechanism of myosin—I: implications for actin-based motility and the evolution of the myosin family of motor proteins. *Cell Struct. Funct.*, 1996, **21**: 351–356.

[17] Stossel, T.P., On the crawling of animal cells. *Science*, 1993, **260**: 1086–1094.

[18] Gail, M.H. and Boone, C.W., The locomotion of mouse fibroblasts in tissue culture. *Biophys. J.*, 1970, **10**: 980–993.

[19] Dunn, G.A., Characterizing a kinesis response: time averaged measures of cell speed and directional persistence. *Agents Actions* (Suppl), 1983, **12**: 14–33.

[20] Stokes, C.L., Lauffenburger, D.A., and William, S.K., Migration of individual microvessel endothelial cells: stochastic model and parameter measurement. *J. Cell Sci.*, 1991, **99**: 419–430.

[21] Dimilla, P., Stone, J., Quinn, J., Albelda, S., and Lauffenburger, D.A., Maximal migration of smooth muscle cells on fibronectin and collagen-IV occurs at an intermediate attachment strength. *J. Cell Biol.*, 1993, **122**: 729–737.

[22] Zigmond, S.H., Klausner, R., Tranquillo, R.T., and Lauffenburger, D.A., Analysis of the requirements for time-averaging of receport occupancy for gradient detection by polymorphonuclear leukocytes, in *Membrane Receptors and Cellular Regulation*, Kahn, C.R., Ed. New York,: Alan R. Liss pp. 347–356, 1985.

[23] Lauffenburger, D.A. and Linderman, J.J., *Receptors: Models for Binding, Trafficking, and Signaling.* New York, NY: Oxford University Press, 1993.

[24] Chan, K.Y., Patton, D.L., and Cosgrove, Y.T., Time-lapse videomicroscopic study of *in vitro* wound closure in rabbit corneal cells. *Invest. Ophthalmol. Visual Sci.*, 1989. **30**: 2488–2498.

[25] Brewitt, H., Sliding of epithelium in experimental corneal wounds. A scanning electron microscopic study. *Acta Ophthalmol.*, 1979, **57**: 945–958.

[26] Sato, Y. and Rifkin, D.B., Autocrine activities of basic fibroblast growth factor: regulation of endothelial cell movement, plasminogen activator synthesis, and DNA synthesis. *J. Cell Biol.*, 1988, **107**: 1199–1205.

[27] Morioka, S., Lazarus, G.S., Baird, J.L., and Jensen, P.J., Migrating keratinocytes express urokinase-type plasminogen activator. *J. Invest. Dermatol.*, 1987, **88**: 418–423.

[28] Ossowski, L., Quigley, J.P., Kellerman, G.M., and Reich, E., Fibrinolysis associated with oncogenic transformation requirement for plasminogen for correlated changes in cellular morphology, colony formation in agar and cell migration. *J. Exp. Med.*, 1973, **138**: 1056–1064.

[29] Baird, A., Schubert, D., Ling, N., and Guillemin, R., Receptor- and heparin-binding domains of basic fibroblast growth factor. *Proc. Natl Acad. Sci. USA* 1988, **70**: 369–373.

[30] Li, W., Fan, J., Chen, M., Guan, S., Sawcer, D. et al., Mechanism of human dermal fibroblast migration driven by type I collagen and platelet-derived growth factor-BB. *Mol. Biol. Cell*, 2004, **15**: 294–309.

[31] Ju, W.D., Schiller, J.T., Kazempour, M.K., and Lowy, D.R., TGF alpha enhances locomotion of cultured human keratinocytes. *J. Invest. Dermatol.*, 1993, **100**: 628–632.

[32] Lorenz, M., Desmarais, V., Macaluso, F., Singer, R.H., and Condeelis, J., Measurement of barbed ends, actin polymerization, and motility in live carcinoma cells after growth factor stimulation. *Cell Motil. Cytoskeleton*, 2004, **57**: 207–217.

[33] Ware, M.F., Wells, A., and Lauffenburger, D.A., Epidermal growth factor alters fibroblast migration speed and directional persistence reciprocally and in a matrix-dependent manner. *J. Cell Sci.*, 1998, **111**: 2423–2432.

[34] Stolz, D.B. and Michalopoulos, G.K., Synergistic enhancement of EGF, but not HGF, stimulated hepatocyte motility by TGF-beta 1 *in vitro. J. Cell. Physiol.*, 1997, **170**: 57–68.

[35] Gabhann, F.M. and Popel, A.S., Model of competitive binding of vascular endothelial growth factor and placental growth factor to VEGF receptors on endothelial cells. *Am. J. Physiol. Heart Circ. Physiol.*, 2004, **286**: H153–H164.

[36] Stoker, M., Gherardi, E., Perryman, M., and Gray, J., Scatter factor is a fibroblast-derived modulator of epithelial cell mobility. *Nature*, 1987, **327**: 239–242.

[37] Nusrat, A., Parkos, C.A., Bacarra, A.E., Godowski, P.J., Delp-Archer, C. et al., Hepatocyte growth factor/scatter factor effects on epithelia. Regulation of intercellular junctions in transformed and nontransformed cell lines, basolateral polarization of c-met receptor in transformed and natural intestinal epithelia, and induction of rapid wound repair in a transformed model epithelium. *J. Clin. Invest.*, 1994, **93**: 2056–2065.

[38] Poomsawat, S., Whawell, S.A., Morgan, M.J., Thomas, G.J., and Speight, P.M., Scatter factor regulation of integrin expression and function on oral epithelial cells. *Arch. Dermatol. Res.*, 2003, **295**: 63–70.

[39] Funasaka, T., Haga, A., Raz, A., and Nagase, H., Tumor autocrine motility factor induces hyperpermeability of endothelial and mesothelial cells leading to accumulation of ascites fluid. *Biochem. Biophys. Res. Commun.*, 2002, **293**: 192–200.

[40] Silletti, S., Paku, S., and Raz, A., Autocrine motility factor and the extracellular matrix. I. Coordinate regulation of melanoma cell adhesion, spreading and migration involves focal contact reorganization. *Int. J. Cancer*, 1998, **76**: 120–128.

[41] Silletti, S., Paku, S., and Raz, A., Autocrine motility factor and the extracellular matrix. II. Degradation or remodeling of substratum components directs the motile response of tumor cells. *Int. J. Cancer*, 1998, **76**: 129–135.

[42] Schor, S.L., Ellis, I.R., Jones, S.J., Baillie, R., Seneviratne, K. et al., Migration-stimulating factor: a genetically truncated onco-fetal fibronectin isoform expressed by carcinoma and tumor-associated stromal cells. *Cancer Res.*, 2003, **63**: 8827–8836.

[43] Hamada, J., Cavanaugh, P.G., Miki, K., and Nicolson, G.L., A paracrine migration-stimulating factor for metastatic tumor cells secreted by mouse hepatic sinusoidal endothelial cells: identification as complement component C3b. *Cancer Res.*, 1993, **53**: 4418–4423.

[44] Schor, S.L. and Schor, A.M., Characterization of migration-stimulating factor (MSF): evidence for its role in cancer pathogenesis. *Cancer Invest.*, 1990, **8**: 665–667.

[45] Postlethwaite, A.E., Keski-Oja, J., Moses, H.L., and Kang, A.H., Stimulation of the chemotactic migration of human fibroblasts by transforming growth factor β. *J. Exp. Med.*, 1987, **165**: 251–256.

[46] Seppä, H., Grotendorst, G., Seppä, S., Schiffmann, E., and Martin, G.R., Platelet-derived growth factor is chemotactic for fibroblasts. *J. Cell Biol.*, 1982, **142**: 1119–1130.

[47] Grotendorst, G.R., Soma, Y., and Takehara, K., EGF and TGF-alpha are potent chemoattractants for endothelial cells and EGF-like peptides are present at sites of tissue regeneration. *J. Cell Physiol.*, 1989, **139**: 617–623.

[48] Wahl, S.M., Hunt, D.A., Wakefield, L.M., Mccart-Ney-Francis, N., Wahl, L.M. et al., Transforming growth factor type β induces monocyte chemotaxis and growth factor production. *Proc. Natl Acad. Sci. USA*, 1987, **84**: 5788–5792.

[49] Grotendorst, G.R., Chemoattractants and growth factors, in *Wound Healing: Biochemical and Clinical Aspects*, Lindblad, W.J., Ed. Philadelphia, Saunders: pp. 237–246, 1992.

[50] Knapp, D.M., Helou, E.F., and Tranquillo, R.T., A fibrin or collagen gel assay for tissue cell chemotaxis: assessment of fibroblast chemotaxis to GRGDSP. *Exp. Cell Res.*, 1999, **247**: 543–553.

[51] Fisher, P.R., Merkl, R., and Gerisch, G., Quantitative analysis of cell motility and chemotaxis in Dictyostelium discoideum by using an image processing system and a novel chemotaxis chamber providing stationary chemical gradients. *J. Cell Biol.*, 1989, **108**: 973–984.

[52] Zigmond, S.H., Ability of polymorphonuclear leukocytes to orient in gradients of chemotactic factors. *J. Cell Biol.*, 1977, **75 Pt 1**: 606–616.

[53] Tranquillo, R.T. and Lauffenburger, D.A., Stochastic model of leukocyte chemosensory movement. *J. Math. Biol. (IYS)*, 1987, **25**: 229–262.

[54] Tranquillo, R.T., Theories and models of gradient perception, in *Biology of the Chemotactic Response*, Lackie, J.M., Ed. Cambridge: Cambridge University Press, pp. 35–75, 1990.

[55] Tranquillo, R.T., Lauffenburger, D.A., and Zigmond, S.H., A stochastic model for leukocyte random motility and chemotaxis based on receptor binding fluctuations. *J. Cell Biol.*, 1988, **106**: 303–309.

[56] Moghe, P.V. and Tranquillo, R.T., Stochastic model of chemoattractant receptor dynamics in leukocyte chemosensory movement. *Bull. Math. Biol.*, 1994, **56**: 1041–1093.

[57] Ruoslahti, E. and Engvall, E., Eds., *Extracellular Matrix Components*. San Diego: Academic Press, 1994.

[58] Bosman, F.T. and Stamenkovic, I., Functional structure and composition of the extracellular matrix. *J. Pathol.*, 2003, **200**: 423–428.

[59] Rodgers, R.J., Irving-Rodgers, H.F., and Russell, D.L., Extracellular matrix of the developing ovarian follicle. *Reproduction*, 2003, **126**: 415–424.

[60] Kanwar, Y.S., Wada, J., Lin, S., Danesh, F.R., Chugh, S.S. et al., Update of extracellular matrix, its receptors, and cell adhesion molecules in mammalian nephrogenesis. *Am. J. Physiol. Renal Physiol.*, 2004, **286**: F202–F215.

[61] Albelda, S.M., Daise, M., Levine, E.M., and Buck, C.A., Identification and characterization of cell–substratum adhesion receptors on cultured human endothelial cells. *J. Clin. Invest.*, 1989, **83**: 1992–2002.

[62] Albelda, S.M. and Buck, C.A., Integrins and other cell adhesion molecules. *FASEB J.*, 1990, **4**: 2868–2880.

[63] Languino, L.R., Gehlsen, K.R., Wayner, E., Carter, W.G., Engvall, E. et al., Endothelial cells use $\alpha_2\beta_1$ integrin as a laminin receptor. *J. Cell Biol.*, 1989, **109**: 2455–2462.

[64] Wu, C., Fields, A.J., Kapteijn, B.A., and Mcdonald, J.A., The role of $\alpha_4\beta_1$ integrin in cell motility and fibronectin matrix assembly. *J. Cell Sci.*, 1995, **108**: 821–829.

[65] Massia, S.P. and Hubbell, J.A., Covalent surface immobilization of Arg–Gly–Asp- and Tyr–Ile–Gly–Ser–Arg-containing peptides to obtain well-defined cell-adhesive substrates. *Anal. Biochem.*, 1990, **187**: 292–301.

[66] Massia, S.P. and Hubbell, J.A., Covalently attached GRGD on polymer surfaces promotes biospecific adhesion of mammalian cells. *Ann. NY Acad. Sci.*, 1990, **589**: 261–270.

[67] Hubbell, J.A., Massia, S.P., Desai, N.P., and Drumheller, P.D., Endothelial cell-selective materials for tissue engineering in the vascular graft via a new receptor. *Biotechnology*, 1991, **9**: 568–572.

[68] Massia, S.P. and Hubbell, J.A., An RGD spacing of 440 nm is sufficient for integrin $\alpha_v\beta_3$-mediated fibroblast spreading and 140 nm for focal contact and stress fiber formation. *J. Cell Biol.*, 1991, **114**: 1089–1100.

[69] Massia, S.P. and Hubbell, J.A., Human endothelial cell interactions with surface-coupled adhesion peptides on a nonadhesive glass substrate and two polymeric biomaterials. *J. Biomed. Mater. Res.*, 1991, **25**: 223–242.

[70] Hubbell, J.A., Massia, S.P., and Drumheller, P.D., Surface-grafted cell-binding peptides in tissue engineering of the vascular graft. *Ann. NY Acad. Sci.*, 1992, **665**: 253.

[71] Massia, S.P., Rao, S.S., and Hubbell, J.A., Covalently immobilized laminin peptide Tyr–Ile–Gly–Ser–Arg (YIGSR) supports cell spreading and co-localization of the 67-kDa laminin receptor with alpha-actinin and vinculin. *J. Biol. Chem.*, 1993, **268**: 8053–8059.

[72] Kouvroukoglou, S., Dee, K.C., Bizios, R., Mcintire, L.V., and Zygourakis, K., Endothelial cell migration on surfaces modified with immobilized adhesive peptides. *Biomaterials*, 2000, **21**: 1725–1733.

[73] Yang, X.B., Roach, H.I., Clarke, N.M., Howdle, S.M., Quirk, R. et al., Human osteoprogenitor growth and differentiation on synthetic biodegradable structures after surface modification. *Bone*, 2001, **29**: 523–531.

[74] Shin, H., Zygourakis, K., Farach-Carson, M.C., Yaszemski, M.J., and Mikos, A.G., Attachment, proliferation, and migration of marrow stromal osteoblasts cultured on biomimetic hydrogels modified with an osteopontin-derived peptide. *Biomaterials*, 2004, **25**: 895–906.

[75] Humphries, M.J., Mould, A.P., and Yamada, K.M., Matrix receptors in cell migration, in *Receptors for Extracellular Matrix*, Mecham, R.P., Ed. San Diego, CA: Academic Press, pp. 195–253, 1991.

[76] Grossi, F.S., Keizer, D.M., Saracino, G.A., Erkens, S., and Romijn, J.C., Flow cytometric analysis and motility response to laminin and fibronectin of four new metastatic variants of the human renal cell carcinoma line RC43. *Prog. Clin. Biol. Res.*, 1992, **378**: 195–205.

[77] Mooradian, D.L., Mccarthy, J.B., Skubitz, A.P., Cameron, J.D., and Furcht, L.T., Characterization of FN-C/H-V, a novel synthetic peptide from fibronectin that promotes rabbit corneal epithelial cell adhesion, spreading, and motility. *Invest. Ophthalmol. Vis. Sci.*, 1993, **34**: 153–164.

[78] Savarese, D.M., Russell, J.T., Fatatis, A., and Liotta, L.A., Type IV collaged stimulates an increase in intracellular calcium. Potential role in tumor cell motility. *J. Biol. Chem.*, 1992, **267**: 21928–21935.

[79] Lin, M.L. and Bertics, P.J., Laminin responsiveness is associated with changes in fibroblast morphology, motility and anchorage-independent growth: cell system for examining the interaction between laminin and EGF signalling pathways. *J. Cell Physiol.*, 1995, **164**: 593–604.

[80] Palecek, S.P., Loftus, J.C., Ginsberg, M.H., Lauffenburger, D.A., and Horwitz, A.F., Integrin–ligand binding properties govern cell migration speed through cell–substratum adhesiveness. *Nature*, 1997, **385**: 537–540.

[81] Schense, J.C. and Hubbell, J.A., Three-dimensional migration of neurites is mediated by adhesion site density and affinity. *J. Biol. Chem.*, 2000, **275**: 6813–6818.

[82] Gobin, A.S. and West, J.L., Cell migration through defined, synthetic ECM analogs. *FASEB J. Exp. Biol.*, 2002, **16**: 751–753.

[83] Holub, A., Byrnes, J., Anderson, S., Dzaidzio, L., Hogg, N. et al., Ligand density modulates eosinophil signaling and migration. *J. Leukocyte Biol.*, 2003, **73**: 657–664.

[84] Goodman, S.L., Risse, G., and Von Der Mark, K., The E8 subfragment of laminin promotes locomotion of myoblasts over extracellular matrix. *J. Cell Biol.*, 1989, **109**: 799–809.

[85] Keely, P.J., Fong, A.M., Zutter, M.M., and Santoro, S.A., Alteration of collagen-dependent adhesion, motility, and morphogenesis by the expression of antisense alpha 2 integrin mRNA in mammary cells. *J. Cell Sci.*, 1995, **108**: 595–607.

[86] Lauffenburger, D.A., A simple model for the effects of receptor-mediated cell–substratuum adhesion on cell migration. *Chem. Eng. Sci.*, 1989, **44**: 1903–1914.

[87] Dimilla, P., Barbee, K., and Lauffenburger, D.A., Mathematical model for the effects of adhesion and mechanics on cell migration speed. *Biophys. J.*, 1991, **60**: 15–37.

[88] Ward, M.D. and Hammer, D.A., A theoretical analysis for the effect of focal contact formation on cell-substrate attachment strength. *Biophys. J.*, 1993, **64**: 936–959.

[89] Schmidt, C.E., Horwitz, A.F., Lauffenburger, D.A., and Sheetz, M.P., Integrin-cytoskeletal interactions in migrating fibroblasts are dynamic, asymmetric, and regulated. *J. Cell Biol.*, 1993, **123**: 977–991.

[90] Lawson, M.A. and Maxfield, F.R., Ca(2+)- and calcineurin-dependent recycling of an integrin to the front of migrating neutrophils. *Nature*, 1995, **376**: 75–79.

[91] Carter, S.B., Principles of cell motility: the direction of cell movement and cancer invasion. *Nature*, 1965, **208**: 1183–1187.

[92] Dickinson, R.B. and Tranquillo, R.T., A stochastic model for adhesion-mediated cell random motility and haptotaxis. *J. Math. Biol.*, 1993, **31**: 563–600.

[93] Bray, D., *Cell Movements*. New York, NY Garland Publishing, Inc., 1992.

[94] Nakatsuji, N. and Johnson, K.E., Experimental manipulation of a contact guidance system in amphibian gastrulation by mechanical tension. *Nature*, 1984, **307**: 453–455.

[95] Oakley, C., Jaeger, N.A., and Brunette, D.M., Sensitivity of fibroblasts and their cytoskeletons to substratum topographies: topographic guidance and topographic compensation by micromachined grooves of different dimensions. *Exp. Cell Res.*, 1997, **234**: 413–424.

[96] Newgreen, D. and Thiery, J.P., Fibronectin in early avian embryos: synthesis and distribution along the migration pathways of neural crest cells. *Cell Tissue Res.*, 1980, **211**: 269–291.

[97] Ronfard, V. and Barrandon, Y., Migration of keratinocytes through tunnels of digested fibrin. *Proc. Natl Acad. Sci. USA*, 2001, **98**: 4504–4509.

[98] Brown, M.J. and Loew, L.M., Electric field-directed fibroblast locomotion involves cell surface molecular reorganization and is calcium independent. *J. Cell Biol.*, 1994, **127**: 117–128.

[99] Gruler, H. and Nuccitelli, R., Neural crest cell galvanotaxis: new data and a novel approach to the analysis of both galvanotaxis and chemotaxis. *Cell Motil. Cytoskeleton*, 1991, **19**: 121–133.

[100] Zhao, M., Agius-Fernandez, A., Forrester, J.V., and Mccaig, C.D., Orientation and directed migration of cultured corneal epithelial cells in small electric fields are serum dependent. *J. Cell Sci.*, 1996, **109**: 1405–1414.

[101] Nuccitelli, R., A role for endogenous electric fields in wound healing. *Curr. Top. Develop. Biol.*, 2003, **58**: 1–26.

[102] Fang, K.S., Farboud, B., Nuccitelli, R., and Isseroff, R.R., Migration of human keratinocytes in electric fields requires growth factors and extracellular calcium. *J. Invest. Dermatol.*, 1998, **111**: 751–756.

[103] Nuccitelli, R., Smart, T., and Ferguson, J., Protein kinases are required for embryonic neural crest cell galvanotaxis. *Cell Motil. Cytoskeleton*, 1993, **24**: 54–66.

[104] Pullar, C.E., Isseroff, R.R., and Nuccitelli, R., Cyclic AMP-dependent protein kinase A plays a role in the directed migration of human keratinocytes in a DC electric field. *Cell Motil. Cytoskeleton*, 2001, **50**: 207–217.

[105] Mcbain, V.A., Forrester, J.V., and Mccaig, C.D., HGF, MAPK, and a small physiological electric field interact during corneal epithelial cell migration. *Invest. Ophthalmol. Visual Sci.*, 2003, **44**: 540–547.

[106] Boyden, S.B., The chemotactic effect of mixtures of antibody and antigen on polymorphonuclear leukocytes. *J. Exp. Med.*, 1962, **115**: 453–466.

[107] Keller, H.U., Borel, J.F., Wilkinson, P.C., Hess, M., and Cottier, H., Reassessment of Boyden's technique for measuring chemotaxis. *J. Immunol. Meth.*, 1972, **1**: 165–168.

[108] Nind, A.F., Neutrophil chemotaxis: technical problems with nitrocellulose filters in Boyden-type chambers. *J. Immunol. Meth.*, 1981, **49**: 39–52.

[109] Glaser, B.M., D'amore, P.A., Seppa, H., Seppa, S., and Schiffmann, E., Adult tissues contain chemoattractants for vascular endothelial cells. *Nature*, 1980, **288**: 483–484.

[110] Pelz, G., Schettler, A., and Tschesche, H., Granulocyte chemotaxis measured in a Boyden chamber assay by quantification of neutrophil elastase. *Eur. J. Clin. Chem. Clin. Biochem.: J.* 1993, **31**: 651–656.

[111] Kohyama, T., Ertl, R.F., Valenti, V., Spurzem, J., Kawamoto, M. et al., Prostaglandin E(2) inhibits fibroblast chemotaxis. *Am. J. Physiol. Lung Cell Mol. Physiol.*, 2001, **281**: L1257–L1263.

[112] Ebrahimzadeh, P.R., Högfors, C., and Braide, M., Neutrophil chemotaxis in moving gradients of fMLP. *J. Leukocyte Biol.*, 2000, **67**: 651–661.

[113] Slattery, M.J. and Dong, C., Neutrophils influence melanoma adhesion and migration under flow conditions. *Int. J. Cancer*, 2003, **106**: 713–722.

[114] Augustin-Voss, H.G. and Pauli, B.U., Quantitative analysis of autocrine-regulated, matrix-induced, and tumor cell-stimulated endothelial cell migration using a silicon template compartmentalization technique. *Exp. Cell Res.*, 1992, **198**: 221–227.

[115] Mignatti, P., Tsuboi, R., Robbins, E., and Rifkin, D.B., *In vitro* angiogenesis on the human amniotic membrane: requirement for basic fibroblast growth factor-induced proteinases. *J. Cell Biol.*, 1989, **108**: 671–682.

[116] Tsuboi, R., Sato, Y., and Rifkin, D.B., Correlation of cell migration, cell invasion, receptor number, proteinase production, and basic fibroblast growth factor levels in endothelial cells. *J. Cell Biol.*, 1990, **110**: 511–517.

[117] Rothman, C. and Lauffenburger, D.A., Analysis of the linear under-agarose leukocyte chemotaxis assay. *Ann. Biomed. Eng.*, 1983, **11**: 451–460.

[118] Rupnick, M.A., Stokes, C.L., Williams, S.K., and Lauffenburger, D.A., Quantitative analysis of random motility of human microvessel endothelial cells using a linear under-agarose assay. *Lab. Invest.*, 1988, **59**: 363–372.

[119] Newton-Nash, D.K., Tonellato, P., Swiersz, M., and Abramoff, P., Assessment of chemokinetic behavior of inflammatory lung macrophages in a linear under-agarose assay. *J. Leukocyte Biol.*, 1990, **48**: 297–305.

[120] Heit, B. and Kubes, P., Measuring chemotaxis and chemokinesis: the under-agarose cell migration assay. *Science's STKE* [electronic resource]: signal transduction knowledge environment. 2003, **2003**: PL5.

[121] Keller, E.F. and Segel, L.A., Model for chemotaxis. *J. Theor. Biol.*, 1971, **30**: 225–234.

[122] Rivero, M.A., Tranquillo, R.T., Buettner, H.M., and Lauffenburger, D.A., Transport models for chemotactic cell populations based on individual cell behavior. *Chem. Eng. Sci.*, 1989, **44**: 2881–2897.

[123] Farrell, B.E., Daniele, R.P., and Lauffenburger, D.A., Quantitative relationships between single-cell and cell-population model parameters for chemosensory migration responses of alveolar macrophages to C5a. *Cell Motil. Cytoskeleton*, 1990, **16**: 279–293.

[124] Buettner, H.M., Lauffenburger, D.A., and Zigmond, S.H., Measurement of leukocyte motility and chemotaxis parameters with the Millipore filter assay. *J. Immunol. Meth.*, 1989, **123**: 25–37.

[125] Cheng, G., Shin, H., Mikos, A.G., and Zygourakis, K., Expansion of marrow stromal osteoblast megacolonies on biomimetic hydrogels: interpreting and evaluating the assay data. *AIChE Annual Meeting* (paper 107cy), 2003.

[126] Dimilla, P.A., Stone, J.A., Quinn, J.A., Albelda, S.M., and Lauffenburger, D.A., Maximal migration of human smooth muscle cells on fibronectin and type IV collagen occurs at an intermediate attachment strength. *J. Cell Biol.*, 1993, **122**: 729–737.

[127] Lee, Y., Mcintire, L.V., and Zygourakis, K., Analysis of endothelial cell locomotion: differential effects of motility and contact inhibition. *Biotechnol. Bioeng.*, 1994, **43**: 622–634.

[128] Demuth, T., Hopf, N.J., Kempski, O., Sauner, D., Herr, M. et al., Migratory activity of human glioma cell lines *in vitro* assessed by continuous single cell observation. *Clin. Exp. Metastasis*, 2000, **18**: 589–597.

[129] Krooshoop, D.J., Torensma, R., Van Den Bosch, G.J., Nelissen, J.M., Figdor, C.G. et al., An automated multi well cell track system to study leukocyte migration. *J. Immunol. Meth.*, 2003, **280**: 89–102.

[130] Dickinson, R.B., Mccarthy, J.B., and Tranquillo, R.T., Quantitative characterization of cell invasion *in vitro*: formulation and validation of a mathematical model of the collagen gel invasion assay. *Ann. Biomed. Eng.*, 1993, **21**: 679–697.

[131] Parkhurst, M.R. and Saltzmann, W.M., Quantification of human neutrophil motility in three-dimensional collagen gels: effect of collagen concentration. *Biophys. J.*, 1992, **61**: 306–315.

[132] Shields, E.D. and Noble, P.B., Methodology for detection of heterogeneity of cell locomotory phenotypes in three-dimensional gels. *Exp. Cell Biol.*, 1987, **55**: 250–256.

[133] Burgess, B.T., Myles, J.L., and Dickinson, R.B., Quantitative analysis of adhesion-mediated cell migration in three-dimensional gels of RGD-grafted collagen. *Ann. Biomed. Eng.*, 2000, **28**: 110–118.

[134] Niggemann, B., Maaser, K., Lü, H., Kroczek, R., Zänker, K.S. et al., Locomotory phenotypes of human tumor cell lines and T lymphocytes in a three-dimensional collagen lattice. *Cancer Lett.*, 1997, **118**: 173–180.

[135] Friedl, P., Noble, P.B., and Zänker, K.S., Lymphocyte locomotion in three-dimensional collagen gels. Comparison of three quantitative methods for analysing cell trajectories. *J. Immunol. Meth.*, 1993, **165**: 157–165.

[136] Friedl, P. and Bröcker, E.B., Reconstructing leukocyte migration in 3D extracellular matrix by time-lapse videomicroscopy and computer-assisted tracking. *Meth. Mol. Biol.*, 2004, **239**: 77–90.

[137] Berg, H.C., *Random Walks in Biology*. Princeton: Princeton University Press, pp. 5–16, 1983.

[138] Peterson, S.C. and Noble, P.B., A two-dimensional random-walk analysis of human granulocyte movement. *Biophys. J.*, 1972, **12**: 1048–1055.

[139] Othmer, H.G., Dunbar, S.R., and Alt, W., Models of dispersal in biological systems. *J. Math. Biol.*, 1988, **26**: 263–298.

[140] Dickinson, R.B., McCarthy, J.B., and Tranquillo, R.T., Quantitative characterization of cell invasion *in vitro*: formulation and validation of a mathematical model of the collagen gel invasion assay. *Ann. Biomed. Eng.*, 1993, **21**: 679–697.

[141] Saltzman, W.M., Parsons-Wingerter, P., Leong, K.W., and Shin, L., Fibroblast and hepatocyte behavior on synthetic polymer surfaces. *J. Biomed. Mater. Res.*, 1991, **25**: 741–759.

[142] Dimilla, P.A., Quinn, J.A., Albelda, S.M., and Lauffenburger, D.A., Measurement of individual cell migration parameters for human tissue cells. *AIChE J.*, 1992, **38**: 1092–1104.

[143] Glasgow, J.E., Farrell, B.E., Fisher, E.S., Lauffenburger, D.A., and Daniele, R.P., The motile response of alveolar macrophages. An experimental study using single-cell and cell population approaches. *Am. Rev. Respir. Dis.*, 1989, **139**: 320–329.

[144] Tan, J., Shen, H., and Saltzman, W.M., Micron-scale positioning of features influences the rate of polymorphonuclear leukocyte migration. *Biophys. J.*, 2001, **81**: 2569–2579.

[145] Lee, Y., Kouvroukoglou, S., Mcintire, L.V., and Zygourakis, K., A cellular automaton model for the proliferation of migrating contact-inhibited cells. *Biophys. J.*, 1995, **69**: 1284–1298.

[146] Boyarsky, A., A Markov chain model for human granulocyte movement. *J. Math. Biol.*, 1975, **2**: 69–78.

[147] Noble, P.B. and Levine, M.D., *Computer-Assisted Analysis of Cell Locomotion and Chemotaxis*. Boca Raton, FL: CRC Press, Inc. pp. 17–48, 1986.

[148] Lee, Y., Mcintire, L.V., and Zygourakis, K., Characterization of endothelial cell locomotion using a Markov chain model. *Biochem. Cell Biol.*, 1995, **73**: 461–472.

[149] Boyarsky, A. and Noble, P.B., A Markov chain characterization of human neutrophil locomotion under neutral and chemotactic conditions. *Can. J. Physiol. Pharmacol.*, 1977, **55**: 1–6.

[150] Noble, P.B. and Bentley, K.C., Locomotory characteristics of human lymphocytes undergoing negative chemotaxis to oral carcinomas. *Exp. Cell Res.*, 1981, **133**: 457–461.

[151] Noble, P.B., Boyarsky, A., and Bentley, K.C., Human lymphocyte migration *in vitro*: charac-terization and quantitation of locomotory parameters. *Can. J. Physiol. Pharmacol.*, 1979, **57**: 108–112.

[152] Papoulis, A., *Probability, Random Variables and Stochastic Processes.* New York, NY: McGraw-Hill, pp. 532–551, 1965.

[153] Ratcliffe, A. and Niklason, L.E., Bioreactors and bioprocessing for tissue engineering. *Ann. NY Acad. Sci.*, 2002, **961**: 210–215.

[154] Lim, J.H.F. and Davies, G.A., A stochastic model to simulate the growth of anchorage dependent cells on flat surfaces. *Biotechnol. Bioeng.*, 1990, **36**: 547.

[155] Zygourakis, K., Bizios, R., and Markenscoff, P., Proliferation of anchorage dependent contact-inhibited cells. I. Development of theoretical models based on cellular automata. *Biotechnol. Bioeng.*, 1991, **38**: 459–470.

[156] Zygourakis, K., Markenscoff, P., and Bizios, R., Proliferation of anchorage dependent contact-inhibited cells. II. Experimental results and comparison to theoretical model predictions. *Biotechnol. Bioeng.*, 1991, **38**: 471–479.

[157] Frame, K.K. and Hu, W.S., A model for density-dependent growth of anchorage-dependent mammalian cells. *Biotechnol. Bioeng.*, 1988, **32**: 1061.

[158] Cherry, R.S. and Papoutsakis, E.T., Modeling of contact-inhibited animal cell growth on flat surfaces and spheres. *Biotechnol. Bioeng.*, 1989, **33**: 300.

[159] Sherratt, J.A., Martin, P., Murray, J.D., and Lewis, J., Mathematical models of wound healing in embryonic and adult epidermis. *IMA J. Math. Appl. Med. Biol.*, 1992, **9**: 177–196.

[160] Sherratt, J.A. and Murray, J.D., Epidermal wound healing: the clinical implications of a simple mathematical model. *Cell Transplant*, 1992, **1**: 365–371.

[161] Dale, P.D., Maini, P.K., and Sherratt, J.A., Mathematical modeling of corneal epithelial wound healing. *Math. Biosci.*, 1994, **124**: 127–147.

[162] Lee, Y., Mcintire, L.V., and Zygourakis, K., Analysis of endothelial cell locomotion: differential effects of motility and contact inhibition. *Biotechnol. Bioeng.*, 1994, **43**: 622–634.

[163] Dallon, J.C. and Othmer, H.G., A discrete cell model with adaptive signalling for aggregation of *Dictyostelium discoideum*. *Phil. Trans. R. Soc. Lond. B Biol. Sci.*, 1997, **352**: 391–417.

[164] Hogeweg, P., Evolving mechanisms of morphogenesis: on the interplay between differential adhesion and cell differentiation. *J. Theor. Biol.*, 2000, **203**: 317–333.

[165] Marée, A.F. and Hogeweg, P., How amoeboids self-organize into a fruiting body: multi-cellular coordination in Dictyostelium discoideum. *Proc. Natl Acad. Sci. USA*, 2001, **98**: 3879–3883.

[166] Palsson, E. and Othmer, H.G., A model for individual and collective cell movement in Dictyostelium discoideum. *Proc. Natl Acad. Sci. USA*, 2000, **97**: 10448–10453.

[167] Dallon, J.C., Sherratt, J.A., and Maini, P.K., Mathematical modelling of extracellular matrix dynamics using discrete cells: fiber orientation and tissue regeneration. *J. Theor. Biol.*, 1999, **199**: 449–471.

[168] Sikavitsas, V.I., Bancroft, G.N., and Mikos, A.G., Formation of three-dimensional cell/polymer constructs for bone tissue engineering in a spinner flask and a rotating wall vessel bioreactor. *J. Biomed. Mater. Res.*, 2002, **62**: 136–148.

[169] Bancroft, G.N., Sikavitsas, V.I., Van Den Dolder, J., Sheffield, T.L., Ambrose, C.G. et al., Fluid flow increases mineralized matrix deposition in 3D perfusion culture of marrow stromal osteoblasts in a dose-dependent manner. *PNAS*, 2002, **99**: 12600–12605.

[170] Belgacem, B.Y., Markenscoff, P., and Zygourakis, K., A computational model for tissue regeneration and wound healing. *Proceedings of the 3rd Chemical Engineering Symposium*, Athens, Greece, Vol. 2, pp. 1133–1136, 2001.

[171] Huttenlocher, A.F., Ginsberg, M.H., and Horwitz, A.F., Modulation of cell migration by integrin-mediated cytoskeletal linkages and ligand-binding affinity. *J. Cell Biol.*, 1996, **134**: 1551–1562.

[172] Palecek, S.P., Loftus, J.C., Ginsberg, M.H., Lauffenburger, D.A., and Horwitz, A.F., Integrin–ligand binding properties govern cell migration speed through cell–substratum adhesiveness. *Nature*, 1997, **385**: 537–540.

[173] Shin, H., Zygourakis, K., Farach-Carson, M.C., Yaszemski, M.J., and Mikos, A.G., Attachment, proliferation, and migration of marrow stromal osteoblasts cultured on biomimetic hydrogels modified with an osteopontin-derived peptide. *Biomaterials*, 2004, **25**: 895–906.

[174] Gosiewska, A., Rezania, A., Dhanaraj, S., Vyakarnam, M., Zhou, J. et al., Development of a three-dimensional transmigration assay for testing cell — polymer interactions for tissue engineering applications. *Tissue Eng.*, 2001, **7**: 267–277.

36

Inflammatory and Immune Responses to Tissue Engineered Devices

James M. Anderson
Case Western Reserve University

36.1 Introduction

Tissue-engineered devices are biologic–biomaterial combinations in which some component of tissue has been combined with a biomaterial to create a device for the restoration or modification of tissue or organ function. Four significant goals must be achieved if these devices are to function adequately and appropriately in the host environment. These four goals are (1) restoration of the target tissue with its appropriate function and cellular phenotypic expression; (2) inhibition of the macrophage and foreign body giant cell foreign body response that may degrade or adversely modify device function; (3) inhibition of scar and fibrous capsule formation that may be deleterious to the function of the device; and (4) inhibition of immune responses that may inhibit the proposed function of the device and ultimately lead to the destruction of the tissue component of the tissue-engineered device. The range of types of tissue-engineered devices is large, yet each device is considered to be unique in its combination of tissue component and biomaterial, thus requiring a unique set of tests to ensure that the four goals are achieved for the lifetime of the device in its *in vivo* environment.

The implantation of a tissue-engineered device activates the host defense systems that include the inflammatory and immune responses. The purpose of this chapter is to provide an overview and fundamental understanding of the inflammatory and immune responses that may be responsive following the *in vivo* implantation of a tissue-engineered device. In general, tissue-engineered devices contain a biomaterials component for which the evaluation of the inflammatory and foreign body reaction is of importance. Tissue-engineered devices also contain an active biological component, that is, proteins and cells, for which evaluation of the immune responses is of importance to the overall safety and efficacy of the tissue-engineered device. In addition, tissue-engineered devices are also considered as combination devices

TABLE 36.1   The Mononuclear Phagocytic System

Tissues	Cells
Implant sites	Inflammatory macrophages, foreign body giant cells
Liver	Kupffer cells
Lung	Alveolar macrophages
Connective tissue	Histiocytes
Bone marrow	Macrophages
Spleen and lymph nodes	Fixed and free macrophages
Serous cavities	Pleural and peritoneal macrophages
Nervous system	Microglial cells
Bone	Osteoclasts
Skin	Langerhans' cells, dendritic cells
Lymphoid tissue	Dendritic cells

and the interaction between the synthetic and biologic components and their interactive inflammatory and immune responses must be considered and evaluated. For clarification, it should be noted that the inflammatory responses are also known as the innate immune system and immune responses are generally considered to be the acquired or adaptive immune system.

The inflammatory and immune systems overlap considerably through the activity and phenotypic expression of macrophages that are derived from blood-borne monocytes. Monocytes and macrophages belong to the mononuclear phagocytic system (MPS) (Table 36.1). Cells in the MPS may be considered as resident macrophages in the respective tissues that take on specialized functions that are dependent on their tissue environment. From this perspective, the host defense system may be seen as blood-borne or circulating inflammatory and immune cells as well as mononuclear phagocytic cells that reside in specific tissues with specialized functions. As will be seen in the overview of the inflammatory and immune responses, the macrophage plays a pivotal role in both the induction and effector phases of these responses.

36.2   Inflammatory Responses

The process of implantation of a biomaterial, prosthesis, medical device, or tissue-engineered device results in injury to tissues or organs and the subsequent perturbation of homeostatic mechanisms that lead to the cellular cascades of wound healing [1–6]. The response to injury is dependent on multiple factors including the extent of injury, the loss of basement membrane structures, blood–material interactions, provisional matrix formation, the extent or degree of cellular necrosis, and the extent of the inflammatory response. These events, in turn, may affect the extent or degree of granulation tissue formation, foreign body reaction, and fibrosis or fibrous capsule development. These host reactions are considered to be tissue-, organ-, and species-dependent. In addition, it is important to recognize that these reactions occur very early, that is, within 2 to 3 weeks of the time of implantation, for biocompatible materials or devices in the normal resolution of the inflammatory and wound healing responses.

Table 36.2 identifies the events in the inflammatory responses and indicates the predominant cell type found in these responses. These characteristic cell types are utilized in histological studies to identify the phase or event in the inflammatory and wound healing sequence of events.

To better appreciate the sequence of inflammatory responses that occur within an implant site, Figure 36.1 illustrates the sequence of events that occur at the tissue/biomaterial interface, that is, foreign body reaction, and the events that occur adjacent to the interfacial foreign body reaction and within the surrounding tissue of the implant site.

Inflammation is generally defined as the reaction of vascularized living tissue to local injury, that is, implantation of a biomaterial, prosthesis, medical device, or tissue-engineered device. Immediately following injury, blood–material interactions occur and a provisional matrix is formed that consists

TABLE 36.2   Principal Cell Types in Inflammatory Responses

Response	Cell type
Acute inflammation	Polymorphonuclear leukocyte (neutrophil)
Chronic inflammation	Monocytes and lymphocytes
Granulation tissue	Fibroblasts and endothelial cells (capillaries)
Foreign body reaction	Macrophages and foreign body giant cells
Fibrous encapsulation	Fibroblasts

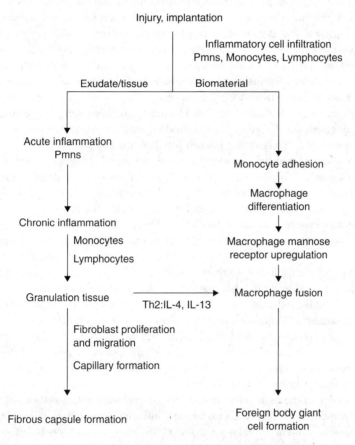

FIGURE 36.1   Inflammation, wound healing and foreign body responses at the implant site. The biomaterial pathway occurs at the surface of the biomaterial, whereas the exudate/tissue pathway occurs in the space surrounding the biomaterial. Both pathways can occur in a simultaneous manner and time frame.

of a platelet/fibrin thrombus/blood clot at the implant surface. As previously indicated, the predominant cell type (Table 36.2) present in the inflammatory response varies with the age of injury. In general, neutrophils (polymorphonuclear leukocytes) predominate during the first several days following injury and then are replaced by monocytes as the predominant cell type. Three factors occur for this change in cell type: neutrophils are short-lived and disintegrate and disappear after 24 to 48 h; neutrophil immigration is of short duration; and chemotactic factors for neutrophil migration are activated early in the inflammatory response. Following immigration from the vasculature, monocytes differentiate into macrophages and these cells are very long-lived (up to months). Monocyte immigration may continue for days to weeks dependent on the injury and implanted device and chemotactic factors for monocytes are activated over longer periods of time. The size, shape, and chemical and physical properties of the biomaterial or device may be responsible for variations in the intensity and duration of the inflammatory and wound-healing processes. Thus, intensity and time duration of the inflammatory reaction may characterize the biocompatibility of the biomaterial or device. Chemical mediators, released from plasma, cells, and injured tissue mediate these responses. These mediators include vasoactive amines, plasma proteases, arachidonic acid metabolites, lysosomal proteases, oxygen-derived free radicals, platelet activating factors, cytokines, and growth factors.

Acute inflammation is dependent on the extent of injury and may be of relatively short duration, lasting from minutes to days. As seen in Figure 36.1, its main characteristics are the formation of a fluid exudate and immigration of polymorphonuclear leukocytes across the endothelial lining of blood vessels and into tissue and the injury (implant) site. Adhesion molecules and receptors present on leukocyte and endothelial cells facilitate this process that is controlled, in part, by chemotaxis. A wide variety of exogenous and endogenous substances have been identified as chemotactic agents. Following localization of leukocytes at the injury (implant) site, phagocytosis and the release of enzymes occur following activation of neutrophils, monocytes, and macrophages. The major role of the polymorphonuclear leukocytes in acute inflammation is to phagocytose microorganisms and foreign materials. Phagocytosis is a three-step process in which the injurious agent undergoes leukocyte attachment, engulfment, and killing or degradation. In regard to biomaterials, phagocytosis and degradation may not occur, depending on the properties of the biomaterial. Biomaterials are not generally phagocytosed by neutrophils or macrophages because of the disparity in size, that is, the surface of the biomaterial is greater than the size of the cell. In general, particles, microcapsules, microspheres, or liposomes less than 10 μm in greatest dimension may undergo phagocytosis. The process of recognition and attachment is expedited when the biomaterial has adsorbed plasma-derived proteins such as immunoglobulin G (IgG) and the complement-activated fragment, C3b. Fibrinogen has also been identified as an adhesion molecule to facilitate leukocyte adhesion to biomaterial surfaces. IgG and C3b are the two major opsonins. These opsonins are naturally occurring serum factors that facilitate inflammatory cell adhesion. This may be significant with tissue-engineered devices in which the synthetic scaffold material or cell encapsulating synthetic membrane is in direct contact with tissue at the time of implantation. Thus, depending on the characteristics of the tissue-engineered device, protein adsorption and cellular adhesion in the inflammatory, wound healing and foreign body responses may be important factors in biocompatibility of the tissue-engineered device as well as its function.

The disparity in size between the biomaterial surface and the adherent cell generally leads to frustrated phagocytosis, which is the release of cellular enzymes, acid and reactive oxygen and nitrogen intermediates by either direct extrusion or exocytosis from the cell [7]. These agents may play significant roles in the biodegradation of biodegradable scaffold materials.

Following resolution of the acute inflammatory response, chronic inflammation with the presence of monocytes and lymphocytes is predominant. Chronic inflammation is characterized by the presence of monocytes, lymphocytes, and macrophages with the proliferation of blood vessels and connective tissue at the implant site. With biocompatible materials, the chronic inflammatory phase is of short duration and usually lasts several days and is seen within the first week to two weeks following implantation. Persistent inflammatory stimuli and motion of the implant may lead to focal chronic inflammation with extended time periods.

Whereas macrophages and lymphocytes play key roles in immune responses, their presence in the early inflammatory response is generally not considered to be an immune reaction. As will be seen later under Immune Responses, specific events in which the macrophages, lymphocytes, and plasma cells participate can lead to immune responses. Macrophages process and present antigens (foreign materials) to immunocompetent cells and thus are key mediators in the development of immune reactions.

In the inflammatory responses, the macrophage is probably the most important cell in chronic inflammation due to the large number of biologically active products that it produces and releases. Important classes of products produced and secreted by macrophages include neutral proteases, chemotactic factors, arachidonic acid metabolites, reactive oxygen metabolites, complement components, coagulation factors, growth-promoting factors, and cytokines. Chemotactic factors, cytokines and growth factors are important in the development of the next phase of the inflammatory and wound healing responses, which is the formation of granulation tissue. Granulation tissue is generally defined as the proliferation of new small blood vessels and the immigration of fibroblasts into the injury site. Depending on the extent of injury, granulation tissue may be seen as early as 3 to 5 days following implantation. As seen in Figure 36.1, at the same time that granulation tissue is being formed, biomaterial adherent macrophages, derived from monocytes, are fusing to form multinucleated foreign body giant cells on the surface of the biomaterial [8,9].

The form and topography of the surface of the biomaterial determines the composition of the foreign body reaction. With biocompatible materials, the composition of the foreign body reaction in the implant site may be controlled by the surface properties of the biomaterial, the form of the implant, and the relationship between the surface area of the biomaterial and the volume of the implant. Porous scaffold materials have high surface-to-volume ratios and can be expected to display large numbers of macrophages and foreign body giant cells. The foreign body reaction consisting mainly of macrophages and foreign body giant cells may persist at the tissue/implant interface for the lifetime of the implant.

Macrophages and foreign body giant cells are capable of releasing acid, enzymes, and reactive oxygen and nitrogen intermediates that can degrade and modify the surfaces to which they are adherent. The foreign body response with macrophages and foreign body giant cells has been identified as the principal cell types responsible for polyurethane biodegradation in clinical devices such as pacemaker leads. It can be anticipated that macrophages and foreign body giant cells at the surfaces of tissue-engineered devices can lead to destruction of the device and its components. For these reasons, mitigation and more preferably, total inhibition, of the foreign body response with macrophages and foreign body giant cells is desirable for tissue-engineered devices. Although the foreign body response may be inhibited through the use of pharmacologic agents, that is, dexamethasone, these agents are broad in their action and may adversely influence other types of cells and events in the normal wound healing response. Genetic engineering approaches to modulate macrophage and foreign body giant cell behavior are scientifically interesting but may provide tortuous and time-consuming regulatory constraints in their development for human application. Approaches targeting macrophage adhesion and activation may be helpful in developing viable tissue-engineered devices. Material surface chemistry may control monocyte adhesion that, of course, would significantly affect subsequent macrophage formation. Also, material surface chemistry may control adherent macrophage apoptosis, that is, programmed cell death, that renders potentially harmful macrophages nonfunctional, while the surrounding environment of the implant remains unaffected [10]. The level of adherent macrophage apoptosis appears to be inversely related to the surface's ability to promote fusion of macrophages into foreign body giant cells. This appears to be a mechanism by which adherent macrophages escape apoptosis.

The end-stage healing response to devices is generally fibrosis or fibrous encapsulation. This, of course, is the replacement of normal or injured tissue by scar or fibrous tissue formation. The replacement of normal or injured tissue by connective tissue that constitutes the fibrous capsule may be deleterious to the function of the tissue-engineered device [11,12]. Well-formed fibrous capsules are both acellular and avascular. The lack of vascularity within the fibrous capsule would certainly indicate that the fibrous encapsulated tissue-engineered device would not be vascularized and cells in the tissue-engineered device would eventually undergo ischemic cell death.

It is clear that the end-stage healing response with fibrous encapsulation of the tissue-engineered device and the presence of the foreign body reaction with macrophages and foreign body giant cells at the interface between the fibrous capsule and the tissue-engineered device would ultimately lead to failure of the tissue-engineered device. To achieve viable and functional tissue-engineered devices, at least until the target tissue or organ has been restored, control of the adverse aspects of the inflammatory and wound healing responses must be achieved. This continues as a challenge for the development of tissue-engineered devices for human application.

The inflammatory (innate) and immune (adaptive) responses have common components. It is possible to have inflammatory responses only with no adaptive immune response. In this situation, both humoral and cellular components that are shared by both types of responses may only participate in the inflammatory response. Table 36.3 indicates the common components to the inflammatory (innate) and immune

TABLE 36.3   Common Components in the Inflammatory
(Innate) and Immune (Adaptive) Responses

Humoral components
    Complement cascade components
    Immunoglobulins

Cellular components
    Macrophages
    NK (natural killer) cells
    Dendritic cells
    Cells with dual phagocytic and antigen presenting capabilities

TABLE 36.4   Cell Types and Function in the Adaptive Immune System

Cell type	Function
Macrophages (APC)	Process and present antigen to immunocompetent T cells phagocytosis Activated by cytokines, that is, IFN-γ, from other immune cells
T cells	Interact with antigen presenting cells (APCs) and are activated through two required cell membrane interactions Facilitate target cell apoptosis Participate in transplant rejection (Type IV hypersensitivity)
B cells	Form plasma cells that secrete immunoglobulins (IgG, IgA, and IgE) Participate in antigen–antibody complex mediated tissue damage (Type III hypersensitivity)
Dendritic cells (APC)	Process and present antigen to immunocompetent T cells Utilize Fc receptors for IgG to trap antigen–antibody complexes
NK (natural killer) cells (Non-T, Non-B lymphocytes)	Innate ability to lyse tumor, virus infected, and other cells without previous sensitization Mediates T and B cell function by secretion of IFN-γ

(adaptive) responses. Macrophages are known as professional antigen presenting cells responsible for the initiation of the adaptive immune response.

36.3   Immune Responses

The acquired or adaptive immune system acts to protect the host from foreign agents or materials and is usually initiated through specific recognition mechanisms and the ability of humoral and cellular components to recognize the foreign agent or material as being "nonself" [11–15]. Generally, the adaptive immune system may be considered as having two components: humoral or cellular. Humoral components include antibodies, complement components, cytokines, chemokines, growth factors, and other soluble mediators. These humoral components are synthesized by cells of the immune response and, in turn, function to regulate the activity of these same cells and provide for communication between different cells in the cellular component of the adaptive immune response. Cells of the immune system arise from stem cells in the bone marrow (B lymphocytes) or the thymus (T lymphocytes) and differ from each other in morphology, function and the expression of cell surface antigens (Table 36.4). They share the common features of maintaining cell surface receptors that assist in the recognition and elimination of foreign materials. Regarding tissue-engineered devices, the adaptive immune response may recognize the biological components, modifications of the biological components, or degradation products of the biological components, commonly known as antigens, and initiate immune response through humoral or cellular mechanisms.

TABLE 36.5   Effector T Lymphocytes in Adaptive Immunity

TH1 helper cells	CD4+
	Proinflammatory
	Activation of macrophages
	Produces IL-2, interferon-γ (IFN-γ), IL-3, tumor necrosis factor-α, GM-CSF, macrophage
	chemotactic factor (MCF), migration inhibitor factor (MIF) induce IgG2a
TH2 helper cells	CD4+
	Anti-inflammatory
	Activation of B cells to make antibodies
	Produces IL-4, IL-5, IL-6, IL-10, IL-3, GM-CSF, and IL-13
	Induce IgG1
Cytotoxic T cells (CTL)	CD8+
	Induce apoptosis of target cells
	Produce IFN-γ, TNF-β, and TNF-α
	Release cytotoxic proteins

Components of the humoral immune system play important roles in the inflammatory responses to foreign materials. Antibodies and complement components C3b and C3bi adhere to foreign materials, act as opsonins and facilitate phagocytosis of the foreign materials by neutrophils and macrophages that have cell surface receptors for C3b. Complement component C5a is a chemotactic agent for neutrophils, monocytes, and other inflammatory cells and facilitates the immigration of these cells to the implant site. The complement system is composed of classic and alternative pathways that eventuate in a common pathway to produce the membrane attack complex (MAC), which is capable of lysing microbial agents. The complement system, that is, complement cascade, is closely controlled by protein inhibitors in the host cell membrane that may prevent damage to host cells. This inhibitory mechanism may not function when nonhost cells are used in tissue-engineered devices.

The T (thymus-derived) lymphocytes are significant cells in the cell-mediated adaptive immune response and their cell-adhesion molecules play a significant role in lymphocyte migration, activation and effector function. The specific interaction of cell membrane adhesion molecules, sometimes also called ligands or antigens, with antigen-presenting cells produce specific types of lymphocytes with specific functions. Table 36.4 indicates cell types and function in the adaptive immune response. Obviously, the functions of these cells are more numerous than indicated in Table 36.4 but the major function of these cells is provided to indicate similarities and differences in the interaction and responsiveness of these cells. Effector T cells (Table 36.5) are produced when their antigen-specific receptors and either the CD4 or the CD8 co-receptors bind to peptide-MHC (major histocompatibility complex) complexes. A second, co-stimulatory signal is also required and this is provided by the interaction of the CD28 receptor on the T cell and the B7.1 and B7.2 glycoproteins of the immunoglobulin superfamily present on antigen-presenting cells. B lymphocytes bind soluble antigens through their cell-surface immunoglobulin and thus can function as professional antigen-presenting cells by internalizing the soluble antigens and presenting peptide fragments of these antigens as MHC:peptide complexes. Once activated, T cells can synthesize the T cell growth factor interleukin-2 and its receptor. Thus, activated T cells secrete and respond to interleukin-2 to promote T cell growth in an autocrine fashion.

Cytokines are the messenger molecules of the immune system. Most cytokines have a wide spectrum of effects, reacting with many different cell types, and some are produced by several different cell types. Table 36.6 presents common categories of cytokines and lists some of their general properties. It should be noted that while cytokines can be subdivided into functional groups, many cytokines such as IL-1, TNF-α, and IFN-γ are pleotropic in their effects and regulate, mediate, and activate numerous responses by numerous cells.

Cytokines produce their effects in three ways. The first type of effect is the autocrine effect in which the cytokine acts on the same cell that produced it. An example is when IL-2 produced by activated T cells promotes T-cell growth. The second way is when a cytokine affects other cells in its vicinity. This

TABLE 36.6   Cytokines and Their Effects

Cytokine	Effect
IL-1, TNF-α, INF-γ, IL-6	Mediate natural immunity
IL-1, TNF-α, IL-6	Initiate nonspecific inflammatory responses
IL-2, IL-4, IL-5, IL-12, IL-15, and TGF-β	Regulate lymphocyte growth, activation, and differentiation
IL-2 and IL-4	Promote lymphocyte growth and differentiation
IL-10 and TGF-β	Down-regulate immune responses
IL-1, INF-γ, TNF-α, and MIF	Activate inflammatory cells
IL-8	Produced by activated macrophages and endothelial cells
	Chemoattractant for neutrophils
MCP-1, MIP-α, and RANTES	Chemoattractant for monocytes and lymphocytes
GM-CSF and G-CSF	Stimulate hematopoiesis
IL-4 and IL-13	Promote macrophage fusion and foreign body giant cell formation

TABLE 36.7   Mechanisms of Immune Mediated Responses

Type	Immune mechanism
TYPE I Anaphylactic	IgE antibodies, produced by B cells, affect the immediate release of basophilic amines and other mediators from basophils and mast cells followed by the recruitment of other inflammatory cells
TYPE II Cytotoxic	Formation and binding of IgG and IgM to antigens on target cell surfaces that facilitate phagocytosis of the target cell or lysis of the target cell by activated complement components
TYPE III Immune complex	Circulating antigen–antibody complexes activate complement whose components are chemotactic for neutrophils that release enzymes and other toxic mediators leading to cellular and tissue injury
TYPE IV Cell-mediated (delayed)	Sensitized T lymphocytes release cytokines and other mediators that lead to cellular and tissue injury

is the paracrine effect and an example is when IL-7 produced by bone marrow stromal cells promotes the differentiation of B-cell progenitors in the bone marrow. The third way is when the cytokine affects many cells systemically. This is the endocrine effect and an example is when circulating IL-1 and TNF-α produce the acute-phase response during inflammation.

This brief and very limited overview of the humoral and cellular mediated immune responses due to space limitations, now provides a basis for understanding mechanisms of immunologic tissue injury, which is also called hypersensitivity reactions. Hypersensitivity reactions can be initiated either by the interaction of antigen with humoral antibody or by cell-mediated immune mechanisms. Table 36.7 lists the four types of hypersensitivity reactions together with a very brief description of their immune mechanism. Type I hypersensitivity (anaphylactic) is generally defined as a rapidly developing immunologic reaction occurring within minutes after the combination of an antigen with antibody bound to mast cells or basophils in individuals previously sensitized to the antigen. Type II hypersensitivity (cytotoxic) is mediated by antibodies directed toward antigens present on the surface of cells or other tissue components. Three different antibody-dependent mechanisms may be involved in this type of reaction: complement-dependent reactions, antibody-dependent cell-mediated cytotoxicity, or antibody-mediated cellular dysfunction. Type III hypersensitivity (immune complex mediated) reaction is induced by antigen-antibody complexes that produce tissue damage as a result of their capacity to activate the complement system. Type IV hypersensitivity (cell-mediated) reactions are initiated by specifically sensitized T lymphocytes. This reaction includes the classic delayed-type hypersensitivity reaction initiated by CD^4+ T cells and direct cell cytotoxicity mediated by CD^8+ T cells. Immunologic reactions that occur with organ transplant rejection also offer insight into potential immune responses to tissue-engineered devices. Mechanisms involved in organ transplant rejection include T cell-mediated reactions by direct and indirect pathways and antibody-mediated reactions. Immune responses may be avoided or diminished by using autologous or isogeneic cells in cell/polymer scaffold constructs. The use of allogeneic or xenogenic cells incorporated into the device require prevention of immune rejection by immune suppression of the host, induction of tolerance in the host, or immunomodulation of the tissue-engineered construct. The development of tissue-engineered constructs by immunoisolation using polymer membranes and the use of nonhost cells have been compromised by immune responses. In this concept, a polymer membrane is used to encapsulate nonhost cells or tissues thus separating them from the host immune system. However, antigens shed by encapsulated cells were released from the device and initiated immune responses [12,16,17].

Although exceptionally minimal and superficial in its presentation, the previously discussed humoral and cell-mediated immune responses demonstrate the possibility that any known tissue-engineered construct may undergo immunologic tissue injury. To date, our understanding of immune mechanisms and their interactions with tissue-engineered constructs is markedly limited. One of the obvious problems is that preliminary studies are generally carried out with nonhuman tissues and immune reactions result when tissue-engineered constructs from one species are used in testing the device in another species. Ideally, tissue-engineered constructs would be prepared from cells and tissues of a given species and subsequently tested in that species. Whereas this approach does not guarantee that immune responses will not be present, the probability of immune responses in this type of situation is markedly decreased.

The following examples provide perspective to these issues. They further demonstrate the detailed and in-depth approach that must be taken to appropriately and adequately evaluate tissue-engineered constructs or devices and their potential adverse responses.

Babensee et al. [18,19] have tested the hypothesis that the biomaterial component of a medical device, by promoting an inflammatory response can recruit antigen-presenting cells (APCs, e.g., macrophages and dendritic cells) and induce their activation, thus acting as an adjuvant in the immune response to foreign antigens originating from the histological component of the device. Utilizing polystyrene and polylactic-glycolic acid microparticles and polylatic-glycolic scaffolds together with their model antigen, ovalbumin, in a mouse model for 18 weeks, Babensee et al. demonstrated that a persistent humoral immune response that was Th2 helper T cell dependent, as determined by the IgG1, was present. These findings indicated that activation of CD^4+ T cells and the proliferation and isotype switching of B-cells had occurred. A Th1 immune response, characterized by the presence of IgG2a was not identified. Moreover, the humoral immune responses for all three types of microparticles were similar indicating that the production of antigen-specific antibodies was not material chemistry-dependent in this model. Babensee suggests that the presence of the biomaterial functions as an adjuvant for initiation and promotion of the immune response and augments the phagocytosis of the antigen with expression of MHC class II and co-stimulatory molecules on APCs with the presentation of antigen to CD^4+ T cells.

Cleland et al. [20] have shown the significance of the use of appropriate animal models in characterizing protein/biodegradable polymer constructs. Utilizing biodegradable PLGA microspheres containing recombinant human growth hormone (rhGH), they used Rhesus monkeys, transgenic mice expressing hGH and normal control (Balb/C) mice in their *in vivo* studies. The Rhesus monkeys were used for serum assays in determining growth hormone release as well as tissue responses to the injected microcapsule formulations. Placebo injection sites were also used and a comparison of the injection sites from rhGH PLGA microspheres and placebo PLGA microspheres demonstrated a normal inflammatory and wound healing response with a normal focal foreign body reaction. To further examine the tissue response and potential for immune reactions, transgenic mice were used to assess the immunogenicity of the rhGH PLGA formulation. Transgenic mice expressing a heterologous protein have been previously used for assessing the immunogenicity of sequence or structural mutant proteins [21]. With the transgenic animals, no detectable antibody response to the rhGH was found. In contrast, the Balb/C control mice had a rapid onset of high titer antibody response to the rhGH PLGA formulation.

Immunotoxicity is any adverse effect on the function or structure of the immune system or other systems as a result of an immune system dysfunction. Adverse or immunotoxic effects occur when humoral or cellular immunity needed by the host to defend itself against infections or neoplastic diseases (immunosuppression) or unnecessary tissue damage (chronic inflammation, hypersensitivity or autoimmunity) is compromised. *In vivo* responses indicating immunotoxicity include histopathological changes, humoral responses, host resistance, clinical symptoms, and cellular responses (T cells, natural killer cells, macrophages, and granulocytes). The inflammatory response considered to be immunotoxic is persistent chronic inflammation. It is this persistent chronic inflammation that is of concern as immune granuloma formation and other serious immunological reactions such as autoimmune disease may occur. In biological response evaluation, it is important to discriminate between the short-lived chronic inflammation that is a component of the normal inflammatory and healing responses vs. long-term, persistent chronic inflammation that may indicate an adverse immunological response.

Immunosuppression may occur when antibody and T cell responses (adaptive immune response) are inhibited. A potentially significant consequence of this type of response is more frequent in serious infections resulting from reduced host defense. Immunostimulation may occur when unintended or inappropriate antigen-specific or nonspecific activation of the immune system is present. From a tissue-engineering perspective, antibody and cellular immune responses to a foreign protein may lead to unintended immunogenicity. Enhancement of the immune response to an antigen by a biomaterial with which it is mixed *ex vivo* or *in situ* may lead to adjuvancy that is a form of immunostimulation. This effect must be considered when biodegradable controlled release systems are designed and developed for use as vaccines. Autoimmunity is the immune response to the body's own constituents that are considered in this response to be autoantigens. An autoimmune response, indicated by the presence of autoantibodies or T lymphocytes that are reactive with host tissue or cellular antigens may, but not necessarily, result in autoimmune disease with chronic, debilitating and sometimes life-threatening tissue and organ injury.

Direct measures of immune system activity by functional assays are the most important types of tests for immunotoxicity [22–25]. Functional assays are generally more important than tests for soluble mediators, which are more important than phenotyping. Functional assays include skin testing, immunoassays (e.g., ELISA), lymphocyte proliferation, plaque-forming cells, local lymph node assay, mixed lymphocyte reaction, tumor cytotoxicity, antigen presentation, and phagocytosis. As with any type of test for biological response evaluation, immunotoxicity tests should be valid and have been shown to provide accurate, reproducible results that are indicative of the effect being studied and are useful in a statistical analysis. This implies that appropriate control groups are also included in the study design.

References

[1] Anderson, J.M., Biological responses to materials, *Ann. Rev. Mater. Res.*, 31, 81, 2001.
[2] Anderson, J.M., Mechanisms of inflammation and infection with implanted devices, *Cardiovasc. Pathol.*, 2, 33S, 1993.
[3] Cotran, R.Z., Kumar, V., and Robbins, S.L., Eds., Inflammation and repair in *Pathologic Basis of Disease*, 6th ed., W.B. Saunders, Philadelphia, 1999, p. 50.
[4] Gallin, J.L. and Snyderman, R., Eds., *Inflammation: Basic Principles and Clinical Correlates*, 3rd ed., Raven Press, New York, 1999.
[5] Babensee, J.E. et al., Host responses to tissue engineered devices, *Adv. Drug Del. Rev.*, 33, 111, 1998.
[6] Anderson, J.M., Multinucleated giant cells, *Curr. Opin. Hematol.*, 7, 40, 2000.
[7] Henson, P.M., The immunologic release of constituents from neutrophil leukocytes: II. Mechanisms of release during phagocytosis, and adherence to nonphagocytosable surfaces, *J. Immunol.*, 107, 1547, 1971.
[8] McNally, A.K. and Anderson, J.M., Beta1 and beta2 integrins mediate adhesion during macrophage fusion and multinucleated foreign body giant cell formation, *Am. J. Pathol.*, 160, 621, 2002.
[9] McNally, A. and Anderson, J.M., Interleukin-4 induces foreign body giant cells from human monocytes/macrophages. Differential lymphokine regulation of macrophage fusion leads to morphological variants of multinucleated giant cells, *Am. J. Pathol.*, 147, 1487, 1995.
[10] Brodbeck, W.G. et al., Influence of biomaterials surface chemistry on apoptosis of adherent cells, *J. Biomed. Mater. Res.*, 55, 661, 2001.

[11] Janeway, C.A. et al., *Immunobiology 5: The Immune System in Health and Disease*, Garland Publishing Inc., New York, 2001, p. 1.

[12] Babensee, J.E. et al., Host response to tissue engineered devices, in *Advanced Drug Delivery Reviews*, Vol. 33, Elsevier, Amsterdam, 1998, p. 111.

[13] Lefell, M.S., Donnenberg, A.D., and Rose, N.R., Eds., *Immunologic Diagnosis of Autoimmune Disease*, CRC Press, Boca Raton, FL, 1997, p. 111.

[14] Cohen, I.R. and Miller, A., Eds., *Autoimmune Disease Models, A Guidebook*, Academic Press, New York, 1994.

[15] Anderson, J.M. and Langone, J.J., Issues and perspectives on the biocompatibility and immunotoxicity evaluation of implanted controlled release systems, *J. Control. Release*, 57, 107, 1999.

[16] Brauker, J.H. et al., Neovascularization of synthetic membranes directed by membrane microarchitecture, *J. Biomed. Mater. Res.*, 29, 1517, 1995.

[17] Brauker, J. et al., Neovascularization of immuno-isolation membranes: the effect of membrane architecture and encapsulated tissue, *Cell Transplant.*, 1, 163, 1992.

[18] Matzelle, M.M. and Babensee, J.E., Humoral immune responses to model antigen co-delivered with biomaterials used in tissue engineering, *Biomaterials*, 25, 295, 2004.

[19] Babensee, J.E., Stein, M.M., and Moore, L.K., Interconnections between inflammatory and immune responses in tissue engineering, *Ann. NY Acad. Sci.*, 961, 360, 2002.

[20] Cleland, J.L. et al., Recombinant human growth hormone poly(lactic-co-glycolic acid) (PLGA) microspheres provide a long lasting effect, *J. Control. Release*, 49, 193, 1997.

[21] Stewart, T.A. et al., Transgenic mice as a model to test the immunogenicity of proteins altered by site-specific mutagenesis, *Mol. Biol. Med.*, 6, 275, 1989.

[22] Rose, N.R., de Mecario, E.C., Folds, J.D., Lane, H.C., and Nakamura, R.M., Eds., *Manual of Clinical Laboratory Immunology*, ASM Press, Washington, DC, 1997.

[23] Smialowicz, R.J. and Holsapple, M.P., Eds., *Experimental Immunotoxicology*, CRC Press, Boca Raton, FL, 1996.

[24] Burleson, G.R., Dean, J.H., and Munson, A.E., Eds., *Methods in Immunotoxicology*, Wiley-Liss, New York, 1995.

[25] Coligan, J.E., Kruisbeek, A.M., Margulies, D.H., Shevach, E.M., and Strober, R., Eds., *Current Protocols in Immunology*, Greene Publishing Associates and Wiley Interscience, New York, 1992.

37

Polymeric Scaffolds for Tissue Engineering Applications

Diana M. Yoon
John P. Fisher
University of Maryland

37.1 Introduction

The incorporation of polymeric scaffolds in tissue regeneration occurred in the early 1980s, and it continues to play a vital role in tissue engineering [1–3]. The function of a degradable scaffold is to act as a temporary support matrix for transplanted or host cells so as to restore, maintain, or improve tissue. Scaffolds may be created from various types of materials, including polymers. There are two main classes of polymers, based upon their source: natural or synthetic. Polymeric scaffolds may be used to support a variety of cells for numerous tissues within the body. The design of a polymeric scaffold plays a significant role in proper cell growth. Therefore, several important properties must be considered: fabrication, structure, biocompatibility, biodegradability, and mechanical strength. This review will discuss natural and synthetic polymers, as well as the properties that scaffolds exhibit.

37.2 Natural Polymers for Scaffold Fabrication

There are two major classes of natural polymers used as scaffolds: polypeptides and polysaccharides (Table 37.1, Figure 37.1). Natural polymers are typically biocompatible and enzymatically biodegradable. The main advantage for using natural polymers is that they contain bio-functional molecules that aid the attachment, proliferation, and differentiation of cells. However, disadvantages of natural polymers do exist. Depending upon the application, the previously mentioned enzymatic degradation may inhibit

TABLE 37.1 Properties of Degradable Natural Homopolymers that have been Utilized in the Fabrication of Tissue Engineering Scaffolds

	Natural polymer	Curing method	Primary degradation method	Primary degradation products	References
A	Agarose	Entanglement	Enzymatic agarases	Oligosaccharides	[4,8]
B	Alginate	Cross-linking	Alginate lyases	Mannuronic acid and guluronic acid	[4,10–13]
C	Hyaluronic acid	Entanglement	Enzymatic hyaluronidase	$\beta(1-4)$ linked glucuronic acid and glucosamine	[4,8,21,22]
D	Chitosan	Cross-linking	Enzymatic chitosanase	Glucosamines	[4,8,22,25,26]
E	Collagen	Cross-linking	Enzymatic collagenase or lysozyme	Various peptides depending on sequence	[8,31–33]
F	Gelatin	Entanglement	Enzymatic collagenases	Various peptides depending on sequence	[4,8,13,22]
G	Silk	Entanglement	Proteolytic proteases	Various peptides depending on sequence	[43]

function. Further, the rate of this degradation may not be easily controlled. Since the enzymatic activity varies between hosts, so will the degradation rate. Therefore it may be difficult to determine the lifespan of natural polymers *in vivo*. Additionally, natural polymers are often weak in terms of mechanical strength but cross-linking these polymers have shown to enhance their structural stability.

37.2.1 Polysaccharides

37.2.1.1 Agarose

Agarose is a polysaccharide polymer extracted from algae (Table 37.1, Figure 37.1). Its molecular structure contains an alternating copolymer linkage of 1,4-linked 3,6 anhydro-α-L-galactose and 1,3-linked β-D-galactose [4]. Agarose is water-soluble due to the presence of hydroxyl groups. Two agarose chains interact with each other through hydrogen bonding to form a double helix. At low temperatures the agarose chains form a thermally reversible gel. Thus, at high temperatures agarose gels may be made water-soluble. Many of the properties of agarose gels, particularly strength and permeability, can be adjusted by altering the concentration of agarose [4]. For example, low concentrations of agarose lead to a highly porous entangled structure with limited mechanical strength. Agarose in its native state is enzymatically degradable by agarases.

For tissue culture systems, agarose hydrogels are widely investigated because they permit growth of cells and tissues in a three-dimensional suspension [5]. Agarose gels have been found to maintain chondrocytes, the predominant cell type in cartilage, in culture for 2 to 6 weeks [6]. Furthermore, agarose hydrogels embedded with chondrocytes allow the expression of type II collagen and proteoglycans [5,7]. These results show promise for using agarose gels in cartilage repair. Additionally, agarose gels have been investigated as a matrix for nerve regeneration [8,9]. Dorsal root ganglia (DRG), a neural cell, has been encapsulated in agarose hydrogels. The influence of increasing porosity and incorporating charged biopolymers (e.g., chitosan) produced an increase in neurite extension of DRG isolated from chicks [9].

37.2.1.2 Alginate

Alginate is a naturally derived water-soluble polysaccharide obtained from algae (Table 37.1, Figure 37.1) [4]. It is a polyanion composed of two repeating monomer units: β-D-mannuronate and α-L-guluronate [10,11]. Alginate is readily degraded at the $\beta(1-4)$ linkage site, located in between the monomer units, by alginate lyases [10]. The physical and mechanical properties of alginate are dependent on the length and proportion of the guluronate block within the chain. Due to alginate's polyelectrolytic nature, it readily forms into an ionotropic cross-linked hydrogel when exposed to divalent ions, the most common being calcium ions [12,13]. Furthermore, alginate gels may be solubilized when these cations are removed

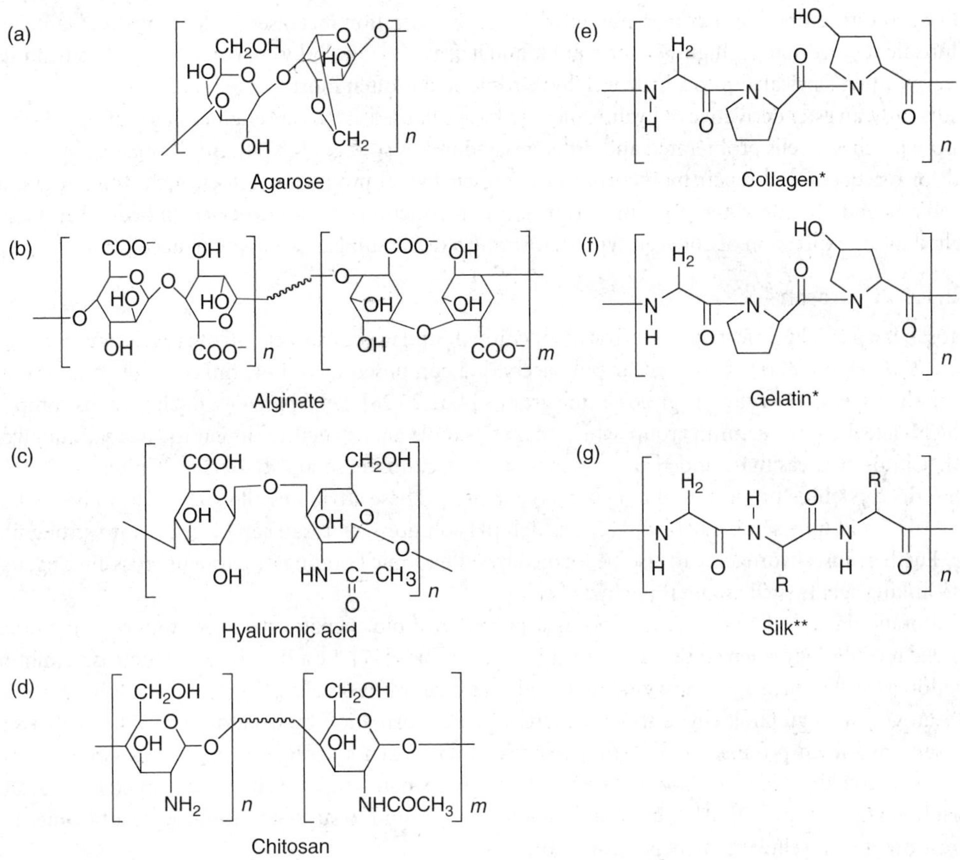

FIGURE 37.1 Repeating structural unit of degradable natural homopolymers under investigation as scaffold materials for tissue engineering applications. (*Collagen and gelatin have variable sequences, but are predominately glycine, proline, and hydroxyproline. **Silks have a glycine rich sequence, with glycine repeating every second or third amino acid residue. The variable residues are primarily alanine or serine.)

or sequestered. This ease in gel reversibility allows alginate to be especially useful for studies requiring the retrieval of encapsulated cells. Alginate does not contain cellular recognition proteins, limiting cell attachment to the natural polymer. By cross-linking alginate with poly(ethylene glycol)-diamine the mechanical properties of alginate can be controlled and even improved [4].

A variety of different cells have been found to maintain their morphology in alginate scaffolds [10,14–17]. The adhesion of fibroblasts in alginate sponges was found not to be affected by the porosity of the scaffold [14]. Chondrocytes embedded in alginate proliferated and expressed type II collagen [18]. Hepatocytes, the functional cell in liver, were also found to grow in alginate scaffolds. When hepatocytes were seeded in three-dimensional porous alginate, albumin was secreted, indicating proper cell function [19]. Other types of cells studied in alginate include cardiomyocytes, rat marrow cells, and Schwann cells [10,17,20].

37.2.1.3 Hyaluronic Acid

Hyaluronic acid (hyaluronan, HA) is a naturally occurring polysaccharide with a $\beta(1-3)$ linkage of two sugar units: D-glucuronate and N-acetyl-D-glucosamine (Table 37.1, Figure 37.1). Hyaluronic acid is an abundant glycosaminoglycan within the extracellular matrix of tissues that promotes early inflammation critical for wound healing [21]. Furthermore, hyaluronic acid is nonimmunogenic and nonadhesive, making it an attractive option for biomedical applications. In dilute concentrations hyaluronic acid has a random coil structure that becomes entangled as its concentration increases [22]. Some disadvantages of hyaluronic acid are that it is highly water-soluble and it degrades rapidly by enzymes, such as hyaluronidase. However, when fabricated into a hydrogel, hyaluronic acid is often more stable [4,8,21].

Currently, an ester derivative of hyaluronic acid has been used as a tissue engineering scaffold [8,23,24]. Adipose precursor cells proliferated and differentiated in HA sponges [23,24]. Additionally, HA has been used for osteochondral repair by incorporating mesenchymal progenitor cells, which differentiate into osteoblasts and chondrocytes [8]. Furthermore, the interaction of chondrocytes embedded in HA has resulted in the expression of collagen type II, forming a tissue similar to native cartilage [23].

37.2.1.4 Chitosan

Chitosan is a partially deacetylated derivative of chitin, found in the exoskeleton of crustaceans and insects (Table 37.1, Figure 37.1). It is a linear polysaccharide composed of $\beta(1-4)$ linked D-glucosamine with randomly dispersed N-acteyl-D-glycosamine groups [4,22,25,26]. Less than 40% of chitosan is composed of the N-acteyl-D-glycosamino group, which makes its molecular structure similar to glycosaminoglycans [4,8]. Chitosan is easily degraded by enzymes such as chitosanase and lysozyme. Chitosan is catonic with semi-crystalline properties of a high charge density. These attributes allow chitosan to be insoluble above pH 7 and fully soluble below pH 5. At high pH solutions, chitosan can be gelled into strong fibers [26]. Furthermore, hydrogels can also be formed by either ionic bonding or covalent cross-linking, using cross-linking agents such as glutaraldehyde [4].

Chitosan is a well-defined matrix and as a porous scaffold, hepatocytes were found to maintain a rounded morphology when cultured within chitosan scaffolds [27]. Results showed an increase in albumin secretion as well as urea synthesis, vital metabolic activities of liver cells [27]. Additionally, cross-linking chitosan gels with glutaraldehyde showed increased urea formation by hepatocytes [28]. Furthermore, chitosan has shown promise as an orthopaedic scaffold. When a sponge form of chitosan was seeded with rat osteoblasts, alkaline phosphatase production was detected, as well as bone spicules, indicating initial bone formation [29]. Also, chitosan scaffolds were found to support chondrocyte attachment and expression of extracellular matrix proteins [30].

37.2.2 Polypeptides

37.2.2.1 Collagen

Collagen is a major component of structural mammalian tissues (Table 37.1, Figure 37.1). Currently, 19 different types of collagen have been found, with the most abundant being type I collagen [31]. Collagen is composed of three polypeptide chains that intertwine with one another to form a triple helix. The polypeptide chains have a repeating sequence of glycine-X–Y, where X and Y are most often found to be proline and hydroxyproline. The chains are held together through hydrogen bonding of the peptide bond in glycine and an adjacent peptide carbonyl group [32]. The presence of adhesion domains allows collagen to display an attractive surface for cell attachment [31]. Some drawbacks in collagen are its high variability due to the numerous forms. Collagen is enzymatically biodegradable, and has a tendency to degrade quickly, limiting its mechanical properties. Cross-linking collagen with glutaraldehyde decreases its degradation rate [33].

Collagen naturally promotes healing wounds by promoting blood coagulation [31]. These attributes allow collagen to be used as a scaffold for cells within the epithelium, such as fibroblasts and keratinocytes [34–36]. Type II collagen is suitable for attaching chondrocytes and aiding in their proliferation and differentiation [37]. Additionally, rat hepatocytes attached onto collagen–chitosan scaffolds secreted albumin, which confirms cell function [38]. Furthermore, corneal keratocytes cultured on collagen sponges synthesized proteoglycans, indicating corneal extracellular matrix formation [39].

37.2.2.2 Gelatin

Gelatin is a collagen derivative acquired by denaturing the triple-helix structure of collagen into single-strand molecules (Table 37.1, Figure 37.1). It is water-soluble, and entangles easily to form into a gel through changes in temperature [4,13]. Gelatin is broken down enzymatically by various collagenases. The primary form of a gelatin scaffold is a hydrogel. Stabilization of gelatin hydrogels occurs through chemical cross-linking with agents such as glutaraldehyde [22].

Gelatin has been used to support cells for orthopaedic applications. Rat marrow stromal osteoblasts encapsulated in gelatin microparticles retained their phenotype [40]. Also, porous gelatin scaffolds supported human adipose derived stem cell attachment and differentiation into a variety of cell lineages. These constructs expressed a chondrogenic phenotype, indicated by the expression of hydroxyproline and glycosaminoglycans, both of which are present in the extracellular matrix of cartilage [41]. Furthermore, nonorthopaedic cell types, such as respiratory epithelial cells and cardiocyocytes, have been shown to attach and form rounded morphologies in gelatin scaffolds [17,42].

37.2.2.3 Silk

Silks are fibers that have a protein polymer basis (Table 37.1, Figure 37.1) [43]. There are two main sources of silks: spiders and silkworms. The primary structure of silks is a repetitive sequence of proteins that are glycine-rich. The secondary structure of silks is a β-sheet, which allows silks to exhibit enormous mechanical strength and is the primary reason for its strong interest as a scaffold. Most types of silks undergo slow proteolytic degradation by proteases, such as chymotrypsin [43]. A drawback for using silks is the potential formation of a granuloma as well as an allergic response. There has been a positive attachment and growth response of fibroblasts on fibroin silks. And recently, osteoblasts seeded on silks have displayed bone growth characteristics [44,45].

37.3 Synthetic Polymers for Scaffold Fabrication

Polymers that are chemically synthesized offer several notable advantages over natural-origin polymers. A major advantage of synthetic polymers is that they can be tailored to suit specific functions and thus exhibit controllable properties. Furthermore, since many synthetic polymers undergo hydrolytic degradation, a scaffold's degradation rate should not vary significantly between hosts. The most common synthetic polymers are polyesters. Other types include polyanhydrides, polycarbonates, and polyphosphazenes (Table 37.2, Figure 37.2). A significant disadvantage for using synthetic polymers is that some degrade into unfavorable products, often acids. At high concentrations of these degradation products, local acidity may increase, resulting in adverse responses such as inflammation or fibrous encapsulation [8,46,47].

37.3.1 Polyesters

37.3.1.1 Poly(glycolic) Acid

Poly(glycolic) acid (PGA) is a linear aliphatic polyester in the family of poly(α-hydroxy esters) (Table 37.2, Figure 37.2). It is formed by ring-opening polymerization of cyclic diesters of glycolide [46]. Due to the crystallinity of glycolide, PGA is a highly crystalline polymer that has a high melting point (185 to 225°C) and low solubility in organic solvents [47,48]. Further, PGA is hydrophilic and undergoes bulk degradation, often leading to a sudden loss in mechanical strength. PGA degrades hydrolytically into glycolic acid, which is metabolized in the body. An unfortunate attribute of glycolic acid is that at high concentrations it lowers the pH of the surrounding tissue, causing inflammation and possible tissue damage [46].

Poly(glycolic) acid polymers have been investigated as a scaffold to support various types of cell growth. Bovine chondrocytes seeded on PGA scaffolds *in vitro* expressed sulfated glycosaminoglycans 25% more than native cartilage [49]. *In vivo* results using a mouse model were comparable to these *in vitro* results. Other studies seeded myofibroblasts and endothelial cells on a PGA fiber matrix. These cells persisted and expressed elastic filaments and collagen, demonstrating the potential use of PGA scaffolds for heart valve engineering [50]. Hepatocytes have also attached to PGA and initiated albumin synthesis [51]. Some

TABLE 37.2 Properties of Degradable Synthetic Homopolymers that have been Utilized in the Fabrication of Tissue Engineering Scaffolds

	Synthetic polymer	Curing method	Primary degradation method	Primary degradation products	References
A	Poly(glycolic acid)	Entanglement	Ester hydrolysis	Glycolic acid	[8,46–48]
B	Poly(L-lactic acid)	Entanglement	Ester hydrolysis	Lactic acid	[8,46–48,53]
C	Poly(D,L-lactic acid-co-glycolic acid)	Entanglement	Ester hydrolysis	Lactic acid and glycolic acid	[8,48,57]
D	Poly(caprolactone)	Entanglement	Ester hydrolysis	Caproic acid	[8,22,48,62–64]
E	Poly(propylene fumarate)	Cross-linking	Ester hydrolysis	Fumaric acid and propylene glycol	[8,67–70]
F	Polyorthoester	Entanglement	Ester hydrolysis	Various acids depending upon R group	[8,22,57,71,72]
G	Polyanhydride	Entanglement	Anhydride hydrolysis	Various acids depending upon R group	[8,75,76]
H	Polyphosphazene	Entanglement	Hydrolysis	Phosphate and ammonia	[8,79]
I	Polycarbonate (tyrosine derived)	Entanglement	Ester and carbonate hydrolysis	Alkyl alcohol and desaminoyrosyl-tyrosine	[53,83,84]
J	Poly(ethylene glycol)/ Polyethylene oxide	Entanglement	Nondegradable	Not applicable	[4,8,32,86–91]
K	Polyurethane	Cross-linking	Ester, urethane, or urea hydrolysis	Diisocyanate and diols	[47,94–96]

investigations have coated PGA with other poly(α-hydroxy esters). Results with these scaffolds have shown that smooth muscle and endothelial cell growth may be supported [52].

37.3.1.2 Poly(L-lactic) Acid

Poly(L-lactic) acid (PLLA) is one of two isomeric forms of poly(lactic acid): D(−) and D,L(−) (Table 37.2, Figure 37.2). Similar to PGA, PLLA is classified as a linear poly(α-hydroxy acid) that is formed by ring-opening polymerization of L-lactide [53]. PLLA is structurally similar to PGA, with the addition of a pendant methyl group. This group increases the hydrophobicity and lowers the melting temperature to 170 to 180°C for PLLA [48]. Additionally, the methyl group hinders the ester bond cleavage of PLLA, and thus decreasing the degradation rate [46]. PLLA typically undergoes bulk, hydrolytic ester-linkage degradation, decomposing into lactic acid. The body is thought to excrete lactic acid in the form of water and carbon dioxide via the respiratory system [47,53]. The hydrophobic nature of PLLA allows for protein absorption and cell adhesion making them suitable as scaffolds.

In recent investigations, results have shown that the hydrophobic surface of PLLA has resulted in decreased adhesion of cells compared to other types of polymers, such as PGA [54]. However, PLLA has been found to support various cell types. Nerve stem cells seeded in PLLA fibers differentiated and expressed positive cues for neurite growth for potential regeneration of neurons [55]. Furthermore, human bladder smooth muscle cells seeded onto PLLA scaffolds also exhibited normal metabolic function and cell growth [16]. There has been similar work done with chondrocytes. The tissue engineered cartilage showed collagen, glycosaminoglycan, and elastin expression, vital for extracellular matrix formation [56].

37.3.1.3 Poly(D,L-lactic acid-co-glycolic acid)

Poly(glycolic acid) and poly(lactic acid) can be copolymerized to form poly(D,L-lactic acid-co-glycolic acid) (PLGA) (Table 37.2, Figure 37.2). This copolymer is amorphous, which decreases the degradation rate and mechanical strength of PLGA compared to PLLA. PLGA typically undergoes bulk degradation by ester hydrolysis. The degradation rate of PLGA can be controlled by adjusting the ratio of PLLA/PGA.

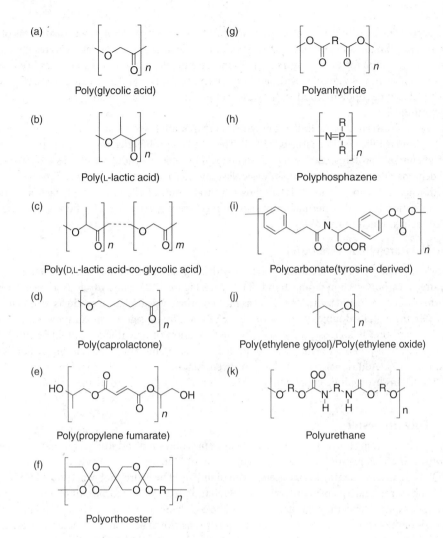

FIGURE 37.2 Repeating structural unit of degradable synthetic homopolymers under investigation as scaffold materials for tissue engineering applications.

However, it is important to note that the copolymer composition is not linearly related to the mechanical and degradation properties of PLGA. For example, a 50 : 50% ratio of PGA and PLLA typically degrades faster than either homopolymer [48,57].

PLGA has been extensively researched as a tissue engineering scaffold and shown to support the growth of a variety of cell types. For instance, PLGA can facilitate human foreskin fibroblasts to regenerate an extracellular matrix [8]. Similar studies has been conducted with chondrocytes and osteoblastic cells [54,58]. Osteoblastic cells seeded on PLGA scaffolds expressed collagen, fibronectin, laminin, and a variety of other extracellular matrix proteins, indicating proper cell function. Furthermore, PLGA promoted smooth muscle cell growth as well as the production of collagen and elastin [59]. Similar works showed enhancement of axon regeneration by murine neural cells seeded on PLGA scaffolds [60]. Additionally, an epithelial layer has been formed on PGLA by seeded enteroctyes derived from intestinal epithelial cells [61].

37.3.1.4 Poly(ε-caprolactone)

Poly(ε-caprolactone) (PCL) is a aliphatic polyester with semi-crystalline properties (Table 37.2, Figure 37.2). PCL has repeating unit of one ester group and five methylene groups. It is highly water-soluble with a melting temperature of 58 to 63°C [22,48]. PCL is formed through ring-opening polymerization, forming a degradable ester linkage. The degradation of PCL occurs by bulk or surface hydrolysis of these ester linkages, resulting in a byproduct of caproic acid. PCL degrades at a slow rate with results showing that it can persist *in vivo* for up to 2 years [48]. To increase the degradation rate, PCL has been copolymerized with collagen, poly(glycolic acid), and poly(lactic acid), polyethylene oxide [62–64]. The ease with which PCL can be copolymerized with a variety of polymers has made it an attractive component of polymeric scaffolds.

PCL has been investigated as a stabilizing polymer on PGA scaffolds to aid in the formation of spherical aggregates by human biliary epithelial cells (hBEC). These hBECs proliferated on the synthetic scaffold and expressed phenotypic proteins, indicating cell stability [63]. Further studies of PCL as a homopolymer has been demonstrated to support human osteoblast and dermal fibroblast cell viability [65,66]. The results with osteoblasts on porous PCL has shown a production of alkaline phosphatase, a marker of bone mineralization [65]. Also, dermal fibroblasts on mechanically stretched PCL films proliferated and maintained their rounded morphology [66].

37.3.1.5 Poly(propylene fumarate)

Poly(propylene fumarate) (PPF) is a linear polyester with a repeating unit containing two ester groups and one unsaturated carbon–carbon double bond (Table 37.2, Figure 37.2). The hydrolysis of the ester bonds in PPF, forms fumaric acid and propylene glycol as the two primary degradation products. Covalent cross-linking of PPF through its double bond allows cured PPF to possess significant compressive and tensile strength. Furthermore, this cross-linking aids in the formation of a synthetic scaffold *in situ* [67,68]. Cross-linked PPF is a potential orthopaedic, especially bone, engineering material due to the strength that it exhibits [67]. Additional research has also been conducted with PPF copolymerized with PEG (PPF-co-PEG). This hydrophilic copolymer has been shown to support endothelial cell attachment and proliferation [69,70].

37.3.1.6 Polyorthoester

A family of surface eroding polyorthoesters (POE) has been synthesized and studied for tissue engineering applications (Table 37.2, Figure 37.2). One particular form of POE has been considered as a scaffold. This type of POE is created by reacting ketene acetals with diols [71]. The hydrophobic nature of POE's surface allows this polymer to undergo primarily surface degradation [8,72]. By incorporating short acid groups, such as glycolic or lactic acid, the degradation rate of the copolymer can be controlled [72]. Furthermore, the hydrolysis of the orthoester linkages in POE is mostly sensitive to acids and is stable in bases [22,57].

The surface eroding characteristics of POE has led to the research of this polymer for bone reconstruction [8,73]. Surface degradation allows a scaffold to sustain mechanical support for the surrounding tissue since the bulk of the material remains structurally intact. In other studies, hepatocytes were grafted onto polyorthoesters and adhered to the surface of the synthetic scaffold [74].

37.3.2 Other Synthetic Polymers

37.3.2.1 Polyanhydride

Polyanhydrides are a class of hydrophobic polymers containing anhydride bonds, which are highly water-reactive (Table 37.2, Figure 37.2) [75]. Polyanhydrides are also crystalline polymers, with a melting temperature of approximately 100°C [76]. Aliphatic polyanhydrides are synthesized by a dehydration reaction between diacids. The instability of the anhydride bond allows polyanhydrides to degrade within a period of weeks. The degradation rate is predictable for polyanhydrides and can be altered through changes in the hydrophobicity of the diacid building blocks [76]. Polyanhydrides are generally thought to degrade following a surface degradation mechanism.

Similar to polyorthoesters, polyanhydrides have been investigated primarily for orthopaedic applications. However, the modest Young's Modulus for entangled polyanhydride networks has limited their application in weight-bearing environments [47]. This limitation resulted in further studies involving the formation of cross-linked polyanhydrides networks with incorporated imides [53,77]. Scaffolds formed from these networks possess significant mechanical properties, such as compressive strength (30–60 MPa), which are in the intermediate range of cortical and trabecular human bone (5–150 MPa) [47,76–78].

37.3.2.2 Polyphosphazene

Polyphosphazenes are a class of polymers formed from an inorganic backbone containing nitrogen and phosphorous atoms (Table 37.2, Figure 37.2). Polyphosphazene is hydrophobic and typically undergoes hydrolytic surface degradation into phosphate and ammonium salt byproducts. There are a variety of polyphosphazenes that may be synthesized, due to the numerous types of hydrolytically labile substituents that can be can be added to the phosphorous atoms [79]. These viable substituents allow the properties of polyphosphazenes to be extremely controllable. Nevertheless, most polyphosphazenes display a slow degradation rate *in vivo* [79].

A number of different polyphosphazenes have been synthesized for use as tissue engineering scaffolds. Due to its high strength and surface degradation properties, it has been particularly investigated as an orthopaedic biomaterial [80]. Osteoblast cells that support skeletal tissue formation has been seeded and proliferated on a three-dimensional polyphosphazene scaffold [81]. Additionally, poly(organo)phosphazenes has been studied as scaffolds for synthetic nerve grafts in peripheral nerve regeneration [82].

37.3.2.3 Polycarbonate

Tyrosine-derived polycarbonate (P(DTR carbonate)) is an amorphous polycarbonate widely studied for biomedical applications (Table 37.2, Figure 37.2). The linear chain of P(DTR carbonate) contains a pendant R group, allowing it to be easily modified [83]. Further, P(DTR carbonate) has three bonds susceptible to hydrolytic degradation: amide, carbonate, and ester [53,83]. The carbonate and ester bonds readily degrade, with the former typically having a faster degradation rate. Nevertheless, the overall degradation time for P(DTR carbonate) can be months to years [84]. The ester bond degrades into carboxylic acid and alcohol, while the carbonate bond releases two alcohols and carbon dioxide [83]. The amide has been found to be relatively stable *in vitro* [83]. Overall, P(DTR carbonate) undergoes bulk degradation and its mechanical properties are determined by the pendant group [53,83].

The slow degradation rate of polycarbonates has led to its investigation in orthopaedic tissue engineering applications. Additionally, P(DTR carbonate) elicits a response for bone ingrowth at the bone-polymer implant interface, supporting the use of P(DTR carbonate) as a bone scaffold [84]. Recent studies have shown that osteoblast cells do attach to the surface of P(DTR carbonate). Results indicate that these osteoblasts maintained their phenotype and rounded cell morphology [85].

37.3.2.4 Poly(ethylene glycol)/Poly(ethylene oxide)

Poly(ethylene glycol) (PEG) is generally a linear-chained polymer consisting of an ethylene oxide repeating unit $(-O-CH_2-CH_2)_n$ (Table 37.2, Figure 37.2). Poly(ethylene oxide) (PEO) has the same backbone as PEG, but an longer chain length and thus a higher molecular weight [86,87]. PEG is hydrophilic and synthesized by a anionic/cationic polymerization [4,8]. The ability of PEG to act as a swelling polymer has primarily led to its function as a hydrogel, and in some instances as an injectable hydrogel. Unfortunately, the linear chain form of PEG leads to rapid diffusion and low mechanical stability [8]. PEG networks may be created by attaching functional groups to the ends of the PEG chain and then initiating covalent cross-linking [8,32,87–90]. PEG is naturally nondegradable. However, PEG may be made degradable by copolymerization with hydrolytically or enzymatically degradable polymers [91].

The ease with which PEG may be modified, whether with cross-linkable groups for network formation or degradable groups for resorbable applications, has probably led to the widespread interest in PEG for tissue engineering or other biomedical applications. For example, PEG has been copolymerized with PLGA as well as alginate to form hydrogels. Results have shown that DNA content of chondrocytes proliferation on copolymerized PLGA-PEG increases as the percentage of degradable components becomes higher [92]. Similarly, islets of Langerhans in alginate–PEG hydrogels retained their viability and expressed function through insulin excretion [93].

37.3.2.5 Polyurethane

Recent investigations have developed polyurethane polymers as scaffold materials. Polyurethane is an elastomeric polymer that is typically nondegradable (Table 37.2, Figure 37.2). Positive attributes, such as flexible mechanical strength and biocompatibility, has led to the synthesis of degradable polyurethanes with nontoxic diisocyanate derivatives [47,94–96]. Studies have shown that polyurethane scaffolds support cell attachment with chondrocytes, bone marrow stromal cells, and cardiomyocytes [96–98].

37.4 Scaffold Design Properties

37.4.1 Fabrication

There are two main considerations in the assembly of a polymeric tissue engineering scaffold. First is the curing method, or the method by which the polymer is assembled into a bulk material. Second is the fabrication strategy. The chemical nature of the polymer often determines both the curing method and fabrication strategy. There are two main curing methods: polymer entanglement and polymer cross-linking. Entanglement usually involves intertwining long, linear polymer chains to form a loosely bound polymer network. An advantage of this type of method is that it is simple, allowing the polymer to be molded into a bulk material using heat, pressure, or both. However, a disadvantage of this process is that the bulk material sometimes lacks significant mechanical strength. The second curing method is cross-linking, which involves the formation of covalent or ionic bonds between individual polymer chains. Typically either a radical or ion is needed to promote cross-linking along with an initiator, such as heat, light, chemical accelerant, or time. The advantages of cross-linked polymers are that they often have significant mechanical properties. Furthermore, cross-linked polymers may be injected into a tissue defect and cured *in situ*. However, one major disadvantage is the possible cytotoxicity issues with cross-linking systems. The multiple components used by cross-linking polymers as well as the necessary chemical reaction may lead to the use of cytotoxic components or the formation of cytotoxic reaction byproducts.

There are two basic strategies of polymeric scaffold fabrication: prefabrication and *in situ*. Prefabrication structures are cured before implantation. This strategy is often preferred since it is formed outside the body, allowing the removal of cytotoxic and nonbiocompatible components prior to implantation. However, the notable disadvantage of prefabricated scaffolds is that it may not properly fit in a tissue defect site, causing gaps between the engineered graft and the host tissue. These void spaces may lead to undesirable results, including fibrous tissue formation. Therefore, the deficiencies of prefabricated scaffolds have led to investigations toward *in situ* fabrication of a scaffold, which involves curing of a polymeric matrix within the tissue defect itself. The deformability of an *in situ* fabricated matrix creates an interface between the scaffold and the surrounding tissue, facilitating tissue integration [99]. Furthermore, the implantation of an *in situ* fabricated scaffold may require as little as a narrow path for injection of the liquid scaffold, allowing minimally invasive surgery techniques to be utilized. A disadvantage of *in situ* fabrication of scaffolds is that the chemical or thermal means of curing the polymer can significantly affect the host tissue as well as any biological component of the engineered graft.

37.4.2 Micro-Structure

Tissue regeneration through cell implantation in scaffolds is dependent on the micro-structure of the scaffold. Since most cells are anchorage dependent, the scaffold should possess properties that aid cell growth and facilitate attachment of a large cell population [46,100]. To this end, a large scaffold surface area is typically favorable. Furthermore, highly porous scaffolds allow for an abundant number of cells to infiltrate the scaffold's void space. Similarly, the continuity of the scaffold's pores is important for proper transport of nutrients and cell migration. It is also generally advantageous for scaffolds to possess a large surface area to volume ratio. This ratio promotes the use of small diameter pores that are larger than the diameter of a cell. However, high porosities compromise the mechanical integrity of the polymeric scaffold. Clearly, balancing a scaffold's surface area, void space, and mechanical integrity is a necessary challenge that must be overcome in the construction of viable tissue engineering scaffolds.

Additionally, a polymer's effectiveness as a scaffolding material is dependent on its interaction with transplanted or host cells. Thus the polymer's surface properties should facilitate their attachment, proliferation, and (possible) differentiation. A strong cell adhesion favors the proliferation of cells, while a rounded morphology promotes their differentiation [46]. The hydrophilic nature of some polymers promotes a highly wettable surface and allows cells to be encapsulated by capillary action [101]. Furthermore, cellular attachment and function on polymeric scaffolds may be enhanced by providing a biomimetic surface through the incorporation of proteins and ligands.

37.4.3 Macro-Structure

A scaffold can be formed into a number of different macro-structures including, fiber meshes, hydrogels, and foams. Fiber meshes are formed by weaving or knitting individual polymeric fibers into a three-dimensional structure and are attractive for tissue engineering as they provide a large surface area for cell attachment [48]. Furthermore, a fiber mesh scaffold structure mimics the properties of the extracellular matrix, allowing the diffusion of nutrients to cells and waste products from cells. A disadvantage to this form is the lack of structural stability. However, fiber bonding, which involves bonding at fiber cross points, has been introduced to create a more stable structure [46,48,102].

Hydrophilic polymers are often formed into hydrogels by physical polymer entanglements, secondary forces, or chemical cross-linking [13,87]. The significant property of hydrogels is their ability to absorb a tremendous amount of water, up to a thousand times their own dry weight [13]. This aqueous environment, ideal for cell encapsulation and drug loading, has encouraged many investigations into hydrogels for biomedical applications. Hydrogels are generally easy to inject or mold, and therefore are often incorporated into strategies involving minimally invasive surgical techniques [32]. Some drawbacks to hydrogels are that they lack strong mechanical properties and they are difficult to sterilize [13,32].

Foam and sponge scaffolds provide a macro-structural template for the cells to form into a three-dimensional tissue structure. There are several different processing techniques for porous constructs, including phase separation, emulsion freeze drying, gas foaming, and solvent casting/particulate leaching [46,103–105]. A recent technology that has become of interest in tissue engineering is rapid prototyping or solid freeform fabrication. These techniques are quite exciting since they allow for the precise construction of scaffold architecture, often based upon a computer-aided design model [106]. The most appropriate scaffold macro-structure is dependent on the type of the polymer utilized and the application (tissue) of interest.

37.4.4 Biocompatibility

One of the most essential properties of an engineered construct is its biocompatibility, or ability to not elicit a significant or prolonged inflammatory response. It is important to know that any injury will elicit some inflammatory response, and this is certainly true with the implantation of a polymeric scaffold. However, this response should be limited and not prolonged.

When a polymeric scaffold is implanted in a tissue, there is typically a three-phase tissue response [107–109]. Phase I incorporates both acute and chronic inflammation, which occurs in a short period of time (1 to 2 weeks). Phase II involves the granulation of tissue, a foreign body reaction, and fibrosis. The rate of phase II is primarily dependent on the degradation rate of the polymeric scaffold. Finally, the fastest step, phase III is when the bulk of the scaffold is lost. These phases are directly influenced by the properties of the polymeric scaffold. Therefore, it is important to evaluate a variety of scaffold properties including synthesis components, fabrication, micro-structure, and macro-structure. It is a general thought that as the complexity of a scaffold system increases, the more likely it will result in a significant response by the body [73].

37.4.5 Biodegradability

Most polymeric scaffolds are designed to provide temporary support and, therefore to be biodegradable. Therefore, the degraded products of the scaffold must have a safe route for removal from the host. The rate of degradation is often affected by the properties of the polymeric scaffold including synthesis components, fabrication, micro-structure, and macro-structure. Most investigations intend for the scaffold degradation rate to closely follow the rate of tissue repair [22,46]. However, this intention may be difficult to implement. An alternative approach is to design the scaffold's degradation rate so that it is quicker than the rate of degradation product removal, in an effort to minimize negative host responses.

There are two types of degradation: surface and bulk [110]. Surface degradation of a scaffold is characterized by a gradual decrease in the dimensions of the scaffold with no change in its mechanical attributes. At a critical point during surface degradation, both size and mechanical properties of the scaffold decrease rapidly. Bulk degradation is characterized by loss of material throughout the scaffold's volume during degradation. Thus, mechanical strength decreases during bulk degradation and is dependent on the degradation rate. Since bulk degradation maintains an intact surface, it may facilitate cell adhesion to a greater extent than surface eroding scaffolds. Natural polymers mainly undergo surface degradation, since enzymes are generally too large to penetrate into the bulk of the scaffold. However, synthetic polymers can degrade by surface, bulk, or both, depending on its composition.

37.4.6 Mechanical Strength

Since many tissues undergo mechanical stresses and strains, the mechanical properties of a scaffold should be considered. This is especially true for the engineering of weight-bearing orthopaedic tissues. In these instances, the scaffold must be able to provide support to the forces applied to both it and the surrounding tissues. Furthermore, the mechanical properties of the polymeric scaffold should be retained until the regenerated tissue can assume its structural role [111]. In cases where mechanical forces are thought to be required for cell growth and phenotype expression, a scaffold which displays surface eroding properties may be preferred. Alternatively, hydrophobic polymers tend to resist water absorption and thus sustain their strength longer than hydrophilic polymers.

37.5   Summary

Tissue engineering has emerged as a growing field for restoring, repairing, and regenerating tissue. Polymeric scaffolds especially have a profound impact on the possibilities of tissue engineering by providing structure for the attachment, proliferation, and differentiation of transplanted or host cells. These constructs have led to exciting and novel clinical options for the repair of tissues, including but not limited to skin, bone, cartilage, kidney, liver, nerve, and smooth muscle. To this end, scaffold properties must be carefully considered for the intended application. Most importantly, the polymeric scaffold must allow invading cells to express proper functionality of the tissue being formed. Thus, tissue engineering research is continuously trying to enhance polymeric scaffold properties to form tissue that closely resembles the native tissue.

References

[1] Langer, R., Tissue engineering, *Mol. Ther.* 2000, 1(1), 12–15.
[2] Bonassar, L.J. and Vacanti, C.A., Tissue engineering: the first decade and beyond, *J. Cell. Biochem. Suppl.* 1998, 30–31, 297–303.
[3] Hutmacher, D.W., Scaffold design and fabrication technologies for engineering tissues — state of the art and future perspectives, *J. Biomater. Sci. Polym. Ed.* 2001, 12(1), 107–124.
[4] Lee, K.Y. and Mooney, D.J., Hydrogels for tissue engineering, *Chem. Rev.* 2001, 101(7), 1869–1879.

[5] Vinall, R.L., Lo, S.H., and Reddi, A.H., Regulation of articular chondrocyte phenotype by bone morphogenetic protein 7, interleukin 1, and cellular context is dependent on the cytoskeleton, *Exp. Cell Res.* 2002, 272(1), 32–44.

[6] Hung, C.T., Lima, E.G., Mauck, R.L., Taki, E., LeRoux, M.A., Lu, H.H., Stark, R.G., Guo, X.E., and Ateshian, G.A., Anatomically shaped osteochondral constructs for articular cartilage repair, *J. Biomech.* 2003, 36(12), 1853–1864.

[7] Rahfoth, B., Weisser, J., Sternkopf, F., Aigner, T., von der Mark, K., and Brauer, R., Transplantation of allograft chondrocytes embedded in agarose gel into cartilage defects of rabbits, *Osteoarthr. Cartil.* 1998, 6(1), 50–65.

[8] Seal, B.L., Otero, T.C., and Panitch, A., Polymeric biomaterials for tissue and organ regeneration, *Mater. Sci. Eng. R-Rep.* 2001, 34(4–5), 147–230.

[9] Dillon, G.P., Yu, X., Sridharan, A., Ranieri, J.P., and Bellamkonda, R.V., The influence of physical structure and charge on neurite extension in a 3D hydrogel scaffold, *J. Biomater. Sci. Polym. Ed.* 1998, 9(10), 1049–1069.

[10] Wang, L., Shelton, R.M., Cooper, P.R., Lawson, M., Triffitt, J.T., and Barralet, J.E., Evaluation of sodium alginate for bone marrow cell tissue engineering, *Biomaterials* 2003, 24(20), 3475–3481.

[11] Davis, T.A., Volesky, B., and Mucci, A., A review of the biochemistry of heavy metal biosorption by brown algae, *Water Res.* 2003, 37(18), 4311–4330.

[12] Rowley, J.A., Madlambayan, G., and Mooney, D.J., Alginate hydrogels as synthetic extracellular matrix materials, *Biomaterials* 1999, 20(1), 45–53.

[13] Hoffman, A.S., Hydrogels for biomedical applications, *Adv. Drug Deliv. Rev.* 2002, 54(1), 3–12.

[14] Shapiro, L. and Cohen, S., Novel alginate sponges for cell culture and transplantation, *Biomaterials* 1997, 18(8), 583–590.

[15] Guo, J.F., Jourdian, G.W., and MacCallum, D.K., Culture and growth characteristics of chondrocytes encapsulated in alginate beads, *Conn. Tissue Res.* 1989, 19(2–4), 277–297.

[16] Pariente, J.L., Kim, B.S., and Atala, A., *In vitro* biocompatibility evaluation of naturally derived and synthetic biomaterials using normal human bladder smooth muscle cells, *J. Urol.* 2002, 167(4), 1867–1871.

[17] Shimizu, T., Yamato, M., Kikuchi, A., and Okano, T., Cell sheet engineering for myocardial tissue reconstruction, *Biomaterials* 2003, 24(13), 2309–2316.

[18] Liu, H., Lee, Y.W., and Dean, M.F., Re-expression of differentiated proteoglycan phenotype by dedifferentiated human chondrocytes during culture in alginate beads, *Biochim. Biophys. Acta* 1998, 1425(3), 505–515.

[19] Glicklis, R., Shapiro, L., Agbaria, R., Merchuk, J.C., and Cohen, S., Hepatocyte behavior within three-dimensional porous alginate scaffolds, *Biotechnol. Bioeng.* 2000, 67(3), 344–353.

[20] Mosahebi, A., Simon, M., Wiberg, M., and Terenghi, G., A novel use of alginate hydrogel as Schwann cell matrix, *Tissue Eng.* 2001, 7(5), 525–534.

[21] Leach, J.B., Bivens, K.A., Patrick, C.W., and Schmidt, C.E., Photocrosslinked hyaluronic acid hydrogels: natural, biodegradable tissue engineering scaffolds, *Biotechnol. Bioeng.* 2003, 82(5), 578–589.

[22] Hayashi, T., Biodegradable polymers for biomedical uses, *Prog. Polym. Sci.* 1994, 19(4), 663–702.

[23] Aigner, J., Tegeler, J., Hutzler, P., Campoccia, D., Pavesio, A., Hammer, C., Kastenbauer, E., and Naumann, A., Cartilage tissue engineering with novel nonwoven structured biomaterial based on hyaluronic acid benzyl ester, *J. Biomed. Mater. Res.* 1998, 42(2), 172–181.

[24] Halbleib, M., Skurk, T., de Luca, C., von Heimburg, D., and Hauner, H., Tissue engineering of white adipose tissue using hyaluronic acid-based scaffolds. I: *in vitro* differentiation of human adipocyte precursor cells on scaffolds, *Biomaterials* 2003, 24(18), 3125–3132.

[25] VandeVord, P.J., Matthew, H.W.T., DeSilva, S.P., Mayton, L., Wu, B., and Wooley, P.H., Evaluation of the biocompatibility of a chitosan scaffold in mice, *J. Biomed. Mater. Res.* 2002, 59(3), 585–590.

[26] Suh, J.K.F. and Matthew, H.W.T., Application of chitosan-based polysaccharide biomaterials in cartilage tissue engineering: a review, *Biomaterials* 2000, 21(24), 2589–2598.

[27] Li, J., Pan, J., Zhang, L., Guo, X., and Yu, Y., Culture of primary rat hepatocytes within porous chitosan scaffolds, *J. Biomed. Mater. Res.* 2003, 67A(3) 938–943.

[28] Kawase, M., Michibayashi, N., Nakashima, Y., Kurikawa, N., Yagi, K., and Mizoguchi, T., Application of glutaraldehyde-crosslinked chitosan as a scaffold for hepatocyte attachment, *Biol. Pharm. Bull.* 1997, 20(6), 708–710.

[29] Seol, Y.J., Lee, J.Y., Park, Y.J., Lee, Y.M., Ku, Y., Rhyu, I.C., Lee, S.J., Han, S.B., and Chung, C.P., Chitosan sponges as tissue engineering scaffolds for bone formation, *Biotechnol. Lett.* 2004, 26(13), 1037–1041.

[30] Nettles, D.L., Elder, S.H., and Gilbert, J.A., Potential use of chitosan as a cell scaffold material for cartilage tissue engineering, *Tissue Eng.* 2002, 8(6), 1009–1016.

[31] Lee, C.H., Singla, A., and Lee, Y., Biomedical applications of collagen, *Int. J. Pharm.* 2001, 221(1–2), 1–22.

[32] Drury, J.L. and Mooney, D.J., Hydrogels for tissue engineering: scaffold design variables and applications, *Biomaterials* 2003, 24(24), 4337–4351.

[33] Ma, L., Gao, C., Mao, Z., Shen, J., Hu, X., and Han, C., Thermal dehydration treatment and glutaraldehyde cross-linking to increase the biostability of collagen–chitosan porous scaffolds used as dermal equivalent, *J. Biomater. Sci. Polym. Ed.* 2003, 14(8), 861–874.

[34] Langer, R. and Vacanti, J.P., Tissue engineering, *Science* 1993, 260(5110), 920–926.

[35] Falanga, V., Margolis, D., Alvarez, O., Auletta, M., Maggiacomo, F., Altman, M., Jensen, J., Sabolinski, M., and Hardin-Young, J., Rapid healing of venous ulcers and lack of clinical rejection with an allogeneic cultured human skin equivalent. Human Skin Equivalent Investigators Group, *Arch. Dermatol.* 1998, 134(3), 293–300.

[36] Noah, E.M., Chen, J., Jiao, X., Heschel, I., and Pallua, N., Impact of sterilization on the porous design and cell behavior in collagen sponges prepared for tissue engineering, *Biomaterials* 2002, 23(14), 2855–2861.

[37] Nehrer, S., Breinan, H.A., Ramappa, A., Hsu, H.P., Minas, T., Shortkroff, S., Sledge, C.B., Yannas, I.V., and Spector, M., Chondrocyte-seeded collagen matrices implanted in a chondral defect in a canine model, *Biomaterials* 1998, 19(24), 2313–2328.

[38] Risbud, M.V., Karamuk, E., Schlosser, V., and Mayer, J., Hydrogel-coated textile scaffolds as candidate in liver tissue engineering: II. Evaluation of spheroid formation and viability of hepatocytes, *J. Biomater. Sci. Polym. Ed.* 2003, 14(7), 719–731.

[39] Orwin, E.J. and Hubel, A., *In vitro* culture characteristics of corneal epithelial, endothelial, and keratocyte cells in a native collagen matrix, *Tissue Eng.* 2000, 6(4), 307–319.

[40] Payne, R.G., Yaszemski, M.J., Yasko, A.W., and Mikos, A.G., Development of an injectable, *in situ* crosslinkable, degradable polymeric carrier for osteogenic cell populations. Part 1. Encapsulation of marrow stromal osteoblasts in surface crosslinked gelatin microparticles, *Biomaterials* 2002, 23(22), 4359–4371.

[41] Awad, H.A., Wickham, M.Q., Leddy, H.A., Gimble, J.M., and Guilak, F., Chondrogenic differentiation of adipose-derived adult stem cells in agarose, alginate, and gelatin scaffolds, *Biomaterials* 2004, 25(16), 3211–3222.

[42] Risbud, M., Endres, M., Ringe, J., Bhonde, R., and Sittinger, M., Biocompatible hydrogel supports the growth of respiratory epithelial cells: Possibilities in tracheal tissue engineering, *J. Biomed. Mater. Res.* 2001, 56(1), 120–127.

[43] Altman, G.H., Diaz, F., Jakuba, C., Calabro, T., Horan, R.L., Chen, J., Lu, H., Richmond, J., and Kaplan, D.L., Silk-based biomaterials, *Biomaterials* 2003, 24(3), 401–416.

[44] Minoura, N., Aiba, S., Gotoh, Y., Tsukada, M., and Imai, Y., Attachment and growth of cultured fibroblast cells on silk protein matrices, *J. Biomed. Mater. Res.* 1995, 29(10), 1215–1221.

[45] Sofia, S., McCarthy, M.B., Gronowicz, G., and Kaplan, D.L., Functionalized silk-based biomaterials for bone formation, *J. Biomed. Mater. Res.* 2001, 54(1), 139–148.

[46] Thomson, R.C., Wake, M.C., Yaszemski, M.J., and Mikos, A.G., Biodegradable polymer scaffolds to regenerate organs, *Biopolymers Ii* 1995, 122, 245–274.

[47] Gunatillake, P.A. and Adhikari, R., Biodegradable synthetic polymers for tissue engineering, *Eur. Cell. Mater.* 2003, 5, 1–16.

[48] Yang, S., Leong, K.F., Du, Z., and Chua, C.K., The design of scaffolds for use in tissue engineering. Part I. Traditional factors, *Tissue Eng.* 2001, 7(6), 679–689.

[49] Freed, L.E., Marquis, J.C., Nohria, A., Emmanual, J., Mikos, A.G., and Langer, R., Neocartilage formation *in vitro* and *in vivo* using cells cultured on synthetic biodegradable polymers, *J. Biomed. Mater. Res.* 1993, 27(1), 11–23.

[50] Shinoka, T., Ma, P.X., Shum-Tim, D., Breuer, C.K., Cusick, R.A., Zund, G., Langer, R., Vacanti, J.P., and Mayer, J.E., Jr., Tissue-engineered heart valves. Autologous valve leaflet replacement study in a lamb model, *Circulation* 1996, 94(9Suppl.), II164–II168.

[51] Kaihara, S., Kim, S., Kim, B.S., Mooney, D.J., Tanaka, K., and Vacanti, J.P., Survival and function of rat hepatocytes cocultured with nonparenchymal cells or sinusoidal endothelial cells on biodegradable polymers under flow conditions, *J. Pediatr. Surg.* 2000, 35(9), 1287–1290.

[52] Mooney, D.J., Mazzoni, C.L., Breuer, C., McNamara, K., Hern, D., Vacanti, J.P., and Langer, R., Stabilized polyglycolic acid fibre-based tubes for tissue engineering, *Biomaterials* 1996, 17(2), 115–124.

[53] Agrawal, C.M. and Ray, R.B., Biodegradable polymeric scaffolds for musculoskeletal tissue engineering, *J. Biomed. Mater. Res.* 2001, 55(2), 141–150.

[54] Ishaug-Riley, S.L., Okun, L.E., Prado, G., Applegate, M.A., and Ratcliffe, A., Human articular chondrocyte adhesion and proliferation on synthetic biodegradable polymer films, *Biomaterials* 1999, 20(23–24), 2245–2256.

[55] Yang, F., Murugan, R., Ramakrishna, S., Wang, X., Ma, Y.X., and Wang, S., Fabrication of nano-structured porous PLLA scaffold intended for nerve tissue engineering, *Biomaterials* 2004, 25(10), 1891–1900.

[56] Park, S.S., Jin, H.R., Chi, D.H., and Taylor, R.S., Characteristics of tissue-engineered cartilage from human auricular chondrocytes, *Biomaterials* 2004, 25(12), 2363–2369.

[57] Middleton, J.C. and Tipton, A.J., Synthetic biodegradable polymers as orthopedic devices, *Biomaterials* 2000, 21(23), 2335–2346.

[58] El-Amin, S.F., Lu, H.H., Khan, Y., Burems, J., Mitchell, J., Tuan, R.S., and Laurencin, C.T., Extra-cellular matrix production by human osteoblasts cultured on biodegradable polymers applicable for tissue engineering, *Biomaterials* 2003, 24(7), 1213–1221.

[59] Kim, B.S., Nikolovski, J., Bonadio, J., Smiley, E., and Mooney, D.J., Engineered smooth muscle tissues: regulating cell phenotype with the scaffold, *Exp. Cell. Res.* 1999, 251(2), 318–328.

[60] Teng, Y.D., Lavik, E.B., Qu, X., Park, K.I., Ourednik, J., Zurakowski, D., Langer, R., and Snyder, E.Y., Functional recovery following traumatic spinal cord injury mediated by a unique polymer scaffold seeded with neural stem cells, *Proc. Natl Acad. Sci. USA* 2002, 99(5), 3024–3029.

[61] Mooney, D.J., Organ, G., Vacanti, J.P., and Langer, R., Design and fabrication of biodegradable polymer devices to engineer tubular tissues, *Cell Transplant* 1994, 3(2), 203–210.

[62] Dai, N.T., Williamson, M.R., Khammo, N., Adams, E.F., and Coombes, A.G., Composite cell support membranes based on collagen and polycaprolactone for tissue engineering of skin, *Biomaterials* 2004, 25(18), 4263–4271.

[63] Barralet, J.E., Wallace, L.L., and Strain, A.J., Tissue engineering of human biliary epithelial cells on polyglycolic acid/polycaprolactone scaffolds maintains long-term phenotypic stability, *Tissue Eng.* 2003, 9(5), 1037–1045.

[64] Park, Y.J., Lee, J.Y., Chang, Y.S., Jeong, J.M., Chung, J.K., Lee, M.C., Park, K.B., and Lee, S.J., Radioisotope carrying polyethylene oxide–polycaprolactone copolymer micelles for targetable bone imaging, *Biomaterials* 2002, 23(3), 873–879.

[65] Ciapetti, G., Ambrosio, L., Savarino, L., Granchi, D., Cenni, E., Baldini, N., Pagani, S., Guizzardi, S., Causa, F., and Giunti, A., Osteoblast growth and function in porous poly epsilon-caprolactone matrices for bone repair: a preliminary study, *Biomaterials* 2003, 24(21), 3815–3824.

[66] Ng, K.W., Hutmacher, D.W., Schantz, J.T., Ng, C.S., Too, H.P., Lim, T.C., Phan, T.T., and Teoh, S.H., Evaluation of ultra-thin poly(epsilon-caprolactone) films for tissue-engineered skin, *Tissue Eng.* 2001, 7(4), 441–455.

[67] Fisher, J.P., Holland, T.A., Dean, D., and Mikos, A.G., Photoinitiated cross-linking of the biodegradable polyester poly(propylene fumarate). Part II. *In vitro* degradation, *Biomacromolecules* 2003, 4(5), 1335–1342.

[68] Peter, S.J., Miller, M.J., Yasko, A.W., Yaszemski, M.J., and Mikos, A.G., Polymer concepts in tissue engineering, *J. Biomed. Mater. Res.* 1998, 43(4), 422–427.

[69] Suggs, L.J. and Mikos, A.G., Development of poly(propylene fumarate-co-ethylene glycol) as an injectable carrier for endothelial cells, *Cell Transplant* 1999, 8(4), 345–350.

[70] Shung, A.K., Behravesh, E., Jo, S., and Mikos, A.G., Crosslinking characteristics of and cell adhesion to an injectable poly(propylene fumarate-co-ethylene glycol) hydrogel using a water-soluble crosslinking system, *Tissue Eng.* 2003, 9(2), 243–254.

[71] Davis, K.A. and Anseth, K.S., Controlled release from crosslinked degradable networks, *Crit. Rev. Ther. Drug Carrier Syst.* 2002, 19(4–5), 385–423.

[72] Heller, J., Barr, J., Ng, S.Y., Abdellauoi, K.S., and Gurny, R., Poly(ortho esters): synthesis, characterization, properties and uses, *Adv. Drug Deliv. Rev.* 2002, 54(7), 1015–1039.

[73] Andriano, K.P., Tabata, Y., Ikada, Y., and Heller, J., *In vitro* and *in vivo* comparison of bulk and surface hydrolysis in absorbable polymer scaffolds for tissue engineering, *J. Biomed. Mater. Res.* 1999, 48(5), 602–612.

[74] Vacanti, J.P., Morse, M.A., Saltzman, W.M., Domb, A.J., Perez-Atayde, A., and Langer, R., Selective cell transplantation using bioabsorbable artificial polymers as matrices, *J. Pediatr. Surg.* 1988, 23(1pt 2) 3–9.

[75] Langer, R., Biomaterials in drug delivery and tissue engineering: one laboratory's experience, *Acc. Chem. Res.* 2000, 33(2), 94–101.

[76] Kumar, N., Langer, R.S., and Domb, A.J., Polyanhydrides: an overview, *Adv. Drug Deliv. Rev.* 2002, 54(7), 889–910.

[77] Uhrich, K.E., Gupta, A., Thomas, T.T., Laurencin, C.T., and Langer, R., Synthesis and characterization of degradable poly(anhydride-co-imides), *Macromolecules* 1995, 28(7), 2184–2193.

[78] Muggli, D.S., Burkoth, A.K., and Anseth, K.S., Crosslinked polyanhydrides for use in orthopedic applications: degradation behavior and mechanics, *J. Biomed. Mater. Res.* 1999, 46(2), 271–278.

[79] Qiu, L.Y. and Zhu, K.J., Novel biodegradable polyphosphazenes containing glycine ethyl ester and benzyl ester of amino acethydroxamic acid as cosubstituents: syntheses, characterization, and degradation properties, *J. Appl. Polym. Sci.* 2000, 77(13), 2987–2995.

[80] Laurencin, C.T., Norman, M.E., Elgendy, H.M., el-Amin, S.F., Allcock, H.R., Pucher, S.R., and Ambrosio, A.A., Use of polyphosphazenes for skeletal tissue regeneration, *J. Biomed. Mater. Res.* 1993, 27(7), 963–973.

[81] Laurencin, C.T., El-Amin, S.F., Ibim, S.E., Willoughby, D.A., Attawia, M., Allcock, H.R., and Ambrosio, A.A., A highly porous 3-dimensional polyphosphazene polymer matrix for skeletal tissue regeneration, *J. Biomed. Mater. Res.* 1996, 30(2), 133–138.

[82] Langone, F., Lora, S., Veronese, F.M., Caliceti, P., Parnigotto, P.P., Valenti, F., and Palma, G., Peripheral nerve repair using a poly(organo)phosphazene tubular prosthesis, *Biomaterials* 1995, 16(5), 347–353.

[83] Tangpasuthadol, V., Pendharkar, S.M., and Kohn, J., Hydrolytic degradation of tyrosine-derived polycarbonates, a class of new biomaterials. Part I: study of model compounds, *Biomaterials* 2000, 21(23), 2371–2378.

[84] Choueka, J., Charvet, J.L., Koval, K.J., Alexander, H., James, K.S., Hooper, K.A., and Kohn, J., Canine bone response to tyrosine-derived polycarbonates and poly(L-lactic acid), *J. Biomed. Mater. Res.* 1996, 31(1), 35–41.

[85] Lee, S.J., Choi, J.S., Park, K.S., Khang, G., Lee, Y.M., and Lee, H.B., Response of MG63 osteoblast-like cells onto polycarbonate membrane surfaces with different micropore sizes, *Biomaterials* 2004, 25(19), 4699–4707.

[86] Cai, J., Bo, S., Cheng, R., Jiang, L., and Yang, Y., Analysis of interfacial phenomena of aqueous solutions of polyethylene oxide and polyethylene glycol flowing in hydrophilic and hydrophobic capillary viscometers, *J. Colloid. Interface Sci.* 2004, 276(1), 174–181.

[87] Gutowska, A., Jeong, B., and Jasionowski, M., Injectable gels for tissue engineering, *Anat. Rec.* 2001, 263(4), 342–349.

[88] Novikova, L.N., Novikov, L.N., and Kellerth, J.O., Biopolymers and biodegradable smart implants for tissue regeneration after spinal cord injury, *Curr. Opin. Neurol.* 2003, 16(6), 711–715.

[89] Sawhney, A.S., Pathak, C.P., and Hubbell, J.A., Bioerodible hydrogels based on photopolymerized poly(ethylene glycol)-co-poly(alpha-hydroxy acid) diacrylate macromers, *Macromolecules* 1993, 26(4), 581–587.

[90] Sims, C.D., Butler, P.E., Casanova, R., Lee, B.T., Randolph, M.A., Lee, W.P., Vacanti, C.A., and Yaremchuk, M.J., Injectable cartilage using polyethylene oxide polymer substrates, *Plast. Reconstr. Surg.* 1996, 98(5), 843–850.

[91] Bourke, S.L. and Kohn, J., Polymers derived from the amino acid L-tyrosine: polycarbonates, polyarylates and copolymers with poly(ethylene glycol), *Adv. Drug Deliv. Rev.* 2003, 55(4), 447–466.

[92] Bryant, S.J. and Anseth, K.S., Controlling the spatial distribution of ECM components in degradable PEG hydrogels for tissue engineering cartilage, *J. Biomed. Mater. Res.* 2003, 64A(1), 70–79.

[93] Desai, N.P., Sojomihardjo, A., Yao, Z., Ron, N., and Soon-Shiong, P., Interpenetrating polymer networks of alginate and polyethylene glycol for encapsulation of islets of Langerhans, *J. Microencapsul.* 2000, 17(6), 677–690.

[94] Ganta, S.R., Piesco, N.P., Long, P., Gassner, R., Motta, L.F., Papworth, G.D., Stolz, D.B., Watkins, S.C., and Agarwal, S., Vascularization and tissue infiltration of a biodegradable polyurethane matrix, *J. Biomed. Mater. Res.* 2003, 64A(2), 242–248.

[95] Gorna, K. and Gogolewski, S., Preparation, degradation, and calcification of biodegradable polyurethane foams for bone graft substitutes, *J. Biomed. Mater. Res.* 2003, 67A(3) 813–827.

[96] Zhang, J., Doll, B.A., Beckman, E.J., and Hollinger, J.O., A biodegradable polyurethane–ascorbic acid scaffold for bone tissue engineering, *J. Biomed. Mater. Res.* 2003, 67A(2) 389–400.

[97] Grad, S., Kupcsik, L., Gorna, K., Gogolewski, S., and Alini, M., The use of biodegradable polyurethane scaffolds for cartilage tissue engineering: potential and limitations, *Biomaterials* 2003, 24(28), 5163–5171.

[98] McDevitt, T.C., Woodhouse, K.A., Hauschka, S.D., Murry, C.E., and Stayton, P.S., Spatially organized layers of cardiomyocytes on biodegradable polyurethane films for myocardial repair, *J. Biomed. Mater. Res.* 2003, 66A(3), 586–595.

[99] Anseth, K.S., Metters, A.T., Bryant, S.J., Martens, P.J., Elisseeff, J.H., and Bowman, C.N., *In situ* forming degradable networks and their application in tissue engineering and drug delivery, *J. Control. Release* 2002, 78(1-3), 199–209.

[100] Kim, B.S., Baez, C.E., and Atala, A., Biomaterials for tissue engineering, *World J. Urol.* 2000, 18(1), 2–9.

[101] Dar, A., Shachar, M., Leor, J., and Cohen, S., Cardiac tissue engineering — optimization of cardiac cell seeding and distribution in 3D porous alginate scaffolds, *Biotechnol. Bioeng.* 2002, 80(3), 305–312.

[102] Sachlos, E. and Czernuszka, J.T., Making tissue engineering scaffolds work. Review: the application of solid freeform fabrication technology to the production of tissue engineering scaffolds, *Eur. Cell. Mater.* 2003, 5, 29–39.

[103] Lu, L., Zhu, X., Valenzuela, R.G., Currier, B.L., and Yaszemski, M.J., Biodegradable polymer scaffolds for cartilage tissue engineering, *Clin. Orthop.* 2001, (391 Suppl), S251–S270.

[104] Chen, G.P., Ushida, T., and Tateishi, T., Development of biodegradable porous scaffolds for tissue engineering, *Mater. Sci. Eng. C-Biomim. Supramol. Syst.* 2001, 17(1-2), 63–69.

[105] Griffith, L.G., Polymeric biomaterials, *Acta Materialia* 2000, 48(1), 263–277.

[106] Yang, S., Leong, K.F., Du, Z., and Chua, C.K., The design of scaffolds for use in tissue engineering. Part II. Rapid prototyping techniques, *Tissue Eng.* 2002, 8(1), 1–11.

[107] Shive, M.S. and Anderson, J.M., Biodegradation and biocompatibility of PLA and PLGA microspheres, *Adv. Drug Deliv. Rev.* 1997, 28(1), 5–24.

[108] Ziats, N.P., Miller, K.M., and Anderson, J.M., *In vitro* and *in vivo* interactions of cells with biomaterials, *Biomaterials* 1988, 9(1), 5–13.

[109] Anderson, J.M. and Miller, K.M., Biomaterial biocompatibility and the macrophage, *Biomaterials* 1984, 5(1), 5–10.

[110] von Burkersroda, F., Schedl, L., and Gopferich, A., Why degradable polymers undergo surface erosion or bulk erosion, *Biomaterials* 2002, 23(21), 4221–4231.

[111] Woodfield, T.B., Bezemer, J.M., Pieper, J.S., van Blitterswijk, C.A., and Riesle, J., Scaffolds for tissue engineering of cartilage, *Crit. Rev. Eukaryot. Gene Expr.* 2002, 12(3), 209–236.

38

Calcium Phosphate Ceramics for Bone Tissue Engineering

P. Quinten Ruhé
Joop G.C. Wolke
Paul H.M. Spauwen
John A. Jansen
*University Medical Center
St. Radboud*

38.1 Introduction

In reconstructive surgery, repair and regeneration of large bone defects is a major challenge. The use of autologous bone is still the gold standard, although concomitant problems as donor site morbidity and limited supply have resulted in worldwide endeavors for the development of bone graft substitutes. Each potential substitute, including tissue engineering approaches with delivery of osteogenic cells or osteoinductive macromolecules, or both is based on an appropriate scaffold biomaterial that is biocompatible, allows bone ingrowth and shows subsequent degradation of the material. In view of this, a biomaterial used for tissue replacement shows by preference a resemblance with the inorganic or organic components of the tissue, or both, to be substituted.

Bone tissue is a living organ composed of an organic and an inorganic component. The organic substance (approx. $\frac{1}{4}$ to $\frac{1}{3}$ of total dry bone weight) consists of more than 90% of collagen and only for a small fraction of cells (2%) and noncollagenous proteins (5%). The inorganic bone mineral (approx. $\frac{2}{3}$ to $\frac{3}{4}$ of total dry bone weight) is composed of specific phases of calcium phosphate (Ca-P), especially carbonate rich hydroxyapatite (HA). In biologically carbonated HA, PO_4 is substituted by CO_3 (so-called type B carbonation). Biological HA also contains other impurity ions as Cl, Mg, Na, K, and F and

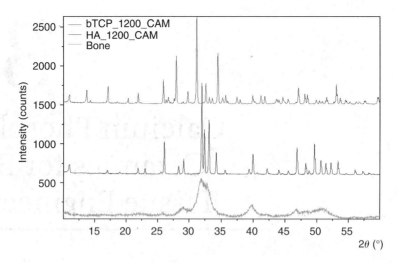

FIGURE 38.1   X-ray diffraction (XRD) pattern of bone, HA and β-tricalcium phosphate, clearly indicating the similarity between HA and bone.

trace elements like Sr and Zn [1]. The apatite in bone mineral is composed of small platelet-like crystals of just 2 to 4 nm in thickness, 25 nm in width, and 50 nm in length [2].

Together with the — organic — collagenous materials, Ca-P materials are among the few biomaterials that show high similarity to natural tissue. Ca-P biomaterials resemble the mineral phase of bone to a higher or lesser extent, depending or their stoichiometry and crystallinity (Figure 38.1). In general, Ca-P biomaterials are crystalline ceramics characterized by a high biocompatibility, the ability of direct bone bonding and osteoconduction, and a variable resorbability. Since the early seventies, Ca-P ceramics are clinically used in dentistry, followed by surgical specialties in the eighties. The various available Ca-P materials differ in their origin (naturally derived or synthetic), chemico-physical composition (calcium to phosphate ratio, crystallinity, [micro]porosity) and preparation process (prefabricated blocks and granules, coatings on other biomaterials, self setting cements and composite materials). In this review, the essential Ca-P characteristics, differences between various Ca-P biomaterials, and proceedings in Ca-P ceramic bone tissue engineering research will be discussed.

38.2   Chemico-Physical Properties of Calcium Phosphate Ceramics

Calcium phosphate (Ca-P) compounds exist in several phases. Discern can be made regarding (1). The crystallinity of various compounds (amorphous vs. various crystalline Ca-P phases), (2). eventual heat treatment of the materials (sintering), and (3). the calcium to phosphate ratio.

38.2.1   Crystallinity

Amorphous Ca-P (ACP) is the first solid phase to appear in solution containing high concentrations of calcium and phosphate. ACP lacks the orderly internal structure of crystalline Ca-P compounds and typically has a spherical morphology [3]. Chemically, it has a Ca : P ratio of around 1.5 and is characterized by the absence of diffraction peaks on x-ray diffraction (XRD) patterns. ACP is unstable in aqueous fluids and transforms into crystalline phases such as octacalciumphosphate (OCP) and apatite. Heating of ACP also results in conversion to poorly crystallized apatite (600°C), β-TCP (800°C, dry heat), or HA (800°C, humid heat) [4]. Therefore, ACP should be considered as a precursor for crystalline Ca-P compounds. There has been, and still is, considerable debate whether or not ACP is substantially present in skeletal tissue. For example, Transmission Electron Microscope (TEM) analysis has never revealed conclusive evidence for the presence of ACP in bone mineral [3].

Other phases of Ca-P than ACP reveal a crystalline structure with characteristic peaks on XRD analysis. There is a broad range in crystal morphology depending on composition and preparation characteristics such as temperature, pH, impurity, and the presence of macromolecules. Impurities, as commonly occur in bone mineral, greatly influence crystallinity (reflecting crystal size and crystal strain) but depend on the type of substitution. For example, type B carbonated apatite (CO_3 for PO_4 substitution) has a lower crystallinity and increased solubility, whereas F substitution (F for OH) give the opposite effects due to a better fit of the F^- ion in the apatite crystal structure.

38.2.2 Sintering

Sintering is the key step in processing of the majority of ceramic materials and conventionally consists of two separate phases: compacting the initial powder and heating the compacted powder up to temperatures only a little lower than their melting points. Thereby, atoms and molecules are set in rapid motion, and the particles coalesce. Fusion of the crystals reduces the porosity and increases the strength and density of the final ceramic product. Currently, several sintering techniques are available, such as continuous hot pressing, microwave sintering, pressureless sintering, and plasma sintering. Obviously, chemical composition of initial powders as well as variation of pressure and temperature influence final structure and composition of the sintered product.

38.2.3 Stoichiometry

The quantitative relationship (stoichiometry) of calcium to phosphate in Ca-P salts is essential for several material characteristics as strength, solubility, and crystal structure. Table 38.1 lists the main Ca-P compounds for biomedical applications. From a crystallographic point of view, the most stable form of Ca-P has a Ca : P ratio of 1.67 (hydroxyapatite). With a decrease of the Ca to P ratio, other Ca-deficient phases occur like tricalcium phosphate (TCP, Ca : P ratio 1.50), octacalcium phosphate (OCP, Ca : P ratio 1.33), dicalcium phosphate anhydrous (DCPA or Monetite, Ca : P ratio 1.00), and dicalcium phosphate dihydrate (DCPD or Brushite, Ca : P ratio 1.00). Most of these calcium deficient compounds are used as raw material for sintering procedures for ceramics, or as ingredients for example, Ca-P cements. TCP and HA will be discussed more in detail, since these materials are most used for biomedical applications.

38.2.3.1 TCP ($Ca_3(PO_4)_2$)

Tricalcium phosphate (TCP) has a Ca : P ratio of 1.5, similar to the amorphous biologic precursors of bone [5]. It can be prepared by sintering Ca deficient apatite (Ca : P ratio 1.5). TCP is a polymorph ceramic and exhibits two phases (α- and β-whitlockite), known as α- and β-TCP. Variation in sintering temperature and humidity determine, which phase is being formed; α-TCP occurs at dry heat $>1300°C$ and subsequent quenching in water [4]. Solubility and resorbability of both forms is much higher compared to HA. However, α-TCP is unstable in water and reacts to produce HA. α-TCP is used mainly as a compound

TABLE 38.1 Ca-P Compounds, Names, Formulas, and Ca : P Ratios

Ca/P	Formula	Name/mineral	Abbreviation
0.5	$Ca(H_2PO_4)_2 \cdot H_2O$	Monocalcium phosphate monohydrate	MCPM
1.0	$CaHPO_4 \cdot 2H_2O$	Hydrated calcium phosphate/brushite	DCP
1.0	$CaHPO_4$	Anhydrous calcium phosphate/Monetite	ADCP
1.33	$Ca_8H_2(PO_4)_6 \cdot 5H_2O$	Octacalcium phosphate	OCP
1.5	$Ca_3(PO_4)_2$	Tricalcium phosphate/whitlockite	TCP
1.67	$Ca_{10}(PO_4)_6(F)_2$	Fluorapatite	FA
1.67	$Ca_{10}(PO_4)_6(OH)_2$	Hydroxylapatite	HA
2.0	$CaO \cdot Ca_3(PO_4)_2$	Tetracalcium phospate/hilgenstockite	TTCP

of some Ca-P cements. β-TCP is less soluble and less reactive than α-TCP. It is used pure as bone substitute, and in combination with HA (biphasic Ca-P ceramic). Due to its solubility, dissolution and reprecipitation occur *in vivo*. This results in gradual phase transition into carbonated apatite, and resorption by macrophages, giant cells, and osteoclasts.

38.2.3.2 Hydroxyapatite ($Ca_{10}(PO_4)_6(OH)_2$)

Hydroxyapatite (HA) is the term commonly used for calcium hydroxyapatite $Ca_{10}(PO_4)_6(OH)_2$, the most stable form of Ca-P under physiological pH and body temperature. With fluorapatite and chlorapatite, hydroxyapatite forms the group of apatite minerals that share a similar hexagonal monoclinic crystal structure and the general formula $A_{10}(PO_4)_6(OH,F,Cl)_2$. The A cation can be several metal ions besides calcium, such as barium, strontium, and magnesium. The phosphate anion can be substituted by a carbonate anion to a limited extent.

HA has a Ca : P ratio of 1.67 which is similar to bone mineral. It can be prepared by sintering of precipitated Ca-P salts in a Ca : P ratio of 1.67 at temperatures above 1000°C. Pure HA is hardly soluble under physiological conditions. Impurities like substitution of Ca^{2+} by other metal ions cause variation in solubility and crystal size due to the differences in ionic radius. With respect to mechanical strength, pure HA materials are superior to other Ca-P materials. *In vivo*, however, pure HA hardly shows any cellular resorption by macrophages, giant cells or osteoclasts unless the particle size is small enough for phagocytosis. As a consequence, HA should be considered as nonresorbable whereas other compositions such as β-TCP show substantial dissolution and resorption.

38.2.4 Strength

Biomechanical properties are a considerable concern in the use of Ca-P ceramics. Compressive strength of cortical and trabecular bone varies, depending on the bone density, from 130 to 180 MPa and 5 to 50 MPa respectively. For tensile strength these values fluctuate from 60 to 160 MPa and 3 to 15 MPa respectively. Dense sintered Ca-P ceramics may reach compressive strengths much higher than cortical bone (300–900 MPa), whereas tensile strengths similar and higher than cortical bone (40–300 MPa) have been reported [6]. Problem, however, is that ceramics do not exhibit substantial elastic or plastic deformation before fracturing. Due to the lack of ductility, virtually all Ca-P ceramics are brittle. The brittleness can be explained by the atomic structure of ceramics. Elasticity is manifested as small reversible changes in the interatomic spacing and stretching of interatomic bonds. Plastic deformation corresponds to breaking of existing bonds and reforming of bonds with new neighboring atoms. In crystalline materials, this occurs in planes by means of atomic slip. As a consequence of the electrically charged nature of the ions, both elastic and plastic deformations in ceramics are limited. The brittleness of ceramics is further enhanced by very small and omnipresent flaws in the material. These microcracks result in local amplification of applied tensile stresses and cause a relatively low fracture strength.

Due to the inferior biomechanical properties, Ca-P ceramics are less suitable for clinical application under weight-bearing conditions compared to, for example, metallic or polymeric biomaterials. Obviously, mechanical properties of porous ceramics deteriorate even further with an increasing porosity. Nevertheless, compressive strengths similar to trabecular bone have been reported [7].

38.2.5 Porosity

Cortical bone has pores ranging from 1 to 100 μm (volumetric porosity 5 to 10%), whereas trabecular bone has pores of 200 to 400 μm (volumetric porosity 70 to 90%). Porosity in bone provides space for nutrients supply in cortical bone and marrow cavity in trabecular bone. As mentioned in the previous paragraph, porosity is devastating for mechanical properties of Ca-P ceramics. On the other hand, it is known that porosity enhances degradation of Ca-P ceramics and determines the nature of ingrowing tissue. Consequently, this delicate equilibrium depends on more factors than mechanical material properties alone, that is, application site (vascularization, weight loading, defect dimensions), biological material properties (biocompatibility, osteoconductivity, and degradation) and other aspects as pore geometry and the use of tissue engineering strategies (addition of osteogenic cells or bioactive factors). Therefore, no general optimal pore size and architecture for all applications and biomaterials can be given.

38.2.5.1 Microporosity

Microporosity covers pores sizes smaller than — an arbitrary — 5 μm: too small for penetration an ingrowth of cells, but sufficient for penetration of fluids. Crystalline Ca-P materials intrinsically exhibit, depending on crystal size and structure, a nano- or microporous structure. However, microporosity of ceramics is highly decreased or virtually absent due to high pressure compaction and (partial) fusion of crystals after sintering. Microporous Ca-P structures have an increased surface area, which influences the biological behavior and the Ca-P dissolution/precipitation characteristics. It has even been reported that microstructure plays a crucial role in osteoinductive properties of ceramics. Yuan et al. [8] observed heterotopic bone formation in macro- and microporous ceramics implanted in the dorsal muscle in dogs, whereas similar implants without microporous structure did not reveal bone formation. They suggested that the increased surface area, resultant of the microporous structure, could have caused accumulation of adsorbed proteins (e.g., BMPs) which could have triggered osteogenesis.

38.2.5.2 Macroporosity

Pores larger than 10 μm can be considered as macropores. Various methods can be used to induce macroporosity in Ca-P material. For example, porous ceramics can be obtained by merging the Ca-P slurry with a polymer sponge-like mold or polymer beads before sintering. During the sintering, the polymer is completely burnt out, which results in a porous ceramic structure. In this way, architecture of porous ceramics can be controlled and a completely interconnected structure with any desirable pore size and pore geometry is feasible. Obviously, interconnection of pores is essential for tissue growth throughout the scaffold. Tsuruga and Kuboki have investigated the influences of pore size and geometry in induced bone formation in ceramics. They reported that for porous sintered HA blocks with pore sizes ranging from 106–212 μm to 500–600 μm, the highest amount of bone was produced in implants with pore sizes of 300 to 400 μm [9]. In another study, Kuboki et al. [10] observed that an optimal vascular ingrowth was achieved in pores with a diameter of 350 μm, and claimed that this was the key factor for effective bone formation. Macroporous dimensions are also reported to play a role in osteoinductive behavior of Ca-P ceramics. In a series of experiments in primates, Ripamonti et al. [11,12] reported that implant geometry is of critical importance for cell shape, cell locomotion and cell differentiation. They hypothesized that concavities in sintered HA mediate intrinsic osteoinduction.

38.3 Ca-P Products

Numerous Ca-P products are currently marketed for bone regenerative purposes. Most frequently used Ca-P products in dentistry and surgery are Ca-P coatings applied to prostheses. Several techniques, such as plasma spraying and RF magnetron sputtering can provide a thin bio-active Ca-P coating on the inert metal prosthesis surface [13]. Consequently, the superior mechanical metal properties can be combined with favorable bone bonding Ca-P properties. Coatings applied usually consist of HA to prevent resorption of the coating in time.

Other Ca-P products are marketed as bone filler and are available in various forms as granules, blocks, and injectable cements. Both granules and blocks are available with a dense or porous structure and several resorption rates. Most synthetic products are composed of β-TCP, HA or a combination of both (so called bi-phasic ceramics [Figure 38.2]). Besides synthetic ceramics, several naturally derived ceramics are commercially available. These and injectable Ca-P cements are being discussed in detail in the next paragraphs.

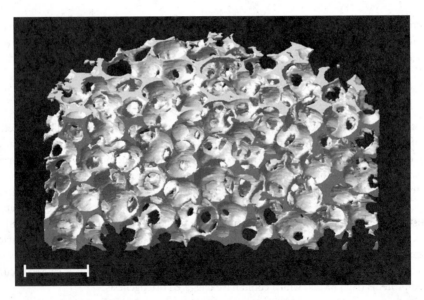

FIGURE 38.2 μCT representation of a highly porous biphasic ceramic implant material (Camceram®, Cam Implants, Leiden, The Netherlands) with a HA : TCP ratio of 60 : 40, porosity of 90%, and macropores ranging from 300 to 500 μm. Bar represents 1 mm.

38.3.1 Natural Ca-P Ceramics

Natural Ca-P biomaterials can be prepared from the inorganic bone mineral matrix of bone. Chemical, or high temperature heat treatment, or both, eliminate organic substances responsible for immunologic response and potential disease transmission (e.g., prions). Chemically treated materials derived from human spongiosa (Puros Tutoplast®, Zimmer Dental, Carslbad, CA, USA) or bovine spongiosa (Ortoss® and Bio-oss®, Geistlich Biomaterials, Geistlich, Switzerland) maintain the macroporous structure of spongious bone as well as the natural small carbonatehydroxyapatite crystal structure. Sintered bovine spongious bone products, such as Osteograf®-N (Dentsply Ceramed, Denver Co, USA) and Endobon® (Biomet Merck, Darmstadt, Germany), also maintain its macroporous structure, but due to the high sintering temperatures (>1100°C) the natural carbonate HA crystals convert into larger HA crystals without CO_3, resembling synthetic HA.

Besides bovine origin, natural Ca-P biomaterials can also be derived from special species of coral (genus Porites and Goniopora). Hydrothermal "replamiform" treatment (260°C; 15.000PSI) of the calcium carbonate (calcite) exoskeletal microstructure of these corals results in conversion into hydroxyapatite [14]. Like natural bone, this hydroxyapatite contains minor elements of Mg, Sr, F, and CO_3. The porous coralline hydroxyapatite is completely interconnected and available in various porosities (Interpore™, Pro Osteon™, Interpore Cross International Inc, Irvine, CA, USA). Different hydrothermal treatment of coral used for Pro Osteon-R results in only partial conversion of the calcium carbonate to HA [5,15]. As a result, the composite of $HA/CaCO_3$ is being resorbed faster than pure HA. Another coral derived bone substitute, which has not been converted into HA at all and therefore cannot be considered as a Ca-P ceramic, shows even faster degradation. This $CaCO_3$ material (Biocoral®, Inoteb, St. Gonnery, France) currently does not have FDA approval, but is available for clinical use in Europe.

38.3.2 Injectable Ca-P Cements

Difficulties with the clinical applicability of preformed ceramic blocks and granules have led to the development of injectable ceramic bone graft substitutes. In the early eighties, Brown and Chow were the first to describe the principles of a self setting Ca-P paste [16,17]. Currently, several different Ca-P cements are commercially available like BoneSource® (Stryker Leibinger, Kalamazoo, MI, USA), Norian® (Synthes, Oberdorf, Switzerland), α-BSM/Biobon® (Etex Corporation, Cambridge, MA, USA), and Calcibon® (Biomet Merck, Darmstadt, Germany). Each cement has a (slightly) different chemical composition, which results in differences in handling properties, setting time, strength and resorbability [18]. The major advantage of Ca-P cements is the injectability of the cement paste. Obviously, this results in favorable moldability of the bone graft, but also it results in immediate, seamless contact of cement to the surrounding bone [19]. Moreover, Ca-P cements have been found to exhibit excellent bone biocompatibility [20,21].

Roughly, the different Ca-P cements can be divided into four distinct groups [17]:

1. Cements composed of a solid Ca-P powder compound with an aqueous liquid component with or without Ca or P ions. After mixing, hardening of the cement is the result of the formation of one or more Ca-P compounds.
2. Cements with a powder component similar to those in (1), but an organic acid as liquid component. Hardening of the cement is the result of complex formation of calcium and the organic acid.
3. Cements similar to those in (2), except that the liquid component is a polymer solution. Cement hardening can be as described in (1) or complex formation of calcium and the polymer solution or both.
4. Cement composites on a polymer basis. Hardening of the cement is based on polymerization of the monomers. The Ca-P compounds present in these materials act as fillers and do not play a significant role in the mechanism of cement hardening.

In this review, we will focus only on the first group, as these cements currently play the most important role in research and clinical applications. The chemico-physical reaction that occurs during and after mixing of the powder and the liquid components is complex. After mixing, soluble compounds dissolve in the aqueous environment and subsequently precipitate, which results in formation and growth of different forms of Ca-P crystals. This crystallization finally results in entanglement of the insoluble Ca-P compounds and hardening of the cement. The setting time and phase transformation depend on the solubility of the various solid compounds, as well as of external factors as pH and temperature [22]. The setting reaction can be accelerated when the liquid phase contains phosphate ions. Therefore, setting time is different for each Ca-P cement formulation and may vary from minutes to hours. After setting, Ca-P cements may have an amorphous appearance under low magnification, but high magnification ($100,000\times$) reveals extremely small crystals. Crystal size and interparticle micropores were observed to grow in time [17]. The final result is a microporous structure of nanometer sized crystals composed of more or less apatitic compounds, resembling the small crystal size of biological apatite.

After setting of the cement, gradual phase transformation of the Ca-P compounds occurs into more apatitic phases. Due to the nonsintered nature and the higher surface area of Ca-P cements, dissolution of calcium and phosphate ions in physiological conditions occurs to a higher extent than in sintered ceramics. However, the relatively large surface area in combination with supersaturated body fluids also results in high Ca-P precipitation. Ishikawa et al. [23] reported that the total precipitation of (B-type) carbonate HA at the surface of Ca-P cement increased the total surface dissolution in simulated blood plasma *in vitro* for a period of 20 weeks. *In vivo*, formation of carbonated HA on cement surface has been reported to occur within 12 h of implantation [24]. This phenomenon could be one of the essential aspects of the exceptionally positive osteoconductive behavior of Ca-P cements.

38.4 *In Vivo* Interactions and Osteoinductivity

In general, Ca-P compounds are found to be biocompatible and favorable for the final bone response [4]. The ability of Ca-P ceramics to bond to bone is a rather unique property. For example, it has been a consistent finding that the larger the ceramic solubility rate, the more pronounced bone ingrowth is observed [25]. Ducheyne et al. hypothesized that the dissolution of Ca-P and precipitation of a carbonated HA layer is essential in the bioactive behavior of ceramics. On the other hand, Davies claimed that microtopography played a crucial role as bone formation at the implant surface was achieved by micromechanical interdigitation of the cement line with the material surface [26].

Protein–biomaterial interactions also play a key role in the biomaterial behavior *in vivo*. Directly after implantation, the surface of a biomaterial is being covered by serum proteins, which determine crucial reactions such as complement activation, thrombogenicity, and cell adhesion. Protein binding capacity depends on the specific ceramic characteristics as well as on the protein involved [27,28]. Ceramic materials exhibit a high binding affinity for proteins. Interestingly, several authors report that the combination of a material with high protein affinity and an appropriate (micro)architecture, can exhibit intrinsic osteoinductive behavior [8,11,12]. In a study in dogs, Yuan et al. observed ectopic bone formation after 3 and 6 months in micro- and macroporous HA, whereas macroporous HA without microporous structure did not reveal bone formation. It was hypothesized that due to the microporosity, total surface area and subsequent protein adsorption was increased, which could have induced bone formation. On the other hand, Ripamonti et al. hypothesized that concave macroporosity was the driving force for intrinsic osteoinduction in ceramics. The findings of intrinsic osteoinductive behavior in ceramic are interesting. However, it must be emphasized that regarding the numerous studies using similar porous ceramics without evidence for intrinsic osteoinduction, these observations currently are a rarity without confirmation of reproducibility.

Protein adsorption on ceramics not only plays an important role in biological processes, it also influences the ceramic itself with respect to dissolution and precipitation of calcium and phosphate ions. Radin et al. [29] reported that in an *in vitro* environment, serum proteins slowed down the dissolution (OHA and β-TCP) and precipitation (carbonated HA) of crystals at the surface of a crystalline multiphasic ceramic coating. A similar observation was done by Ong et al. [30], who reported an initial decrease in dissolution of phosphate molecules from Ca-P coatings in the presence of proteins with a high binding affinity. Combes et al. [31] investigated the interference of protein adsorption and HA maturation in detail and found that, depending on the concentration, serum albumin can exhibit a dual role and act as a promotor or inhibitor of nucleation and growth of (octa)Ca-P crystals. The energy needed for the first step in the precipitation process, nucleation, was lower when adsorbing molecules were present. Therefore, multiplication of nuclei occurred as a consequence of protein adsorption. The subsequent steps, growth to critical nuclei and formation of Ca-P crystals, were slowed down by a protein coating. However, at low serum albumin concentrations, the mineral surface could not be efficiently coated and crystal growth occurred faster than in the absence of albumin due to the larger number of nuclei and their greater reactivity. At high — physiological — serum albumin concentration, the mineral surface was efficiently coated slowing down the ionic diffusion to the crystal surface and inhibiting crystal growth [31].

38.5   Calcium Phosphate Ceramics for Bone Tissue Engineering

For reconstruction of large bone defects, implantation of osteoconductive porous scaffold materials alone is not sufficient for complete bone regeneration. Therefore, osteogenesis needs to be induced throughout the scaffold material. In the tissue engineering paradigm, osteogenic cells or osteoinductive macromolecules or both are being delivered to a suitable scaffold material. Many prerequisites have been postulated for the ideal scaffold material but none of the current materials meet all the demands. Porous ceramics are potential scaffold materials for bone tissue engineering due to their outstanding osteocompatible properties, especially with respect to osteoconduction and gradual resorption. In the recent years, a variety of researchers have investigated Ca-P ceramic scaffold materials for cellular as well as growth factor based tissue engineering.

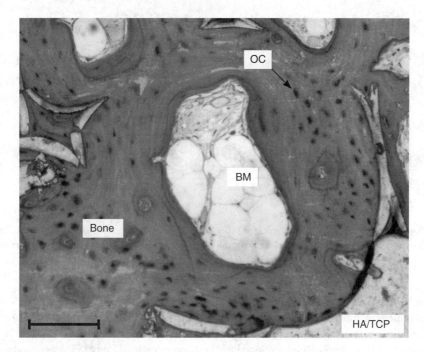

FIGURE 38.3 Bone formation in rat bone marrow stromal cell loaded porous HA/TCP implants (Camceram®), implanted in muscular flaps in rats for 8 weeks. Direct apposition of bone on the ceramic surface and bone marrow formation in the remaning porosity is observed. OC = osteocyte, BM = bone marrow. Bar represents 100 μm. Light microscopical undecalcified section stained with methylene blue and basic fuchsin (original magnification 10×). Printed with permission from Hartman et al. (Unpublished work, 2004).

38.5.1 Ca-P Ceramics and Osteogenic Cells

In 1988, Maniatopoulos et al. published a study on harvesting and culturing of rat bone marrow stromal cells (BMSCs) *in vitro* [32]. Through this method, the small number of undifferentiated progenitor cells present in bone marrow could be isolated, expanded, and differentiated into the osteoblastic lineage. Currently, the essence of this technique is still in use to administer osteoprogenitor cells to various scaffold materials for cell-based bone engineering. Many studies in rodent animal studies have shown the validity of this concept in conjunction with ceramic scaffold materials as coralline HA, porous HA, porous HA/β-TCP and porous β-TCP [33–38] (Figure 38.3). Less studies, however, have investigated the bone forming capacities of large BMSC loaded ceramic implants in higher mammals. This is in particular challenging, as the living constructs are transposed from ideal cell culture conditions to an *in vivo* environment where oxygen supply prior to capillary ingrowth is only provided by (limited) diffusion. Vitality of the BMSCs within ceramic scaffold material was shown to be essential for osteogenicity [39]. Despite the potential jeopardy of cell death, bone formation was observed in the studies investigating ectopic implants in dogs and goats [40,41], or critical size defects in dogs, goats, and sheep [41–46]. In most of these studies, bone formation was also observed in the center of the implants where the unloaded controls did not show osteogenesis. This indicates that possibly even a small number of surviving progenitor cells may be sufficient to result in significant bone formation. Also, it emphasizes that future tissue engineering research should also focus on multicomponent constructs, in which BMSCs are being combined with bone- and vasculature inducing growth factors.

38.5.2 Ca-P Ceramics and Osteoinductive Growth Factors

During the last decade, several strategies have been developed to deliver growth factors to the desired site. Basically, the proteins can be delivered directly via a carrier/delivery vehicle, or by gene therapy

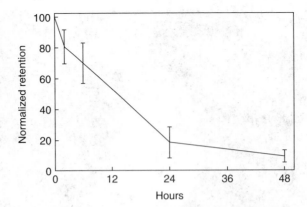

FIGURE 38.4   Retention of ^{131}I rhBMP-2 injected subcutaneously in rats. Over 80% of rhBMP-2 was cleared from the application site within 24 h, underlining the short residence time of rhBMP-2 after release from a carrier material. Error bars represent means $\pm$ standard deviation for $n = 6$.

techniques, in which a growth factor encoding gene is delivered to host cells via a viral factor or plasmid. Through this method, transfected cells start secreting growth factor. Cells can be transfected *in vitro*, prior to transplantation to the desired site, or directly *in vivo*. In this review, only direct delivery of proteins will be discussed as this approach has developed furthest and recently has led to FDA approval for specific clinical applications [47].

The growth factor loaded ceramic has a twofold function; first, it serves as a scaffold material, which enables and stimulates bone and blood vessel ingrowth; second, it serves as a carrier or delivery vehicle for the inductive factor, which should result in most favorable biopresentation and optimal activity of the protein. The role of ceramics on the bioactivity of growth factors is not completely clear. The ceramic might potentiate the activity of BMP by binding the protein and presenting it to target cells in a "bound" form [48,49]. On the other hand, the ceramic can act as vehicle for factor delivery to the surrounding tissues. Released protein may provide a supra-physiological concentration of free protein in the vicinity of the implant, what may attract target cells to the implant-site by chemotaxis [50]. It is hypothesized that for optimal bioactivity, initial burst release chemotactically recruits osteoprogenitor cells, and following sustained release — or retained factor — differentiates these cells toward the desired phenotype [51]. To our judgment, however, no convincing evidence provides further specification of this partition. Moreover, optimal pharmacokinetics are presumably specific for each surgical site.

38.5.2.1   Growth Factor Release from Ca-P Ceramics

The correlation between factor bioactivity and release or retention is a delicate issue. Since the protein needs to induce bone locally and not systemically, the released protein only has a short time to attract cells before it is being cleared from the application site. For example, a depot of 5 μg rhBMP-2 injected subcutaneously in the back in rats is cleared from the application site for more than 80% within 24 h (Figure 38.4). After clearance, the proteins are being metabolized by the body and excreted through the urinary tract [52]. The systemic exposure to released rhBMP-2 is reported to be neglectible [52].

The specific parameters resulting in protein release or retention are the driving factors behind the final clinical efficacy of a carrier system. Unfortunately, only few researchers have investigated these phenomena for ceramics. In a series of experiments in a rat ectopic model, Uludag et al. [53,54] have shown that growth factor retention depend on carrier- as well as on factor characteristics. Proteins with a higher isoelectric point (pI) show higher implant retention and higher retention of BMP yields higher osteoinductive activity. Various rhBMP-2 loaded ceramic implants (TCP cylinders and coral derived HA cylinders) show initial burst release of approximately 70% within three hours after implantation, which is followed by a slower second phase release and a final retention of approximately 6% of the initial dose after 14 days. In another study carried out by Louis-Ugbo et al. [52], initial burst release from HA/TCP granules (60 : 40) was less than 20% within the first day in a rabbit spinal fusion model. After 2 weeks 27 ± 9% of rhBMP-2 was still retained in this model. Li et al. [55] determined the release kinetics of rhBMP-2 mixed through Ca-P cement (α-BSM) and injected in a rabbit ulnar defect. Within the first day, approximately 40% of the initial factor was released. After 14 days, 15 ± 7% of the initial factor was still present in the cement. The differences in release and retention rates between these studies could be explained by variations in surgical site, dose, adsorption procedures, material surface area and chemico-physical interactions between material and growth factor. Overall, ceramics exhibit multiphasic release kinetics *in vivo* with a decrease of release in time and a certain retention for several weeks. It has been hypothesized, that ceramic surface area plays the key role in protein binding [56].

As previously mentioned, Ca-P ceramic materials show a high binding affinity for proteins. Conformational changes of proteins upon adsorption on Ca-P surface have been observed [30]. Protein conformation is of great importance for the accessibility of the specific binding sites and subsequent protein-cell interaction [57,58]. As a result, protein-biomaterial bonding may directly effect the protein's intrinsic function due to orientation or conformational changes. To evaluate the bioactivity of retained proteins, cells can be cultured on the surface of protein loaded ceramics *in vitro* [59]. A complicating factor is that no material exhibits a 100% retention [54]. For a true differentiation between activity expressed by retained protein vs. presently released protein, control groups have to correct for the released fraction bioactivity. In an *in vitro* model, Santos et al. [59] investigated the bioactivity of rhBMP-2 adsorbed onto a Ca-P layer on bioactive glass-gel (Xerogel S70) in comparison with the activity of "free" rhBMP-2 present in cell culture medium. The osteogenic response of osteoblast like cells seeded on the Ca-P surface was found significantly higher in the adsorbed rhBMP-2 group. The authors suggested that the biomaterial could generate, maintain, or even concentrate an effective level of growth factor.

38.5.2.2   Growth Factor Loading in Ca-P Ceramics

In view of the previous paragraph, discern has to be made between proteins/growth factors adsorbed at the ceramic surface and proteins/growth factors mixed through the material during preparation. For sintered ceramic materials, the latter is impossible as sintering temperatures would result in complete protein destruction. For the self setting Ca-P cements though, mixing of proteins during setting reaction has been described [60–62]. Due to physical entrapment by cement particles, the majority of the protein binding sites will be unavailable until the protein is released from the cement. This situation is quite similar to bioactive macromolecules entrapped in polymeric drug delivery vehicles, where protein release is the main focus [63–68]. However, a frequently neglected issue is that mixing of proteins through ceramics can influence the crystallization process during the setting reaction. This can modify the *in vivo* dissolution and/or degradation properties of the formed material.

For the growth factors entrapped within a Ca-P ceramic material, bioactivity is likewise expected only after release from its carrier. Bioactivity of released protein can be demonstrated through *in vitro* models where sensible cells are being exposed to the released protein [55,64,68]. To evaluate loss of activity, the induced biological response should be compared to the response to similar protein directly suspended in the culture medium [55]. *In vivo*, however, this comparison is difficult and most authors just examine whether or not the protein expresses (part of its) bioactivity.

38.5.2.3   Osteoinductive Capacity of Growth Factor Loaded Ca-P Ceramics

Osteogenic differentiation induced by BMPs is dependent on the regulating growth factor as well as on the carrier specifications. Murata et al. [69] observed that in a synthetic HA carrier, BMP induced ossification was predominantly intramembranous, whereas enchondral bone formation was observed in a nonceramic carrier. Direct bone formation on BMP loaded Ca-P ceramics was also observed by others [70–73].

However, the osteogenic behavior of growth factor loaded Ca-P ceramics is not as straightforward as suggested, because a wide variety of material compositions, animal models, surgical sites and factor dosage have been used in various studies. Another complicating factor is that physiological bone regeneration is induced by a cascade of growth factors, whereas most tissue engineered concepts investigate osteoinduction by single factors only. Consequently, most research in the recent years has focused on BMPs, like rhBMP-2

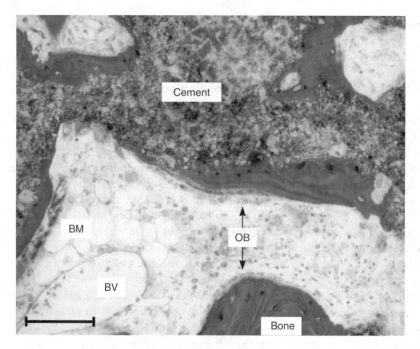

FIGURE 38.5 Bone formation in rhBMP-2 loaded porous Ca-P cement implants, implanted subcutaneously in rabbits for 10 weeks. Macroporosity in the cement (Calcibon®, Biomet Merck, Darmstadt, Germany) was induced by formation of CO_2 during setting of the cement, after which a dosage of 5 μg rhBMP-2 was applied. OB = osteoblasts, BM = bone marrow, BV = blood vessel. Bar represents 100 μm. Light microscopical undecalcified section stained with methylene blue and basic fuchsin (original magnification 10×). (From Kroese-Deutman, H.C., Ruhe, P.Q., Spauwen, P.H., and Jansen, J.A. *Biomaterials*, in press: 2004. With permission.)

and rhBMP-7 (OP-1). Due to the numerous parameters, there is no such thing as one ideal dosage or scaffold composition. Most animal studies investigating growth factor loaded ceramics have been carried out in smaller animals as rats [9,10,53,54,69,70,72,74–78] and rabbits [52,55,73,79–85] (Figure 38.5) whereas only few studies were performed in larger animals as minipigs [86,87], dogs [71,88,89], and primates [90–92]. Generally speaking for all carrier materials, the relative dosage of growth factor needed for bone induction raises with the animal size [51]. However, the dosages applied to ceramics vary substantially within similar animal models as well as between different species. For rhBMP-2, dosages applied for effective osteoinduction varied from 0.03 to 0.46 mg/ml implants in rats [9,54,75] to 0.004 to 2.1 mg/ml implant in rabbits [55,73,80,81,83,85], whereas in canine and primate models dosages have been used from 0.15 to 1.2 mg/ml [71] and 1.35 to 2.7 mg/ml [92] respectively. A dose–response relation for BMP loaded ceramics has been reported in some studies in rodents [75,80,83], but was absent or even reciprocal in studies with larger animal models [71,91,92]. Yet, it seems likely that in the dose–response relation, there is first a certain threshold dosage to achieve consistent results [92], followed by a linear dose–response interval and finalized by a certain saturation effect.

Besides BMPs, other growth factors like transforming growth factor-β (TGF-β) and insulin-like growth factor-I (IGF-I) have been investigated. TGF-β may potentiate the osteoinductivity of BMPs, but its overall osteoinductive capacity when applied alone is weak compared to BMPs [93]. IGF-I has also been applied to TCP ceramic carriers, which resulted in increased osteogenesis in an orthotopic implantation site four weeks after implantation [94]. Similarly, Damien et al. [95] reported that IGF-I loaded porous hydroxyapatite accelerated orthotopic bone ingrowth during an implantation period up to three weeks.

The synergism of various growth factors, as present in the physiological bone regeneration cascade, has only been investigated in few studies with Ca-P ceramics. Ono et al. investigated the role of prostaglandin E_1 (PGE_1) and basic fibroblast growth factor (bFGF) loaded on porous hydroxyapatite and observed that PGE$_1$ as well as bFGF acted synergistically with rhBMP-2 [80,83,96]. Meraw et al. prepared a true growth factor cocktail and reported that orthotopic bone formation in a canine model was enhanced by a combination of extremely low dosages of TGF-β, bFGF, BMP-2, and PDGF mixed through a calcium phosphate cement [89].

38.6   Conclusion and Future Perspective

Like all scaffolds materials currently under investigation for bone tissue engineering applications, Ca-P ceramics reveal both advantages and disadvantages. Intrinsic brittleness of Ca-P ceramics unquestionably is the greatest shortcoming of these materials, whereas their biocompatibility, osteoconductivity and resorption potential are virtues of an ideal scaffold material. Future research should further clarify the importance of release and retention of growth factors, optimize their delivery and investigate dose–response relation for the various factors and applications. Furthermore, the potentials of multicomponent constructs, in which various bone- and vasculature inducing growth factors or cultured bone marrow stromal cells or both are being combined, should be investigated to come to a successful alternative for autologous bone grafting.

References

[1] LeGeros, R.Z. Properties of osteoconductive biomaterials: calcium phosphates. *Clin. Orthop.* 81–98, 2002.

[2] Dorozhkin, S.V. and Epple, M. Biological and medical significance of calcium phosphates. *Angew. Chem. Int. Ed. Engl.* 41: 3130–3146, 2002.

[3] Eanes, E.D. Amorphous calcium phosphate. *Monogr. Oral Sci.* 18: 130–147, 2001.

[4] LeGeros, R.Z. Calcium phosphates in oral biology and medicine. *Monogr. Oral Sci.* 15: 1–201, 1991.

[5] Vaccaro, A.R. The role of the osteoconductive scaffold in synthetic bone graft. *Orthopedics* 25: s571–s578, 2002.

[6] Ravaglioli, A. and Krajewski, A. *Bioceramics.* London: Chapman & Hall, 1992.

[7] Le Huec, J.C., Schaeverbeke, T., Clement, D., Faber, J., and Le Rebeller, A. Influence of porosity on the mechanical resistance of hydroxyapatite ceramics under compressive stress. *Biomaterials* 16: 113–118, 1995.

[8] Yuan, H., Kurashina, K., de Bruijn, J.D., Li, Y., de Groot, K., and Zhang, X. A preliminary study on osteoinduction of two kinds of calcium phosphate ceramics. *Biomaterials* 20: 1799–1806, 1999.

[9] Tsuruga, E., Takita, H., Itoh, H., Wakisaka, Y., and Kuboki, Y. Pore size of porous hydroxyapatite as the cell-substratum controls BMP-induced osteogenesis. *J. Biochem. (Tokyo)* 121: 317–324, 1997.

[10] Kuboki, Y., Jin, Q., and Takita, H. Geometry of carriers controlling phenotypic expression in BMP-induced osteogenesis and chondrogenesis. *J. Bone Joint Surg. Am.* 83-A (Suppl 1): 105–115, 2001.

[11] Ripamonti, U., Crooks, J., and Kirkbride, A.N. Sintered porous hydroxyapatites with intrinsic osteoinductive activity: geometric induction of bone formation. *S. Afr. J. Sci.* 95: 335–343, 1999.

[12] Ripamonti, U. Smart biomaterials with intrinsic osteoinductivity: Geometric control of bone differentiation. In *Bone Engineering*, ed. Davies, J.E., Toronto: EM Squared Incorporated, 2000, pp. 215–222.

[13] Jansen, J.A., Wolke, J.G., Swann, S., van der Waerden, J.P., and de Groot, K. Application of magnetron sputtering for producing ceramic coatings on implant materials. *Clin. Oral. Implants Res.* 4: 28–34, 1993.

[14] Roy, D.M. and Linnehan, S.K. Hydroxyapatite formed from coral skeletal carbonate by hydrothermal exchange. *Nature* 247: 220–222, 1974.

[15] Truumees, E. and Herkowitz, H.N. Alternatives to autologous bone harvest in spine surgery. *Univ. Penn. Orthop. J.* 12: 77–88, 1999.

[16] Brown, W.E. and Chow, L.C. Dental restorative cement pastes. U.S. Patent (4,518,430), 1985.

[17] Chow, L.C. Calcium phosphate cements. *Monogr. Oral Sci.* 18: 148–163, 2001.

[18] Schmitz, J.P., Hollinger, J.O., and Milam, S.B. Reconstruction of bone using calcium phosphate bone cements: a critical review. *J. Oral Maxillofac. Surg.* 57: 1122–1126, 1999.

[19] Ooms, E.M., Wolke, J.G., van de Heuvel, M.T., Jeschke, B., and Jansen, J.A. Histological evaluation of the bone response to calcium phosphate cement implanted in cortical bone. *Biomaterials* 24: 989–1000, 2003.

[20] Comuzzi, L., Ooms, E., and Jansen, J.A. Injectable calcium phosphate cement as a filler for bone defects around oral implants: an experimental study in goats. *Clin. Oral Implants Res.* 13: 304–311, 2002.

[21] Ooms, E.M., Wolke, J.G., van der Waerden, J.P., and Jansen, J.A. Trabecular bone response to injectable calcium phosphate (Ca-P) cement. *J. Biomed. Mater. Res.* 61: 9–18, 2002.

[22] Driessens, F.C., Boltong, M.G., Bermudez, O., and Planell, J.A. Formulation and setting times of some calcium orthophosphate cements: a pilot study. *J. Mater. Sci. Mater. Med.* 4: 503–508, 1993.

[23] Ishikawa, K., Takagi, S., Chow, L.C., Ishikawa, Y., Eanes, E.D., and Asaoka, K. Behavior of a calcium phosphate cement in simulated blood plasma *in vitro. Dent. Mater.* 10: 26–32, 1994.

[24] Takagi, S., Chow, L.C., Markovic, M., Friedman, C.D., and Costantino, P.D. Morphological and phase characterizations of retrieved calcium phosphate cement implants. *J. Biomed. Mater. Res.* 58: 36–41, 2001.

[25] Ducheyne, P. and Qiu, Q. Bioactive ceramics: the effect of surface reactivity on bone formation and bone cell function. *Biomaterials* 20: 2287–2303, 1999.

[26] Davies, J.E. Mechanisms of endosseous integration. *Int. J. Prosthodont.* 11: 391–401, 1998.

[27] Rosengren, A., Pavlovic, E., Oscarsson, S., Krajewski, A., Ravaglioli, A., and Piancastelli, A. Plasma protein adsorption pattern on characterized ceramic biomaterials. *Biomaterials* 23: 1237–1247, 2002.

[28] Rosengren, A., Oscarsson, S., Mazzocchi, M., Krajewski, A., and Ravaglioli, A. Protein adsorption onto two bioactive glass-ceramics. *Biomaterials* 24: 147–155, 2003.

[29] Radin, S., Ducheyne, P., Berthold, P., and Decker, S. Effect of serum proteins and osteoblasts on the surface transformation of a calcium phosphate coating: a physicochemical and ultrastructural study. *J. Biomed. Mater. Res.* 39: 234–243, 1998.

[30] Ong, J.L., Chittur, K.K., and Lucas, L.C. Dissolution/reprecipitation and protein adsorption studies of calcium phosphate coatings by FT-IR/ATR techniques. *J. Biomed. Mater. Res.* 28: 1337–1346, 1994.

[31] Combes, C. and Rey, C. Adsorption of proteins and calcium phosphate materials bioactivity. *Biomaterials* 23: 2817–2823, 2002.

[32] Maniatopoulos, C., Sodek, J., and Melcher, A.H. Bone formation *in vitro* by stromal cells obtained from bone marrow of young adult rats. *Cell Tissue Res.* 254: 317–330, 1988.

[33] Hanada, K., Dennis, J.E., and Caplan, A.I. Stimulatory effects of basic fibroblast growth factor and bone morphogenetic protein-2 on osteogenic differentiation of rat bone marrow-derived mesenchymal stem cells. *J. Bone Miner. Res.* 12: 1606–1614, 1997.

[34] Okumura, M., Ohgushi, H., Dohi, Y., Katuda, T., Tamai, S., Koerten, H.K., and Tabata, S. Osteoblastic phenotype expression on the surface of hydroxyapatite ceramics. *J. Biomed. Mater. Res.* 37: 122–129, 1997.

[35] Boo, J.S., Yamada, Y., Okazaki, Y., Hibino, Y., Okada, K., Hata, K., Yoshikawa, T., Sugiura, Y., and Ueda, M. Tissue-engineered bone using mesenchymal stem cells and a biodegradable scaffold. *J. Craniofac. Surg.* 13: 231–239, 2002.

[36] Dong, J., Uemura, T., Shirasaki, Y., and Tateishi, T. Promotion of bone formation using highly pure porous beta-TCP combined with bone marrow-derived osteoprogenitor cells. *Biomaterials* 23: 4493–4502, 2002.

[37] Uemura, T., Dong, J., Wang, Y., Kojima, H., Saito, T., Iejima, D., Kikuchi, M., Tanaka, J., and Tateishi, T. Transplantation of cultured bone cells using combinations of scaffolds and culture techniques. *Biomaterials* 24: 2277–2286, 2003.

[38] Hartman, E.H., Ruhe, P.Q., Spauwen, P.H., and Jansen, J.A. Ectopic bone formation in rats: comparison of biphasic ceramic implants seeded with cultured rat bone marrow cells in a pedicled and a revascularised muscle flap. Unpublished work, 2004.

[39] Kruyt, M.C., de Bruijn, J.D., Wilson, C.E., Oner, F.C., van Blitterswijk, C.A., Verbout, A.J., and Dhert, W.J. Viable osteogenic cells are obligatory for tissue-engineered ectopic bone formation in goats. *Tissue Eng.* 9: 327–336, 2003.

[40] Kadiyala, S., Young, R.G., Thiede, M.A., and Bruder, S.P. Culture expanded canine mesenchymal stem cells possess osteochondrogenic potential *in vivo* and *in vitro*. *Cell Transplant* 6: 125–134, 1997.

[41] Kruyt, M.C., Dhert, W.J., Yuan, H., Wilson, C.E., van Blitterswijk, C.A., Verbout, A.J., and de Bruijn, J.D. Bone tissue engineering in a critical size defect compared to ectopic implantations in the goat. *J. Orthop. Res.* 22: 544–551, 2004.

[42] Schliephake, H., Knebel, J.W., Aufderheide, M., and Tauscher, M. Use of cultivated osteoprogenitor cells to increase bone formation in segmental mandibular defects: an experimental pilot study in sheep. *Int. J. Oral Maxillofac. Surg.* 30: 531–537, 2001.

[43] Bruder, S.P., Kraus, K.H., Goldberg, V.M., and Kadiyala, S. The effect of implants loaded with autologous mesenchymal stem cells on the healing of canine segmental bone defects. *J. Bone Joint Surg. Am.* 80: 985–996, 1998.

[44] Kon, E., Muraglia, A., Corsi, A., Bianco, P., Marcacci, M., Martin, I., Boyde, A., Ruspantini, I., Chistolini, P., Rocca, M., Giardino, R., Cancedda, R., and Quarto, R. Autologous bone marrow stromal cells loaded onto porous hydroxyapatite ceramic accelerate bone repair in critical-size defects of sheep long bones. *J. Biomed. Mater. Res.* 49: 328–337, 2000.

[45] Petite, H., Viateau, V., Bensaid, W., Meunier, A., De Pollak, C, Bourguignon, M., Oudina, K., Sedel, L., and Guillemin, G. Tissue-engineered bone regeneration. *Nat. Biotechnol.* 18: 959–963, 2000.

[46] Shang, Q., Wang, Z., Liu, W., Shi, Y., Cui, L., and Cao, Y. Tissue-engineered bone repair of sheep cranial defects with autologous bone marrow stromal cells. *J. Craniofac. Surg.* 12: 586–593, 2001.

[47] Nakashima, M. and Reddi, A.H. The application of bone morphogenetic proteins to dental tissue engineering. *Nat. Biotechnol.* 21: 1025–1032, 2003.

[48] Reddi, A.H. and Cunningham, N.S. Initiation and promotion of bone differentiation by bone morphogenetic proteins. *J. Bone Miner. Res.* 8: 499–502, 1993.

[49] Uludag, H., Gao, T., Porter, T.J., Friess, W., and Wozney, J.M. Delivery systems for BMPs: factors contributing to protein retention at an application site. *J. Bone Joint Surg. Am.* 83-A: 128–135, 2001.

[50] Cunningham, N.S., Paralkar, V., and Reddi, A.H. Osteogenin and recombinant bone morphogenetic protein 2B are chemotactic for human monocytes and stimulate transforming growth factor beta 1 mRNA expression. *Proc. Natl Acad. Sci. USA* 89: 11740–11744, 1992.

[51] Li, R.H. and Wozney, J.M. Delivering on the promise of bone morphogenetic proteins. *Trends Biotechnol.* 19: 255–265, 2001.

[52] Louis-Ugbo, J., Kim, H.S., Boden, S.D., Mayr, M.T., Li, R.C., Seeherman, H., D'Augusta, D., Blake, C., Jiao, A., and Peckham, S. Retention of 125I-labeled recombinant human bone morphogenetic protein-2 by biphasic calcium phosphate or a composite sponge in a rabbit posterolateral spine arthrodesis model. *J. Orthop. Res.* 20: 1050–1059, 2002.

[53] Uludag, H., D'Augusta, D., Golden, J., Li, J., Timony, G., Riedel, R., and Wozney, J.M. Implantation of recombinant human bone morphogenetic proteins with biomaterial carriers: a correlation between protein pharmacokinetics and osteoinduction in the rat ectopic model. *J. Biomed. Mater. Res.* 50: 227–238, 2000.

[54] Uludag, H., D'Augusta, D., Palmer, R., Timony, G., and Wozney, J. Characterization of rhBMP-2 pharmacokinetics implanted with biomaterial carriers in the rat ectopic model. *J. Biomed. Mater. Res.* 46: 193–202, 1999.

[55] Li, R.H., Bouxsein, M.L., Blake, C.A., D'Augusta, D., Kim, H., Li, X.J., Wozney, J.M., and Seeherman, H.J. rhBMP-2 injected in a calcium phosphate paste (alpha-BSM) accelerates healing in the rabbit ulnar osteotomy model. *J. Orthop. Res.* 21: 997–1004, 2003.

[56] Herr, G., Hartwig, C.H., Boll, C., and Kusswetter, W. Ectopic bone formation by composites of BMP and metal implants in rats. *Acta Orthop. Scand.* 67: 606–610, 1996.

[57] Kirsch, T., Sebald, W., and Dreyer, M.K. Crystal structure of the BMP-2-BRIA ectodomain complex. *Nat. Struct. Biol.* 7: 492–496, 2000.

[58] Nickel, J., Dreyer, M.K., Kirsch, T., and Sebald, W. The crystal structure of the BMP-2 : BMPR-IA complex and the generation of BMP-2 antagonists. *J. Bone Joint Surg. Am.* 83-A: 7–14, 2001.

[59] Santos, E.M., Radin, S., Shenker, B.J., Shapiro, I.M., and Ducheyne, P. Si–Ca–P xerogels and bone morphogenetic protein act synergistically on rat stromal marrow cell differentiation *in vitro*. *J. Biomed. Mater. Res.* 41: 87–94, 1998.

[60] Blom, E.J., Klein-Nulend, J., Yin, L., van Waas, M.A., and Burger, E.H. Transforming growth factor-beta1 incorporated in calcium phosphate cement stimulates osteotransductivity in rat calvarial bone defects. *Clin. Oral Implants Res.* 12: 609–616, 2001.

[61] Lee, D.D., Tofighi, A., Aiolova, M., Chakravarthy, P., Catalano, A., Majahad, A., and Knaack, D. Alpha-BSM: a biomimetic bone substitute and drug delivery vehicle. *Clin. Orthop.* 396–405, 1999.

[62] Li, R.H., D'Augusta, D., Blake, C., Bouxsein, M., Wozney, J.M., Li, J., Stevens, M., Kim, H., and Seeherman, H. rhBMP-2 delivery and efficacy in an injectable calcium phosphate based matrix. *The 28th International Symposium on Controlled Release of Bioactive Materials,* San Diego, 2001.

[63] Isobe, M., Yamazaki, Y., Oida, S., Ishihara, K., Nakabayashi, N., and Amagasa, T. Bone morphogenetic protein encapsulated with a biodegradable and biocompatible polymer. *J. Biomed. Mater. Res.* 32: 433–438, 1996.

[64] Lu, L., Yaszemski, M.J., and Mikos, A.G. TGF-beta1 release from biodegradable polymer microparticles: its effects on marrow stromal osteoblast function. *J. Bone Joint Surg. Am.* 83-A (Suppl 1): 82–91, 2001.

[65] Miyamoto, S., Takaoka, K., Okada, T., Yoshikawa, H., Hashimoto, J., Suzuki, S., and Ono, K. Polylactic acid–polyethylene glycol block copolymer. A new biodegradable synthetic carrier for bone morphogenetic protein. *Clin. Orthop.* 333–343, 1993.

[66] Oldham, J.B., Lu, L., Zhu, X., Porter, B.D., Hefferan, T.E., Larson, D.R., Currier, B.L., Mikos, A.G., and Yaszemski, M.J. Biological activity of rhBMP-2 released from PLGA microspheres. *J. Biomech. Eng.* 122: 289–292, 2000.

[67] Pean, J.M., Venier-Julienne, M.C., Boury, F., Menei, P., Denizot, B., and Benoit, J.P. NGF release from poly(D,L-lactide-co-glycolide) microspheres. Effect of some formulation parameters on encapsulated NGF stability. *J. Control. Release.* 56: 175–187, 1998.

[68] Peter, S.J., Lu, L., Kim, D.J., Stamatas, G.N., Miller, M.J., Yaszemski, M.J., and Mikos, A.G. Effects of transforming growth factor beta1 released from biodegradable polymer microparticles on marrow stromal osteoblasts cultured on poly(propylene fumarate) substrates. *J. Biomed. Mater. Res.* 50: 452–462, 2000.

[69] Murata, M., Inoue, M., Arisue, M., Kuboki, Y., and Nagai, N. Carrier-dependency of cellular differentiation induced by bone morphogenetic protein in ectopic sites. *Int. J. Oral Maxillofac. Surg.* 27: 391–396, 1998.

[70] Ripamonti, U., Ma, S., and Reddi, A.H. The critical role of geometry of porous hydroxyapatite delivery system in induction of bone by osteogenin, a bone morphogenetic protein. *Matrix* 12: 202–212, 1992.

[71] Sumner, D.R., Turner, T.M., Urban, R.M., Turek, T., Seeherman, H., and Wozney, J.M. Locally delivered rhBMP-2 enhances bone ingrowth and gap healing in a canine model. *J. Orthop. Res.* 22: 58–65, 2004.

[72] Kuboki, Y., Saito, T., Murata, M., Takita, H., Mizuno, M., Inoue, M., Nagai, N., and Poole, A.R. Two distinctive BMP-carriers induce zonal chondrogenesis and membranous ossification, respectively; geometrical factors of matrices for cell-differentiation. *Connect. Tissue. Res.* 32: 219–226, 1995.

[73] Kroese-Deutman, H.C., Ruhe, P.Q., Spauwen P.H., and Jansen J.A. Bone inductive properties of rhBMP-2 loaded porous calcium phosphate cement implants inserted at an ectopic site in rabbits. *Biomaterials* 26: 1131–1138, 2005.

[74] Kuboki, Y., Takita, H., Kobayashi, D., Tsuruga, E., Inoue, M., Murata, M., Nagai, N., Dohi, Y., and Ohgushi, H. BMP-induced osteogenesis on the surface of hydroxyapatite with geometrically feasible and nonfeasible structures: topology of osteogenesis. *J. Biomed. Mater. Res.* 39: 190–199, 1998.

[75] Ohura, K., Hamanishi, C., Tanaka, S., and Matsuda, N. Healing of segmental bone defects in rats induced by a beta-TCP-MCPM cement combined with rhBMP-2. *J. Biomed. Mater. Res.* 44: 168–175, 1999.

[76] Glass, D.A., Mellonig, J.T., and Towle, H.J. Histologic evaluation of bone inductive proteins complexed with coralline hydroxylapatite in an extraskeletal site of the rat. *J. Periodontol.* 60: 121–126, 1989.

[77] Herr, G., Wahl, D., and Kusswetter, W. Osteogenic activity of bone morphogenetic protein and hydroxyapatite composite implants. *Ann. Chir. Gynaecol. Suppl.* 207: 99–107, 1993.

[78] Clarke, S.A., Brooks, R.A., Lee, P.T., and Rushton, N. Bone growth into a ceramic-filled defect around an implant. The response to transforming growth factor beta1. *J. Bone Joint Surg. Br.* 86: 126–134, 2004.

[79] Ono, I., Ohura, T., Murata, M., Yamaguchi, H., Ohnuma, Y., and Kuboki, Y. A study on bone induction in hydroxyapatite combined with bone morphogenetic protein. *Plast. Reconstr. Surg.* 90: 870–879, 1992.

[80] Ono, I., Inoue, M., and Kuboki, Y. Promotion of the osteogenetic activity of recombinant human bone morphogenetic protein by prostaglandin E1. *Bone* 19: 581–588, 1996.

[81] Ono, I., Gunji, H., Kaneko, F., Saito, T., and Kuboki, Y. Efficacy of hydroxyapatite ceramic as a carrier for recombinant human bone morphogenetic protein. *J. Craniofac. Surg.* 6: 238–244, 1995.

[82] Ono, I., Gunji, H., Suda, K., Kaneko, F., Murata, M., Saito, T., and Kuboki, Y. Bone induction of hydroxyapatite combined with bone morphogenetic protein and covered with periosteum. *Plast. Reconstr. Surg.* 95: 1265–1272, 1995.

[83] Ono, I., Tateshita, T., and Kuboki, Y. Prostaglandin E1 and recombinant bone morphogenetic protein effect on strength of hydroxyapatite implants. *J. Biomed. Mater. Res.* 45: 337–344, 1999.

[84] Koempel, J.A., Patt, B.S., O'Grady, K., Wozney, J., and Toriumi, D.M. The effect of recombinant human bone morphogenetic protein-2 on the integration of porous hydroxyapatite implants with bone. *J. Biomed. Mater. Res.* 41: 359–363, 1998.

[85] Ruhe, P.Q., Kroese-Deutman, H.C., Wolke, J.G., Spauwen, P.H., and Jansen, J.A. Bone inductive properties of rhBMP-2 loaded porous calcium phosphate cement implants in cranial defects in rabbits. *Biomaterials* 25: 2123–2132, 2004.

[86] Terheyden, H., Warnke, P., Dunsche, A., Jepsen, S., Brenner, W., Palmie, S., Toth, C., and Rueger, D.R. Mandibular reconstruction with prefabricated vascularized bone grafts using recombinant human osteogenic protein-1: an experimental study in miniature pigs. Part II: transplantation. *Int. J. Oral Maxillofac. Surg.* 30: 469–478, 2001.

[87] Terheyden, H., Knak, C., Jepsen, S., Palmie, S., and Rueger, D.R. Mandibular reconstruction with a prefabricated vascularized bone graft using recombinant human osteogenic protein-1: an experimental study in miniature pigs. Part I: prefabrication. *Int. J. Oral Maxillofac. Surg.* 30: 373–379, 2001.

[88] Sumner, D.R., Turner, T.M., Purchio, A.F., Gombotz, W.R., Urban, R.M., and Galante, J.O. Enhancement of bone ingrowth by transforming growth factor-beta. *J. Bone Joint Surg. Am.* 77: 1135–1147, 1995.

[89] Meraw, S.J., Reeve, C.M., Lohse, C.M., and Sioussat, T.M. Treatment of peri-implant defects with combination growth factor cement. *J. Periodontol.* 71: 8–13, 2000.

[90] Ripamonti, U., Ramoshebi, L.N., Matsaba, T., Tasker, J., Crooks, J., and Teare, J. Bone induction by BMPs/OPs and related family members in primates. *J. Bone Joint Surg. Am.* 83-A (Suppl 1): 116–127, 2001.

[91] Ripamonti, U., Crooks, J., and Rueger, D.C. Induction of bone formation by recombinant human osteogenic protein-1 and sintered porous hydroxyapatite in adult primates. *Plast. Reconstr. Surg.* 107: 977–988, 2001.

[92] Boden, S.D., Martin, G.J., Jr., Morone, M.A., Ugbo, J.L., and Moskovitz, P.A. Posterolateral lumbar intertransverse process spine arthrodesis with recombinant human bone morphogenetic protein 2/hydroxyapatite-tricalcium phosphate after laminectomy in the nonhuman primate. *Spine* 24: 1179–1185, 1999.

[93] Lane, J.M., Tomin, E., and Bostrom, M.P. Biosynthetic bone grafting. *Clin. Orthop.* 107–117, 1999.

[94] Laffargue, P., Fialdes, P., Frayssinet, P., Rtaimate, M., Hildebrand, H.F., and Marchandise, X. Adsorption and release of insulin-like growth factor-I on porous tricalcium phosphate implant. *J. Biomed. Mater. Res.* 49: 415–421, 2000.

[95] Damien, E., Hing, K., Saeed, S., and Revell, P.A. A preliminary study on the enhancement of the osteointegration of a novel synthetic hydroxyapatite scaffold *in vivo*. *J. Biomed. Mater. Res.* 66A: 241–246, 2003.

[96] Ono, I., Tateshita, T., Takita, H., and Kuboki, Y. Promotion of the osteogenetic activity of recombinant human bone morphogenetic protein by basic fibroblast growth factor. *J. Craniofac. Surg.* 7: 418–425, 1996.

39

Biomimetic Materials

Andrés J. García
Georgia Institute of Technology

Over the last decade, considerable advances in the engineering of biomaterials that elicit specific cellular responses have been attained by exploiting biomolecular recognition. These biomimetic engineering approaches focus on integrating recognition and structural motifs from biological macromolecules with synthetic and natural substrates to generate bio-inspired, biofunctional materials. These strategies represent a paradigm shift in biomaterials development from conventional approaches which deal with purely synthetic or natural materials, and provide promising schemes for the development of novel bioactive substrates for enhanced tissue replacement and regeneration. Because of the central roles that extracellular matrices (ECMs) play in tissue morphogenesis, homeostasis, and repair, these natural scaffolds provide several attractive characteristics worthy of "copying" or mimicking to convey functionality for molecular control of cell function, tissue structure, and regeneration. Four ECM "themes" have been targeted (i) motifs to promote cell adhesion, (ii) growth factor binding sites that control presentation and delivery, (iii) protease-sensitive sequences for controlled degradation, and (iv) structural motifs to convey mechanical properties.

39.1 Extracellular Matrices: Nature's Engineered Scaffolds

ECMs comprise a complex, insoluble, three-dimensional mixture of secreted macromolecules, including collagens and noncollagenous proteins, such as elastin and fibronectin, glycosaminoglycans, and proteoglycans that are present between cells. In addition, provisional fibrin-based networks constitute specialized matrices for wound healing and tissue repair. ECMs function to provide structure and order in the extracellular space and regulate multiple functions associated with the establishment, maintenance, and remodeling of differentiated tissues [1]. Matrix components, such as fibronectin and laminin, mediate adhesive interactions that support anchorage, migration, and tissue organization and activate signaling pathways directing cell survival, proliferation, and differentiation. ECM components also interact with growth and differentiation factors, chemotropic agents, and other soluble factors that regulate cell cycle progression and differentiation to control their availability and activity. By immobilizing and ordering these ligands, ECMs control the spatial and temporal profiles of these signals and generate gradients necessary for vectorial responses. Moreover, structural elements within ECMs, namely collagens, elastin, and proteoglycans, contribute to the mechanical integrity, rigidity, and viscoelasticity of skin, cartilage, vasculature, and other tissues. Finally, the composition and structure of ECMs are dynamically modulated by the cells within them, reflecting the highly regulated and bidirectional communication between cells and ECMs.

39.2 Bioadhesive Materials

Following the identification of adhesion motifs in ECM components, such as the arginine–glycine–aspartic acid (RGD) tri-peptide for fibronectin [2] and tyrosine–isoleucine–glycine–serine–arginine (YIGSR) oligopeptide for laminin [3], numerous groups have tethered short bioadhesive peptides onto synthetic or natural substrates and three-dimensional scaffolds to produce biofunctional materials that bind adhesion receptors and promote adhesion and migration in various cell types (as reviewed in References 4 to 6) (Figure 39.1). Nonfouling supports, such as poly(ethylene glycol), poly(acrylamide), and alginate, are often used to reduce nonspecific protein adsorption and background adhesion. The density of tethered peptide is an important design parameter as cell adhesion, focal adhesion assembly, spreading and migration [7–10], neurite extension and neural differenitiation [11,12], smooth muscle cell activities [13], and osteoblast and myoblast differentiation [14,15] exhibit peptide density-dependent effects. More importantly, tethering of bioadhesive ligands onto biomaterial surfaces and scaffolds enhances *in vivo* responses, such as bone formation and integration [16–18], nerve regeneration [19,20], and corneal tissue repair [21].

These results indicate that functionalization of biomaterials with short adhesive oligopeptides significantly enhances cellular activities. In addition to conveying biospecificity while avoiding unwanted interactions with other regions of the native ligand, short bioadhesive peptides allow facile incorporation into synthetic backbones and enhanced stability of the tethered motif. These strategies, however, are limited by (i) low activity of oligopeptides compared to native ligand due to the absence of modulatory domains, (ii) limited specificity for adhesion receptors and cell types, and (iii) inability to bind certain receptors due to conformational differences compared to the native ligand. Conformationally constrained (e.g., cyclic) RGD [22], oligopeptides mixtures [23,24], and recombinant protein fragments spanning the binding domains of native ligands [25]

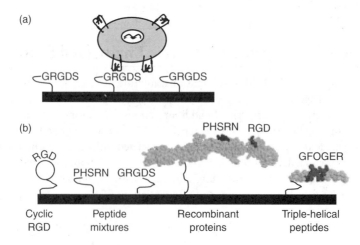

FIGURE 39.1 Biomimetic materials supporting cell adhesion. (a) Basic strategy focusing on RGD tethering to promote binding of cell adhesion receptors. (b) Biomolecular approaches to improve ligand activity and specificity.

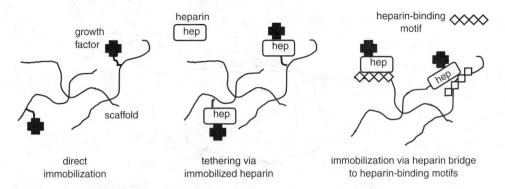

FIGURE 39.2 Biomimetic strategies for controlled growth factor interactions.

have been explored to improve ligand activity. Similarly, substrates presenting RGD in combination with other peptides, such as heparan sulfate-binding lyrine–arginine–serine–arginine (KRSR) [26] and Phenylalanine–histidine–arginine–arginine–isoleucine–lysine–alanine (FHRRIKA) [27], display improved cell adhesion and selectivity over materials modified with RGD alone. Finally, self-assembling peptides reconstituting the triple helical structure of type I collagen have been used to target collagen integrin receptors and promote enhanced osteoblastic differentiation and mineralization on biomaterial supports [28,29]. The improved activity and selectivity of these "second generation" biomolecular materials are expected to reconstitute additional features of natural ECMs and promote enhanced cellular activities.

39.3   Materials Engineered to Interact with Growth Factors

Natural ECMs interact with soluble growth and differentiation factors to control their activity by regulating their presentation, delivery kinetics, and stability [1]. Three general strategies have been pursued to convey growth factor activity to synthetic materials (Figure 39.2). Covalent immobilization of growth factors onto biomaterial supports, either via conventional peptide chemistry or enzymatic cross-linking, results in enhanced signaling activity [30,31]. Furthermore, enzyme-regulated release of tethered growth factors by incorporating protease-sensitive sequences in the tether has been applied to modulate release kinetics [32,33] and shown to improve blood vessel growth [34]. Mimicking the natural affinity of ECM glycosaminoglycans for heparin-binding growth factors, heparin has been covalently immobilized onto scaffolds to control the presentation and release kinetics of heparin-binding growth factors, such as basic fibroblast growth factor [35,36] and transforming growth factor-β [37]. Similarly, engineering of basic heparin-binding motifs, such as phenylalanine–alanine–lysine–leucine–alanine–alanine–arginine–lysine–tyrosine–arginine–lysine–alanine (FAKLAARLYRKA) and tyrosine–lysine–lysine–isoleucine–lysine–lysine–leucine (YKKIIKKL), into scaffolds and sequestering of heparin-binding growth factors via a heparin bridge results in enhanced delivery kinetics and nerve regeneration [38,39].

39.4   Protease-Degradable Materials

Cell-mediated local degradation of ECMs is critical to tissue development, maintenance, and remodeling [40]. To mimic this behavior, proteolytically sensitive substrate motifs specific for natural ECM enzymes, including matrix metalloproteinases and plasmin, have been incorporated into biomaterial scaffolds [41] (Figure 39.3). Consistent with migration behaviors in collagen and fibrin ECMs [40], cell migration and neurite extension through engineered networks require protease activity specific for the incorporated protease substrate motifs [42,43]. Structure–function analyses of cell invasion into synthetic hydrogels have shown that the extent of invasion depends on protease substrate activity, adhesion ligand concentration,

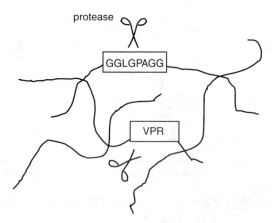

FIGURE 39.3   Enzyme-sensitive materials incorporating protease substrate motifs.

and network cross-linking density [44]. Furthermore, poly(ethylene glycol)-based hydrogels containing RGD oligopeptides and substrates for matrix metalloproteinases engineered to deliver BMP-2 to bone defects exhibit enhanced healing compared to standard treatments [44]. Bone regeneration in this model is dependent on the proteolytic sensitivity of the matrices and their architecture.

39.5   Artificial Proteins as Building Elements for Matrices

Artificial analogues of ECM proteins incorporating structural motifs to reconstitute secondary structures (e.g., coiled coil, α-helix) and convey controlled mechanical properties have been engineered via both synthetic routes and recombinant DNA technology [45]. These artificial proteins provide opportunities to generate novel hybrid macromolecules with additional or new functionalities and enhanced cost-efficiency, while overcoming limitations associated with natural ECMs, such as a restricted range in mechanical properties, processability, batch-to-batch variability, and the potential of pathogen transmission. For example, artificial proteins consisting of terminal leucine zipper domains flanking a central polyelectrolyte segment produce coiled-coil domains that render the material into a reversible, self-assembling hydrogel [46]. Polymers containing the glycine–valine–glycine–valine–proline (GVGVP) repeat from elastin have been designed to mimic the mechanical behavior of elastin [47]. These materials can be formulated as fibers and networks to create artificial ECMs [48,49]. Moreover, combination of elastin and fibronectin motifs has resulted in novel materials with biological and mechanical properties similar to those from natural ECMs [50]. Engineering of biofunctionalized and synthetic glycosaminoglycan polymers represents another promising avenue to artificial ECMs [51–53].

39.6   Conclusions and Outlook

Biomimetic materials incorporating bioactive motifs from natural ECMs have emerged as promising, novel biofunctional materials for tissue maintenance, repair, and regeneration. Although considerable progress has been attained in mimicking particular characteristics of ECMs, next-generation, bio-inspired materials must incorporate multiple characteristics from biological matrices to recapitulate the robust activities associated with these natural scaffolds. Furthermore, advances in materials engineering should provide routes for integrating multiple ligands, ligand gradients, nanoscale clustering, and dynamic, environment-responsive interfacial, and bulk properties. Finally, these biomimetic materials must be designed to support the activities of multiple cell types to successfully mimic desired tissue behavior and function.

References

[1] Reichardt, L.F., Introduction: extracellular matrix molecules, in *Guidebook to the Extracellular Matrix, Anchor, and Adhesion Proteins*, 2nd ed., Oxford University Press, New York, 1999, p. 335.

[2] Ruoslahti, E. and Pierschbacher, M.D., New perspectives in cell adhesion: RGD and integrins, *Science*, 238, 491, 1987.

[3] Graf, J. et al., A pentapeptide from the laminin B1 chain mediates cell adhesion and binds the 67,000 laminin receptor, *Biochemistry*, 26, 6896, 1987.

[4] Hubbell, J.A., Bioactive biomaterials, *Curr. Opin. Biotechnol.*, 10, 123, 1999.

[5] Shakesheff, K., Cannizzaro, S., and Langer, R., Creating biomimetic micro-environments with synthetic polymer–peptide hybrid molecules, *J. Biomater. Sci. Polym. Ed.*, 9, 507, 1998.

[6] Hubbell, J.A., Materials as morphogenetic guides in tissue engineering, *Curr. Opin. Biotechnol.*, 14, 551, 2003.

[7] Massia, S.P. and Hubbell, J.A., An RGD spacing of 440 nm is sufficient for integrin alpha v beta 3-mediated fibroblast spreading and 140 nm for focal contact and stress fiber formation, *J. Cell Biol.*, 114, 1089, 1991.

[8] Maheshwari, G. et al., Cell adhesion and motility depend on nanoscale RGD clustering, *J. Cell Sci.*, 113, 1677, 2000.

[9] Shin, H., Jo, S., and Mikos, A.G., Modulation of marrow stromal osteoblast adhesion on biomimetic oligo[poly(ethylene glycol) fumarate] hydrogels modified with Arg-Gly-Asp peptides and a poly(ethyleneglycol) spacer, *J. Biomed. Mater. Res.*, 61, 169, 2002.

[10] Sagnella, S.M. et al., Human microvascular endothelial cell growth and migration on biomimetic surfactant polymers, *Biomaterials*, 25, 1249, 2004.

[11] Schense, J.C. and Hubbell, J.A., Three-dimensional migration of neurites is mediated by adhesion site density and affinity, *J. Biol. Chem.*, 275, 6813, 2000.

[12] Silva, G.A. et al., Selective differentiation of neural progenitor cells by high-epitope density nanofibers, *Science*, 303, 1352, 2004.

[13] Mann, B.K. and West, J.L., Cell adhesion peptides alter smooth muscle cell adhesion, proliferation, migration, and matrix protein synthesis on modified surfaces and in polymer scaffolds, *J. Biomed. Mater. Res.*, 60, 86, 2002.

[14] Rezania, A. and Healy, K.E., The effect of peptide surface density on mineralization of a matrix deposited by osteogenic cells, *J. Biomed. Mater. Res.*, 52, 595, 2000.

[15] Rowley, J.A. and Mooney, D.J., Alginate type and RGD density control myoblast phenotype, *J. Biomed. Mater. Res.*, 60, 217, 2002.

[16] Ferris, D.M. et al., RGD-coated titanium implants stimulate increased bone formation *in vivo*, *Biomaterials*, 20, 2323, 1999.

[17] Eid, K. et al., Effect of RGD coating on osteocompatibility of PLGA-polymer disks in a rat tibial wound, *J. Biomed. Mater. Res.*, 57, 224, 2001.

[18] Alsberg, E. et al., Engineering growing tissues, *Proc. Natl Acad. Sci. USA*, 99, 12025, 2002.

[19] Schense, J.C. et al., Enzymatic incorporation of bioactive peptides into fibrin matrices enhances neurite extension, *Nat. Biotechnol.*, 18, 415, 2000.

[20] Yu, X. and Bellamkonda, R.V., Tissue-engineered scaffolds are effective alternatives to autografts for bridging peripheral nerve gaps, *Tissue Eng.*, 9, 421, 2003.

[21] Li, F. et al., Cellular and nerve regeneration within a biosynthetic extracellular matrix for corneal transplantation, *Proc. Natl Acad. Sci. USA*, 100, 15346, 2003.

[22] Humphries, J.D. et al., Molecular basis of ligand recognition by integrin alpha5beta 1. II. Specificity of arg-gly-Asp binding is determined by Trp157 of the alpha subunit, *J. Biol. Chem.*, 275, 20337, 2000.

[23] Kao, W.J. et al., Fibronectin modulates macrophage adhesion and FBGC formation: the role of RGD, PHSRN, and PRRARV domains, *J. Biomed. Mater. Res.*, 55, 79, 2001.

[24] Dillow, A.K. et al., Adhesion of alpha5beta1 receptors to biomimetic substrates constructed from peptide amphiphiles, *Biomaterials*, 22, 1493, 2001.

[25] Cutler, S.M. and García, A.J., Engineering cell adhesive surfaces that direct integrin alpha5beta1 binding using a recombinant fragment of fibronectin, *Biomaterials*, 24, 1759, 2003.

[26] Dee, K.C., Andersen, T.T., and Bizios, R., Design and function of novel osteoblast-adhesive peptides for chemical modification of biomaterials, *J. Biomed. Mater. Res.*, 40, 371, 1998.

[27] Rezania, A. and Healy, K.E., Biomimetic peptide surfaces that regulate adhesion, spreading, cyto-skeletal organization, and mineralization of the matrix deposited by osteoblast-like cells, *Biotechnol. Prog.*, 15, 19, 1999.

[28] Reyes, C.D. and García, A.J., Engineering integrin-specific surfaces with a triple-helical collagen-mimetic peptide, *J. Biomed. Mater. Res.* 65A, 511, 2003.

[29] Reyes, C.D. and García, A.J., $\alpha2\beta1$ integrin-specific collagen-mimetic surfaces that support osteoblastic differentiation, *J. Biomed. Mater. Res.*, 69A, 591, 2004.

[30] Kuhl, P.R. and Griffith-Cima, L.G., Tethered epidermal growth factor as a paradigm for growth factor-induced stimulation from the solid phase, *Nat. Med.*, 2, 1022, 1996.

[31] Zisch, A.H. et al., Covalently conjugated VEGF — fibrin matrices for endothelialization, *J. Control. Release*, 72, 101, 2001.

[32] Kopecek, J., Controlled biodegradability of polymers — a key to drug delivery systems, *Biomaterials*, 5, 19, 1984.

[33] Sakiyama-Elbert, S.E., Panitch, A., and Hubbell, J.A., Development of growth factor fusion proteins for cell-triggered drug delivery, *FASEB J.*, 15, 1300, 2001.

[34] Ehrbar, M. et al., Cell-demanded liberation of VEGF121 from fibrin implants induces local and controlled blood vessel growth, *Circ. Res.*, 94, 1124, 2004.

[35] Edelman, E.R. et al., Controlled and modulated release of basic fibroblast growth factor, *Biomaterials*, 12, 619, 1991.

[36] Wissink, M.J. et al., Binding and release of basic fibroblast growth factor from heparinized collagen matrices, *Biomaterials*, 22, 2291, 2001.

[37] Schroeder-Tefft, J.A., Bentz, H., and Estridge, T.D., Collagen and heparin matrices for growth factor delivery, *J. Control. Release*, 49, 291, 1997.

[38] Sakiyama-Elbert, S.E. and Hubbell, J.A., Development of fibrin derivatives for controlled release of heparin-binding growth factors, *J. Control. Release*, 65, 389, 2000.

[39] Sakiyama-Elbert, S.E. and Hubbell, J.A., Controlled release of nerve growth factor from a heparin-containing fibrin-based cell ingrowth matrix, *J. Control. Release*, 69, 149, 2000.

[40] Chang, C. and Werb, Z., The many faces of metalloproteases: cell growth, invasion, angiogenesis and metastasis, *Trends Cell Biol.*, 11, S37, 2001.

[41] West, J.L. and Hubbell, J.A., Polymeric biomaterials with degradation sites for proteases involved in cell migration, *Macromolecules*, 32, 241, 1999.

[42] Gobin, A.S. and West, J.L., Cell migration through defined, synthetic ECM analogs, *FASEB J.*, 16, 751, 2002.

[43] Halstenberg, S. et al., Biologically engineered protein-graft-poly(ethylene glycol) hydrogels: a cell adhesive and plasmin-degradable biosynthetic material for tissue repair, *Biomacromolecules*, 3, 710, 2002.

[44] Lutolf, M.P. et al., Synthetic matrix metalloproteinase-sensitive hydrogels for the conduction of tissue regeneration: engineering cell-invasion characteristics, *Proc. Natl Acad. Sci USA*, 100, 5413, 2003.

[45] van Hest, J.C. and Tirrell, D.A., Protein-based materials, toward a new level of structural control, *Chem. Commun. (Camb.)*, 1897, 2001.

[46] Petka, W.A. et al., Reversible hydrogels from self-assembling artificial proteins, *Science*, 281, 389, 1998.

[47] Lee, J., Macosko, C.W., and Urry, D.W., Elastomeric polypentapeptides cross-linked into matrixes and fibers, *Biomacromolecules*, 2, 170, 2001.

[48] Nagapudi, K. et al., Photomediated solid-state cross-linking of an elastin-mimetic recombinant protein polymer, *Macromolecules*, 35, 1730, 2002.

[49] Trabbic-Carlson, K., Setton, L.A., and Chilkoti, A., Swelling and mechanical behaviors of chemically cross-linked hydrogels of elastin-like polypeptides, *Biomacromolecules*, 4, 572, 2003.

[50] Welsh, E.R. and Tirrell, D.A., Engineering the extracellular matrix: a novel approach to polymeric biomaterials. I. Control of the physical properties of artificial protein matrices designed to support adhesion of vascular endothelial cells, *Biomacromolecules*, 1, 23, 2000.

[51] Baskaran, S. et al., Glycosaminoglycan-mimetic biomaterials. 3. Glycopolymers prepared from alkene-derivatized mono- and disaccharide-based glycomonomers, *Bioconjug. Chem.*, 13, 1309, 2002.

[52] Dong, C.M. et al., Synthesis and characterization of glycopolymer-polypeptide triblock copolymers, *Biomacromolecules*, 5, 224, 2004.

[53] Shu, X.Z. et al., Attachment and spreading of fibroblasts on an RGD peptide-modified injectable hyaluronan hydrogel, *J. Biomed. Mater. Res.*, 68A, 365, 2004.

40

Nanocomposite Scaffolds for Tissue Engineering

Amit S. Mistry
Xinfeng Shi
Antonios G. Mikos
Rice University

40.1 Introduction

In recent years, a great deal of attention has been directed toward nanotechnology and the potential benefits that this growing field may bring to a wide variety of engineering applications. One of the many applications of nanotechnology toward the biomedical sciences is the advancement of biomaterials designed for tissue engineering, especially those intended for biological tissues with complex properties. Nanoscience will be particularly useful in tissue engineering since the interactions between cells and biomaterials occur in the nanoscale and the components of biological tissues are nanomaterials themselves.

Bone tissue, for example, is a nanocomposite composed of rigid hydroxyapatite (HA) nanocrystals (60%) precipitated onto collagen fibers (30%) (Figure 40.1) [1]. Hydroxyapatite, which occurs as small plates that are tens of nanometers in length and width and 2–3 nm in depth, impart compressive strength to bone. Collagen fibrils (1.5–3.5 nm in diameter) form triple helices and bundle into fibers (50–70 nm diameter) responsible for the unique tensile properties of composite bone tissue [2]. The unique and complex mechanical properties of bone tissue arise from the interaction of these two components in the nanoscale [3].

Similarly, nanomaterials possessing superior properties compared to conventional materials are capable of imparting some of their properties onto macroscopic materials to form nanocomposites. In this manner, biomaterials may gain enhanced properties for medical applications with the addition of nanomaterials. Biodegradable polymers, for example, are generally too weak for load-bearing tissue applications. However, the incorporation of nanofillers into the polymer matrix can greatly improve the polymer's

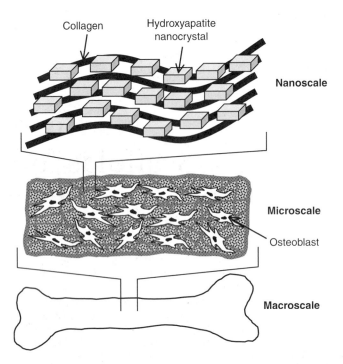

FIGURE 40.1 Nanocomposite structure of bone. The interaction between collagen fibers and HA nanocrystals in the nanoscale gives rise to the complex mechanical properties of bone tissue observed in the macroscale. Cells operating on this collagen/hydroxyapatite nanocomposite continually remodel bone on the microscale.

properties. More specifically, nanofillers have been shown to improve a composite material's flexural modulus [4], tensile strength, stiffness, toughness [5–8], fatigue resistance [9], wear resistance [10], thermal stability [11,12], and gas permeability properties [13]. Nanophase ceramic materials have been shown to also improve bone cell functions [14] and can impart osteoconductivity and improved biocompatibility to synthetic polymers [15,16]. Alternatively, HA nanocrystals can improve the osteoconductivity and biocompatibility of natural polymers, such as collagen, by mimicking the natural composition of bone [17–19]. The present chapter highlights current efforts toward nanocomposite scaffolds for tissue engineering applications.

40.2 Nanocomposite Materials

40.2.1 Nanomaterials Overview

Nanomaterials, as described here, are defined as materials with at least one of three dimensions <100 nm. Spherical nanoparticles, such as alumoxanes or silica nanoparticles, are nano-sized in all three dimensions. Nanotubes (carbon nanotubes), rods, or needles (HA) have two nanometer-sized dimensions. Nanosheets, such as layered silicates, have only one dimension in the nanoscale. Each of these nanomaterials offers mechanical reinforcement or osteoconductivity by dispersing into a matrix and chemically interacting with the macroscopic material. However, these particles are typically hydrophilic while the macroscopic material into which they are dispersed is usually hydrophobic. Thus, nanomaterial dispersion and promotion of interactions between the nanofillers and the macroscopic material are the two primary challenges for nanocomposite development.

Table 40.1 describes some of the many different nanomaterials currently being investigated for biomedical scaffolds. Each section of this chapter discusses the synthesis of a nanomaterial as well as the fabrication

TABLE 40.1   Nanomaterials for Biomedical Composites

Nanomaterial	Chemical formula	Composite materials for biomedical applications	References
Carboxylate Alumoxane	$[Al(O)_x(OH)_y(O_2CR)_z]_n$	PPF	Horch et al. [4]
Montmorillonite	$M_x(Al_{4-x}Mg_x)Si_8O_{20}(OH)_4$	PLLA	Lee et al. [11]
		Polyurethanes	Xu et al. [26]
Hydroxyapatite	$Ca_{10}(PO_4)_6(OH)_2$	PMMA	Fang et al. [39]
		PEG, PMMA, PBMA, PHEMA, PEG/PBT	Liu et al. [40–42]
		Chitosan	Hu et al. [43]
		PPF	Lewandrowskiet al. [44]
		Collagen	Zhang et al. [45]
Silica	SiO_2	PMMA, PCL	Rhee et al. [16, 46–47]
			Yoo et al. [48]
Alumina	Al_2O_3	Ce-TZP	Nawa et al. [8,49]
			Tanaka et al. [10]
			Uchida et al. [50]
Carbon nanotube	C	PMMA	Cooper et al. [65]
		PLA	Supronowicz et al. [67]

of nanocomposites from this material. A brief description of relevant issues and results of physical and biological testing is also included for each material.

40.2.2 Functionalized Alumoxane Nanocomposites

Carboxylate-alumoxanes are alumina-based nanoparticles developed as inorganic ceramic fillers for a variety of engineering applications. Alumoxanes are prepared directly from boehmite mineral in a "top-down" synthesis involving acid hydrolysis [20]. Nanoparticle size is controlled by conditions during synthesis and particles are easily functionalized based on the type of carboxylic acid used during synthesis [21]. Certain functional groups can be added to the hydrophilic alumoxane nanoparticles to aid in dispersion and covalent interaction with the composite medium. Vogelson et al. [6] modified alumoxanes with lysine and p-hydroxybenzoic acid to reinforce organic epoxy resins and yield sizable increases in thermal stability and tensile strength over blank resin [6].

In our laboratory, we have studied the effects of various surface-modified alumoxane nanoparticles on the mechanical properties of a biodegradable polymer for load-bearing bone tissue applications [4]. Alumoxane nanoparticles with three different surface modifications were tested — "activated" alumoxanes possessing two reactive double bonds available for interaction with the cross-link network of the polymer; "surfactant" alumoxanes modified with long fatty acid chains to aid in dispersion within the hydrophobic polymer; and "hybrid" alumoxanes modified with a surfactant chain and a reactive double bond within the same substituent (Figure 40.2). These nanoparticles were incorporated into a biodegradable poly(propylene fumarate)-based (PPF) system and the nanocomposites were tested for flexural and compressive mechanical properties.

Unmodified boehmite particle composites showed no significant improvement in mechanical properties compared to polymer resin alone and demonstrated a significant decrease in flexural fracture strength with increased loading. This is explained by the formation of large aggregates within the hydrophobic polymer, which promote crack formation (Figure 40.3a). The activated alumoxane nanocomposites were expected to covalently interact with the PPF matrix, but instead tended to aggregate into micron-sized clusters, which decreased flexural fracture strength with increased loading. Surfactant alumoxane nanocomposites demonstrated significant improvements in flexural modulus over blank polymer resin due to the fine dispersion of nanoparticles within the polymer matrix as determined by scanning electron microscopy (SEM). The hybrid alumoxane nanocomposites performed the best out of all materials by

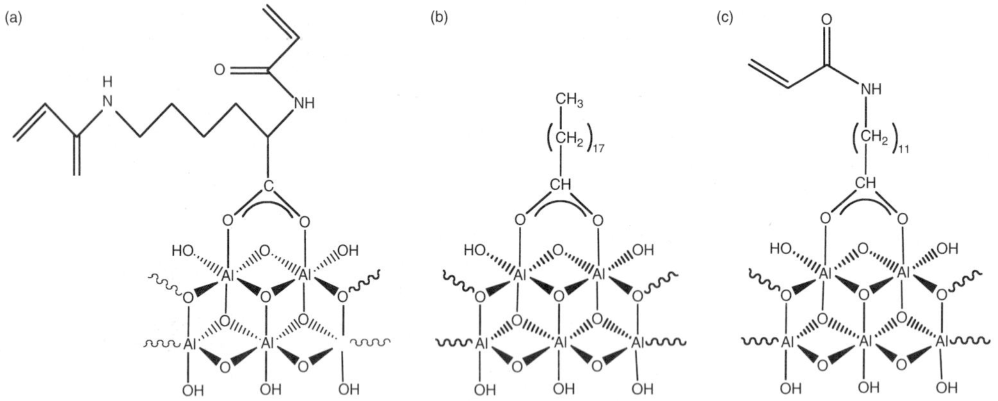

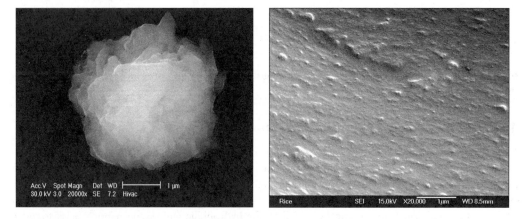

FIGURE 40.2 Chemical structures of modified alumoxanes: (a) diacryloyl lysine–alumoxane (activated), (b) stearic acid–alumoxane (surfactant), and (c) acryloyl undecanoic amino acid–alumoxane (hybrid).

FIGURE 40.3 SEM images of fracture planes of nanocomposite samples after mechanical testing: (a) unmodified boehmite crystals in polymer, bar is 1 μm; (b) hybrid alumoxane nanocomposite, bar is 1 μm.

improving the flexural modulus of PPF at loading concentrations between 0.5 and 5 wt.%. At a 1 wt.% loading, the flexural modulus reached 5410 $\pm$ 460 MPa, a factor of 3.5 greater than polymer alone (Figure 40.4a). Additionally, hybrid nanocomposites caused no significant loss of flexural or compressive fracture strength up to 5 wt. % loading (Figure 40.4b). SEM images revealed that the surfactant chain within the functional group of hybrid alumoxanes aided in dispersion within the polymer (Figure 40.3b) while the significant increase in mechanical properties may be explained by covalent interaction between PPF polymer and alumoxane nanoparticles. Thus, surface modification of alumoxane nanoparticles significantly increased the flexural modulus of polymer nanocomposites without a detrimental effect on fracture strength.

40.2.3 Polymer-Layered Silicate Nanocomposites

Layered silicates, derived from smectite clays, are commonly used as fillers for polymeric materials for many different applications as their chemistries have been extensively studied [22]. Polymer-layered silicate nanocomposites have shown improvements in mechanical, thermal, optical, physicochemical, and barrier properties as well as fire resistance compared to pure polymers or conventional composites (composed of micron-sized particles) [5,12].

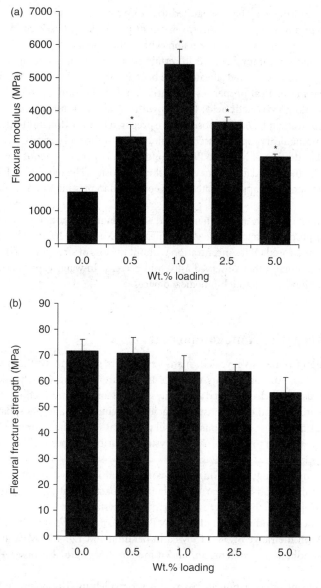

FIGURE 40.4 Flexural testing of hybrid alumoxanes. Flexural modulus (a) and flexural fracture strength (b) of hybrid alumoxane nanocomposites as a function of nanoparticle loading weight percentage. Error bars represent mean ± standard deviation for $n = 5$. The symbol "*" indicates a statistically significant difference compared to the pure polymer resin ($p < .05$).

These materials, unlike the other nanophase materials described in this chapter, are nano-sized in only one dimension and thereby act as nanoplatelets that sandwich polymer chains in composites. Montmorillonite (MMT) is a well-characterized layered silicate that can be made hydrophobic through either ionic exchange or modification with organic surfactant molecules to aid in dispersion [5,23]. Polymer-layered silicates may be synthesized by exfoliation adsorption, *in situ* intercalative polymerization, and melt intercalation to yield three general types of polymer/clay nanocomposites. Intercalated structures are characterized as alternating polymer and silicate layers in an ordered pattern with a periodic space between layers of a few nanometers [13]. Exfoliated or delaminated structure occurs when silicate layers are uniformly distributed throughout the polymer matrix. In some cases, the polymer does not intercalate the layers of silicate, resulting in a phase-separated structure containing micron-sized clusters of multiple silicate layers [5]. Typically, the greatest improvement of properties is observed in exfoliated structures based on the degree of layered-silicate dispersion within the polymer [13,24,25], though intercalated systems show more significant improvements in certain properties such as fracture behavior [23].

For biomedical applications, layered silicates have been incorporated into biodegradable lactide-based polymers to improve mechanical properties for hard-tissue applications. Lee et al. [11] incorporated MMT nanoplatelets into poly(L-lactic acid) (PLLA) with the aim of improving the intrinsic stiffness of porous polymer scaffolds. Exfoliated composites were prepared by the exfoliation-adsorption process and thermal and tensile mechanical properties were examined. The authors observed decreased glass transition temperatures with the addition of MMT to PLLA along with a larger amorphous region, which may have a positive effect on the biodegradation behavior of the composite. The tensile modulus of PLLA loaded with 5.79 wt.% MMT increased approximately 40% compared to pristine PLLA while maintaining more than 90% porosity.

Biomedical polyurethanes have also been modified with organically modified layered silicates (OLS) to improve mechanical properties and reduce gas permeability. Xu et al. [26] demonstrated an increase in tensile modulus with increased OLS concentration without the loss of strength and ductility that is typical for filler systems. Additionally, they observed a fivefold decrease in water vapor permeability, which is a major advantage for blood-contacting biomedical devices.

40.2.4 Hydroxyapatite Nanocomposites

As the nanostructure of bone was revealed, many researchers started to synthesize nanoscale HA and investigate its properties. Among various methods to prepare HA, the wet chemical method is most commonly used because it is well developed and easily adjusted for mass production [27]. Briefly, solutions of either calcium hydroxide and orthophosphoric acid or calcium salts and phosphate salts are mixed in a Ca/P ratio of 5:3. Under these conditions, HA will precipitate from the solution [28]. Researchers can finely tune this simple method to make HA nanocrystals in various shapes such as spheres, rods, needles, and plates [28–33].

Due to its low flexural strength and toughness, commercial HA powders (of micron-sized particles) are usually limited to use as non-load-bearing implants or bioactive coatings on stronger materials, such as titanium alloys, to promote bone ingrowth [34]. Nanocrystalline HA with an average grain size of 100 nm possesses superior bending strength (182 MPa) and compressive strength (879 MPa) compared to conventional HA (in the range of 38–113 MPa in bending and 120–800 MPa in compression) [35]. Improved osteoblast adhesion, proliferation, and mineralization were also observed on the surface of nanoscale HA [14,36–38].

It is very attractive to introduce nanoscale HA as a filler for widely used biopolymers to improve bioactive and mechanical properties. As mentioned previously, however, the major challenge is achieving uniform dispersion of hydrophilic HA nanoparticles throughout hydrophobic polymer matrixes. Surfactants, such as lecithin, can be used to prevent aggregation of HA nanocrystals and homogeneously distribute them into poly(methylmethacrylate) (PMMA) polymer [39]. Liu et al. [40,41] successfully modified the surface of HA nanocrystals with poly(ethylene glycol) (PEG), PMMA, poly(butyl methacrylate) (PBMA), and poly(hydroxyethyl methacrylate) (PHEMA) to produce chemical bonding between the filler and matrix [40,41]. In another study, tensile strength and modulus of composites were significantly enhanced by the improved interface of HA nanocrystals and PEG/poly(butylenes terephthalate) (PEG/PBT) block copolymer [42].

Natural polymers have also been investigated for nanocomposites. In fact, a biodegradable chitosan/HA nanocomposite made by *in situ* hybridization exhibited higher bending strength and modulus than PMMA [43]. Moreover, nanoscale HA fillers can reduce water absorption, thus retaining material mechanical properties under moisture conditions for the potential application of internal fixation of bone fractures [43].

In an *in vivo* study, the biocompatibility and osteointegration of biodegradable PPF polymer grafts were improved when nanoscale HA was employed as opposed to micron-sized particles [44]. In another study, HA nanocrystals were reported to grow on the surface of self-assembled collagen triple helices along the longitudinal axes of their fibrils [45]. This designed hierarchical structure is very close to the actual nanostructure of bone. Thus, HA nanocomposites provide significant advantages for successful orthopaedic and dental applications in that they closely mimic natural bones and improve the bioactivity of many materials.

40.2.5 Other Ceramic Nanocomposites

In an effort to enhance the osteoconductivity of PMMA bone cement, Rhee and Choi [16,46] incorporated silica nanoparticles into the polymer. This composite was synthesized by sol–gel processing with the goal of improving binding at the bone-implant interface. The authors observed high mechanical properties in addition to crystalline apatite formation on implants in simulated body fluid.

While PMMA is useful as a bone cement, it is not ideal for tissue engineering applications as it is nondegradable. Researchers incorporated the same type of silica nanoparticles into the biodegradable poly(ε-caprolactone) (PCL) and also observed apatite formation and favorable mechanical properties [47,48].

Another noteworthy effort at nanocomposite fabrication applied ceramic nanoparticles to a ceramic material to enhance osteoconductivity and mechanical performance. Nawa et al. [49] developed a ceria-stabilized tetragonal zirconia polycrystal (Ce-TZP) ceramic and incorporated alumina (Al_2O_3) nanocrystals into it via wet chemistry methods for load-bearing bone applications. Further studies of this material investigated its ability to induce apatite formation [50], *in vivo* biocompatibility, and resistance to wear [10] with favorable results.

40.2.6 Carbon Nanotube Nanocomposites

Carbon nanotubes are among the strongest materials known because of their almost defect-free graphite architecture with the sp^2 type of carbon–carbon covalent bond, which is one of the strongest chemical bonds in nature [51,52]. There are two types of carbon nanotubes: multiwalled carbon nanotubes (MWNTs), first discovered in 1991 [53], and single-walled carbon nanotubes (SWNTs), first reported in 1993 [54,55]. Depending on the quality of nanotubes, elastic moduli can be as high as 1 TPa for SWNTs and 0.3 to 1 TPa for MWNTs, while strength ranges from 50 to 500 GPa for SWNTs and 10 to 60 GPa for MWNTs [56]. Owing to their very small diameters (ranging from 0.42 nm to dozens of nanometers) and lengths of more than several micrometers, the aspect ratio (length-to-diameter ratio) of carbon nanotubes can be more than 1000, while those of conventional carbon fibers are only about 100 [57]. Therefore, carbon nanotubes could become the best reinforcing fiber for composite materials.

Both types of carbon nanotubes are synthesized by three methods involving gas phase processing, namely, arc-discharge, laser ablation, and chemical vapor deposition (CVD) [58]. Subsequent purification procedures are required to remove impurities, such as catalyst particles, amorphous carbon, and nontubular fullerenes, from the nanotubes [59].

One of the greatest challenges for developing carbon nanotube nanocomposites is separating nanotube bundles, which aggregate into ropes due to strong inter-tube van der Waals attractions. This makes it quite difficult to obtain a uniform dispersion of individual nanotubes into a matrix material. Another significant challenge is effectively transferring load from a matrix to nanotubes, which have atomically smooth surfaces. The main dispersion methods include mechanical procedures, sonication of nanotubes in solvents and surfactants, and surface functionalization [60]. Among them, surface functionalization seems superior in that functional groups on the surfaces can not only isolate individual nanotubes from each other and therefore achieve uniform distribution throughout a matrix, but can also provide possible sites for covalent bonding between nanotubes and matrix to facilitate load transfer. Dyke and Tour [61] added various functional moieties to the surfaces of SWNTs by diazonium-based reactions and were able to separate bundles into individual nanotubes. Mitchell et al. [62] showed that such functionalized SWNTs demonstrated much better dispersion in polymer than nonfunctionalized ones.

Many researchers have reported significant improvements of mechanical properties in thermoplastics and epoxy resins by the addition of MWNTs or SWNTs [63,64]. Cooper et al. [65] found that impact strengths of both types of carbon nanotubes in PMMA were significantly improved compared to pure polymer. Carbon nanotubes provide another opportunity for creating dense ceramic composites with enhanced mechanical properties by absorbing energy through their highly flexible elastic behavior during deformation [66]. With the addition of 5 or 10% well-dispersed MWNTs, both the strength and fracture toughness of alumina were greatly increased [56]. In addition to their exceptional mechanical properties, carbon nanotubes also possess superior electric properties [58]. In an *in vitro* study, current-conducting composites of polylactic acid (PLA) and multiwalled carbon nanotubes were effectively used as substrates to expose osteoblasts to electrical stimulation, which promotes cellular functions for new bone formation [67]. Though carbon nanotubes are a relatively new material for biomedical applications, they show great potential for engineering biomaterials for hard tissue scaffolds.

40.3   Conclusions

As is evident by the described studies, a great deal of progress has been made toward improving biomaterials for tissue engineering through nanotechnology. Nanocomposite scaffolds have demonstrated enhanced mechanical properties and improved osteoconductivity of polymers as well as other materials. The challenge remains to design a nanocomposite scaffold with mechanical properties suitable for hard, cortical bone regeneration therapies. Future studies of nanocomposites should focus on answering an important question: How do these novel materials perform *in vivo*? The *in vivo* biocompatibility and osteoconductivity must be well characterized before the high potential of nanocomposite scaffolds for tissue engineering can be achieved.

Acknowledgments

This work was supported by the National Institutes of Health (R01 AR48756) (AGM) and the Nanoscale Science and Engineering Initiative of the National Science Foundation (EEC-0118001). ASM acknowledges the support of the NIH Biotechnology Training Grant (5 T32 GMO 08362).

References

[1] Athanasiou, K.A. et al., Fundamentals of biomechanics in tissue engineering of bone, *Tissue Eng.*, 6, 361, 2000.

[2] Rho, J.Y., Kuhn-Spearing, L., and Zioupos, P., Mechanical properties and the hierarchical structure of bone, *Med. Eng. Phys.*, 20, 92, 1998.

[3] Taton, T.A., Nanotechnology. Boning up on biology, *Nature*, 412, 491, 2001.

[4] Horch, R.A. et al., Nanoreinforcement of poly(propylene fumarate)-based networks with surface modified alumoxane nanoparticles for bone tissue engineering, *Biomacromolecules*, 5, 1990, 2004.

[5] Alexandre, M. and Dubois, P., Polymer-layered silicate nanocomposites: preparation, properties and uses of a new class of materials, *Mat. Sci. Eng. R*, 28, 1, 2000.

[6] Vogelson, C.T. et al., Inorganic–organic hybrid and composite resin materials using carboxylate-alumoxanes as functionalized cross-linking agents, *Chem. Mater.*, 12, 795, 2000.

[7] Kumar, S. et al., Synthesis, structure, and properties of PBO/SWNT composites, *Macromolecules*, 35, 9039, 2002.

[8] Nawa, M. et al., Tough and strong Ce-TZP/alumina nanocomposites doped with titania, *Ceram. Int.*, 24, 497, 1998.

[9] Bellare, A. et al., Improving the fatigue properties of poly(methyl methacrylate) orthopaedic cement containing radiopacifier nanoparticles, *Mater. Sci. Forum*, 426-4, 3133, 2003.

[10] Tanaka, K. et al., Ce-TZP/Al_2O_3 nanocomposite as a bearing material in total joint replacement, *J. Biomed. Mater. Res.*, 63, 262, 2002.

[11] Lee, J.H. et al., Thermal and mechanical characteristics of poly(L-lactic acid) nanocomposite scaffold, *Biomaterials*, 24, 2773, 2003.

[12] Torre, L. et al., Processing and characterization of epoxy-anhydride-based intercalated nanocomposites, *J. Appl. Polym. Sci.*, 90, 2532, 2003.

[13] Krook, M. et al., Barrier and mechanical properties of montmorillonite/polyesterarnide nanocomposites, *Polym. Eng. Sci.*, 42, 1238, 2002.

[14] Webster, T.J. et al., Enhanced functions of osteoblasts on nanophase ceramics, *Biomaterials*, 21, 1803, 2000.

[15] Liu, Q., de Wijn, J.R., and van Blitterswijk, C.A., Nano-apatite/polymer composites: mechanical and physicochemical characteristics, *Biomaterials*, 18, 1263, 1997.

[16] Rhee, S.H. and Choi, J.Y., Preparation of a bioactive poly(methyl methacrylate)/silica nanocomposite, *J. Am. Ceram. Soc.*, 85, 1318, 2002.

[17] Kikuchi, M. et al., Porous body preparation of hydroxyapatite/coliagen nanocomposites for bone tissue regeneration, *Key Eng. Mater.*, 254-2, 561, 2004.

[18] Du, C. et al., Three-dimensional nano-HAp/collagen matrix loading with osteogenic cells in organ culture, *J. Biomed. Mater. Res.*, 44, 407, 1999.

[19] Cui, F.Z. et al., Biodegradation of a nano-hydroxyapatite/collagen composite by peritoneal monocyte-macrophages, *Cells Mater.*, 6, 31, 1996.

[20] Callender, R.L. et al., Aqueous synthesis of water soluble alumoxanes: environmentally benign precursors to alumina and aluminum-based ceramics, *Chem. Mater.*, 9, 2418, 1997.

[21] Vogelson, C.T. and Barron, A.R., Particle size control and dependence on solution pH of carboxylate-alumoxane nanoparticles, *J. Non-Cryst. Solids*, 290, 216, 2001.

[22] Theng, B.K.G., *Formation and Properties of Clay–Polymer Complexes*, Elsevier Scientific Pub. Co., New York, 1979.

[23] Zerda, A.S. and Lesser, A.J., Intercalated clay nanocomposites: morphology, mechanics, and fracture behavior, *J. Polym. Sci. Polym. Phys.*, 39, 1137, 2001.

[24] Burnside, S.D. and Giannelis, E.P., Synthesis and properties of new poly(dimethylsiloxane) nanocomposites, *Chem. Mater.*, 7, 1597, 1995.

[25] Akelah, A. et al., Organophilic rubber — montmorillonite nanocomposites, *Mater. Lett.*, 22, 97, 1995.

[26] Xu, R. et al., Low permeability biomedical polyurethane nanocomposites, *J. Biomed. Mater. Res.*, 64, 114, 2003.

[27] Aoki, H., *Science and Medical Applications of Hydroxyapatite*, Ishiyaku EuroAmerica, St. Louis, MO, 1991.

[28] Pang, Y.X. and Bao, X., Influence of temperature, ripening time and calcination on the morphology and crystallinity of hydroxyapatite nanoparticles, *J. Eur. Ceram. Soc.*, 23, 1697, 2003.

[29] Li, Y. et al., Shape change and phase transition of needle-like non-stochiometric apatite crystals, *J. Mater. Sci.: Mater. Med.*, 5, 263, 1994.

[30] Li, Y. et al., Preparation and chracterization of nano-grade osteoapatite-like rod crystals, *J. Mater. Sci.: Mater. Med.*, 5, 252, 1994.

[31] Hsieh, M.F. et al., Organic–inorganic hybrids of collagen or biodegradable polymers with hydroxyapatite, *Key Eng. Mater.*, 254-2, 473, 2004.

[32] Liou, S.C. et al., Structural characterization of nano-sized calcium deficient apatite powders, *Biomaterials*, 25, 189, 2004.

[33] Wang, Y.F. et al., Preparation and characterization of nano hydroxyapatite sol, *T Nonferr. Metal. Soc.*, 14, 29, 2004.

[34] Catledge, S.A. et al., Nanostructured ceramics for biomedical implants, *J. Nanosci. Nanotechnol.*, 2, 293, 2002.

[35] Ahn, E. et al., Properties of nanostructured hydroxyapatite-based bioceramics, *Transactions of the Sixth World Biomaterials Congress*, p. 643, 2000.

[36] Webster, T.J. et al., Specific proteins mediate enhanced osteoblast adhesion on nanophase ceramics, *J. Biomed. Mater. Res.*, 51, 475, 2000.

[37] Webster, T.J., Siegel, R.W., and Bizios, R., Osteoblast adhesion on nanophase ceramics, *Biomaterials*, 20, 1221, 1999.

[38] Webster, T.J., Siegel, R.W., and Bizios, R., Nanoceramic surface roughness enhances osteoblast and osteoclast functions for improved orthopaedic/dental implant efficacy, *Scr. Mater.*, 44, 1639, 2001.

[39] Fang, L.R. et al., Preparation of nano-sized hydroxyapatite in chloroform medium, *J. Inorg. Mater.*, 18, 801, 2003.

[40] Liu, Q. et al., Surface modification of nano-apatite by grafting organic polymer, *Biomaterials*, 19, 1067, 1998.

[41] Liu, Q., de Wijn, J.R., and van Blitterswijk, C.A., Covalent bonding of PMMA, PBMA, and poly(HEMA) to hydroxyapatite particles, *J. Biomed. Mater. Res.*, 40, 257, 1998.

[42] Liu, Q., de Wijn, J.R., and van Blitterswijk, C.A., Composite biomaterials with chemical bonding between hydroxyapatite filler particles and PEG/PBT copolymer matrix, *J. Biomed. Mater. Res.*, 40, 490, 1998.

[43] Hu, Q.L. et al., Preparation and characterization of biodegradable chitosan/hydroxyapatite nano-composite rods via *in situ* hybridization: a potential material as internal fixation of bone fracture, *Biomaterials*, 25, 779, 2004.

[44] Lewandrowski, K.U. et al., Enhanced bioactivity of a poly(propylene fumarate) bone graft substitute by augmentation with nano-hydroxyapatite, *Bio-Med. Mater. Eng.*, 13, 115, 2003.

[45] Zhang, W., Liao, S.S., and Cui, F.Z., Hierarchical self-assembly of nano-fibrils in mineralized collagen, *Chem. Mater.*, 15, 3221, 2003.

[46] Rhee, S.H. and Choi, J.Y., Synthesis of a bioactive poly(methyl methacrylate)/silica hybird, *Bioceramics* 14, 218-2, 433, 2002.

[47] Rhee, S.H., Effect of calcium salt content in the poly(epsilon-caprolactone)/silica nanocomposite on the nucleation and growth behavior of apatite layer, *J. Biomed. Mater. Res.*, 67A, 1131, 2003.

[48] Yoo, J.J. and Rhee, S.H., Evaluations of bioactivity and mechanical properties of poly (epsilon-caprolactone)/silica nanocomposite following heat treatment, *J. Biomed. Mater. Res.*, 68A, 401, 2004.

[49] Nawa, M. et al., The effect of TiO_2 addition on strengthening and toughening in intragranular type of $12Ce$-TZP/Al_2O_3 nanocomposites, *J. Eur. Ceram. Soc.*, 18, 209, 1998.

[50] Uchida, M. et al., Apatite-forming ability of a zirconia/alumina nano-composite induced by chemical treatment, *J. Biomed. Mater. Res.*, 60, 277, 2002.

[51] Jin, Z. et al., Dynamic mechanical behavior of melt-processed multi-walled carbon nan-otube/poly(methyl methacrylate) composites, *Chem. Phys. Lett.*, 337, 43, 2001.

[52] Bernholc, J. et al., Mechanical and electrical properties of nanotubes, *Annu. Rev. Mater. Res.*, 32, 347, 2002.

[53] Iijima, S., Helical microtubules of graphitic carbon, *Nature*, 354, 56, 1991.

[54] Iijima, S. and Ichihashi, T., Single-shell carbon nanotubes of 1-nm diameter, *Nature*, 363, 603, 1993.

[55] Bethune, D.S. et al., Cobalt-catalyzed growth of carbon nanotubes with single-atomic-layerwalls, *Nature*, 363, 605, 1993.

[56] Ajayan, P.M., Schadler, L.S., and Braun, P.V., *Nanocomposite Science and Technology*, Wiley-VCH Verlag, New York, 2003.

[57] Calvert, P., Nanotube composites — a recipe for strength, *Nature*, 399, 210, 1999.

[58] Terrones, M., Science and technology of the twenty-first century: synthesis, properties and applications of carbon nanotubes, *Annu. Rev. Mater. Res.*, 33, 419, 2003.

[59] Haddon, R.C. et al., Purification and separation of carbon nanotubes, *Mrs Bull.*, 29, 252, 2004.

[60] Hilding, J. et al., Dispersion of carbon nanotubes in liquids, *J. Disper. Sci. Technol.*, 24, 1, 2003.

[61] Dyke, C.A. and Tour, J.M., Unbundled and highly functionalized carbon nanotubes from aqueous reactions, *NanoLetters*, 3, 1215, 2003.

[62] Mitchell, C.A. et al., Dispersion of functionalized carbon nanotubes in polystyrene, *Macromolecules*, 35, 8825, 2002.

[63] Qian, D. et al., Load transfer and deformation mechanisms in carbon nanotube–polystyrene composites, *Appl. Phys. Lett.*, 76, 2868, 2000.

[64] Zhu, J. et al., Improving the dispersion and integration of single-walled carbon nanotubes in epoxy composites through functionalization, *NanoLetters*, 3, 1107, 2003.

[65] Cooper, C.A. et al., Distribution and alignment of carbon nanotubes and nanofibrils in a polymer matrix, *Comp. Sci. Technol.*, 62, 1105, 2002.

[66] Yakobson, B.I. and Avouris, P., Mechanical properties of carbon nanotubes, *Carbon Nanotubes*, 80, 287, 2001.

[67] Supronowicz, P.R. et al., Novel current-conducting composite substrates for exposing osteoblasts to alternating current stimulation, *J. Biomed. Mater. Res.*, 59, 499, 2002.

41

Roles of Thermodynamic State and Molecular Mobility in Biopreservation

Alptekin Aksan

University of Minnesota
Center for Engineering in
Medicine/Surgical Services
Harvard Medical School
Massachusetts General Hospital
Shriners Hospital for Children

Mehmet Toner

Center for Engineering in
Medicine/Surgical Services
Harvard Medical School
Massachusetts General Hospital
Shriners Hospital for Children

In a very broad sense, preservation can be defined as the process of reversibly arresting the biochemical reactions and therefore the metabolism of an organism (in a state of suspended animation [1]) in order to sustain function after a "prolonged" exposure to otherwise lethal conditions. The lethal conditions are created by the inadequacy of the surrounding medium in supplying nutrients and removing by-products, exposure to draught, or the extremes of temperature that would disturb the biochemical processes vital to the organism.

The rates of biochemical reactions are dependent on the proximity and mobility of the reactants. Mobility is determined by the mutual interactions of the solvent with the solutes. The state of water (the solvent) determines the mobility of the solutes and in return, the solutes change the structural organization of nearby water molecules through hydrophilic and hydrophobic interactions. In the cytoplasm, the thermodynamic state of the medium (and therefore the molecular mobility) determines the rate of metabolic activity.

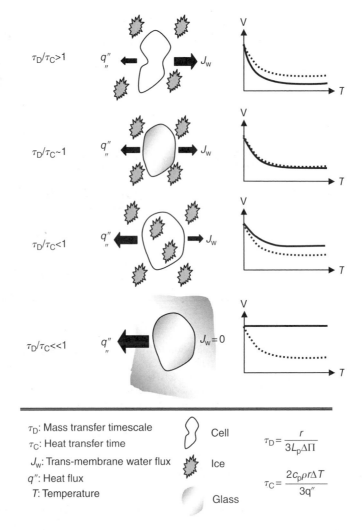

FIGURE 41.1   Effect of timescales on cell response.

In this chapter, the mechanisms enabling preservation of biological systems will be examined from the perspective of "molecular mobility" exploring the effects of the timescales for cooling, freezing, crystallization, vitrification, structural relaxation, and diffusion. Following example underlines the importance of timescales in preservation.

The timescales of biochemical reactions and the preservation conditions applied to the organism play crucial roles in determining the success of preservation. For example, the ratio of the timescale of water diffusion, τ_D, across the cell membrane ($\tau_D = r/3L_p\Delta\Pi$, where r, L_p, and $\Delta\Pi$ are the cell radius, membrane permeability, and osmotic pressure differential, respectively) to the timescale of cooling the cell experiences, τ_C ($\tau_C = (2c_p\rho r\Delta T)/(3q'')$, where c_p, ρ, q'', and ΔT are the specific heat, mass density, heat flux, and temperature differential, respectively) determines the fate of a cell during freezing such that (Figure 41.1):

- $\tau_D/\tau_C > 1$ causes excessive dehydration of the cell.
- $\tau_D/\tau_C \sim 1$ establishes an intra/extracellular equilibrium such that the intracellular water transported across the membrane balances the extracellular osmotic increase induced by freezing (the solute-concentration effect [2]) minimizing the amount of intracellular free water.

- $\tau_D/\tau_C < 1$ results in rapid cooling (faster than the cell can reach equilibrium with its surroundings) inducing Intracellular Ice Formation (IIF) known to be lethal to most cells (see Figure 41.2 Toner [3], for the correlation between IIF and post-thaw viability of mammalian cells).
- $\tau_D/\tau_C \ll 1$ theoretically, yields to ultrafast cooling without ice crystallization (if as an additional constraint $\tau_\alpha/\tau_C \ll 1$ where, τ_α is the timescale of structural relaxations) enabling vitrification of the extracellular medium, and more importantly the cytosol.

41.1 Water–Solute Interactions and Intracellular Transport

Water is the most abundant substance in and around an organism, yet it is the least understood in terms of its role in biological function and preservation. Water has unique physical and chemical properties [4] (for a complete review, see Franks [5], for an extensive collection of the properties and the anomalies of water, see the excellent electronic source by Chaplin [6]). Hydrogen bonds ($E_a = 4$ to 7 kJ/mol [7]) with bond energies similar to the local thermal fluctuations are continuously formed and broken between neighboring water molecules organizing them into flickering clusters of minimum free energy. These loosely bonded hydrogen clusters have very short life spans ($\tau_W = 10^{-11}$ to 10^{-12} sec) and are quickly destroyed just to form new ones in a never-ending cycle. This behavior establishes the basis of molecular mobility of water such that even in pure liquid form, a single water molecule is not independent in its motion but, at any instant of time, moves in coordination with a cluster of molecules. It is therefore widely believed that for water a cluster (rather than an individual water molecule) is the elementary structural unit and the interactions of clusters are responsible for its unique chemical and physical properties [8].

There is a continuous tug-of-war between the hydrogen bonds trying to stabilize the network of water molecules and the temperature dependent random motions breaking these bonds. With decreasing temperature, the magnitude of local thermal fluctuations decrease, increasing the lifetime of the hydrogen

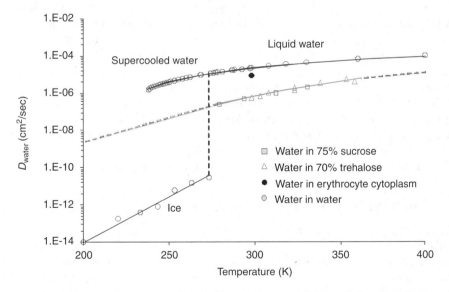

FIGURE 41.2 Self-diffusivity of water. Data of water diffusivity in 70% trehalose solution: NMR by Ekdawi-Sever et al. [112], NMR by Rampp et al. [42] and DMS by Conrad and de Pablo [41]; water diffusivity in 75% sucrose solution: Ekdawi-Sever et al. [112]; water diffusivity in the supercooled region: DMS by Paschek and Geiger [113] and NMR by Price et al. [114]; water diffusivity in ice: Onsager and Runnels [115] and Petrenko and Whitworth [116]; water diffusivity in liquid phase by Mills [117], NMR by Harris and Newitt [118]; water diffusivity in 75% sucrose: NMR by Moran et al. [119].

bonds among water molecules (i.e., the number of available neighboring hydrogen bonding sites per water molecule at any given time decreases). Water mobility (and its self-diffusion coefficient, D_w, as shown in Figure 41.2) therefore decreases [9,10] while the water clusters they participate in get more densely packed and grow [7]. Water mobility is not only a function of temperature but also the thermodynamic state. For example, D_w of liquid water decreases only by an O(2) over a range of 150 K whereas it drops by an O(6) upon freezing at 0°C (Figure 41.2). In the frozen state, each water molecule makes hydrogen bonds with only four neighboring molecules in a three-dimensional tetrahedron-like configuration. The degree of tetrahedricity (perfectness of the tetrahedral configuration) increases with decreasing temperature [10]. The strong interations between water molecules also cause an unexpected decrease in D_w when the density is decreased by increasing hydrostatic pressure. In water, density decrease lowers the hydrogen bonding possibility, therefore reduces mobility. In other liquids however, mobility is increased due to the increase in the free volume.

Any surface (hydrophilic or hydrophobic) or solute (charged or uncharged) disrupts the bonding patterns of the water molecules in its near vicinity causing local polarization and altering the life cycles of the surrounding water clusters [6,11]. This results in variations in water mobility, which can be detected by methods such as Nuclear Magnetic Resonance (NMR) and Fourier Transform Infrared Spectroscopy (FTIR). Close to a hydrophilic surface exerting a higher attraction force, water mobility decreases (the water molecules make stronger bonds with the surface and they are less available to join in a cluster). This causes depression of the freezing temperature and is the origin of the "unfreezable water" concept frequently used by the cryobiologists. Similarly, in close proximity to a hydrophobic surface or a solute, in this case entirely due to geometrical factors limiting hydrogen bonding possibility (that the water molecules can not make bonds with the hydrophobic surface), in the direction perpendicular to the surface, water mobility and therefore diffusion decreases. Parallel to the hydrophobic surface however, water diffusivity is not different from that of free water [12]. The coexistence of hydrophobic and hydrophilic surfaces on most proteins therefore creates large spatial gradients of water mobility, which may be closely related to protein function (e.g., the alternating regions of high and low water mobility within the hydration shells of actin filaments are thought to be contributing to the movement of myosin along these filaments [13]). Ions also affect nearby water molecules and alter their mobility [14]. For example, structure-breaking solutes such as urea [15] and large ions such as I^- and Cs^+ [14] increase the mobility of the water molecules in their immediate vicinity. Small ions such as Mg^{++} and F^-, on the other hand, have the opposite effect on their hydration layer. Interactions with nearby surfaces and solutes change the lifetime and the stability of each vicinal water cluster and change their physical properties (e.g., low mobility vicinal water has lower mass density, lower freezing point, and higher specific heat than bulk water).

The interaction of water with solids and surfaces is mutual. Water is not only a solvent but is also a react-ant itself. It is a substance functioning in cooperation with the solutes [16] altering their charge, conforma-tion, and reactivity. The range of water–solute interactions (the distance a water molecule should be from a surface or a solute to be fully isolated from its effects) is one of the most controversial topics in the literature, however it is widely accepted that vicinal water layers do not extend beyond 1 to 10 water molecules.

41.1.1 Intracellular Water and Molecular Mobility

In isotonic conditions, approximately 70% of the cell's volume is water. However, it would be wrong to think that the intracellular solutes and macromolecules bathe in a dilute solution. It has long been known that most, if not all, of the intracellular water exhibits physical properties unlike those in the bulk [17] (see the D_w in erythrocytes in Figure 41.2). This is attributed to the presence of high concentrations of proteins (200 to 300 g/l) [18], ions, amino acids, fatty acids, sugars, and other small solutes in the cytoplasm enmeshed in a network of cytoskeletal macromolecules (actin filaments, microtubules, and intermediate filaments). In individual organelles (such as mitochondria) the protein concentration may be even higher [19]. Within the cytoplasm, at any given time, water molecules are either a part of a tight cluster (bulk water) or in the close vicinity (vicinal water) of a surface (cell or organelle membrane) or a solute (a macromolecule, ion, or amino acid). There is not a consensus in the literature on the relative populations of vicinal and bulk water within the cytosol. The estimates vary in a range of 0 to 100% of the total intracellular water (for details, see Clegg [17] and the references therein). Similarly, the names given to the various subpopulations of water molecules in the close proximity of surfaces/solutes also vary from one source to another (hydration, bound, vicinal, essential, structural, ordered, unfreezable, osmotically inactive, etc.).

Overall cytosolic mobility is directly related to the metabolism and function of a cell [20,21]. However, the mobility of water in the cytosol is not spatially homogeneous [22,23] as evidenced by the presence of compartmentalization inside the cytoplasm (regions of solute aggregation and variable water mobility) using Fluorescence Recovery After Photobleaching (FRAP) [24] and Raman Scattering Microscopy (RSM) [25]. It is postulated that the intracellular mobility gradients determine the active and resting states of cells [26,27] and are altered in response to osmotic stress [28] and in the presence of carcinogens [26].

As opposed to dilute solutions, where the chemical reactions are transition-state-limited [29], most of the biochemical reactions in crowded environments are diffusion-limited. However, the diffusion mechanism in the cytoplasm is different from that in a dilute solution and is altered by the increased frequency of close-range interactions such as binding of and collisions between solutes and surfaces. In order to determine the hydrodynamic properties of the cytosol (translational, rotational diffusion coefficients and viscosity) various techniques have been utilized (NMR, FRAP, Electron Spin Resonance (ESR), etc. See Table 41.1 for details). The values reported in the literature lie in a very broad range (e.g., cytosolic viscosity values vary from 0.5 to 5 times that of water) and contradict each other (see reviews by Luby-Phelps et al. [24] and Arrio-Dupont et al. [30] for cytosolic diffusivity measurements using different methods and tracer molecules). The main reason for the discrepancy among the reported values is believed to be originating from the differences in the methodologies applied (such as the measurement of the translational diffusivity of a very large number of tracer molecules over a large volume [~1/10 to 1/20 of the volume of an attached cell] with FRAP or the shortcoming of NMR in distinguishing the signals from the intermolecular and intramolecular bonds and the requirement for relatively long acquisition times [31]), the characteristics of the tracer used (e.g., its size [24]), and inability of most of these methods to distinguish among different molecular interactions (free diffusion, binding, or collision) in this crowded environment [32]. The differences observed between the cytoplasmic viscosity values measured by rotational vs. translational diffusion of tracers indicate that physical interactions (such as binding and

TABLE 41.1 Most Common Methods for Measurement of Molecular Mobility

Method	Quantity measured	Range/limitations
Nuclear magnetic resonance (NMR)	Relaxation times T_1, T_2 of proton (^{1}H) and carbon (^{13}C) nuclei of water–carbohydrate samples	Cannot distinguish between the intermolecular and intramolecular bond signals. Measurement times are higher than the measured relaxation times
Dielectric spectroscopy	Complex dielectric permittivity	Water dipole moment relaxations in the kHz–GHz range
Differential scanning calorimetry (DSC)	Specific heat change $\Delta C_p\vert_{T=T_g}$	May be used in the 100–1500 K range. Measures the glass transition temperature of the bulk sample
Fluorescence recovery after photobleaching (FRAP)	Translational diffusivity of the tracer molecule	Measures mobility of very large number of molecules in a large area ($\sim 1\ \mu m^3$). Measurements in a glass are not feasible due to photobleaching
Electron spin resonance (ESR)	Spin relaxation of molecular probes (such as tempol)	Rotational mobility range [110]: $t = 10^{-12}$–10^{-8} sec (continuous-wave EPR), $t = 10^{-7}$–10^3 sec (saturation tranfser EPR). Probe properties change with hydration level [111]
Fourier Transform Infrared Spectroscopy (FTIR)	Molecular bond vibration	Strong absorption of IR light by water
Circular dichroism		
Quasielastic neutron scattering (QNS)		Measurement time $\sim 10^{-12}$ sec, Measurement distance ~ 1A [17]

collisions) present a higher obstacle to diffusion when compared to fluid phase viscosity (see e.g., Figure 1 in Mastro and Keith [33]). Crowding and solute concentration affect larger macromolecules more than the small solutes and ions, and it is therefore not feasible to assign a single parameter for mobility. Even though the viscosity of the cytosol is not significantly higher than water, some large macromolecules do not diffuse at all in the timescale of hours [34]. This would limit the reaction rates of some of the intracellular biochemical processes, if they depended on diffusion only. Nature overcomes this problem by crowding certain reactants in small regions (compartmentalization) of the cytoplasm [35], which also explains the spatial heterogeneity of water mobility observed intracellularly [22,23].

41.1.2 Transmembrane Water Transport Effects

The cell membrane shows very low resistance to water transport. However, it is the biggest obstacle to the transport of solutes. Membrane permeability to solutes depends on the size, charge, and the hydrogen bonding characteristics of the solute (for a review of membrane transport phenomena, see McGrath [36]). Transport across the cell membrane in response to osmotic gradients is at the cornerstone of biopreservation studies since it is directly related to administration of preservation agents and to the amount and mobility of the intracellular water. Water is transported into the cell by three different methods (a) diffusive transport across the membrane, ($L_p \sim 2$–50×10^4 cm/sec), (b) facilitated transport through membrane channels ($L_p \sim 200 \times 10^4$ cm/sec), and (c) cotransport through glucose transporters and ion channels ($L_p \sim 4 \times 10^4$ cm/sec) [37]. Methods for quantifying membrane transport are reviewed by Verkman [38].

Both desiccation and freezing (as well as their complementary processes; rehydration and thawing) induce very high osmotic gradients across the cell membrane. Cells are capable of responding to mild osmotic gradients by adjusting their volume, mainly by water transport. Applying an osmotic gradient almost all of the free water (called the osmotically active water) in a cell can be removed temporarily without any permanent damage. The water of hydration (participating in the osmotically inactive volume) on the other hand, is tightly associated with the solutes and surfaces and upon removal causes polarization of surfaces, aggregation and denaturation of the macromolecules [20,21].

41.2 Molecular Mobility in Preservation

In a dilute, nonreacting, binary solution diffusivities of the solvent and the solute depend on their relative molecular sizes [39] as well as their concentrations and temperature. For this system, Stokes–Einstein relationship correlates the hydrodynamical properties of the solution as,

$$D_{\text{translational}} = \frac{kT}{n\pi r\eta}, \tag{41.1}$$

where, D, k, T, r, and η are the diffusivity, Boltzmann's constant, absolute temperature, hydrodynamic radius of the diffusing particle (van der Waals radius), and the viscosity, respectively. The constant n, takes the value of 6 for a "stick (hydrophilic) boundary" condition and the value of 4, for a "slip (hydrophobic) boundary" condition. With increased solute concentration, diffusion becomes more restricted and different interactions such as collisions with other solutes and binding between molecules start to dominate and deviations from the Stokes–Einstein relationship is observed.

For a supersaturated solution, crystallization is the energetically most favorable path. However, if the concentration increases very rapidly (or the temperature drops very fast) a meta-stable "glassy" form can be reached. For a glass-forming system, the transition from a dilute to a concentrated solution diffusion mechanism is determined by the concentration corresponding to the crossover temperature, T_c, predicted by the Mode Coupling Theory [40]. At the crossover temperature there is a transition from liquid-like to solid-like dynamics. Note that $T_c \sim (1.14$–$1.6)\,T_g$ for most glass-forming solutions, where T_g is the glass transition temperature. Diffusion in very high concentration solutions (close to glass transition

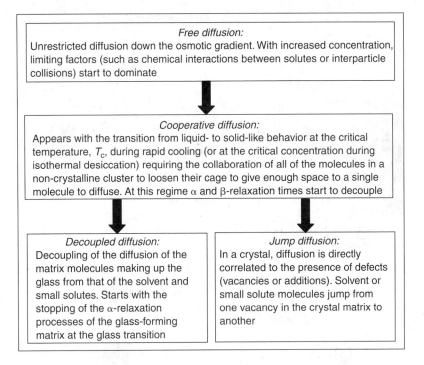

FIGURE 41.3 Mechanisms of diffusion.

temperature) is governed by the frequency of jumping between the cages surrounding the tagged molecule (either the solvent or a small solute) and is comparable to the time the molecule spends entrapped in the cage rattling (β-relaxation) [41]. This is similar to the mechanism of diffusion in crystalline systems, where the diffusing molecule jumps between the crystal defects (vacancies). Frequency of jumping is inversely related to the structural relaxation (α-relaxation) time, τ_α of the matrix. Temperature dependence of τ_α distinguishes between the "fragile" and "strong" glasses, where the variation in τ_α with temperature is steeper in the former case. In Figure 41.3 changes in the mechanism of diffusion with the thermodynamic state of the system is summarized.

In a concentrated and crowded environment such as in the cytosol, the motion of a small solute can be divided into two main components (Figure 41.4a) (1) the translational diffusive motion (governed by the α-relaxation timescale of the system), which results in a net displacement of the molecule down its osmotic gradient and (2) the random motion, which does not result in a net displacement. The random motion is governed by the physical and chemical interactions with the solvent and the surrounding solutes and is characterized by the β-relaxation timescale of the system, which includes rotation and Brownian motion. When the solvent is frozen, as a function of the storage temperature and the perfectness of the crystal structure formed, α-relaxation timescale increases. Depending on the relative magnitudes of the solvent and the solute molecules (and the size of the pores formed) β-relaxation may still continue (Figure 41.4b). Note the unfrozen bound water molecules in close proximity to the protein surface with lower mobility. If the system is desiccated (to a point where some of the water molecules in the hydration layer is also removed), both α and β-relaxations of the system may be stopped completely, however, due to removal of the hydration layer, the protein may denature and its active site may not be available for the binding of the ligand (Figure 41.4c). If denaturation of the protein is irreversible, even after rehydration (when molecular mobility is restored) the ligand can still not bind to the protein. Carbohydrates may be administered in order to prevent the denaturation of the protein while water is removed from the system lowering the mobility within the medium forming a glass (Figure 41.4d,e).

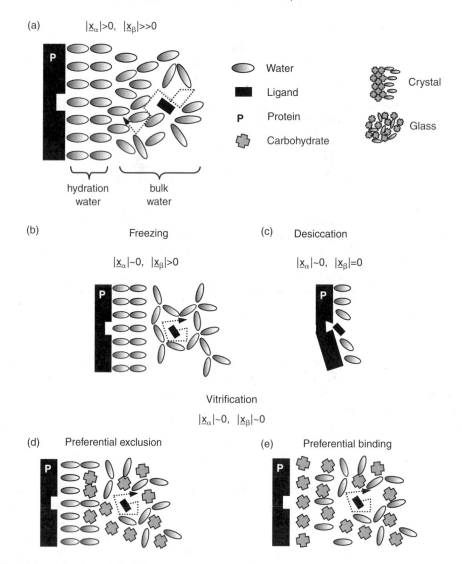

FIGURE 41.4   Molecular mobility in biopreservation.

For high solute concentrations in the absence of crystallization, Vogel–Tammann–Fulcher (VTF) equation predicts the changes in the timescales of molecular motion as:

$$\tau = \tau_0\, e^{-(BT_0)/(T-T_0)}, \tag{41.2}$$

where τ is the timescale of molecular motion, T_0 is the Kauzmann temperature corresponding to the zero mobility state, τ_0 is the timescale of motion at the Kauzmann temperature (usually taken to be in the order of 10^{17} sec), and B is a constant related to the energy of activation of the relaxation process. The values of B, for different carbohydrate solutions can be found in Rampp et al. [42].

41.2.1 Molecular Mobility in Supercooling and Phase Change

At temperatures below the freezing temperature (0°C, 1 atm) water may exist as a supercooled liquid or ice. The theoretical limit for the presence of free water in the liquid form is −40°C, where homogeneous crystallization is initiated. For freezing to occur at any given temperature, certain number of water clusters should form at the same time and reach a critical size (known as the formation of a nucleation embryo). With decreasing temperature, the critical number of water molecules required to form a nucleation embryo for the initiation of freezing decreases (from approximately 16,000 at −10°C to 120 at −40°C [5]) and at −40°C, it becomes statistically impossible for free water to remain in the liquid phase. In biological systems, due to the presence of small hydrophobic solutes with low surface energy (such as ice nucleating proteins in certain plants and bacteria that survive freeze injury), ice nucleation in the supercooled state is initiated well before the theoretical limit is reached. This is believed to help protect against the freeze-induced damage by minimizing compartmentalization and creating a more uniform ice structure.

With decreasing temperature, the diffusivity of liquid water decreases (approximately O(2) 370 to 240 K, see Figure 41.2) due to change in the mechanism of diffusion from unrestricted to cooperative (Figure 41.3). Upon freezing, the drop in water diffusivity becomes even more significant (approximately O(6) as shown in Figure 41.2). The reduction in water mobility with supercooling and liquid-to-solid phase change in addition to the decrease in most chemical reaction rates at low temperatures, makes cryopreservation feasible.

41.2.2 Cryopreservation

Certain organisms are known to synthesize carbohydrates upon exposure to cold and desiccation (such as trehalose synthesis by *Escherichia coli* [43], yeast [44], and nematodes [45]), which is crucial for their survival [46]. It was discovered (by accident) that glycerol also protects against freeze injury. These findings have fueled researchers to explore ways to use these chemical agents (cryoprotectants) for the preservation of biological organisms, which are normally not freeze or desiccation resistant. Over the years, this has led to the discovery of other cryoprotectants such as dimethylsulfoxide (DMSO) and ethylene glycol.

Cryoprotectants traditionally are divided into two main groups as membrane permeable and impermeable. Most effective and widely used cryoprotectants, DMSO [47], ethylene glycol, and glycerol are highly membrane permeable whereas most of the carbohydrates (trehalose, hydroxyethyl starch, dextran, etc.), proteins, and polymers are normally not. Exposure to membrane impermeable (or low permeability when compared to that of water) cryoprotectants creates an osmotic gradient across the membrane, to which a cell responds by shrinking. If a membrane permeable cryoprotectant is present on the other hand, after initial shrinkage, with prolonged exposure and penetration of the chemical, the cell recovers to its original volume. Similarly after thawing, to remove intracellular cryoprotectants, the cells are exposed to hypotonic solutions. This results in swelling of the cell followed by return to its isotonic volume. It is widely accepted that a significant part of freeze damage is related to the uncontrolled swelling response during thawing, that the membrane stretches beyond its mechanical limit and ruptures. The volume response of the cell to cryoprotectants creates changes in the cytoplasmic molecular mobility due to the changes in (a) the amount of cytoplasmic free water present at any time, (b) the intracellular solute concentration, and (c) the changes in the electrical potential gradients due to proximity of macromolecular surfaces. Additionally, during freezing, depending on the freezing-rate-dependent solute concentration (as presented previously in the first part of this chapter) volume of the cell changes responding to osmotic gradients (Figure 41.1). Briefly, damage to cells during cryopreservation is attributed to various factors directly or indirectly correlated to the presence of intra/extracellular ice (such as solute concentration, membrane potential change, mechanical damage by ice crystals, steep electrical potential, and osmotic gradients, etc.), however the exact mechanism of freeze injury is not known.

Cryopreservation is a process, which inherently disrupts intra/extracellular continuum and introduces heterogeneity within the cytoplasm. During freezing of a complex solution, there always is a mutual interaction between the two phases present simultaneously: the frozen liquid phase, which rejects solids and the supercooled liquid phase, which cannot freeze due to the increased concentration of the solutes rejected by the ice. Presence of solutes depresses the freezing temperature of the water, as a function of their mole fraction. The tug-of-war between these two phases introduces compartmentalization yielding to very high osmotic and electrical gradients within the cytosol. This may explain the low survival rates recorded at relatively high subzero temperatures.

To this date numerous post-thaw viability and function experiments have been performed with virtually every kind of cell using cryoprotectants at different concentrations, freezing/thawing rates, and storage conditions. Interested readers are directed to reviews by Mazur [48] and McGrath [36]. Interestingly, the mechanism of cryoprotection offered by the most widely used chemicals, for example DMSO and glycerol, is not known [49,50] beyond the colligative action (that they replace the water molecules in the cytosol) and their "strong interaction potential with water" at low temperatures. The colligative action of cryopreservatives in the absence of water can be divided into the space-filling effect, which prevents structural collapse and the osmotic effect, which presents the cryoprotectant as an alternative solvent reducing solute concentration. DMSO has a very high hydrogen bonding affinity toward water creating a nonideal mixture behavior (e.g., even though the freezing point of water and DMSO are 0 and 18.6°C respectively, the freezing point of a 1 : 3 molar ratio DMSO–water solution is −70°C).

Given that, DMSO is toxic at high temperatures [51] and has been shown to cause gene activation (for a review, see Ashwood-Smith [52]) and have mutagenic potential [53] at high concentrations, it is surprising that it works so well for preservation at low temperatures in spite of its biological inadequacy: an indication that the preservation phenomena is directly related to the thermodynamical properties of most cryoprotectants (freezing point depression), their effects on the structure of water (such as eliminating ice crystallization), and to the degree of molecular mobility reduction they offer (e.g., DMSO increases cytoplasmic viscosity [50]).

A mechanism offered to explain the protective potential of membrane permeable cryoprotectants and certain solutes introduced artificially into the cell (such as carbohydrates) is that they have the ability to retard ice formation by replacing water and imposing an ordered water structure resistant to crystallization. Raman Scattering, NMR, dynamic molecular modeling, and Quasi Elastic Neutron Scattering data indicate that especially trehalose, even at low concentrations breaks the structure of adjacent water molecules and slows down their mobility [54,55] and therefore makes them more resistant to crystallization at low temperatures [56]. Similarly, DMSO can alter the structure and the rotational and translational mobilities of water (e.g., 10% DMSO reduces the self-diffusion coefficient of water by half [50]) as a function of its concentration and environmental temperature [57]. Analysis of osmotic stress injury to frozen cells [58] in the presence of DMSO, glycerol, and ethylene glycol [59] also point to different reasons to explain the protective mechanism offered by these cryoprotectants beyond their colligative action.

Even though the chemical reaction rates are expected to slow at low temperatures following Arrhenius kinetics, due to freeze concentration, which decreases the distance between reactants and changes the pH of the medium in addition to the possible catalytic effects of ice crystals [60] (and given that proton mobility is higher in ice than in water due to the organized crystal structure), some enzyme-catalyzed chemical reaction rates do increase by orders of magnitude in the frozen state as compared to supercooled state [61]. Combined with the detrimental effects of IIF, the factors stated above formed the scientific reasoning behind development of an alternative preservation method: preservation of cells in an undercooled state [62]. It is known that with the addition of each mole of solute to one liter of water suppresses the freezing temperature by approximately 2°C by increasing the entropy of the liquid phase. It was shown that if structural stability at subzero temperatures could be ensured so that the probability of intra/extracellular ice formation is at a minimum, short-term storage could be feasible for certain cells. This can be achieved for example, by adding ice nucleation retarding solutes, applying high pressures, or using smaller water volumes with minimum peripheral contact (such as utilization of small water droplets suspended in oil).

The intracellular ice formation (IIF) has been thought to be the main source of viability loss for preserved biological systems. It is postulated that the ice crystals in the cytosol mechanically disrupt the cytoskeleton and the macromolecules in addition to causing very high localized solute concentrations due to solute rejection from the frozen phase. It is also suggested that IIF can not form by itself and is usually induced by Extracellular Ice Formation (EIF) breaching the cell membrane through membrane pores, enlarging them and causing the membrane to rupture.

It was therefore suggested that if IIF and EIF can be eliminated altogether (in spite of the disadvantages of having to load very high concentrations of cryoprotectants into the cells and keeping them at liquid nitrogen temperatures) then the preservation of cells, organs, and even whole human bodies would be possible in a vitrified state [63]. With high cryoprotectant concentrations (as high as 9 M [63]) and low temperature storage, ice formation within the cells can be completely eliminated and also an intracellular amorphous (or glassy?) state may be reached. This line of work however, is not supported by detailed theoretical, experimental, and numerical analysis of molecular motion confirming the presence of intracellular glass. Given that the glass transition temperatures for DMSO, glycerol, and ethylene glycol (at 100% w/w) are -122.2, -187, and $-115°C$, respectively [64] when compared to that of pure water ($-135°C$) even if their primary mechanism of action in preservation at high concentration is by vitrification, then their only role is relaxing the high cooling rate (10^6 K/sec) requirement for the vitrification of water. Actually, for a 5 M solution of DMSO in water, the critical cooling rate for vitrification (the cooling rate at which crystal formation is minimum) is approximately 10 K/sec. This is achievable, however the critical warming rate is still unattainable (10^8 K/sec) [65].

41.2.3 Vitrification

The discovery of the presence of a vitrified state in the cytoplasms of desiccated plant seeds [66], Artemia cysts, and fungal spores started extensive research for desiccation preservation of mammalian cells and tissues. For plants and certain animals, it was shown that the transition to the glassy state was enabled through the accumulation of certain carbohydrates (glucose, sucrose, raffinose, and stachyose in plants, and trehalose in microorganisms and animals making up about 15 to 25% of their dry weight). Having the same chemical groups (–OH) as water, carbohydrates are hypothesized to replace the hydrogen bonds formed between water molecules and the macromolecules in the cytoplasm and the lipid membranes stabilizing their conformations in the absence of water [5]. This has formed the basis of the "water replacement hypothesis" [67] that was offered as an explanation for the protective capacity of certain carbohydrates against freezing and desiccation damage. Another theory proposed is based on the "preferential exclusion" of carbohydrates from macromolecule surfaces [68,69]. This theory predicts that when water is scarce in the cytoplasm (as would be the case during desiccation or freezing), water molecules in the hydration shell of the macromolecules remain undisturbed while the void left by the removed free water is filled by the carbohydrates eliminating structural collapse. It is not known to this date which one of these hypotheses explains the protection mechanism responsible for reducing macromolecule and membrane denaturation during desiccation.

Additionally, a recently introduced hypothesis based on molecular mobility measurements suggests that the main protective effect of carbohydrates is by breaking the structure of the surrounding water molecules (especially at low water concentrations) and creating more structured water clusters, therefore enabling encapsulation of biological macromolecules in a rigid matrix [70]. This hypothesis is in agreement with the additional claim made by the first two hypotheses that upon removal of the free water, a cytosolic glass with reduced molecular mobility is formed, virtually stopping all biochemical processes. In addition to carbohydrates, certain solutes abundant in the cytosol (such as proteins, amino acids, ions, and salts) are also thought to be participating in the formation of the cytoplasmic glass [71] (for a recent review, see Buitink et al. [72]). It should be noted that the glass transition temperature of an ideal mixture is determined by the glass transition temperatures of its constituents. Since it has a very low glass transition temperature ($T_g = -135°C$), water significantly reduces the glass transition temperature of carbohydrates as a function of its concentration.

Chemical reaction rates have been shown to decrease in the presence of high concentrations of carbohydrates, facilitating protein dynamics studies [73,74], slowing down oxygen diffusion therefore increasing the stability of fluorescent molecules [73], reducing degradation of enzymes [75,76] and proteins [74,77], and enabling lyophilization of bacteria [78] and viruses [79] supporting the cytosolic vitrification hypothesis by experimental evidence. However, contradicting reports also exist, where researchers did not find any difference between the state diagrams (glass transition temperature as a function of water content) of desiccation tolerant and intolerant plants [80]. This has been offered as the basis of why cytosolic vitrification alone can not be responsible for preservation in the desiccated state.

It was shown that for the carbohydrates to protect against desiccation damage, they should be present on both sides of the membrane [81]. Almost all of the glass-forming carbohydrates and polymers are membrane impermeable and should be introduced artificially with the exception of glucose. Currently applied reversible membrane breaching methods are microinjection [82], osmotic shock [83], electroporation [84,85], thermal shock [86], acoustical exposure [87,88], endocytosis [89], and transport through switchable membrane pores [90,91]. For details of these methods, see Acker et al. [81]. An alternative method utilized is the genetic modification of mammalian cells to express genes for coding carbohydrates intracellularly [92]. It is still perceived as a challenge to upload mammalian cells with high concentrations (0.2 to 0.3 M) of carbohydrates required for preservation.

A glass is a metastable liquid with very low molecular mobility of its main structural ingredient, which forms an amorphous matrix rather than an energetically more favorable crystal. Whether achieved by rapid cooling, desiccation, addition of cryoprotectants or carbohydrates, amorphous to glassy phase transition is characterized by a sharp discontinuity in the temperature–density curve. As an indication of very compact packing in the molecular arrangement in the glassy phase, density is a very weak function of temperature. At the glass transition temperature, specific heat also decreases significantly since a higher percentage of the thermal energy transferred to the system causes a temperature change without being dissipated by the exceedingly confined molecular motions of the matrix molecules. Even though vitrification is characterized by a very significant change in viscosity ($O(7–9)$), and the stopping of α-relaxation processes, depending on the relative sizes of the matrix molecules and the solvent remaining in the system, molecular motion does not completely stop [42]. During drying of thin films or small droplets of high molecular weight polymer and carbohydrate solutions for example, evaporation continues even though early on a glassy film is formed on the surface. The decoupling of matrix mobility from that of the solvent at glass transition may present a challenge that the diffusion of the solvent and the small solutes can not be prevented during storage of biological materials. The glass transition temperature increases with increasing molecular weight. Therefore, with increasing molecular weight of the matrix, the mobility of the solvent at matrix glass transition also increases [93,94]. This has led some researchers [95] to conclude that a glassy matrix (actin embedded in a glass formed by dextran, a very high molecular weight carbohydrate) can not protect against desiccation damage. Apparently, in this particular case even though the matrix was glassy, decoupling of matrix and solvent (and small solute) mobilities were very significant resulting in denaturation of actin.

It would be wrong to conclude however, that the diffusion of small solutes and the solvent in a glassy matrix would not be affected by the presence of the glass. With increasing solute concentration, the mobility of the solvent is increasingly limited and therefore the solvent switches from the free, unrestricted diffusion to jump-diffusion (Figure 41.3) between the cages formed by the glassy matrix [96]. There is evidence that the transition in the diffusion mode of water coincides with the point, where the carbohydrates have been shown to form a three-dimensional hydrogen bonded network [97]. The diffusion constant shows an Arrhenius type dependence on temperature above and below the glass transition temperature (with different activation energies) indicating decoupling of the solvent and the carbohydrate matrix mobility [98–100]. For example, during desiccation diffusivity of water in the Artemia cysts decreases with decreasing water content, however below a critical water content corresponding to 0.15 $g_{water}/g_{drymatter}$ [101], it starts to increase.

As opposed to diffusion in a glassy matrix, where translational mobility is dictated by cooperative diffusion, in cryopreservation, diffusion is dependent on the presence of defects in the crystalline structure (and the presence of grain boundaries). In a perfect crystal (without any defects or grain boundaries), mobility of the solvent and small solutes are exceedingly hindered (Figure 41.2).

For glass-forming liquids, with increasing cooling rate, the probability of reaching the glassy state increases (when compared to crystallization). However, since a glass is intrinsically a liquid with a higher energy than its crystal, given enough time (depending on the characteristics of the carbohydrate and the storage conditions this could be weeks, years, or even centuries) it will crystallize.

In the absence of chemical and electrical interactions, the size of a molecule determines its mobility in a glassy matrix. In dextran solutions, for example with increasing molecular weight of the dextran, water mobility at glass transition increases. For successful storage therefore, the size of the molecules to be preserved should be larger than that of the molecules making up the glassy matrix and the free volume of the matrix they form. Rigidity of the glassy matrix may also contribute to its storage potential by reducing solvent mobility. For example, it was shown by Elastic Incoherent Neutron Scattering measurements that the glassy matrix formed by trehalose (which is known to be superior in terms of its protective potential) is more rigid than the glasses formed by maltose and sucrose [102]. If the preserved molecules are polar, their mobility may further be reduced since they can form strong hydrogen bonds with the glassy matrix. Due to the facts presented above, we may conclude that a high glass transition temperature alone is not sufficient in determining the storage potential offered by a particular glass former. Even though dextran has a higher glass transition temperature than trehalose and sucrose, it has been repeatedly shown to have inferior protective capacity against desiccation and freezing damage. One reason for its low protective capacity may be its large size making it less flexible and therefore its hydration sites less accessible. However, there is reason to believe that the main factor is the high pore size of the glassy matrix it forms presenting lower resistance to the diffusion of solutes and solvents. With the technological advances making it feasible to measure molecular mobility in the glassy state, this hypothesis can be put to test.

41.2.4 Vitrification by Ultrafast Cooling

If the kinetic energy can be reduced faster than the rotational and translational diffusion timescales at any temperature, then vitrification without crystallization can be achieved for an aqueous glass former at any water content. If it can be cooled fast enough (10^6 to $10^7 °C$/sec), even water can be vitrified at a temperature of $-135°C$. For biological materials, these cooling rates can not be achieved using conventional techniques such as liquid nitrogen immersion. However, methods utilizing cooling with simultaneous heating are promising [103]. Ultrafast cooling, if achieved, does not expose cells to osmotic and dehydration stresses and therefore also eliminates compartmentalization (Figure 41.1). However, if storage at noncryogenic temperatures is desired, methods to reduce mobility at high temperatures should be developed.

41.2.5 Vitrification by Desiccation

During isothermal drying, the glass transition temperature of the solution increases. Evaporation of the solvent causes a decrease in the free volume increasing the viscosity and the structural relaxation times. Mode Coupling Theory [40] predicts a crossover temperature located at approximately 40 to 50 K above the glass transition temperature of a glass-forming solution, where there is a transition from liquid-like to solid-like molecular dynamics. The structural relaxation time, τ_α, is related to the collective motion of a group of molecules to loosen up the cage they form around a single molecule and enable it to make a translational diffusive motion. The short timescale relaxation time, τ_β, however involves the temperature dependent vibrational motion of a single molecule, which also involves rotation. τ_α reaches a value of 10^2 sec ($\tau_\alpha = 10^{-7}$ sec at the crossover temperature) very close to glass transition (for an extensive review, see Novikov, 2003 [104]). The O(9) decrease in the structural relaxation time with proximity to glassy state (each evaporating water molecule making it more difficult for the next one in the solution to evaporate) is thought to make vitrification improbable in the experimental timescales considered. However, vitrification of carbohydrate solutions can be accelerated using a cocktail of carbohydrates [105] and salts [120].

41.2.6 Lyophilization

Cryopreservation (either in the frozen or the vitrified state) requires very low temperatures for storage and transportation and therefore is not economical for many purposes. An alternative to cryopreservation is lyophilization, where the reduction of molecular mobility reached at low temperatures by cryopreservation can be achieved at relatively high temperatures by the removal of water (the universal plasticizer), thus increasing the glass transition temperature [106]. The product to be stored is initially frozen in the presence of cryoprotectants and carbohydrates. Then, by the application of vacuum, frozen water is sublimated at progressively increasing temperatures. Removal of water increases the glass transition temperature of the product and establishes stability at ambient temperatures. In the pharmaceutical and food industries, lyophilization is widely used for the preservation of proteins, enzymes, bacteria, and foodstuff.

The main advantage of lyophilization over desiccation is in minimizing the exposure to osmotic stresses. During diffusive or convective drying, by the removal of water, the solutes concentrate and the product to be preserved is exposed to increasing osmotic stresses over long periods of time. In lyophilization, the product is first frozen and then the water is removed, minimizing osmotic stress buildup. However, the removal of water from the frozen structure leaves pores within the protective matrix and the product. These pores in time may collapse and the structural integrity of the product may be lost. In order to prevent this during lyophilization, the primary and secondary drying temperatures are kept above the collapse temperature of the matrix. Certain high molecular weight carbohydrates (such as dextran) are also incorporated to increase the structural stability of the matrix.

41.3 Storage

During storage the preserved organism does not need a steady supply of nutrients (and removal of the by-products). On the down side, it does not have the metabolic activity to repair the accumulating damage. In the preserved state, the harmful environmental factors are, to a degree, physically isolated from the organism by the surrounding matrix (the frozen liquid crystal structure in cryopreservation or an amorphous matrix of carbohydrates during desiccation) reducing the amount of accumulated damage.

Regardless of the processing method, the final thermodynamic state of the product and the molecular mobility at that state determine the storage stability as a function of storage parameters (primarily humidity, temperature, and pressure). If at the storage condition, the product is not at equilibrium (internally or externally with the environment), the chemical processes will continue even at slow rates toward the minimum energy state. For example in vitrification, since the glass formed is inherently at a higher energy state it will crystallize in time. Crystallization is accompanied by compartmentalization [105] and heteregeneous devitrification, resulting in an increase in mobility. It also creates high mechanical stresses that can damage the product. The structural mobility of the glass determines its crystallization lifetime, while the mobilities of the solvents and small solutes within the glass determine the degradation of the stored product. One way to eliminate crystallization is to use cocktails of carbohydrates and salts. For example, raffinose and stachyose are very effective in inhibiting sucrose crystallization [107]. The presence of small solutes and proteins in the cytoplasm may also help reduce crystallization of sugars [108]. In cryopreservation, the grain boundaries between the frozen sections and the interfaces between the ice crystals and the solutes rejected during freezing have higher free energy and therefore mobility. Molecular mobility in these regions determine the stability of the stored product.

Vitrified products can be stored at higher temperatures, however their storage conditions still need to be regulated carefully since molecular mobility increases significantly with increasing water content. For a trehalose glass the glass transition temperature decreases by 50 K by a very slight change in the water content (0.05 $g_{water}/g_{drymatter}$). If the water activity in the environment is higher than that in glass, the product absorbs water and the molecular mobility within increases. On the opposite end, if the environmental water activity is lower, the stored product may desiccate further, losing its hydration water. For most lyophilized bacteria, it has been shown that irrespective of the preservation agent used, for successful revival, the water content within the product should not drop below a certain limit.

The other important factors that need to be considered for successful storage in vitrified state are oxygen and light. Free oxygen radicals have very high diffusivity and are extremely reactant. Even at very low mobility environments, they may jump-start enzymatic reactions. Some carbohydrates, such as trehalose are known to prevent oxygen radical damage [109] as well.

41.4 Summary

The "molecular mobility" hypothesis analyzed here suggests that, if all of the reactants in an organism can be reversibly immobilized in their native configuration, the biochemical processes can be stopped and preservation can be achieved (Figure 41.4). The condition set forth by the hypothesis is sufficient to halt the diffusion-limited biochemical reactions, which dominate in a crowded, confined environment such as in the cytoplasm [29]. However, not all of the chemical reactions in an organism is governed by diffusion. In order to respond to sudden changes in its environment (under certain conditions, the metabolic rate has been known to increase up to 35 times), the mammalian cell has devised strategies to accelerate certain reactions without being limited by diffusion timescales, for example by accumulating reactants in aggregates (compartmentalization), reducing the degree-of-freedom of the reactants (such as the case with membrane proteins) and advection (bulk mixing due to cell motion). The effects of the currently applied and proposed biopreservation methods on this kind of chemical reactions remain to be researched.

The important points that are highlighted in this chapter are:

(1) Glass transition is a collaborative phenomena involving the solvent and the solute. With increasing difference in the molecular sizes of the solvent and the solute mobility of the solute molecules making up the glassy matrix and that of the solvent (or other small solutes suspended in the solvent) decouple strongly at glass transition. Mobility of the solvent may be significantly higher than that of the matrix, even below the glass transition temperature of the system, enabling certain chemical reactions to proceed. High molecular weight carbohydrates increase the glass transition temperature of the system, however they do not necessarily decrease the solvent (or small solute) mobility in the same degree.

(2) If noncryogenic temperature storage is desired, the mobility within and surrounding the preserved product should be lowered. This may be achieved by loading high amounts of protectants (cryoprotectant solvents such as glycerol, DMSO, etc. or carbohydrates, proteins, etc.) into the product to displace water or change the properties of the intracellular water. It is unlikely that any organism can be successfully preserved by vitrification at conditions requiring complete removal of all of its water. The "essential water" in the product upon removal causes irreversible damage. This quantity is not easily measurable. The water affinities of the macromolecules and membranes in the preserved product and that of the added protectant are different and also change with the decrease in the availability of water. Decreasing the water content of the overall system comprised of the product to be preserved and the surrounding protectant matrix (frozen, amorphous, or glassy) does not necessarily mean that the water contents of the matrix and the product are equally reduced.

(3) The importance of diffusion-limited reactions for the metabolic activity of the product should be established. Reduction of mobility within the medium is most likely to reduce the diffusion of any size molecule, however there is increasingly more evidence collected showing that the majority of the biochemical reactions do not depend on diffusion alone. For preservation to be successful, mobility of all molecules in all size scales should be stopped without irreversibly disrupting their native configurations.

(4) The state of intracellular water is directly related to the metabolism and functioning of an organism. All of the chemical agents known to have protective capacity against freezing and desiccation damage modify the structure of the intracellular water. More research is required to establish the role of water in organisms in order to develop successful preservation methods and to increase the efficiency of the currently applied ones.

Acknowledgments

The authors thank Dr. James Clegg, Dr. John Bischof, and Dr. Xiang-Hong Liu for careful reading of the manuscript and their constructive feedback. This work was supported by the National Institutes of Health grants.

References

[1] Crowe, J.H. and Cooper, A.F., Cryptobiosis, *Sci. Am.*, 225, 30, 1971.

[2] Mazur, P., Leibo, S., and Chu, E.H.Y., A two-factor hypothesis of freezing injury, *Exp. Cell Res.*, 71, 345, 1972.

[3] Toner, M., Nucleation of ice crystals inside biological cells, in *Advances in Low-Temperature Biology*, Steponkus, P.L., Ed., JAI Press Ltd, Greenwich CN, 1993.

[4] Sastry, S., Order and oddities, *Nature*, 409, 300, 2001.

[5] Franks, F., *Water: A Matrix of Life*, Royal Society of Chemistry, Cambridge, UK, 2000.

[6] Chaplin, M., *Www.Lsbu.Ac.Uk/water/index.Html*, 2004.

[7] Szasz, A. et al., Water states in living systems: I. Structural aspects, *Physiol. Chem. Phys. Med. NMR*, 26, 299, 1994.

[8] Franks, F., *Water: A Comprehensive Treatise*, Plenum Press, New York, 1979.

[9] Sciortino, F., Geiger, A., and Stanley, H.E., Network defects and molecular mobility in liquid water, *J. Chem. Phys.*, 96, 3857, 1992.

[10] Geiger, A. et al., Mechanisms of the molecular mobility of water, *J. Mol. Liq.*, 106, 161, 2003.

[11] Granick, S., Motions and relaxations of confined liquids, *Science*, 253, 1374, 1991.

[12] Jensen, M.O., Mouritsen, O.G., and Peters, G.H., The hydrophobic effect: molecular dynamics simulations of water confined between extended hydrophobic and hydrophilic surfaces, *J. Chem. Phys.*, 120, 9729, 2004.

[13] Kabir, S.R. et al., Hyper-mobile water is induced around actin filaments, *Biophys. J.*, 85, 3154, 2003.

[14] Hribar, B. et al., How ions affect the structure of water, *J. Am. Chem. Soc.*, 124, 12302, 2002.

[15] Tovchigrechko, A., Rodnikova, M., and Barthel, J., Comparative study of urea and tetramethylurea in water by molecular dynamics simulations, *J. Mol. Liq.*, 79, 187, 1999.

[16] Watterson, J.G., A role of water in cell structure, *Biochem. J.*, 248, 615, 1987.

[17] Clegg, J.S., Intracellular water and the cytomatrix: some methods of study and current views, *J. Cell Biol.*, 99, 167S, 1984.

[18] Zimmerman, S.B. and Trach, S.O., Estimation of macromolecule concentrations and excluded volume effects for the cytoplasm of *Escherichia coli*, *J. Mol. Biol.*, 222, 599, 1991.

[19] Scalettar, B.A., Abney, J.R., and Hackenbrock, C.R., Dynamics, structure and function are coupled in the mitochondrial matrix, *Proc. Natl Acad. Sci. USA*, 88, 8057, 1991.

[20] Cayley, S. and Record, M.T., Roles of cytoplasmic osmolytes, water and crowding in the response of *Escherichia coli* to osmotic stress: biophysical basis of osmoprotection by glycine betaine, *Biochemistry*, 42, 12595, 2003.

[21] Clegg, J.S., Properties and metabolism of the aqueous cytoplasm and its boundaries, *Am. J. Physiol.*, 246, R133, 1984.

[22] Sehy, J.V., Ackerman, J.J.H., and Neil, J.J., Apparent diffusion of water, ions, and small molecules in the xenopus oocyte is consistent with brownian displacement, *Magn. Reson. Med.*, 48, 42, 2002.

[23] Ovádi, J. and Saks, V., On the origin of intracellular compartmentation and organized metabolic systems, *Mol. Cell. Biochem.*, 256/257, 5, 2004.

[24] Luby-Phelps, K., Taylor, D.L., and Lanni, F., Probing the structure of cytoplasm, *J. Cell Biol.*, 102, 2015, 1986.

[25] Potma, E.O. et al., Real-time visualization of intracellular hydrodynamics in single living cells, *Proc. Natl Acad. Sci. USA*, 98, 1577, 2001.

[26] Wiggins, P.M., High and low density water and resting, active and transformed cells, *Cell Biol. Int.*, 20, 429, 1996.

[27] Beall, P.T., Hazlewood, C.F., and Rao, P.N., Nuclear magnetic resonance patterns of intracellular water as a function of hela cell cycle, *Science*, 192, 904, 1976.

[28] Cameron, I.L., et al., A mechanistic view of the non-ideal osmotic and motional behavior of intracellular water, *Cell Biol. Int.*, 21, 99, 1997.

[29] Ellis, R.J., Macromolecular crowding: an important but neglected aspect of the intracellular environment, *Curr. Opin. Struct. Biol.*, 11, 114, 2001.

[30] Arrio-Dupont, M. et al., Translational diffusion of globular proteins in the cytoplasm of cultured muscle cells, *Biophys. J.*, 78, 901, 2000.

[31] Garcia-Martin, M.L., Ballesteros, P., and Cerdan, S., The metabolism of water in cells and tissues as detected by NMR methods, *Prog. Nucl. Magn. Reson. Spectrosc.*, 39, 41, 2001.

[32] Kao, H.P., Abney, J.R., and Verkman, A.S., Determinant of the translational mobility of a small solute in cell cytoplasm, *J. Cell Biol.*, 120, 175, 1993.

[33] Mastro, A.M. and Keith, A.D., Diffusion in aqueous compartment, *J. Cell Biol.*, 99, 180s, 1984.

[34] Welch, G.R. and Clegg, J.S., *The Organization of Cell Metabolism*, Welch, G.R. and Clegg, J.S., Eds., Plenum Press, New York, 1986.

[35] Minton, A.P., The influence of macromolecular crowding and macromolecular confinement on biochemical reactions in physiological media, *J. Biol. Chem.*, 276, 10577, 2001.

[36] McGrath, J.J., Membrane transport properties, in *Low Temperature Biotechnology*, McGrath, J.J. and Diller, K.R., Eds., ASME, New York, NY, 1988.

[37] Fettiplace, R. and Haydon, D.A., Water permeability of lipid membranes, *Physiol. Rev.*, 60, 510, 1980.

[38] Verkman, A.S., Water permeability measurement in living cells and complex tissues, *J. Membr. Biol.*, 173, 73, 2000.

[39] Bhattacharyya, S. and Bagchi, B., Anomalous diffusion of small particles in dense liquids, *J. Chem. Phys.*, 106, 1757, 1997.

[40] Gotze, W., Recent tests of the mode coupling theory for glassy dynamics, *J. Phys.: Condens. Matter*, 11, A1, 1999.

[41] Conrad, P.B. and de Pablo, J.J., Computer simulation of cryoprotectant disaccharide α,α-trehalose in aqueous solution, *J. Phys. Chem. A*, 103, 4049, 1999.

[42] Rampp, M., Buttersack, C., and Lüdemann, H.-D., C, t-Dependence of the viscosity and the self-diffusion coefficients in some aqueous carbohydrate solutions, *Carbohydr. Res.*, 328, 561, 2000.

[43] Kandror, O., DeLeon, A., and Goldberg, A.L., Trehalose synthesis is induced upon exposure of *Escherichia coli* to cold and is essential for viability at low temperatures., *Proc. Natl Acad. Sci. USA*, 99, 9727, 2002.

[44] Attfield, P.V., Trehalose accumulates in *Saccharomyces cerevisiae* during exposure to agents that induce heat shock response, *FEBS Lett.*, 225, 259, 1987.

[45] Madin, K.A.C. and Crowe, J.H., Anhydrobiosis in nematodes: carbohydrate and lipid metabolism during dehydration, *J. Exp. Zool.*, 193, 335, 1975.

[46] Crowe, J.H., Hoekstra, F.A., and Crowe, L.M., Anhydrobiosis, *Ann. Rev. Physiol.*, 54, 579, 1992.

[47] Arakawa, T. et al., The basis for toxicity of certain cryoprotectants — a hypothesis, *Cryobiology*, 27, 401, 1990.

[48] Mazur, P., Principles of cryobiology, in *Life in the Frozen State*, Fuller, B.J., Lane, N., and Benson, E.E., Eds., CRC Press, Boca Raton, FL, 2004.

[49] Murthy, S.S.N., Phase behavior of the supercooled aqueous solutions of dimethyl sulfoxide, ethylene glycol, and methanol as seen by dielectric spectroscopy, *J. Phys. Chem. B*, 101, 6043, 1997.

[50] Yu, Z.W. and Quinn, P.J., The modulation of membrane structure and stability by dimethyl sulphoxide (review), *Mol. Membr. Biol.*, 15, 59, 1998.

[51] Fahy, G.M., The relevance of cryoprotectant toxicity to cryobiology, *Cryobiology*, 23, 1, 1986.

[52] Ashwood-Smith, M.J., Genetic damage is not produced by normal cryopreservation procedures involving either glycerol or dimethyl sulfoxide: a cautionary note, however, on possible effects of dimethyl sulfoxide, *Cryobiology*, 22, 427, 1985.

[53] Preisler, H.D. and Lyman, G., Differentiation of erythroleukemia cells *in vitro* — properties of chemical inducers, *Cell Differ.*, 4, 179, 1975.

[54] Magazu, S. et al., Diffusive dynamics in trehalose aqueous solutions by qens, *Physica B*, 276, 475, 2000.

[55] Bordat, P. et al., Comparative study of trehalose, sucrose and maltose in water solutions by molecular modelling, *Europhys. Lett.*, 65, 41, 2004.

[56] Branca, C. et al., A,α-trehalose-water solutions. 3. Vibrational dynamics studies by inelastic light scattering, *J. Phys. Chem. B*, 103, 1347, 1999.

[57] Packer, K.J. and Tomlinson, D.J., Nuclear spin relaxation and self-diffusion in the binary system, dimethylsulfoxide (DMSO) + water, *Trans. Faraday Soc.*, 67, 1302, 1971.

[58] Takashashi, T., Hammett, M.F., and Cho, M.S., Multifaceted freezing injury in human polymorphonuclear cells at high subfreezing temperatures, *Cryobiology*, 22, 215, 1985.

[59] Takashashi, T. et al., Effect of cryoprotectants on the viability and function of unfrozen human polymorphonuclear cells, *Cryobiology*, 22, 336, 1985.

[60] Takenaka, N. et al., Acceleration mechanism of chemical reaction by freezing: the reaction of nitrous acid with dissolved oxygen, *J. Phys. Chem.*, 100, 13874, 1996.

[61] Hatley, R.H.M., Franks, F., and Mathias, S.F., The stabilization of labile biochemicals by undercooling, *Process Biochem.*, 22, 171, 1987.

[62] Mathias, S.F., Franks, F., and Hatley, R.H.M., Preservation of viable cells in the undercooled state, *Cryobiology*, 22, 537, 1985.

[63] Fahy, G.M. et al., Vitrification as an approach to cryopreservation, *Cryobiology*, 21, 407, 1984.

[64] Murthy, S.S.N., Some insight into the physical basis of the cryoprotective action of dimethyl sulfoxide and ethylene glycol, *Cryobiology*, 36, 84, 1998.

[65] Baudot, A., Lawrence, L., and Boutron, P., Glass-forming tendency in the system water–dimethyl sulfoxide, *Cryobiology*, 40, 151, 2000.

[66] Williams, R.J. and Leopold, A.C., The glassy state in corn embryos, *Plant Physiol.*, 89, 977, 1989.

[67] Webb, S.J., *Bound Water in Biological Integrity*, Charles C. Thomas Publisher, Springfield, IL, 1965.

[68] Xie, G. and Timasheff, S.N., Mechanism of the stabilization of ribonuclease a by sorbitol: preferential hydration is greater for the denatured than for the native protein, *Protein Sci.*, 6, 211, 1997.

[69] Arakawa, T. and Timasheff, S.N., Stabilization of protein structure by sugars, *Biochemistry*, 21, 6536, 1982.

[70] Migliardo, F., Magazu, S., and Migliardo, M., INS investigation on disaccharide/H_2O mixtures, *J. Mol. Liq.*, 110, 11, 2004.

[71] Sun, W.Q. and Leopold, A.C., Cytoplasmic vitrification and survival of anhydrobiotic organisms, *Compar. Biochem. Physiol.*, 117A, 327, 1997.

[72] Buitink, J. and Leprince, O., Glass formation in plant anhydrobiotes: survival in the dry state, *Cryobiology*, 48, 215, 2004.

[73] Mei, E. et al., Motions of single molecules and proteins in trehalose glass, *J. Am. Chem. Soc.*, 125, 2730, 2003.

[74] Sastry, G.M. and Agmon, N., Trehalose prevents myoglobin collapse and preserves its internal mobility, *Biochemistry*, 36, 7097, 1997.

[75] DePaz, R.A. et al., Effects of drying methods and additives on the structure, function and storage stability of subtilisin: role of protein conformation and molecular mobility, *Enzyme Microb. Technol.*, 21, 765, 2002.

[76] Miller, D.P., Anderson, R.E., and de Pablo, J.J., Stabilization of lactate dehydrogenase following freeze-thawing and vacuum-drying in the presence of trehalose and borate, *Pharma. Res.*, 15, 1215, 1998.

[77] Allison, S.D. et al., Hydrogen bonding between sugar and protein is responsible for inhibition of dehydration-induced protein folding, *Arch. Biochem. Biophys.*, 223, 289, 1999.

[78] Conrad, P.B. et al., Stabilization and preservation of *Lactobacillus acidophilus* in saccharide matrices, *Cryobiology*, 41, 17, 2000.

[79] Bieganski, R.M. et al., Stabilization of active recombinant retroviruses in an amorphous dry state with trehalose, *Biotechnol. Prog.*, 14, 615, 1998.

[80] Sun, W.Q., Irving, T.C., and Leopold, A.C., The role of sugar, vitrification and membrane phase transition in seed desiccation tolerance, *Physiol. Plant*, 90, 621, 1994.

[81] Acker, J.P. et al., Engineering desiccation tolerance in mammalian cells: tools and techniques, in *Life in the Frozen State*, Fuller, B.J., Lane, L., and Benson, E.E., Eds., CRC Press, Boca Raton, FL, 2004.

[82] Eroglu, A., Toner, M., and Toth, T.L., Beneficial effect of microinjected trehalose on the cryosurvival of human oocytes, *Fertil. Steril.*, 77, 152, 2002.

[83] Wolkers, W.F. et al., Temperature dependence of fluid phase endocytosis coincides with membrane properties of pig platelets, *Biochem. Biophys. Acta — Biomembr.*, 1612, 154, 2003.

[84] Mussauer, H., Sukhorukov, V.L., and Zimmermann, U., Trehalose improves survival of electrotransfected mammalian cells, *Cytometry*, 45, 2001.

[85] Shirakashi, R. et al., Intracellular delivery of trehalose into mammalian cells by electropermeabilization, *J. Membr. Biol.*, 189, 45, 2002.

[86] Puhlev, I. et al., Desiccation tolerance in human cells, *Cryobiology*, 42, 207, 2001.

[87] Lee, S. and Doukas, A.G., Laser-generated stress waves and their effects on the cell membrane, *IEEE J. Select. Top. Quant. Electron.*, 5, 997, 1999.

[88] Kodama, T., Hamblin, M.R., and Doukas, A.G., Cytoplasmic molecular delivery with shock waves: importance of impulse, *Biophys. J.*, 79, 1821, 2000.

[89] Oliver, A.E. et al., Loading human mesenchymal stem cells with trehalose by fluid-phase endocytosis, *Cell Preserv. Technol.*, 2, 35, 2004.

[90] Russo, M.J., Bayley, H., and Toner, M., Reversible permeabilization of plasme membranes with an engineered switchable pore, *Nat. Biotechnol.*, 15, 278, 1997.

[91] Eroglu, A. et al., Intracellular trehalose improves the survival of cryopreserved mammalian cells, *Nat. Biotechnol.*, 18, 163, 2000.

[92] Guo, N. et al., Trehalose expression confers desiccation tolerance on human cells, *Nat. Biotechnol.*, 18, 168, 2000.

[93] van den Dries, I.J. et al., Effects of water content and molecular weight on spin probe and water mobility in malto-oligamer glasses, *J. Phys. Chem. B*, 1004, 10126, 2000.

[94] Cicerone, M.T., Blackburn, F.R., and Ediger, M.D., How do molecules move near tg — molecular rotation of 6 probes in o-terphenyl across 14 decades in time, *J. Chem. Phys.*, 102, 471, 1995.

[95] Allison, S.D. et al., Effects of drying methods and additives on structure and function of actin: mechanisms of dehydration-induced damage and its inhibition, *Arch. Biochem. Biophys.*, 358, 171, 1998.

[96] Magazu, S., Maisano, G., and Majolino, D., Diffusive properties of alpha,alpha-trehalose-water solutions, *Prog. Theoret. Phys. Suppl.*, 195, 1997.

[97] Molinero, V., Çagin, T., and Goddard III, W.A., Mechanisms of nonexponential relaxation in supercooled glucose solutions: the role of water facilitation, *J. Phys. Chem. A*, 108, 3699, 2004.

[98] Tromp, R.H., Parker, R., and Ring, S.G., Water diffusion in glasses of carbohydrates, *Carbohydr. Res.*, 303, 199, 1997.

[99] Parker, R. and Ring, S.G., Diffusion in maltose–water mixtures at temperatures close to the glass-transition, *Carbohydr. Res.*, 273, 147, 1995.

[100] Aldous, B.J., Franks, F., and Greer, A.L., Diffusion of water within an amorphous carbohydrate, *J. Mater. Sci.*, 32, 301, 1997.

[101] Clegg, J.S. et al., Cellular response to extreme water loss: the water-replacement hypothesis, *Cryobiology*, 19, 306, 1982.

[102] Migliardo, F., Magazu, S., and Mondelli, C., Elastic incoherent neutron scattering studies on glass forming hydrogen-bonded systems, *J. Mol. Liq.*, 110, 7, 2004.

[103] Fowler, A.J. and Toner, M., Prevention of hemolysis in rapidly frozen erythrocytes by using a laser pulse, *Ann. NY Acad. Sci.*, 858, 245, 1998.

[104] Novikov, V.N. and Sololov, A.P., Universality of the dynamic crossover in glass-forming liquids: a "magic" relaxation time, *Phys. Rev. E*, 67, 031507, 2003.

[105] Aksan, A. and Toner, M., Isothermal desiccation and vitrification kinetics of trehalose–dextran solutions, *Langmuir*, 20, 5521, 2004.

[106] Rey, L. and May, J.C., *Freeze-Drying/Lyophilization of Pharmaceutical and Biological Products*, Rey, L. and May, J.C., Eds., New York, Marcel Dekker, Drugs and the pharmaceutical sciences, 1999.

[107] Smythe, B.M., Sucrose crystal growth, *Aust. J. Chem.*, 20, 1097, 1967.

[108] Sarciaux, J.M. et al., Influence of bovine somatotropin (BST) concentration on the physical/chemical stability of freeze-dried sucrose/BST formulations, *Pharmac. Res.*, 12, S, 1995.

[109] Benaroudj, N., Lee, D.H., and Goldberg, A.L., Trehalose accumulation during cellular stress protects cells and cellular proteins from damage by oxygen radicals, *J. Biol. Chem.*, 276, 24261, 2001.

[110] Buitink, J., Hemminga, M.A., and Hoekstra, F.A., Characterization of molecular mobility in seed tissues: an electron paramagnetic spin probe study, *Biophys. J.*, 76, 3315, 1999.

[111] Le Meste, M. and Voilley, A., Influence of hydration on rotational diffusivity of solutes in model systems, *J. Phys. Chem.*, 92, 1612, 1988.

[112] Ekdawi-Sever, N. et al., Diffusion of sucrose and α,α-trehalose in aqueous solutions, *J. Phys. Chem. A*, 107, 936, 2003.

[113] Paschek, D. and Geiger, A., Simulation study on the diffusive motion in deeply supercooled water, *J. Phys. Chem. B*, 103, 4139, 1999.

[114] Price, W.S., Ide, H., and Arata, Y., Self-diffusion of supercooled water to 238 K using PGSE NMR diffusion measurements, *J. Phys. Chem. A*, 103, 448, 1999.

[115] Onsager, L. and Runnels, L.K., Diffusion and relaxation phenomena in ice, *J. Chem. Phys.*, 50, 1089, 1969.

[116] Petrenko, V.F. and Whitworth, R.W., *Physics of Ice*, Oxford University Press Inc., New York, NY, 1999.

[117] Mills, R., Self-diffusion in normal and heavy water in the range 1–45°C, *J. Phys. Chem.*, 77, 685, 1973.

[118] Harris, K.R. and Newitt, P.J., Self-diffusion of water at low temperatures and high pressure, *J. Chem. Eng. Data*, 42, 346, 1997.

[119] Moran, G.R. and Jeffrey, K.R., A study of the molecular motion in glucose/water mixtures using deuterium nuclear magnetic resonance, *J. Chem. Phys.*, 110, 3472, 1999.

[120] Miller, D.P., dePablo, J.J., and Corti, H.R., Viscosity and glass transition temperature of aqueous mixtures of trehalose with borax and sodium chloride, *J. Phys. Chem. B*, 103, 10243–10249, 1999.

42

Drug Delivery

C. Becker
A. Göpferich
University of Regensburg

42.1 Introduction

42.1.1 Significance

The science of tissue engineering takes an integrated approach to replacing nonfunctional or missing tissue by gathering input from many different scientific disciplines [1]. An integral part of the emergence of a mature tissue from cells both *in vitro* and *in vivo* involves guiding cells through their development. Apart from the choice of materials used for cell and tissue culture, the use of pharmacologically active substances such as cytokines and growth factors has emerged as an important tool in tissue engineering research and development in recent years [2–4]. By taking advantage of these substances at the right time and in the right context, cells can be induced to proliferate, differentiate, or to migrate in a controlled way. The positive impact of growth factors, such as vascular endothelial growth factor (VEGF) and basic fibroblast growth factor (bFGF), which both stimulate the vascularization of tissue *in vivo*, and members of the bone morphogenic protein family, used to enhance bone formation, illustrate how useful drug-delivery strategies have been for tissue engineering applications in recent years [5,6].

Although many drugs can simply be added to cell- and tissue culture media or administered *in vivo* in the form of an injectable solution, we can take better advantage of many compounds, when they are administered in a controlled way. Protein and peptide drugs, for example, have short half-lives [7] and must, therefore, be administered continuously, which can be very cumbersome for large volumes of solution. In addition, undesired side effects may arise when substances intended for local delivery to a specific tissue are not spatially contained. It is obvious that for these and for many other reasons it has been deemed necessary to administer drugs according to regimes that cannot solely be achieved through the administration of solutions. The field of drug-delivery research has emerged over the last 30 years to overcome such limitations. In recent years, tissue engineering has profited tremendously from integrating drug-delivery technology into more traditional design schemes [8].

It is the goal of this chapter to elucidate the significance of drug delivery within the field of tissue engineering. We first review a number of definitions and basic drug-delivery technologies with a special focus on drug release mechanisms. We then briefly describe the fundamentals of tissue engineering within the realm of drug delivery. We then have a look at the specifics of drugs that are attractive for tissue engineering applications. Thereafter, we address classical drug-carrier systems that have already been used to deliver drugs to cells and tissues and concomitantly give an outlook on systems that hold great promise for similar applications in the future. We then give an overview over the area of using cell carriers for drug delivery. Finally, we review the specifics of some growth factors that have special requirements with respect to stability and pharmacokinetics. At the end, we provide a brief glance at the challenges that have still to be addressed, in an attempt to give an outlook on the further developments that are currently under way. More information can be found in a number of excellent reviews on related topics [9–12].

42.1.2 Goals of Drug Delivery

Defining the term "drug delivery" is not an easy task, because a plethora of definitions can be found in the contemporary literature. They range from brief statements such as "method and route used to provide medication" [13] to more detailed ones, such as "systems of administering drugs through controlled delivery so that an optimum amount reaches the target site. Drug-delivery systems encompass the carrier, route, and target." [14]. Some of them already imply that there is a close relation to tissue engineering research: "delivering agents to specific cells, tissues, or organs" [15].

While all of the definitions make it very clear that drug delivery is intended to control the kinetics of drug release, it is not at all obvious, why one should do so. The reasons are manifold and some of them date back more than 100 years to when Paul Ehrlich (*1854–†1915) coined the term of the "magic bullet" [16]. Since then it has been a well-accepted fact by the scientific community that hitting a biological target with high precision has significant advantages. While Ehrlich intended to avoid side effects during an antibacterial therapy by targeted drug delivery, we nowadays have more incentive than "only" avoiding collateral damage to control the delivery of drug in a biological environment. Thus, the pharmacokinetics, that is, the kinetics of drug resorption, distribution, and elimination processes, may force us to finely dose a drug over a defined time interval to account for its rapid clearance from an application site. Another motivation involves the short tissue half-lives of therapeutic agents, especially of protein and peptide drugs, which are frequently inactivated by proteases and peptidases [17,18] and need, therefore, to be substituted continuously by "fresh" compound from the drug-delivery device's reservoir. These are just a few of the many reasons that may illustrate the need for drug delivery. It is easy to imagine that in the post genomic era, when the number of drug candidates dramatically increases with continuing progress in proteomics [19], even more reasons may arise, leading us to use controlled drug-delivery devices for tissue engineering applications.

Drug delivery is often linked to the concepts of "sustained release" or "controlled release," meaning that a pharmaceutical compound is released over a certain period of time or in a somehow predetermined way, respectively. While "sustained" suggests only that the drug is released over an extended period of time, "controlled" suggests that the kinetics are well defined, but does not necessarily imply that the release runs over long time periods.

42.2 Mechanisms of Drug Delivery

The means that we can exploit to release a drug in a controlled way and which are an indispensable part of a drug-delivery device are manifold and different in nature. We can roughly classify them into three major mechanisms: diffusion, erosion, and swelling [20–23]. Besides these three major instruments that we have in our hands, a plethora of additional strategies have been used [24–27]. Among them are electric fields [28–30] that allow for the transport of charged molecules, osmosis whereby molecules are "squeezed" out of a reservoir due to a build up in osmotic pressure [31–33], convection by which the drug is moved along some stream of gas or fluid [34,35], or even the mechanical stimulation of a drug carrier [36,37]. This list of examples is not nearly complete, but it is beyond the scope of this chapter to describe all of them. As excellent reviews on the topic can be found in the contemporary literature [38–42], we only further describe the most important mechanisms with respect to applications in tissue engineering.

42.2.1 Diffusion

Diffusion is one of the most important transport mechanisms in drug-delivery applications. It is a thermodynamically driven process with well understood kinetics [43,44]. Diffusion is caused by Brownian motion, which is a random walk of particles that are typically micrometer-sized or smaller. Macroscopically, we observe that the particles appear to move along a concentration gradient. Fick's second law of diffusion describes the net transport of particles in time and space:

$$\frac{\partial C(x, y, z, t)}{\partial t} = \frac{\partial^2 C}{\partial x^2} + \frac{\partial^2 C}{\partial y^2} + \frac{\partial^2 C}{\partial z^2}$$

For this partial differential equation, numerous algebraic and numerical solutions have been derived, two of which are depicted in Figure 42.1. The solutions depend strongly on the initial conditions (such as the drug concentration inside a drug-delivery device) as well as the boundary conditions (such as the geometry of a drug-delivery device) of the diffusion problem. An advantage of diffusion controlled drug-delivery systems is certainly that we can usually predict the kinetics of drug release very well. One of its major disadvantages is that the flux (the mass transport per unit area and time) out of a device is usually, according to above outlined nature of the process, concentration dependent. Therefore, as the release progresses, the process can lead to a break down of concentration gradients and, as a result, the release

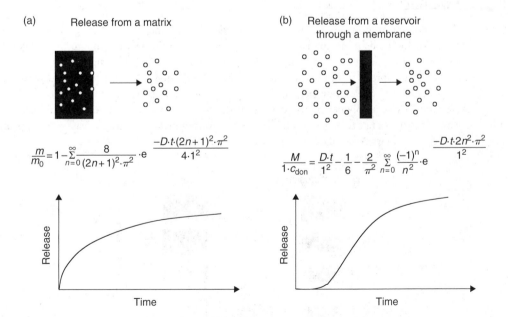

(a) Release from a matrix

$$\frac{m}{m_0} = 1 - \sum_{n=0}^{\infty} \frac{8}{(2n+1)^2 \cdot \pi^2} \cdot e^{\frac{-D \cdot t \cdot (2n+1)^2 \cdot \pi^2}{4 \cdot 1^2}}$$

(b) Release from a reservoir through a membrane

$$\frac{M}{1 \cdot c_{don}} = \frac{D \cdot t}{1^2} - \frac{1}{6} - \frac{2}{\pi^2} \sum_{n=0}^{\infty} \frac{(-1)^n}{n^2} \cdot e^{\frac{-D \cdot t \cdot 2n^2 \cdot \pi^2}{1^2}}$$

Release / Time

Release / Time

FIGURE 42.1 Drug release profiles resulting from diffusion controlled release. Equations represent exemplery solutions of Fick's second law of diffusion in one dimension describing release profiles (a) from a matrix type device, (b) via diffusion through a membrane.

rates may decline. This is usually the case whenever we release a substance from a monolithic system (Figure 42.1a).

A method that allows the system to maintain a fairly constant flux over an extended period of time utilizes release through a membrane. In that case, an almost constant release over time is possible, especially when the drug reservoir contains large amounts of substance (Figure 42.1b). This is the more the case when the drug reservoir hosting the substance is oversaturated, so that a constant drug concentration can be maintained over an extended period of time.

42.2.2 Erosion

The materials and design of a drug carrier may be chosen to either encourage or hinder release via erosion. A carrier that erodes over time either precludes the necessity of postapplication removal or does not persist at the application site, which is an additional advantage for applications in tissue engineering.

Erosion is usually defined as the sum of all processes leading to a mass loss from a drug-delivery device [45]. In some cases, the material can simply dissolve in an aqueous environment, while in other cases, like with lipophilic degradable polymers, the material degrades into water soluble oligomers that allow for the initiation of matrix erosion. Polymers that are insoluble in water have been classified according to their erosion mechanism into surface-eroding and bulk-eroding materials [46,47]. While in the case of the first class, erosion phenomena are confined to the material surface [48], bulk-eroding materials tend to degrade over extended periods of time until a critical degree of degradation is reached, after which the whole material bulk is undergoing erosion (Figure 42.2) [49].

It is obvious that surface-eroding polymers allow for the control of drug release via the erosion process, which usually proceeds at constant velocity. A classification of polymers as surface and bulk eroding can be made based mainly on the nature of the bond between the monomers. As a rule of thumb, one can assume that the faster a bond is cleaved (usually by hydrolysis) the more the material is likely to undergo surface erosion. In recent years, models have been developed that allow for the calculation of a dimensionless "erosion number" that predicts the erosion mechanism of a polymer device [50].

42.2.3 Swelling

The swelling phenomena of polymers has widely been used to control the release of drugs from a device [46,51]. The major mechanism thereby is an increase of polymer chain mobility due to the uptake of water, which lowers the glass transition temperature of the polymer [52,53]. Drugs that are trapped inside a polymer matrix profit from the resulting increase in flexibility by an enhanced diffusivity and consequently an enhanced release rate [54]. In many cases, one can observe the formation of swelling fronts that separate a glassy polymer matrix core from the swollen polymer surface. It is obvious that diffusion plays a major overall role, as both the process of water uptake and drug release are diffusion controlled. Excellent reviews are available that provide more detail [55–57].

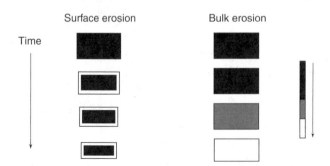

FIGURE 42.2 Schematic illustration of surface erosion and bulk erosion. (Reprinted from Gopferich, A. and Tessmar, J., *Adv. Drug Deliv. Rev.*, 54, 911, 2002.)

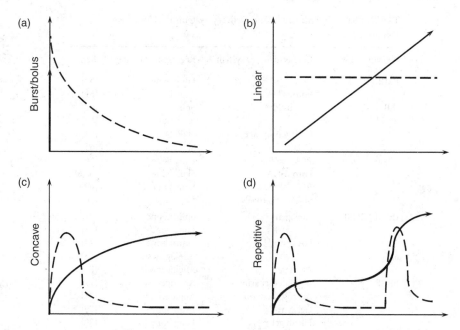

FIGURE 42.3 Schematic illustration of release profiles (closed lines) and resulting tissue concentrations (broken line). (a) Pulsatile release, (b) constant (zero order) release, (c) concave release kinetics, (d) repeated pulsatile release kinetics.

42.2.4 Competing Mechanisms and Overall Kinetics

In many drug-delivery systems, the mechanisms outlined above compete with one another. Release from a degradable polymer, for example, is usually a complex mixture of all three pathways of drug-release control. However, from a design point of view, it is highly desirable that one of the mechanisms dominates the overall release kinetics, as otherwise unfavorable release profiles may result.

A plethora of release profiles are available to choose from, ranging from the continuous delivery of a drug over an extended period of time to pulsatile release kinetics, by which an incorporated compound is set free according to a preprogrammed pattern [58]. Excellent overviews on the multitude of release kinetics can be found in the literature [59]. Figure 42.3 illustrates schematically typical drug-release profiles and the resulting tissue concentrations that one may expect, assuming that the substance is cleared from the application site according to first order kinetics, that is, in a concentration dependent way.

The kinetics that one should choose depends on the biological needs of the specific application. In tissue engineering, this may for example be defined by a desired cell phenotype or by the pharmacokinetics of the drug when applied to a tissue or administered *in vivo*. Typically, more continuous release profiles will lead to more constant tissue levels *in vivo*, while the pulsatile application of a drug will result in concentration peaks that rapidly fall.

42.3 Protein Drug Properties

Prior to a detailed look at the various drug-delivery strategies, it seems necessary to have a glance at the properties of active compounds that are currently in use for tissue engineering applications. Most of these drugs are growth factors and, therefore, peptides or proteins. A brief list of compounds that have been formulated to drug-delivery systems for the use in tissue engineering applications is given in Table 42.1.

TABLE 42.1   Growth Factor and Delivery Systems that have been Developed

Growth factor	Carrier/delivery system	Regenerated tissue	Ref.
BMP	PLA	Long bone	[60]
	Porous HA	Skull bone	[61]
rhBMP-2	Porous PLA	Spinal bone	[62]
		Skull bone	[63]
	Collagen sponge	Skull bone	[64]
	Gelatin	Skull bone	[65]
	PLA-coating	Long bone	[66]
	Porous HA	Skull bone	[67,68]
	PLA–PEG copolymer	Long bone	[69]
	Si–Ca–P xerogels		[70]
rhBMP-7/ OP-1	Collagen	Spinal bone	[71,72]
		Long bone	[73]
	HA	Spinal bone	[74]
aFGF	PVA	Angiogenesis	[75]
	Alginate	Angiogenesis	[76]
bFGF	Alginate/heparin	Angiogenesis	[77]
	Agarose/heparin	Angiogenesis	[78]
	Gelatin	Skull bone	[79]
	Fibrin gel	Long bone	[80]
	Chitosan	Dermis	[81]
	Collagen	Cartilage	[82]
EGF	Gelatin	Dermis	[83]
TGF-β1	Alginate	Cartilage	[84]
	Poloxamer; PEO gel	Dermis	[85]
	PLGA	Skull bone	[86]
	Collagen	Dermis	[87]
PDGF	Fibrin	Ligament	[88]
	CMC gel	Dermis	[89]
VEGF	Alginate	Angiogenesis	[90]
	Collagen	Angiogenesis	[91]
	PLGA scaffold	Angiogenesis	[92]
	Fibrin mesh	Angiogenesis	[93]
VEGF/PDGF	PLGA scaffold	Angiogenesis	[94]
NGF	PLGA	Nerve	[95]
	Collagen minipellet	Nerve	[96]

BMP, bone morphogenic protein; rhBMP; recombinant human bone morphogenic protein; OP-1, osteogenic protein 1; aFGF, acidic fibroblast growth factor; bFGF, basic fibroblast growth factor; EGF, endothelial growth factor; TGF-β1, transforming growth factor beta 1; PDGF, platelet derived growth factor; VEGF, vascular endothelial growth factor; NGF, nerve growth factor; PLA, poly lactic acid; PLGA, poly(lactic-co-glycolic) acid copolymer; PEG, poly(ethylene glycol); HA, hydroxyapatite; PVA, poly(vinyl alcohol).

In the case of these proteins we have to deal with highly efficient substances with often substantially limited stability, such as in physiological fluids, due to proteolytic enzyme activity [97]. The choice of an appropriate delivery system for these substances is, therefore, not only a matter of the intended therapeutic use or the pharmacokinetics but also of the physicochemical properties of the drug. Special attention must be paid to the chemical stability and physical integrity of a protein drug even during the formulation process. Examples for chemical and physical instabilities are deamidation, redox reactions, hydrolysis, and aggregation. These and other instability mechanisms have been extensively reviewed by numerous authors [98–100]. In addition environmental effects like pH, organic acids, metal ions, detergents, and temperature can induce a denaturation of proteins [101].

Another source of inactivation is the biological environment that we expose a protein to. Even if a growth factor of choice can be stabilized during formulation and inside a delivery system the biological environment can pose another severe threat. Half-lives of growth factors are typically in the range of minutes due to degradation by peptidases. Intravenous injections are indicative of this problem [102]. Platelet-derived growth factor (PDGF), bFGF, and VEGF, for example, have plasma half-lives of 2 [103], 3 [104], and 50 [105] minutes respectively. Besides rapid degradation, unfavorable distribution [104] or elimination by glomerular filtration [97] are problematic after intravenous administration. Direct systemic administration of growth factors, therefore, requires substantial drug doses that may lead to side effects [2,106], or if direct injection into the target site is possible, repeated administration to achieve biological efficacy is required. Prolonging the half-life of growth factors is, therefore, an important research goal. A promising approach to increase half-life is to conjugate proteins with poly(ethyleneglycol) (PEG) chains. Pegylation seems to cause a significant reduction of protein clearance from plasma [107–109]. The pegylation of growth hormone-releasing hormone (GRF) analogues, for example, led to an enhanced *in vivo* stability with acceptable biological activity [110]. In addition pegylation seems to reduce the velocity of enzymatic degradation [111]. Detailed reviews on protein and peptide pegylation can be found in the literature [112–115].

The incorporation of proteins into a controlled release drug-delivery device can protect it from inactivation, but the formulation process is sometimes another source of protein inactivation. One class of problem that occurs frequently is related to the interaction of proteins with interfaces. Considering the small quantities that have to be handled when growth factors are formulated to applicable systems, physical phenomena like protein adsorption to solid–liquid or liquid–liquid interfaces and subsequent denaturation can lead to massive protein loss in some instances [116–118]. Approaches to minimize protein adsorption to glass or plastic include competitive "coating" with bovine serum albumin [119,120], the use of PEG and glycerol solutions or the application of surfactants [121,122]. Enhanced denaturation and aggregation of proteins at interfaces have been observed under certain conditions like the application of mechanical forces [123]. It has, for example, been shown that simple vortex mixing of a 0.5 mg/ml porcine growth hormone solution for 1 min can lead to a loss of 70% of the protein due to aggregation [124,125]. Unfortunately the problem of adsorption on solid surfaces is not the only one that can occur during formulation. When microparticles are prepared by using emulsion techniques [126], for example, there is frequently the need for the use of organic solvent and vigorous mixing. The liquid–liquid interfaces and the high shear forces are two factors that may lead to denaturation and hence activity loss [125,127,128]. Moreover during the degradation of polymers a very harsh microclimate can be created [129] in which even chemical reactions such as an acylation of proteins and peptides can occur [130,131]. To stabilize proteins in polymers numerous approaches have been tried [132–135], many of them being very specific for an individual drug-delivery system.

The unfavorable interactions of growth factors with synthetic materials made many groups have a closer look at how they are created and stored in their natural biological environment. Transcription of genes encoding for growth factors create unstable mRNA [136–138], which leads to short half-life and only limited growth factor synthesis. Growth factors are released by cells either for instant signalling or are stored in the extracellular matrix (ECM). Some growth factors such as transforming growth factor beta (TGF-β) are secreted as biologically inactive latent precursors [139]. The release of growth factors from the ECM is controlled by matrix degradation. This natural environment provides a dynamic and responsive growth factor delivery system which can react according to specific cellular requirements and can, therefore, also serve as a cell guidance system [2,139,140]. This led various research groups to the development and use of ECM [141] derived materials for the design of controlled delivery systems for growth factors. Especially gel like systems can simulate the interaction of growth factors and the extracellular matrix [142,143] and can, therefore, provide similar stabilizing effects like the natural ECM. Interestingly, it was found that the bioactivity of vascular endothelial growth factor (VEGF) delivered from alginate microspheres was higher than VEGF alone [144]. It was speculated that that effect was due to stabilization of the factor in the system over alginate interaction. A detailed review about on the interactions between growth factors and the ECM can be found in the literature [145].

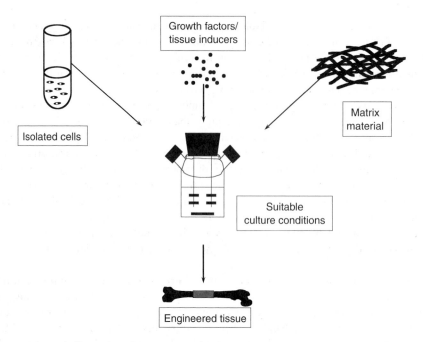

FIGURE 42.4   Schematic illustration of components of tissue engineering.

42.4 Drug Delivery in Tissue Engineering

It is certainly beyond the scope of this chapter to provide the reader with a complete overview of tissue engineering; however, it is necessary that we review several aspects that may be crucial (or beneficial) for a better understanding of drug-delivery applications in this field.

In the early days of tissue engineering, pioneers like Langer and Vacanti stressed its interdisciplinary character in their definitions [1]. At that time four fundamental components of tissue engineering were identified (Figure 42.4):

1. Cells that will form the desired type of tissue
2. A matrix that allows for cell proliferation and differentiation
3. Suitable cell culture conditions
4. Finally the use of cytokines and other drugs

While each of these components alone may be sufficient for an application, it is obvious that for *in vivo* as well as *in vitro* approaches it is important to guide cell- and tissue development into the right direction. Cytokines and growth factors have therefore emerged in recent years as precious substances for tissue engineering applications. That a controlled delivery of these and other pharmacologically active substances is very beneficial for tissue engineering applications is well accepted in the field.

The strategies to deliver a drug to cells or tissues are diverse. However, we can classify them into four major categories, which follow immediately from the blue print of tissue engineering as depicted in Figure 42.4.

A first strategy, which is all too obvious, is to use classical established technology for the delivery of substances either in cell culture media or near a tissue site *in vivo* (Figure 42.5a).

Doing so has the advantage that we can use systems that have been developed and described thoroughly in the contemporary literature [38,146–148]. Among these systems, we find essentially everything that has been developed for the parenteral application of drugs, such as implants, microspheres, and injectable gels, just to name a few. Despite their advantages, they may also cause some problems. They must always be administered in addition to tissue engineering specific components, such as cells and cell carriers.

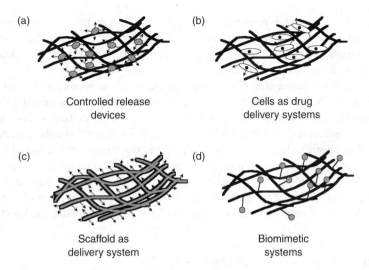

FIGURE 42.5 Drug-delivery strategies for tissue engineering applications: (a) Use of "classical" controlled delivery devices such as microspheres or monolithic systems incorporated into a cell carrier, (b) genetically altered cells serving for protein and peptide drug expression, (c) the cell carrier itself serving as a drug-delivery system, (d) covalent attachment of drugs to the polymer surface.

Moreover, they may not unequivocally allow for a homogeneous distribution in the tissue and may thereby cause undesirable drug concentration gradients.

A second approach is to deliver drugs via cells (Figure 42.5b) [149]. It is possible to genetically alter a portion of the cells or all of them to produce a certain protein or peptide drug. For this approach, numerous viral and nonviral gene delivery approaches are available [150–154].

A third approach is to use the scaffolds intended for cell attachment and proliferation as a drug-delivery system (Figure 42.5c). Many of these materials provide tremendous opportunities to control the release of drugs. Especially biodegradable polymers and hydrogel materials have been used extensively as porous scaffolds to allow for erosion controlled drug or DNA release.

Finally, we can implement the pharmacologically active substances that we want to use for signaling to cells into the design of materials that are used for cell proliferation and differentiation. In this scheme, drugs and cytokines are tethered to the surface of a material [155] (Figure 42.5d). The term "biomimetic" has been coined in recent years to describe materials that have been modified in this way [156,157]. There are numerous publications that illustrate the principle behind and advantages of this strategy [158–162].

In the following pages, we focus on aspects of classical drug-delivery systems and on the use of scaffolds as release systems, as the other two delivery strategies are covered in the sections on gene delivery and biomimetic materials of the handbook. We try to give a brief overview of the vast number of devices that have already been used for the delivery of drugs in tissue engineering applications and some of the more recent trends, such as the use of scaffolds concomitantly as a cell carrier and for the delivery of a drug.

42.4.1 The Use of Classical Drug-Delivery Systems

When designing a drug-delivery device for an application in tissue engineering, there are numerous aspects to be considered beyond the pharmacological aspects that are usually linked to the nature of the drug to be administered. Of utmost significance is the pharmacokinetics of the drug. The clearance rate from the site of application, in particular, should be determined as this, together with the drug efficacy and the intended time of application, dictates the dosing regimen. Once the required dosage is known, the corresponding release kinetics may be determined. The type of drug-delivery system to be used may then be chosen, taking the drug loading and release into account. Thereafter, further fundamental questions, such as, which material provides a maximum of drug stability, biocompatibility, and functionality with respect to a desired controlled-release pattern or with respect to biodegradability, can be addressed. Once these questions are answered, more individual aspects such as shaping the material to defect sites or to a specific type of application such as via injection may be considered.

Unfortunately, the information needed to address all of the problems listed above is often unavailable. In particular, there is usually little known about newly formulated compounds besides the pharmacological effect of the substance. At that stage of development, one goal of drug delivery is frequently to provide release systems that are capable of stabilizing and releasing the drug over an as long a period of time as possible. Controlled release technology can then help to find out if long-term applications are beneficial and what the reaction of a tissue to such an exposure is. In the case of proteins, this is usually not a trivial task. In the following section, we try to illustrate the options that we currently have to deliver drugs for tissue engineering applications. The reader should be aware that this is just a brief glance at the field that hosts a plethora of systems and technologies. To allow for better orientation, we classify the field roughly into:

- Monolithic systems of macroscopic geometries
- Particulate systems comprising microparticles and colloids with a size range from 1 to 1000 μm and from 1 to 1000 nm respectively
- Gel-like systems

42.4.1.1 Monolithic Systems

The foundations for the controlled release of bioactive substances especially of protein and peptide drugs from monolithic systems were laid in the 1970s when Folkman and Langer described the use of polymeric membrane systems made of poly(ethylene-co-vinyl acetate) (EVAc) for the release of bovine serum albumin, which served as a model compound. These delivery systems were among the first that achieved a controlled-release pattern for protein drugs [163]. Although these systems allowed for an excellent control of drug release [164,165], one of their major limitations was that they were not degradable. Since the 1980s a number of degradable polymer materials have been synthesized with the goal of enhancing the *in vivo* performance of devices made thereof. A plethora of polymer classes, such as poly(a-hydroxyesters) [42], polyanhydrides [166], and poly(orthoesters) [167], have been developed for this purpose, to mention just a few. More materials are described in the literature [46,168,169]. Materials that undergo biodegradation are typically significantly more complex than nondegradable materials, as they add several new variables to the already intricate system. In poly(lactic acid) (PLA) and poly(lactic-co-glycolic acid) (PLGA) matrices, for example, the degradation of the material can cause the pH of the surrounding region to drop below 2 [170], the osmotic pressure inside aqueous pores to increase far above physiological values [171], and chemical reactions between degradation products and peptides have been reported as well [172].

The first delivery systems that were made of these materials were monolithic matrices because they are easy to manufacture by techniques such as solvent casting, extrusion, or injection molding and usually provide excellent control over drug release. Furthermore, these matrices are able to carry large doses of drug and the release can be tailored to a required direction by changing the matrix material, drug loading, or use of co-dispersants [164]. The release of drug in nondegradable systems is primarily controlled by diffusion processes. The degradable systems, in contrast, offer the possibility of erosion-controlled release. Thus, there are more variables that may be adjusted in degradable systems, leading to more control over the release rate. In PLA/PLGA, for example, the degradation rate is influenced by factors such as crystallinity, copolymer composition [173,174], and molecular weight [175].

The materials that have been used for the manufacture of monolithic matrix-type delivery systems for tissue engineering have mainly been made of cross-linked hydrogels. Lipophilic degradable materials, such as PLA or PLGA, would also be suitable, however, over long time periods they are sometimes detrimental to the stability of a protein. Thus, gelatin has been used extensively for the manufacture of matrices by cross-linking gels either with glutaraldehyde or water-soluble carbodiimide [176]. Cross-linking can also be used with other hydrogel materials, such as alginate [177] or collagen. The latter has been used extensively for the manufacture of drug-delivery systems. Fujioka et al. extensively reviewed collagen-based systems that were developed for the delivery of cytokines and growth factors [178].

42.4.1.1.1 Particulate Systems

A major disadvantage of monolithic systems is the problem of application. A surgical procedure is usually needed for implantation. In the last 20 years, micro- and nanoparticulate systems have been developed as an alternative to facilitate the application of substances in a minimally invasive way. An excellent overview of the use of biodegradable microspheres has been given in recent reviews [179,180]. An advantage of the use of microparticles in tissue engineering is that they can be evenly distributed either in a tissue by injection or in a cell suspension, which guarantees that drug gradients, which often result from the application of monolithic systems, are avoided. An additional advantage for tissue engineering is the use of microencapsulation technology for the encapsulation of cells [181,182]. In addition to microparticles, nanoparticles and liposomes have found their way into tissue engineering applications [183,184], but we will focus on microparticulate systems in the next section because the have been applied more frequently.

Particulate systems have been used intensively in the past to deliver growth factors with the intention to regenerate tissue. Thus, Haller et al. reviewed efforts to deliver nerve growth factors [185]. The authors conclude that polymeric NGF release systems are useful for supporting cellular therapies for the treatment of neurodegenerative diseases. They found that microparticles made of EVAc and PLGA are suited for the release of nerve growth factor (NGF) [186]. Lipophilic degradable polymers have been especially popular for the delivery of protein drugs [179] and a multitude of further applications can be found in the contemporary literature, in many cases leading to very successful drug-delivery applications [179,180,187–189]. Despite the advantages that lipophilic degradable polymers such as PLA and PLGA and others offer, however, they are problematic materials for the reasons outlined above. De Weert et al. [190] summarized the problems with a special emphasis on the stability of protein drugs in an excellent review, in which they identify problems related to protein loading, microsphere formation, and drying. Despite the numerous countermeasures used to stabilize protein in these polymers, mounting problems led to tremendous research efforts to develop alternative systems.

Hydrogels, in particular, have emerged as a class of material that hold great promise for the release of sensitive protein and peptide drugs from microsphere systems. Among the first systems that were used are alginate beads, which can be manufactured by dropping or spraying alginate solutions into solutions containing divalent cations, such as calcium [191]. The ease of manufacture allows for a simple procedure to load growth factors. Gu et al. [192] could show, for example, that VEGF can be released at a fairly constant rate over a period of two weeks. Collagen and gelatin emerged as promising materials, as they can be considered biocompatible and biodegradable. Usually these materials are first processed in a gel state to microparticles, are then cross-linked to stabilize their geometry and finally loaded with proteins by immersion into a protein solution [193]. Tabata et al. [194] used this technology to deliver bFGF for de novo adipogenesis following subcutaneous microparticle injection into mice.

A problem that can exist with hydrogel-based microparticles is that they frequently require cross-linking procedures that can be detrimental to the stability of protein drugs. Therefore, alternative materials, such as lipids, have been intensively studied in the past to encapsulate protein and peptide drugs as well [195]. Like lipophilic degradable polymer microspheres, these substances offer the advantage that they can release drugs over an extended period of time [196]. Cortesi et al. [197] describe the manufacture of lipid microspheres from triglycerides and monoglycerides using emulsion and melt dispersion techniques. Reithmeier et al. achieved the manufacture of lipid microspheres that are able to release a tripeptide over a period of a few days [198] and insulin over a period of several days [199].

42.4.1.1.2 Gel-Like Systems

Like particulate systems, the ease of application of gel-like systems provides a significant benefit. Many systems have already been developed and have become precious materials for tissue engineering applications [200]. Gels offer the advantage of a fairly good compatibility with sensitive protein and peptide drugs. A disadvantage of these systems can be that they allow for drug release only over a short period of time.

Numerous systems with outstanding properties have been developed in recent years. In many cases, hydrogels have served as drug-delivery carriers for the delivery of growth factors. Cross-linked gelatin, for example, has served as a carrier for BMP-2 [201] and TGF-β1 [202], while cross-linked amylopectin was used to release bFGF [203]. Zisch et al. [204] reviewed the use of hydrogels for the release of angiogenic factors in more detail. A closer look at the literature reveals that more and more sophisticated systems have been developed in recent years. Kim et al., for example, has described a block copolymer that consists of poly(ethylene oxide), poly(L-lactic acid), and a urethane unit that exhibited a sol–gel transition at 37°C and was able to release dextrans that served as high molecular weight model compounds over a period of several days [205]. Similar principles can be used in tissue engineering applications to lift cells or tissues off of culture surfaces by decreasing the temperature below the lower critical solution temperature of the system at which the solidified gel to which the tissue is attached becomes liquid, leading to the detachment of cells from the culture plate [206]. Zisch et al. [207] describe the synthesis of a hydrogel network that consists essentially of branched PEG molecules that are linked by peptides; this material was then used as a substrate for matrix metalloproteinases. VEGF, which was covalently attached to this network, is liberated when tissue grows into the hydrogel, supporting tissue vascularization. Other systems take advantage of the binding of growth factors to heparin, which allows for the development of delivery systems in which heparin regulates the release of the protein by slowly releasing it from the complex [208].

42.4.2 The Delivery of Drugs via Cell Carriers

While the examples given above depend on the use of controlled-delivery devices in addition to a cell carrier, the carrier itself can serve as a delivery system. This can happen in two ways: we can either use a drug-delivery system, such as microspheres, and process it together with another material into a scaffold, or we can incorporate the drug directly into it. The use of multicomponent systems has the advantage that we can rely on off-the-shelf technology for the stabilization of a drug and for the control of its release. Doing so has, however, the disadvantage of being more complicated than loading a matrix directly with a drug.

42.4.2.1 Cell Carriers Loaded with Drug-Delivery systems

Holland et al. proposed the use of gelatin microspheres that have previously been developed for the delivery of proteins, such as bFGF [143,209], for the controlled release of transforming growth factor-β1 (TGF-β1) from oligo(poly(ethylene glycol) fumarate) (OPF) [210,211]. The authors took advantage of the fact that the polymer can be dissolved in water and suspend the microspheres therein. Upon chemical cross-linking, the particles were trapped inside the hydrogel and released the factor over a period of several weeks *in vitro*. The system can thus be used as an injectable scaffold material that also delivers a growth factor. Concomitantly, while gelatin degrades over time, this property allows cells to migrate into the biomaterial. Alternatively, such materials might be loaded with cells prior to cross-linking. Hollinger et al. [212] report a technique that allowed them to incorporate proteins into PLGA microparticles and to incorporate them into PLGA scaffolds.

42.4.2.2 Cell Carriers Loaded with Drugs

While the opportunities to incorporate a complete release system into a cell carrier are limited by the nature of the complexity of the endeavor, there are many options to incorporate a drug directly. Figure 42.6 gives an overview of the possibilities that we can choose from.

The choice of drug-loading method depends on the circumstances, such as the stability of the drug, the dose that we need, and the desired release kinetics, to mention just a few. In this section we will try to give a few examples that shed some light on the advantages and disadvantages of the individual approaches.

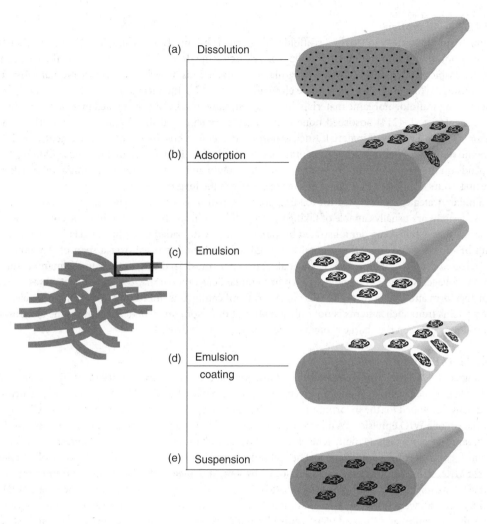

FIGURE 42.6 Schematic illustration of drug-loading strategies for cell carriers (further details provided in the text). (a) Dissolution of drug in the matrix material, (b) adsorption of drug to the matrix surface, (c) incorporation via emulsion droplets, (d) coating with drug–matrix emulsions, (e) suspension of drug inside the matrix.

42.4.2.2.1 Dissolution of Drug

In the simplest case, we can simply dissolve the drug in the bulk material prior to processing. This requires, however, that we find a solvent that dissolves both the matrix material and the drug. Kim et al. [213] describe the incorporation of ascorbate-2-phophate (AsAP) and dexamethasone into poly(D,L-lactic acid) (PLGA). Both drugs have been used to enhance the differentiation of mesenchymal stem cells to an osteoblastic phenotype. While dexamethasone dissolved in a PLGA, AsAP formed a suspension. The whole dispersion was then processed via solvent casting particulate leaching techniques. Both substances were released over a period of several weeks and enhanced the mineralization of the cells, which can be regarded as a differentiation marker.

Whenever we use hydrogels we have a fair chance that we will be able to dissolve them together with the drug in an aqueous solution. This is especially attractive when we intend to deliver a protein drug, which usually has very good stability in an aqueous environment. Lee et al. [141] used cross-linked alginate gels to control the release of VEGF. They could show that the mechanical stimulation of matrices lead to a significant increase in the release velocity.

42.4.2.2.2 Adsorption

Another simple strategy to "load" a scaffold with a drug is by simply adsorbing it to the material surface or incorporating it into the material bulk. The release of the drug is then controlled by the desorption kinetics, which are controlled by the drug/material interactions as well as transport mechanisms, such as diffusion. While polymers offer ample alternative options for the incorporation of drugs into a tissue engineering scaffold, inorganic materials, in particular, can typically only be loaded by adsorption. In one case, Ziegler et al. [214] adsorbed bone morphogenic protein 4 (BMP-4) and basic fibroblast growth factor (FGF) to a variety of materials, such as porous tricalcium phosphate ceramic and a neutralized glass ceramic (GB9N) as well as a composite of the latter with PLGA. They found that the adsorption behavior depends on the nature of both the material and the protein and that a phase of fast initial release during the first hours is followed by a phase of slow release from the investigated carriers.

Similar strategies can be used for loading polymer hydrogels after cross-linking as described earlier. These systems are usually capable of taking up drugs from solution by diffusion into the cross-linked gel. This has successfully been demonstrated by Tabata [215], who loaded cross-linked gelatin microspheres with bFGF. He could show that the release of growth factor takes place over a span of days and that the released drug is still bioactive. Ueda et al. [216] later transferred this strategy to the manufacture of porous collagen sponges. It could be shown in a cranial defect model that the growth factor was released in active form and that bone repair was enhanced significantly. It is interesting to note that the release of the proteins from such systems is not only a matter of diffusion, but also dependent on the electrostatic interactions between the charge protein carrier and the protein drug.

42.4.2.2.3 Emulsion Techniques

Whang et al. [217] describe a method that allows for the incorporation of a drug into lipophilic biodegradable polymer scaffolds made of poly(D,L-lactic-co-glycolic acid) (PLGA). This technique, which was originally developed for the incorporation of hydrophilic drugs into lipophilic microspheres, relies on the formation of a W/O emulsion. While the drug is dissolved in the aqueous phase, the polymer is dissolved in organic solvents such as methylene chloride. Porous polymer scaffolds were manufactured from the liquid formulation by lyophilization. The technology was successfully applied to the controlled release of rhBMP2 [218]. Another approach developed by Jang and Shea [219] uses a multiple emulsion technique to manufacture PLA microspheres loaded with DNA. The particles that were made via a W/O/W technique [220] were fused to a porous scaffold by mixing with sodium chloride crystals compressed into discs by incubation at 37°C and 95% relative humidity. After drying in a pressurized CO_2 atmosphere, the particles were leached in water. The scaffolds released the DNA over a period of more than 3 weeks.

An approach related to the use of emulsions as a raw material for scaffolding is the use of emulsions for coating. Sohier et al. [221] used a W/O emulsion of poly(ethylene glycol) terephthalate/poly(butylene terephthalate) multiblock copolymer loaded with lysozyme as a model protein to coat porous scaffolds made of the same material. They could release the protein over several days and were able to show that the activity of lysozyme was maintained. While the use of emulsions has the advantage of creating an even distribution of drugs inside the material, in some cases, sensitive drugs may not be stable in such an emulsion system [222–224].

42.4.2.2.4 Suspension of the Drug and Physical Mixtures

Drug suspensions and mixtures can be especially useful for the manufacture of a cell carrier. While the matrix material is dissolved in a solvent, the drug obviously needs to be insoluble in this mixture. This is especially attractive for the incorporation of proteins into lipophilic polymers, because proteins exhibit an extraordinary stability against organic solvents when they are in the solid state [225].

Physical mixtures have also been of interest to scientists working in tissue engineering. In this case, the matrix material and the drug are mixed in the solid state and subsequently processed into porous cell carriers. This process has been used by Shea et al. [226] to load PLGA scaffolds with plasmid DNA. For their studies, they used PLGA granules and suspended them in an aqueous solution of plasmid DNA at pH 7.4 in 10 M HEPES buffer containing mannitol, which was used as a lyophilization constituent. After freeze drying, the mixture was compressed with NaCl particles into discs, the polymer particles fused using pressurized CO_2 and the porogen finally removed by leaching in water. The porous scaffolds allowed for the delivery of DNA over several weeks and showed excellent transfection efficiency.

42.5 Outlook

The field of tissue engineering has profited significantly from controlled release research and technology. Numerous growth factors and cytokines have been successfully applied via controlled drug-delivery devices in recent years. Despite this progress, there are numerous challenges ahead of us. First of all, we have to develop release systems that are on the one hand very flexible with respect to controlled drug release and that are on the other hand able to stabilize sensitive drugs, such as proteins and peptides.

Furthermore, more research will be needed on delivery systems that target intracellular compartments, cells, and tissues. This would allow for the delivery of DNA as well as drugs more specifically and safely.

We must also take better advantage of progress in medicinal chemistry, which will provide us with low molecular weight ligands that have a high affinity for well-defined targets. So far our efforts in tissue engineering research have profited only minimally from the opportunities that low molecular weight drugs offer.

Currently, release systems suffer from an inability to adequately mimic biology, in that typically only one drug is delivered. Guided by an increasingly better understanding of cell biology, drug-delivery systems that release several drugs according to a well-defined time pattern hold great promise.

Continuing progress will depend significantly on the availability of new materials for the development of drug-delivery systems. Biomimetic materials or materials that respond to biological stimuli are good examples. We have to overcome the problem that the rate-limiting step for the bench to beside process is not solely determined by our scientific progress, but also by tedious regulatory hurdles that new materials have to overcome.

References

[1] Langer, R. and Vacanti, J.P., Tissue engineering, *Science*, 260, 920, 1993.
[2] Chen, R.R. and Mooney, D.J., Polymeric growth factor delivery strategies for tissue engineering, *Pharm. Res.*, 20, 1103, 2003.
[3] Tabata, Y., Tissue regeneration based on growth factor release, *Tissue Eng.*, 9, S5, 2003.
[4] Boontheekul, T. and Mooney, D.J., Protein-based signaling systems in tissue engineering, *Curr. Opin. Biotechnol.*, 14, 559, 2003.
[5] Nomi, M. et al., Principals of neovascularization for tissue engineering, *Mol. Aspects Med.*, 23, 463.
[6] Nakashima, M. and Reddi, A.H., The application of bone morphogenetic proteins to dental tissue engineering, *Nat. Biotechnol.*, 21, 1025, 2003.
[7] Baldwin, S.P. and Mark Saltzman, W., Materials for protein delivery in tissue engineering, *Adv. Drug Deliv. Rev.*, 33, 71, 1998.
[8] Rose, F.R.A.J., Hou, Q., and Oreffo, R.O.C., Delivery systems for bone growth factors — the new players in skeletal regeneration, *J. Pharm. Pharmacol.*, 56, 415, 2004.
[9] Langer, R. and Peppas, N.A., Advances in biomaterials, drug delivery, and bionanotechnology, *AIChE J.*, 49, 2990, 2003.
[10] Crommelin, D.J.A. et al., Shifting paradigms: biopharmaceuticals versus low molecular weight drugs, *Int. J. Pharm.*, 266, 3, 2003.
[11] Gittens, S.A. and Uludag, H., Growth factor delivery for bone tissue engineering, *J. Drug Target.*, 9, 407, 2001.
[12] LaVan, D.A., McGuire, T., and Langer, R., Small-scale systems for *in vivo* drug delivery, *Nat. Biotechnol.*, 21, 1184, 2003.
[13] Definition drug delivery, *www.dictionarybarn.com*, 2004.

[14] Definition drug delivery systems, *www.dictionarybarn.com*, 2004.

[15] You, H.B. and Sung, W.K., Drug delivery, in *Frontiers in Tissue Engineering*, Patrick, C.W., Mikos, A.G., and McIntire, L.V., Eds., Pergamon, 261–277, 1998.

[16] Schwartz, R.S., Perspective: Paul Ehrlich's magic bullets, *N. Engl. J. Med.*, 350, 1079, 2004.

[17] Li, W. et al., Lysyl oxidase oxidizes basic fibroblast growth factor and inactivates its mitogenic potential, *J. Cell. Biochem.*, 88, 152, 2002.

[18] Klagsbrun, M. et al., Multiple forms of basic fibroblast growth factor: amino-terminal cleavages by tumor cell- and brain cell-derived acid proteinases, *Proc. Natl Acad. Sci. USA*, 84, 1839, 1987.

[19] Cunningham, M.J., Genomics and proteomics. The new millennium of drug discovery and development, *J. Pharmacol. Toxicol. Meth.*, 44, 291, 2001.

[20] Siepmann, J. and Gopferich, A., Mathematical modeling of bioerodible, polymeric drug delivery systems, *Adv. Drug Deliv. Rev.*, 48, 229, 2001.

[21] Gopferich, A., Mechanisms of polymer degradation and erosion, *Biomaterials*, 17, 103, 1996.

[22] Gopferich, A., Erosion of composite polymer matrices, *Biomaterials*, 18, 397, 1997.

[23] Gopferich, A. and Tessmar, J., Polyanhydride degradation and erosion, *Adv. Drug Deliv. Rev.*, 54, 911, 2002.

[24] Wright, S. and Huang, L., Antibody-directed liposomes as drug-delivery vehicles, *Adv. Drug Deliv. Rev.*, 3, 343, 1989.

[25] Wissing, S.A., Kayser, O., and Muller, R.H., Solid lipid nanoparticles for parenteral drug delivery, *Adv. Drug Deliv. Rev.*, 56, 1257, 2004.

[26] Mitragotri, S. and Kost, J., Low-frequency sonophoresis: a review, *Adv. Drug Deliv. Rev.*, 56, 589, 2004.

[27] Kalia, Y.N. et al., Iontophoretic drug delivery, *Adv. Drug Deliv. Rev.*, 56, 619, 2004.

[28] Sawahata, K. et al., Electrically controlled drug delivery system using polyelectrolyte gels, *J. Control. Release*, 14, 253, 1990.

[29] Murdan, S., Electro-responsive drug delivery from hydrogels, *J. Control. Release*, 92, 1, 2003.

[30] Gangarosa, S. and Hill, J.M., Modern iontophoresis for local drug delivery, *Int. J. Pharm.*, 123, 159, 1995.

[31] Verma, R.K., Krishna, D.M., and Garg, S., Formulation aspects in the development of osmotically controlled oral drug delivery systems, *J. Control. Release*, 79, 7, 2002.

[32] Santus, G. and Baker, R.W., Osmotic drug delivery: a review of the patent literature, *J. Control. Release*, 35, 1, 1995.

[33] Thombre, A.G., Zentner, G.M., and Himmelstein, K.J., Mechanism of water transport in controlled porosity osmotic devices, *J. Membr. Sci.*, 40, 279, 1989.

[34] Hamilton, J.F. et al., Heparin coinfusion during convection-enhanced delivery (CED) increases the distribution of the glial-derived neurotrophic factor (GDNF) ligand family in rat striatum and enhances the pharmacological activity of neurturin, *Exp. Neurol.*, 168, 155, 2001.

[35] Bankiewicz, K.S. et al., Convection-enhanced delivery of AAV vector in Parkinsonian monkeys; *in vivo* detection of gene expression and restoration of dopaminergic function using pro-drug approach, *Exp. Neurol.*, 164, 2, 2000.

[36] Qiu, Y. and Park, K., Environment-sensitive hydrogels for drug delivery, *Adv. Drug Deliv. Rev.*, 53, 321, 2001.

[37] Lee, K.Y., Peters, M.C., and Mooney, D.J., Controlled drug delivery from polymers by mechanical signals, *Adv. Mater. (Weinheim, Germany)*, 13, 837, 2001.

[38] Sah, H. and Chien, Y.W., Rate control in drug delivery and targeting: fundamentals and applications to implantable systems, in *Drug Delivery and Targeting*, Hillary, A.M., Llyod, A.W., and Swarbrick, J., Eds., London, Taylor & Francis Ltd., 83–115, 2001.

[39] Kalia, Y.N. et al., Iontophoretic drug delivery, *Adv. Drug Deliv. Rev.*, 56, 619, 2004.

[40] Huang, X. and Brazel, C.S., On the importance and mechanisms of burst release in matrix-controlled drug delivery systems, *J. Control. Release*, 73, 121, 2001.

[41] Kamath, K.R. and Park, K., Biodegradable hydrogels in drug delivery, *Adv. Drug Deliv. Rev.*, 11, 59, 1993.

[42] West, J.L., Drug delivery: pulsed polymers, *Nat. Mater.*, 2, 709, 2003.

[43] Cussler, E.L., *Diffusion, Mass Transfer in Fluid Systems*, p. 525, 1984.

[44] Gehrke, S.H. and Cussler, E.L., Mass transfer in pH-sensitive hydrogels, *Chem. Eng. Sci.*, 44, 559, 1989.

[45] Zhang, M. et al., Simulation of drug release from biodegradable polymeric microspheres with bulk and surface erosions, *J. Pharm. Sci.*, 92, 2040, 2003.

[46] Gombotz, W.R. and Pettit, D.K., Biodegradable polymers for protein and peptide drug delivery, *Bioconjug. Chem.*, 6, 332, 1995.

[47] Kumar, N. et al., Biodegradation of polyanhydrides, in *Biopolymers*, Matsamura, S. and Steinbuechel, A., Eds., Wiley-VCH Verlag GmbH, Weinheim, 2003, chap 9, 2003.

[48] Heller, J., Controlled drug release from poly(ortho esters) — a surface eroding polymer, *J. Control. Release*, 2, 167, 1985.

[49] Goepferich, A., Polymer bulk erosion, *Macromolecules*, 30, 2598, 1997.

[50] von Burkersroda, F., Schedl, L., and Gopferich, A., Why degradable polymers undergo surface erosion or bulk erosion, *Biomaterials*, 23, 4221, 2002.

[51] Rao, K.V.R. and Devi, K.P., Swelling controlled-release systems: recent developments and applications, *Int. J. Pharm.*, 48, 1, 1988.

[52] Kranz, H. et al., Physicomechanical properties of biodegradable poly(D,L-lactide) and poly(D,L-lactide-co-glycolide) films in the dry and wet states, *J. Pharm. Sci.*, 89, 1558, 2000.

[53] Bouillot, P., Petit, A., and Dellacherie, E., Protein encapsulation in biodegradable amphiphilic microspheres. I. Polymer synthesis and characterization and microsphere elaboration, *J. Appl. Polym. Sci.*, 68, 1695, 1998.

[54] Lee, W.F. and Chen, Y.J., Studies on preparation and swelling properties of the N-isopropylacrylamide/chitosan semi-IPN and IPN hydrogels, *J. Appl. Polym. Sci.*, 82, 2487, 2001.

[55] Colombo, P. et al., Swellable matrixes for controlled drug delivery: gel-layer behavior, mechanisms and optimal performance, *Pharm. Sci. Technol. Today*, 3, 198, 2000.

[56] Peppas, N. and Khare, A.R., Preparation, structure and diffusional behavior of hydrogels in controlled release, *Adv. Drug Deliv. Rev.*, 11, 1, 1993.

[57] Yoshida, T. et al., Newly designed hydrogel with both sensitive thermoresponse and biodegradability, *J. Polym. Sci., Part A: Polym. Chem.*, 41, 779, 2003.

[58] Vogelhuber, W. et al., Programmable biodegradable implants, *J. Control. Release*, 73, 75, 2001.

[59] Fan, L.S.S., *Controlled Release: A Quantitative Treatment*, Springer-Verlag, New York, 1989.

[60] Heckman, J.D. et al., The use of bone morphogenetic protein in the treatment of non-union in a canine model, *J. Bone Joint Surg. Am.*, 73, 750, 1991.

[61] Ono, I. et al., A study on bone induction in hydroxyapatite combined with bone morphogenetic protein, *Plast. Reconstr. Surg.*, 90, 870, 1992.

[62] Muschler, G.F. et al., Evaluation of human bone morphogenetic protein 2 in a canine spinal fusion model, *Clin. Orthop. Relat. Res.*, 308, 229, 1994.

[63] Kenley, R. et al., Osseous regeneration in the rat calvarium using novel delivery systems for recombinant human bone morphogenetic protein-2, *J. Biomed. Mater. Res.*, 28, 1139, 1994.

[64] Zellin, G. and Linde, A., Importance of delivery systems for growth-stimulatory factors in combination with osteopromotive membranes. An experimental study using rhBMP-2 in rat mandibular defects, *J. Biomed. Mater. Res.*, 35, 181, 1997.

[65] Hong, L. et al., Comparison of bone regeneration in a rabbit skull defect by recombinant human BMP-2 incorporated in biodegradable hydrogel and in solution, *J. Biomater. Sci., Polym. Ed.*, 9, 1001, 1998.

[66] Miyamoto, S. et al., Evaluation of polylactic acid homopolymers as carriers for bone morphogenetic protein, *Clin. Orthop. Relat. Res.*, 278, 274, 1992.

[67] Ripamonti, U., Yeates, L., and van den Heever, B., Initiation of heterotopic osteogenesis in primates after chromatographic adsorption of osteogenin, a bone morphogenetic protein, onto porous hydroxyapatite, *Biochem. Biophys. Res. Commun.*, 193, 509, 1993.

[68] Ripamonti, U. et al., Osteogenin, a bone morphogenetic protein, adsorbed on porous hydroxyapatite substrata, induces rapid bone differentiation in calvarial defects of adult primates, *Plast. Reconstr. Surg.*, 90, 382.

[69] Miyamoto, S. et al., Polylactic acid–polyethylene glycol block copolymer. A new biodegradable synthetic carrier for bone morphogenetic protein, *Clin. Orthop. Relat. Res.*, 294, 333, 1993.

[70] Santos, E.M. et al., Si–Ca–P xerogels and bone morphogenetic protein act synergistically on rat stromal marrow cell differentiation *in vitro*, *J. Biomed. Mater. Res.*, 41, 87, 1998.

[71] Cook, S.D. et al., *In vivo* evaluation of recombinant human osteogenic protein (rhOP-1) implants as a bone graft substitute for spinal fusions, *Spine*, 19, 1655, 1994.

[72] Grauer, J.N. et al., 2000 Young investigator research award winner. Evaluation of OP-1 as a graft substitute for intertransverse process lumbar fusion, *Spine*, 26, 127, 2001.

[73] Cook, S.D. et al., Effect of recombinant human osteogenic protein-1 on healing of segmental defects in non-human primates, *J. Bone Joint Surg. Am.*, 77, 734, 1995.

[74] Blattert, T.R. et al., Successful transpedicular lumbar interbody fusion by means of a composite of osteogenic protein-1 (rhBMP-7) and hydroxyapatite carrier: a comparison with autograft and hydroxyapatite in the sheep spine, *Spine*, 27, 2697, 2002.

[75] Fajardo, L.F. et al., The disc angiogenesis system, *Lab. Invest.*, 58, 718, 1988.

[76] Downs, E.C. et al., Calcium alginate beads as a slow-release system for delivering angiogenic molecules *in vivo* and *in vitro*, *J. Cell. Physiol.*, 152, 422, 1992.

[77] Laham, R.J. et al., Local perivascular delivery of basic fibroblast growth factor in patients undergoing coronary bypass surgery: results of a phase I randomized, double-blind, placebo-controlled trial, *Circulation*, 100, 1865, 1999.

[78] Edelman, E.R. et al., Controlled and modulated release of basic fibroblast growth factor, *Biomaterials*, 12, 619, 1991.

[79] Tabata, Y. et al., Bone regeneration by basic fibroblast growth factor complexed with biodegradable hydrogels, *Biomaterials*, 19, 807, 1998.

[80] Kawaguchi, H. et al., Stimulation of fracture repair by recombinant human basic fibroblast growth factor in normal and streptozotocin-diabetic rats, *Endocrinology*, 135, 774, 1994.

[81] Mizuno, K. et al., Effect of chitosan film containing basic fibroblast growth factor on wound healing in genetically diabetic mice, *J. Biomed. Mater. Res.*, 64A, 177, 2003.

[82] Fujisato, T. et al., Effect of basic fibroblast growth factor on cartilage regeneration in chondrocyte-seeded collagen sponge scaffold, *Biomaterials*, 17, 155, 1996.

[83] Ulubayram, K. et al., EGF containing gelatin-based wound dressings, *Biomaterials*, 22, 1345, 2001.

[84] Mierisch, C.M. et al., Transforming growth factor-beta in calcium alginate beads for the treatment of articular cartilage defects in the rabbit, *Arthroscopy: Journal of Arthroscopic & Related Surgery: Official Publication of the Arthroscopy Association of North America and the International Arthroscopy Association*, 18, 892, 2002.

[85] Puolakkainen, P.A. et al., The enhancement in wound healing by transforming growth factor-b1 (TGF-b1) depends on the topical delivery system, *J. Surg. Res.*, 58, 321, 1995.

[86] Gombotz, W.R. et al., Controlled release of TGF-b1 from a biodegradable matrix for bone regeneration, *J. Biomater. Sci., Polym. Ed.*, 5, 49, 1993.

[87] Mustoe, T.A. et al., Accelerated healing of incisional wounds in rats induced by transforming growth factor-b, *Science (Washington, DC, United States)*, 237, 1333, 1987.

[88] Hildebrand, K.A. et al., The effects of platelet-derived growth factor-BB on healing of the rabbit medial collateral ligament. An *in vivo* study, *Am. J. Sports Med.*, 26, 549, 1998.

[89] Nagai, M.K. and Embil, J.M., Becaplermin: recombinant platelet derived growth factor, a new treatment for healing diabetic foot ulcers, *Expert Opin. Biol. Ther.*, 2, 211, 2002.

[90] Lee, K.Y., Peters, M.C., and Mooney, D.J., Comparison of vascular endothelial growth factor and basic fibroblast growth factor on angiogenesis in SCID mice, *J. Control. Release*, 87, 49, 2003.

[91] Tabata, Y. et al., Controlled release of vascular endothelial growth factor by use of collagen hydrogels, *J. Biomater. Sci., Polym. Ed.*, 11, 915, 2000.

[92] Peters, M.C., Polverini, P.J., and Mooney, D.J., Engineering vascular networks in porous polymer matrices, *J. Biomed. Mater. Res.*, 60, 668, 2002.

[93] Kipshidze, N., Chawla, P., and Keelan, M.H., Fibrin meshwork as a carrier for delivery of angiogenic growth factors in patients with ischemic limb, *Mayo Clin. Proc.*, 74, 847, 1999.

[94] Richardson, T.P. et al., Polymeric system for dual growth factor delivery, *Nat. Biotechnol.*, 19, 1029, 2001.

[95] Camarata, P.J. et al., Sustained release of nerve growth factor from biodegradable polymer microspheres, *Neurosurgery*, 30, 313, 1992.

[96] Yamamoto, S. et al., Protective effect of NGF atelocollagen mini-pellet on the hippocampal delayed neuronal death in gerbils, *Neurosci. Lett.*, 141, 161, 1992.

[97] Robinson, S.N. and Talmadge, J.E., Sustained release of growth factors, *In Vivo*, 16, 535, 2002.

[98] Wang, W., Instability, stabilization, and formulation of liquid protein pharmaceuticals, *Int. J. Pharm.*, 185, 129, 1999.

[99] Manning, M.C., Patel, K., and Borchardt, R.T., Stability of protein pharmaceuticals, *Pharm. Res.*, 6, 903, 1989.

[100] Schwendeman, S.P. et al., Stability of proteins and their delivery from biodegradable polymer microspheres, in *Microparticulate Systems for Delivery of Proteins and Vaccines*, New York, Dekker, 1–49, 1996 1996.

[101] Tanford, C., Protein denaturation, *Adv. Protein Chem.*, 23, 121, 1968.

[102] Kubiak, T.M. et al., Position 2 and position 2/Ala15-substituted analogs of bovine growth hormone-releasing factor (bGRF) with enhanced metabolic stability and improved *in vivo* bioactivity, *J. Med. Chem.*, 36, 888, 1993.

[103] Bowen-Pope, D.F. et al., Platelet-derived growth factor *in vivo*: levels, activity, and rate of clearance, *Blood*, 64, 458, 1984.

[104] Edelman, E.R., Nugent, M.A., and Karnovsky, M.J., Perivascular and intravenous administration of basic fibroblast growth factor: vascular and solid organ deposition, *Proc. Natl Acad. Sci. USA*, 90, 1513, 1993.

[105] Lazarous, D.F. et al., Comparative effects of basic fibroblast growth factor and vascular endothelial growth factor on coronary collateral development and the arterial response to injury, *Circulation*, 94, 1074, 1996.

[106] Yancopoulos, G.D. et al., Vascular-specific growth factors and blood vessel formation, *Nature (London)*, 407, 242, 2000.

[107] Yang, B.B. et al., Polyethylene glycol modification of filgrastim results in decreased renal clearance of the protein in rats, *J. Pharm. Sci.*, 93, 1367, 2004.

[108] Eliason, J.F., Pegylated cytokines. Potential application in immunotherapy of cancer, *BioDrugs*, 15, 705, 2001.

[109] Edwards, C.K., III, PEGylated recombinant human soluble tumor necrosis factor receptor type I (r-Hu-sTNF-RI): novel high affinity TNF receptor designed for chronic inflammatory diseases, *Ann. Rheum. Dis.*, 58, I73, 1999.

[110] Archimbaud, E., Clinical trials of pegylated recombinant human megakaryocyte growth and development factor (PEG-rHuMGDF), *Haematol. Blood Transfus.*, 39, 343, 1998.

[111] Molineux, G., PEGylation: engineering improved pharmaceuticals for enhanced therapy, *Cancer Treat. Rev.*, 28, 13, 2002.

[112] Sato, H., Enzymatic procedure for site-specific pegylation of proteins, *Adv. Drug Deliv. Rev.*, 54, 487, 2002.

[113] Roberts, M.J., Bentley, M.D., and Harris, J.M., Chemistry for peptide and protein PEGylation, *Adv. Drug Deliv. Rev.*, 54, 459, 2002.

[114] Zalipsky, S., Chemistry of polyethylene glycol conjugates with biologically active molecules, *Adv. Drug Deliv. Rev.*, 16, 157, 1995.

[115] Veronese, F.M. and Harris, J.M., Introduction and overview of peptide and protein pegylation, *Adv. Drug Deliv. Rev.*, 54, 453, 2002.

[116] Zhdanov, V.P. and Kasemo, B., Monte Carlo simulations of the kinetics of protein adsorption, *Surf. Rev. Lett.*, 5, 615, 1998.

[117] Norde, W., Adsorption of proteins from solution at the solid–liquid interface, *Adv. Colloid Interface Sci.*, 25, 267, 1986.

[118] Malmsten, M., Protein adsorption at the solid–liquid interface, in *Protein Architecture*, Lvov, Y. and Moehwald, H., Eds., New York, Marcel Dekker, 1–23, 2000.

[119] Felgner, P.L. and Wilson, J.E., Hexokinase binding to polypropylene test tubes. Artifactual activity losses from protein binding to disposable plastics, *Anal. Biochem.*, 74, 631, 1976.

[120] Beyerman, H.C. et al., On the instability of secretin, *Life Sci.*, 29, 885, 1981.

[121] Kramer, K.J. et al., Purification and characterization of the carrier protein for juvenile hormone from the hemolymph of the tobacco hornworm *Manduca sexta* Johannson (Lepidoptera: Sphingidae), *J. Biol. Chem.*, 251, 4979, 1976.

[122] Suelter, C.H. and DeLuca, M., How to prevent losses of protein by adsorption to glass and plastic, *Anal. Biochem.*, 135, 112, 1983.

[123] Katakam, M. and Banga, A.K., Use of poloxamer polymers to stabilize recombinant human growth hormone against various processing stresses, *Pharm. Dev. Technol.*, 2, 143, 1997.

[124] Charman, S.A., Mason, K.L., and Charman, W.N., Techniques for assesing the effects of pharmaceutical excipients on the aggregation of porcine growth hormone, *Pharm. Res.*, 10, 954, 1993.

[125] Oliva, A. et al., Effect of high shear rate on stability of proteins: kinetic study, *J. Pharm. Biomed. Anal.*, 33, 145, 2003.

[126] Spenlehauer, G., Spenlehauer-Bonthonneau, F., and Thies, C., Biodegradable microparticles for delivery of polypeptides and proteins, *Prog. Clin. Biol. Res.*, 292, 283, 1989.

[127] van Erp, S.H., Kamenskaya, E.O., and Khmelnitsky, Y.L., The effect of water content and nature of organic solvent on enzyme activity in low-water media. A quantitative description, *Eur. J. Biochem./FEBS*, 202, 379, 1991.

[128] Khmelnitsky, Y.L. et al., Denaturation capacity: a new quantitative criterion for selection of organic solvents as reaction media in biocatalysis, *Eur. J. Biochem./FEBS*, 198, 31, 1991.

[129] Brunner, A., Mader, K., and Gopferich, A., The chemical microenvironment inside biodegradable microspheres during erosion, *Proceedings of the International Symposium on Controlled Release of Bioactive Materials*, Vol. 25, p. 154, 1998.

[130] Lucke, A. et al., The effect of poly(ethylene glycol)–poly(D,L-lactic acid) diblock copolymers on peptide acylation, *J. Control. Release*, 80, 157, 2002.

[131] Lucke, A., Kiermaier, J., and Gopferich, A., Peptide acylation by poly(.alpha.-hydroxy esters), *Pharm. Res.*, 19, 175, 2002.

[132] Schwendeman, S.P., Recent advances in the stabilization of proteins encapsulated in injectable PLGA delivery systems, *Crit. Rev. Ther. Drug Carrier Syst.*, 19, 73, 2002.

[133] Zhu, G., Mallery, S.R., and Schwendeman, S.P., Stabilization of proteins encapsulated in injectable poly(lactide-co-glycolide), *Nat. Biotechnol.*, 18, 52, 2000.

[134] Lam, X.M., Duenas, E.T., and Cleland, J.L., Encapsulation and stabilization of nerve growth factor into poly(lactic-co-glycolic) acid microspheres, *J. Pharm. Sci.*, 90, 1356, 2001.

[135] Pean, J.M. et al., Why does PEG 400 co-encapsulation improve NGF stability and release from PLGA biodegradable microspheres? *Pharm. Res.*, 16, 1294, 1999.

[136] Tang, B., Wang, M., and Wise, C., Nerve growth factor mRNA stability is controlled by a cis-acting instability determinant in the 3′-untranslated region, *Mol. Brain Res.*, 46, 118, 1997.

[137] Shaw, G. and Kamen, R., A conserved AU sequence from the 3′ untranslated region of GM-CSF mRNA mediates selective mRNA degradation, *Cell*, 46, 659, 1986.

[138] Schiavi, S.C., Belasco, J.G., and Greenberg, M.E., Regulation of proto-oncogene mRNA stability, *Biochim. Biophys. Acta*, 1114, 95, 1992.

[139] Nimni, M.E., Polypeptide growth factors: targeted delivery systems, *Biomaterials*, 18, 1201, 1997.

[140] Davis, G.E. and Camarillo, C.W., Regulation of endothelial cell morphogenesis by integrins, mechanical forces, and matrix guidance pathways, *Exp. Cell Res.*, 216, 113, 1995.

[141] Lee, K.Y. et al., Controlled growth factor release from synthetic extracellular matrices, *Nature*, 408, 998, 2000.

[142] Wallace, D.G. and Rosenblatt, J., Collagen gel systems for sustained delivery and tissue engineering, *Adv. Drug Deliv. Rev.*, 55, 1631, 2003.

[143] Drury, J.L. and Mooney, D.J., Hydrogels for tissue engineering: scaffold design variables and applications, *Biomaterials*, 24, 4337, 2003.

[144] Peters, M.C. et al., Release from alginate enhances the biological activity of vascular endothelial growth factor, *J. Biomater. Sci., Polym. Ed.*, 9, 1267, 1998.

[145] Taipale, J. and Keski-Oja, J., Growth factors in the extracellular matrix, *FASEB J.*, 11, 51, 1997.

[146] Langer, R. and Tirrell, D.A., Designing materials for biology and medicine, *Nature (London, United Kingdom)*, 428, 487, 2004.

[147] Majeti, N.V. and Ravi Kumar, M.N.V., Nano and microparticles as controlled drug delivery devices, *J. Pharm. Pharm. Sci. [online computer file]*, 3, 234, 2000.

[148] Lopez, V.C. and Snowden, M.J., The role of colloidal microgels in drug delivery, *Drug Deliv. Syst. Sci.*, 3, 19, 2003.

[149] Saltzman, W.M., Delivering tissue regeneration, *Nat. Biotechnol.*, 17, 534, 1999.

[150] Xu, R. et al., Diabetes gene therapy: potential and challenges, *Curr. Gene Ther.*, 3, 65, 2003.

[151] Merdan, T., Kopecek, J., and Kissel, T., Prospects for cationic polymers in gene and oligonucleotide therapy against cancer, *Adv. Drug Deliv. Rev.*, 54, 715, 2002.

[152] Lollo, C.P., Banaszczyk, M.G., and Chiou, H.C., Obstacles and advances in non-viral gene delivery, *Curr. Opin. Mol. Ther.*, 2, 136, 2000.

[153] Johnson-Saliba, M. and Jans, D.A., Gene therapy: optimising DNA delivery to the nucleus, *Curr. Drug Targets*, 2, 371, 2001.

[154] Bout, A. and Crucell, L., Gene therapy, in *Pharmaceutical Biotechnology*, 2nd ed., Commelin, D.J.A. and Sindelar, R.D., Eds., London, Taylor & Francis Ltd., 175–192, 2002.

[155] Kuhl, P.R. and Griffith-Cima, L.G., Tethered epidermal growth factor as a paradigm for growth factor-induced stimulation from the solid phase, *Nat. Med.*, 2, 1022, 1996.

[156] Blunk, T., Goepferich, A., and Tessmar, J., Special issue biomimetic polymers, *Biomaterials*, 24, 4335, 2003.

[157] Aldersey-Williams, H., Towards biomimetic architecture, *Nat. Mater.*, 3, 277, 2004.

[158] Ito, Y., Tissue engineering by immobilized growth factors, *Mater. Sci. Eng. C: Biomimetic Mater., Sensors Syst.*, C6, 267, 1998.

[159] Shakesheff, K.M., Cannizzaro, S.M., and Langer, R., Creating biomimetic micro-environments with synthetic polymer–peptide hybrid molecules, *J. Biomater. Sci., Polym. Ed.*, 9, 507, 1998.

[160] Thayumanavan, S. et al., Towards dendrimers as biomimetic macromolecules, *C. R. Chimie*, 6, 767, 2003.

[161] Hoffman, A.S. et al., Design of "smart" polymers that can direct intracellular drug delivery, *Polym. Adv. Technol.*, 13, 992, 2002.

[162] Peppas, N.A. and Huang, Y., Polymers and gels as molecular recognition agents, *Pharm. Res.*, 19, 578, 2002.

[163] Langer, R. and Folkman, J., Polymers for the sustained release of proteins and other macromolecules, *Nature*, 263, 797.

[164] Saltzman, W.M. and Langer, R., Transport rates of proteins in porous materials with known microgeometry, *Biophys. J.*, 55, 163, 1989.

[165] Bawa, R. et al., An explanation for the controlled release of macromolecules from polymers, *J. Control. Release*, 1, 259, 1985.

[166] Leong, K.W. et al., Polyanhydrides for controlled release of bioactive agents, *Biomaterials*, 7, 364, 1986.

[167] Heller, J., Controlled drug release from poly(ortho esters) — a surface eroding polymer, *J. Control. Release*, 2, 167, 1985.

[168] Goepferich, A., Mechanisms of polymer degradation and erosion, *Biomaterials*, 17, 103, 1996.

[169] Goepferich, A., Polymer degradation and erosion. Mechanisms and applications, *Eur. J. Pharm. Biopharm.*, 42, 1, 1996.

[170] Fu, K. et al., Visual evidence of acidic environment within degrading poly(lactic-co-glycolic acid) (PLGA) microspheres, *Pharm. Res.*, 17, 100, 2000.

[171] Brunner, A., Mader, K., and Gopferich, A., pH and osmotic pressure inside biodegradable microspheres during erosion, *Pharm. Res.*, 16, 847, 1999.

[172] Lucke, A., Kiermaier, J., and Gopferich, A., Peptide acylation by poly(a-hydroxy esters), *Pharm. Res.*, 19, 175, 2002.

[173] Athanasiou, K.A. et al., Orthopaedic applications for PLA–PGA biodegradable polymers, *Arthroscopy: The Journal of Arthroscopic and Related Surgery: Official Publication of the Arthroscopy Association of North America and the International Arthroscopy Association*, 14, 726, 1998.

[174] Biggs, D.L. et al., *In vitro* and *in vivo* evaluation of the effects of PLA microparticle crystallinity on cellular response, *J. Control. Release: Official Journal of the Controlled Release Society*, 92, 147, 2003.

[175] Sandor, M. et al., Effect of protein molecular weight on release from micron-sized PLGA microspheres, *J. Control. Release*, 76, 297, 2001.

[176] Tabata, Y. and Ikada, Y., Protein release from gelatin matrixes, *Adv. Drug Deliv. Rev.*, 31, 287, 1998.

[177] Gombotz, W.R. and Wee, S., Protein release from alginate matrixes, *Adv. Drug Deliv. Rev.*, 31, 267, 1998.

[178] Fujioka, K. et al., Protein release from collagen matrixes, *Adv. Drug Deliv. Rev.*, 31, 247, 1998.

[179] Sinha, V.R. and Trehan, A., Biodegradable microspheres for protein delivery, *J. Control. Release*, 90, 261, 2003.

[180] Sinha, V.R. et al., Poly-e-caprolactone microspheres and nanospheres: an overview, *Int. J. Pharm.*, 278, 1, 2004.

[181] Orive, G. et al., Cell microencapsulation technology for biomedical purposes: novel insights and challenges, *Trends Pharmacol. Sci.*, 24, 207, 2003.

[182] Orive, G., Hernandez, R.M., Gascón, A.R., and Pedraz, J.L., Challenges in cell encapsulation, in *Cell Immobilization Biotechnology. Part II. Applications*, Nedović, N. and Willaert, R., Eds., "Focus on Biotechnology" series, Dordrecht, The Netherlands, Kluwer, 9999, 1991.

[183] Giannoni, P. and Hunziker, E.B., Release kinetics of transforming growth factor beta1 from fibrin clots, *Biotechnol. Bioeng.*, 83, 121, 2003.

[184] Collier, J.H. and Messersmith, P.B., Phospholipid strategies in biomineralization and biomaterials research, *Ann. Rev. Mater. Res.*, 31, 237, 2001.

[185] Haller, M.F. and Saltzman, W.M., Nerve growth factor delivery systems, *J. Control. Release*, 53, 1, 1998.

[186] Saltzman, W.M. et al., Intracranial delivery of recombinant nerve growth factor: release kinetics and protein distribution for three delivery systems, *Pharm. Res.*, 16, 232, 1999.

[187] Lee, J.E. et al., Effects of the controlled-released TGF-b1 from chitosan microspheres on chondrocytes cultured in a collagen/chitosan/glycosaminoglycan scaffold, *Biomaterials*, 25, 4163, 2004.

[188] Cleland, J.L. et al., Recombinant human growth hormone poly(lactic-glycolic acid) (PLGA) microspheres provide a long lasting effect, *J. Control. Release*, 49, 193, 1997.

[189] Cleland, J.L., Protein delivery from biodegradable microspheres, *Pharm. Biotechnol.*, 10, 1, 1997.

[190] Van de Weert, M., Hennink, W.E., and Jiskoot, W., Protein instability in poly(lactic-co-glycolic acid) microparticles, *Pharm. Res.*, 17, 1159, 2000.

[191] Tonnesen, H.H. and Karlsen, J., Alginate in drug delivery systems, *Drug Dev. Ind. Pharm.*, 28, 621, 2002.

[192] Gu, F., Amsden, B., and Neufeld, R., Sustained delivery of vascular endothelial growth factor with alginate beads, *J. Control. Release*, 96, 463, 2004.

[193] Mladenovska, K. et al., BSA-loaded gelatin microspheres: preparation and drug release rate in the presence of collagenase, *Acta Pharm. (Zagreb, Croatia)*, 52, 91, 2002.

[194] Tabata, Y. et al., *De novo* formation of adipose tissue by controlled release of basic fibroblast growth factor, *Tissue Eng.*, 6, 279, 2000.

[195] Bummer, P.M., Physical chemical considerations of lipid-based oral drug delivery — solid lipid nanoparticles, *Crit. Rev. Ther. Drug Carrier Syst.*, 21, 1, 2004.

[196] Maschke, A. et al., Lipids: an alternative material for protein and peptide release, *ACS Symp. Ser.*, 879, 176, 2004.

[197] Cortesi, R. et al., Production of lipospheres as carriers for bioactive compounds, *Biomaterials*, 23, 2283, 2002.

[198] Reithmeier, H., Herrmann, J., and Gopferich, A., Lipid microparticles as parenteral controlled release device for peptides, *J. Control. Release*, 73, 339, 2001.

[199] Reithmeier, H., Gopferich, A., and Herrmann, J., Preparation and characterization of lipid micro-particles containing thymocartin, an immunomodulating peptide, *Proceedings of the International Symposium on Controlled Release of Bioactive Materials*, Vol. 26, p. 681, 1999.

[200] Lee, K.Y. and Mooney, D.J., Hydrogels for tissue engineering, *Chem. Rev.*, 101, 1869, 2001.

[201] Yamamoto, M., Takahashi, Y., and Tabata, Y., Controlled release by biodegradable hydrogels enhances the ectopic bone formation of bone morphogenetic protein, *Biomaterials*, 24, 4375, 2003.

[202] Yamamoto, M. et al., Bone regeneration by transforming growth factor b1 released from a biodegradable hydrogel, *J. Control. Release*, 64, 133, 2000.

[203] Tabata, Y., Matsui, Y., and Ikada, Y., Growth factor release from amylopectin hydrogel based on copper coordination, *J. Control. Release*, 56, 135, 1998.

[204] Zisch, A.H., Lutolf, M.P., and Hubbell, J.A., Biopolymeric delivery matrices for angiogenic growth factors, *Cardiovasc. Pathol.*, 12, 295, 2003.

[205] Jeong, B. et al., Biodegradable block copolymers as injectable drug-delivery systems, *Nature*, 388, 860, 1997.

[206] Ebara, M. et al., Temperature-responsive cell culture surfaces enable "On-Off" affinity control between cell integrins and RGDS ligands, *Biomacromolecules*, 5, 505, 2004.

[207] Zisch, A.H. et al., Cell-demanded release of VEGF from synthetic, biointeractive cell-ingrowth matrices for vascularized tissue growth, *FASEB J.*, 17, 2260, 2003.

[208] Sakiyama-Elbert, S.E. and Hubbell, J.A., Controlled release of nerve growth factor from a heparin-containing fibrin-based cell ingrowth matrix, *J. Control. Release*, 69, 149, 2000.

[209] Kimura, Y. et al., Adipose tissue engineering based on human preadipocytes combined with gelatin microspheres containing basic fibroblast growth factor, *Biomaterials*, 24, 2513, 2003.

[210] Holland, T.A., Tabata, Y., and Mikos, A.G., *In vitro* release of transforming growth factor-b1 from gelatin microparticles encapsulated in biodegradable, injectable oligo(poly(ethylene glycol) fumarate) hydrogels, *J. Control. Release*, 91, 299, 2003.

[211] Holland, T.A. et al., Transforming growth factor-b1 release from oligo(poly(ethylene glycol) fumarate) hydrogels in conditions that model the cartilage wound healing environment, *J. Control. Release*, 94, 101, 2004.

[212] Hu, Y., Hollinger, J.O., and Marra, K.G., Controlled release from coated polymer microparticles embedded in tissue-engineered scaffolds, *J. Drug Target.*, 9, 431, 2001.

[213] Kim, H., Kim, H.W., and Suh, H., Sustained release of ascorbate-2-phosphate and dexa-methasone from porous PLGA scaffolds for bone tissue engineering using mesenchymal stem cells, *Biomaterials*, 24, 4671, 2003.

[214] Ziegler, J. et al., Adsorption and release properties of growth factors from biodegradable implants, *J. Biomed. Mater. Res.*, 59, 422, 2002.

[215] Tabata, Y. and Ikada, Y., Vascularization effect of basic fibroblast growth factor released from gelatin hydrogels with different biodegradabilities, *Biomaterials*, 20, 2169, 1999.

[216] Ueda, H. et al., Use of collagen sponge incorporating transforming growth factor-beta1 to promote bone repair in skull defects in rabbits, *Biomaterials*, 23, 1003, 2002.

[217] Whang, K., Goldstick, T.K., and Healy, K.E., A biodegradable polymer scaffold for delivery of osteotropic factors, *Biomaterials*, 21, 2545, 2000.

[218] Whang, K. et al., Ectopic bone formation via rhBMP-2 delivery from porous bioabsorbable polymer scaffolds, *J. Biomed. Mater. Res.*, 42, 491, 1998.

[219] Jang, J.H. and Shea, L.D., Controllable delivery of non-viral DNA from porous scaffolds, *J. Control. Release*, 86, 157, 2003.

[220] Brunner A., Gopferich, A., *Characterization of Polyanhydride Microspheres*, p. 169, 1996.

[221] Sohier, J. et al., A novel method to obtain protein release from porous polymer scaffolds: emulsion coating, *J. Control. Release*, 87, 57, 2003.

[222] Li, X. et al., Influence of process parameters on the protein stability encapsulated in poly-DL-lactide-poly(ethylene glycol) microspheres, *J. Control. Release*, 68, 41, 2000.

[223] Crotts, G. and Park, T.G., Protein delivery from poly(lactic-co-glycolic acid) biodegradable microspheres: release kinetics and stability issues, *J. Microencapsul.*, 15, 699, 1998.

[224] Jiang, G. et al., Assessment of protein release kinetics, stability and protein polymer interaction of lysozyme encapsulated poly(D,L-lactide-co-glycolide) microspheres, *J. Control. Release*, 79, 137, 2002.

[225] Sirotkin, V.A. et al., Calorimetric and Fourier transform infrared spectroscopic study of solid proteins immersed in low water organic solvents, *Biochim. Biophys. Acta*, 1547, 359, 2001.

[226] Shea, L.D. et al., DNA delivery from polymer matrices for tissue engineering, *Nat. Biotechnol.*, 17, 551, 1999.

43

Gene Therapy

J.M. Munson
W.T. Godbey
Tulane University

43.1 Introduction

Gene therapy is the delivery of genetic material into cells for the purpose of altering cellular function. This seemingly straightforward definition encompasses a variety of situations that can at times seem unrelated. The delivered genetic material can be composed of deoxyribonucleic acid (DNA) or RNA, or even involve proteins in some cases. The alteration in cellular function can be an increase or decrease in the amount of a native protein that is produced, or the production of a protein that is foreign. The delivery of the genetic material can occur directly, as is the case with microinjection, or involve carriers that interact with cell membranes or membrane-bound proteins as a part of cellular entry. Polynucleotides can be single or double stranded, and can code for a message, or not (as is the case for antisense gene delivery). Even the location of cells at the time of gene delivery is not restricted. Cells can be part of a living organism, can exist as a culture on a plate, or can be removed from an organism, transfected, and replaced into the same or a different organism at a later time.

Gene therapy came into being after the development of recombinant DNA technology and initially moved forward using viruses to target sites *in vitro* [1]. With the understanding of retroviruses and their possible uses as vectors for delivery, gene therapy progressed to applications involving mammalian organisms during the 1980s [1]. Since then, new techniques for gene delivery have been developed that utilize both viral and nonviral carriers. These techniques have been successful enough that proposed disease treatments have evolved to the clinical trial stage with encouraging success. Although many cellular processing mechanisms remain unclear and the search for the ideal gene delivery vector remains ongoing, the tools and methods for gene therapy have provided a strong base from which to build.

43.2 Nucleotides for Delivery

43.2.1 DNA (deoxyribonucleic acid)

DNA is the building block of life and as such it remains a staple in the delivery of genetic material to the cell. There are many strategies as to how the DNA will interact with the existing genome and what is the best way to produce the desired effect.

43.2.1.1 Plasmids

A plasmid is a circular piece of DNA. Extrachromosomal plasmids can be replicated or transcribed independently of the rest of the DNA in the nucleus. This attribute makes plasmids an ideal tool for gene therapy. Plasmids can include a selectable marker for identification of transfectants/transductants, a multiple cloning site for ease of inserting/deleting additional nucleotide strands, the exon(s) of interest, and regulatory/binding elements such as promoters and enhancers. A common promoter used in gene therapy is the cytomegalovirus immediate early promoter (CMV_{ie}), used because of its strength in transcription initiation in nearly every mammalian cell. However, several other promoters have been investigated, such as the glucose-related protein promoter [2] and many cell-specific promoters. Enhancers include the simian virus 40 (SV_{40}) enhancer as well as long terminal repeats (LTRs) [2]. The exons that are delivered may code for necessary cell-specific proteins, engineered protein polymers [3], or what has become a common objective in cancer cell research: suicide genes [4].

43.2.1.2 Nucleotide Decoys

DNA and RNA decoys are small oligonucleotide fragments that mimic the start sequences of potentially harmful genes. By doing so, the decoys can effectively trap the transcriptional and translational machinery, thereby causing a sharp decrease in mRNA or protein production. There has been success with this approach in human immunodeficiency virus (HIV) research. DNA and RNA decoys have been used to halt the function of REV proteins, which are responsible for making late transcripts of RNA and exporting them to the cytoplasm [5], and the TAT protein, which binds and activates the natural promoter for HIV-1 [6].

43.2.2 RNA

RNA also holds a valuable place in gene therapy because it can be used to alter cellular function. Two examples of RNA use in gene therapy are antisense RNA and small interfering RNA (siRNA). Antisense RNA provides functional alterations in cells by acting on host gene products post-transcriptionally. Antisense RNA functions by binding to cellular mRNA transcripts, which prevents ribosomal binding and therefore translation. Antisense RNAs have been investigated for their use in applications such as beta-globin gene inhibition as a possible treatment for sickle cell anemia [7], bcr/abl interference in myeloid leukemia research [8], and CXCR4 disruption for HIV-1 gene therapy [9], among others. The use of siRNA can interfere directly with genomic DNA transcription. First described by Elbashir et al. [10] in 2001, siRNAs have very high specificity that can be used to target a single-nucleotide polymorphism (SNP) on a single mutant allele [11,12]. The result would be to silence the mutant allele while permitting continued transcription of the wild type gene. This technology has been used *in vivo* to successfully target spinocerebellar ataxia type 3 and frontotemporal dementia [13].

43.3 Gene Delivery

Simply administering naked genetic material in the vicinity of cell exteriors is usually not sufficient to bring about the desired cellular response at adequate levels. Carriers have been employed to aid in the transfer of genetic material from the cell exterior to the cytoplasm or nucleus. There is a wide variety of carriers available, each with links back to one of the main branches of natural science: biology, chemistry,

TABLE 43.1 Examples of Virus Families and Members Used for Gene Delivery

Family	Example	References
Adenoviridae	Adenovirus	[14]
Baculoviridae	Baculovirus	[15]
Herpesviridae	Pseudorabies virus	[16]
	Simplex virus	[17]
Parvoviridae	Adeno-associated	[18]
	Parvovirus	[19]
Poxviridae	Vaccinia	[20]
	Yaba monkey tumor virus	[21]
Retroviridae	Human immunodeficiency virus 1 and 2	[22,23]
	Lentivirus	[24]
	Murine leukemia virus	[25]
	Retrovirus	[26]

and physics. It is possible for hybrid systems that combine two or more basic technologies to exist, but the individual classifications will be discussed separately for clarity.

43.3.1 Biological Delivery Methods

Because they are a product of millions of years of biologic evolution, viruses are included here as the biological forms of gene delivery in spite of the fact that viruses are not technically alive (they do not respire). Viruses are the most efficient vectors for large-scale gene delivery. Some also offer permanent expression of delivered genes through the integration of genetic material into the transduced organism's genome. Table 43.1 lists some of the major viral families and specific members that have been used in gene therapy. Many of the references in the table cite review articles of the specific virus classification for further reading.

Currently, herpes simplex virus (HSV) is being used to transduce cells in the central nervous system. By altering the genome of the virus, researchers have been able to decrease cytotoxicity and increase transfection efficiency [27]. HSV is also desirable because it is relatively large to allow packaging of larger plasmids, does not integrate its DNA into the host genome which avoids the deleterious effects that are possible with random integration, and is easily deliverable into the brain due to its ability to actively travel towards the nuclei of the neurons through the axons in the peripheral nervous system. HSV has also been applied to the transduction of skeletal muscle. Recent reports have described successful HSV-mediated gene transfer into skeletal muscle cells *in vitro* and *in vivo* and outlined possible applications for the delivery of large genes such as that coding for dystrophin [28].

In the liver, the virus Ac*M*NPV (of the family baculoviridae) has yielded promising transfection efficiencies [29]. The YABA-like virus, which exhibits very similar attributes to the vaccinia virus but does not produce immune responses in the host, has successfully targeted and treated ovarian cancer in mice [30].

Adeno-associated virus (AAV) requires coinfection with a helper virus (typically adenovirus) to be productive. AAV offers an advantage to the gene therapist in that it has been reported to provide permanent expression of delivered genes. *In utero* experiments in mice and nonhuman primates indicate that recombinant AAVs can successfully alter the genome of the host organism to produce stable transductants [31]. Adeno-associated viruses are commonly used and successful in targeting the central nervous system [32]. Although repeated viral transduction is associated with inflammatory and immunological responses in the host, it has been reported that these responses can be reduced by carefully balancing recombinant AAV dosing with prudent timing [33].

Retroviruses offer good transduction efficiencies *in vivo*. Hallmarks of retroviral transduction are that RNA is delivered into cells as opposed to DNA, cDNA is made using viral reverse transcriptase, and this cDNA is introduced into the host genome via the protein integrase to produce stable transfectants. Immunodeficiency viruses are commonly investigated retroviruses, and include HIV and feline immunodeficiency virus (FIV). Investigations into retroviral genome alterations, such as self-inactivation via promoter deletion, are being conducted in an attempt to render HIV-1 a safe vector for gene transfer [34]. Use of FIV has shown efficient transduction of nondividing cells without many of the inherent risks associated with delivering recombinant HIV to humans [35]. Lentivirus, which belongs to the same family as HIV and FIV, has been developed to produce concurrent regulated multiple gene delivery upon transduction [36].

43.3.2   Chemical Delivery Methods

Many chemical methods of transfection have been engineered and utilized in the past 20 years. The use of synthetic gene delivery vehicles, such as polymers or cationic lipids, offers several advantages. Nonviral gene delivery is not restricted to plasmid DNA sizes based upon the ability to fit into a viral head of finite size, as is evidenced by successful delivery of a 2.3 Mb artificial human chromosome using poly(ethylenimine)(PEI) [37], and a 60 Mb artificial chromosome into Chinese hamster ovary cells using liposomes [38]. Although nonviral gene delivery usually results in transient gene expression, an advantage of this characteristic is that there is little or no risk of random integration into host genomes. Random integration poses a problem in that it can knock out a vital gene such as a housekeeping gene or a tumor suppressor gene. An additional advantage of nonviral gene delivery is the reduced threat of immune response *in vivo* versus repeated viral injections.

Several cationic polymers exist that exhibit strong transfection qualities. Many of these polymers are based on polypeptide chains containing multiple lysine, histidine, or arginine residues. Historically, poly(L-lysine) has been the most commonly used peptide transfection agent. However, several arginine-based combinations of peptides have been formed into polyplexes of varying sizes and charge ratios which may yield better transfection results than the previously used polypeptide chains composed of a single amino acid [39]. Histidine–lysine polyplexes have also produced good transfection results that positively correlated with the amount of histidine in the complex [40]. There are also additions that can be made to these complexes in order to increase transfection efficiency and lower cytotoxic effects. These include ligands such as nerve growth factor, and hydrophilic polymers such as polyethylene glycol (PEG), which has been shown to increase transfection efficiency and lower cytotoxicity of poly(L-lysine) both *in vitro* and *in vivo* [41].

PEI is a highly cationic polymer that is available in both linear and branched forms. Each form of the polymer has a repeating [–CH$_2$–CH$_2$–N<] structure, with each nitrogen taking the form of a primary (end group), secondary (middle of a straight chain), or tertiary (branch point) amine (Figure 43.1). The groups attached to secondary and tertiary amines are typically additional [–CH$_2$–CH$_2$–N<], although terminal amines can be modified through the attachment of moieties for targeting or degradation purposes. Because of the large number of amines present in PEI, many of which carry a positive charge at physiological pH, DNA and RNA easily bind with the polymer via electrostatic interactions to form stable complexes. The transfection efficiency of branched PEI correlates with its molecular weight, with weight-average molecular weights of approximately 25,000 Da working best [42,43]. PEGylation of PEI polymers can, as was also the case for poly(L-lysine), increase transfection efficiency; this has been indicated in delivery of complexes to the central nervous system *in vivo* [44]. PEI has also been successfully used in *in vitro* transfections of rat endothelia and chicken embryonic neurons as well as *in vivo* in mice [45]. Conjugates of PEI are also being developed, such as silica microspheres coated with the polymer–DNA complexes. These conjugates have been used successfully for *in vitro* transfection, and offer the potential for relatively simple covalent surface modifications [46].

Dendrimers are highly branched polymers built around a single atom or molecule. Poly(amidoamine) (PAMAM) dendrimers are often used for gene delivery because of their high nitrogen content which aids in DNA binding and condensation. With a central atom of nitrogen, these polymers are built by the addition of amine-containing molecules, such as [CH$_2$–CH$_2$–NH$_2$] (Figure 43.1). The result is a maximally branched molecule of known molecular weight; a sort of controlled version of PEI. PAMAM dendrimers, sometimes referred to as starburst dendrimers, have shown good transfection efficiencies in

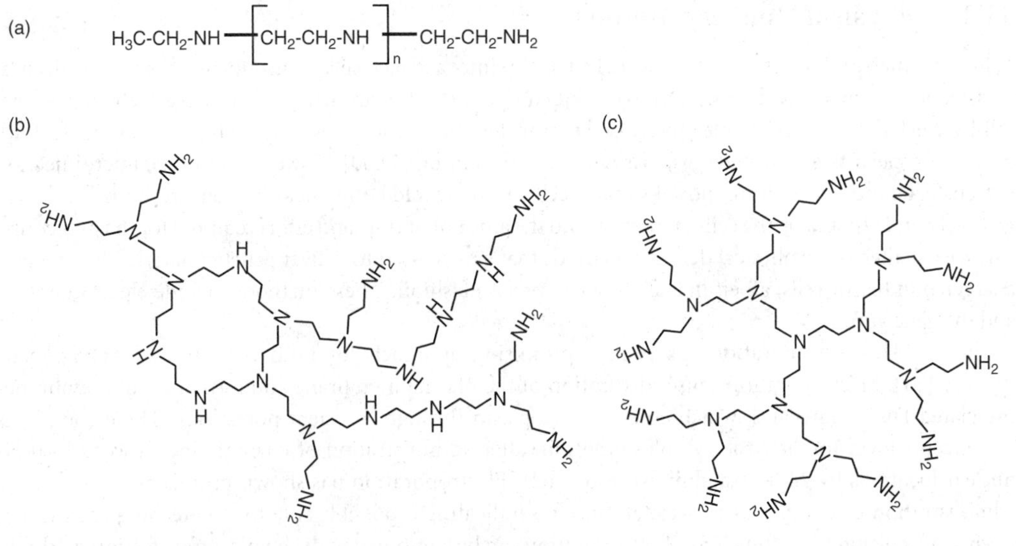

(a)

H_3C-CH_2-NH —[CH_2-CH_2-NH]_n— CH_2-CH_2-NH_2

(b)

(c)

FIGURE 43.1 Three polymers based upon the [–CH2–CH2–N<] basic unit. Amines are shown in the uncharged state for clarity. (A) *Linear PEI*; (B) *An example of a branched PEI*. The polymerization permits 2° amines and one cyclization via a back biting reaction. The polymer is somewhat irregular; (C) Third *generation PAMAM dendrimer*. All amines are tertiary amines (except for chain termini).

mammalian cells with little or no cytotoxicity *in vitro* [47]. A current application of this dendrimer is its coupling with an Epstein–Barr virus-based plasmid for suicide gene therapy in cancer cells [48].

Chitosan is another polymer that has been well characterized for use in transfection [49]. This natural nontoxic polysaccharide lends DNAase-resistance to its cargo while condensing the DNA to form stronger complexes [50]. The efficiency of chitosan is thought to rely upon its ability to swell and burst endolysosomes, which allows the delivered DNA to continue its path to the nucleus [51].

Alginate, a polycationic polysaccharide that can be used in the form of a hydrogel, has been used alone for transfection [52], as well as in combination with poly(L-lysine) complexes to form an oligonucleotide "sponge" [53]. Through slow degradation, these gels were shown to release embedded oligonucleotides over time. Possible applications of these gels to deliver antisense RNA are currently being pursued [53].

Microgels are similar to the alginate complex just mentioned. A thermosensitive microgel, composed of poly[ethylene glycol-(D, L-lactic acid-co-glycol acid)-ethylene glycol] (PEG–PLGA–PEG) triblock copolymers, has been created to have the property of being a liquid at room temperature but solidifying at 37°C. Once solidified, the gel slowly degrades over the course of 30 days, releasing its component oligonucleotides to the surrounding cells. Possible applications of this gel system to wound healing are being pursued [54].

Lipids, particularly cationic lipids, have been used for gene delivery in a process termed lipofection. Several lipofection agents have been used for successful transfection of cells both *in vitro* and *in vivo*. Because of the aqueous environment inside cells and tissues, the hydrophobic tails of the lipids will coalesce to form hollow micelles, the interiors of which can contain oligonucleotides for cellular delivery. The combination of more than one hydrophobic entity can often yield higher transfection efficiencies than using a single type of lipid. In primary cortical neurons, a combination of *N*-[1-(2,3-dioleoyloxy)propyl]-*N,N,N*-trimethyl-ammonium methylsulfate and cholesterol (DOTAP : Chol) shows high transfection efficiency [55]. Using intraveneous administration of *N*-[1-(2,3-dioleoyloxy)propyl]-*N,N,N*-trimethylammonium chloride–Tween 80 (DOTMA-Tween 80) complexes with high DOTMA : DNA ratios, transient transfection to several organs has also been accomplished [56]. The use of helper lipids such as cholesterol or dioleoyl phosphatidylethanolamine (DOPE) can increase transfection efficiency significantly through endosomal membrane destabilization [57].

43.3.3 Physical Delivery Methods

A highly efficient way of transferring naked DNA into a select cell or group of cells is via physical transfection methods. Microinjection by a skilled operator offers nearly perfect delivery efficiency on a cell-by-cell basis. This technique can be used to transfer oligonucleotides to cell cytoplasms or nuclei [58], or entire nuclei into enucleated eggs, as is the case with cloning [59,60]. However, the use of microinjection to transfect hundreds or thousands of somatic cells *in vivo* would be an infeasible venture, both in terms of getting to and visualizing the cells of interest, and the amount of time and effort required for the procedure. There exist alternative physical delivery methods that can be used to deliver genetic material directly into a larger number of cells, albeit in a slightly less precise fashion. These methods include electroporation and the gene gun.

Since 1982, electroporation has been a promising approach for both *in vitro* and *in vivo* gene delivery [61]. Electroporation causes disruption of the plasma membrane and formation of membrane-associated DNA aggregates, which enter the cytoplasm through transient pores [62]. These complexes have been shown to enter the cytoplasm 30 min after administration of current, and proceed to peri-nuclear locations by 24 h postadministration [62]. Electroporation has shown promising results in the administration of complexes to skeletal muscles, indicating a possible role for the technique in future *in vivo* muscular applications [63]. Electroporation can be combined with chemical transfection methods, including dendrimers, to increase the overall efficiency of transfection [64]. A similar approach, termed nucleofection, utilizes an electrical current in conjunction with specific solutions to deliver DNA not only into the cell but also into the cell nucleus [65].

The gene gun provides a ballistic means of transporting genetic material into cells. A typical application of the gene gun would entail attaching DNA to gold particles that are on the order of 1 μm in diameter. The coated gold is then loaded onto a cartridge or onto a disc and propelled down the barrel of the gun via pressurized helium at a force on the order of 200 to 300 psi. The end of the gun barrel is too small for the disk to exit, so its motion is halted abruptly before exit. The coated gold colloids detach from the disc and continue their path, passing through or becoming embedded within cells. When passing through cell membranes, cytoskeletons, and other structures, some of the DNA can become dislodged and remain within the cells for processing. This method provides good transfection of tissue surface layers and offers an advantage over microinjection in that many cells in a specified area are quickly transfected. However, cell damage and depth of gold penetration are two limiting factors of this method. The gene gun has been used successfully *in vivo* to transfect murine tumors with cytokines, successfully restricting cell growth [66]. Direct gene gun transfer of gold-adhered DNA particles has also been used in successful transfections of beating hearts with genes encoding the green fluorescent protein [67].

43.4 Intracellular Pathways

The mechanisms governing the transport of nonviral gene delivery complexes into the cytoplasm and on into the nucleus vary between different vectors. Endocytosis is the primary means for cellular import of nonviral gene carriers, which makes complex modification through the addition of specific ligands beneficial. Endocytosed complexes enter the cytoplasm in endosomes, which mature from early to late endosomes before meeting up with lysosomes to form endolysosomes. As this vesicle maturation occurs, membrane bound H^+/ATPases create an acidic environment within the compartments. It is this acidic environment which allows lysosomal enzymes (acid hydrolases) to remain active and potentially degrade the endocytosed material. The endolysosome therefore presents a major obstacle to nonvirally mediated gene therapy, as evidenced by increases in transfection efficiency in the presence of the lysosomotrophic agent chloroquine [68–70]. Research into lysosomal disruption has produced a peptide that can degrade the membrane of the late endosome, based on its cholesterol content. This method has reportedly increased the transfection efficiency of parenchymal liver by 30-fold [71].

PEI has been hypothesized to serve as a proton acceptor within endolysosomes, serving to buffer the pH of the endolysosome while additional H^+ is pumped in. According to this hypothesis, Cl^- ions will leak into the vesicles to alleviate the electric gradient, thereby creating an osmotic gradient which will be offset by an influx of water molecules into the endolysosomes. The result will be swelling and bursting of the endolysosomes [45]. PEI has been shown to enter cells via endocytosis, and the endosomes have been shown to swell within a period of under 6 h [72]. However, there exists a question of the degree of lysosomal involvement during PEI-mediated transfection. PEI/DNA-containing endosomes have been imaged while passing through lysosomal beds without lysosomal interaction [73]. In addition, PEI has been reported to utilize microtubules of the cytoskeleton as a direct pathway to the nuclear envelope, thereby eluding lysosomes [74]. It is perhaps the large excess of positive charges in PEI/DNA complexes that help direct the complexes in a seemingly atypical fashion during cellular processing. More research is required to elucidate the complete cellular mechanism of PEI-mediated transfection.

If the delivered genetic material is DNA, and the desired outcome of the transfection is expression of the delivered gene, then the next major hurdle to successful transfection is getting the delivered DNA into the cell nucleus for transcription. Many studies have monitored the effect of cell cycle stage upon transfection efficiency. Some viral vectors show strong transduction during all phases of the cell cycle because of their strong nuclear-importation machinery [75]. However, polyplex and lipoplex carriers show optimal transfection if they are administered during the G1 or S phases of the cell cycle [75]. It is known that the nuclear envelope is dismantled during late mitosis, hence perhaps these findings can be explained by the length of time required for transfection complexes to proceed from endocytosis to the outer nuclear membrane being roughly equal to the amount of time needed for the cell to progress from G1 or S phase to late mitosis. Other work indicates the barrier to transfection presented by the nuclear envelope through results that reveal very low transfection efficiencies in nondividing cells when cationic lipid-mediated vectors were used [76].

Aside from entering the nucleus by virtue of location during mitotic nuclear membrane disruption, genes and gene delivery complexes can be delivered to the nucleus via import. Possible mechanisms for nuclear import include interactions between the complexes and other proteins bound for nuclear import and interactions between the complexes and nuclear import receptors themselves. Proteins in the cytoplasm that are bound for nuclear import typically have a conserved peptide sequence that is recognized by the cell as a nuclear localization signal (NLS). Such signals can be manufactured in the laboratory for inclusion as an integral part of the gene delivery complexes [77,78]. Many factors govern the success of NLS-mediated nuclear import: the type of NLS, the manner in which the NLS is incorporated, DNA form, and the proper definition of the complexes [79].

43.5   Cell and Tissue Targeting

Each of the physical delivery methods listed in Section 43.3.3 is an excellent way to deliver genes to a specific region. Certainly, microinjection is a very straightforward way to introduce genes into a single cell of interest. However, physical delivery methods can be technically difficult, insubstantial in the number of cells that are transfected, or impossible for delivery to remote areas of the body. To provide feasible alternatives when such challenges exist, molecular targeting methods have been developed, yielding encouraging results.

The use of cell-specific ligands or receptors to target extracellular attributes is a good method for gene delivery to specific cell types or classes. Neuronal cells have been targeted for transduction via a neuron-specific viral envelope in conjunction with specific glycoproteins, leaving nonneuronal cells unaffected [80]. Other examples of ligands that have been used include LOX-1 to potentially target endothelial cells [81], the human hepatitis B virus preS1 peptide to target hepatocytes [82], plus transferrin [83], folate [84], anti-CD34 [85], and galactose [86], among others. The list of potential and realized target ligands is very large, which suggests the utility of this targeting technique.

Using cell-specific transcription regulation sequences (binding elements such as promoters or enhancers) is another way to target cells without modification of the gene delivery vehicle, which allows for cell targeting with known delivery and release kinetics without having to repeat the same work for modified vectors. This type of targeting, known as promoter or expression-targeting, works on the principle that many cell types could take up the delivered genes, but only the cells of interest will transcribe them because the transcriptional machinery that binds to the utilized promoters is present only in the target cells. This type of targeting has been used to target megakaryocytes via the promoter for integrin αIIβ (for a possible treatment for platelet disorders) [87]. Targeting liver cells has been achieved by using the promoter for liver-type pyruvate kinase and SV40 enhancer [88]. Expression-targeting has also been used to target an entire class of cells (Cox-2 overexpressing cells), which could be an important technique in the treatment of carcinomas or inflammation [89]. The use of two specific binding elements, a promoter/enhancer combination, has been employed to deliver the suicide gene for thymidine kinase to prostate tumors [90]. Expression-targeted gene delivery could prove to be a valuable tool in clinical gene therapy, alone or in conjunction with ligand-targeted systems.

43.6   Applications

43.6.1   *In Vitro*

In 1977, a chemically created somatostatin gene was fused to an *Escherichia coli* β-galactosidase gene and introduced into a bacterium resulting in expression of the gene [91]. The alteration of both cells and cellular functions has expanded greatly since then to produce many new experimental applications. *In vitro* modeling is valuable in learning more about living systems without the involvement of animals, while potentially leading to *in vivo* applications. For example, liposomal delivery of the gene for adenomatous polyposis coli (APC), delivered to produce a potential anticancer agent, has produced excellent results in diminishing a human duodenal cancer in the presence of bile *in vitro* [92].

The proliferation of cells *in vitro* not only serves as a model for *in vivo* studies but also serves as a valuable component of most *ex vivo* applications. However, it is often the case that cell behavior differs between *in vitro* and *in vivo* environments. Hematopoietic stem cells show this characteristic, displaying substantial proliferation *in vivo* but dividing at a more conservative rate *in vitro*. Building on the retroviral overexpression of the homeobox B4 gene, a 40-fold increase in *in vitro* growth has been observed in mouse bone marrow cells [93]. However, the difference between cell behavior inside and outside the living organism along with the involvement of a wider array of cell types and cellular proteins continue to be significant barriers to scientific research, and are reasons why *in vitro* investigations are not enough to produce treatments ready for the clinic. *In vitro* research is still important because it allows greater control over experimental conditions for molecular studies and reduces the need for research animals.

In vitro gene therapy also has applications in the creation of regulation vehicles for the complexes needed *in vivo*. The delivery of L-dopa and dopamine to the nervous system by genetically altered cells can be regulated by embedding the cells in hydrogels, created and currently being tested *in vitro*, and implanting these systems into the affected area [94]. Another regulation device has been created from freeze-dried PEI/DNA complexes along with sucrose and PLGA to create a porous medium filled with encapsulated transfection complexes [95]. *In vitro*, the use of this PLGA sponge has caused expression of a reporter gene in adherent fibroblasts for 15 days.

Besides delivery regulation mechanisms there are *in vitro* transfection applications that treat cells as microfactories to create pharmaceutical products. An example of using gene delivery to utilize cells as manufacturing plants is the injection of engineered plasmids into silkworm eggs for the production of type III procollagen [96]. This application is a useful way of producing protein-based polymers with high sequence specificity and low polydispersity. This technology could be used to create scaffolds for cell-seeding in tissue engineering applications.

43.6.2   *Ex Vivo*

Ex vivo gene therapy involves the methods of *in vitro* cell therapy coupled with the reintroduction of the altered cells into an organism. Likely candidates for this approach are bone marrow progenitor cells of the adult (mesenchymal and hematopoetic) embryonic and adult stem cells. Delivery of the transfecting (or transducing) gene can be accomplished via any of the methods mentioned previously in this chapter. There has been much success with this application of gene therapy, which has progressed to the clinical trial stage. Transplantation of nerve growth factor (NGF)-producing grafts of neural progenitor cells into the septum and nucleus basalis of the rat cerebrum has been shown to diminish the atrophy of the brain associated with aging [97]. Several more *ex vivo* investigations are outlined in Section 43.7 of this chapter.

43.6.3 *In Vivo*

To transport gene delivery complexes into living organisms, there exist several strategies that do not entail surgery. The first method that might come to mind is injection via syringe. Injections can be very simple, entailing introduction of complexes into a vein [98], into the peritoneum [99], or directly into a tissue such as muscle [98] or tumor [100]. Even the blood–brain barrier can be circumvented via direct injection [101] or injection into the jugular vein using the brain-specific promoter GFAP [102]. Additional approaches for gene delivery to the central nervous system include injection into the cranial nerves for retrograde transport of PEI/DNA complexes into the brainstem [103], and intraveneous administration of lipoplexes conjugated with transferrin to effectively cross the blood–brain barrier via its transferrin receptors [104]. Permanent transfection via nonrandom integration has even been achieved via high-pressure tail vein injection, in which plasmids coding for bacteriophage φC31 integrase were co-injected with plasmids containing attB and a gene for human factor IX to yield site-specific genomic integration of the factor IX gene in rat hepatocytes at native pseudo attP sites [105]. This concept could be applied to achieve permanent transfection in many nonviral applications, which lend themselves to IV administration.

Another method of complex administration *in vivo* is through inhalation. Inhalation of aerosols is an intuitive choice for gene delivery to the respiratory system. In mice, aerosol administration of a liposome–DNA complex has yielded transfection results that persisted for 21 days [106]. More recently, aerosol delivery of adeno-associated viral vectors through the nasal cavity produced positive transfection that was apparent in the bloodstream in addition to that in the lungs [107]. Aerosol delivery is a logical method of delivering transfection complexes to the lungs, while intravenous delivery might be better suited for organs such as the spleen or liver, as demonstrated by results from a recent study that compared the two delivery methods for PEI/DNA transfection complexes [108].

Mucosal administration of gene delivery complexes by oral or rectal routes is another option for *in vivo* gene therapy. Mice that were fed chitosan-coated plasmid particles showed expression of the delivered gene in the intestinal epithelium [109]. Another delivery method involves particle-mediated gene delivery directly into the oral mucosa [110]. In the cited study, several marker and cancer-targeting genes were delivered and shown to be expressed in the oral cavities of canines. Transrectal complex administration (enema) has also been used to deliver genes to canines, where a recombinant adenovirus vector carrying a marker gene (β-galactosidase) was used to demonstrate successful transduction in the colon [111].

43.7 Clinical Applications

To date, over 900 reported gene therapy clinical trials are underway worldwide; approximately 2% of these are phase III investigations [112]. Well over half of the current trials utilize viruses as the gene delivery vehicle. Physical and chemical (especially liposomal) delivery methods are also represented. Over half of the current trials are cancer investigations [112]. Following is an overview of some of the more visible trials.

Severe combined immunodeficiency (SCID) was the first clinical application of gene therapy to go into human trials, commencing in 1990. The treatment involved removing bone marrow stem cells, altering them by exposure to healthy T-cells in culture, and then reintroducing the differentiated marrow-derived cells to the host organism [113]. Another malady involving immunocompromise is the HIV infection, a retrovirally caused disease that affects T-helper cells and can eventually lead to acquired immunodeficiency syndrome (AIDS). Phase I, II, and III clinical trials are currently underway for several applications of HIV-related gene therapy. *Ex vivo* manipulation of T lymphocytes with ribozymes, followed by reintroduction of the cells into the host, shows promise in that the T-cells have a greater survival time and are clinically safe for the subject [114]. A separate study conducted on twins was completed in 2002, and showed the safety and efficacy of *ex vivo* lymphocyte manipulation for expression of an anti-HIV gene (revTD) [115].

Clinical investigations for tissue- or organ-related maladies are also underway. Ischemic heart disease is the result of poor circulatory perfusion of cardiac muscle, commonly from coronary artery blockage. The delivery of vascular endothelial growth factor (VEGF), first described as a tumor-produced vascular permeability factor, has been shown to stimulate angiogenesis in several tissues including cardiac muscle [116]. Phase I studies have indicated that direct injection of naked [117] or adenovirally delivered [118] plasmids encoding VEGF into cardiac tissue yields both safe and effective transfection/transduction.

Cystic fibrosis is another tissue/organ malady. The disease is the result of a mutation in a gene encoding a cellular cAMP-mediated chloride channel, known as the cystic fibrosis transmembrane conductance regulator (CFTR). With inadequate chloride transport capabilities, affected cells will develop an osmotic gradient that is relieved by internalization of water from the extracellular environment. In cells that are bathed in mucus, such as lung airway epithelia, the result is a loss of water from the coating mucus, raising mucus viscosity and lowering the body's ability to transport it via ciliary movement. Bacterial colonization is often the result of such stasis. Clinical trials for the treatment of cystic fibrosis have been conducted using different target administrations. A trial of liposome-mediated transfection for cystic fibrosis patients showed the efficacy and safety of delivery of the CFTR gene to nasal epithelium cells [119]. Aerosolized adenoviral particles carrying CFTR cDNA have also been used clinically for transduction in the lungs [120].

Neurologic disorders have also been the target of clinical gene therapy trials. A phase I study of Alzheimer's disease involved the removal of primary fibroblasts from subjects, effectively transducing the harvested cells with nerve growth factor and reintroducing the cells into the brain [121] (also reviewed in Reference 122). The use of nerve growth factor to target the cholinergic neurons was employed with the aim of preventing neural degradation and elevating levels of acetylcholine transferase.

Gene therapy applications for cancer treatment are very well represented in the group of clinical trial investigations. Phase I and II trials directed at malignant gliomas are using a modified herpes virus to target glioma cells in order to cause an immune response to diminish the number of cancerous cells [123]. The referenced study is currently focused on drug dose amount in subjects with recurrent glioblastoma. A phase II study of ovarian cancer commenced in the year 2000 to determine the safety and efficacy of genetically altered herpes simplex thymidine kinase-producing cells (HSV-TK) delivered into cancer-affected ovaries [124]. The amount of cancer research that is underway is too large to allow a proper presentation of the area in sufficient detail here.

43.8 Summary

Gene therapy is a very diverse and rapidly growing field. Researchers in many areas, including biology, chemistry, physics, engineering, and medicine can find new applications for their creations and discoveries in gene therapeutics. Since molecular biology and genetic recombination laid the foundation for controlled genetic alteration, the field of gene therapy has expanded dramatically. The ability to alter cellular function through the introduction of exogenous genetic material has drawn considerable hope that this technology can be used to discover new disease treatments as well as explicate some of the mysteries of life at the level of basic science. As laboratory and clinical trials proceed and knowledge of the area becomes more rational and objective within the general public, gene therapy should prove to deliver beneficial and lasting advances from the world of biomolecular science.

References

[1] Wolff, J. and Lederberg, J., An early history of gene transfer and therapy, *Hum. Gene Ther.*, 5, 469, 1994.

[2] Little E., et al., The glucose-regulated proteins (GRP78 and GRP94): functions, gene regulation, and applications, *Crit. Rev. Eukaryot. Gene Expr.*, 4, 1–18, 1994.

[3] Haider, M., Megeed, Z., and Ghandehari, H., Genetically engineered polymers: status and prospects for controlled release, *J. Control. Release*, 95, 1, 2004.

[4] Sun, X., Wu, Z., and Hu, J., Suicide gene therapy of hepatocellular carcinoma and delivery procedure and route of therapeutic gene *in vivo*, *HPBD Int.*, 1, 373, 2003.

[5] Nakaya, T. et al., Decoy approach using RNA–DNA chimera oligonucleotides to inhibit the regulatory function of human immunodeficiency virus type 1 Rev protein, *Antimicrob. Agents Chemother.*, 41, 319, 1997.

[6] Browning, C. et al., Potent inhibition of human immunodeficiency virus type 1 (HIV-1) gene expression and virus production by an HIV-2 Tat activation-response RNA decoy, *J. Virol.*, 73, 5191, 1999.

[7] Pace, B.S., Qian, X., and Ofori-Acquah, S.F., Selective inhibition of beta-globin RNA transcripts by antisense RNA molecules, *Cell. Mol. Biol.*, 50, 43, 2004.

[8] Li, M.J. et al., Specific killing of Ph+ chronic myeloid leukemia cells by a lentiviral vector-delivered anti-bcr/abl small hairpin RNA, *Oligonucleotides*, 13, 401, 2003.

[9] Anderson, J. et al., Potent suppression of HIV type 1 infection by a short hairpin anti-CXCR4 siRNA, *AIDS Res. Hum. Retroviruses*, 19, 699, 2003.

[10] Elbashir, S.M., Lendeckel, W., and Tuschl, T., RNA interference is mediated by 21- and 22-nucleotide RNAs, *Genes Dev.*, 15, 188, 2001.

[11] Elbashir, S.M. et al., Duplexes of 21-nucleotide RNAs mediate RNA interference in cultured mammalian cells, *Nature*, 411, 494, 2001.

[12] Miller, V.M. et al., Allele-specific silencing of dominant disease genes, *Proc. Natl Acad. Sci. USA*, 100, 7195, 2003.

[13] Miller, V. et al., Allele-specific silencing of dominant disease genes, *Proc. Natl Acad. Sci. USA*, 100, 7195, 2003.

[14] Douglas, J.T., Adenovirus-mediated gene delivery: an overview, *Meth. Mol. Biol.*, 246, 3, 2004.

[15] Huser, A. and Hofmann, C., Baculovirus vectors: novel mammalian cell gene-delivery vehicles and their applications, *Am. J. Pharmacogenom.*, 3, 53, 2003.

[16] Boldogkoi, Z. and Nogradi, A., Gene and cancer therapy — pseudorabies virus: a novel research and therapeutic tool? *Curr. Gene Ther.*, 3, 155, 2003.

[17] Goins, W.F. et al., Delivery using herpes simplex virus: an overview, *Meth. Mol. Biol.*, 246, 257, 2004.

[18] Lu, Y., Recombinant adeno-associated virus as delivery vector for gene therapy — a review, *Stem Cells Dev.*, 13, 133 2004.

[19] Gafni, Y. et al., Gene therapy platform for bone regeneration using an exogenously regulated, AAV-2-based gene expression system, *Mol. Ther.*, 9, 587, 2004.

[20] Hodge, J.W. et al., Modified vaccinia virus ankara recombinants are as potent as vaccinia recombinants in diversified prime and boost vaccine regimens to elicit therapeutic antitumor responses, *Cancer Res.*, 63, 7942, 2003.

[21] Hu, Y. et al., Yaba-like disease virus: an alternative replicating poxvirus vector for cancer gene therapy. *J. Virol.*, 75, 10300, 2001.

[22] Cockrell, A.S. and Kafri, T., HIV-1 vectors: fulfillment of expectations, further advancements, and still a way to go, *Curr. HIV Res.*, 1, 419, 2003.

[23] Cheng, L. et al., Human immunodeficiency virus type 2 (HIV-2) vector-mediated *in vivo* gene transfer into adult rabbit retina, *Curr. Eye Res.*, 24, 196, 2002.

[24] Kafri, T., Gene delivery by lentivirus vectors an overview, *Meth. Mol. Biol.*, 246, 367, 2004.

[25] Wolkowicz, R., Nolan, G.P., and Curran, M.A., Lentiviral vectors for the delivery of DNA into mammalian cells, *Meth. Mol. Biol.*, 246, 391, 2004.

[26] Rainov, N.G. and Ren, H., Clinical trials with retrovirus mediated gene therapy — what have we learned? *J. Neuro-oncol.*, 65, 227, 2003.

[27] Lilley, C. et al., Multiple immediate-early gene-deficient herpes simplex virus vectors allowing efficient gene delivery to neurons in culture and widespread gene delivery to the central nervous system *in vivo*, *J. Virol.*, 75, 4343, 2001.

[28] Cao, B. and Huard, J., Gene transfer to skeletal muscle using herpes simplex virus-based vectors, *Meth. Mol. Biol.*, 246, 301, 2004.

[29] Billelo, J. et al., Transient disruption of intercellular junctions enables baculovirus entry into nondividing hepatocytes, *J. Virol.*, 75, 9857, 2001.

[30] Hu, Y. et al., Yaba-like disease virus: an alternative replicating poxvirus vector for cancer gene therapy, *J. Virol.*, 75, 10500, 2001.

[31] Garrett, D. et al., In utero recombinant adeno-associated virus gene transfer in mice, rats, and primates, *BMC Biotech.*, 3, 16, 2003.

[32] Ahmed, B. et al., Efficient delivery of Cre-recombinase to neurons *in vivo* and stable transduction of neurons using adeno-associated and lentiviral vectors, *BMC Neurosci.*, 5, 4, 2004.

[33] Mastakov, M. et al., Immunological aspects of recombinant adeno-associated virus delivery to the mammalian brain, *J. Virol.*, 76, 8446, 2002.

[34] Zufferey, R., Self-inactivating lentivirus vector for safe and efficient *in vivo* gene delivery, *J. Virol.*, 72, 9873, 1998.

[35] Curran, M. et al., Efficient transduction of nondividing cells by optimized feline immunodeficiency virus vectors, *Mol. Ther.*, 1, 31, 2000.

[36] Reiser, J. et al., Development of multigene and regulated lentivirus vectors, *J. Virol.*, 74, 10589, 2000.

[37] Marschall, P., Malik, N., and Larin, Z., Transfer of YACs up to 2.3 Mb intact into human cells with polyethylenimine, *Gene Ther.*, 6, 1634, 1999.

[38] Vanderbyl, S., MacDonald, N., and de Jong, G., A flow cytometry technique for measuring chromosome-mediated gene transfer, *Cytometry*, 44, 100, 2001.

[39] Rossenberg, S. van. et al., Stable polyplexes based on arginine-containing oligopeptides for *in vivo* gene delivery, *Nature*, 11, 457, 2004.

[40] Chen, Q. et al., Branched co-polymers of histidine and lysine are efficient carriers of plasmids, *Nucleic Acids Res.*, 29, 1334, 2001.

[41] Toncheva V. et al., Novel vectors for gene delivery formed by self-assembly of DNA with poly(-lysine) grafted with hydrophilic polymers, *Biochim. Biophys. Acta*, 1380, 354, 1998.

[42] Godbey, W., Wu, K., and Mikos A., Size matters: molecular weight affects the efficiency of poly(ethylenimine) as a gene delivery vehicle, *J. Biomed. Mater. Res.*, 45, 268, 1999.

[43] Fischer, D. et al., A novel non-viral vector for DNA delivery based on low molecular weight, branched polyethylenimine: effect of molecular weight on transfection efficiency and cytotoxicity, *Pharm. Res.*, 16, 1273, 1999.

[44] Tang, G. et al., Polyethylene glycol modified polyethylenimine for improved CNS gene transfer: effects of PEGylation extent, *Biomaterials*, 24, 2351, 2004.

[45] Boussif, O. et al., A versatile vector for gene and oligonucleotide transfer into cells in culture and *in vivo*: polyethylenimine, *Proc. Natl Acad. Sci. USA*, 92, 7297, 1995.

[46] Manuel, W., Zheng, J., and Hornsby, P., Transfection by polyethyleneimine-coated microspheres, *J. Drug Target.*, 9, 15, 2001.

[47] Kuskowska-Latallo, J. et al., Efficient transfer of genetic material into mammalian cells using Starburst polyamidoamine dendrimers, *Proc. Natl Acad. Sci. USA*, 93, 4897, 1996.

[48] Maruyama-Tabata, H. et al., Effective suicide gene therapy *in vivo* by EBV-based plasmid vector coupled with polyamidoamine dendrimer, *Gene Ther.*, 7, 53, 2000.

[49] Mao, H.Q. et al., Chitosan-DNA nanoparticles as gene carriers: synthesis, characterization and transfection efficiency, *J. Control. Release*, 70, 399, 2001.

[50] Mansouri, S. et al., Chitosan-DNA nanoparticles as non-viral vectors in gene therapy: strategies to improve transfection efficacy, *Eur. J. Pharm. Biopharm.*, 57, 1, 2004.

[51] Ishii, T., Okahata, Y., and Sato, T., Mechanism of cell transfection with plasmid/chitosan complexes, *Biochim. Biophys. Acta*, 1514, 51, 2001.

[52] Padmanabhan, K. and Smith, T.A., Preliminary investigation of modified alginates as a matrix for gene transfection in a HeLa cell model, *Pharm. Dev. Technol.*, 7, 97, 2002.

[53] Gonzalez Ferreiro M. et al., Characterization of alginate/poly-L-lysine particles as antisense oligonucleotide carriers, *Int. J. Pharm.*, 239, 47 2002.

[54] Li, Z. et al., Controlled gene delivery system based on thermosensitive biodegradable hydrogel, *Pharm. Res.*, 20, 884, 2003.

[55] Girao Da Cruz, M., Simoes, S., and Pedroso De Lima, M., Improving lipoplex-mediated gene transfer into C6 glioma cells and primary neurons, *Exp. Neurol.*, 187, 65, 2004.

[56] Liu, F., Huang, L., and Liu, D., Factors controlling the efficiency of cationic lipid-mediated transfection *in vivo* via intravenous administration, *Gene Ther.*, 4, 517, 1997.

[57] Farhood, H., Serbina, N., and Huang, L., The role of dioleoyl phosphatidylethanolamine in cationic liposome mediated gene transfer, *Biochim. Biophys. Acta*, 1235, 289, 1995.

[58] King, R., Gene delivery to mammalian cells by microinjection, *Meth. Mol. Biol.*, 245, 167, 2004.

[59] Wilmut, I. et al., Viable offspring derived from fetal and adult mammalian cells, *Nature*, 385, 810, 1997.

[60] Hosaka, K. et al., Cloned mice derived from somatic cell nuclei, *Hum. Cell*, 13, 237, 2000.

[61] Neumann, E. et al., Gene transfer into mouse myeloma cells by electroporation in high electric fields, *EMBO J.*, 1, 841, 1982.

[62] Golzio, M., Teissié, J., and Rols, M., Direct visualization at the single-cell level of electrically mediated gene delivery, *Proc. Natl Acad. Sci. USA*, 99, 1292, 2002.

[63] Mir, L. et al., High-efficiency gene transfer into skeletal muscle mediated by electric pulses, *Proc. Natl Acad. Sci USA*, 96, 4262, 1999.

[64] Wang, Y. et al., Combination of electroporation and DNA/dendrimer complexes enhances gene transfer into murine cardiac transplants, *Am. J. Transplant.*, 1, 334, 2001.

[65] Schakowski, F. et al., Novel non-viral method for transfection of primary leukemia cells and cell lines, *Genet. Vaccines Ther.*, 2, 1, 2004.

[66] Sun, W. et al., *In vivo* cytokine gene transfer by gene gun reduces tumor growth in mice, *Proc. Natl Acad. Sci. USA*, 92, 2889, 1995.

[67] Matsuno Y. et al., Nonviral gene gun mediated transfer into the beating heart, *ASAIO J.*, 49, 641, 2003.

[68] Jeon, E., Kim, H.D., and Kim, J.S., Pluronic-grafted poly-(L)-lysine as a new synthetic gene carrier, *J. Biomed. Mater. Res.*, 66A, 854, 2003.

[69] Joubert, D. et al., A note on poly-L-lysine-mediated gene transfer in HeLa cells, *Drug Deliv.*, 10, 209, 2003.

[70] Tan, P.H. et al., Transferrin receptor-mediated gene transfer to the corneal endothelium, *Transplantation*, 71, 552, 2001.

[71] Van Rossenberg S.M. et al., Targeted lysosome disruptive elements for improvement of parenchymal liver cell-specific gene delivery, *J. Biol. Chem.*, 277, 45803, 2002.

[72] Godbey, W., Wu, K., and Mikos, A., Tracking the intracellular path of poly(ethylenimine)/DNA complexes for gene delivery, *Proc. Natl Acad. Sci. USA*, 96, 5177, 1999.

[73] Godbey, W.T. et al., Poly(ethylenimine)-mediated transfection: a new paradigm for gene delivery, *J. Biomed. Mater. Res.*, 51, 321, 2000.

[74] Suh, J., Wirtz, D., and Hanes, J., Efficient active transport of gene nanocarriers to the cell nucleus, *Proc. Natl Acad. Sci. USA*, 100, 3878, 2003.

[75] Brunner, S. et al., Cell cycle dependence of gene transfer by lipoplex, polyplex and recombinant adenovirus, *Gene Ther.*, 7, 7401, 2000.

[76] Escriou, V. et al., Critical assessment of the nuclear import of plasmid during cationic lipid-mediated gene transfer, *J. Gene Med.*, 3, 179, 2001.

[77] Zanta, M. et al., Gene delivery: a single nuclear localization signal peptide is sufficient to carry DNA to the cell nucleus, *Proc. Natl Acad. Sci. USA*, 96, 91, 1999.

[78] Aronsohn, A.I. and Hughes, J.A., Nuclear localization signal peptides enhance cationic liposome-mediated gene therapy, *J. Drug Target.*, 5, 163, 1998.

[79] Bremner, K. et al., Factors influencing the ability of nuclear localization sequence peptides to enhance nonviral gene delivery, *Bioconjug. Chem.*, 15, 152, 2004.

[80] Parveen, Z. et al., Cell-type-specific gene delivery into neuronal cells *in vitro* and *in vivo*, *Virology*, 314, 74, 2003.

[81] White, S.J. et al., Identification of peptides that target the endothelial cell-specific LOX-1 receptor, *Hypertension*, 37, 449, 2001.

[82] Argnani, R. et al., Specific targeted binding of herpes simplex virus type 1 to hepatocytes via the human hepatitis B virus preS1 peptide, *Gene Ther.*, 2004.

[83] Voinea, M., Binding and uptake of transferrin-bound liposomes targeted to transferrin receptors of endothelial cells, *Vascul. Pharmacol.*, 39, 13, 2002.

[84] Zhao, X.B. and Lee, R.J., Tumor-selective targeted delivery of genes and antisense oligodeoxyribonucleotides via the folate receptor, *Adv. Drug Deliv. Rev.*, 56, 1193, 2004.

[85] Yang, Q. et al., Development of novel cell surface CD34-targeted recombinant adenoassociated virus vectors for gene therapy, *Hum. Gene Ther.*, 9, 1929, 1998.

[86] Kunath, K. et al., Galactose–PEI–DNA complexes for targeted gene delivery: degree of substitution affects complex size and transfection efficiency, *J. Control. Release*, 88, 159, 2003.

[87] Wilcox, D.A. et al., Integrin alphaIIb promoter-targeted expression of gene products in megakaryocytes derived from retrovirus-transduced human hematopoietic cells, *Proc. Natl Acad. Sci. USA*, 96, 9654, 1999.

[88] Park, C. et al., Targeting of therapeutic gene expression to the liver by using liver-type pyruvate kinase proximal promoter and the SV40 viral enhancer active in multiple cell types, *Biochem. Biophys. Res. Commun.*, 314, 131, 2004.

[89] Godbey, W.T. and Atala, A., Directed apoptosis in Cox-2-overexpressing cancer cells through expression-targeted gene delivery, *Gene Ther.*, 10, 1519, 2003.

[90] Ikegami, S. et al., Treatment efficiency of a suicide gene therapy using prostate-specific membrane antigen promoter/enhancer in a castrated mouse model of prostate cancer, *Cancer Sci.*, 95, 367, 2004.

[91] Itakura, K. et al., Expression in *Escherichia coli* of a chemically synthesized gene for the hormone somatostatin, *Science*, 198, 1056, 1977.

[92] Lee, J. et al., *In vitro* model for liposome-mediated adenomatous polyposis coli gene transfer in a duodenal model, *Dis. Col. Rec.*, 47, 219, 2004.

[93] Krosl, J., *In vitro* expansion of hematopoietic stem cells by recombinant TAT-HOXB4 protein, *Nat. Med.*, 9, 1428, 2003.

[94] Li, R.H. et al., Dose control with cell lines used for encapsulated cell therapy, *Tissue Eng.*, 5, 453, 1999.

[95] Huang, Y.C. et al., Fabrication and *in vitro* testing of polymeric delivery system for condensed DNA, *J. Biomed. Mat. Res.*, 67A, 1384, 2003.

[96] Tomita, M. et al., Transgenic silkworms produce recombinant human type III procollagen in cocoons, *Nat. Biotechnol.*, 21, 52, 2003.

[97] Martínez-Serrano, A. et al., *Ex vivo* nerve growth factor gene transfer to the basal forebrain in presymptomatic middle-aged rats prevents the development of cholinergic neuron atrophy and cognitive impairment during aging, *Proc. Natl Acad. Sci. USA*, 95, 1858, 1998.

[98] Magin-Lachmann, C. et al., *In vitro* and *in vivo* delivery of intact BAC DNA — comparison of different methods, *J. Gene Med.*, 6, 195, 2004.

[99] Brown, C.B., Use of the peritoneal cavity for therapeutic delivery, *Perit. Dial. Int.*, 19, 512, 1999.

[100] Shariat, S.F., Adenovirus-mediated transfer of inducible caspases: a novel "death switch" gene therapeutic approach to prostate cancer, *Cancer Res.*, 61, 2562, 2001.

[101] Xia, C.F. et al., Kallikrein gene transfer protects against ischemic stroke by promoting glial cell migration and inhibiting apoptosis, *Hypertension*, 43, 452, 2004.

[102] Shi, N. et al., Brain-specific expression of an exogenous gene after i.v. administration, *Proc. Natl Acad. Sci. USA*, 98, 12754, 2001.

[103] Wang, S. et al., Transgene expression in the brain stem effected by intramuscular injection of polyethylenimine/DNA complexes, *Mol. Ther.*, 3, 658, 2001.

[104] Shi, N. and Pardridge, W., Noninvasive gene targeting to the brain, *Proc. Natl Acad. Sci. USA*, 97, 7567, 2000.

[105] Olivares, E.C. et al., Site-specific genomic integration produces therapeutic factor IX levels in mice, *Nat. Biotechnol.*, 20, 1124, 2002.

[106] Stribling, R. et al., Aerosol gene delivery *in vivo*, *Proc. Natl Acad. Sci. USA*, 89, 11277, 1992.

[107] Auricchio, A. et al., Noninvasive gene transfer to the lung for systemic delivery of therapeutic proteins, *J. Clin. Invest.*, 110, 499, 2002.

[108] Koshkina, N.V. et al., Biodistribution and pharmacokinetics of aerosol and intravenously administered DNA-polyethyleneimine complexes: optimization of pulmonary delivery and retention, *Mol. Ther.*, 8, 249, 2003.

[109] Chen, J. et al., Transfection of mEpo gene to intestinal epothelium *in vivo* mediated by oral delivery of chitosan-DNA nanoparticles, *World J. Gastroenterol.*, 10, 112, 2004.

[110] Keller, E.T. et al., *In vivo* particle-mediated cytokine gene transfer into canine oral mucosa and epidermis, *Cancer Gene Ther.*, 3, 186, 1996.

[111] Weld, K.J. et al., Transrectal gene therapy of the prostate in the canine model, *Cancer Gene Ther.*, 9, 189, 2002.

[112] *Journal of Gene Medicine* Website, http://www.wiley.co.uk/genmed/clinical, Accessed 10/18/2005.

[113] Cavazzana-Calvo, M. et al., Gene therapy of human severe combined immunodeficiency (SCID)-X1 disease, *Science*, 288, 627, 2000.

[114] Wong-Staal, F., Poeschla, E.M., and Looney, D.J., A controlled, phase 1 clinical trial to evaluate the safety and effects in HIV-1 infected humans of autologous lymphocytes transduced with a ribozyme that cleaves HIV-1 RNA, *Hum. Gene Ther.*, 9, 2407, 1998.

[115] Twins Study of Gene Therapy for HIV Infection, National Human Genome Research Institute (NHGRI).

[116] Senger, D.R. et al., Tumor cells secrete a vascular permeability factor that promotes accumulation of ascites fluid, *Science*, 219, 983, 1983.

[117] Losordo, D. et al., Gene therapy for myocardial angiogenesis: initial clinical results with direct myocardial injection of phVEGF165 as sole therapy for myocardial ischemia, *Circulation*, 98, 2800, 1998

[118] Rosengart, T.K. et al., Six-month assessment of a phase I trial of angiogenic gene therapy for the treatment of coronary artery disease using direct intramyocardial administration of an adenovirus vector expressing the VEGF121 cDNA, *Ann. Surg.*, 230, 466, 1999.

[119] Sorscher, E., Study chair, Phase I Study of Liposome-Mediated Gene Transfer in Patients with Cystic Fibrosis, University of Alabama.

[120] Moss, R.B. et al., Repeated adeno-associated virus serotype 2 aerosol-mediated cystic fibrosis transmembrane regulator gene transfer to the lungs of patients with cystic fibrosis: a multicenter, double-blind, placebo-controlled trial, *Chest*, 125, 509, 2004.

[121] Tuszynski, M., Prin. invest., Gene therapy for Alzheimer's Disease Clinical Trial, University of California, San Diego.

[122] Tuszynski, M.H. and Blesch, A., Nerve growth factor: from animal models of cholinergic neuronal degeneration to gene therapy in Alzheimer's disease, *Prog. Brain Res.*, 146, 441, 2004.

[123] de Haan, Hans, Prin. invest., Gene Therapy in Treating Patients with Recurrent Malignant Glioma, University of Alabama at Birmingham Comprehensive Cancer Center, Birmingham, AL.

[124] Link, C., Prin. invest., Gene Therapy in Treating Women With Refractory or Relapsed Ovarian Epithelial Cancer, Fallopian Tube Cancer, or Peritoneal Cancer, Human Gene Therapy Research Institute, Des Moines, Iowa.

44

Tissue Engineering Bioreactors

Jose F. Alvarez-Barreto
Vassilios I. Sikavitsas
University of Oklahoma

44.1 Introduction

The main goal of tissue engineering is the creation of artificial tissue having the ability to repair or simply replace lost or damaged tissue. Common tissue engineering strategies involve the extraction of cells from a small piece of tissue and their *in vitro* culture for later implantation using a carrier that allows the formation of new tissue (Figure 44.1) [1]. Most approaches in this field are based on common bioactive factors, consisting of cells (generally stem cells, or progenitor cells), a scaffolding material, and growth and differentiation factors [2]. The *in vitro* creation of an efficient construct can be accelerated by applying certain stimuli that can elicit specific responses to the cells. Stimulation can be done in two major ways: chemically and electro/mechanically.

Chemical stimulation is carried out by using growth and differentiation factors specific for different responses. Growth factors play a major role in cell division, matrix synthesis, and tissue differentiation [3]. Examples of these proteins are: bone morphogenetic proteins (BMPs), which have been demonstrated to induce the differentiation of mesenchymal stem cells into an osteoblastic lineage (BMP-2 and BMP-7), and the vascular endothelial growth factor that greatly enhances angiogenesis [4,5]. The need for *in vitro* mechanical stimulation in tissue engineering is drawn from the fact that most tissues function under specific biomechanical environments *in vivo*. These environments play a key role in tissue remodeling and regeneration. The stresses can be translated into different kinds of forces that range from load bearing to hydrodynamic forces due to fluid flow [6]. Thus, the mechanochemical microenvironment that progenitor

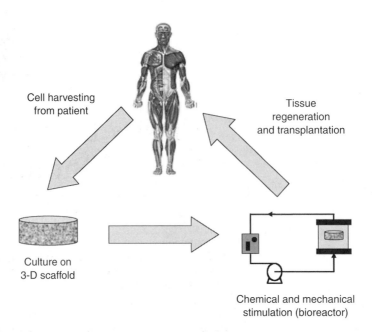

Cell harvesting
from patient

Tissue
regeneration
and transplantation

Culture on
3-D scaffold

Chemical and mechanical
stimulation (bioreactor)

FIGURE 44.1   Basic steps in the process of tissue engineering: cells are harvested from the patient and proliferated in a three-dimensional environment, followed by the application of mechanical and chemical stimuli in a bioreactor prior to implantation.

cells grow into is expected to control the fate of these cells while undergoing differentiation toward different lineages.

A bioreactor is generally defined as a device capable of creating the proper environment for the creation of a certain biological product [21]. Therefore, a bioreactor is described as a simulator, a device in which biological as well as biochemical processes can be carried out. In tissue engineering, bioreactors are used to impart certain forces that imitate different electromagnetic and mechanical stimuli occurring in the body. However, these devices are not limited to the sole application of electromechanical stimuli; they must meet other requirements in order to create grafts that, when implanted, will lead to the regeneration of damaged organs. A bioreactor must efficiently transport nutrients and oxygen to the construct, maintaining an appropriate concentration in solution. In most tissue engineering applications, a scaffold is seeded with cells and supports the formation of extracellular matrix (ECM). Consequently, the bioreactor has to induce a homogeneous cell distribution throughout these structures in order to generate a uniformly distributed ECM. Tissue engineering bioreactors can be used for cell seeding and long-term cultures.

This chapter describes some of the most popular bioreactor designs available for the engineering of different tissues. Hydrodynamic conditions and transport phenomena considerations are addressed, as well as applications to functional tissues and unique devices for specific applications. Design considerations, challenges, and new directions are also presented.

44.2   Most Common Bioreactors in Tissue Engineering

The choice of a bioreactor to cultivate three-dimensional constructs depends upon the tissue to be engineered and its functional biomechanical environment. Emulation of physiological conditions is the main objective when developing these kinds of systems, and this issue has been addressed in different ways. The incorporation of convective forces has become a common characteristic among most bioreactors. In this section, we describe some of the most common bioreactors found in the engineering of several functional tissues such as bone, cartilage, and cardiovascular applications, among others.

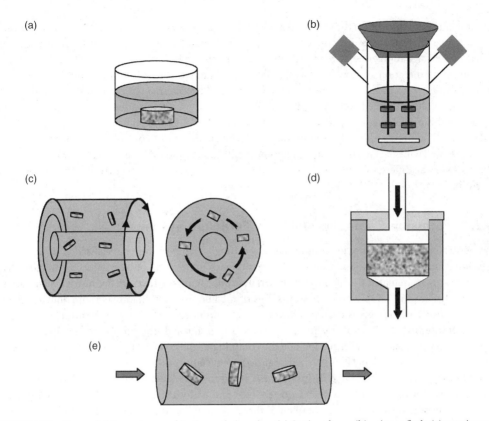

FIGURE 44.2 Common bioreactors used in tissue engineering. (a) Static culture, (b) spinner flask, (c) rotating wall, (d) perfusion system, and (e) perfused column.

44.2.1 Spinner Flask

The spinner flask (Figure 44.2b) represents one of the simplest bioreactor models. It was first designed with the idea to use convection in order to maintain a well-mixed system. The scaffolds are threaded into needles connected to the cover of the flask, and submerged in the culture medium. Convection is generated through the usage of a magnetic stir bar or a shaft that continuously mixes the media surrounding the scaffolds, providing a practically homogenous distribution of oxygen and nutrients [7,8]. The fluid dynamic environment at the external surface of the scaffolds is turbulent and characterized by the existence of eddies that may enhance the transport of nutrients into the porosity, and locally expose cells residing at the exterior of the construct to relatively high shear forces. The magnitude of the shear stresses can vary significantly between different locations; therefore, not all the cells are exposed to the same shear stresses. The presence of convective forces external to the scaffolds may not suppress concentration gradients appearing deep inside large three-dimensional constructs, where diffusion is the controlling mechanism of nutrient transport [9,25].

44.2.2 Rotating-Wall Vessels

Initially designed by NASA as a microgravity environment for cell culture, the rotating-wall bioreactor (Figure 44.2c) is now widely used in the formation of engineered bone, cartilage, and other tissues [7,8,10–12]. This device consists of two concentric cylinders whose annular space contains the cell culture medium [13]. The inner cylinder is static and permeable to allow gas exchange for oxygen supply. The outer cylinder, on the other hand, is impermeable and horizontally rotates at a speed that causes centrifugal forces that can balance, if tuned properly, the gravitational forces; thus, generating a pseudo microgravity environment [7,13,14]. Unlike the spinner flask, in the rotating-wall vessel the fluid flow is mostly laminar and the range of shear forces experienced by the cells at the outer surface is relatively narrow, with the existence of a stagnation zone at the upstream edge. As reported by Williams et al. [15], shear stresses decrease in the direction of flow and no significant variations from scaffold to scaffold are observed. Medium can be recirculated between the annular space and an external gas membrane. A modification of the original design, called rotating-wall perfused-vessel bioreactor, includes the rotation of the inner cylinder. In this model, media is perfused from the vessel's end cap to the pores of the inner cylinder [14].

The conditions of operation of a rotating-wall vessel must be carefully controlled. Large rotation speeds of the outer wall will affect mass transport since most of the inlet fluid bypasses the vessel volume, whereas an increase on the differential rotation enhances the radial and axial distribution of the fluid at low mean shear stresses [14].

44.2.3 Perfusion Chambers and Flow Perfusion Systems

Flow perfusion bioreactors provide continuous flow through chambers were the scaffolds are located. The perfusion column (Figure 44.2e) was one of the first designs of this kind of bioreactors. Culture medium is continuously recirculated through the chamber, thus improving the transport of nutrients and oxygen to the constructs [16,17,22]. Nevertheless, the flow of medium in these chambers is distributed between the inner network of the construct and its surroundings, minimizing convective flow through the scaffold [18]. To ensure that the flow of medium occurs exclusively through the porosity of the material, new designs of flow perfusion bioreactors include the confining of the construct in chambers (Figure 44.2d). In this way, a more controllable flow is achieved and nutrient transport limitations are virtually eliminated. Internal flow can also expose the cells inside the scaffold to fluid shear forces that have been known to be stimulatory for some cell types such as osteoblasts and endothelial cells [19,20]. A standard design of this kind of reactors does not exist, but all of them are based on the same principle. A more detailed description of a perfusion system is given later in this chapter.

44.3 Cell Seeding in Bioreactors

The first step to culturing cells in a three-dimensional environment is the seeding of scaffolds [21]. Along with the characteristics of the material, this process plays a crucial role in the development of efficient constructs for tissue engineering. Seeding of scaffolds determines the initial number of cells in the construct, as well as their spatial distribution throughout the matrix. Consequently, proliferation, migration, and the specific phenotypic expression of the engineered tissue will be affected by the utilized seeding technique [22]. In the case of tissues that require a fibrous or porous material, static seeding has been the most widely used method of cell seeding (Figure 44.2a). Burg et al. [26] compared different seeding techniques using rat aortic cells in polyglycolide fibrous meshes. Static seeding produced the poorest cellular distribution. In addition to preventing a homogeneous spatial distribution of the cells, static seeding also produces a low yield [23,26]. Holy et al. [23] reported a 25% efficiency of attachment after seeding 0.5 to 10×10^6 cells on porous PLGA 75/25 scaffolds. A low yield diminishes the development of specific functions related to cell–cell interactions and increases the required amount of cells; therefore, the usage of new seeding techniques becomes imperative.

In order to address these issues, researchers have incorporated convection into the process of cell seeding, suppressing some of the mass transfer limitations encountered in the static procedure. Spinner flask bioreactors (Figure 44.2b) have been implemented to create convection and, thereby, hydrodynamic forces that could help increase mass transport. Poly(glycolic acid) (PGA) scaffolds were threaded onto needles and chondrocytes suspensions with a total number of cells between 2×10^6 and 10×10^6 were used. A yield of 60% was obtained after 2 h of seeding. A more uniform distribution of the cells in the scaffold was seen (compared to the static seeding); nonetheless, the concentration of cells in the outer layer of the construct was 60 to 70% higher than that in the bulk [24]. This behavior may be due to the poor convection to the interior of the scaffold, making migration the only way for cells to reach the interior of the scaffold.

It has been reported that, in the spinner flask, the shear forces at the external surface of the scaffold are highly nonuniform. Such variability may influence the homogeneity of the seeded cells even when considering only the external surface area [25]. To avoid such problem, Mauney et al. rotated the scaffold every 2 h for the first 6 h of seeding so that each face of the construct could be exposed to the flow field, reaching a homogenous distribution of the cells and a higher efficiency than that of the static methodology. However, despite the high efficiency of seeding achieved with the spinner flask bioreactor, a more homogeneous distribution of the cells throughout the construct volume is still desired.

One way to guarantee mass transfer to the interior of the scaffold and a better distribution of cells is by applying perfusion [26,27]. In this technique, the construct is press fitted into a chamber, and the cell suspension is flowed through it (Figure 44.2c). Li et al. used a depth filtration system to seed poly (ethylene terephthalate) matrices at a rate of 1 ml/min. The cell suspension was recycled to increase the yield. Cell density increased along with the inoculation cell number, with an efficiency of about 65%, while with the static seeding, the yield stayed constant and lower than that achieved with the perfusion [22]. Similarly, Kim et al. seeded hepatocytes on polymeric matrices using a flow perfusion system. A suspension of rat hepatocytes at a density of 5×10^6 cells/ml was pumped through decellularized bone matrices at a flow rate of 1.5 ml/min for 4 h. A total of approximately 4.4×10^6 cells were attached to the matrix, which was considered successful. Furthermore, scanning electron microscopy and histology confirmed a uniform distribution of hepatocytes throughout the scaffold.

Wendt et al. [27] monitored seeding efficiency and uniformity of static, spinner flask, and perfusion systems. Using the same inoculation concentrations, there was not statistical significance among the efficiencies of the static and perfused techniques, both producing a larger yield than the spinner flask. Uniformity, however, was optimized by the perfusion apparatus, while the static and the spinner flask generated cell-scaffold constructs with low spatial uniformity [27].

44.4 Bioreactor Applications in Functional Tissues

After being seeded with the specific type of cells needed for the application, scaffolds must be subjected to longer periods of culture under the desired physical stimuli. The appropriate stimulation relies on the mechanical, biological, and ultrastructural characteristics of the native tissue. Bioreactors for engineered vascular grafts must mimic the natural fluid dynamic conditions of blood flow, including relatively high flow rates and pulsatile flow [42]. Bone tissue has also been shown to be stimulated by fluid flow [19]. Engineered ligaments and tendons need mechanical loading to emulate the conditions that they normally experience [87]. In this section we highlight some of the most important bioreactor applications in the engineering of different tissues; different designs and their efficiency in the development of inductive constructs are discussed.

44.4.1 Tissues of the Cardiovascular System

Several types of bioreactors have been used for the regeneration of tissues from the cardiovascular system. Spinner flasks and rotating-wall vessels have been employed in the regeneration of heart tissue. Cardiac myocytes were cultured on PGA scaffolds in a spinner flask, rotating-wall vessels and perfusion systems [28,29]. After 14 days of culture, the medium in the rotating-wall vessels showed higher levels of oxygen. The cell number in the spinner flask and rotating-wall reactor was larger than that of the static culture. Likewise, the uniformity of extracellular matrix throughout the scaffold was more homogeneous in the rotating-wall vessels. The engineered constructs had similar structural characteristics to that of the native tissue, and the cultured cells secreted proteins related to mature cardiac myocytes (myosin, troponin-T, tropomyosin, etc.). However, the cell density was always lower in the interior of the constructs [29].

44.4.1.1 Vascular Grafts

The emulation of physiological conditions in tissue-engineered vascular grafts is extremely important. Factors affecting the successful generation of a vascular graft include the selection of the appropriate scaffolding material, the cell type (smooth muscle cells, endothelial cells, and fibroblasts), and the culturing conditions [30,35]. Evaluation of mechanical properties is necessary to determine the quality of the engineered construct. Mechanical strength is directly related to the matrix structure, especially to the alignment of smooth muscle cells and collagen fibers [30,31].

Blood experiences rapid pulsating flow in the body with a velocity of about 33 cm/sec in the aorta and 0.33 mm/sec in capillaries [32]. Moreover, the conditions of flow will determine the differentiation path and properties of endothelial cells [6,33]. The extracellular matrix organization and mechanical properties of the graft, such as burst pressure and suture retention, are determinant factors of the graft quality [34]. Different systems with pulsatile flow have been designed in order to achieve these goals [35–38].

Static culture of endothelial cells seeded on different synthetic or natural polymers resulted in grafts with poor mechanical properties and morphological characteristics different from that of the native tissue [39]. In an attempt to mimic the natural environment of blood vessels, fluid flow has been employed during *in vitro* culture of smooth muscle cells seeded on PGA scaffolds. Incorporation of pulsation improved the mechanical properties of the constructs and their histological appearance resembled that of native arteries. It is important to point out that plain pulsation generated grafts with inferior mechanical properties [40]. The implementation of biomimetic bioreactors that utilize pulsatile flow in the physiological range appears to stimulate the formation of an organized matrix similar to that of the native tissue [41,42].

An example of a pulsatile-flow bioreactor for vascular grafts is shown in Figure 44.3. This design, used in the Laboratory of Cardiovascular Tissue Engineering at the University of Oklahoma, resembles the shell and tube concept of some heat exchangers. Flow circuits are separated into shell-side and tube-side to monitor (and control) system pressure and flow rates independently. Control valves downstream

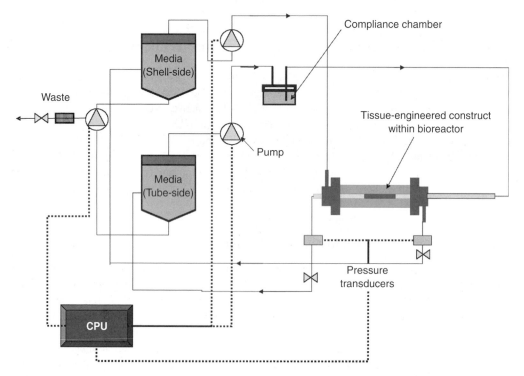

FIGURE 44.3 Shell–tube bioreactor for vascular grafts. (Courtesy of Dr. P. McFetridge from the School of Chemical Engineering and Materials Science, University of Oklahoma Bioengineering.)

of the bioreactor can be adjusted automatically in response to pressure variation. Typically, vascular bioreactors require different cell types seeded onto each side of the construct; as such, the dual-circuit-process flow allows different media types (endothelial and smooth muscle cell) to be run independently. Media is recirculated until nutrients, antibiotics, and pH require correction to remain within physiological parameters.

In another model designed by Thompson et al. [35], pressure is created by cyclical air inflow and the amount of pressure introduced in the system is controlled by a check valve. The air comes into contact with the culture medium in the so-called driving shaft. Tubing with medium is connected to the unit where the constructs are placed; this unit is called the manifold. Constructs can be accommodated in series or parallel, with a capacity of six scaffolds. Real-time flow and pressure can be monitored using an in-line flow meter and pressure transducer [35]. Hoerstrup et al. [43] designed a similar system in which the pulsatile flow is generated by the inflation/deflation of an elastic membrane.

Pulsatile flow, however, is not the only stimulation that has been used in the formation of tissue-engineered blood vessels. Selitkar et al. [44] designed a bioreactor to apply cyclic strain to cell-seeded scaffolds. After seeding aortic rat SMCs and culturing them for 8 days, circumferential orientation and a homogeneous distribution was observed in the scaffold. Collagen fibers were also produced in an organized fashion, forming bound assemblies. Mechanical properties were improved compared to unstrained constructs, achieving an ultimate stress of 58 kPa and modulus of 142 kPa, which are much greater than those achieved without any stimulation (16 and 68 kPa, respectively) [44].

Different stimuli have also been combined in order to enhance the formation of the extracellular matrix and mechanical properties. Peng et al. [45] used both cyclic stretching and pulsatile flow with perfusion to culture vascular cells. Endothelial cells were grown in distensible silastic tubes and subjected to pulse pressures and shear stresses comparable to the physiological values (up to 150 mmHg and 15 dyn/cm^2). Cells aligned in the direction of higher pulsation, almost parallel to the flow. Actin fibers showed a peripheral longitudinal orientation at greater pulsatilities.

44.4.1.2 Heart Valves

The environment in which heart valves perform is mechanically complex. Heart valves must operate at a frequency of approximately 1Hz, undergoing shear and bending stresses caused by blood flow [46,47]. Hoerstup et al. designed a pulsatile-flow system for the engineering of heart valves. This bioreactor basically consists of two chambers with a silicone diaphragm between them. The lower chamber maintains air, while the upper one is the culture medium chamber. Air is pumped, using a ventilator, into the lower chamber to displace the diaphragm and create the pulsation. Pulsatile flows from 50 to 2000 ml/min and systemic pressures from 10 to 240 mmHg can be achieved using this system [38]. Dumont et al. [37] designed a similar bioreactor for the formation of engineered aortic heart valves. This apparatus consists of a left ventricle (LV) made out of a silicone and an after-load with a compliance chamber and a resistance. The stroke and frequency of the machine is controlled by a piston that compresses and decompresses the LV. In this design, air is also incorporated in a compliance chamber, being pumped under conditions that resemble the standard systolic and diastolic pressures. The tissue-engineered aortic heart valve is placed between the left ventricle and the compliance chamber [37].

Schenke-Layland et al. [48] cultured endothelial cells and myofibroblasts on decellularized porcine heart valves under static and pulsatile conditions. Increased cellularity, collagen and elastin content, and mechanical strength were observed when the heart valves were cultured under pulsatile flow. The level of pulsation is also a critical parameter in the formation of functional heart valves, as demonstrated by Mol et al. [49].

44.4.2 Bone

Bone is a hard connective tissue that provides mechanical support to the human body and is a frame for locomotion. Bone grafts have been generated under a wide variety of culturing conditions, including static and dynamic systems. Among the most popular dynamic systems are spinner flasks, rotating-wall vessels, and perfusion systems [20,24,50,51]. As for every tissue, before deciding upon the kind of bioreactor to be used, considerations concerning the carrier matrix, cells (osteoblasts, mesenchymal stem cells, etc.), and growth factors must be taken into account. In the case of bone, the matrix to be used must be osteoconductive, provide mechanical support, deliver cells and allow their attachment, growth, migration, and osteoblastic differentiation [52]. Synthetic and natural polymers have been implemented. Among the synthetic polymers poly-α-hydroxy esters, poly(ε-caprolactone), poly(propylene fumarate), poly(sebacic acid), and their copolymers have been widely used. Materials such as ceramics and titanium have also been used for bone replacement [53,54]. Cell number and calcium deposition are good markers to evaluate the evolution of bone matrix. Furthermore, alkaline phosphatase activity (ALP) is used to assess early differentiation activity of osteoblastic cells. Production of extracellular matrix proteins such as osteocalcin, osteopontin, and bone sialoprotein is also taken into consideration [55].

As mentioned before, static culture was one of the first attempts to produce bone matrix. Ishaug et al. [56] seeded marrow stromal cells on top of poly (DL-lactic-co-glycolic acid) (PLGA) foams of different pore sizes at different densities. Cell proliferation was supported by the scaffold, and high level of ALP activity and calcium matrix deposition were observed. It was found that the depth of mineralized tissue increased over time, but the maximum penetration was only around 240 μm, resulting in a nonhomogeneous cell and matrix distribution [56].

Improvement in the development of bone matrix *in vitro* has been achieved with the addition of convection in the *in vitro* culture stage, which ultimately translates in a better transport of nutrients and gases. After statically seeding 1×10^6 marrow stromal cells on 75 : 25 PLGA scaffolds, Sikavitsas et al. [7] cultured these constructs under three different conditions: statically, in a spinner flask and in a rotating-wall vessel. The culture was carried out for 21 days, and samples were analyzed at 7, 14, and 21 days. Scaffolds cultured in the spinner flask bioreactor showed the largest number of cells at all time points, followed by the static culture. At the end of the culture period, constructs in the spinner flask presented higher calcium contents than those encountered in the static and rotating-wall vessel [7].

Shea et al. [57] also utilized a spinner flask to culture poly(lactic acid) foams seeded with MC3T3-E1 preosteoblasts and evaluated their differentiation. Cells were seeded statically and cultured for 12 weeks. Proliferation was observed over time; however, their distribution throughout the scaffold lacked homogeneity. Cells were densely located only at a thin layer of 200 μm near the scaffold's surface. The density dramatically decreased deeper into the construct. The same behavior was seen for the formation of extracellular matrix and calcium deposition.

It has been shown that mechanical stimulation augments the production of alkaline phosphatase, osteoblast proliferation, and mineral deposition in osteoblastic cells seeded on different scaffolding materials [58]. Osteoblastic cells have been shown to be responsive to shear stress induced by fluid flow. The stimulatory effect of shear stresses has shown to induce an increase in the release of important regulatory factors such as nitric oxide and prostaglandin E2 [59–61]. Interestingly, osteoblasts have been found to be more responsive to fluid shear forces than mechanical strain [62]. A question arises then, what is the physiological relevance of the stimulatory effect of fluid flow on bone cells? It has been hypothesized that mechanical strains on bone tissue cause fluid flow in the lacunar–canalicular porosity of bone [63–65]. Consequently, the incorporation of fluid flow through the porous network is desired in order to stimulate a faster and more efficient formation of bone matrix. This goal has been reached with the implementation of flow perfusion bioreactors [20,66,67].

Bancroft et al. [8] developed a perfusion system (Figure 44.4) where medium is pumped through the scaffold, thereby maintaining mechanical stimulation and transport of nutrients through the pores. The scaffolds are tightly fit into cassettes in order to ensure fluid flow exclusively through the porous network. Constructs are later placed in flow chambers that are capped and secured with o-rings to restrict the flow around them (Figure 44.4a). The medium is pumped from a flask to the top of the chamber and sent to another reservoir from the bottom. This direction of flow helps avoiding the entrance of air bubbles into the flow chamber. Both flasks are connected so that the medium is in continuous recirculation. The main body of the reactor consists of a total of six chambers and is made out of Plexiglas to allow the visualization and monitoring of the flow inside the chambers. Each chamber corresponds to an independent circuit

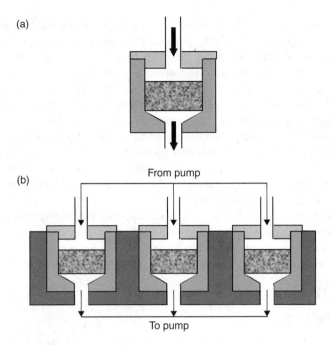

FIGURE 44.4 Schematics of a flow perfusion bioreactor. (a) Close up of the perfusion chamber where the scaffold is press fitted. (b) Lateral view of the main body of the bioreactor.

using one of the heads of a peristaltic pump that produces flow rates from 0.1 to 10 ml/min (Figure 44.4b). The tubing permits the exchange of carbon dioxide and oxygen with the atmosphere in the incubator. A complete change of medium can be done due to the two-reservoir set up [18].

To study how the shear rate affects the growth of bone matrix *in vitro*, Bancroft et al. [19] varied the flow rate when culturing titanium fiber meshes seeded with rat marrow stromal cells for 16 days. Controls have been cultured under static conditions, and the flow rates used in the perfusion culture were 0.3, 1.0, and 3.0 ml/min. It was found that the deposition of calcium was greatly increased in the flow perfusion culture as compared with the static conditions. It was also observed that increased medium flow improves the distribution of extracellular matrix throughout the construct volume [19]. The increased calcium deposition could have been due to the increased shear forces or increased chemotransport in the porosity of the scaffolds when higher flow rates were employed. To isolate the effects of shear forces from the mass transport effects, the shear forces were changed by varying the viscosity of the culture medium under constant flow rate [68]. An increase in viscosity, which translates into greater shear forces, was found to enhance the deposition of mineral matrix and the ECM distribution throughout the construct, demonstrating the importance of fluid-flow induced shear forces on the creation of bone tissue-engineered grafts.

Meinel et al. [67] cultured human mesenchymal stem cells on silk scaffolds for 5 weeks in a flow perfusion chamber (at 0.2 ml/min) and a spinner flask. Scaffolds cultured under flow perfusion showed a more homogenous distribution of the mineralized matrix throughout the construct although those cultured in the spinner flask produced a greater amount of deposited calcium.

Other kinds of stimulation include mechanical strain and electrical current. A bioreactor was developed that allowed the continuous exposure of cells to continuous cyclic stretching [69]. Primary osteoblast-like cells were seeded on silicone rubbers and subjected to 1000 microstrains at 1 Hz either continuously or in periods of 60 min. Cellularity and calcium deposition were enhanced under the presence of mechanical strain and the intermittent procedure was the most efficient of them [70]. Another bioreactor that can expose cells to mechanical load has been developed by Shimko et al. [71]. Unlike the previous study, mechanical loading had a negative impact in the mineral deposition.

Electrical current has been shown to stimulate bone regeneration and enhance its healing [72–75]. Bioreactors have been designed to electrically stimulate cells seeded on conductive surfaces [75]. After culturing calvarial osteoblasts under an electric field with 10 μA and 10 Hz for 6 h/day, the cell number was higher by 46% and the amount of calcium deposited was raised by 307% after 21 days, compared to nonstimulated cells. Upregulation of mRNA expression for collagen type I was also observed.

As demonstrated by several studies, the usage of flow perfusion greatly enhances the formation of bone matrix. By doing this, mechanotransduction mechanisms related to the differentiation of osteoblastic cells are potentially activated. Great challenges are still encountered however. What are the actual mechanisms that transduce the external shear forces and influence the cellular behavior? Currently, only estimates of the shear rates at the interior of three-dimensional scaffolds have been provided, and detailed mathematical modeling needs to be conducted. This will allow the determination of the actual values of the shear rate inside the constructs and their spatial distribution.

Using larger scaffolds can represent another problem; is it possible to achieve a completely homogeneous distribution of matrix in larger constructs? What would be the necessary culturing conditions to achieve this? How long must the cells be cultured to produce an osteoinductive enough matrix? And how long and under what conditions must the cells be precultured prior to the application of mechanical forces to avoid their detachment?

44.4.3 Cartilage

Cartilage is a tissue with limited capabilities of regeneration when damaged. Between the two general types of cartilage, articular cartilage is continuously exposed to mechanical forces and needs to dissipate loads under physiological conditions. On the other hand, in other parts of the body the elastic properties of the cartilage are more important. Cartilaginous tissue has been engineered using spinner flasks, rotating-wall bioreactors, perfusion systems, and compression bioreactors that better mimic the physiological environment of the cartilage tissue. The most widely used cell types for the regeneration of cartilage are mesenchymal stem cells or primary chondrocytes. Regarding the scaffold, different materials have been used; synthetic and natural hydrogels are among the most popular choices, including collagen, poly α-hydroxy esters, and their copolymers. Fibrinogen-based and glycosaminoglycan (GAG)-based matrices are also being employed [76,77]. Some of the markers used to evaluate the formation of cartilaginous matrix are cellularity, production of collagen type II, and production of GAGs [8]. It has to be pointed out that the synthesis of native cartilage dramatically varies in different locations of the body.

Vunjak-Novakovic et al. [10] compared the performance of different bioreactors (static, spinner flask, and rotating wall) in the formation of cartilaginous matrix. Highly porous PGA scaffolds were seeded with chondrocytes and cultured statically, in a spinner flask, and a rotating-wall vessel for 6 weeks. At the end of the culture period, GAG and collagen type II levels were five times greater than the values obtained in early culture. The spinner flask induced a larger production of GAGs and collagen type II; however, an even greater difference was observed in the rotating bioreactor compared to the static culture. Histomorphometric studies revealed the formation of tissue in the periphery of the constructs cultured statically, while those in the spinner flask had an outer fibrous capsule in spite of the increment in mass transport. Scaffolds cultured in the rotating-wall bioreactor, on the other hand, showed a better distribution of the matrix, but a gradient in concentration of GAGs was observed in all the constructs.

Gooch et al. [78] studied the effect of shear stress on the formation of cartilage matrix in a spinner flask and compared it with a static culture. Chondrocytes were dynamically seeded for 3 days on fibrous PGA matrices with a fiber diameter of 13 μm using a spinner flask bioreactor. Cultivation was carried out for 42 days at different mixing intensities. Production of GAGs was greater in the spinner flask, and increased along with the mixing intensity. Collagen production showed a similar behavior although no significant difference was observed among the different mixing intensities.

The effect of shear stress has also been conducted in a rotating-wall vessel [11]. Variation of the rotation speed of the mobile wall when culturing chondrocytes in poly(lactic acid) (PLA) foams for 28 days did not cause a change in cell density among scaffolds cultured at different rotation rates although they were larger than those found in static conditions. However, the deposition of matrix GAGs decreased at higher shear rates, whereas the collagen production showed a contrary behavior. The production of collagen increased along with the shear rate and time of cultivation, showing a more dramatic dependence on the rotation speed.

It is important to point out that the shear stress induced in a rotating-wall bioreactor occurs only at the surface of the scaffold; therefore, perfused cartridges have been used to produce stress stimulation at the interior of the construct. Pazzano et al. [79] cultured calf chondrocytes seeded on PGA matrices for 4 weeks under static and flow perfusion conditions. Not only did the perfusion system increase the amount of GAGs by 180% compared with the static conditions, but it also created an organized, homogeneous matrix. After the 4 weeks of culture, chondrocytes were aligned in the direction of flow, creating a structure similar to that of some regions of native articular cartilage [80].

Native articular cartilage withstands up to 20 MPa due to compression *in vivo*; therefore, bioreactors using this kind of stimulus have been implemented obtaining promising results [6,81–84]. Mizuno et al. [85] used a culture system that consisted of a perfusion column and a pressurizer. Medium is peristaltically pumped through the perfusion column were the scaffolds are kept. Downstream from the column there is a back-pressure regulator. Cyclic pressure was controlled by using a needle valve and a computer-controlled spring. Chondrocytes were statically seeded in porous collagen matrices for 3 days. Posteriorly, the sponges were introduced in the perfusion chamber, and flow was started at the rate of 0.33 ml/min. The culture conditions were pure perfusion, cyclic compression (0.015 Hz) 2.8 MPa, and constant compression at 2.8 MPa of hydrostatic fluid pressure. Production of GAGs and collagen type II were enhanced by the application of pressure load even though there were no significant differences in cellularity. Hydrostatic pressure produced about 3.1 times more sulfated GAGs than the controls, whereas the cyclic pressure produced 2.7 times more sulfated GAGs than the controls. In addition, a native-like matrix was observed, containing lacunae that entrapped the chondrocytes and a uniform spatial distribution [85]. Carver et al. [86] had found similar results when comparing the influences of cyclic pressure, flow perfusion, and culture in spinner flasks, in the formation of cartilaginous matrix. They found that the combination of flow perfusion and intermittent pressurization seemed to accelerate the matrix formation. In agreement with these findings, Hung et al. [84] reported the production of cartilage-like tissue after culturing chondrocytes seeded on agarose gels for 8 weeks under physiologic deformational loading.

The variability in the synthesis and the mechanical properties of cartilage in different locations of the body and zones of the same location introduces a great challenge in the regeneration of cartilage tissue. Is the mechanical environment the controlling factor in the formation of zone and location-specific ECM? Or in different locations of the body, are chondrocytes preprogrammed with different genetic information to generate a specific type of extracellular matrix? How do chondrocytes in the growth plate cartilage recognize a differentiation pattern that leads to bone formation? The elucidation of these questions will provide valuable information to cartilage tissue engineers.

44.4.4 Anterior Cruciate Ligament and Tendons

Ligaments and tendons operate in the presence of various types and levels of mechanical strains that are expected to influence the behavior of cells residing in these tissues. Mesenchymal stem cells (MSCs) have been shown to preferentially differentiate into ligament fibroblasts in the presence of mechanical forces when cultured in bioreactors that generated mechanical strains that resemble the native ligament stretching conditions [87].

The most widely used material as scaffolding for the regeneration of anterior cruciate ligament (ACL) and tendon is collagen; other materials such as polymeric fibrous matrices have been utilized [88]. However, the mechanical properties of collagen bundles are considerably inferior to those of the native tissue. This problem can be partially overcome by preferentially orienting the collagen fibers of the matrix through the seeding of cells and the application of mechanical strain [89].

The principle of a bioreactor that can mimic the biomechanical conditions of ligament and tendons is shown in Figure 44.5. The construct is attached to a moving platform that produces mechanical strain

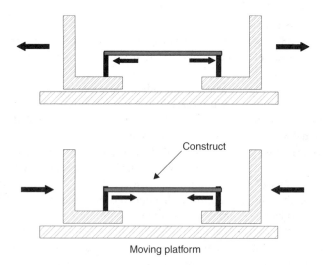

FIGURE 44.5   Principle of cyclic strain bioreactor for ligament and tendon engineering.

through stretching. Langelier et al. [89] designed a cyclic traction device that can produce these mechanical strains on cell-seeded constructs. This machine consists of an actuating unit that controls the cyclic motion frequency (0.01 to 1 cycle/min) and amplitude (0 to 2 cm) for collagenous matrices with a length between 2 and 10 cm. A transmission unit connects the actuating unit to the testing unit, and its purpose is to transmit motion to the testing unit through a rotating shaft. The testing compartment unit, shown in Figure 44.4, is where the matrix is located. The two walls at both extremes are made out of stainless steel, and the material chosen for the other surfaces was acrylic to allow visualization of the construct. The top of the compartment is a removable acrylic plate screwed to the walls and is removed when the scaffold needs to be manipulated. Generally, the collagen gel is formed over two bone anchors for adequate mechanical attachment to the traction machine [89]. The construct can be subjected to cyclic stretching at a frequency of up to 1 Hz and amplitude from 0 to 30 mm for any extended period of time. The system is controlled via special software, and the experimental conditions of stretching and amplitude can be easily changed [90].

MSCs seeded on collagen gels were cultured under translational and rotational strain concurrently. After 21 days of culture, a ligament-like morphology was observed in the constructs, with elongated, well-organized collagen types I and III in the longitudinal direction. Unlike the constructs cultured statically, those under mechanical strain presented an ECM that contained tenascin-C, which is a marker of ligament ECM [87]. A similar behavior was observed by Awad et al. [91] when MSC-seeded collagen scaffolds were cultured under a continuously strained environment; formation of organized collagen bundles was also observed.

Cyclic stretching has been also implemented in tendon tissue engineering and has demonstrated a significant effect on the alignment of collagen bundles [92]. Avian tendon internal fibroblasts were incorporated into type-I collagen matrices at a rate of 2×10^5 cells per scaffold. Mechanical loading was applied 1 h per day with 1% elongation and 1 Hz for up to 11 days. Loaded constructs presented aligned cells that spread throughout the matrix, with elongated nuclei and cytoplasmic extensions. Moreover, the modulus of elasticity of the mechanically loaded constructs was 2.9 times greater than those of the nonstimulated controls [92].

One of the challenges in tendon and ligament tissue engineering is the selection of cell source for their repair. Although MSCs have been shown to have the ability to differentiate into tendon and ligament cells in the presence of mechanical forces, the use of specific growth factor combinations that can initiate the differentiation toward these phenotypes in regular cell cultures would minimize the time of tissue regeneration in bioreactors. In addition to that, the specific cellular mechanisms that transduce the mechanical signals to these cells and control their behavior are not yet clearly understood.

44.4.5 Other Tissues

Apart from the previously mentioned applications where bioreactors have been widely utilized, bioreactors have been used for the culture of cell types involved in the regeneration of other tissues, including hepatocytes and neuronal cells. The high metabolic requirements of hepatic cells make the use of perfusion systems for their culture ideal. Powers et al. [93] cultured hepatocytes in the presence of continuous flow perfusion and the cells remained viable for up to 2 weeks. The use of electromagnetic fields in neuronal tissue regeneration has also provided elegant ways for the alignment of neuronal cells in the guided regrowth of axons [94].

44.5 Design Considerations

When designing a bioreactor, the first factor that must be taken into account is the kind of stimulation to be emulated. Therefore, the apparatus must be able to cause similar effects to those found physiologically and at matching conditions, in addition to ensuring proper transportation of nutrients. A temperature of $37^{\circ}C$ and a humid atmosphere with 5% CO_2 are required [95]. Other important factors are:

1. Easy handling and assembling, lowering risks of contamination
2. Sterilizability
3. Fit into an incubator and operate at the given conditions
4. Allow change of culture medium aseptically
5. Facilitate monitoring of tissue formation
6. Automatically operated in order to ensure reproducibility of operation conditions
7. Ability to produce several constructs at the same time
8. Ease of scaling up

44.6 Challenges in Bioreactor Technologies

Implementation of bioreactors in the process of tissue engineering has been driven by the need to mimic the physiological conditions in which cells operate at different locations of the human body. Most bioreactors in reality are biomimetic environments that induce morphological arrangements similar to those found in native tissues. To a certain degree, the new technologies have been successful in achieving the initial goals: creation of native tissue-like matrices; nevertheless, many obstacles are yet to be overcome in order to produce efficient and practical constructs that can be used for the regeneration of damaged or lost organs.

The transport of nutrients and oxygen still remains an issue in the processing of many tissues. Some cells have a high metabolic demand; such is the case of hepatic tissue, thus requiring an efficient transportation of these components to the place of growth. As discussed in this chapter, part of this problem has been overcome by the utilization of perfusion systems. However, scaling up the size of the construct may pose new challenges. When increasing the dimensions of the scaffolding, other interrogatives arise. Would it still be possible to obtain a homogeneous distribution of cells and ECM throughout the scaffold? What is the flow rate necessary to guarantee the delivery of oxygen and nutrients to the interior of the construct?

Cell source is a factor that has not been studied in detail. It is not clear, for the engineering of some tissues, whether cells extracted from different locations could have different responses under identical stimulation. In the case of bone the question arises, as to whether cells extracted from an area that is not load bearing respond in similar fashion to those harvested from a load-bearing site like the femur? Similar questions are unanswered for cartilage and ligaments.

Bone, cartilage, vascular grafts, and ligaments, among others, require potent mechanical properties that have not been matched by the engineered constructs to this day. Establishing effective mechanical properties depends not only on the biomaterial used but also in the bioreactor design and time of culture.

Mechanical stimulations have proved to be the path to generate mechanically efficient implants, but not all biomaterials can be exposed to mechanical strains without generating some degree of structural damage.

Standard criteria for the evaluation of the quality of the final construct are necessary from a mechanical, chemical, biological, and morphological point of view. Large variations on the conditions of operation and culture in different bioreactor designs to engineer a given tissue prevent the comparison of different studies and thereby the drawing of definite conclusions regarding the optimization of these conditions. In addition, histological evaluation of the regenerated tissue (or *in vitro* generated graft) should always be complemented by appropriate mechanical tests.

Time also represents a significant concern when engineering tissue grafts. Given the fact that the engineered constructs will ultimately be transplanted into diseased patients, the time of production becomes a critical factor. The ultimate goal is to produce, in a short period of time, a construct that can induce the formation of new tissue *in vivo*. It is obvious that the definition of a "short period of time" depends upon the tissue being engineered and the urgency for a replacement. Some tissues like bone or cartilage could offer some flexibility in the time of production depending on the type of injury, but in life-threatening situations, such as failing heart valves, it is important to rapidly produce a construct. Consequently, tissue engineering strategies should always attempt to minimize the time of production.

The answer to shortening the time of generation of engineered tissues may lie in the combination of mechanical and chemical signals. Both principles have been studied separately; certain growth factors such as bone morphogenetic proteins, vascular endothelial growth factor, and insulin like growth factors, among others, have been shown to greatly help the formation of tissues *in vitro* and *in vivo*. Therefore, it is expected that the combination of growth factors and mechanical stimulation in a bioreactor could generate mature matrices at a faster pace. It is important as well to determine what the intracellular mechanisms related to the signaling pathways are. A better understanding of the biological mechanisms involved in the mechanosensing processes will give a new perspective in the design of new experiments and improvement of those already existent. Moreover, new directions could be taken based on these mechanisms.

Acknowledgment

We would like to acknowledge the Seed Grant Program of the Bioengineering Center at the University of Oklahoma.

References

[1] Bonassar, J. and Vacanti, C. Tissue engineering: the first decade and beyond. *J. Cell Biochem. Suppl.* 30/31, 297, 1998.

[2] Boden, S.D. Bioactive factors for bone tissue engineering. *Clin. Orthop.*, 367S, S84, 1999.

[3] Lieberman, J.R., Daluiski, A., and Einhorn, T.A. The role of growth factors in the repair of bone. *J. Bone Joint Surg.*, 84-A, 1032, 2002.

[4] Wang, E.A. et al. Recombinant human bone morphogenetic protein induces bone formation. *Proc. Natl Acad. Sci. USA*, 87, 2220, 1990.

[5] Trivedi, N. et al. Improved vascularization of planar diffusion devices following continuous infusion of vascular endothelial growth factor (VEGF). *Cell Transplant*, 8, 175, 1999.

[6] Stoltz, J.F. et al. Influence of mechanical forces on cells and tissues. *Biotechnology*, 37, 3, 2000.

[7] Sikavitsas, V.I., Bancroft, G.N., and Mikos, A.G. Formation of three-dimensional cell/polymer constructs for bone tissue engineering in a spinner flask bioreactor and a rotating wall Bessel bioreactor. *J. Biomed. Mater. Res.*, 62, 136, 2002.

[8] Darling, E.M. and Athanasiou, K.A. Articular cartilage bioreactors and bioprocesses. *Tissue Eng.*, 9, 9, 2003.

[9] Goldstein, A.S. et al. Effect of convection on osteoblastic cell growth and function in biodegradable polymer foam scaffolds. *Biomaterials*, 22, 1279, 2001.

[10] Vunjak-Novakovic, G., Obradovic, B., and Free, L.E. Bioreactor studies of native and tissue engineered cartilage. *Biorheology*, 39, 259, 2002.

[11] Saini, S. and Wick, T.M. Concentric cylinder bioreactor for production of tissue engineered cartilage: effect of cell density and hydrodynamic loading on construct development. *Biotechnol. Prog.*, 19, 510, 2003.

[12] Sutherland F.W. et al. Advances in the mechanisms of cell delivery to cardiovascular scaffolds: comparison of two rotating cell culture systems. *ASAIO J.*, 48, 346, 2002.

[13] Vunjak-Novakovic, G. et al. Microgravity studies of cells and tissues. *Ann. N Y Acad. Sci.*, 974, 504, 2002.

[14] Begley, C.M. and Kleis, S.J. The fluid dynamic and shear environment in the NASA/JSC rotating wall perfused-vessel bioreactor. *Biotechnol. Bioeng.*, 70, 32, 2000.

[15] Williams, K.A. et al. Computational fluid dynamics modeling of steady-state momentum and mass transport in a bioreactor for cartilage tissue engineering. *Biotechnol. Prog.*, 18, 951, 2002.

[16] Mizuno, S., Allemann, F., and Glowacki, J. Effects of medium perfusion on matrix production by bovine chondrocytes in three-dimensional collagen sponges. *J. Biomed. Mater. Res.*, 56, 368, 2001.

[17] Navarro, F.A. et al. Perfusion of medium improves growth of human oral neomucosal tissue constructs. *Wound Repair Regen.*, 9, 507, 2001.

[18] Bancroft, G.N., Sikavitsas, V.I., and Mikos, A.G. Design of a flow perfusion bioreactor system for bone–tissue engineering applications. *Tissue Eng.*, 9, 549, 2003.

[19] Bancroft, G.N. et al. Fluid flow increases mineralized matrix deposition in 3D perfusion culture of marrow stromal osteoblasts in a dose-dependent manner. *Proc. Natl Acad. Sci. USA*, 99, 12600, 2002.

[20] Cartmell, S.H. et al. Effects of medium perfusion rate on cell seeded three-dimensional bone constructs *in vitro*. *Tissue Eng.*, 9, 1197, 2003.

[21] Martin, I., Wendt, D., and Herberer, M. The role of bioreactors in tissue engineering. *Trends Biotechnol.*, 22, 80–86, 2004.

[22] Li, Y. Effects of filtration seeding on cell density, spatial distribution, and proliferation in nonwoven fibrous matrices. *Biotechnol. Prog.*, 17, 935, 2001.

[23] Holy, C.E., Shoichet, M.S., and Davies, J.E. Engineering three-dimensional bone tissue *in vitro* using biodegradable scaffolds: investigating initial cell-seeding density and culture period. *J. Biomed. Mater. Res.*, 51, 376, 2000.

[24] Vunjak-Novakovic, G. et al. Dynamic cell seeding of polymer scaffolds for cartilage tissue engineering. *Biotechnol. Prog.*, 14, 193, 1998.

[25] Sucosky, P. et al. Fluid mechanics of a spinner-flask bioreactor. *Biotechnol. Bioeng.*, 85, 34, 2004.

[26] Burg, K.J.L. et al. Comparative study of seeding methods for three-dimensional polymeric scaffolds. *J. Biomed. Mater. Res.*, 51, 642, 2000.

[27] Wendt, D. et al. Oscilating perfusion of cell suspensions through three-dimensional scaffolds enhances cell seeding efficiency and uniformity. *Biotechnol. Bioeng.*, 84, 205, 2003.

[28] Sodian, R. et al. Tissue-engineering bioreactors: a new combined cell-seeding and perfusion system for vascular tissue engineering. *Tissue Eng.*, 8, 863, 2002.

[29] Carrier, R.L. et al. Cardiac tissue engineering: cell seeding, cultivation parameters, and tissue construct characterization. *Biotechnol. Bioeng.*, 64, 580, 1999.

[30] Tranquillo, R. The tissue-engineered small-diameter artery. *Ann. N Y Acad. Sci.*, 961, 251, 2002.

[31] L'Heureux, N. et al. A completely biological tissue-engineered human blood vessel. *FASEB J.*, 12, 47, 1998.

[32] Guyton, A. and Hall, J. *Textbook of Medical Physiology*, 10th ed., Saunders Company, 2000, p. 145.

[33] Braddock, M. et al. Fluid shear stress modulation of gene expression in endothelial cells. *New Physiol. Sci.*, 13, 241, 1998.

[34] Nerem, R. and Sliktar, D. Vascular tissue engineering. *Annu. Rev. Biomed. Eng.*, 3, 225, 2001.

[35] Thompson, C.A. et al. A novel pulsatile, laminar flow bioreactor for the development of tissue-engineered vascular structures. *Tissue Eng.*, 8, 1083, 2002.

[36] Sodian, R. et al. New pulsatile bioreactor for fabrication of tissue-engineered patches. *J. Biomed. Mater. Res. (Appl. Biomater.)*, 58, 401, 2001.

[37] Dumont, K. et al. Design of new pulsatile bioreactor for tissue engineered aortic heart valve formation. *Artif. Organs*, 26, 710, 2002.

[38] Hoerstrup, S.P. et al. New pulsatile bioreactor for *in vitro* formation of tissue engineered heart valves. *Tissue Eng.*, 6, 75, 2000.

[39] Weinberg, C.B. and Bell, E. A blood vessel model constructed from collagen and cultured vascular cells. *Science*, 23, 397, 1986.

[40] Niklason, L.E. et al. Functional arteries grown *in vitro*. *Science*, 284, 489, 1999.

[41] Lian, X. and Howard, P.G. Blood vessels, in *Principles of Tissue Engineering*, Lanza, R., Langer, R., and Vacanti, J. (Eds.), 2nd ed., Academic Press, New York, 2000, chap. 32.

[42] Niklason L.E. and Langer, R.S. Advances in tissue engineering of blood vessels and other tissues. *Transp. Immunol.*, 5, 303, 1997.

[43] Hoerstrup, S.P. et al. Tissue engineering of small caliber vascular grafts. *Eur. J. Cardiothorac. Surg.*, 20, 164, 2001.

[44] Selitkar, D. et al. Dynamic mechanical conditioning of collagen–gel blood vessel constructs induces remodeling *in vitro*. *Ann. Biomed. Eng.*, 28, 351, 2000.

[45] Peng, X. et al. *In vitro* system to study realistic pulsatile flow and stretch signaling in cultured vascular cells. *Am. J. Physiol. Cell Physiol.*, 279, C797, 2000.

[46] Barron, V. et al. Bioreactors for cardiovascular cell and tissue growth: a review. *Ann. Biomed. Eng.*, 31, 1017, 2003.

[47] Mann, B.K. and West, J.L. Tissue engineering in the cardiovascular system: progress toward a tissue engineered heart. *Anat. Rec.*, 263, 367, 2001.

[48] Schenke-Layland, K. Complete dynamic repopulation of decellularized heart valves by application of defined physical signals — an *in vitro* study. *Cardiovasc. Res.*, 60, 497, 2003.

[49] Mol, A. The relevance of large strains in functional tissue engineering of heart valves. *Thorac. Cardiovasc. Surg.*, 51, 78, 2003.

[50] Goldstain, A.S. et al. Effect of osteoblastic culture conditions on the structure of poly(DL-Lactic-co-Glycolic acid) foam scaffolds. *Tissue Eng.*, 5, 421, 1999.

[51] Botchwey, E.A. et al. Bone tissue engineering in a rotating bioreactor using a microcarrier matrix system. *J. Biomed. Mater. Res.*, 55, 242, 2001.

[52] Bancroft, G.N. and Mikos, A.G. Bone tissue engineering by cell transplantation, in *Polymer Based Systems on Tissue Engineering, Replacement and Regeneration*, Reis, R.L. and Cohn, D. (Eds.), Kluwer Academic Publishers, Boston, 2002, p. 251.

[53] Nam, Y.S., Yoon, J.J., and Park, T.G. A novel fabrication method of macroporous biodegradable polymer scaffolds using gas foaming salt as a porogen additive. *J. Biomed. Mater. Res. (Appl. Biomater.)*, 53, 1, 2000.

[54] Hollinger, J.O. and Battistone, G.C. Biodegradable bone repair materials. Synthetic polymers and ceramics. *Clin. Orthop. Relat. Res.*, 207, 290, 1986.

[55] Nefussi, J.R. et al. Sequential expression of bone matrix proteins during rat calvaria osteoblast differentiation and bone nobule formation *in vitro*. *J. Histochem. Cytochem.*, 45, 493, 1997.

[56] Ishaug, S.L. et al. Bone formation by three-dimensional stromal osteoblast culture in biodegradable polymer scaffolds. *J. Biomed. Mater. Res.*, 36, 17, 1997.

[57] Shea, L. et al. Engineered bone development from pre-osteoblast cell line on three-dimensional scaffold. *Tissue Eng.*, 6, 605, 2000.

[58] Pavlin D. et al. Mechanical loading stimulates differentiation of periodontal osteoblasts in a mouse osteoinduction model: effect on type I collagen and alkaline phosphatase genes. *Calcif. Tissue Int.*, 67, 163, 2002.

[59] Sikavitsas, V.I., Temenoff, J.S., and Mikos, A.G. Biomaterials and bone mechanotransduction. *Biomaterials*, 22, 2581, 2001.

[60] Reich, K.M. and Frangos, J.A. Effect of flow on prostaglandin E2 inositol trisphosphate levels in osteoblasts. *Am. J. Physiol.*, 261, C429, 1991.

[61] Klein-Nulend, J. et al. Nitric oxide response to shear stress by human bone cell cultures is endothelial nitric oxide synthase dependent. *Biochem. Biophys. Res. Commun.*, 250, 108, 1998.

[62] Owan, I. et al. Mechanotransduction in bone: osteoblasts are more responsive to fluid forces than mechanical strain. *Am. J. Physiol.*, 273, C810, 1997.

[63] Knothe-Tate, M.L., Knothe, U., and Niederer, P. Experimental elucidation of mechanical load-induced fluid flow and its potential role in bone metabolism and functional adaptation. *Am. J. Med. Sci.*, 316, 189, 1998.

[64] Burger, E.H. and Klein-Nulend, J. Mechanotransduction in bone: role of the lacuno-canalicular network. *FASEB J.*, 13S, S101, 1997.

[65] Cowin, S.C. Bone poroelasticity. *J. Biomech.*, 32, 217, 1999.

[66] Van den Dolder, J. et al. Flow perfusion culture of marrow stromal osteoblasts in titanium fiber mesh. *J. Biomed. Mater. Res.*, 64A, 235, 2003.

[67] Meinel, L. et al. Bone tissue engineering using human mesenchymal stem cells: effects of scaffold material and medium flow. *Ann. Biomed. Eng.*, 32, 112, 2004.

[68] Sikavitsas, V.I. et al. Mineralized matrix deposition by marrow stromal osteoblasts in 3D perfusion culture increases with increasing fluid shear forces. *Proc. Natl Acad. Sci. USA*, 100, 14683, 2003.

[69] Neidlinger-Wilke, C., Wilke, H.J., and Claes, L. Cyclic stretching of human osteoblasts affects proliferation and metabolism: a new experimental method and its application. *J. Orthop. Res.*, 12, 70, 1994.

[70] Winter, L.C. et al. Intermittent versus continuous stretching effects on osteoblast-like cells *in vitro*. *J. Biomed. Mater. Res.*, 67A, 1269, 2003.

[71] Shimko, D. et al. A device for long term, *in vitro* loading of three-dimensional natural and engineered tissues. *Ann. Biomed. Eng.*, 31, 1347, 2003.

[72] Yonernori, K. Early effects of electrical stimulation on osteogenesis. *Bone*, 19, 173, 1996.

[73] Brighton, C.T. et al. Signal transduction in electrically stimulated bone cells. *J. Bone Joint Surg. Am.*, 83-A, 1514, 2003.

[74] Bassett, C.A., Pawluk, R.J., and Pilla, A.A. Augmentation of bone repair by inductively coupled electromagnetic fields. *Science*, 184, 575–577, 1984.

[75] Supronowicz, P.R. et al. Novel current-conducting composite substrates for exposing osteoblasts to alternating current stimulation. *J. Biomed. Mater. Res.*, 59, 499, 2002.

[76] Temenoff, J.S. and Mikos, A.G. Review: tissue engineering for regeneration of articular cartilage. *Biomaterials*, 21, 431, 2000.

[77] Hendrickson, D.A. et al. Chondrocyte-fibrin matrix transplants for resurfacing extensive articular cartilage defects. *J. Orthop. Res.*, 12, 485, 1994.

[78] Gooch, K.J. et al. Effects of mixing intensity on tissue-engineered cartilage. *Biotechnol. Bioeng.*, 72, 402, 2001.

[79] Pazzano, D. et al. Comparison of chondrogenesis in static and perfused bioreactor culture. *Biotechnol. Prog.*, 16, 893, 2000.

[80] Kuettner, K.E. Biochemistry of articular cartilage in health and disease. *Clin. Biochem.*, 25, 155, 1992.

[81] Shieh, A.C. and Athanasiou, K.A. Principles of cell mechanics for cartilage tissue engineering. *Ann. Biomed. Eng.*, 31, 1, 2003.

[82] Buschmann, M.D. et al. Stimulation of aggrecan synthesis in cartilage explants by cyclic loading is localized to regions of high interstitial fluid flow. *Arch. Biochem. Biophys.*, 366, 1, 1999.

[83] Guilak, F. et al. The effects of matrix compression on PG metabolism in articular cartilage explants. *Osteoarthr. Cartil.*, 2, 91, 1994.

[84] Hung, C. et al. A paradigm for functional tissue engineering of articular cartilage via applied physiologic deformational loading. *Ann. Biomed. Eng.*, 32, 35, 2004.

[85] Mizuno, S. et al. Hydrostatic fluid pressure enhances matrix synthesis and accumulation by bovine chondrocytes in three-dimensional culture. *J. Cell Physiol.*, 39, 319, 2002.

[86] Carver, S.E. and Heath, C.A. Influence of intermittent pressure, fluid flow, and mixing on the regenerative properties of articular chondrocytes. *Biotechnol. Bioeng.*, 65, 274, 1999.

[87] Altman, G.H. et al. Cell differentiation by mechanical stress. *FASEB J.*, 16, 270, 2002.

[88] Goh, J.C. et al. Tissue-engineering approach to the repair and regeneration of tendons and ligaments. *Tissue Eng.*, 9, S31, 2003.

[89] Langelier, E. et al. Cyclic traction machine for long-term culture of fibroblast-populated collagen gels. *Ann. Biomed. Eng.*, 27, 67, 1999.

[90] Goulet, F. et al. Tendons and ligaments, in *Principles of Tissue Engineering*, Lanza, R., Langer, R., and Vacanti, J. (Eds.), 2nd ed., Academic Press, New York, 2000, chap. 50.

[91] Awad, H.A. et al. *In vitro* characterization of mesenchymal stem cell-seeded collagen scaffolds for tendon repair: effects of initial seeding density on contraction kinetics. *J. Biomed. Mater. Res.*, 51, 233, 2000.

[92] Garvin et al. Novel system for engineering bioartificial tendons and application of mechanical load. *Tissue Eng.*, 9, 130–132, 2003.

[93] Powers, M.J. et al. A microfabricated array bioreactor for perfused 3D liver cultures. *Biotechnol. Bioeng.*, 78, 257, 2002.

[94] Eguchi, Y., Ogiue-Ikeda, M., and Ueno, S. Control of orientation of rat Schwann cells using an 8-T static magnetic field. *Neurosci. Lett.*, 351, 130, 2003.

[95] Miller, W.M. Bioreactor design considerations for cell therapies and tissue engineering. In *WTEC Workshop on Tissue Engineering Research in the United States, Proceedings*, MD: International Technology Research Institute, Loyola College, Baltimore, 2000, p. 5.

45

Animal Models for Evaluation of Tissue-Engineered Orthopedic Implants

Lichun Lu
Esmaiel Jabbari
Michael J. Moore
Michael J. Yaszemski
Mayo Clinic College of Medicine

45.1 Introduction

Animal models are an indispensable tool in tissue engineering research as they provide important inform-ation that may lead to eventual development of clinically useful treatment of diseases. Current tissue engineering strategies often involve three main components: cells, scaffolds, and bioactive factors for the repair or regeneration of a specific tissue type. Research in animal models thus bridges the gap between *in vitro* studies (such as scaffold degradation, cell–scaffold interactions, and scaffold toxicity) and human clinical trials. Animal models have been and will continue to be used to develop an understanding of each of the primary components separately, in combination, and ultimately in pathologic orthopedic conditions.

As an example, the appropriate sequence of studies for the development of a new biodegradable bone regeneration material might be (1) biomaterial synthesis and structural characterization; (2) scaffold fabrication and measurements of mechanical and degradation properties *in vitro*; (3) biocompatibility and bone formation assessed by cell culture *in vitro*; (4) biocompatibility and degradation of the material *in vivo*, typically by subcutaneous implantation in a lower-level animal model such as a rat; (5) if no significant toxic effect is observed, the material is then evaluated for its intended application such as an appropriate bone defect model in a higher-level animal such as a rabbit; (6) if the material functions well in small animals, then a well-controlled study in large animals such as primates may be considered before human clinical trials.

In this chapter, we first discuss the general considerations when selecting an animal model and the most commonly used animals in orthopedic research. Then, specific animal models for testing the biocompatibility and biodegradation of tissue-engineered constructs are described. Well-established animal models for the evaluation of osteogeneic or chondrogenic potential of these constructs are introduced. Finally, the experimental design and evaluation methods involved in the animal studies are reviewed.

45.2   Animal Model Selection

Studies using animal models may be deemed necessary if there are no other *in vitro* alternatives, the knowledge gained can be applied for the benefit of humans or animals, and the procedure does not cause extreme pain or disability to the animals. In an ideal animal model, the anatomy and physiology should be suitable for the specific study design, the pathogenesis and disease progression should parallel that of humans, and there should be a similar histopathologic response to that seen in humans [1]. The preclinical animal models in which the tissue-engineered constructs are tested should mimic the clinical situation as closely as possible.

The use of animals in tissue engineering research has become a scientific as well as an ethical issue. Generally, the use of invertebrates is preferred over vertebrates and the use of rats, rabbits, goats, and sheep are preferred over dogs and cats due to their pet status. All animal protocols should be approved by the researcher's Institutional Animal Care and Use Committee to ensure that the experiments are appropriately designed, the number of animals is justified, and the animal procedures comply with the Animal Welfare Act.

From a practical perspective, animals of a particular species, strain, type, age, or weight should be easily available for the entire experimental study [1]. It is preferable that the local animal research facility has the capacity to house these animals. The animals should also be easy to handle in terms of transportation, housing, peri-operative care, specimen handling, and disposal. The susceptibility of animals to disease is also an important consideration especially for long-term survival studies. Finally, the costs of animal purchasing, transportation, time for quarantine, housing, surgical supply, and special equipment should be carefully calculated before the project begins. Generally, larger animals impose more housing and handling difficulties than small animals such as rats and rabbits, and are more expensive.

45.3   Commonly Used Animals

Although a lower level vertebrate, the rat is among the most popular animal subjects in tissue engineering orthopedic research and often the first to consider for a new study due to its low cost and easy care and handling. Rats have a mean healthy life span of 21 to 24 months. After bone elongation ceases by the age of 6 to 9 months, considerable useful lifespan remains for experimental evaluation [1]. Rats have been used extensively in studies of biocompatibility [2], fracture [3], and bone defect repair [4]. The mouse, also a small rodent, has gained popularity in tissue engineering research because its genome can be easily manipulated and investigated. Both regular and immunocompromised nude mice have been widely used for osteogenesis [5] and chondrogenesis [6] in subcutaneous tissue.

Rabbits are another commonly used animal in tissue engineering research. They are a relatively higher vertebrate, with an appropriate size for surgical operation and analysis. Rabbits are suitable for studies of bone defect repair [7], articular cartilage repair [8], ligament reconstruction [9], and spine fusion [10]. The dog, a higher-level vertebrate, has also played a dominant role in orthopedic research and has been extensively used in studies of bone defect repair [11], cartilage repair [12], ligament reconstruction [9], and meniscus repair [13].

Goats have become increasingly popular in tissue engineering research. They have been used for studies of biocompatibility [14], bone repair [15], cartilage repair [16], meniscus repair [17], ligament reconstruction [9], and spine fusion [18]. Sheep are large animals similar to goats, but less literature is available for their application in tissue engineering research. They have been used in studies of bone defect repair [19], cartilage defect repair [20], meniscus repair [13], and ligament reconstruction [9].

Pigs have been used in studies such as osteonecrosis of the femoral head [21] and fractures of cartilage and bone [22]. A miniature pig articular cartilage defect model has also been established [23]. Horses have been used mainly for the studies of cartilage and joint conditions due to their rich cartilage tissue [24]. Primates would be ideal for tissue engineering research because they are the closest to humans; however, due to lack of availability and high cost, they are only chosen when absolutely necessary as a step before human clinical trials. They have been used in studies of bone repair [25], cartilage repair [26], and spinal conditions [27].

Other animals in orthopedic research, though less frequently used, include hamsters for implant infection, chickens for scoliosis and tendon repair, turkeys for bone remodeling, emus for osteonecrosis of the femoral head, cats for osteoarticular transplantation, and guinea pigs for osteoarthritis [1].

45.4 Specific Animal Models

45.4.1 Biocompatibility

The biocompatibility study, as the first *in vivo* step of biomaterial evaluation, is typically performed by subcutaneous or intramuscular implantation in rats or rabbits. The rat is more economical and offers about a 15 month observation period, while the rabbit is used for longer-term evaluations of up to 6 months. Discs of 10 mm in diameter and 1 mm in thickness are commonly inserted in the dorsal subcutaneous tissue or back muscles (up to six implants per rat and eight to ten per rabbit) [28]. Alternatively, porous discs, biomaterials with seeded or encapsulated cells, and biomaterials contained in a stainless steel wire mesh cage have been studied [29,30].

The factors that determine the biocompatibility of a biomaterial include its chemistry, structure, morphology, and degradation. Biomaterial implantation often induces an inflammatory response through the activation of macrophages. The degree of fibrosis and vascularization of the tissue reaction dictate the nature of the response [29]. For instance, a mature fibrous capsule was observed after 12 weeks surrounding the implanted poly(propylene fumarate)/beta-tricalcium phosphate (PPF/beta-TCP) scaffolds in rats. Photocrosslinked PPF scaffolds also elicited a mild inflammatory response in rabbits [31]. The soft tissue response to oligo(poly(ethylene glycol)fumarate) (OPF) hydrogels was affected by the block length of poly(ethylene glycol) in a rabbit model [32]. In a granular tissue reaction, fibrovascular tissue ingrowth into porous poly(L-lactic acid) (PLLA) scaffolds was found to depend on the pore size [33].

A wide range of other biodegradable materials have also been assessed for their biocompatibility including commonly used poly(lactic acid) (PLA), poly(glycolic acid) (PGA), and their copolymers [34], as well as natural materials such as crosslinked gelatin [35] and hyaluronic acid [36].

45.4.2 Biodegradation

Biodegradable materials should be fully characterized for their degradation properties *in vitro*, but these studies cannot substitute for *in vivo* evaluation of degradation. Often, the rate of material degradation is significantly different *in vivo* compared to the *in vitro* condition. For example, poly(DL-lactic-co-glycolic acid) (PLGA) foams [37] and injectable PPF/beta-TCP composites [2] were both found to degrade more rapidly *in vivo* than *in vitro*. Differences in degradation rate *in vivo* vs. *in vitro* may be due to the extent of perfusion, pH levels, enzymatic or inflammatory mechanisms, or mechanical loading. Moreover, the apparent biocompatibility of a material may be confounded by greater toxicity of degradation products or material fragments.

Initial *in vivo* biodegradation studies may be undertaken in models similar or identical to those addressed in Section 45.4.1. Typically, discs, rods, foams, or other constructs are implanted in mice or rabbits and evaluated at multiple time intervals for changes in dry mass, molecular weight, mechanical properties, dimensions, and geometry. Standardization of sample geometry and dimensions is desirable to allow for comparison among research groups [28]. Samples may be implanted in various soft tissue locations, including the subdermal or subcutaneous space, intramuscular regions, or in the mesentery or intraperitoneal cavity.

Tests under loading conditions similar to the target tissue are ideal to include effects of mechanical loading on material degradation. If the material in question will have contact with bone, soft tissue evaluation must be followed or replaced by evaluation in bony tissue. Bone defect models are numerous [28], and generally involve drilled or otherwise excised bone segments. For example, self-reinforced PLLA and poly(DL-lactic acid) (PDLLA) [38] have been evaluated by implantation in mandibular bone or a femoral cavity of Sprague-Dawley rats. Because bone naturally remodels, it exhibits great healing capacity, and for this reason, critical sized defects are often necessary for long-term evaluation. These are defects that will predictably not heal spontaneously.

The choice of animal model to evaluate biodegradation *in vivo* also depends on the duration of the bio-degradation study. For 1 to 6-month implantation studies, mice, rats, or rabbits can be used. Subdermal or subcutaneous implantation for up to 90 days in Sprague-Dawley rats has been used to evaluate bio-degradation of poly(carbonate urethane), poly(ether urethane) [39], poly(ester amides) [40], poly(ether carbonates) [30], and poly(tetrahydrofuran) [41]. However, for long-term implantation studies, larger animals such as goats, sheep, or dogs should be used. As an example, sheep have been used as a model to evaluate biodegradation of self-reinforced poly(L-lactide) screws for up to 3 years *in vivo* [42,43].

45.4.3 Osteogenesis

In bone tissue engineering applications, after promising *in vitro* cell culture results are revealed, it is often a first step to use a heterotopic animal model for testing *in vivo* osteogenesis of the constructs. The major heterotopic models include the subcutaneous model, intramuscular model, intraperitoneal model, and mesentery model. Tissue-engineered constructs, either alone or placed in diffusion chambers can be implanted in mice, rats, rabbits, dogs, pigs, goats, or primates [44]. The rat subcutaneous model is the most frequently used. For example, bone formation was observed by marrow stromal osteoblast transplantation in a porous ceramic [45]. Ectopic bone formation was also demonstrated by transplantation of PLGA foams to the rat mesentery [46].

Although the heterotopic models are useful to provide some information helping to bridge the gap of *in vitro* and *in vivo* studies, the results obtained may not be the same once the constructs are implanted in actual bone defects. Therefore, further studies must be performed in bone defect models. Among them, the rabbit calvarial defect model is a very popular and reproducible bone defect model [44]. The calvarial bone is a plate which allows creation of a uniform defect that enables convenient radiographic and histological analysis. The calvarial bone has an appropriate size for easier surgical procedures and specimen handling. Because of the support by the dura and the overlying skin, no fixation is needed. This model has recently been used to evaluate the osteogenicity of a composite scaffold of PPF and PLGA [47], and growth-factor-coated PPF scaffolds [48].

Common long bone defect models include the rabbit radial model (most popular), rat femoral model, and the dog radial model. A composite bone scaffold consisting of nano-hydroxyapatite, collagen, and PLA was found to integrate the rabbit radial defect after 12 weeks [49]. The effect of bone morphogenetic protein was evaluated in the rat femoral defect model [4]. It should be noted that the rat model requires either internal or external fixation. In the dog model, ulnae fractures may occur, resulting in unexpected loss.

Due to the regenerative capability of bone defects, it is typical in tissue engineering research to consider critical sized defects. The critical size of the defect (CSD), defined as the smallest size that does not heal by itself if left untreated over a certain period of time, is 15 mm in diameter for adult New Zealand white rabbit calvarial defect model. The rat calvarial model is also popular with a CSD of 8 mm in diameter. A bone biomimetic device consisting of a porous biodegradable scaffold of poly(DL-lactide) and type I collagen, human osteoblast precursor cells, and rhBMP-2 was shown to promote bone regeneration in this model [50]. The CSD of long bones is at least two times the bone diameter (e.g., 12 to 15 mm for rabbit radial model and 5 to 10 mm for rat femoral model).

45.4.4 Chondrogenesis

Similar to bone tissue engineering, the first step to test the chondrogenic potential of tissue-engineered cartilage constructs *in vivo* is to use heterotopic models by subcutaneous, intramuscular, or intraperitoneal implantation in nude mice, syngeneic mice, rats, or rabbits. Among them, implantation of the constructs in dorsal subcutaneous pouches of nude mice is the most popular. For example, constructs containing genetically engineered chondrocytes were implanted into nude mice to demonstrate transgene expression and synthesis of glycosaminoglycan [51].

Commonly used cartilage defect models include partial-thickness (chondral) and full-thickness (osteochondral) defects in rabbits and dogs [52]. The rabbit distal femoral defect model is a well-established, reproducible model. Creating a partial-thickness defect can be challenging because the cartilage thickness in the rabbit femoral condyles is only 0.25 to 0.75 mm (compared to 2.2 to 2.4 mm in humans) [53]. The dog distal femur defect model, by contrast, offers a larger defect size with which to work. Besides species, the age of the animal is also an important consideration since the potential for cartilage repair as well as the response to various treatments varies with different animals [53]. Skeletal maturity of the commonly used New Zealand white rabbits typically occurs between 4 and 6 months.

Tissue-engineered articular cartilage is generally anchored to a defect by press fitting, suture, fibrin glue, or by using a periosteal flap. The local mechanical environment is well known to influence chondrogenesis and tissue healing. In the rabbit knee model, a defect created on the distal femoral surface is considered weight bearing, while a defect in the intercondylar groove is partial weight bearing [52]. The type of postoperative treatment should also be considered; the use of continuous passive motion can enhance cartilage healing [54] whereas joint immobilization may lead to decreased articular cartilage regeneration [55].

Many naturally derived and synthetic polymers are currently used as scaffolds for regeneration of articular cartilage [56]. They function not only as a vehicle for the delivery and retention of chondrogenic cells, but also as a substrate for cell attachment and matrix production. Natural polymeric materials such as collagen, hyaluronic acid, alginate, and fibrin glue have been extensively studied, as well as many synthetic polymers including PLA, PGA, and poly(ethylene oxide) (PEO) [53]. More recently, a new synthetic hydrogel based on oligopolyethylene glycol fumarate (OPF) was developed for cartilage tissue engineering [57].

45.5 Experimental Studies

45.5.1 Experimental Design

The experimental design includes the experimental groups to be used, sample size, sampling error, and control groups. The number of animals depends on the intrinsic variability among the animals, the consistency of the surgical procedure, the accuracy of the evaluation methods, and the choice of statistical method for data analysis. The number of animals needed in a study can often be determined from the results of a preliminary pilot study. For example, six to eight animals can be used in a preliminary study with histomorphometry or mechanical testing as the evaluation methods [58,59]. From this preliminary study, the standard deviation of the mean, coefficient of variation, and mean difference among the groups are determined. The sample size is affected by the desired power, the acceptable significance level, and the expected effect size. To reduce the interanimal variance, the animals should be of the same strain, sex, age, and weight. Some of the experimental animal models such as Sprague-Dawley rats and New Zealand white rabbits have identical genetic traits, but dogs and cats are relatively heterogeneous [60]. Therefore larger numbers of animals are often required for studies employing dogs or cats. The number of animals also depends on the evaluation methods.

Sampling error reflects the inherent uncertainty of results about a population based on information gained from sample data, which is a subset of the population. Two sampling procedures used in biomedical research are random and stratified sampling [61,62]. In simple random sampling, each element of a population has an equal probability of being included. In stratified sampling, the elements are divided into nonoverlapping blocks, and specimens are chosen from each block by simple random sampling. Stratified sampling provides greater control over the distribution of specimens.

Controls in an experimental study include normal controls, treatment controls, and time controls. Unilateral, bilateral, unicortical, and bicortical bone models are being used in bone tissue engineering studies. Because of more efficient comparison between control and experimental groups, bilateral models are extensively used for evaluating biocompatibility and function of foreign materials in bones [63,64]. When major procedures are performed involving a joint, a unilateral model should be designed to allow the animal to heal over time. The bilateral cortical model is a design that doubles the number of specimens for testing if it is appropriate from animal use perspective [65,66].

45.5.2 Evaluation Methods

The evaluation method should be valid and capable of measuring the parameter of interest. The development of new evaluation methods requires assessment of its accuracy. Sources of error in an evaluation method are inadequate surgical procedures or specimen preparation, systemic error of testing systems, and data collection error. Clinical evaluation, necroscopy, morphological or structural analysis, biochemical evaluation, mechanical testing, and the use of specialized devices are used in orthopedic research for evaluation. The most commonly used methods in orthopedic animal research are clinical observation, radiography, histological evaluation, and mechanical testing [60].

One method of biocompatibility evaluation is the implantation of disk-shaped samples of the material into the right and left epididymal fat pads or the right and left rear haunch subcutaneous tissue [67]. The following are removed at autopsy: the implant with its surrounding capsule, skin and subcutaneous tissue, the axillary and popliteal lymph nodes, heart, kidneys, lungs, liver, spleen, brain, and aorta, as well as any macroscopically unusual findings in the stomach, bowels, and mesenteric lymph nodes [68,69]. For evaluation of bone growth in explanted skeletal specimens, the total cross-sectional area of newly formed trabecular bone is determined on sequential longitudinal sections [70–72]. Confocal microscopy is utilized for cell visualization and morphology [73]. Alkaline phosphatase activity and calcium content are measured to assess the extent of mineralization in newly formed bone [74,75]. Western analyses of the newly synthesized collagen types I, II, and IX from the explanted samples are done using monoclonal antibodies and chemiluminescent substrate [76,77].

The explanted bone samples should be tested intact to establish reference mechanical properties [78]. Loads should be applied in a manner that minimizes focal loading of the specimen, so that accurate, representative material properties are measured. Preconditioning the specimens by cyclic loading, over several complete load-unload cycles, to a peak compressive force of approximately one average body weight (70 kg) is reasonable to do. This technique tends to smooth out variability in the data, and increases the likelihood of obtaining reproducible data.

References

[1] An, Y.H. and Friedman, R.J., Animal selections in orthopaedic research, in *Animal Models in Orthopaedic Research*, An, Y.H. and Friedman, R.J. (Eds.), CRC Press, Boca Raton, FL, 1999, p. 39.

[2] Peter, S.J. et al., *In vivo* degradation of a poly(propylene fumarate)/beta-tricalcium phosphate injectable composite scaffold, *J. Biomed. Mater. Res.* 41, 1, 1998.

[3] An, Y. et al., Production of a standard closed fracture in the rat tibia, *J. Orthop. Trauma* 8, 111, 1994.

[4] Yasko, A.W. et al., The healing of segmental bone defects, induced by recombinant human bone morphogenetic protein (rhBMP-2). A radiographic, histological, and biomechanical study in rats, *J. Bone Joint Surg. Am.* 74, 659, 1992.

[5] Miyazawa, K., Kawai, T., and Urist, M.R., Bone morphogenetic protein-induced heterotopic bone in osteopetrosis, *Clin. Orthop. Relat. Res.* 324, 259, 1996.

[6] Paige, K.T. et al., *De novo* cartilage generation using calcium alginate-chondrocyte constructs, *Plast. Reconstr. Surg.* 97, 168, 1996.

[7] Roy, T.D. et al., Performance of degradable composite bone repair products made via three-dimensional fabrication techniques, *J. Biomed. Mater. Res.* 66A, 283, 2003.

[8] Wakitani, S. et al., Repair of large full-thickness articular cartilage defects with allograft articular chondrocytes embedded in a collagen gel, *Tissue Eng.* 4, 429, 1998.

[9] Carpenter, J.E. and Hankenson, K.D., Animal models of tendon and ligament injuries for tissue engineering applications, *Biomaterials* 25, 1715, 2004.

[10] Boden, S.D., Biology of lumbar spine fusion and use of bone graft substitutes: present, future, and next generation, *Tissue Eng.* 6, 383, 2000.

[11] Johnson, K.D. et al., Evaluation of ground cortical autograft as a bone graft material in a new canine bilateral segmental long bone defect model, *J. Orthop. Trauma* 10, 28, 1996.

[12] Lee, C.R. et al., Effects of a cultured autologous chondrocyte-seeded type II collagen scaffold on the healing of a chondral defect in a canine model, *J. Orthop. Res.* 21, 272, 2003.

[13] Buma, P. et al., Tissue engineering of the meniscus, *Biomaterials* 25, 1523, 2004.

[14] Mendes, S.C. et al., Biocompatibility testing of novel starch-based materials with potential application in orthopaedic surgery: a preliminary study, *Biomaterials* 22, 2057, 2001.

[15] Kruyt, M.C. et al., Optimization of bone–tissue engineering in goats, *J. Biomed. Mater. Res.* 69B, 113, 2004.

[16] Butnariu-Ephrat, M. et al., Resurfacing of goat articular cartilage by chondrocytes derived from bone marrow, *Clin. Orthop. Relat. Res.* 330, 234, 1996.

[17] Port, J. et al., Meniscal repair supplemented with exogenous fibrin clot and autogenous cultured marrow cells in the goat model, *Am. J. Sports Med.* 24, 547, 1996.

[18] Kruyt, M.C. et al., Bone tissue engineering and spinal fusion: the potential of hybrid constructs by combining osteoprogenitor cells and scaffolds, *Biomaterials* 25, 1463, 2004.

[19] Viljanen, V.V. et al., Xenogeneic mouse (*Alces alces*) bone morphogenetic protein (mBMP)-induced repair of critical-size skull defects in sheep, *Int. J. Oral Maxillofac. Surg.* 25, 217, 1996.

[20] Homminga, G.N. et al., Repair of sheep articular cartilage defects with a rabbit costal perichondrial graft, *Acta Orthop. Scand.* 62, 415, 1991.

[21] Seiler, J.G., III et al., Posttraumatic osteonecrosis in a swine model. Correlation of blood cell flux, MRI and histology, *Acta Orthop. Scand.* 67, 249, 1996.

[22] Tomatsu, T. et al., Experimentally produced fractures of articular cartilage and bone. The effects of shear forces on the pig knee, *J. Bone Joint Surg. Br.* 74, 457, 1992.

[23] Hunziker, E.B., Driesang, I.M., and Morris, E.A., Chondrogenesis in cartilage repair is induced by members of the transforming growth factor-beta superfamily, *Clin. Orthop. Relat. Res.* 391S, S171, 2001.

[24] Litzke, L.E. et al., Repair of extensive articular cartilage defects in horses by autologous chondrocyte transplantation, *Ann. Biomed. Eng.* 32, 57, 2004.

[25] Cancian, D.C. et al., Utilization of autogenous bone, bioactive glasses, and calcium phosphate cement in surgical mandibular bone defects in *Cebus apella* monkeys, *Int. J. Oral Maxillofac. Implants* 19, 73, 2004.

[26] Buckwalter, J.A. et al., Osteochondral repair of primate knee femoral and patellar articular surfaces: implications for preventing post-traumatic osteoarthritis, *Iowa Orthop. J.* 23, 66, 2003.

[27] Boden, S.D., Grob, D., and Damien, C., Ne-osteo bone growth factor for posterolateral lumbar spine fusion: results from a nonhuman primate study and a prospective human clinical pilot study, *Spine* 29, 504, 2004.

[28] An, Y.H. and Friedman, R.J., Animal models for testing bioabsorbable materials, in *Animal Models in Orthopaedic Research*, An, Y.H. and Friedman, R.J. (Eds.), CRC Press, Boca Raton, FL, 1999, p. 219.

[29] Babensee, J.E. et al., Host response to tissue engineered devices, *Adv. Drug Deliv. Rev.* 33, 111, 1998.

[30] Dadsetan, M. et al., *In vivo* biocompatibility and biodegradation of poly(ethylene carbonate), *J. Control. Release* 93, 259, 2003.

[31] Fisher, J.P. et al., Soft and hard tissue response to photocrosslinked poly(propylene fumarate) scaffolds in a rabbit model, *J. Biomed. Mater. Res.* 59, 547, 2002.

[32] Shin, H. et al., *In vivo* bone and soft tissue response to injectable, biodegradable oligo(poly(ethylene glycol) fumarate) hydrogels, *Biomaterials* 24, 3201, 2003.

[33] Wake, M.C., Patrick, C.W., Jr., and Mikos, A.G., Pore morphology effects on the fibrovascular tissue growth in porous polymer substrates, *Cell Transplant* 3, 339, 1994.

[34] Behravesh, E. et al., Synthetic biodegradable polymers for orthopaedic applications, *Clin. Orthop. Relat. Res.* 367S, S118, 1999.

[35] Hong, S.R. et al., Biocompatibility and biodegradation of cross-linked gelatin/hyaluronic acid sponge in rat subcutaneous tissue, *J. Biomater. Sci. Polym. Ed.* 15, 201, 2004.

[36] Baier Leach, J. et al., Photocrosslinked hyaluronic acid hydrogels: natural, biodegradable tissue engineering scaffolds, *Biotechnol. Bioeng.* 82, 578, 2003.

[37] Lu, L. et al., *In vitro* and *in vivo* degradation of porous poly(DL-lactic-co-glycolic acid) foams, *Biomaterials* 21, 1837, 2000.

[38] Majola, A. et al., Absorption, biocompatibility, and fixation properties of polylactic acid in bone tissue: an experimental study in rats, *Clin. Orthop. Relat. Res.* 268, 260, 1991.

[39] Christenson, E.M. et al., Poly(carbonate urethane) and poly(ether urethane) biodegradation: *in vivo* studies, *J. Biomed. Mater. Res.* 69A, 407, 2004.

[40] Tsitlanadze, G. et al., Biodegradation of amino-acid-based poly(ester amide)s: *in vitro* weight loss and preliminary *in vivo* studies, *J. Biomater. Sci. Polym. Ed.* 15, 1, 2004.

[41] Pol, B.J. et al., *In vivo* testing of crosslinked polyethers. I. Tissue reactions and biodegradation, *J. Biomed. Mater. Res.* 32, 307, 1996.

[42] Jukkala-Partio, K. et al., Biodegradation and strength retention of poly-L-lactide screws *in vivo*. An experimental long-term study in sheep, *Ann. Chir. Gynaecol.* 90, 219, 2001.

[43] Suuronen, R. et al., A 5-year *in vitro* and *in vivo* study of the biodegradation of polylactide plates, *J. Oral Maxillofac. Surg.* 56, 604, 1998.

[44] An, Y.H. and Friedman, R.J., Animal models of bone defect repair, in *Animal Models in Orthopaedic Research*, An, Y.H. and Friedman, R.J. (Eds.), CRC Press, Boca Raton, FL, 1999, p. 241.

[45] Gao, J. et al., Tissue-engineered fabrication of an osteochondral composite graft using rat bone marrow-derived mesenchymal stem cells, *Tissue Eng.* 7, 363, 2001.

[46] Ishaug-Riley, S.L. et al., Ectopic bone formation by marrow stromal osteoblast transplantation using poly(DL-lactic-co-glycolic acid) foams implanted into the rat mesentery, *J. Biomed. Mater. Res.* 36, 1, 1997.

[47] Dean, D. et al., Poly(propylene fumarate) and poly(DL-lactic-co-glycolic acid) as scaffold materials for solid and foam-coated composite tissue-engineered constructs for cranial reconstruction, *Tissue Eng.* 9, 495, 2003.

[48] Vehof, J.W. et al., Bone formation in transforming growth factor beta-1-coated porous poly(propylene fumarate) scaffolds, *J. Biomed. Mater. Res.* 60, 241, 2002.

[49] Liao, S.S. et al., Hierarchically biomimetic bone scaffold materials: nano-HA/collagen/PLA composite, *J. Biomed. Mater. Res.* 69B, 158, 2004.

[50] Winn, S.R. et al., Tissue-engineered bone biomimetic to regenerate calvarial critical-sized defects in athymic rats, *J. Biomed. Mater. Res.* 45, 414, 1999.

[51] Madry, H. et al., Gene transfer of a human insulin-like growth factor I cDNA enhances tissue engineering of cartilage, *Hum. Gene Ther.* 13, 1621, 2002.

[52] An, Y.H. and Friedman, R.J., Animal models of articular cartilage defect, in *Animal Models in Orthopaedic Research*, An, Y.H. and Friedman, R.J. (Eds.), CRC Press, Boca Raton, FL, 1999, p. 309.

[53] Reinholz, G.G. et al., Animal models for cartilage reconstruction, *Biomaterials* 25, 1511, 2004.

[54] O'Driscoll, S.W. and Salter, R.B., The repair of major osteochondral defects in joint surfaces by neo-chondrogenesis with autogenous osteoperiosteal grafts stimulated by continuous passive motion. An experimental investigation in the rabbit, *Clin. Orthop. Relat. Res.* 208, 131, 1986.

[55] Vanwanseele, B., Lucchinetti, E., and Stussi, E., The effects of immobilization on the characteristics of articular cartilage: current concepts and future directions, *Osteoarthr. Cartil.* 10, 408, 2002.

[56] Temenoff, J.S. and Mikos, A.G., Injectable biodegradable materials for orthopedic tissue engineering, *Biomaterials* 21, 2405, 2000.

[57] Holland, T.A. et al., Transforming growth factor-beta1 release from oligo(poly(ethylene glycol) fumarate) hydrogels in conditions that model the cartilage wound healing environment, *J. Control Release* 94, 101, 2004.

[58] Munro, B.H., Jacobson, B.J., and Braitman, L.E., Introduction to inferential statistics and hypothesis testing, in *Statistical Methods for Health Care Research*, 2nd ed., Munro, B.H. and Page, E.B. (Eds.), Lippincott, Philadelphia, 1993.

[59] Matthews, D.E. and Farewell, V.T., *Using and Understanding Medical Statistics*, 3rd ed, Basel Karger, London, 1996.

[60] An, Y.H. and Bell, T.D., Experimental design, evaluation methods, data analysis, publication, and research ethics, in *Animal Models in Orthopaedic Research*, An, Y.H. and Friedman, R.J. (Eds.), CRC Press, Boca Raton, FL, 1999, p. 15.

[61] Manly, B.J., *The Design and Analysis of Research Studies*, Cambridge University Press, Cambridge, 1992.

[62] Forthofer, R.N. and Lee, E.S., *Introduction to Biostatistics. A Guide to Design, Analysis, and Discovery*, Academic Press, San Diego, CA, 1995.

[63] Laberge, M. and Powers, D.L., Scientific basis for bilateral animal models in orthopaedics, *J. Invest. Surg.* 4, 109, 1991.

[64] An, Y.H. et al., Fixation of osteotomies using bioabsorbable screws in the canine femur, *Clin. Orthop. Relat. Res.* 355, 300, 1998.

[65] Thomas, K.A. and Cook, S.D., An evaluation of variables influencing implant fixation by direct bone apposition, *J. Biomed. Mater. Res.* 19, 875, 1985.

[66] Thomas, K.A. et al., The effect of surface treatments on the interface mechanics of LTI pyrolytic carbon implants, *J. Biomed. Mater. Res.* 19, 145, 1985.

[67] Kidd, K.R. et al., A comparative evaluation of the tissue responses associated with polymeric implants in the rat and mouse, *J. Biomed. Mater. Res.* 59, 682, 2002.

[68] Nary Filho, H. et al., Comparative study of tissue response to polyglecaprone 25, polyglactin 910 and polytetrafluorethylene structure materials in rats, *Braz. Dent. J.* 13, 86, 2002.

[69] Eltze, E. et al., Influence of local complications on capsule formation around model implants in a rat model, *J. Biomed. Mater. Res.* 64A, 12, 2003.

[70] Lewandrowski, K.U. et al., Effect of a poly(propylene fumarate) foaming cement on the healing of bone defects, *Tissue Eng.* 5, 305, 1999.

[71] Schantz, J.T. et al., Induction of ectopic bone formation by using human periosteal cells in combination with a novel scaffold technology, *Cell Transplant* 11, 125, 2002.

[72] Yasin, M. and Tighe, B.J., Polymers for biodegradable medical devices. VIII. Hydroxybutyrate-hydroxyvalerate copolymers: physical and degradative properties of blends with polycaprolactone, *Biomaterials* 13, 9, 1992.

[73] Behravesh, E. and Mikos, A.G., Three-dimensional culture of differentiating marrow stromal osteo-blasts in biomimetic poly(propylene fumarate-co-ethylene glycol)-based macroporous hydrogels, *J. Biomed. Mater. Res.* 66A, 698, 2003.

[74] Temenoff, J.S. et al., *In vitro* osteogenic differentiation of marrow stromal cells encapsulated in biodegradable hydrogels, *J. Biomed. Mater. Res.* 70A, 235, 2004.

[75] Temenoff, J.S. et al., Thermally cross-linked oligo(poly(ethylene glycol) fumarate) hydrogels support osteogenic differentiation of encapsulated marrow stromal cells *in vitro*, *Biomacromolecules* 5, 5, 2004.

[76] Adkisson, H.D. et al., *In vitro* generation of scaffold independent neocartilage, *Clin. Orthop. Relat. Res.* 391S, S280, 2001.

[77] Gibson, G. et al., Type X collagen is colocalized with a proteoglycan epitope to form distinct morphological structures in bovine growth cartilage, *Bone* 19, 307, 1996.

[78] Elder, S. et al., Biomechanical evaluation of calcium phosphate cement-augmented fixation of unstable intertrochanteric fractures, *J. Orthop. Trauma* 14, 386, 2000.

46

The Regulation of Engineered Tissues: Emerging Approaches

Kiki B. Hellman
The Hellman Group, LLC

David Smith
Teregenics, LLC

46.1 Introduction

A critical step in translating tissue engineering research into product applications for the clinic and marketplace is understanding the strategies developed by government agencies for providing appropriate regulatory oversight. Since the eventual goal is the establishment of a global industry with the ability of companies to market products across national boundaries, a harmonized international regulatory approach would be ideal. However, while groups actively work toward that end, and, recognizing that market acceptance can be influenced by local cultural, ethical, and legal concerns, it is essential to recognize and appreciate the approaches of the regulatory agencies of those countries where engineered tissue research is already moving into product development and clinical application. While the science in the field is now worldwide in scope [1], we will limit our discussion to the regulatory approaches of the United States, with attention to emerging trends in Europe and Japan.

The U.S. Food and Drug Administration (FDA) has recognized that an important segment of the products it regulates arises from applications of new technology such as tissue engineering, and that, the product applications pose unique and complex questions. As a result, the agency has devoted considerable resources, from the 1990s on, to the regulatory considerations of what have been termed human cellular and tissue-based products (HCT/Ps).

In February 1997, FDA proposed a comprehensive approach (the "Proposed Approach") for regulation of these products, which was tier-based with the level of product review proportionate to the degree of risk [2]. Tissues recovered and processed by methods which did not change tissue function or characteristics (i.e., tissues which have not been more than "minimally manipulated") did not require premarket application review and approval. These "banked" human tissues, such as cornea, skin, umbilical cord blood stem cells, cartilage, and bone would be regulated under Section 361 of the Public Health Service (PHS) Act (42 USC §264), under which the agency is empowered to take action to prevent the spread of infectious disease. All other products would be regulated as medical products for which clinical testing and premarket applications would be required, with the expectation that most would be classified as either biological drugs ("biologics") (Section 351 of the PHS Act) [3] or medical devices ("devices") [Food, Drug and Cosmetic (FD&C) Act, 1976 Amendments] [4]. Specific jurisdiction over biologics and devices is generally assigned within the FDA to the Center for Biologics Evaluation and Research (CBER) or the Center for Devices and Radiological Health (CDRH), respectively, two of the agency's internal medical product review centers.

However, as these products typically consist of more than one component, such as biomolecules, cells, or tissues combined with a biomaterial, they are considered "Combination Products" and regulated under the jurisdiction of CBER, CDRH, or the FDA's third medical product review center, the Center for Drug Evaluation and Research (CDER). A determination of the product's primary mode of action dictates the jurisdictional authority for the product and the primary reviewing center; other centers act as consultants in the review process.

The FDA followed its issue of the Proposed Approach with a series of proposed rules to begin the process of translating its thinking about the regulation of HCT/Ps into law. In May 1998, the agency published two proposed rules to implement aspects of the proposed approach which would (1) create a unified system for registering establishments that manufacture HCT/Ps and for the listing of their products [5]. The following year it released a proposed rule to require most cell and tissue donors to be tested for relevant communicable diseases [6]. A proposed rule to require compliance with current good tissue practice by manufacturers of Human Cellular and Tissue-Based Products and to provide for inspection and enforcement was issued in 2001 [7]. Over the last few years, FDA has converted these proposed rules into final rules and new regulations having the force of law (Table 46.1). The last of these final rules, regarding donor eligibility and current good tissue pracices, became effective as of May 25, 2005.

Because of the continuing concern of communicable disease transmission, the FDA is now in the process of establishing a comprehensive new system for HCT/Ps formerly considered as "banked" human tissue. New regulations would require manufacturers of HCT/Ps to follow current good tissue practices (cGTP), such as proper product handling, processing, storage and labeling, as well as recordkeeping and establishment of a quality program [7]. In addition, manufacturers would be subject to inspection and enforcement activity by the agency.

46.2 FDA Regulation

Broad authority to control the distribution and sale of medical products in the United States has been granted to the FDA under the federal Food, Drug, and Cosmetic Act (FD&C Act) and the Public Health Service Act (PHS Act). The FD&C Act contains numerous provisions regarding the development and distribution of medical products classifiable as "drugs" or "devices." The PHS Act contains just two sections of particular importance to FDA regulation of medical products, especially those derived through tissue engineering: §351 prohibits the distribution of unlicensed "biological products" and establishes criteria and procedures the FDA shall observe in issuing such licenses; and §361 empowers the FDA to prevent the spread of communicable diseases.

TABLE 46.1   Key FDA Documents Concerning Regulation of Human Tissue and Cell Therapies[a]

1.   FDA Notice: Application of Current Statutory Authorities to Human Somatic Cell Therapy Products and Gene Therapy Products (58 FR 53248; October 14, 1993)
2.   FDA Notice of Interim Rule: Human Tissue Intended for Transplantation (58 FR 65514; December 14, 1993)
3.   FDA Notice of Public Hearing: Products Comprising Living Autologous Cells Manipulated *ex vivo* and Intended for Implantation for Structural Repair or Reconstruction (60 FR 36808; July 18, 1995)
4.   FDA Final Rule: Elimination of Establishment License Application for Specified Biotechnology and Specified Synthetic Biological Products (61 FR 24227; May 14, 1996)
5.   FDA Notice: Availability of Guidance on Applications for Products Comprising Living Autologous Cells … (etc.) (61 FR 26523; May 28, 1996)
6.   FDA Guidance on Applications for Products Comprised of Living Autologous Cells Manipulated of *ex vivo* and Intended for Structural Repair or Reconstruction (61 FR 24227; May 14, 1996)
7.   FDA Proposed Approach to Regulation of Cellular and Tissue-Based Products (February 28, 1997)
8.   FDA Notification of Proposed Regulatory Approach Regarding Cellular and Tissue-Based Products (62 FR 9721; March 4, 1997)
9.   FDA Final Rule: Human Tissue Intended for Transplantation (62 FR 40429; July 29, 1997)
10.   FDA Notice: Availability of Guidance on Screening and Testing of Donors of Human Tissue Intended for Transplantation (62 FR 40536; July 29, 1997)
11.   FDA Guidance to Industry: Screening and Testing of Donors of Human Tissue Intended for Transplantation (July 29, 1997)
12.   FDA Guidance for Industry: Guidance for Human Somatic Cell Therapy and Gene Therapy (March, 1998)
13.   FDA Proposed Rule: Establishment Registration and Listing for Manufacturers of Human Cellular and Tissue-Based Products (63 FR 26744; May 14, 1998)
14.   FDA Proposed Rule: Eligibility Determination for Donors of Human Cellular and Tissue-Based Products (64 FR 52696; September 30, 1999)
15.   FDA Proposed Rule: Current Good Tissue Practice for Manufacturers of Human Cellular and Tissue-Based Products; Inspection and Enforcement (66 FR 1508; January 8, 2001)
16.   FDA Final Rule: Human Cells, Tissues, and Cellular and Tissue-Based Products; Establishment Registration and Listing (66 FR 5447; January 19, 2001)
17.   FDA Final Rule: Human Cells, Tissues, and Cellular and Tissue-Based Products; Establishment Registration and Listing; Delay of Effective Date (68 FR 2689; January 21, 2003)
18.   FDA Interim Final Rule: Human Cells, Tissues, and Cellular and Tissue-Based Products; Establishment Registration and Listing (69 FR 3823; January 27, 2004)
19.   FDA Final Rule: Eligibility Determination for Donors of Human Cellular and Tissue-Based Products (69 FR 29786; May 25, 2004)
20.   FDA Final Rule: Current Good Tissue Practice for Human Cell, Tissue and Cellular Tissue-Based Product Establishments: Inspection and Enforcement (69 FR 68612; November 24, 2004)

[a]With the exception of Document #1, each document listed here can be obtained through the FDA Web site (www.fda.gov/cber). While provisions of the FD&C and PHS Acts and the Final Rules, codified as part of the Code of Federal Regulations (CFR), promulgated thereunder by the FDA, have the force of law and are binding on the agency, FDA guidance documents are not. Nevertheless, guidances are clearly helpful in anticipating the agency's response to particular marketing approval and other regulatory issues.

Exercising its authority under these statutes, the FDA has adopted a set of regulations that control virtually every aspect of the development and marketing of a medical product according to the potential risk of harm the product may pose to patients or the public health. Thus, the FDA regulates the introduction, manufacture, advertising, labeling, packaging, marketing and distribution of, and record-keeping for, such products.

As a rule, the FDA requires a sponsor of a new medical product to submit a formal application for approval to market the product after the completion of preclinical studies and phased clinical trials that demonstrate to the agency's satisfaction that the product is safe and effective. The form and review of that request to initiate human trials and the subsequent marketing application vary according to the classification of the product with reference to categories established in the statutes granting regulatory authority to the FDA.

46.2.1 Classification of Medical Products

Under current federal law, every medical product is classifiable as a drug, device, biological product (a "biologic"), or "combination product" (i.e., a combination device/drug, device/biologic, etc.). The classification of the product determines the particular processes of review and approval the FDA may employ in determining the safety and efficacy of the product for human use.

Under the FD&C Act (at §201(g)(1)), a "*drug*" is broadly defined as

> *[an article] intended for use in the diagnosis, cure, mitigation, treatment, or prevention of disease ... [or] ... intended to affect the structure or any function of the body.*

The FD&C Act (at §201(h)) defines a "*device*" largely by what it is not (i.e., neither a drug nor a biologic):

> *an instrument, apparatus, implement, machine, contrivance, implant, in vitro reagent, or other similar related article ... intended for use in the diagnosis of disease or other conditions, or in the cure, mitigation, treatment or prevention of disease ... or intended to affect the structure or any function of the body ... and which does not achieve any of its primary intended purposes through chemical action within or on the body ... and which is not dependent upon being metabolized for the achievement of any of its primary intended purposes.[Emphasis added.]*

Finally, the PHS Act (at §351(a)) defines a "*biologic*" as

> *any virus, therapeutic serum, toxin, antitoxin, vaccine, blood, blood component or derivative, allergenic product, or analogous product" applicable to the prevention, treatment or cure of diseases or injuries.*

Not surprisingly, the advance of medical technology has generated products not readily classifiable as drugs, devices, or biologics as those terms have been defined by federal statute. To provide for the expanding varieties of products expressing features of more than one of those classifications, the FDA has been authorized to recognize "combination products." A combination product is classified, assigned to a particular center, and regulated as a drug, device, or biologic according to its "primary mode of action," as determined by the FDA. Disputes over the classification of a combination product between a sponsor and the FDA or between centers are submitted to the FDA's ombudsman in the Office of the Combination Products for resolution. In fact, the FDA's current approach to the regulation of engineered tissue products began with the ombudsman's consideration of the classification of the Carticel™ autologous cartilage repair service developed by Genzyme Tissue Repair in 1995.

The Office of the Combination Products was established under the aegis of the Medical Device User Fee and Modernization Act of 2002. This office has responsibilities over the regulatory life cycle of combination products, and (1) assigns the FDA Center for primary review jurisdiction of the product; (2) works with FDA Centers to develop regulatory guidance and clarify regulation of these products; and (3) serves as a focal point for combination product-related issues for internal and external stakeholders.

With respect to engineered tissue products, the consequences inuring to the device and biologic classifications deserve particular attention. First, and most importantly, a medical product cannot be a device if its therapeutic or diagnostic benefit is obtained through metabolization, a limitation in the statutory definition of a device that might appear to exclude any product incorporating and depending on the function of any living human tissues. Nevertheless, allogeneic skin products such as Organogenesis's Apligraf have been classified and granted market approval as devices. They were considered interactive wound and burn dressings and, hence, classified as devices, since CDRH has regulating jurisdiction over wound and burn dressings. As engineered tissue products become less "structural" and more "functional" that is, more interactive with the host or require metabolism by the host, in nature, a "device" classification may become more difficult to square with the current statutory definition.

46.2.2 Special Product Designations

The FD&C Act recognizes that demand for all new medical products is not equally large or robust, such that the cost of obtaining marketing approval for a given product may be prohibitive in view of the relatively small size of the population it will benefit. To reduce the likelihood that a financial cost–benefit analysis applied to rarer diseases will leave them untreated, the FDA is authorized to grant special considerations and exceptions to reduce the economic burden upon developers of products under such conditions. Thus, the FDA may be petitioned to grant a "humanitarian device exemption" for certain devices (FD&C Act, §520(m)) or to recognize certain drugs or biologics as "orphan drugs" (FD&C Act, §525, et. seq.). However, the significance or value of these designations — especially for sponsors of tissue products — varies considerably according to the classification of the product in question.

Humanitarian use devices are those intended to treat a disease or condition that affects fewer than 4000 people in the United States. The FDA is authorized to exempt a sponsor from the obligation to demonstrate the effectiveness of such a device to obtain marketing approval; however, the sponsor is precluded from selling the product for more than the cost to develop and produce it.

Orphan drugs are those intended to treat a disease or condition affecting fewer than 200,000 persons in the United States, or for which there is little likelihood that the cost of developing and distributing it in the United States will be recovered from sales of the drug in the United States. The orphan drug designation was established through an amendment of the FD&C Act by the 1982 Orphan Drug Act (ODA) prior to the creation of the humanitarian device exemption. In contrast to the humanitarian use device designation, the orphan drug designation could be important to sponsors of certain engineered tissue products classifiable as biologics, illustrating the larger implications of the classification process. An orphan drug is defined to include biologics specifically licensed under §351 of the PHS Act, a distinction which may be relevant under the FDA's proposed plan for regulating engineered tissue products (see below). The FDA is empowered, under certain conditions, to grant marketing exclusivity for an orphan drug in the United States for a period of seven years from the date the drug is approved for clinical use; this exclusivity is stronger than and far less expensive to maintain than that provided by a patent. Additional benefits of the orphan drug designation include: certain tax credits for clinical research expenses; cash grant support for clinical trials; and waiver of the expensive prescription drug filing fee. A petition for orphan drug designation must be filed before any application for marketing approval.

46.2.3 Human Cellular and Tissue-Based Products

While a broad range of potential therapeutic applications for engineered tissues is being developed, they fall into two general categories, those providing either a structural/mechanical or a metabolic function. Structural/mechanical applications include approaches for skin, musculoskeletal, cardiovascular, and central nervous systems, among them, while metabolic applications include therapies for conditions such as diabetes and liver disease.

The FDA defines an HCT/P as a "product containing or consisting of human cells or tissue that is intended for implantation, transplantation, infusion, or transfer into a human recipient" and, in addition to those indicated previously, includes cadaveric ligaments, dura mater, heart valves, manipulated autologous chondrocytes, and spermatozoa [7]. Since determining the regulatory process for certain HCT/Ps may be complicated, the agency will rely on the Tissue Reference Group (TRG) composed of representatives from CBER, CDRH, and Office of Combination Products in the Office of the Commissioner to provide a single reference point and make recommendations to the center directors regarding product jurisdiction of specific tissue products.

Much of the regulatory framework for engineered tissues has been promulgated by the FDA through formal, binding, rule-making procedures. Previously the FDA had issued a number of documents which, while not binding upon the Agency, provide the public with a formal expression of its evolving thinking regarding the future regulation of human cellular or tissue-based products (see Table 46.1). Of these documents, by far the most important has been the Proposed Approach to Regulation of Cellular and Tissue-Based Products ("Proposed Approach") that the FDA issued on February 28, 1997.

The Proposed Approach outlined a plan of regulatory oversight, which may include a premarket approval requirement for such tissue products based upon a matrix ranking the products, classified by certain characteristics, within identified areas of regulatory concern. These tissue products would be classified according to the relationship between the donor and the recipient of the biological material used to produce the tissue product; the degree of *ex vivo* manipulation of the cells comprising the tissue product; and whether the tissue product is intended for a homologous use, for metabolic or structural purposes, or is to be combined with a device, drug, or another biologic.

Since issuing the Proposed Approach more than seven years ago, the FDA has been working to formalize its regulation of human tissue and cell therapies through a rule-making process to amend the U.S. Code of Federal Regulations ("CFR"). This process was completed as of May 25, 2005, when the last of the regulations implementing the proposed approach went into effect (see Table 46.1).

In introducing the February 1997 "Proposed Approach," the FDA identified five areas of regulatory concern raised by the development of new medical products derived from the manipulation of human biological materials: communication of infectious disease; processing and handling; clinical safety and efficacy; indicated uses and promotional claims; and monitoring and education (Table 46.2).

The FDA has proposed that autologous tissue that is banked, processed, or stored should be tested for infection agents and it will require companies to keep appropriate records to assure that patient tissues are not mismatched or commingled. The agency proposes that allogeneic tissue be tested for infection agents, that donors be screened, and that appropriate records be kept. Periodic submissions to the agency showing compliance with the testing or record-keeping requirements will not be necessary; the FDA assumes that a company's observation of these requirements will be assured through the accreditation they can be expected to maintain with professional tissue banking or processing societies.

The extent of the FDA's regulatory intervention in the areas of processing and handling and clinical safety and efficacy according to the characteristics of the particular tissue product in question. To the extent that a tissue product undergoes more than minimal manipulation in processing, is intended for a non-homologous use, is combined with nontissue components, or is intended to achieve a metabolic outcome, the agency will require a greater demonstration of safety and efficacy through appropriate clinical trials.

"Manipulation," in the agency's regulatory salience, is a measure of the extent to which the biological characteristics of a tissue have been changed *ex vivo*. The FDA has stated it presently considers cell selection or separation, or the cutting, grinding, or freezing of tissue, to constitute minimal manipulation. Cell expansion and encapsulation are examples of more than minimal manipulation.

To the extent that the tissue product only undergoes minimal manipulation, is intended for a homologous application to achieve a structural outcome (or reproductive or metabolic outcome, as between family members related by blood), and does not combine with nontissue components, the FDA will expect "good tissue practices" to be observed but will not impose any reporting duties or, consistent with its authority under §361 of the PHS Act, any product licensing or premarket approval requirements. Any other tissue product requires submission of appropriate chemistry, manufacturing, and controls information and BLA approval for any tissue product that does not incorporate nontissue components. Tissue products that are combinations of tissue and devices or tissue and drugs may be regulated according to established premarket approval (PMA or PDP) or new drug application (NDA) schemes.

Regulations now in effect compel the registration of sponsors and other persons engaged in production and distribution of such products, to screen donors of tissues used to produce HCT/Ps, and to observe Good Tissue Practices in their manufacturing or processing of such products.

46.2.4 Marketing Review and Approval Pathways

As discussed above, the particular program(s) of regulatory review applicable to a medical product are predetermined according to its FDA classification. Thus, the FD&C Act requires a sponsor to submit a device Pre-Market Application (PMA) or Product Development Protocol (PDP) to market a device, or

TABLE 46.2 First HCT/Ps Approved in the United States

HCT/P (Sponsor)	Approval	Approved indicated use	Composition; mode of action	Pivotal clinical studies
Dermagraft (Advanced Tissue Science, Inc.)	September 28, 2001 (approved as a Device)	Treatment of full-thickness diabetic foot ulcers	Cryopreserved human fibroblast-derived dermal substitute; it is composed of neonatal foreskin fibroblasts, extracellular matrix, and a bioabsorbable scaffold. Fibroblasts proliferate to fill the interstices of this scaffold and secrete human dermal collagen, matrix proteins, growth factors, and cytokines, to create a three-dimensional human dermal substitute containing metabolically active, living cells	595 Patients (2 Studies: 281/142 Control; 314/151 Control)
Cultured composite skin (Ortec, Inc.)	February 2, 2001 (approved as a Device under HDE Designation)	Adjunct to standard autograft procedures for covering wounds and donor sites created after the surgical release of hand contractions	Collagen matrix in which allogeneic human skin cells (i.e., epidermal keratinocytes and dermal fibroblasts) are cultured in two distinct layers. Designed to enhance wound healing in part by release of cytokines	145 Patients (63 control)
Apligraf (Organogenesis, Inc.)	May 22, 1998 (approved as a Device)	Standard therapeutic compression for the treatment of noninfected partial and full-thickness skin ulcers	Viable, bilayered, skin construct, which contains Type I bovine collagen, extracted and purified from bovine tendons and viable allogeneic human fibroblast and keratinocyte cells isolated from human infant foreskin	297 Patients (136 control)
Carticel (Genzyme Corporation)	August 22, 1997 (approved as a Biologic)	Repair of clinically significant, symptomatic, cartilaginous defects of the femoral condyle (medial, lateral, or trochlear) caused by acute or repetitive trauma	Used in conjunction with debridement, placement of a periosteal flap, and rehabilitation. The independent contributions of the autologous cultured chondrocytes and other components of the therapy to outcome are unknown	Retrospective analysis of Swedish Study (153 Patients) and US Registry data (241 Patients)

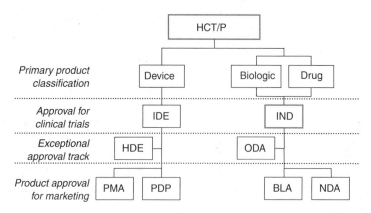

FIGURE 46.1   Product approval pathways.

a new drug application (NDA) to market a drug. The PHS Act provides that marketing approval for a biologic shall be obtained through the submission of a Biologics License Application (BLA). Certain drugs or biologics may qualify for special designation as orphan drugs under the Orphan Drug Act.

In addition, the FDA requires that sponsors of regulated products must first obtain preliminary approval for the clinical trials on humans that will support a subsequent application for full marketing approval. Clinical trials in support of a PMA application or as part of a PDP for a device may be conducted only after the FDA has issued an investigational device exemption (IDE); clinical trials in support of an application for marketing approval of a drug or biologic cannot be initiated until the FDA has approved an investigational new drug (IND) application (Figure 46.1).

46.2.4.1   Devices

The FDA has divided devices into three classes to identify the level of regulatory control applicable to them. The highest category, Class III, includes those devices for which premarket approval is or will be required to determine the safety and effectiveness of the device (21 CFR, §860.3(c); 21 U.S.C., §360c(a)(1)(C)). Absent a written statement of reasons to the contrary, the FDA classifies any "implant" or "life-supporting or life-sustaining device" as Class III (21 CFR, §860.93; 21 U.S.C., §360c(c)(2)(C)).

There are two primary pathways by which the FDA permits a medical device to be marketed: premarket clearance by means of a 510(k) notification, or premarket approval by means of a PMA ("Premarket Approval Application") or PDP ("Product Development Protocol") submission.

A sponsor may seek clearance for a device by filing a 510(k) premarket notification with the FDA, which demonstrates that the device is "substantially equivalent" to a device that has been legally marketed or was marketed before May 28, 1976, the enactment date of the Medical Device amendments to the FD&C act. The sponsor may not place the device into commercial distribution in the United States until the FDA issues a substantial equivalence determination notice. This notice may be issued within 90 days of submission but usually takes longer. The FDA, however, may determine that the proposed device is not substantially equivalent, or require further information such as additional test data or clinical data, or require a sponsor to modify its product labeling, before it will make a finding of substantial equivalence.

If a sponsor cannot establish to the FDA's satisfaction that a new device is substantially equivalent to a legally marketed device, it will have to seek approval to market the device through the PMA or PDP process. This process involves preclinical studies and clinical trials to demonstrate that the device is safe and effective.

FDA regulations (21 CFR, §860.7(d)) provide that, based on "valid scientific evidence," a device shall be found to be "safe"

> *… when it can be determined … that the probable benefits to health from use of the device for its intended uses and conditions of use … outweigh any probable risks[,]*

and that a device shall be found to be "effective"

> ... when it can be determined ... that in a significant portion of the target population, the use of the device for its intended uses and conditions of use ... will provide clinically significant results.

Testing in humans to obtain clinical data demonstrating these qualities in support of a PMA or pursuant to a PDP must be conducted pursuant to an investigational device exemption (IDE). The IDE is the functional equivalent of the IND that governs clinical trials of drugs and biologics. As with other medical products, clinical testing is typically conducted in multiple phases, with the earliest phases primarily intended to demonstrate safety and later phases addressing both safety and effectiveness considerations. The sponsor of the device must also demonstrate compliance with applicable current good manufacturing practices (cGMPs, now also known as Quality System Regulations) before the FDA may approve the product for marketing by granting the PMA or accepting the completion of the PDP.

46.2.4.2 Biologics

Until recently, permission to market a biologic required two applications: one to obtain a product license application (PLA) for the biologic itself and another for approval of the facility where the biologic would be prepared, that is, an establishment license application. The 1997 FDA Modernization Act amended the PHS Act by eliminating the separate product and establishment license applications in favor of a single biologics license application (BLA), which, like the PMA or PDP for devices, includes an evaluation of compliance with appropriate quality controls and current cGMP as part of the assessment of the safety and efficacy of the product in question.

§351 of the PHS Act directs the FDA to approve a BLA on the basis of a determination that the biologic in question is "safe, pure, and potent." Those terms are defined in FDA regulations promulgated to give effect to that statutory authority:

> safety means the relative freedom from harmful effect to persons affected, directly or indirectly, by a product when prudently administered, taking into consideration the character of the product in relation to the condition of the recipient at the time[;]

> purity means relative freedom from extraneous matter in the finished product, whether or not harmful to the recipient or deleterious to the product . . . [and] includes but is not limited to relative freedom from residual moisture or other volatile substances and pyrogenic substances[;]

> potency is interpreted to mean the specific ability or capacity of the product, as indicated by appropriate laboratory tests or by adequately controlled clinical data obtained through the administration of the product in the manner intended, to effect a given result.

Testing in humans to obtain clinical data demonstrating these qualities in support of a BLA must be conducted pursuant to an investigational new drug application (IND). The IND is the functional equivalent of the IDE that governs clinical trials of devices. As with other medical products, clinical testing is typically conducted in multiple phases, with the earliest phases primarily intended to demonstrate safety, and later phases intended to address both safety and efficacy considerations.

The emphasis given to process by the earlier requirement of a separate approval of the manufacturing facility illuminates the dual nature of the regulatory authority created under the PHS Act and ultimately exercised by the FDA. Besides assuring that only safe, pure, and potent biologics are marketed in the United States, the FDA is also charged with a general duty to prevent the introduction, transmission, or spread of communicable disease (PHS Act, §361(a)). While the BLA is an amalgam of product and process quality criteria, a particular emphasis upon the authority to eliminate sources of dangerous infection reappears in the context of the FDA's proposed regulatory triage for engineered tissues.

46.3   Regulation of Pharmaceutical/Medical Human Tissue Products in Europe

Regulation of medical products incorporating viable human tissue products among or within the member states of the European Union (EU) is marked by inconsistency but is presently the subject of substantial discussion and debate. As part of the overall coordination of national laws and governmental activities within the EU, the regulation of the marketing of certain medical products by national authorities is being consolidated within designated EU agencies, especially the European Medicines Evaluation Agency (EMEA). Within the scope of what medical products are considered pharmaceutical and regulated, there are two broad subcategories, medicinal products and medical devices.

The EMEA was established in 1993 by the European Economic Community (EEC, now EU) Council Regulation No. 2309/93 to implement procedures to give effect to a single market for "medicinal products" among the member states. In conjunction with three directives adopted concurrently (Council Directives 93/39EEC, 93/40EEC, and 93/41EEC), the regulation authorized EMEA to manage a "centralized procedure" for an EEC authorization to market medicinal products for either human or veterinary use. The directives also established a "mutual recognition procedure" for marketing authorization of medicinal products based upon the principle of mutual recognition of authorizations granted by national regulatory bodies. These procedures came into effect on January 1, 1995, with a three-year transition period until December 31, 1997. As of January 1, 1998, the independent authorization procedures of the member states are strictly limited to the initial phase of mutual recognition (i.e., granting marketing authorization by the "reference Member State") and to medicinal products that are not marketed in more than one member state. Consequently, sponsors seeking marketing authorization for medicinal products throughout the EU are obliged to seek such approval through the centralized procedure administered by EMEA.

The concept of a "medicinal product" in EEC legislation substantially predated the organization of EMEA. Council Directive 65/65EEC of January 26, 1965, defined the term medicinal product to include

any substance or combination of substances presented for treating or preventing disease in human beings or animals.

[and]

any substance or combination of substances which may be administered to human beings or animals with a view to making a medical diagnosis or to restoring, correcting or modifying physiological functions in human beings or in animals ... .

A "substance" is further defined to include "[a]ny matter irrespective of origin which may be human ... animal ... vegetable ... [or] chemical" (Directive 65/65/EEC, Article 1). However, the directive also makes clear that its regulation of medicinal products (and, through amendments to the directive recognizing the authority of EMEA, the "centralized procedure") does not apply to products "intended for research and development trials" (Directive 65/65/EEC, Article 2).

Sponsors of medical products derived through tissue engineering have reported substantial inconsistency among the regulatory bodies of EU member states regarding the classification of such products for purposes of determining the applicability of national or EU marketing authorization requirements (see Table 8.2). A determination that engineered tissue products are "medicinal products" subject to the centralized procedure for authorization administered by EMEA will substantially clarify and rationalize the process by which such products may be marketed throughout the European Community.

The EMEA has in place a Biotechnology Working Party that has considered, among other things, safety issues in the delivery of human somatic cell therapies and a definition of a "cell therapy medicinal product"

(CPMP/BWP/41450/98 draft). This definition would consider engineered human tissues to be "medicinal products" within the meaning of Directive 65/65/EEC, provided the engineered tissue was the product of both the following:

> a. ... *an industrial manufacturing process carried out in dedicated facilities. The process encompasses expansion or more than minimal manipulation designed to alter the biological or physiological characteristics of the resulting cells, and*
> b. ... *further to such manipulation, the resulting cell product is definable in terms of qualitative and quantitative composition including biological activity.*

Points to Consider on Human Somatic Cell Therapy, CPMP/BWP/41450/98 draft, page 3/9.

The Biotechnology Sector of EMEA is likely to have primary responsibility for considering the authorization of engineered tissue products in the event they are classifiable as "medicinal products" [8].

Human tissue and cellular products may not be presently definable as "medicinal products" subject to regulation, to the extent that they are the result of modest manipulation of autologous tissues in the course of treating a fairly small patient population. Under these circumstances, the regulation of such cellular products is more likely to remain with the competent authorities of the Member States (with substantial variability in the classification and resulting regulation of such products, as outlined in Table 8.2). Nevertheless, an EMEA decision to accept an engineered tissue product as a "medicinal product" could occur in response to a petition from a sponsor of such a product. To be successful, such a petition should probably stress the "industrial" nature of the fabrication process and the extent of manipulation of the human biological material to develop the engineered tissue product. Assuming an engineered tissue product could be established to be a "medicinal product," there does not appear to be any EU rule that could limit the ability of EMEA to grant market authorization according to the type or source of tissue from which the product had been derived.

EMEA is aligned with Enterprise DG (formerly DG III; the department of the European Commission primarily responsible for establishing and implementing rules promoting the Single Market for products). A unit of Enterprise DG oversees application of EU directives regulating marketing authorization of medical devices. Providing for engineered tissue products could require some reconsideration of the specific areas of responsibility of the units or agencies involved in regulating medical products.

46.4 Regulation of Pharmaceutical/Medical Human Tissue Products in Japan

It appeared at the time of the World Technology Evaluation Center (WTEC) panel's visit to Japan that the Government of Japan was only beginning to focus on codifying regulation of engineered human tissue products within its scheme of regulating other medical products [1]. The WTEC panel was unable within the scope of this study to provide an analysis of Japan's medical product approval process as potentially applied to engineered human tissue products. However, presented here is an outline of Japan's process and agencies responsible for regulation of medical products generally.

The Pharmaceutical and Medical Safety Bureau (PMSB) has primary responsibility within the Japanese Ministry of Health, Labour and Welfare for administering the requirements established for the safety and efficacy of medical products under Japan's Pharmaceutical Affairs Law. This legislation was substantially amended in 1996 (with the reforms made effective in April 1997) to provide for the present medical product review and approval system.

Applications for approval of new drugs and medical devices are referred by PMSB to the Central Pharmaceutical Affairs Council (CPAC) to obtain its recommendation. The CPAC, in turn, is advised by the Pharmaceutical and Medical Devices Evaluation Center (PMDEC), an expert body organized in July 1997 to evaluate the quality, efficacy, and safety of medical products administered to humans. Specific authority within PMSB to approve recommendations received from CPAC regarding the discrete aspects of the clinical testing, licensing, and use of new medical products is distributed among relevant divisions, such as the Evaluation and Licensing Division (premarketing and supplemental application approvals) and the Safety Division (adverse reaction measures). A regulatable medical product in Japan is classified as either a medical device or a pharmaceutical.

Advice concerning the design and conduct of clinical trials, as well as the adequacy of applications for approval of pharmaceuticals, is provided to PMDEC and to the product sponsor by the Drug Organization, a quasi-governmental agency established in 1979 as a fund to support patients experiencing adverse drug reactions. It is not clear whether the Drug Organization serves a similar function with respect to medical devices, or if there exists an equivalent medical device organization. However, applications for approval of "copy-cat" devices are referred to the Japan Association for the Advancement of Medical Equipment for a determination of the equivalence of the new device to devices already approved for clinical use. For a more detailed description of Japan's general medical product approval process, see, for example, Hirayama [9] and Yamada [10].

46.5 Other Considerations Relevant to Engineered Tissues

46.5.1 FDA Regulation and Product Liability

Protection from product liability lawsuits, in the form of an immunity from such litigation, may come from satisfying the federal regulations which govern the design and manufacture of, as well as the warnings to be supplied with, medical products.

By virtue of the Supremacy Clause of the Constitution, the federal government is permitted to regulate certain affairs free of state interference. State civil litigation is a form of regulation, so it is a form of interference. If Congress elects to exclusively regulate certain conduct, then litigation under state law regarding the same conduct is prohibited, as it may produce inconsistent or conflicting standards regulating that conduct.

The public policy arguments in favor of federal preemption with respect to the regulation of medical products are readily discernible: while both state and federal regulation would have the enhancement of public health and safety as their goal, the establishment of nationwide labeling and design criteria for medical products will promote uniformity and regularity in the interpretation of applicable regulations and will ensure enforcement of these regulations is conducted in the public interest, rather than through isolated lawsuits that may produce inconsistent results. In addition, the natural preeminence of a federal administration administering such regulations will simplify and improve communication between the regulators and the medical product sponsors. Federal preemption, then, is not a shield for bad medical products; rather, it protects a process of reasoned, scientific inquiry.

Congressional and FDA silence on the question of preemption in statutes and regulations governing drugs and biologics going back to the earliest federal Food and Drug Acts has meant that sponsors of these products have been left to argue only "implied" or "conflict" preemption with largely inconsistent — though often disappointing — results.

The situation for sponsors of devices would seem to be decidedly different. When Congress passed the 1976 Medical Device Amendments to the FD&C Act, it explicitly authorized preemption of any state requirement as to the safety or effectiveness of a medical device in favor of FDA regulations governing the same product. Because of the high degree of scrutiny to which Class III devices are subjected through the FDA's premarket approval (PMA) process, courts have shown a general willingness to recognize that personal injury litigation regarding these devices has been preempted. However, the FDA may also permit the marketing of devices which have been shown to be "substantially equivalent" to devices either previously approved or marketed before the enactment of the Medical Device Amendments in 1976. This "510(k)" clearance involves significantly less regulatory review of the device than would have been given to a PMA application.

In *Medtronic v. Lohr*, though, the U.S. Supreme Court concluded that the apparent preemption language of the Medical Device Amendments does not actually preclude product liability actions against sellers of "510(k)" devices. The court reasoned that the 510(k) premarket clearance process did not involve a comprehensive, in-depth analysis of the safety, efficacy, and labeling of a medical product prior to clinical use. While a number of justices suggested they might not reach the same conclusion regarding "PMA" devices, the *Lohr* decision has weakened — but certainly has not obliterated — a major defense of those engineered tissue products which may be classified and regulated as devices. Indeed, to the extent the further viability of the preemption defense is predicated upon the degree to which the FDA has given specific attention to and approval of the design of the device in question, premarket approval by means of the PDP process would seem to offer the greatest chance of immunity from product liability litigation.

46.5.2 Ownership of Human Tissues

While critical to the general advance of medical research, access to human tissues for research or product development is highly sensitive to public disclosure of practices where tissues are taken or used without consent or under circumstances suggesting a commercial market in body parts. The absence of comprehensive federal or state legislation governing "research" tissues deprives the biomedical community of clear, consistent guidelines to follow in acquiring and using tissues, while simultaneously representing a legislative vacuum that may be filled with substantial adverse unintended consequences if done suddenly in response to some public outcry. Absent effective coordination, the initiatives of individual federal agencies to establish policies for research involving human tissues or subjects may impose conflicting requirements or expectations.

Significant advances in medical research over the past several years has contributed substantially to the commercial utility of human biological materials. Consequently, the source of such materials used in the creation of engineered tissue products may become important for reasons beyond — and certainly removed from — the possible transfer of adventitious agents or the management of immunological responses. Simply put, the use of allogeneic materials raises issues of ownership, donation, and consent not to be found with respect to autologous tissues.

The common law of the United States recognizes a severely restricted property interest in human bodies or organs. In a broad sense, a "property interest" in something may be thought of as a "bundle of rights" to possess, to use, to profit from, to dispose of, and to deal in that thing. Courts have granted next of kin nothing more than a "quasiproperty" right — or right of sepulcher — in a decedent's body for the purposes of burial or other lawful disposition. In place of an exegesis of the religious or cultural prohibitions against recognizing a property interest in a dead body, it is clear that the limited right which has been fashioned by the courts has been intended to offer nothing more than that some interested person may ensure the remains are disposed of with dignity.

Organ transplantation has certainly created the conditions for a market for human body parts. In response, Congress and state legislatures have enacted statutes prohibiting the sale of any human organ. The National Organ Transplant Act was passed to regulate the availability of organs for transplantation through voluntary donation exclusively by explicitly prohibiting organ purchases. The same prohibition has been passed into law by the 15 states, to date, which have adopted the Uniform Anatomical Gift Act (1987) [11]. Other state statutes have imposed criminal penalties for the purchase of organs or tissue from either living or cadaveric providers.

These federal and state statutes effectively banning purchases of human organs were enacted in the mid-1980s in immediate response to the prospect of a widespread trade in these body parts to supply the growing demand for transplant material. The vision of a vendor selling livers and kidneys — or worse, a patient harvesting one of his or her own organs for money clearly hovered over the debate leading to the passage of this legislation. But that vision imagined people selfdismantling for cash; it did not really allow for a trade in renewable body parts, especially cells.

46.6 Conclusion

No part of the process of bringing new biomedical products from the laboratory to the patient occurs in isolation from or independent of all of the other aspects of organizing and maintaining that technology development effort: including intellectual property protection and financing market and end user acceptance, and public perception just to mention a few. While FDA premarket approval is the most obvious form of external control over the introduction of new medical products in the United States, it is not the only one; healthcare reimbursement under U.S. centers for Medicare and Medicaid Services (CMS) regulations and private insurer practices is critical, and the evidence necessary to secure reimbursement should be considered in planning clinical trials for FDA approval. The approach to FDA regulatory oversight itself requires careful analysis of product classification (including special designation) options. The novelty, variety, and potential complexity of forms of tissue engineering compel strategic analysis of external controls over the commercial development of human cellular and tissue-based products.

The FDA has adopted a cooperative approach across appropriate FDA Centers and the Office of Commissioner in developing its regulatory strategies for engineered tissue products. These strategies have attempted to simplify and facilitate the administrative process for evaluating products and for resolving product regulatory jurisdiction questions. However, it is apparent that, just as the science continues to evolve, so too must the regulatory approaches. As new and different research directions are pursued, such as the apparent shift toward the use of stem cell technology [12] new and different products will be developed, with the expectation of unique product-specific issues. The FDA, given its legislative authority and regulatory responsibility will certainly continue to build on current initiatives, apply lessons learned from previous products as applicable, and look to the best scientific minds and methods to achieve innovative, flexible, and appropriate resolutions that are transparent to the research and industrial community as well as the public. The challenge for the tissue engineering community is to maintain awareness of the regulatory landscape in the United States and abroad and to be an active voice for articulating issues in order to maintain a productive dialogue with the regulatory agencies and consumers so that engineered tissue products find their proper place in clinical medicine.

References

[1] Hellman, K.B. and Heineken, F.G. Introductory letter. In *World Technology Evaluation Center (WTEC) Panel Report on Tissue Engineering Research*, McIntyre, J.L. et al. (Eds.), Academic Press, San Diego, CA, 2003.

[2] Reinventing the Regulation of Human Tissue: A Proposed Approach to Regulation of Cellular and Tissue-based Products (the "Proposed Approach") (62 FR 9721) March 4, 1997.

[3] PHS Act. Effective 1999. Public Health Service Act, 42 U.S. Code Section 201. See also FDA website: http://www.fda.gov/opacom/laws/phsvcact/phsvcact.htm

[4] U.S. Government. *Food, Drug, and Cosmetic Act* (as amended by the FDA Modernization Act of 1997). See also http://www.fda.gov/opacom/laws/fdcact/fdctoc.htm

[5] Establishment Registration and Listing for Manufacturers of Human Cellular and Tissue-based Products (63 FR 26744), May 14, 1998.

[6] Suitability Determination for Donors of Human Cellular and Tissue-based Products (64 FR 52696), September 30, 1999.

[7] Current Good Tissue Practice for Manufacturers of Human Cellular and Tissue-based Products: Inspection and Enforcement.

[8] EMEA Biotechnology Working Party, *Points to Consider on Human Somatic Cell Therapy*, *CPMP/BWP/41450/98 draft.*

[9] Hirayama, Y. Changing the review process: the view of the Japanese Ministry of Health and Welfare. *Drug Inform. J.* 1998; 32:111–117.

[10] Yamada, M. The approval system for biological products in Japan. *Drug Inform. J.* 1997; 3:1385–1393.

[11] *Uniform Anatomical Gift Act of 1987*, Section 10. Reproduced at 8A Uniform Laws Annotated 58 (Master Edition, 1993).

[12] Lysaght, M. *Tissue Engineering: Great Expectations; Presentation at Engineering Tissue Growth Conference and Exposition*, Pittsburgh, PA, March 17–20, 2003.

47
Bioengineering of Human Skin Substitutes

Dorothy M. Supp
*Shriners Hospital for Children
Cincinnati Burns Hospital*

Steven T. Boyce
University of Cincinnati

47.1 Introduction

The field of tissue engineering has grown in response to the many medical needs for tissue replacement. For the skin, two distinctly different types of wounds have stimulated the development of various tissue-engineered skin substitutes. On one end of the spectrum are burn wounds, which represent an acute injury to the skin. Over 1 million burn injuries occur annually, resulting in over 50,000 acute hospital admissions and more than 5,000 deaths [1]. Partial-thickness wounds have the capacity to heal without the need for tissue replacement from stem cells present in skin appendages. However, full-thickness burn wounds require grafting of skin to replace the destroyed tissue. The grafting of split-thickness autologous skin has been the prevailing standard for permanent closure of excised full-thickness burn wounds. This can be accomplished in patients with relatively small wounds, but in patients with massive burns involving a large total body surface area (TBSA), permanent wound closure is problematic because of the lack of donor sites for skin autografting. Delayed wound coverage increases the likelihood of infection and sepsis, major causes of burn mortality [2].

On the other end of the spectrum are chronic wounds, which tend to involve a relatively small area of skin, but represent a major medical need because they affect a large population of patients. The most common chronic wounds include pressure ulcers and leg ulcers, which are estimated to affect over 2 million people in the United States alone [3]. This figure may be expected to rise as the average age of the population increases. In some patients, wound closure can be enhanced with topical agents, such as growth factors to stimulate healing and antimicrobial agents to minimize infection. However, a large percentage of patients require grafting for permanent closure of chronic wounds. Autograft may not be a feasible option in these patients due to underlying deficiencies in wound healing, which compromise healing of donor sites.

The need for timely wound closure in these diverse clinical settings has led to the development of skin substitutes as alternatives to split-thickness or full-thickness autograft. Although none of the skin substitutes currently available can replace all of the structures and functions of native skin, they can be used to provide wound coverage and facilitate healing of both acute and chronic wounds. Further, the technologies that have yielded skin substitutes for grafting have also been used to produce materials for *in vitro* irritancy and toxicology studies.

47.2   Objectives of Skin Substitutes

Normal human skin performs a wide variety of protective, perceptive, and regulatory functions that help the body maintain homeostasis. The outermost layer of the skin, the epidermis, is comprised mainly of keratinocytes, which provide the barrier function of the skin. Other epidermal cells and structures include adnexal cells that comprise the glands, hair, and nails; melanocytes, which contribute pigment; Langerhans cells of the immune system; and sensory structures of nerves. The epidermis contains only very small amounts of extracellular matrix, predominantly carbohydrate polymers and stratum corneum lipids that form a barrier to permeability of aqueous fluids [4–6]. In contrast, the underlying dermis consists mainly of extracellular matrix molecules, including collagens, elastin, reticulin, and polysaccharides, that give mechanical strength to the skin. Dermal cells include fibroblasts, which synthesize collagen and other matrix components; vascular components, such as endothelial cells and smooth muscle cells; nerve cells; and mast cells of the immune system.

To be useful in a clinical setting, the primary goal for any skin substitute is restoration of skin barrier, normally a function of the epidermis, which helps to minimize protein and fluid loss and prevent infection [7]. As outlined in Table 47.1, there are many products that meet this need, but most provide only temporary wound coverage or partial skin replacement. Currently, limitations of bioengineered skin substitutes, compared with native skin grafts, include: reduced rates of engraftment, increased microbial contamination, mechanical fragility, increased time to healing, increased requirement for regrafting, and very high cost [59–63]. These complications may increase, rather than decrease, the risks to patients and delay recovery. Therefore, the use of skin substitutes may be suitable as an adjunctive therapy in cases without other alternatives, such as very large burns or chronic wounds that have failed to respond to conventional treatments.

Ideally, skin replacements should promote permanent engraftment without the need for regrafting; allow rapid healing to replace both dermal and epidermal layers; be ready to use when needed; achieve acceptable functional and cosmetic outcome; and be free from risk of disease transmission and immunological reaction [2]. These many goals have not yet been satisfied by any skin substitute, but ongoing research in biomedical and genetic engineering may someday make an "off-the-shelf" skin replacement a reality.

47.3   Composition of Skin Substitutes

Skin substitutes currently available vary in complexity, ranging from temporary synthetic wound dressings to permanent skin replacements, either with or without incorporation of cultured skin cells (Table 47.1). Some of the acellular materials have components that incorporate into the wound bed and may become populated with dermal cells from the host. These dermal substitutes replace the dermal component of the

TABLE 47.1 Bioengineered Skin Substitutes

Skin substitute	Dermal component	Epidermal component	Indications for use	Refs.
AlloDerm® (LifeCell Corp.)	Allogeneic acellular human dermis	None	Burn wounds; repair of soft tissue defects	[8–11]
Apligraf® (Novartis)	Collagen gel with allogeneic fibroblasts	Allogeneic keratinocytes	Burn wounds; chronic foot ulcers; venous leg ulcers; epidermolysis bullosa	[12–20]
Biobrane® (Bertek Pharmaceuticals)	Nylon mesh coated with collagen	Semipermeable silicone membrane	Partial-thickness burn wounds and donor sites	[21–24]
Cultured Skin Substitutes (Univ. Cincinnati/Shriners Hospitals	Collagen-based polymer with autologous fibroblasts	Autologous keratinocytes	Burn wounds; congenital nevi; chronic wounds (using allogeneic cells)	[25–29]
Dermagraft® (Smith and Nephew)	Polyglactin mesh scaffold with allogeneic fibroblasts	None	Chronic/diabetic foot ulcers	[30–32]
Epicel® (Genzyme Biosurgery)	None	Autologous keratinocyte sheet	Burn wounds; congenital nevi	[33–36]
Epiderm™ (MatTek Corporation)	Collagen coated cell culture insert	Allogeneic keratinocytes	In vitro assessment for irritancy and toxicology testing	[37–40]
EpidermFT™ (MatTek Corporation)	Allogeneic fibroblasts on cell culture insert	Allogeneic keratinocytes	In vitro testing model for assessment of dermal–epidermal interactions	
Epidex™ (Modex Therapeutics)	None	Autologous keratinocytes with silicone membrane support	Chronic leg ulcers	[41,42]
Integra® (Integra Life Sciences)	Collagen-chondroitin-6-sulfate matrix	Silicone polymer coating	Burn wounds	[43–49]
Melanoderm™ (MatTek Corporation)	Collagen coated cell culture insert	Allogeneic keratinocytes and melanocytes	In vitro testing model for assessment of pigmentation	
OrCel® (OrTec International)	Collagen sponge with allogeneic fibroblasts	Allogeneic keratinocytes	Donor sites in burn patients; epidermolysis bullosa	[50,51]
SkinEthic® (SkinEthic Laboratories)	Cell culture insert	Allogeneic keratinocytes (without or with melanocytes)	In vitro testing model	[52–54]
SureDerm (Hans Biomed)	Allogeneic acellular human dermis	None	Burn wounds; repair of soft tissue defects	
TranCell (CellTran Limited)	None	Autologous keratinoctyes on acrylic acid polymer	Chronic diabetic foot ulcers	[55]
TransCyte® (Smith and Nephew)	Nylon mesh with dermal matrix secreted by allogeneic fibroblasts (cells nonviable at grafting)	None	Burn wounds	[56–58]

skin, but may require grafting of autologous epidermis in a second surgical procedure. Skin substitutes that contain allogeneic cells have greater similarity to native skin at grafting than acellular materials, but these are considered temporary skin substitutes [64]. The allogeneic cells are eventually replaced by host-derived cells [7]. Allogeneic skin substitutes containing cells can secrete extracellular matrix and growth factors that improve healing, and can provide wound coverage until autograft is available. For small wounds, such as chronic wounds, allogeneic skin substitutes may stimulate healing from the wound bed and margins, without further grafting. These characteristics, coupled with essentially immediate availability, are advantages of the allogeneic skin substitutes. However, for permanent closure of large wounds grafting of autologous skin or engineered skin containing autologous cells is required. A disadvantage of bioengineered skin substitutes containing autologous cells is the increased time required for cell culture and graft preparation [65]. However, they can act as permanent skin replacements once engraftment is achieved. Therefore, the increased time required for preparation may be offset by a reduction in the number of surgical procedures required for permanent wound closure [66].

Skin replacements can be used as adjunctive therapies in patients who are also receiving conventional skin grafts to facilitate wound closure [25–27,67,68]. By increasing availability of skin grafts, skin substitutes can provide several advantages over conventional therapy, including reduced donor site area required to close wounds permanently, decreased number of surgical procedures and hospitalization time, and reduced scarring [66,69].

47.3.1 Acellular Skin Substitutes

Biobrane, an acellular biocomposite dressing, has been used for over two decades for treatment of partial-thickness burn wounds [21,70]. It has been shown to control pain and reduce frequency of dressing changes, decrease the length of hospitalization, and improve healing times [21,23,70]. Biobrane is composed of a collagen peptide-coated nylon mesh material attached to a semipermeable silicone membrane. It is applied to clean, debrided wounds with the mesh side down; the mesh adheres to the wound, and the material is removed after the underlying tissue has healed. Integra is also a synthetic acellular skin replacement, but one that combines both temporary and permanent components. It consists of a cross-linked collagen–glycosaminoglycan membrane as a dermal matrix, and a silastic coating that provides a synthetic epidermal structure for barrier replacement [43,44]. It has been widely used for coverage of excised burn wounds. The artificial dermis does not contain cells at the time of grafting, but within a few weeks it becomes populated with cells from the wound bed and is vascularized. Thus, the dermal component incorporates into the wound, generating a neodermis; the temporary silastic coating can then be removed and replaced with a thin sheet of split-thickness skin [45,46].

Another example of a bilayer temporary skin substitute is TransCyte, which has been used for coverage of partial-thickness wounds during re-epithelialization, or for full-thickness wounds prior to autograft placement. Transcyte is comprised of a synthetic semipermeable epidermal layer, and a dermal nylon mesh layer seeded with allogeneic human fibroblasts [56–58]. The fibroblasts are allowed to proliferate within the synthetic dermal construct, where they secrete extracellular matrix components and growth factors that can facilitate wound healing. Prior to grafting, the material is frozen, without cryoprotection of the cells. Thus, at the time of grafting, Transcyte does not contain any viable cells.

AlloDerm is an acellular dermal matrix derived from donated human skin [8]. The skin is processed to remove cells, circumventing tissue rejection but preserving much of the dermis's three-dimensional dermal structure. Vascular channels with basement membrane are present, even though the cells have been destroyed, facilitating graft vascularization [10]. It has been most useful for soft tissue replacement, such as abdominal wall reconstruction [10]. For treatment of burn wounds, it has been used in conjunction with split-thickness autograft to yield results similar to split-thickness grafts of greater thickness [8].

47.3.2 Allogeneic Cellular Skin Substitutes

Other temporary wound covers, such as Dermagraft, Apligraf, and OrCel, contain viable cells at the time of grafting. Because the cells are allogeneic, typically isolated from donated human neonatal foreskin, these products are considered temporary skin substitutes rather than permanent skin replacements. Dermagraft is composed of a polymer mesh scaffold seeded with allogeneic fibroblasts [30–32]. Apligraf and OrCel both contain allogeneic keratinocytes and fibroblasts, coupled with a biopolymer consisting of either a bovine type I collagen gel or collagen sponge, respectively [12,13,51]. Grafts that contain allogeneic cells provide wound coverage and supply growth factors that facilitate wound repair, but the allogeneic cells do not persist on the patient after healing is complete. It is generally believed that allogeneic cells are replaced within 1 to 6 weeks after grafting by the patient's own cells.

Cultured skin models containing allogeneic cells have been developed for *in vitro* testing purposes [37,40,52–54]. SkinEthic Laboratories has developed a Reconstituted Human Epidermis model, comprised of stratified epidermal keratinocytes supplied on cell culture inserts, for *in vitro* test applications [52–54]. In addition, several tissue-specific models of Reconstructed Human Epithelium have been prepared. These include models of oral, vaginal, corneal, and alveolar epithelium. Similar models designed for *in vitro* toxicology testing include EpiDerm, a differentiated model of human epidermis, and Melanoderm, a stratified coculture of human melanocytes and keratinocytes [37]. EpiDermFT (EpiDerm "Full Thickness") is comprised of neonatal foreskin-derived fibroblasts and keratinocytes grown on cell culture inserts. These skin models closely parallel human skin at the ultrastructural level, and can be reproducibly manufactured, offering attractive alternatives to *in vivo* animal testing for irritancy, toxicology, and gene expression studies.

47.3.3 Autologous Cellular Skin Substitutes

Autologous keratinocytes and fibroblasts have generally been derived from biopsies of the patient's uninjured skin [71–73]. Recently, keratinocytes have been isolated from the outer root sheath of plucked hair follicles [41,42]. The cells can be expanded in culture and used to populate skin substitutes *in vitro*. Grafted as epithelial sheets or as composites of biopolymers and cells, these are theoretically permanent skin substitutes once engraftment is achieved [25–27,33,41].

Relatively few commercial skin substitutes contain autologous cells. Epicel was the first commercial product comprised of cultured autologous cells for wound transplantation. It is indicated for use in burn patients with very large deep partial-thickness or full-thickness wounds and in congenital nevi patients [33,36,74]. Also referred to as cultured epithelial autograft (CEA), Epicel consists of a sheet of autologous keratinocytes that are grown in culture and transplanted to patients with a petrolatum gauze backing. The keratinocytes are isolated from a full-thickness biopsy of the patient's uninjured skin, and grafts are generally ready within 3 weeks time [74]. Epicel can be grafted on top of vascularized allogeneic dermis or directly onto debrided wounds; however, engraftment is higher when used in conjunction with allodermis [34,74]. A major problem encountered with Epicel has been epidermal blistering. Small blisters may resolve spontaneously, but larger blisters result in graft failure [34]. This phenomenon has been attributed to absence of dermal–epidermal junction components at grafting. Despite this limitation, the availability of Epicel has provided a much needed treatment option for patients with massive burns where donor skin for autograft is extremely limited [34].

A similar product, EpiDex, is a cultured epidermal sheet graft that is indicated for the treatment of small chronic wounds. The unique aspect of EpiDex is that the keratinocytes are not cultured from skin biopsies, but from scalp hair follicles [42]. For preparation of grafts, hair is plucked from the patient and the outer root sheath cells are placed in explant culture [42]. The keratinocytes that are cultured in this fashion are highly proliferative, apparently regardless of donor age [41]. After approximately 5 weeks of cell expansion, a secondary culture is initiated for preparation of epithelial sheet grafts. These are transplanted to wounds as discs measuring approximately 1 cm diameter, attached to a silicone backing to facilitate handling. Early clinical results have been favorable, though the wound areas treated with EpiDex are relatively small [41].

A limitation of these autologous skin replacements is that they contain only keratinocytes, and thus they supply only an epidermal layer. For large full-thickness wounds, such as burns, replacement of both dermal and epidermal layers is beneficial, to reduce scarring and improve the functional and cosmetic outcome. This can be accomplished by combining dermal substitutes and epidermal skin replacements, but this generally requires multiple surgical procedures. A composite cultured skin substitute (CSS) that contains both autologous keratinocytes and fibroblasts *in vitro* is currently in clinical trials [26,27,67,68,75]. CSS are comprised of bovine collagen-glycosaminoglycan sponges that are populated with autologous fibroblasts and keratinocytes (Figure 47.1) [76,77]. The most extensive experience with autologous CSS has

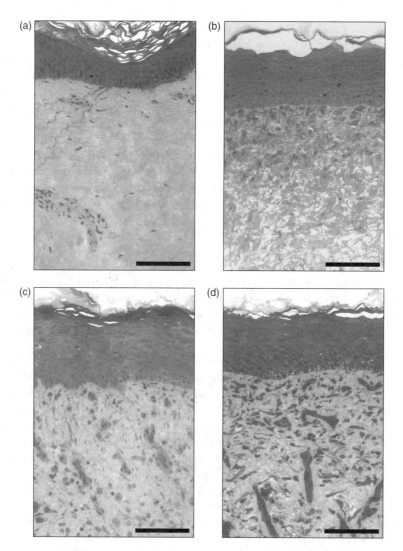

FIGURE 47.1   Histological comparison of native skin and cultured skin substitute prepared for treatment of pediatric burn patient. (a) Native human skin. (b) Cultured skin substitute *in vitro*, shown after 6 days of incubation. Graft was transplanted to patient after 10 days of *in vitro* incubation. (c),(d) Healed autograft (c), and healed cultured skin substitute (d), biopsied 3 weeks after grafting to excised full-thickness burn wounds. Scale bars = 0.1 mm.

been in the treatment of patients with burns affecting greater than 50% TBSA. In these patients, donor sites for autografting are extremely limited and adjunctive treatments for wound coverage are required. For preparation of CSS, primary cultures of keratinocytes and fibroblasts are isolated using standard techniques from a small split-thickness skin biopsy that is usually taken during a patient's first autografting procedure [26,27,71,72,78,79]. Selective *in vitro* culture of keratinocytes and fibroblasts stimulates exponential increases in cell numbers, resulting in very large populations of cells in only 2 to 3 weeks of culture [78]. Grafting to patients can generally be performed within 2 weeks of inoculation of CSS, which corresponds to 4 to 5 weeks after the initial patient biopsy. Because the CSS contains both dermal and epidermal layers and develops a functional basement membrane *in vitro*, grafting of CSS can replace both skin layers in a single surgical procedure (Figure 47.1) [80]. Culture of CSS at the air–liquid interface promotes development of a stratified epidermal layer with functional barrier properties *in vitro*, providing protection of the wound immediately after grafting [68,80,81]. CSS have been used with favorable results as an adjunctive treatment for the healing of large burn wounds, and have been shown to significantly reduce the requirement for autograft and shorten the number of surgical procedures needed for definitive wound closure [27,67,68]. CSS have also been used to a limited extent for treatment of chronic wounds and congenital giant nevi [28,29].

47.4 Clinical Considerations

Multiple clinical factors can determine whether treatment of wounds with engineered skin substitutes will result in skin repair. Modifications of care protocols for wounds must be used to compensate for the anatomic and physiologic deficiencies in engineered skin. Currently available skin substitutes are avascular, tend to heal more slowly than skin autograft, and may be mechanically fragile. Factors that affect the clinical outcome with bioengineered skin replacements include, but are not limited to: composition at the time of grafting; wound bed preparation; control of microbial contamination; dressings and nursing care; and survival of transplanted cells during vascularization of grafts.

Attachment of cultured epithelium to a dermal substitute *in vitro* is advantageous because both epidermal and dermal components can be applied in a single procedure, similar to skin autograft. Culture conditions can be optimized to promote deposition of basement membrane proteins at the dermal–epidermal junction prior to grafting, thereby eliminating the problem of blistering that is frequently observed after grafting of epithelial sheets [33,80]. Alternatively, dermal and epidermal components of skin substitutes may be applied in two stages: first, application of a dermal substitute followed by vascularization; and second, grafting of an autologous epidermal substitute [45,82,83]. This two-step approach increases the density of blood vessels and extracellular matrix in the wound bed, and has been reported to improve engraftment of cultured keratinocyte sheets. However, it requires two surgical procedures to achieve permanent wound closure.

The lack of a vascular plexus is a major limitation of all skin replacements currently available. Split-thickness skin contains a vascular plexus and adheres to debrided wounds by coagulum. Inosculation of vessels in the graft to vessels in the wound occurs within 2 to 3 days [84]. In the absence of microbial contamination or mechanical damage, autograft skin is generally engrafted and reperfused within 1 week after transplantation. In contrast, current clinical models of engineered skin substitutes are avascular, requiring reperfusion from *de novo* angiogenesis. The time required for perfusion is proportional to the thickness of the dermal component of the skin substitute, and is longer than perfusion of split-thickness skin. Vascularization can be accelerated by secretion of angiogenic factors from engineered skin containing keratinocytes and fibroblasts, but growth factors alone cannot compensate for the lack of a vascular plexus prior to grafting [85,86]. The additional time required for vascularization may contribute to epithelial loss from microbial destruction and nutrient deprivation.

Due to the delayed vascularization of skin replacements, control of contamination is critical for engraftment. Topical antimicrobials are more effective for control of wound contamination than parenteral agents [87]. Topical treatments must provide effective coverage of a broad spectrum of microorganisms, but must have low cytotoxicity to allow healing to proceed. It is also important to avoid overlap of topical agents with parenteral drugs used for treatment of sepsis, which could facilitate development of resistant organisms. Several studies have identified individual agents, and mixtures of multiple agents, which are effective against common wound organisms but are not inhibitory to proliferation of keratinocytes and fibroblasts [88–90].

An additional limitation of engineered skin substitutes is mechanical fragility, which contributes to graft failure due to shear and maceration. For delicate grafts, a backing material can facilitate handling and attachment to the wound. For example, CEA are routinely attached to petrolatum-impregnated gauze for surgical application [91]. However, this material may not be compatible with wet dressings used to manage infection. CSS may be handled and stapled to wounds with a backing of N-Terface™, a relatively strong, nonadherent, highly porous material [25,26]. Porous dressings do not interfere with the delivery of topical solutions and permit drainage of wound exudate.

An important practical obstacle to the routine clinical use of skin substitutes, as with any engineered tissue, remains the high cost of their preparation and care. Estimates for the cost of keratinocyte sheets range from $1,000 to $13,000 for each percent of absolute TBSA [63,92]. If a dermal substitute is also included, the cost can be expected to approximately double [8,45]. Therefore, expense can become a limiting factor for treatment of very large wounds, such as those seen in severely burned patients. Unfortunately, these are the patients most in need of skin substitutes. Although the use of skin substitutes can theoretically reduce the number of surgeries required to heal large burns, which should decrease the total time of hospitalization, there are currently no studies that clearly demonstrate a decrease in costs by use of skin substitutes of any kind. Engineered skin grafts remain an important adjunct to conventional skin grafting, particularly in the treatment of burns, but cannot be used as a primary modality of wound closure except in the most extreme cases [61].

47.5 Assessment

The outcome after treatment of wounds with bioengineered skin substitutes must be measured to determine whether the benefits justify any risks associated with the therapy. Qualitative outcome, which relies heavily on the trained eye of the clinician, can be assessed through clinical evaluation integrating multiple properties of the wound. For example, the Vancouver Scale is used for assessment of burn scar by trained clinicians, and provides an ordinal score for properties of skin including pigmentation, vascularity, pliability, and scar height [93]. Such scales assign quantitative values to qualitative measurements and can provide a relative comparison for evaluation, but they are inherently subjective and dependent on the examiner.

Objectivity may be increased by use of noninvasive instruments to measure biophysical properties of skin, including vascular perfusion, epidermal barrier, pliability, color, and surface pH. Quantitative assessment of skin substitutes can highlight deficiencies compared to normal skin or split-thickness autograft, or can be used to assess the advantage of skin substitutes to the patient without interfering with recovery. Although no single biophysical property is definitive, multiple measurements can provide a general assessment for evaluation of outcome. For example, measurements of surface electrical capacitance (SEC) can be used to define the degree of skin barrier development [94]. SEC is measured using a dermal phase meter, an instrument that is easily used in a clinical setting, with minimal pain or discomfort for the patient [95]. Pigmentation of grafted wounds treated with engineered skin substitutes can be measured using a chromameter. Multiple parameters of skin function must be measured to quantify overall benefit from treatment with skin substitutes.

47.6 Regulatory Issues

In the United States, it is the responsibility of the Food and Drug Administration (FDA) to protect the public from health risks associated with new medical therapies. FDA approval requires that new therapies be safe and effective, and that the probable benefits to health outweigh the probable risks of the therapy or of the untreated disease or condition [96]. Safety considerations for engineered skin substitutes must take several factors into account, including media composition, tissue acquisition, graft fabrication and storage, and sterility testing of the final product [96]. For example, cell culture media must be of the highest purity and free from toxic contaminants. Cells derived from allogeneic donors must test negative for transmissible pathogens. Autologous cells must be handled carefully as well. Because autologous tissues are not routinely screened for pathogens, universal precautions to protect laboratory personnel must be practiced. Xenogeneic components, such as bovine collagen, must not only be free from pathogens that can cross species boundaries, but must also be nonimmunogenic. If xenogeneic cells, such as irradiated 3T3 mouse fibroblasts, are used to facilitate initiation of keratinocytes cultures, compliance with safety standards for xenogeneic transplantation must be assured [97]. Although these common cells are generally thought to be free from risk of disease transmission, unknown risks may exist, and hence patients are excluded from future donation of blood or body parts [36,98].

Bioengineered skin substitutes may be regulated as either devices or biologics, depending on their composition and "primary mode of action." Skin substitutes consisting of autologous cells only, or an acellular human tissue matrix, may not require collection of effectiveness data for regulatory approval. Living autologous cell populations intended for structural repair are considered to be inherently efficacious [99]. However, if no effectiveness data are collected, no claims of effectiveness can be made. Skin substitutes that combine cells with biopolymers are currently considered class III (significant risk) devices that require demonstration of effectiveness in addition to safety [96].

47.7 Future Directions

Despite encouraging clinical results with bioengineered skin for the adjunctive treatment of burns, chronic wounds, and other skin deficiencies, skin substitutes containing just two cell types are limited by anatomic and physiologic deficiencies compared to split-thickness skin autograft. Several areas of preclinical investigation suggest that skin substitutes can be further engineered to increase homology to native human skin. These include the incorporation of additional cell types to improve functional and cosmetic outcome, and the use of genetically modified skin cells to enhance performance after grafting.

47.7.1 Pigmentation

Normal skin pigmentation results from the appropriate epidermal distribution and function of melanocytes. The most critical function of melanocytes is protection from ultraviolet irradiation, but they have psychological importance as well, as a patient's body image and personal identity can impact recovery from massive skin injury [100–102]. Pigmentation of cultured skin may result from transplantation of "passenger" melanocytes, which may persist in selective cultures of epidermal keratinocytes [67,79]. Melanocytes can survive under conditions used for keratinocyte culture, though they proliferate at slower rates and are depleted upon serial passage or cryopreservation [103–105]. In CSS grafted to excised burns, pigmented areas resulting from passenger melanocytes have been observed as individual foci within two months after transplantation [79]. By 1 to 2 years after healing, the foci increase in area, occasionally fusing together to form larger pigmented regions. Uniform pigmentation was demonstrated in preclinical studies with CSS deliberately populated with selectively cultured human melanocytes [106–108]. Future studies will be needed to address regulation of the level of pigmentation in uniformly pigmented cultured skin.

47.7.2 *In Vitro* Angiogenesis

The absence of a vascular plexus in bioengineered skin necessitates vascularization to occur *de novo*, rather than through inosculation of the graft with the wound, increasing the time of nutrient deprivation and susceptibility to microbial contamination after grafting. This limitation can be indirectly addressed in a clinical setting by irrigating the graft with solutions of nutrients and antimicrobial agents for several days after transplantation [27,67,109]. A direct approach would be to initiate angiogenesis in the skin substitutes *in vitro*, prior to grafting. This would permit vascularization to occur through both inosculation of existing vessels and also neovascularization, as occurs for grafted split-thickness skin [84].

Initiation of angiogenesis *in vitro* requires the addition of endothelial cells to the engineered skin. Endothelial cells may organize into vascular structures in culture with the aid of biomaterial supports and coculture with accessory cells. For example, engineered blood vessels have been constructed *in vitro* using mixed cultures of fibroblasts, human umbilical vein endothelial cells (HUVEC), and vascular smooth muscle cells in a collagen matrix [110]. In preclinical studies, transplantation of engineered blood vessels constructed by culture of HUVEC in three-dimensional collagen/fibronectin gels has been reported [111]. More recently, a composite cultured skin containing HUVEC and keratinocytes in a human dermal matrix was reported, which displayed evidence of perfusion after grafting to mice [112]. These studies illustrate the feasibility of grafting synthetic vessels in cultured skin, but overexpression of Bcl-2 through retroviral modification was required to promote survival of the transplanted endothelial cells [111]. In addition, another potential limitation of these studies that will impede their clinical application is the reliance on nondermal or nonautologous endothelial cells. Ideally, multiple cell types (keratinocytes, fibroblasts, and human dermal microvascular endothelial cells, or HDMEC) could be derived from a single autologous skin sample. Transplantation of HDMEC in a composite skin substitute containing isogenic keratinocytes and fibroblasts was demonstrated in an athymic mouse model, though perfusion was not observed [113]. The transplantation of HDMEC in a clinically relevant cultured skin model showed the feasibility of preparing autologous cultured skin containing HDMEC, but future studies must demonstrate inosculation of vessels in the graft with vessels in the wound bed to yield improved performance after grafting.

47.7.3 Cutaneous Gene Therapy

Keratinocytes and fibroblasts are amenable to genetic modification *in vitro* by a variety of methods. Genetically modified cells can be used to populate engineered skin substitutes. This is termed *"ex vivo"* gene therapy because cells are removed from the body and genetically modified in culture before being transplanted back to the recipient. There has been a great deal of interest in the use of genetically modified skin substitutes for the treatment of cutaneous diseases. For example, preclinical studies suggest that *ex vivo* gene therapy can be useful for treatment of lamellar ichthyosis, a condition characterized by defective epidermal barrier, and the blistering skin disease junctional epidermolysis bullosa (JEB) [114–116]. Theoretically, genetically modified keratinocytes can be transplanted for secretion of circulating factors to treat systemic diseases. Keratinocytes have been genetically modified to secrete human growth hormone and clotting factor IX, but therapeutic protein levels have been difficult to obtain after grafting [117–121].

Another application of cutaneous gene therapy is the regulation of wound healing. Hypothetically, genetic modification may be used to overcome anatomic limitations or to enhance their biological activity. For example, keratinocytes modified to overexpress the mesenchymal cell mitogen Platelet Derived Growth Factor-A (PGDF-A), seeded on an acellular dermal matrix, showed increased cellularity, vascularization, and collagen deposition after grafting to mice, suggesting improved function due to PDGF-A overexpression [122]. In other studies, keratinocytes were genetically modified by retroviral transduction to overexpress the angiogenic cytokine Vascular Endothelial Growth Factor (VEGF) [85,86]. After transplantation to athymic mice, skin substitutes containing fibroblasts and VEGF-modified keratinocytes showed enhanced and accelerated vascularization, decreased contraction, and increased engraftment compared to control grafts containing unmodified cells [85,86]. Thus, genetic modification of keratinocytes can hypothetically be used to overcome the lack of a vascular plexus in engineered skin grafts.

A particularly promising avenue of research involves the genetic modification of cells in cultured skin grafts to reduce or eliminate immune rejection. Preclinical studies have shown that reduced expression of major histocompatibility complex (MHC) class I and II antigens can prolong engraftment of skin grafts in mouse allograft models [123]. In one study, fetal skin was used because it exhibited substantially reduced MHC class I and II expression compared with neonatal skin. In another study, keratinocytes were genetically modified to overexpress indoleamine 2,3-deoxygenase (IDO), a tryptophan-catalyzing enzyme that functions to prevent fetal rejection during pregnancy [124]. Increased IDO expression in keratinocytes led to a down-regulation of MHC class I expression. These studies suggest a possible mechanism for preparation of allogeneic skin substitutes that would escape immune rejection, and may someday lead to universal donor cultured skin grafts.

47.8 Conclusions

Technological advances in the fabrication of biomaterials and the culture of skin cells have permitted the production of bioengineered skin substitutes. These have provided improved therapeutic options for patients suffering from acute or chronic wounds, and offer the promise of new treatments for inherited cutaneous diseases. Continued research will be needed to identify more efficient methods to utilize precious autologous tissue, which will provide greater amounts of skin substitutes for grafting as well as shorten the time required for their preparation. Increasing the complexity of skin substitutes, from acellular biopolymers to composite materials with multiple cell types, will result in continued improvements in anatomy and physiology, working toward greater homology to native human skin. These improvements will lead to enhanced performance of engineered skin grafts, greater clinical efficacy, and reduction of morbidity and mortality for patients with wounds or cutaneous disease.

References

[1] Brigham, P. and McLoughlin, E., Burn incidence and medical care use in the United States: estimates, trends, and data sources, *J. Burn Care Rehabil.*, 17, 95, 1996.

[2] Berthod, F. and Damour, O., *In vitro* reconstructed skin models for wound coverage in deep burns, *Br. J. Dermatol.*, 136, 809, 1997.

[3] Phillips, T.J., Chronic cutaneous ulcers: etiology and epidemiology, *J. Invest. Dermatol.*, 102, 38S, 1994.

[4] Sorrell, J.M., Caterson, B., Caplan, A.I., Davis, B., and Schafer, I.A., Human keratinocytes contain carbohydrates that are recognized by keratan sulfate-specific monoclonal antibodies, *J. Invest. Dermatol.*, 95, 347, 1990.

[5] Schurer, N.Y. and Elias, P.M., The biochemistry and role of epidermal lipid synthesis, *Adv. Lipid Res.*, 24, 27, 1991.

[6] Elias, P.M., Stratum corneum architecture, metabolic activity and interactivity with subjacent cell layers, *Exp. Dermatol.*, 5, 191, 1996.

[7] Gallico, G.G.I., Biologic skin substitutes, *Clin. Plast. Surg.*, 17, 519, 1990.

[8] Wainwright, D., Madden, M., Luterman, A., Hunt, J., Monafo, W., Heimbach, D., Kagan, R., Sittig, K., Dimick, A., and Herndon, D., Clinical evaluation of an acellular allograft dermal matrix in full-thickness burns, *J. Burn Care Rehabil.*, 17, 124, 1996.

[9] Sheridan, R., Choucair, R., Donelan, M., Lydon, M., Petras, L., and Tompkins, R., Acellular allodermis in burns surgery: 1-year results of a pilot trial, *J. Burn Care Rehabil.*, 19, 528, 1998.

[10] Menon, N.G., Rodrigues, E.D., Byrnes, C.K., Girotto, J.A., Goldberg, N.H., and Silverman, R.P., Revascularization of human acellular dermis in full-thickness abdominal wall reconstruction in the rabbit model, *Ann. Plast. Surg.*, 50, 523, 2003.

[11] Lorenz, R.R., Dean, R.L., Hurley, D.B., Chuang, J., and Citardi, M.J., Endoscopic reconstruction of anterior and middle cranial fossa defects using acellular dermal allograft, *Laryngoscope*, 113, 496, 2003.

[12] Falanga, V., Margolis, D.J., Alvarez, O., Auletta, M., Maggiacomo, F., Altman, M., Jensen, J., Sabolinski, M., and Hardin-Young, J., Rapid healing of venous ulcers and lack of clinical rejection with an allogeneic cultured human skin equivalent, *Arch. Dermatol.*, 134, 293, 1998.

[13] Eaglstein, W.H., Iriondo, M., and Laszlo, K., A composite skin substitute (Graftskin) for surgical wounds: a clinical experience, *Dermatol. Surg.*, 21, 839, 1995.

[14] Sams, H.H., Chen, J., and King, L.E., Graftskin treatment of difficult to heal diabetic foot ulcers: one center's experience, *Dermatol. Surg.*, 28, 698, 2002.

[15] Curran, M.P. and Plosker, G.L., Bilayered bioengineered skin substitute (Apligraf): a review of its use in the treatment of venous leg ulcers and diabetic foot ulcers, *BioDrugs*, 16, 439, 2002.

[16] Phillips, T.J., Manzoor, J., Rojas, A., Isaacs, C., Carson, P., Sabolinski, M., Young, J., and Falanga, V., The longevity of a bilayered skin substitute after application to venous ulcers, *Arch. Dermatol.*, 138, 1079, 2002.

[17] Falabella, A.F., Schachner, L.A., Valencia, I.C., and Eaglstein, W.H., The use of tissue-engineered skin (Apligraf) to treat a newborn with epidermolysis bullosa, *Arch. Dermatol.*, 135, 1219, 1999.

[18] Falabella, A.F., Valencia, I.C., Eaglstein, W.H., and Schachner, L.A., Tissue-engineered skin (Apligraf) in the healing of patients with epidermolysis bullosa wounds, *Arch. Dermatol.*, 136, 1225, 2000.

[19] Ozerdem, O.R., Wolfe, S.A., and Marshall, D., Use of skin substitutes in pediatric patients, *J. Craniofac. Surg.*, 14, 517, 2003.

[20] Fivenson, D.P., Scherschun, L., and Cohen, L.V., Apligraf in the treatment of severe mitten deformity associated with recessive dystrophic epidermolysis bullosa, *Plast. Reconstr. Surg.*, 112, 584, 2003.

[21] Tavis, M.N., Thornton, N.W., Bartlett, R.H., Roth, J.C., and Woodroof, E.A., A new composite skin prosthesis, *Burns*, 7, 123, 1980.

[22] Purdue, G.F., Hunt, J.L., Gillespie, R.W., Hansbrough, J.F., Dominic, W.J., Robson, M.C., Smith, D.J., MacMillan, B.G., Waymack, J.P., Heradon, D.N. et al., Biosynthetic skin substitute versus frozen human cadaver allograft for temporary coverage of excised burn wounds, *J. Trauma*, 27, 155, 1987.

[23] Lal, S., Barrow, R.E., Wolf, S.E., Chinkes, D.L., Hart, D.W., Heggers, J.P., and Herndon, D.N., Biobrane improves wound healing in burned children without increased risk of infection, *Shock*, 14, 314, 2000.

[24] Arevalo, J.M. and Lorente, J.A., Skin coverage with Biobrane biomaterial for the treatment of patients with toxic epidermal necrolysis, *J. Burn Care Rehabil.*, 20, 406, 1999.

[25] Hansbrough, J.F., Boyce, S.T., Cooper, M.L., and Foreman, T.J., Burn wound closure with cultured autologous keratinocytes and fibroblasts attached to a collagen–glycosaminoglycan substrate, *JAMA*, 262, 2125, 1989.

[26] Boyce, S.T., Greenhalgh, D.G., Kagan, R.J., Housinger, T., Sorrell, J.M., Childress, C.P., Rieman, M., and Warden, G.D., Skin anatomy and antigen expression after burn wound closure with composite grafts of cultured skin cells and biopolymers, *Plast. Reconstr. Surg.*, 91, 632, 1993.

[27] Boyce, S.T., Goretsky, M.J., Greenhalgh, D.G., Kagan, R.J., Rieman, M.T., and Warden, G.D., Comparative assessment of cultured skin substitutes and native skin autograft for treatment of full-thickness burns, *Ann. Surg.*, 222, 743, 1995.

[28] Boyce, S.T., Glatter, R., and Kitzmiller, W.J., Treatment of chronic wounds with cultured cells and biopolymers: a pilot study, *Wounds*, 7, 24, 1995.

[29] Passaretti, D., Billmire, D., Kagan, R., Corcoran, J., and Boyce, S., Autologous cultured skin substitutes conserve donor site autograft in elective treatment of congenital giant melanocyte nevus, *Plast. Reconstr. Surg.* 114, 1523, 2004.

[30] Cooper, M.L., Hansbrough, J.F., Spielvogel, R.L., Cohen, R., Bartel, R.L., and Naughton, G., *In vivo* optimization of a living dermal substitute employing cultured human fibroblasts on a biodegradable polyglycolic or polyglactin mesh, *Biomaterials*, 12, 243, 1991.

[31] Hansbrough, J.F., Dore, C., and Hansbrough, W.B., Clinical trials of a living dermal tissue replacement placed beneath meshed, split-thickness skin grafts on excised wounds, *J. Burn Care Rehabil.*, 13, 519, 1992.

[32] Hanft, J.R. and Surprenant, M.S., Healing of chronic foot ulcers in diabetic patients treated with a human fibroblast-derived dermis, *J. Foot Ankle Surg.*, 41, 291, 2002.

[33] Carsin, H., Ainaud, P., Le Bever, H., Rives, J., Lakhel, A., Stephanazzi, J., Lambert, F., and Perrot, J., Cultured epithelial autografts in extensive burn coverage of severely traumatized patients: a five year single-center experience with 30 patients, *Burns*, 26, 379, 2000.

[34] Gobet, R., Raghunath, M., Altermatt, S., Meuli-Simmen, C., Benathan, M., Dietl, A., and Meuli, M., Efficacy of cultured epithelial autografts in pediatric burns and reconstructive surgery, *Surgery*, 121, 654, 1997.

[35] Compton, C.C., Current concepts in pediatric burn care: the biology of cultured epithelial autografts: an eight-year study in pediatric burn patients, *Eur. J. Pediatr. Surg.*, 2, 216, 1992.

[36] Gallico III, G.G., O'Connor, N.E., Compton, C.C., Remensynder, J.P., Kehinde, O., and Green, H., Cultured epithelial autografts for giant congenital nevi, *Plast. Reconstr. Surg.*, 84, 1, 1989.

[37] Koria, P., Brazeau, D., Kirkwood, K., Hayden, P., Klausner, M., and Andreadis, S.T., Gene expression profile of tissue engineered skin subjected to acute barrier disruption, *J. Invest. Dermatol.*, 121, 368, 2003.

[38] Oren, A., Ganz, T., Liu, L., and Meerloo, T., In human epidermis, beta-defensin 2 is packaged in lamellar bodies, *Exp. Mol. Pathol.*, 74, 180, 2003.

[39] Liu, L., Roberts, A.A., and Ganz, T., By IL-1 signaling, monocyte-derived cells dramatically enhance the epidermal antimicrobial response to lipopolysaccharide, *J. Immunol.*, 170, 575, 2003.

[40] Liebsch, M., Traue, D., Barrabas, C., Spielmann, H., Uphill, P., Wilkins, S., McPherson, J.P., Wiemann, C., Kaufmann, T., Remmele, M., and Holzhutter, H.-G., The ECVAM prevalidation study on the use of EpiDerm for skin corrosivity testing, *ATLA*, 28, 371, 2000.

[41] Limat, A., Mauri, D., and Hunziker, T., Successful treatment of chronic leg ulcers with epidermal equivalents generated from cultured autologous outer root sheath cells, *J. Invest. Dermatol.*, 107, 128, 1996.

[42] Yang, J.S., Lavker, R.M., and Sun, T.T., Upper human hair follicle contains a subpopulation of keratinocytes with superior *in vitro* proliferative potential, *J. Invest. Dermatol.*, 101, 652, 2003.

[43] Yannas, I.V. and Burke, J.F., Design of an artificial skin. I. Basic design principles, *J. Biomed. Mater. Res.*, 14, 65, 1980.

[44] Yannas, I.V., Burke, J.F., Gordon, P.L., Huang, C., and Rubenstein, R.H., Design of an artificial skin. II. Control of chemical composition, *J. Biomed. Mater. Res.*, 14, 107, 1980.

[45] Heimbach, D., Luterman, A., Burke, J.F., Cram, A., Herndon, D., Hunt, J., Jordon, M., McManus, W., Solem, L., Warden, G., and Zawacki, B., Artificial dermis for major burns; a multi-center randomized clinical trial, *Ann. Surg.*, 208, 313, 1988.

[46] Sheridan, R.L., Hegarty, M., Tompkins, R.G., and Burke, J.F., Artificial skin in massive burns — results to ten years, *Eur. J. Plast. Surg.*, 17, 91, 1994.

[47] Heimbach, D.M., Warden, G.D., Luterman, A., Jordan, M.H., Ozobia, N., Ryan, C.M., Voigt, D.W., Hickerson, W.L., Saffle, J.R., DeClement, F.A., Sheridan, R.L., and Dimick, A.R., Multicenter postapproval clinical trial of Integra dermal regeneration template for burn treatment, *J. Burn Care Rehabil.*, 24, 42, 2003.

[48] Wisser, D. and Steffes, J., Skin replacement with a collagen based dermal substitute, autologous keratinocytes and fibroblasts in burn trauma, *Burns*, 29, 375, 2003.

[49] Kopp, J., Magnus, N.E., Rubben, A., Merk, H.F., and Pallua, N., Radical resection of giant congenital melanocyte nevus and reconstruction with meek-graft covered integra dermal template, *Dermatol. Surg.*, 29, 653, 2003.

[50] Stephens, R., Wilson, K., and Silverstein, P., A premature infant with skin injury successfully treated with bilayered cell matrix, *Ostomy Wound Manage.*, 48, 34, 2002.

[51] Still, J., Glat, P., Silverstein, P., Griswold, J., and Mozingo, D., The use of a collagen spong/living cell composite material to treat donor sites in burn patients, *Burns*, 29, 837, 2003.

[52] Doucet, O., Robert, C., and Zastrow, L., Use of a serum-free reconstituted epidermis as a skin pharmacological model, *Toxicol. In Vitro*, 10, 305, 1996.

[53] De Fraissinette, A.D.B., Picarles, V., Chibout, S.D., Kolopp, M., Medina, J., Burtin, P., Ebelin, M.-E., Osborne, S., Mayer, F.K., Spake, A., Rosdy, M., De Wever, B., Ettline, R.A., and Cordier, A., Predictivity of an *in vitro* model for acute and chronic skin irritation (SkinEthic) applied to the testing of topical vehicles, *Cell Biol. Toxicol.*, 15, 121, 1999.

[54] Medina, J., Elsaesser, C., Picarles, V., Grenet, O., Kolopp, M., Chibout, S.D., and De Fraissinette, A.D.B., Assessment of the phototoxic potential of compounds and finished topical products using a human reconstructed epidermis, *In Vitro Mol. Toxicol.*, 14, 157, 2001.

[55] Higham, M.C., Dawson, R., Szabo, M., Short, R., Haddow, D.B., and MacNeil, S., Development of a stable chemically defined surface for the culture of human keratinocytes under serum-free conditions for clinical use, *Tissue Eng.*, 9, 919, 2003.

[56] Hansbrough, J.F., Mozingo, D.W., Kealey, G.P., Davis, M., Gidner, A., and Gentzkow, G.D., Clinical trials of a biosynthetic temporary skin replacement, Dermagraft-transitional covering, compared

with cryopreserved human cadaver skin for temporary coverage of excised burn wounds, *J. Burn Care Rehabil.*, 18, 43, 1997.

[57] Purdue, G.F., Hunt, J.L., Still Jr, J.M., Law, E.J., Herndon, D.N., Goldfarb, I.W., Schiller, W.R., Hansbrough, J.F., Hickerson, W.L., Himel, H.N., Kealey, G.P., Twomey, J., Missavage, A.E., Solem, L.D., Davis, M., Totoritis, M., and Gentzkow, G.D., A multicenter clinical trial of a biosynthetic skin replacement, Dermagraft-TC, compared with cryopreserved human cadaver skin for temporary coverage of excised burn wounds, *J. Burn Care Rehabil.*, 18, 52, 1997.

[58] Noordenbos, J., Dore, C., and Hansbrough, J.F., Safety and efficacy of TransCyte for the treatment of partial-thickness burns, *J. Burn Care Rehabil.*, 20, 275, 1999.

[59] Odessey, R., Addendum: multicenter experience with cultured epithelial autografts for treatment of burns, *J. Burn Care Rehabil.*, 13, 174, 1992.

[60] Pittelkow, M.R. and Scott, R.E., New techniques for the *in vitro* culture of human skin keratinocytes and perspectives on their use for grafting of patients with extensive burns, *Mayo Clin. Proc.*, 61, 771, 1986.

[61] Desai, M.H., Mlakar, J.M., McCauley, R.L., Abdullah, K.M., Rutan, R.L., Waymack, J.P., Robson, M.C., and Herndon, D.N., Lack of long term durability of cultured keratinocyte burn wound coverage: a case report, *J. Burn Care Rehabil.*, 12, 540, 1991.

[62] Williamson, J., Snelling, C., Clugston, P., Mac Donald, I., and Germann, E., Cultured epithelial autograft: five years of clinical experience with twenty-eight patients, *J. Trauma*, 39, 309, 1995.

[63] Rue, L.W., Cioffi, W.G., McManus, W.F., and Pruitt, B.A., Wound closure and outcome in extensively burned patients treated with cultured autologous keratinocytes, *J. Trauma*, 34, 662, 1993.

[64] Arons, M.S., Management of giant congenital nevi, *Plast. Reconstr. Surg.*, 110, 352, 2002.

[65] Boyce, S.T., Cultured skin substitutes: a review, *Tissue Eng.*, 2, 255, 1996.

[66] Boyce, S.T. and Warden, G.D., Principles and practices for treatment of cutaneous wounds with cultured skin substitutes, *Am. J. Surg.*, 183, 445, 2002.

[67] Boyce, S.T., Kagan, R.J., Meyer, N.A., Yakuboff, K.P., and Warden, G.D., *The 1999 Clinical Research Award*, Cultured skin substitutes combined with Integra to replace native skin autograft and allograft for closure of full-thickness burns, *J. Burn Care Rehabil.*, 20, 453, 1999.

[68] Boyce, S.T., Kagan, R.J., Yakuboff, K.P., Meyer, N.A., Rieman, M.T., Greenhalgh, D.G., and Warden, G.D., Cultured skin substitutes reduce donor skin harvesting for closure of excised, full-thickness burns, *Ann. Surg.*, 235, 269, 2002.

[69] Lukish, J.R., Eichelberger, M.R., Newman, K.D., Pao, M., Nobuhara, K., Keating, M., Golonka, N., Pratsch, G., Misra, V., Valladares, E., Johnson, P., Gilbert, J.C., Powell, D.M., and Hartman, G.E., The use of a bioactive skin substitute decreases length of stay for pediatric burn patients, *J. Pediatr. Surg.*, 36, 1118, 2001.

[70] Klein, R.L., Rothmann, B.F., and Marshall, R., Biobrane — a useful adjunct in the therapy of outpatient burns, *J. Pediatr. Surg.*, 19, 846, 1984.

[71] Boyce, S.T. and Ham, R.G., Cultivation, frozen storage, and clonal growth of normal human epidermal keratinocytes in serum-free media, *J. Tissue Cult. Meth.*, 9, 83, 1985.

[72] Boyce, S.T., Methods for serum-free culture of keratinocytes and transplantation of collagen-GAG based composite grafts, in *Methods in Tissue Engineering*, Morgan, J.R. and Yarmush, M., Eds., Humana Press, Inc., Totowa, NJ, 1998, p. 365.

[73] Boyce, S.T., Methods for the serum-free culture of keratinocytes and transplantation of collagen-GAG-based skin substitutes, in *Methods in Molecular Medicine, Vol. 18: Tissue Engineering Methods and Protocols*, Morgan, J.R. and Yarmush, M.L., Eds., Humana Press Inc., Totowa, NJ, 2001, p. 365.

[74] Munster, A.M., Cultured skin for massive burns: a prospective, controlled trial, *Ann. Surg.*, 224, 372, 1996.

[75] Boyce, S.T., Foreman, T.J., English, K.B., Stayner, N., Cooper, M.L., Sakabu, S., and Hansbrough, J.F., Skin wound closure in athymic mice with cultured human cells, biopolymers, and growth factors, *Surgery*, 110, 866, 1991.

[76] Boyce, S.T., Cultured skin for wound closure, in *Skin Substitute Production by Tissue Engineering: Clinical and Fundamental Applications*, Rouahbia, M., Ed., R.G. Landes, Austin, TX, 1997, p. 75.

[77] Boyce, S.T., Skin substitutes from cultured cells and collagen-GAG polymers, *Med. Biol. Eng. Comp.*, 36, 791, 1998.

[78] Boyce, S.T. and Ham, R.G., Calcium-regulated differentiation of normal human epidermal keratinocytes in chemically defined clonal culture and serum-free serial culture, *J. Invest. Dermatol.*, 81 (Suppl 1), 33s, 1983.

[79] Harriger, M.D., Warden, G.D., Greenhalgh, D.G., Kagan, R.J., and Boyce, S.T., Pigmentation and microanatomy of skin regenerated from composite grafts of cultured cells and biopolymers applied to full-thickness burn wounds, *Transplantation*, 59, 702, 1995.

[80] Boyce, S.T., Supp, A.P., Swope, V.B., and Warden, G.D., Vitamin C regulates keratinocyte viability, epidermal barrier, and basement membrane formation *in vitro*, and reduces wound contraction after grafting of cultured skin substitutes, *J. Invest. Dermatol.*, 118, 565, 2002.

[81] Boyce, S.T., Supp, A.P., Harriger, M.D., Pickens, W.L., Wickett, R.R., and Hoath, S.B., Surface electrical capacitance as a noninvasive index of epidermal barrier in cultured skin substitutes in athymic mice, *J. Invest. Dermatol.*, 107, 82, 1996.

[82] Cuono, C., Langdon, R., Birchall, N., Barttelbort, S., and McGuire, J., Composite autologous-allogeneic skin replacement: development and clinical application, *Plast. Reconstr. Surg.*, 80, 626, 1987.

[83] Burke, J.F., Yannas, I.V., Quinby, W.C., Bondoc, C.C., and Jung, W.K., Successful use of a physiologically acceptable skin in the treatment of extensive burn injury, *Ann. Surg.*, 194, 413, 1981.

[84] Young, D.M., Greulich, K.M., and Weier, H.G., Species-specific *in situ* hybridization with fluorochrome-labeled DNA probes to study vascularization of human skin grafts on athymic mice, *J. Burn Care Rehabil.*, 17, 305, 1996.

[85] Supp, D.M., Supp, A.P., Bell, S.M., and Boyce, S.T., Enhanced vascularization of cultured skin substitutes genetically modified to overexpress Vascular Endothelial Growth Factor, *J. Invest. Dermatol.*, 114, 5, 2000.

[86] Supp, D.M. and Boyce, S.T., Overexpression of vascular endothelial growth factor accelerates early vascularization and improves healing of genetically modified cultured skin substitutes, *J. Burn Care Rehabil.*, 23, 10, 2002.

[87] Monafo, W.W. and West, M.A., Current treatment recommendations for topical burn therapy, *Drugs*, 40, 364, 1990.

[88] Boyce, S.T. and Holder, I.A., Selection of topical antimicrobial agents for cultured skin for burns by combined assessment of cellular cytotoxicity and antimicrobial activity, *Plast. Reconstr. Surg.*, 92, 493, 1993.

[89] Boyce, S.T., Warden, G.D., and Holder, I.A., Cytotoxicity testing of topical antimicrobial agents on human keratinocytes and fibroblasts for cultured skin grafts, *J. Burn Care Rehabil.*, 16, 97, 1995.

[90] Boyce, S.T., Warden, G.D., and Holder, I.A., Non-cytotoxic combinations of topical antimicrobial agents for use with cultured skin, *Antimicrob. Agents Chemother.*, 39, 1324, 1995.

[91] Compton, C.C., Wound healing potential of cultured epithelium, *Wounds*, 5, 97, 1993.

[92] Munster, A.M., Weiner, S.H., and Spence, R.J., Cultured epidermis for coverage of burn wounds: a single center experience, *Ann. Surg.*, 211, 676, 1990.

[93] Sullivan, T., Smith, H., Kermode, J., McIver, E., and Courtemanche, D.J., Rating the burn scar, *J. Burn Care Rehabil.*, 11, 256, 1990.

[94] Supp, A.P., Wickett, R.R., Swope, V.B., Harriger, M.D., Hoath, S.B., and Boyce, S.T., Incubation of cultured skin substitutes in reduced humidity promotes cornification *in vitro* and stable engraftment in athymic mice, *Wound Repair Regen.*, 7, 226, 1999.

[95] Goretsky, M.J., Supp, A.P., Greenhalgh, D.G., Warden, G.D., and Boyce, S.T., *The 1995 Young Investigator Award:* Surface electrical capacitance as an index of epidermal barrier properties of composite skin substitutes and skin autografts, *Wound Repair Regen.*, 3, 419, 1995.

[96] Boyce, S.T., Regulatory issues and standardization, in *Methods of Tissue Engineering*, Atala, A. and Lanza, R., Eds., Academic Press, San Diego, 2001, p. 3.

[97] US Food and Drug Administration, Guidance for industry: precautionary measures to reduce the possible risk of transmission of zoonoses by blood and blood products from xenotransplantation product recipients and their contacts, *Fed. Regist.*, 64, 73562, 1999.

[98] Rheinwald, J.G. and Green, H., Serial cultivation of strains of human epidermal keratinocytes: the formation of keratinizing colonies from single cells, *Cell*, 6, 331, 1975.

[99] US Food and Drug Administration, Guidance on applications for products comprised of living autologous cells manipulated *ex vivo* and intended for structural repair or reconstruction, *Fed. Regist.*, 61, 26523, 1996.

[100] Abdel-Malek, Z.A., Endocrine factors as effectors of integumental pigmentation, *Dermatol. Clin.*, 6, 175, 1988.

[101] Nordlund, J.J., Abdel-Malek, Z.A., Boissy, R.E., and Rheins, L.A., Pigment cell biology: an historical review, *J. Invest. Dermatol.*, 92, 53S, 1989.

[102] Fauerbach, J.A., Heinberg, L.J., Lawrence, J.W., Munster, A.M., Palombo, D.A., Richter, D., Spence, R.J., Stevens, S.S., Ware, L., and Muehlberger, T., Effect of early body image dissatisfaction on subsequent psychological and physical adjustment after disfiguring injury, *Psychosom. Med.*, 62, 576, 2000.

[103] Compton, C.C., Gill, J.M., Bradford, D.A., Regauer, S., Gallico G.G., and O'Connor, N.E., Skin regenerated from cultured epithelial autografts on full-thickness burn wounds from 6 days to 5 years after grafting, *Lab. Invest.*, 60, 600, 1989.

[104] DeLuca, M., Franzi, A., D'Anna, F., Zicca, A., Albanese, E., Bondanza, S., and Cancedda, R., Co-culture of human keratinocytes and melanocytes: differentiated melanocytes are physiologically organized in the basal layer of the cultured epithelium, *Eur. J. Cell Biol.*, 46, 176, 1988.

[105] Compton, C.C., Warland, G., and Kratz, G., Melanocytes in cultured epithelial autografts are depleted with serial subcultivation and cryopreservation: implications for clinical outcome, *J. Burn Care Rehabil.*, 19, 330, 1998.

[106] Boyce, S.T., Medrano, E.E., Abdel-Malek, Z.A., Supp, A.P., Dodick, J.M., Nordlund, J.J., and Warden, G.D., Pigmentation and inhibition of wound contraction by cultured skin substitutes with adult melanocytes after transplantation to athymic mice, *J. Invest. Dermatol.*, 100, 360, 1993.

[107] Swope, V.B., Supp, A.P., Cornelius, J.R., Babcock, G.F., and Boyce, S.T., Regulation of pigmentation in cultured skin substitutes by cytometric sorting of melanocytes and keratinocytes, *J. Invest. Dermatol.*, 109, 289, 1997.

[108] Swope, V.B., Supp, A.P., and Boyce, S.T., Regulation of cutaneous pigmentation by titration of human melanocytes in cultured skin substitutes grafted to athymic mice, *Wound Repair Regen.*, 10, 378, 2002.

[109] Boyce, S.T., Supp, A.P., Harriger, M.D., Greenhalgh, D.G., and Warden, G.D., Topical nutrients promote engraftment and inhibit wound contraction of cultured skin substitutes in athymic mice, *J. Invest. Dermatol.*, 104, 345, 1995.

[110] L'Heureux, N., Germian, L., Labbe, R., and Auger, F.A., *In vitro* construction of a human blood vessel from cultured vascular cells: a morphologic study, *J. Vasc. Surg.*, 14, 499, 1993.

[111] Schechner, J.S., Nath, A.K., Zheng, L., Kluger, M.S., Hughes, C.C.W., Sierra-Honigmann, M.R., Lorber, M.I., Tellides, G., Kashgarian, M., Bothwell, A.L.M., and Pober, J.S., *In vivo* formation of complex microvessels lined by human endothelial cells in an immunodeficient mouse, *Proc. Natl Acad. Sci. USA*, 97, 9191, 2000.

[112] Schechner, J.S., Crane, S.K., Wang, F., Szeglin, A.M., Tellides, G., Lorber, M.I., Bothwell, A.L., and Pober, J.S., Engraftment of a vascularized human skin equivalent, *FASEB J.*, 17, 2250, 2003.

[113] Supp, D.M., Wilson-Landy, K., and Boyce, S.T., Human dermal microvascular endothelial cells form vascular analogs in cultured skin substitutes after grafting to athymic mice, *FASEB J.*, 16, 797, 2002.

[114] Choate, K.A., Medalie, D.A., Morgan, J.R., and Khavari, P.A., Corrective gene transfer in the human skin disorder lamellar ichthyosis, *Nat. Med.*, 2, 1263, 1996.

[115] Vailly, J., Gagnouz-Palacios, L., Dell'Ambra, E., Romero, C., Pinola, M., Zambruno, G., De Luca, M., Ortonne, J.P., and Meneguzzi, G., Corrective gene transfer of keratinoyctes from patients with junctional epidermolysis bullosa restores assembly of hemidesmosomes in reconstructed epithelia, *Gene Ther.*, 5, 1322, 1998.

[116] Dellambra, E., Vailly, J., Pellegrini, G., Bondanza, S., Golisano, O., Macchia, C., Zambruno, G., Meneguzzi, G., and De Luca, M., Corrective transduction of human epidermal stem cells in laminin-5-dependent junctional epidermolysis bullosa, *Hum. Gene Ther.*, 9, 1359, 1998.

[117] Vogt, P.M., Thompson, S., Andree, C., Liu, P., Breuing, K., Hatzis, D., Brown, H., Mulligan, R.C., and Ericksson, E., Genetically modified keratinocytes transplanted to wounds reconstitute the epidermis, *Proc. Natl Acad. Sci. USA*, 91, 9307, 1994.

[118] Morgan, J.R., Barrandon, Y., Green, H., and Mulligan, R.C., Expression of an exogenous growth hormone gene in transplantable human epidermal cells, *Science*, 237, 1476, 1987.

[119] Gerrard, A.J., Hudson, D.L., Brownlee, G.G., and Watt, F.M., Towards gene therapy for haemophilia B using primary human keratinocytes, *Nat. Gen.*, 3, 180, 1993.

[120] Page, S.M. and Brownlee, G.G., An *ex vivo* keratinocyte model for gene therapy of hemophilia B, *J. Invest. Dermatol.*, 108, 139, 1997.

[121] White, S.J., Page, S.M., Margaritis, P., and Brownlee, G.G., Long-term expression of human clotting factor IX from retrovirally transduced primary human keratinocytes *in vivo*, *Hum. Gene Ther.*, 9, 1187, 2002.

[122] Eming, S.A., Medalie, D.A., Tompkins, R.G., Yarmush, M.L., and Morgan, J.R., Genetically modified human keratinocytes overexpressing PDGF-A enhance the performance of a composite skin graft, *Hum. Gene Ther.*, 9, 529, 1998.

[123] Erdag, G. and Morgan, J.R., Survival of fetal skin grafts is prolonged on the human peripheral blood lymphocyte reconstituted-severe combined immunodeficient mouse/skin allograft model, *Transplantation*, 73, 519, 2002.

[124] Li, Y., Tredget, E.E., and Ghahary, A., Cell surface expression of MHC class I antigen is suppressed in indoleamine 2,3-dioxygenase genetically modified keratinoycytes: implications in allogeneic skin substitute engraftment, *Hum. Immunol.*, 65, 114, 2004.

48

Nerve Regeneration: Tissue Engineering Strategies

Jennifer B. Recknor
Surya K. Mallapragada
Iowa State University

48.1 Introduction

The nervous system of the adult mammal is divided into two main components: the peripheral nervous system (PNS) and central nervous system (CNS). The PNS, consisting of cranial and spinal nerves and their associated ganglia, has the intrinsic ability for repair and regeneration. However, the adult mammalian central nervous system (CNS), consisting of the brain and spinal cord, is viewed as largely incapable of self-repair or regeneration of correct axonal and dendritic connections after injury [1–3]. When a peripheral nerve is injured and the nerve retracts, or tissue is lost, preventing an end-to-end repair, grafting is a commonly performed. Grafting methods, involving autografts and allografts, provide trophic factors and guidance for regenerating axons [4,5]. However, there are major limitations to grafting including multiple surgeries, lack of donor tissue, and immune rejection. The CNS is a more complex environment that proves to be not as amenable to healing as the PNS. Adult CNS injury is typically followed by neuronal degeneration, cell death, and the breakdown of synaptic connections. It is established that fish, amphibia, mammalian peripheral nerves as well as developing central nerves respond differently to injury than the adult mammalian CNS. In these systems, functional axons can regrow after they have been damaged [1]. However, currently, in the mammalian CNS, there is no treatment for the restoration of human nerve function due to the intricate series of events that must take place in order for regeneration to occur.

Growth across the PNS–CNS transition zone has not been successful in many regeneration attempts [6]. The limitations with current strategies for repair of the PNS and CNS can eventually be minimized using tissue-engineering applications to restore biological function by providing a permissive environment for regeneration. The purpose of this chapter is to review recent research applications involving guidance and molecular and cellular strategies for nerve repair that have demonstrated the use of neural tissue engineering to achieve therapeutic goals for nervous system regeneration.

48.2   Neural Regeneration

Injured axons in the PNS are capable of regenerating long distances and have the capacity to establish connections with their targets. In adult mammals, injury to the CNS does not usually result in regeneration. When nerve damage occurs, the portion of the axon isolated from the cell body is referred to as the distal segment. The portion connected to the cell body is the proximal segment. The response of the native environment surrounding these segments following injury is the key reason behind the inherent capacity of the PNS for regeneration, which is not characteristic of the CNS.

48.2.1   Peripheral Nervous System

Nerve injury results in a characteristic chain of degenerative and regenerative events. Complete transection of a nerve is the most severe PNS injury. At the site of nerve damage, the myelin and axons break up, triggering the migration of phagocytic cells, Schwann cells and macrophages, into the PNS to clean up debris. After an axon is transected, the proximal segment of the nerve swells and experiences retrograde degeneration near the wound site. After myelin is cleared and the Schwann cells and macrophages remove debris, the proximal end begins to sprout axons and growth cones emerge [7]. After transection, Wallerian degeneration occurs distal to the injury within hours. The axons and myelin degenerate completely but the endoneurium is left intact forming natural conduits [8]. The endoneurial channel directs the axon regrowth in the reparative phase, and axons of surviving neurons grow into the endoneurial tube. Axons of the proximal segment can regenerate back to previous synaptic sites as long as their cell bodies remain alive and the proximal axons have made successful contact with neurolemmocytes in the endoneurial channel. The proliferation of Schwann cells at this time retains the endoneurial tube structure as these cells form ordered columns. Neurotrophic factors are also produced by Schwann and macrophages, and growth-promoting substances are upregulated providing an optimal environment for axon growth. In humans, regeneration proceeds at approximately 2 mm/d in the smaller nerve and 5 mm/d in the larger nerve. Functional reinnervation only occurs when axons find the Schwann cell column and reach their distal target or effector organ. Successful axonal regeneration depends on the distance of the lesioned site from the cell body, the nature of the injury and axonal contact with neurolemmocytes in the distal segment. For additional reviews on peripheral nerve regeneration, refer to Fawcett and Keynes [9].

48.2.2   Central Nervous System

CNS axons do not regenerate due to a lack of support by the endogenous environment following injury. In the CNS of mammals, axonal regeneration is limited by inhibitory influences of the glial and extracellular environment [10]. The CNS environment is inhibitory in nature making axonal regrowth from adult neurons nearly impossible. Myelin-associated inhibitors of neurite growth, astrocytes, oligodendrocytes, oligodendrocyte precursors, and microglia migrate to the injury site making the environment nonpermissive for axonal growth. In the distal axonal segment, degeneration is slower in the CNS compared to the PNS, and inhibitory myelin and axonal debris are not cleared away as quickly. The axons that survive axotomy are surrounded by unfavorable glial reactions at the lesion site, known as the glial scar. Neurons cannot regenerate beyond the glial scar where axonal outgrowth is essentially stopped [11]. Proximal axons initially demonstrate a spontaneous attempt to regenerate, but the surrounding environment rapidly hinders growth [12]. Consequently, regenerating axons in the CNS cannot reach synaptic targets and reestablish their original connections. Mechanisms for removing or neutralizing the inhibitory components of cellular debris cannot be found in the CNS. However, severed mammalian CNS axons will regrow in more permissive environments [13–15]. They are able to recognize target areas and to re-establish functional synapses with target neurons [16,17]. There has been much recent evidence that suggests that the mature CNS is a less hostile environment for regeneration than was previously thought. If the axons can transverse the injury site, there is possibility of regrowth in the unscarred areas and of functional recovery [18,19]. The use of scaffolds [18,20–23], cell implantation and replacement therapies involving neural stem [20,24], Schwann [25,26] and olfactory ensheathing cells [27], as well as delivery of growth factors [28,29] have provided greater potential for production of new neurons and the repair of injured CNS regions. For additional reviews on central nervous system regeneration, refer to Fry [3] and Schwab [30].

48.3 Guidance Strategies for Regeneration

For successful regeneration, damaged axons must be prevented from dying, the sprouting axons from the proximal nerve stump must extend axons toward their targets, across the injury site, into the distal nerve stump and make synaptic connections to the correct target regions. Common repair techniques facilitating regeneration include grafting using natural materials and entubulization using nerve conduits or scaffolds. These methods connect proximal and distal nerve stumps using a synthetic or biologically derived conduit. Such conduits optimize regeneration by allowing for both physical and chemical guidance and reducing cellular invasion and scarring of the nerve. Entubulization minimizes unregulated axonal growth at the site of injury by providing a distinct environment, and allows for diffusion of trophic factors emitted from the distal stump to reach the proximal segment, which enhances physiological conditions for nerve regeneration. The transplantation of tissue engineered nerve conduits based on polymers and alternative methods to engineer an artificial environment to mimic natural physical and chemical stimulus promotes nerve regeneration and minimizes difficulties associated with grafting.

48.3.1 Autografts

A nerve autograft (or autologous tissue graft) is the transfer of nerve segments from an uninjured part of the body to another. This graft tissue provides endoneurial tubes that enable guided regeneration of axons. Autologous nerve grafts are currently used in the treatment of peripheral nerve injuries where the gap of a transected nerve is large [31]. This method for restoring tissue results in partial deinnervation of the donor site to repair the injury site. Tissue availability is a concern as well as the need for multiple surgeries and potential differences in size and shape leading to difficulties with scale-up.

The capacity of the CNS axons to regrow in a permissive environment has been demonstrated using autologous PNS tissue grafts to bridge the adult rat medulla oblongata and the spinal cord following injury to the CNS. Axons from neurons at the medulla and spinal cord levels grew along the bridge. However, the axons did not re-enter the host tissue [14]. So and Aguayo [32] also demonstrated that transected axons of retinal ganglion cells could regrow into autologous PNS segments grafted directly into the rat retina. Regenerating axons were able to recognize target areas and re-establish functional synapses with target neurons [16,17]. Such autologous PNS grafts provide essential components for the facilitation of growth and functional recovery that are not found in the native CNS.

48.3.2 Allografts and Acellular Nerve Matrices

Allografts involve the transfer of nerve tissue from donor to recipient. These nerve grafts make use of allogenic and xenogeneic tissues to replace lost function. Allografts eliminate the need for harvesting patient tissue. However, tissue rejection involving an undesirable immune response and lack of donor tissue are two major disadvantages of using allografts. Disease transmission is also a risk. Using allografts with immunosuppression has been considered. However, results obtained with allografts have not matched the performance observed with autografts [33].

Acellular nerve matrix allografts have also been observed as useful biomaterials for nerve regeneration [34]. These allografts preserve extracellular matrix (ECM) components and, therefore, mimic the ECM of peripheral nerves mechanically and physically. In this way, acellular nerve matrices aid in the reconstruction of the peripheral nerve. However, decellularization techniques, such as thermal decellularization, can damage the ECM structure and fail to extract all cellular components leading to inflammation upon implantation [35].

48.3.3 Entubulization Using Nerve Conduits

Current limitations with autografts and allografts have led to exploration of possible alternatives for the repair of nerve injury. Tissue-engineered nerve conduits based on polymers have been created for implantation mimicking the three-dimensional and biological environment that is necessary for enhanced regeneration. While bridging the gap between nerve segments, these conduits can preserve neurotropic and neurotrophic communication between the nerve stumps, repel external inhibitory molecules, and provide physical guidance for the regenerating axons similar to the grafts (Figure 48.1) [36]. The spatial cues provided by conduits also induce a change in tissue-architecture cabling cells within the microconduit [37]. Polymers are being extensively investigated to help facilitate nerve regeneration and provide physical and chemical stimulus to regenerating axons [38,39]. These materials vary in composition from entirely synthetic to naturally derived biomaterials. Synthetic conduits are fabricated from metals and ceramics, biodegradable (i.e., poly(esters), such as poly(lactic acid) [40–42], poly(lactic-co-glycolic acid) [42,43], and poly(caprolactone) [44,45], or polyhydroxybutarate [46]) and nonbiodegradable (i.e., methacrylate-based hydrogels [47], polystyrene [48], silicone [49,50], expanded poly(tetrafluoroethylene) or ePTFE (Gore-Tex®: W.L. Gore & Associates, Flagstaff, AZ) [51,52] or poly(tetrafluroethylene) (PTFE) [53]) synthetic polymers. These materials are especially advantageous because specific chemical and physical properties can be readily changed depending on the application for which they are used. Such properties include microgeometry, degradation rate, porosity, and mechanical strength. Biologically derived materials include proteins and polysaccharides (i.e., ECM-based proteins including fibronectin [54], laminin [55] and collagen [56,57], fibrin and fibrinogen [58–60], hyaluronic acid derivatives [61], and agarose [62]). Collagen has been the most widely used natural polymer [57]. These natural materials are biocompatible and enhance migration of support cells [33]. However, batch-to-batch variability needs to be considered when using biological materials such as these. Selecting the appropriate material for a particular application is an essential part of the scaffold design. There are also certain physical properties and that are most desirable for nerve conduits (Figure 48.2) [63]. General requirements for scaffold design are typically followed, which include being biocompatible, having a high surface area/volume ratio with sufficient mechanical integrity and having the ability to provide a suitable environment for axonal growth that can integrate with the surrounding neural environment. These biomaterial-based (synthetic or natural) conduits can also be environmentally enhanced with chemical stimulants, such as laminin and nerve growth factor (NGF), biological or cellular cues such as from neural stem cells as well as Schwann cells and astrocytes, the satellite cells of the peripheral and central nervous systems, and lastly, physical guidance cues.

48.4 Enhancing Neural Regeneration Using Entubulization Strategies

...iding a permissive environment for damaged neural tissues that have suffered trauma is essential ... regeneration of the injured nervous system. In order to generate an environment that supports ...tion, physical, chemical, and biological manipulations must be made. Guidance cues must be ...that aid in control of nerve outgrowth and navigate neuronal growth cones to distant targets

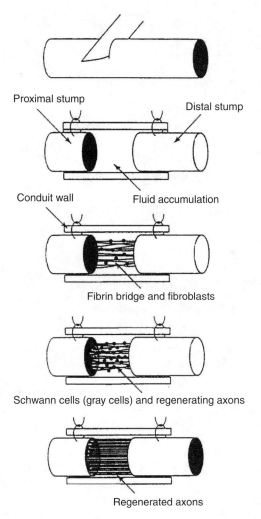

FIGURE 48.1 Silicone-chamber model showing the progression of events during peripheral-nerve rgeneration. After bridging the proximal and distal nerve stumps, the silicone tube becomes filled with serum and other extracellular fluids. A fibrin bridge containing a variety of cell types connects the two stumps. Schwann cells and axons processes migrate from the proximal end to the distal stump along the bridge. The axons continue to regenerate through the distal stump to their final contacts. (Reproduced from Heath, C. and Rutkowski, G.E. *Trends Biotechnol.*, 16, 163–168, 1998. With permission.)

in vivo. "Intelligent" nerve conduits having the appropriate combination of such cues will provide insight into the mechanisms behind axon growth and regeneration in nervous system. These scaffolds can enhance regeneration and help repair severed or injured neural tissue.

48.4.1 Physical Modifications

48.4.1.1 Microtexturing

Scaffolds are extremely useful for evaluating nerve regeneration processes for many reasons. Among these is that the properties of these conduits can be physically altered to optimize nerve regeneration. The microtexture of the surface of the lumen within the conduit affects the outgrowth of neurons and regulates regeneration. Smooth inner surfaces allow the formation of an organized, discrete nerve cable having many myelinated axons. In contrast, inside rough inner surfaces, nerve fascicles are dispersed throughout

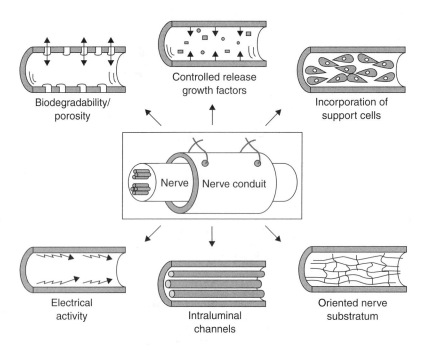

FIGURE 48.2 Properties of the ideal nerve conduit. The desired physical properties of a nerve conduit include (*clockwise from top left*): a biodegradable and porous channel wall; the ability to deliver bioactive factors, such as growth factors; the incorporation of support cells; an internal oriented matrix to support cell migration; intraluminal channels to mimic the structure of nerve fascicles; and electrical activity. (Reproduced from Hudson, T.W., Evans, G.R.D., and Schmidt, C.E. *Clin. Plast. Surg.*, 26, 617, 1999. With permission.)

the lumen and unorganized resulting in little regeneration. When comparing expanded microfibrillar poly(tetrafluroethylene) (Gore–Tex®: W.L. Gore & Associates, Flagstaff, AZ) tubes having different inter-nodal distances (1, 5, and 10 μm) to smooth-walled, impermeable PTFE tubes, it was discovered that rougher the texture of the surface, the greater the spread of nerve fascicles [64]. Furthermore, the molecular and cellular makeup of the regenerating tissue is affected the stability of the wall structure [41] and channel geometry [65].

48.4.1.2   Micropatterning

In addition to texture, scaffolds can exert control over other aspects of the neural environment. The structure of these scaffolds can be precisely defined for a particular application. Relying on knowledge of structure and function of cells and tissues in the nervous system, specific biomaterial "architecture" can be created and applied to the reconstruction of tissue function. The susceptibility of a cell to topographical structure is determined by the organization of the cytoskeleton, cell adhesion, and cell-to-cell interactions [66]. Cell growth can be controlled at the cellular level through the fabrication of microgrooves and other patterns on substrate surfaces [67]. The development of microfabrication and nanofabrication techniques involving photolithography and reactive ion etching has allowed precise control over patterned features using a variety of materials. Recent developments in manufacturing techniques have included the move from silicon-based fabrication to polymer-based biomaterial scaffolds and the creation of three-dimensional constructs based on success with two-dimensional fabrication methods. Isolating large numbers of individual cells and having control over their shape and distribution is extremely valuable in the analyzing functional changes in individual cells and their relationship with their environment in culture. Fabrication techniques producing substrates with various feature shapes and dimensions are used to study cell behavior and morphology *in vitro* before integrating similar techniques into a scaffold design. In the recent past, micropatterned biodegradable and nonbiodegradable substrates have been developed using microfabrication and transfer patterning techniques [48,68–70]. Microcontact printing techniques involving elastomeric polydimethylsiloxane (PDMS) stamps have been used to create adhesive islands for the control of cell shape, growth, and function [71,72]. Microfluidic patterning has also been used for developing topographical cues on substrates [73]. The effects of the microenvironment on cell behavior has been studied on different substrate materials, including Perspex [66,67,74], silicon wafers [75–77], quartz [78,79], and polymers such as polystyrene [48,80] and biodegradable polymers, including poly (lactide-*co*-glycolide) and poly(DL-lactide) [69,70].

Cell adhesion and proliferation has also been examined using various shapes and feature sizes with several neural cell types. Rectangular shapes [68,81], hexagonal [76], as well as circular features [82] have been successful in controlling cellular behavior. In experiments using lithographically patterned quartz, hippocampal neurites grew parallel to deep, wide grooves but perpendicular to those that were shallow and narrow. Neurites also grew faster in the favored direction of orientation and turned through large angles to align on grooves [81]. The shape and expression of a differentiated phenotype of retinal pigment epithelium (RPE) was controlled using octadecyltrichlorosilane (OTS)-modified glass micropatterned substrates [82]. Webb et al. [79] demonstrated that rat optic nerve astrocytes aligned on surface features as small as 100 nm depths with 260 nm pattern spacing on quartz discs. The oligodendrocyte lineage displayed a high degree of sensitivity to topography as well [79]. Schwann cell and neurite alignment has been demonstrated on micropatterned biodegradable substrates with evidence that groove depth affects the proportion of neurites aligned. Deeper grooves have a stronger effect on cellular behavior [68,70]. Furthermore, these micropatterned biodegradable polymer films were inserted inside poly(D,L-lactide) (PDLA) conduits. The micropatterned surfaces were pre-seeded with Schwann cells in order to provide guidance to axons at the cellular level. Over 95% alignment of the axons and Schwann cells was observed on the micropatterned surfaces with laminin selectively attached to the microgrooves [68]. Mechanisms of contact guidance as well as the intracellular distribution of cytoskeletal elements such as microtubules, microfilaments, intermediate filaments, and adhesive structures on cells as they respond to various geometric configurations, including pillars, columns, and spikes, has been analyzed on microfabricated substrates [73,83].

48.4.2 Biochemical Modifications: Creating an "Active" Nerve Conduit

Eliciting a desirable reaction from the host tissue after nerve injury has a profound influence on the regenerative capacity of the nervous tissue. It has been determined that the response of the host tissue is related to not only the mechanical and physical properties of the implanted biomaterial but the chemical properties also play a strong role in promoting a beneficial response from the native environment [38]. Manipulating the natural repair process of the nervous system by engineering a specific biochemical response from the matrix within the conduit or through delivery of growth and neurotrophic factors is an attractive strategy for enhanced nerve regeneration.

48.4.2.1 Chemical Patterning

Providing an adhesive substrate for cells and neurites to grow on is an important mechanism for guidance. To control cell adhesion, migration as well as tissue growth and repair, scaffolds for neural tissue engineering incorporate specific bioactive chemicals. Several studies have been performed using different methods for generating patterns of adhesive domains on various materials. These studies have largely consisted of two-dimensional substrates where adhesive areas are patterned adjacent to nonadhesive areas. However, chemical patterning of three-dimensional substrates has also been demonstrated. The techniques developed for these *in vitro* studies are then applied to create precise patterns of adhesive domains in conduits [84] to be used in *in vivo* experimentation. Patterning techniques manipulating surface chemistry and using photolithographic photomasks have aided in the reproducible creation of desired patterns of biological molecules on surfaces. Microstamping hexadecanethiol on gold in a self-assembled monolayer (SAM) has been used to create islands of various shapes that support the adsorption of many proteins [72]. Similar methods have been used to print poly-L-lysine, laminin, and bovine serum albumin directly on surfaces using texturized silicone stamps dipped in protein, dried, and transferred onto chemically modified substrates [85,86]. Microfabrication techniques have also been used in the photolithographic patterning of organosilanes to silicon wafers [75,76], quartz, and standard glass [82,87]. Several chemicals and proteins have been employed to create regions of two-dimensional patterns of adhesive domains: laminin [88]; nerve growth factor [89]; fibronectin; collagen; albumin; and laminin paired with other chemicals including laminin–denatured laminin, laminin–albumin, polylysine-conjugated laminin [90], and laminin–collagen [91]. Results from cell experimentation have suggested that biochemical patterning might play a stronger role in inducing cellular response (i.e., attachment, spreading, and alignment) than topography. Therefore, efforts have been made to combine multiple guidance cues by chemically patterning three-dimensional substrates [48,69,70]. For more information on the topographical and biochemical patterning of scaffolds see Flemming et al. [92]; Curtis and Wilkinson [93]; Craighead et al. [73]; and Bhatia and Chen [84].

48.4.2.2   Matrices Within Polymer Conduits

Neural tissue-engineering applications focus on mimicking the nerve and the supporting extracellular matrix (ECM) in order to repair or regenerate axons following damage or disease. Experimentation with ECM molecules [94] and the tailoring of matrices within conduits has led to support of axonal regrowth following injury. Evidence has been presented that the basement membrane protein laminin provides pathways of adhesiveness in both peripheral and central nervous system tissues [95]. This ECM protein is capable of initiating and supporting neurite extension on glass and biodegradable polymers of poly (lactide-*co*-glycolide) and poly(DL-lactide) [68,87] as well as glial cell outgrowth on polystyrene [48] (Figure 48.3). Agarose gels derivatized with laminin oligopeptides have enabled three-dimensional neurite outgrowth *in vitro* from cells containing receptors to the laminin peptides [96]. Regeneration of transected peripheral nerves was enhanced using agarose gels having specific laminin peptides inside the scaffold lumen [97,98]. These gel matrices provide support, create an environment that supports growth and incorporate materials that alter surface area. Collagen, fibronectin, and fibrin have also been used to enhance cell-substrate interaction [55–57,99–103]. Gels using magnetic fields have been shown to orient fibers of collagen within the gels. Compared to randomly oriented fibers, these gels promoted neurite extension both *in vitro* and *in vivo* [56]. Magnetically aligned fibrin gels (MAFGs) having different fibril diameters but similar alignment (Figure 48.4) resulted in drastic changes in the contact guidance response of neurites. In gels formed in 1.2 mM Ca^{2+} and having a smaller fibril diameter, there was no response from chick dorsal root ganglia. However, a strong response in gels formed in 12 and 30 mM Ca^{2+} with a larger fibril diameter enhanced neurite length twofold [103]. Inosine, a purine analog that promotes axonal extension, was loaded into PLGA conduits for controlled release during sciatic nerve regeneration. Inosine-loaded PLGA foams were fashioned into cylindrical nerve guidance channels using a novel low-pressure injection molding technique. After ten weeks, a higher percentage cross-sectional area composed of neural tissue was found in the inosine-loaded conduits compared with controls [104]. Furthermore, nerve conduits can be filled with specific bioactive molecules to elicit new axonal growth following injury. Such molecules including axon guidance and pathfinding molecules (netrins, semaphorins, ephrins, Slits) [105], cell adhesion molecules (CAMs) that promote neurite growth (NCAM, L1, *N*-cadherin, tenascin) [106,107], as well as proteins involved in synaptic differentiation (agrin, laminin beta 2, and ARIA) [108] have numerous applications for nerve regeneration *in vivo*.

Synthetic hydrogels have served as artificial matrices for neural tissue reconstruction, for the delivery of cells and for the promotion of axonal regeneration required for successful neurotransplantation. Cultured neurons were found to attach to hydrogel substrates prepared from poly (2-hydroxyethylmethacrylate) (PHEMA) but grow few nerve fibers unless fibronectin, collagen, or nerve growth factor was incorporated into the hydrogel. This provides a mechanism to provide controlled growth on hydrogel surfaces [109]. Hydrogels have been created with bioactive characteristics for neural cell adhesion and growth [110]. Arg–Gly–Asp (RGD) peptides were synthesized and chemically coupled to the bulk of poly (*N*-(2-hydroxypropyl) methacrylamide) (PHPMA) based polymer hydrogels. These RGD-grafted polymers implanted into the striata of rat brains promoted and supported the growth and spread of glial tissue

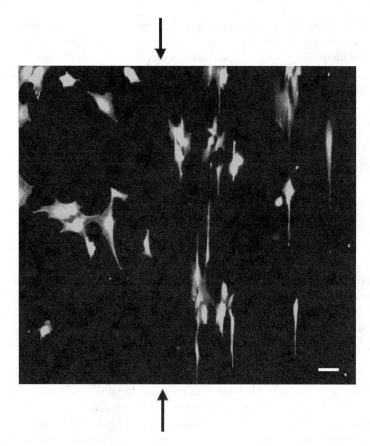

FIGURE 48.3 Astrocytes cultured on a laminin (LAM)-coated (0.01 mg/ml in EBSS) PS substrate. On the 10/20/3 μm LAM-PATTERN/LAM–NO PATTERN substrate, astrocytes are aligned in the direction of the groove on the patterned side (grooves at 90°; right of the arrows) while astrocytes were oriented randomly on the nonpatterned side (left of the arrows) of the substrate. Astrocytes were stained with CFDA SE in cell suspension prior to seeding. Images were taken from PS substrate fixed 24 h after seeding. Scale bar = 30 μm. (Reproduced from Recknor, J.B. et al. *Biomaterials*, 25, 2753–2767, 2004. With permission.)

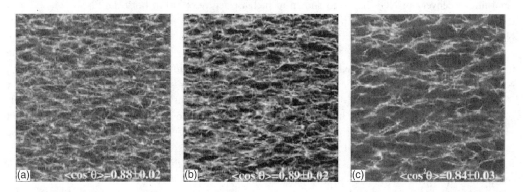

FIGURE 48.4 Confocal fluorescence images of aligned fibrin gels for varied Ca^{2+} concentration. Representative confocal images are shown along with the calculated fibrin fibril alignment parameter for magnetically aligned fibrin gels (MAFGs) formed for three different Ca^{2+} concentrations used in the fibrin-forming solution: (a) 1.2 mM, (b) 12 mM, and (c) 30 mM. Fibril diameter and inter-fibril spacing (porosity) is seen to increase with increasing Ca^{2+} concentration. (Reproduced from Dubey, N., Letourneau, P.C., and Tranquillo, R.T., *Biomaterials*, 22, 1065–1075, 2001. With permission.)

onto and into the hydrogels [111]. Cultured Schwann cells, neonatal astrocytes or cells dissociated from embryonic cerebral hemispheres were also dispersed within PHPMA hydrogel matrices and found to promote cellular ingrowth *in vivo* [112]. These polymer hydrogel matrices were found to have neuroinductive and neuroconductive properties and the potential to repair tissue defects in the central nervous system by promoting the formation of a tissue matrix and axonal growth by replacing lost tissue [47,113–115]. Furthermore, in the injured adult and developing rat spinal cord, these biocompatible porous hydrogels (NeuroGels) promoted axonal growth within the hydrogels, and supraspinal axons migrated into the reconstructed cord segment [116].

48.4.2.3 Neurotrophins

Neurotrophins are proteins in the nervous system that regulate neuronal survival and outgrowth, synaptic connectivity and neurotransmission. These growth-promoting factors are used to functionalize guidance conduits and create a desired response from the regenerating neural environment. Manipulation of polymer conduits for growth factor administration may be a useful treatment for neurodegenerative diseases, such as Alzheimer's disease or Parkinson's disease, which are characterized by the degeneration of neuronal cell populations. There is also much potential for overcoming severe tissue loss using growth factors released from nerve conduits in cases where there is a large gap as a result of axotomy. Various neurotrophic factors, including nerve growth factor (NGF), brain- derived neurotrophic factor (BDNF), neurotrophin-3 (NT-3), and neurotrophin-4/5 (NT-4/5) as well as other important growth factors and cytokines, including ciliary neurotrophic factor (CNTF), glial cell line-derived growth factor (GDNF), and acidic and basic fibroblast growth factor (aFGF, bFGF), have been "trapped" inside polymer conduits that control their release. For further information on these neurotrophic factors and their effects on neural regeneration, refer to Blesch et al. [117]; Jones et al. [119]; Terenghi [118]; Stichel and Muller [120].

Nerve growth factor (NGF) was one of the earliest neurotrophic factors identified and is one of the most thoroughly studied neurotrophins. In early experiments incorporating NGF into silicone chambers, the effects of NGF on nerve regeneration were positive but limited. This was attributed to the rapid decline in NGF concentrations in the conduit due to degradation in aqueous media and leakage from the conduit [121]. The method of delivery of these factors is a challenge and such limitations were overcome by providing controlled release of NGF. Controlled-release polymer delivery systems may be an important technology in enabling the prevention of neuronal degeneration, or even the stimulation of neuronal regeneration, by providing a sustained release of growth factors to promote the long-term survival of endogenous or transplanted cells [122]. Polymeric implants providing controlled release of NGF for one month were developed and found to improve neurite extension in cultured PC12 cells [123]. Continuous delivery of NGF has been shown to increase regeneration in both the PNS [124,125] and the CNS [126,127]. Furthermore, in an effort to readily provide for prolonged, site-specific delivery of NGF to the tissue, without adverse effects on the conduit, biodegradable polymer microspheres of poly (L-lactide) *co*-glycolide containing NGF were fabricated. Biologically active NGF was released from the microspheres, as assayed by neurite outgrowth in a dorsal root ganglion tissue culture system [128–130]. NGF co-encapsulated in PLGA microspheres along with ovalbumin was found to be bioactive for over 90 days [131]. Sustained release of NGF within nerve guide conduits has also been tested. NGF release from biodegradable poly(phosphoester) microspheres produced using a double emulsion technique exhibited a lower burst effect but similar protein entrapment levels and efficiencies when compared with those made of PLGA [132]. These NGF-loaded poly(phosphoester) microspheres were successfully implanted to bridge a 10 mm gap in a rat sciatic nerve model. Furthermore, the exogenous NGF had long-term morphological regeneration effects in the sciatic nerve [133].

Basic fibroblast growth factor (b-FGF) has been shown to enhance the *in vitro* survival and neurite extension of various types of neurons including dorsal root ganglia. One of the earliest studies involved controlled release of b-FGF and alpha-1 glycoprotein (α1-GP) from synthetic nerve guidance channels fabricated using the dip molding technique. After an initial burst in the first day, linear release was obtained from the conduits for a period of at least 2 weeks afterward. Only the tubes releasing b-FGF or b-FGF and alpha 1-GP displayed regenerated cables bridging both nerve stumps, which contained nerve fascicles with myelinated and unmyelinated axons [134]. Biodegradable polymer foams modified with a-FGF and used for controlled release and the provision of a permissive environment for spinal cord regeneration were formed using freeze-drying techniques [135]. Furthermore, evidence has been shown that a-FGF and b-FGF promote angiogenesis and may aid in the repair of damaged nerves [136].

Other neurotrophic factors such as GDNF, BDNF, and NT-3 have been released from synthetic guidance channels. In an effort to study facial nerve regeneration, the effects of the cytokine growth factor, GDNF, and NT-3 on nerve regeneration were assessed after rat facial nerve axotomy. Nerve cables regenerated in the presence of GDNF showed a large number of myelinated axons while no regenerated axons were observed in the absence of growth factors, demonstrating that GDNF, as previously described for the sciatic nerve, a mixed sensory and motor nerve, is also very efficient in promoting regeneration of the facial nerve, an essentially pure motor nerve [137]. Exogenous BDNF and NT-3 were delivered simultaneously into Schwann cell-grafted semipermeable guidance channels by an Alzet minipump to test the ability of these neurotrophins to promote axonal regeneration. This novel experiment elegantly demonstrated that BDNF and NT-3 infusion enhanced propriospinal axonal regeneration and enhanced axonal regeneration of specific distant populations of brain stem neurons into grafts in the adult rat spinal cord [138].

A pharmacotectonics concept, in which drug-delivery systems were arranged spatially in tissues to shape concentration fields for potent agents, has been presented. NGF-releasing implants placed within 1 to 2 mm of the treatment site enhanced the biological function of cellular targets, whereas identical implants placed approximately 3 mm from the target site of treatment produced no beneficial effect [139]. Due to certain limitations with controlled-delivery systems, alternatives such as the encapsulation of cells that secrete these factors are discussed in the next section.

48.4.3   Cellular Modifications

Due to certain limitations with the control of growth factor delivery systems, cells have been manipulated for the direct delivery of certain neurotrophic factors using a variety of therapeutic strategies. Genetic engineering has been used to modify cells for neurotrophic factor delivery [140]. (For a review of gene therapy, refer to Tresco et al. [141] and Tinsley and Eriksson [142]) Cells that produce specific neurotrophic and growth factors have been encapsulated using polymeric biomaterials. Other experiments have involved the direct seeding of cells known to secrete neurotrophic factors, such as Schwann cells, olfactory ensheathing cells (OECs) and neural stem cells (NSCs), into nerve conduits.

48.4.3.1   Cell Encapsulation

Implanting polymer-encapsulated cells for secreting growth and neurotrophic factors has been used for treatment for neurodegenerative disorders and to promote nerve regeneration. As an experimental therapy for Parkinsonian patients, enhanced benefit from neural transplantation can be provided through the combination of grafting with trophic factor treatment. This strategy ultimately results in improved survival and growth of grafted embryonic dopaminergic neurons. It has been demonstrated that the implantation of polymer-encapsulated cells genetically engineered to continuously secrete glial cell line-derived neurotrophic factor to the adult rat striatum improves dopaminergic graft survival and function. This shows that polymer encapsulation of cells can be used as an effective vehicle for long-term trophic factor supply [143]. A number of proteins have specific neuroprotective activities *in vitro*; however, the local delivery of these factors into the central nervous system over the long term at therapeutic levels has been difficult to achieve. Direct administration at the target site is a logical alternative, particularly in the central nervous system, but the limits of direct administration have not been defined clearly. For instance NGF must be delivered within several millimeters of the target to be effective in treating Alzheimer's disease [139]. Cells engineered to express the neuroprotective proteins, encapsulated in immunoisolation polymeric devices and implanted at the site of lesions have the potential to alter the progression of neurodegenerative disorders. The polymers used for encapsulation should allow transport of nutrients and oxygen to the cells, but also afford immunoprotection. Long-term cell viability *in vivo* in these constructs due to diffusional limitations has been the major drawback of this approach.

Ciliary neurotrophic factor (CNTF) decreases naturally occurring and axotomy-induced cell death and has been evaluated as a treatment for neurodegenerative disorders such as amyotrophic lateral sclerosis (ALS) and Huntington's disease [144]. Effective administration of this protein to motoneurons has been hampered by the exceedingly short half-life of CNTF, and the inability to deliver effective concentration into the central nervous system after systemic administration *in vivo*. BHK cells stably transfected with a plasmid construct containing the gene for human or mouse CNTF were encapsulated in polymer fibers and found to continuously release CNTF and slow down motoneuron degeneration following axotomy [145]. Implantation of polymer-encapsulated cells genetically engineered to continuously secrete GDNF to the adult rat striatum was found to improve dopaminergic graft survival and function [143]. Therefore cell encapsulation is a potentially important method in nerve regeneration, and can be used alone or in conjunction with other methods such as entubulization. For a review on the microencapsulation of neuroactive compounds and living cells producing these substances, see Maysinger and Morinville [146].

48.4.3.2 Cell Implantation

48.4.3.2.1 Schwann Cells

Schwann cells play an important role in supporting axonal regeneration after damage or disease. These cells clean debris from the injury site and secrete regulatory proteins that aid in neuronal survival and axonal growth. In the PNS and CNS, Schwann cells organize the regenerating environment through the myelination of axons, production of ECM, CAMs, and neurotrophins as well as aiding in the guidance of regenerating axons. The use of PNS grafts in the CNS by David and Aguayo [14] in the early 1980s distinguished Schwann cells as essential for CNS repair [14]. Conduits incorporating these cells have enhanced PNS regeneration [147]. CNS regeneration has also been induced after implantation of the semipermeable polyacrylonitrile/polyvinylchloride (PAN/PVC) and Matrigel conduits seeded with Schwann cells into the transected rat spinal cord [26,148]. Poly (α-hydroxy acids) with seeded Schwann cells or Schwann cell grafts were also found to be effective candidates for spinal cord regeneration [22,149]. However, limited regeneration has been demonstrated between the implant and the distal end of the host spinal cord [150] and myelination beyond the injury site has not been observed [151]. Recent research has shown that rolled Schwann cell monolayer grafts implanted into the transected rat sciatic nerve increased functional regeneration compared to acellular controls [152]. Research applicable to human applications has demonstrated that implantation of human Schwann cells in the nude (T cell deficient) rat spinal cord allowed axonal growth across the graft and re-entry into the spinal cord. For reviews of these and other Schwann cell therapies, see Jones et al. [119] and Bunge [150].

48.4.3.2.2 Olfactory Ensheathing Cells

Olfactory bulb ensheathing cells (OECs) are the primary glial cells found in both the PNS and CNS of the olfactory system. This system differs from other CNS tissues in that axons continue to grow throughout adulthood. These cells share characteristics with astrocytes of the CNS and Schwann cells from the PNS. Like astrocytes, these cells express glial fibrillary acidic protein (GFAP), yet they ensheath and myelinate axons and support axonal regrowth, which are features of Schwann cells. Most work in this area has involved OEC transplantations performed to promote remyelination of demyelinated rat spinal cord axons [153,154] and foster regeneration of damaged axons in the mature CNS [27,155–157]. Incorporating OECs into conduits has promoted axonal regeneration in both the PNS [158] and CNS [156] using Schwann cell-filled guidance channels. The results from these transplantations have demonstrated a distinct advantage of these cells over Schwann cells in creating a regenerative environment within the CNS.

48.4.3.2.3 Neural Stem Cells

Neural stem cells (NSCs) that have the potential to produce new neurons and glia are present in the mammalian CNS. These cells can remain in certain regions of the adult CNS after development even though neurogenesis no longer occurs in most areas after birth. Neural stem cells are described as generating neural tissue or being derived from the neural system, having capacity for self-renewal, and they are multipotent or possess the ability to adopt a variety of cellular fates. Neural progenitors with more limited capacities in terms of growth and differentiation have been known to proliferate throughout life in a variety of

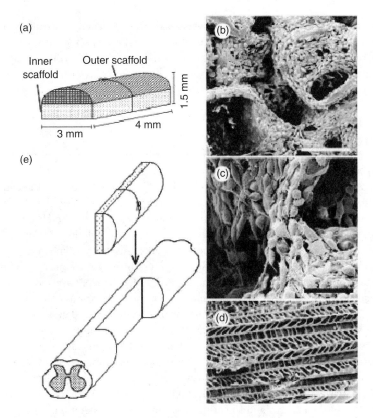

FIGURE 48.5   (a) Schematic of the scaffold design showing the inner and outer scaffolds. (b) and (c) Inner scaffolds seeded with NSCs. (Scale bars: 200 and 50 μm, respectively.) The outer section of the scaffold was created by means of a solid–liquid phase separation technique that produced long, axially oriented pores for axonal guidance as well as radial pores to allow fluid transport and inhibit the ingrowth of scar tissue. (d) Scale bar, 100 μm. (e) Schematic of surgical insertion of the implant into the spinal cord. (Reproduced from Teng, Y.D. et al., *Proc. Natl Acad. Sci. USA*, 99, 3024–3029, 2002. With permission.)

mammalian species, including humans [159,160]. NSCs were seeded into a dual scaffold structure made of biodegradable polymers to address the issues of spinal cord injury. Unique biodegradable polymer scaffolds were fabricated where the general design of the scaffold was derived from the structure of the spinal cord with an outer section that mimics the white matter with long axial pores to provide axonal guidance and an inner section seeded with neural stem cells for cell replacement and mimic the general character of the gray matter (Figure 48.5) [161]. The seeded scaffold improved functional recovery as compared with the lesion control or cells alone following spinal cord injury. Implantation of the scaffold-neural stem cells unit into an adult rat hemisection model of spinal cord injury promoted long-term improvement in function that was persistent up to one year in some animals, relative to a lesion-control group [18].

Human embryonic stem (hES) cells hold promise as an unlimited source of cells for transplantation therapies [162]. However, control of their proliferation and differentiation into complex, viable 3D tissues is challenging. Combining physical support with chemical cues created a supportive environment for the control of differentiation and organization of hES cells. Langer et al. developed biodegradable poly(lactic-*co*-glycolic acid)/poly(L-lactic acid) polymer scaffolds to promote hES cell growth and differentiation and formation of 3D structures. Complex structures with features of various committed embryonic tissues were generated *in vitro* using early differentiating hES cells and using the supportive three-dimensional environment to further induce differentiation. Growth factors such as retinoic acid, transforming growth factor β activin-A, or insulin-like growth factor directed hES cell differentiation and organization within the scaffold resulting in the formation of structures with characteristics of developing neural tissues, cartilage, or liver as well as the formation of a 3D vessel-like network. These constructs were transplanted into severe combined immunodeficient mice and continued to express specific human proteins in defined differentiated structures. This recent study presents a novel mechanism for creating viable human tissue structures for therapeutic applications [20]. For a review on stem cells in tissue engineering, refer to Bianco and Robey [163].

48.5 Conclusions

Engineering regeneration in the nervous system presents many challenges. Many strategies that may enhance regeneration in the PNS cannot be applied directly to the CNS due to the complexity of the environment. Novel tissue-engineering strategies and mechanisms, including the use of three dimensional polymer constructs with or without biological components (i.e., cells) and products fabricated for the induction of specific responses (i.e., regeneration), and the manipulation of biological cells *in vitro* (i.e., stem cells or cells for neuronal support), hold much promise for the enhancement of functional repair and replacement of tissue function. The successful use of polymeric nerve conduits in facilitating peripheral nerve regeneration has been demonstrated and polymers have shown great promise in addressing spinal cord injuries as well. This regeneration process, with various polymers, both degradable as well as nondegradable, has been enhanced further by promoting directed growth and by the addition of chemical cues such as ECM molecules, nerve growth factors and neurotrophins and other agents incorporated in the conduits to be released in a controlled fashion. Polymers have also played an important role in encapsulating cells and in the transplantation of neuronal support cells that release factors to promote nerve regeneration. Multidiscliplinary tissue-engineering approaches involving such biomaterials to mimic the native neural environment of the body have resulted in significant progress in gaining some understanding of the systems and signals involved in nerve regeneration. Incorporating multiple guidance cues and experimental strategies will allow further opportunities to elucidate the mechanisms behind nerve regeneration and specific considerations for the efficient repair of the nervous system.

Acknowledgments

The authors would like to acknowledge NSF (BES-9983735) and USDOD for funding.

References

[1] Horner, P.J. and Gage, F.H., Regenerating the damaged central nervous system, *Nature* 407, 963–970, 2000.

[2] Bjorklund, A. and Lindvall, O., Cell replacement therapies for central nervous system disorders, *Nat. Neurosci.* 3, 537–544, 2000.

[3] Fry, E.J., Central nervous system regeneration: mission impossible? *Clin. Exp. Pharmacol. Physiol.* 28, 253–258, 2001.

[4] Keeley, R.T., Atagi, T., Sabelman, E., Padilla, J., Kadlcik, S., Keeley, A., Nguyen, K., and Rosen, J., Peripheral nerve regeneration across 14-mm gaps: a comparison of autograft and entubulation repair methods in the rat, *J. Reconstruc. Microsurg.* 9, 349–358, 1993.

[5] Wang, G., Hirai, K., and Shimada, H., The role of laminin, a component of Schwann cell basal lamina, in rat sciatic nerve regeneration within antiserum-treated nerve grafts, *Brain Res.* 570, 116–125, 1992.

[6] Carlstedt, T., Nerve fibre regeneration across the peripheral-central transitional zone, *J. Anat.* 190, 51–56, 1997.

[7] Goodrum, J.F. and Bouldin, T.W., The cell biology of myelin degeneration and regeneration in the peripheral nervous system, *J. Neuropathol. Exp. Neurol.* 55, 943–953, 1996.

 [8] Tortora, G.J., *Principles of Human Anatomy: Nervous System*, 6th ed. Harper Collins, New York, 1992, pp. 459–466.

 [9] Fawcett, J.W. and Keynes, R.J., Peripheral nerve regeneration, *Annu. Rev. Neurosci.* 13, 43–60, 1990.

[10] Bahr, M. and Bonhoeffer, F., Perspectives on axonal regeneration in the mammalian CNS, *Trends Neurosci.* 17, 473–479, 1994.

[11] Silver, J. and Miller, J.H., Regeneration beyond the glial scar, *Nat. Rev. Neurosci.* 5, 146–156, 2004.

[12] Tatagiba, M., Brosamle, C., and Schwab, M.E., Regeneration of injured axons in the adult mammalian central nervous system, *Neurosurgery* 40, 541–546, 1997.

[13] Bray, G.M., Villegasperez, M.P., Vidalsanz, M., and Aguayo, A.J., The use of peripheral-nerve grafts to enhance neuronal survival, promote growth and permit terminal reconnections in the central-nervous-system of adult-rats, *J. Exp. Biol.* 132, 5–19, 1987.

[14] David, S. and Aguayo, A.J., Axonal elongation into peripheral nervous-system bridges after central nervous-system injury in adult-rats, *Science* 214, 931–933, 1981.

[15] Villegas-Perez, M.P., Vidal-Sanz, M., Bray, G.M., and Aguayo, A.J., Influences of peripheral nerve grafts on the survival and regrowth of axotomized retinal ganglion cells in adult rats, *J. Neurosci.* 8, 265–280, 1988.

[16] Aguayo, A.J., Vidalsanz, M., Villegasperez, M.P., and Bray, G.M., Growth and connectivity of axotomized retinal neurons in adult-rats with optic nerves substituted by Pns grafts linking the eye and the midbrain, *Anna. NY Acad. Sci.* 495, 1–9, 1987.

[17] Keirstead, S.A., Rasminsky, M., Fukuda, Y., Carter, D.A., Aguayo, A.J., and Vidalsanz, M., Electrophysiologic responses in hamster superior colliculus evoked by regenerating retinal axons, *Science* 246, 255–257, 1989.

[18] Teng, Y.D., Lavik, E.B., Qu, X., Park, K.I., Ourednik, J., Zurakowski, D., Langer, R., and Snyder, E.Y., Functional recovery following traumatic spinal cord injury mediated by a unique polymer scaffold seeded with neural stem cells, *Proc. Natl Acad. Sci. USA* 99, 3024–3029, 2002.

[19] Neumann, S. and Woolf, C.J., Regeneration of dorsal column fibers into and beyond the lesion site following adult spinal cord injury, *Neuron* 23, 83–91, 1999.

[20] Levenberg, S., Huang, N.F., Lavik, E., Rogers, A.B., Itskovitz-Eldor, J., and Langer, R., Differentiation of human embryonic stem cells on three-dimensional polymer scaffolds, *Proc. Natl Acad. Sci. USA* 100, 12741–12746, 2003.

[21] Vacanti, M.P., Leonard, J.L., Dore, B., Bonassar, L.J., Cao, Y., Stachelek, S.J., Vacanti, J.P., O'Connell, F., Yu, C.S., Farwell, A.P., and Vacanti, C.A., Tissue-engineered spinal cord, *Transplant Proc.* 33, 592–598, 2001.

[22] Gautier, S.E., Oudega, M., Fragoso, M., Chapon, P., Plant, G.W., Bunge, M.B., and Parel, J.M., Poly(alpha-hydroxyacids) for application in the spinal cord: resorbability and biocompatibility with adult rat Schwann cells and spinal cord, *J. Biomed. Mater. Res.* 42, 642–654, 1998.

[23] Holmes, T.C., de Lacalle, S., Su, X., Liu, G.S., Rich, A., and Zhang, S.G., Extensive neurite outgrowth and active synapse formation on self-assembling peptide scaffolds, *Proc. Natl Acad. Sci. USA* 97, 6728–6733, 2000.

[24] Park, K.I., Teng, Y.D., and Snyder, E.Y., The injured brain interacts reciprocally with neural stem cells supported by scaffolds to reconstitute lost tissue, *Nat. Biotechnol.* 20, 1111–1117, 2002.

[25] Xu, X.M., Zhang, S.X., Li, H.Y., Aebischer, P., and Bunge, M.B., Regrowth of axons into the distal spinal cord through a Schwann-cell-seeded mini-channel implanted into hemisected adult rat spinal cord, *Eur. J. Neurosci.* 11, 1723–1740, 1999.

[26] Xu, X.M., Chen, A., Guenard, V., Kleitman, N., and Bunge, M.B., Bridging Schwann cell transplants promote axonal regeneration from both the rostral and caudal stumps of transected adult rat spinal cord, *J. Neurocytol.* 26, 1–16, 1997.

[27] Li, Y., Field, P.M., and Raisman, G., Repair of adult rat corticospinal tract by transplants of olfactory ensheathing cells, *Science* 277, 2000–2002, 1997.

[28] Menei, P., Montero-Menei, C., Whittemore, S.R., Bunge, R.P., and Bunge, M.B., Schwann cells genetically modified to secrete human BDNF promote enhanced axonal regrowth across transected adult rat spinal cord, *Eur. J. Neurosci.* 10, 607–621, 1998.

[29] Teng, Y.D., Mocchetti, I., Taveira-DaSilva, A.M., Gillis, R.A., and Wrathall, J.R., Basic fibroblast growth factor increases long-term survival of spinal motor neurons and improves respiratory function after experimental spinal cord injury, *J. Neurosci.* 19, 7037–7047, 1999.

[30] Schwab, M.E., Increasing plasticity and functional recovery of the lesioned spinal cord, *Prog. Brain Res.* 137, 351–359, 2002.

[31] Lundborg, G., *Nerve Injury and Repair*, Longman Group, UK, New York, 1988.

[32] So, K.F. and Aguayo, A.J., Lengthy regrowth of cut axons from ganglion-cells after peripheral-nerve transplantation into the retina of adult-rats, *Brain Res.* 328, 349–354, 1985.

[33] Evans, G.R.D., Challenges to nerve regeneration, *Semin. Surg. Oncol.* 19, 312–318, 2000.

[34] Kim, B.-S. and Atala, A., Periperal nerve regeneration, in *Methods of Tissue Engineering*, Atala, A. and Lanza, R. (Eds.), Academic Press, New York, 2002, pp. 1135–1142.

[35] Frerichs, O., Fansa, H., Schicht, C., Wolf, G., Schneider, W., and Keilhoff, G., Reconstruction of peripheral nerves using acellular nerve grafts with implanted cultured Schwann cells, *Microsurgery*, 22, 311–315, 2002.

[36] Heath, C.A. and Rutkowski, G.E., The develpoment of bioartifical nerve grafts for peripheral-nerve regeneration, *Trends Biotechnol.* 16, 163–168, 1998.

[37] Pearson, R.G., Molino, Y., Williams, P.M., Tendler, S.J., Davies, M.C., Roberts, C.J., and Shakesheff, K.M., Spatial confinement of neurite regrowth from dorsal root ganglia within nonporous microconduits, *Tissue Eng.* 9, 201–208, 2003.

[38] Bellamkonda, R. and Aebischer, P., Review: tissue engineering in the nervous system, *Biotechnol. Bioeng.* 43, 543–556, 1994.

[39] Schmidt, C.E. and Leach, J.B., Neural tissue engineering: strategies for repair and regeneration, *Annu. Rev. Biomed. Eng.* 5, 293–347, 2003.

[40] Evans, G.R., Brandt, K., Katz, S., Chauvin, P., Otto, L., Bogle, M., Wang, B., Meszlenyi, R.K., Lu, L., Mikos, A.G., and Patrick, C. W., Jr., Bioactive poly(L-lactic acid) conduits seeded with Schwann cells for peripheral nerve regeneration, *Biomaterials* 23, 841–848, 2002.

[41] Evans, G.R.D., Brandt, K., Widmer, M.S., Lu, L., Meszlenyi, R.K., Gupta, P.K., Mikos, A.G., Hodges, J., Williams, J., and Gurlek, A., *In vivo* evaluation of poly(-lactic acid) porous conduits for peripheral nerve regeneration, *Biomaterials* 20, 1109–1115, 1999.

[42] Hadlock, T., Elisseeff, J., Langer, R., Vacanti, J., and Cheney, M., A tissue-engineered conduit for peripheral nerve repair, *Arch. Otolaryngol. Head Neck Surg.* 124, 1081–1086, 1998.

[43] Widmer, M.S., Gupta, P.K., Lu, L., Meszlenyi, R.K., Evans, G.R., Brandt, K., Savel, T., Gurlek, A., Patrick, C.W., Jr., and Mikos, A.G., Manufacture of porous biodegradable polymer conduits by an extrusion process for guided tissue regeneration, *Biomaterials* 19, 1945–1955, 1998.

[44] Nicoli Aldini, N., Fini, M., Rocca, M., Giavaresi, G., and Giardino, R., Guided regeneration with resorbable conduits in experimental peripheral nerve injuries, *Int. Orthop.* 24, 121–125, 2000.

[45] Nicoli Aldini, N., Perego, G., Cella, G.D., Maltarello, M.C., Fini, M., Rocca, M., and Giardino, R., Effectiveness of a bioabsorbable conduit in the repair of peripheral nerves, *Biomaterials* 17, 959–962, 1996.

[46] Hazari, A., Wiberg, M., Johansson-Ruden, G., Green, C., and Terenghi, G., A resorbable nerve conduit as an alternative to nerve autograft in nerve gap repair, *Br. J. Plast. Surg.* 52, 653–657, 1999.

[47] Woerly, S., Pinet, E., De Robertis, L., Bousmina, M., Laroche, G., Roitback, T., Vargova, L., and Sykova, E., Heterogeneous PHPMA hydrogels for tissue repair and axonal regeneration in the injured spinal cord, *J. Biomater. Sci. Polym. Ed.* 9, 681–711, 1998.

[48] Recknor, J.B., Recknor, J.C., Sakaguchi, D.S., and Mallapragada, S.K., Oriented astroglial cell growth on micropatterned polystyrene substrates, *Biomaterials* 25, 2753–2767, 2004.

[49] Danielsen, N., Pettmann, B., Vahlsing, H.L., Manthorpe, M., and Varon, S., Fibroblast growth factor effects on peripheral nerve regeneration in a silicone chamber model, *J. Neurosci. Res.* 20, 320–330, 1988.

[50] Lundborg, G., Dahlin, L.B., Danielsen, N., Gelberman, R.H., Longo, F.M., Powell, H.C., and Varon, S., Nerve regeneration in silicone chambers — influence of gap length and of distal stump components, *Exp. Neurol.* 76, 361–375, 1982.

[51] Pitta, M.C., Wolford, L.M., Mehra, P., and Hopkin, J., Use of gore-tex tubing as a conduit for inferior alveolar and lingual nerve repair: experience with 6 cases, *J. Oral Maxillofac. Surg.* 59, 493–496, 2001.

[52] Miloro, M., Halkias, L.E., Mallery, S., Travers, S., and Rashid, R.G., Low-level laser effect on neural regeneration in Gore-Tex tubes, *Oral Surg. Oral Med. Oral Pathol. Oral Radiol. Endodontics* 93, 27–34, 2002.

[53] Tong, Y.W. and Shoichet, M.S., Enhancing the interaction of central nervous system neurons with poly(tetrafluoroethylene-co-hexafluoropropylene) via a novel surface amine-functionalization reaction followed by peptide modification, *J. Biomater. Sci. Polym. Ed.* 9, 713–729, 1998.

[54] Ahmed, Z. and Brown, R.A., Adhesion, alignment, and migration of cultured Schwann cells on ultrathin fibronectin fibres, *Cell Motil. Cytoskel.* 42, 331–343, 1999.

[55] Toba, T., Nakamura, T., Lynn, A.K., Matsumoto, K., Fukuda, S., Yoshitani, M., Hori, Y., and Shimizu, Y., Evaluation of peripheral nerve regeneration across an 80-mm gap using a polyglycolic acid (PGA) — collagen nerve conduit filled with laminin-soaked collagen sponge in dogs, *Int. J. Artif. Organs* 25, 230–237, 2002.

[56] Dubey, N., Letourneau, P.C., and Tranquillo, R.T., Guided neurite elongation and Schwann cell invasion into magnetically aligned collagen in simulated peripheral nerve regeneration, *Exp. Neurol.* 158, 338–350, 1999.

[57] Tong, X.J., Hirai, K.I., Shimada, H., Mizutani, Y., Izumi, T., Toda, N., and Yu, P., Sciatic-nerve regeneration navigated by laminin–fibronectin double coated biodegradable collagen grafts in rats, *Brain Res.* 663, 155–162, 1994.

[58] Ahmed, Z., Underwood, S., and Brown, R.A., Low concentrations of fibrinogen increase cell migration speed on fibronectin/fibrinogen composite cables, *Cell Motil. Cytoskel.* 46, 6–16, 2000.

[59] Herbert, C.B., Nagaswami, C., Bittner, G.D., Hubbell, J.A., and Weisel, J.W., Effects of fibrin micromorphology on neurite growth from dorsal root ganglia cultured in three-dimensional fibrin gels, *J. Biomed. Mater. Res.* 40, 551–559, 1998.

[60] Schense, J.C., Bloch, J., Aebischer, P., and Hubbell, J.A., Enzymatic incorporation of bioactive peptides into fibrin matrices enhances neurite extension, *Nat. Biotechnol.* 18, 415–419, 2000.

[61] Seckel, B.R., Jones, D., Hekimian, K.J., Wang, K.K., Chakalis, D.P., and Costas, P.D., Hyaluronic acid through a new injectable nerve guide delivery system enhances peripheral nerve regeneration in the rat, *J. Neurosci. Res.* 40, 318–324, 1995.

[62] Balgude, A.P., Yu, X., Szymanski, A., and Bellamkonda, R.V., Agarose gel stiffness determines rate of DRG neurite extension in 3D cultures, *Biomaterials* 22, 1077–1084, 2001.

[63] Hudson, T.W., Evans, G.R.D., and Schmidt, C.E., Engineering strategies for peripheral nerve repair, *Clin. Plastic Surg.* 26, 617–628, 1999.

[64] Valentini, R.F., Nerve guidance channels, in *The Biomedical Engineering Handbook*, 2nd ed., Bronzino, J.D. Ed., CRC Press, Boca Raton, FL, 2000, pp. 135-1–135-12.

[65] Sundback, C., Hadlock, T., Cheney, M., and Vacanti, J., Manufacture of porous polymer nerve conduits by a novel low-pressure injection molding process, *Biomaterials* 24, 819–830, 2003.

[66] Clark, P., Connolly, P., Curtis, A.S.G., Dow, J.A.T., and Wilkinson, C.D.W., Topographical control of cell behaviour: II. Multiple grooved substrata, *Development* 108, 635–644, 1990.

[67] Clark, P., Connolly, P., Curtis, A.S.G., Dow, J.A.T., and Wilkinson, C.D.W., Topographical control of cell behaviour. I. Simple step cues, *Development* 99, 439–448, 1987.

[68] Miller, C., Jeftinija, S., and Mallapragada, S., Synergistic effects of physical and chemical guidance cues on neurite alignment and outgrowth on biodegradable polymer substrates, *Tissue Eng.* 8, 367–378, 2002.

[69] Miller, C.A., Jeftinija, S., and Mallapragada, S.K., Micropatterned Schwann cell-seeded biodegradable polymer substrates significantly enhance neurite alignment and outgrowth, *Tissue Eng.* 7, 705–715, 2001.

[70] Miller, C., Shanks, H., Witt, A., Rutkowski, G., and Mallapragada, S., Oriented Schwann cell growth on micropatterned biodegradable polymer substrates, *Biomaterials* 22, 1263–1269, 2001.

[71] Chen, C., Mrkisch, M., Huang, S., Whitesides, G., and Ingber, D., Geometric control of life and death, *Science* 276, 1425–1428, 1997.

[72] Singhvi, R., Kumar, A., Lopez, G., Stephanopoulous, G., Wang, D.I.C., Whitesides, G., and Ingber, D., Engineering cell shape and function, *Science* 264, 696–698, 1994.

[73] Craighead, H.G., Turner, S.W., Davis, R.C., James, C., Perez, A.M., St. John, P.M., Isaacson, M.S., Kam, L., Shain, W., Turner, J. N., and Banker, G., Chemical and topographical surface modification for control of central nervous system cell adhesion, *Biomed. Microdev.* 1, 49–64, 1998.

[74] Clark, P., Cell and neuron growth cone behavior on micropatterned surfaces, in *Nanofabrication and Biosystems: Integrating Materials, Science, Engineering, and Biology*, Hoch, H.C., Jelinski, L.W., and Craighead, H.G. (Eds.), Cambridge University Press, New York, 1996, pp. 356–366.

[75] Kleinfeld, D., Kahler, K., and Hockberger, P., Controlled outgrowth of dissociated neurons on patterned substrates, *J. Neurosci.* 8, 4098–4120, 1988.

[76] Kam, L., Shain, W., Turner, J.N., and Bizios, R., Correlation of astroglial cell function on micropatterned surfaces with specific geometric parameters, *Biomaterials* 20, 2343–2350, 1999.

[77] Brunette, D.M., Fibroblasts on micromachined substrata orient hierarchically to grooves of different dimensions, *Exp. Cell Res.* 164, 11–26, 1986.

[78] Kawana, A., Formation of a simple model brain on microfabricated electrode arrays, in *Nanofabrication and Biosystems: Integrating Materials, Science, Engineering, and Biology*, Hoch, H.C., Jelinski, L.W., and Craighead, H.G. Ed., Cambridge University Press, New York, 1996, pp. 258–275.

[79] Webb, A., Clark, P., Skepper, J., Compston, A., and Wood, A., Guidance of oligodendrocytes and their progenitors by substratum topography, *J. Cell Sci.* 108, 2747–2760, 1995.

[80] Ohara, P.T. and Buck, R.C., Contact guidance *in vitro*. A light, transmission, and scanning electron microscopic study, *Exp. Cell Res.* 121, 235–249, 1979.

[81] Rajnicek, A., Britland, S., and McCaig, C., Contact guidance of CNS neurites on grooved quartz: influence of groove dimensions, neuronal age and cell type, *J. Cell Sci.* 110, 2905–2913, 1997.

[82] Lu, L., Kam, L., Hasenbein, M., Nyalakonda, K., Bizios, R., Gopferich, A., Young, J.F., and Mikos, A.G., Retinal pigment epithelial cell function on substrates with chemically micropatterned surfaces, *Biomaterials* 20, 2351–2361, 1999.

[83] Turner, A.M.P., Dowell, N., Turner, S.W.P., Kam, L., Isaacson, M., Turner, J.N., Craighead, H.G., and Shain, W., Attachment of astroglial cells to microfabricated pillar arrays of different geometries, *J. Biomed. Mater. Res.* 51, 430–441, 2000.

[84] Bhatia, S.N. and Chen, C.S., Tissue engineering at the micro-scale, *Biomed. Microdev.* 2, 131–144, 1999.

[85] Wheeler, B.C., Corey, J.M., Brewer, G.J., and Branch, D.W., Microcontact printing for precise control of nerve cell growth in culture, *J. Biomech. Eng.-Trans. ASME* 121, 73–78, 1999.

[86] Bernard, A., Delamarche, E., Schmid, H., Michel, B., Bosshard, H.R., and Biebuyck, H., Printing patterns of proteins, *Langmuir* 14, 2225–2229, 1998.

[87] Clark, P., Britland, S., and Connolly, P., Growth cone guidance and neuron morphology on micropatterned laminin surfaces, *J. Cell Sci.* 105, 203–212, 1993.

[88] Tai, H.C. and Buettner, H.M., Neurite outgrowth and growth cone morphology on micropatterned surfaces, *Biotechnol. Prog.* 14, 364–370, 1998.

[89] Gundersen, R.W., Sensory neurite growth cone guidance by substrate adsorbed nerve growth factor, *J. Neurosci. Res.* 13, 199–212, 1985.

[90] Kam, L., Shain, W., Turner, J.N., and Bizios, R., Axonal outgrowth of hippocampal neurons on micro-scale networks of polylysine-conjugated laminin, *Biomaterials* 22, 1049–1054, 2001.

[91] Buettner, H.M., Microcontrol of neuronal outgrowth, in *Nanofabrication and Biosystems: Integrating Materials, Science, Engineering, and Biology*, Hoch, H.C., Jelinski, L.W., and Craighead, H.G. (Eds.), Cambridge University Press, New York, 1996, pp. 300–314.

[92] Flemming, R.G., Murphy, C.J., Abrams, G.A., Goodman, S.L., and Nealey, P.F., Effects of synthetic micro- and nano-structured surfaces on cell behavior, *Biomaterials* 20, 573–588, 1999.

[93] Curtis, A. and Wilkinson, C., Topographical control of cells, *Biomaterials* 18, 1573–1583, 1998.

[94] Grimpe, B. and Silver, J., The extracellular matrix in axon regeneration, *Prog. Brain Res.* 137 (Spinal Cord Trauma), 333–349, 2002.

[95] Letourneau, P.C., Madsen, A.M., Palm, S.L., and Furcht, L.T., Immunoreactivity for laminin in the developing ventral longitudinal pathway of the brain, *Develop. Biol.* 125, 135–144, 1988.

[96] Bellamkonda, R., Ranieri, J.P., and Aebischer, P., Laminin oligopeptide derivatized agarose gels allow 3-dimensional neurite extension *in-vitro*, *J. Neurosci. Res.* 41, 501–509, 1995.

[97] Yu, X.J. and Bellamkonda, R.V., Tissue-engineered scaffolds are effective alternatives to autografts for bridging peripheral nerve gaps, *Tissue Eng.* 9, 421–430, 2003.

[98] Yu, X.J., Dillon, G.P., and Bellamkonda, R.V., A laminin and nerve growth factor-laden three-dimensional scaffold for enhanced neurite extension, *Tissue Eng.* 5, 291–304, 1999.

[99] Itoh, S., Takakuda, K., Kawabata, S., Aso, Y., Kasai, K., Itoh, H., and Shinomiya, K., Evaluation of cross-linking procedures of collagen tubes used in peripheral nerve repair, *Biomaterials* 23, 4475–4481, 2002.

[100] Yoshii, S. and Oka, M., Peripheral nerve regeneration along collagen filaments, *Brain Res.* 888, 158–162, 2001.

[101] Chen, Y.S., Hsieh, C.L., Tsai, C.C., Chen, T.H., Cheng, W.C., Hu, C.L., and Yao, C.H., Peripheral nerve regeneration using silicone rubber chambers filled with collagen, laminin and fibronectin, *Biomaterials* 21, 1541–1547, 2000.

[102] Ceballos, D., Navarro, X., Dubey, N., Wendelschafer-Crabb, G., Kennedy, W.R., and Tranquillo, R.T., Magnetically aligned collagen gel filling a collagen nerve guide improves peripheral nerve regeneration, *Exp. Neurol.* 158, 290–300, 1999.

[103] Dubey, N., Letourneau, P.C., and Tranquillo, R.T., Neuronal contact guidance in magnetically aligned fibrin gels: effect of variation in gel mechano-structural properties, *Biomaterials* 22, 1065–1075, 2001.

[104] Hadlock, T., Sundback, C., Koka, R., Hunter, D., Cheney, M., and Vacanti, J., A novel, biodegradable polymer conduit delivers neurotrophins and promotes nerve regeneration, *Laryngoscope* 109, 1412–1416, 1999.

[105] Dickson, B.J., Molecular mechanisms of axon guidance, *Science* 298, 1959–1964, 2002.

[106] Webb, K., Budko, E., Neuberger, T.J., Chen, S., Schachner, M., and Tresco, P.A., Substrate-bound human recombinant L1 selectively promotes neuronal attachment and outgrowth in the presence of astrocytes and fibroblasts, *Biomaterials* 22, 1017–1028, 2001.

[107] Thanos, P.K., Okajima, S., and Terzis, J.K., Ultrastructure and cellular biology of nerve regeneration, *J. Reconstruct. Microsurg.* 14, 423–436, 1998.

[108] Ruegg, M.A., Agrin, laminin beta 2 (s-laminin) and ARIA: their role in neuromuscular development, *Curr. Opin. Neurobiol.* 6, 97–103, 1996.

[109] Carbonetto, S.T., Gruver, M.M., and Turner, D.C., Nerve fiber growth on defined hydrogel substrates, *Science* 216, 897–899, 1982.

[110] Woerly, S., Hydrogels for neural tissue reconstruction and transplantation, *Biomaterials* 14, 1056–1058, 1993.

[111] Woerly, S., Laroche, G., Marchand, R., Pato, J., Subr, V., and Ulbrich, K., Intracerebral implantation of hydrogel-coupled adhesion peptides: tissue reaction, *J. Neural Transplant Plast.* 5, 245–255, 1995.

[112] Woerly, S., Plant, G.W., and Harvey, A.R., Cultured rat neuronal and glial cells entrapped within hydrogel polymer matrices: a potential tool for neural tissue replacement, *Neurosci. Lett.* 205, 197–201, 1996.

[113] Woerly, S., Doan, V.D., Evans-Martin, F., Paramore, C.G., and Peduzzi, J.D., Spinal cord reconstruction using NeuroGel implants and functional recovery after chronic injury, *J. Neurosci. Res.* 66, 1187–1197, 2001.

[114] Woerly, S., Doan, V.D., Sosa, N., de Vellis, J., and Espinosa, A., Reconstruction of the transected cat spinal cord following NeuroGel implantation: axonal tracing, immunohistochemical and ultrastructural studies, *Int. J. Dev. Neurosci.* 19, 63–83, 2001.

[115] Woerly, S., Petrov, P., Sykova, E., Roitbak, T., Simonova, Z., and Harvey, A.R., Neural tissue formation within porous hydrogels implanted in brain and spinal cord lesions: ultrastructural, immunohistochemical, and diffusion studies, *Tissue Eng.* 5, 467–488, 1999.

[116] Woerly, S., Pinet, E., de Robertis, L., Van Diep, D., and Bousmina, M., Spinal cord repair with PHPMA hydrogel containing RGD peptides (NeuroGel™), *Biomaterials* 22, 1095–1111, 2001.

[117] Blesch, A., Lu, P., and Tuszynski, M.H., Neurotrophic factors, gene therapy, and neural stem cells for spinal cord repair, *Brain Res. Bull.* 57, 833–838, 2002.

[118] Terenghi, G., Peripheral nerve regeneration and neurotrophic factors, *J. Anatomy* 194, 1–14, 1999.

[119] Jones, L.L., Oudega, M., Bunge, M.B., and Tuszynski, M.H., Neurotrophic factors, cellular bridges and gene therapy for spinal cord injury, *J. Physiol. (Lond.)* 533, 83–89, 2001.

[120] Stichel, C.C. and Muller, H.W., Experimental strategies to promote axonal regeneration after traumatic central nervous system injury, *Prog. Neurobiol.* 56, 119–148, 1998.

[121] Hollowell, J.P., Villadiego, A., and Rich, K.M., Sciatic nerve regeneration across gaps within silicone chambers: long-term effects of NGF and consideration of axonal branching, *Exp. Neurol.* 110, 45–51, 1990.

[122] Haller, M.F. and Saltzman, W.M., Nerve growth factor delivery systems, *J. Control. Release* 53, 1–6, 1998.

[123] Powell, E.M., Sobarzo, M.R., and Saltzman, W.M., Controlled release of nerve growth factor from a polymeric implant, *Brain Res.* 515, 309–311, 1990.

[124] Fine, E.G., Decosterd, I., Papaloizos, M., Zurn, A.D., and Aebischer, P., GDNF and NGF released by synthetic guidance channels support sciatic nerve regeneration across a long gap, *Eur. J. Neurosci.* 15, 589–601, 2002.

[125] Bloch, J., Fine, E.G., Bouche, N., Zurn, A.D., and Aebischer, P., Nerve growth factor- and neurotrophin-3-releasing guidance channels promote regeneration of the transected rat dorsal root, *Exp. Neurol.* 172, 425–432, 2001.

[126] Ramer, M.S., Priestley, J.V., and McMahon, S.B., Functional regeneration of sensory axone into the adult spinal cord, *Nature* 403, 312–316, 2000.

[127] Nakahara, Y., Gage, F.H., and Tuszynski, M.H., Grafts of fibroblasts genetically modified to secrete NGF, BDNF, NT-3, or basic FGF elicit differential responses in the adult spinal cord, *Cell Transplant* 5, 191–204, 1996.

[128] Camarata, P.J., Suryanarayanan, R., Turner, D.A., Parker, R.G., and Ebner, T.J., Sustained release of nerve growth factor from biodegradable polymer microspheres, *Neurosurgery* 30, 313–319, 1992.

[129] Pean, J.M., Boury, F., Venier-Julienne, M.C., Menei, P., Proust, J.E., and Benoit, J.P., Why does PEG 400 co-encapsulation improve NGF stability and release from PLGA biodegradable microspheres? *Pharm. Res.* 16, 1294–1299, 1999.

[130] Pean, J.M., Venier-Julienne, M.C., Boury, F., Menei, P., Denizot, B., and Benoit, J.P., NGF release from poly(D,L-lactide-co-glycolide) microspheres. Effect of some formulation parameters on encapsulated NGF stability, *J. Control. Release* 56, 175–187, 1998.

[131] Cao, X. and Schoichet, M.S., Delivering neuroactive molecules from biodegradable microspheres for application in central nervous system disorders, *Biomaterials* 20, 329–339, 1999.

[132] Xu, X., Yu, H., Gao, S., Ma, H.Q., Leong, K.W., and Wang, S., Polyphosphoester microspheres for sustained release of biologically active nerve growth factor, *Biomaterials* 23, 3765–3772, 2002.

[133] Xu, X., Yee, W.C., Hwang, P.Y., Yu, H., Wan, A.C., Gao, S., Boon, K.L., Mao, H.Q., Leong, K.W., and Wang, S., Peripheral nerve regeneration with sustained release of poly(phosphoester) microencapsulated nerve growth factor within nerve guide conduits, *Biomaterials* 24, 2405–2412, 2003.

[134] Aebischer, P., Salessiotis, A.N., and Winn, S.R., Basic fibroblast growth factor released from synthetic guidance channels facilitates peripheral nerve regeneration across long nerve gaps, *J. Neurosci. Res.* 23, 282–289, 1989.

[135] Maquet, V., Martin, D., Scholtes, F., Franzen, R., Schoenen, J., Moonen, G., and Jerme, R., Poly(D,L-lactide) foams modified by poly(ethylene oxide)-block-poly(D,L-lactide) copolymers and a-FGF: *in vitro* and *in vivo* evaluation for spinal cord regeneration, *Biomaterials* 22, 1137–1146, 2001.

[136] Friesel, R.E. and Maciag, T., Molecular mechanisms of angiogenesis — fibroblast growth-factor signal-transduction, *FASEB J.* 9, 919–925, 1995.

[137] Barras, F.M., Pasche, P., Bouche, N., Aebischer, P., and Zurn, A.D., Glial cell line-derived neurotrophic factor released by synthetic guidance channels promotes facial nerve regeneration in the rat, *J. Neurosci. Res.* 70, 746–755, 2002.

[138] Xu, X.M., Guenard, V., Kleitman, N., Aebischer, P., and Bunge, M.B., Combination of Bdnf and Nt-3 promotes supraspinal axonal regeneration into Schwann-cell grafts in adult-rat thoracic spinal-cord, *Exp. Neurol.* 134, 261–272, 1995.

[139] Mahoney, M.J. and Saltzman, W.M., Millimeter-scale positioning of a nerve-growth-factor source and biological activity in the brain, *Proc. Natl Acad. Sci. USA.* 96, 4536–4539, 1999.

[140] Grill, R., Murai, K., Blesch, A., Gage, F.H., and Tuszynski, M.H., Cellular delivery of neurotrophin-3 promotes corticospinal axonal growth and partial functional recovery after spinal cord injury, *J. Neurosci.* 17, 5560–5572, 1997.

[141] Tresco, P.A., Biran, R., and Noble, M.D., Cellular transplants as sources for therapeutic agents, *Adv. Drug Deliv. Rev.* 42, 3–27, 2000.

[142] Tinsley, R. and Eriksson, P., Use of gene therapy in central nervous system repair, *Acta. Neurol. Scand.* 109, 1–8, 2004.

[143] Sautter, J., Tseng, J.L., Braguglia, D., Aebischer, P., Spenger, C., Seiler, R.W., Widmer, H.R., and Zurn, A.D., Implants of polymer-encapsulated genetically modified cells releasing glial cell line-derived neurotrophic factor improve survival, growth, and function of fetal dopaminergic grafts, *Exp. Neurol.* 149, 230–236, 1998.

[144] Emerich, D.F., Winn, S.R., Hantraye, P.M., Peschanski, M., Chen, E.Y., Chu, Y., McDermott, P., Baetge, E.E., and Kordower, J.H., Protective effect of encapsulated cells producing neurotrophic factor CNTF in a monkey model of Huntington's disease, *Nature* 386, 395–399, 1997.

[145] Tan, S.A., Deglon, N., Zurn, A.D., Baetge, E.E., Bamber, B., Kato, A.C., and Aebischer, P., Rescue of motoneurons from axotomy-induced cell death by polymer encapsulated cells genetically engineered to release CNTF, *Cell Transplant* 5, 577–587, 1996.

[146] Maysinger, D. and Morinville, A., Drug delivery to the nervous system, *Trends Biotechnol.* 15, 410–418, 1997.

[147] Guenard, V., Kleitman, N., Morrissey, T.K., Bunge, R.P., and Aebischer, P., Syngeneic Schwann-cells derived from adult nerves seeded in semipermeable guidance channels enhance peripheral-nerve regeneration, *J. Neurosci.* 12, 3310–3320, 1992.

[148] Xu, X.M., Guenard, V., Kleitman, N., and Bunge, M.B., Axonal regeneration into Schwann cell-seeded guidance channels grafted into transected adult-rat spinal-cord, *J. Comp. Neurol.* 351, 145–160, 1995.

[149] Oudega, M., Gautier, S.E., Chapon, P., Fragoso, M., Bates, M.L., Parel, J.M., and Bunge, M.B., Axonal regeneration into Schwann cell grafts within resorbable poly(alpha-hydroxyacid) guidance channels in the adult rat spinal cord, *Biomaterials* 22, 1125–1136, 2001.

[150] Bunge, M.B., Bridging areas of injury in the spinal cord, *Neuroscientist* 7, 325–339, 2001.

[151] Franklin, R.J.M. and Barnett, S.C., Do olfactory glia have advantages over Schwann cells for CNS repair? *J. Neurosci. Res.* 50, 665–672, 1997.

[152] Hadlock, T.A., Sundback, C.A., Hunter, D.A., Vacanti, J.P., and Cheney, M.L., A new artificial nerve graft containing rolled Schwann cell monolayers, *Microsurgery* 21, 96–101, 2001.

[153] Franklin, R.J.M., Gilson, J.M., Franceschini, I.A., and Barnett, S.C., Schwann cell-like myelination following transplantation of an olfactory bulb-ensheathing cell line into areas of demyelination in the adult CNS, *Glia* 17, 217–224, 1996.

[154] Imaizumi, T., Lankford, K.L., Waxman, S.G., Greer, C.A., and Kocsis, J.D., Transplanted olfactory ensheathing cells remyelinate and enhance axonal conduction in the demyelinated dorsal columns of the rat spinal cord, *J. Neurosci.* 18, 6176–6185, 1998.

[155] Ramon-Cueto, A. and Nietosampedro, M., Regeneration into the spinal-cord of transected dorsal-root axons is promoted by ensheathing glia transplants, *Exp. Neurol.* 127, 232–244, 1994.

[156] Ramon-Cueto, A., Plant, G.W., Avila, J., and Bunge, M.B., Long-distance axonal regeneration in the transected adult rat spinal cord is promoted by olfactory ensheathing glia transplants, *J. Neurosci.* 18, 3803–3815, 1998.

[157] Navarro, X., Valero, A., Gudino, G., Fores, J., Rodriguez, F.J., Verdu, E., Pascual, R., Cuadras, J., and Nieto-Sampedro, M., Ensheathing glia transplants promote dorsal root regeneration and spinal reflex restitution after multiple lumbar rhizotomy, *Ann. Neurol.* 45, 207–215, 1999.

[158] Verdu, E., Navarro, X., Gudino-Cabrera, G., Rodriguez, F.J., Ceballos, D., Valero, A., and Nieto-Sampedro, M., Olfactory bulb ensheathing cells enhance peripheral nerve regeneration, *Neuroreport* 10, 1097–1101, 1999.

[159] Temple, S., The development of neural stem cells, *Nature* 414, 112–117, 2001.

[160] Lowenstein, D.H. and Parent, J.M., Brain, heal thyself, *Science* 283, 1126–1127, 1999.

[161] Lavik, E., Teng, Y.D., Zurakowski, D., Qu, X., Snyder, E., and Langer, R., Functional recovery following spinal cord hemisection mediated by a unique polymer scaffold seeded with neural stem cells, *Materials Research Society Symposium Proceedings* 662 (Biomaterials for Drug Delivery and Tissue Engineering), OO1.2/1-OO1.2/5, 2001.

[162] Thomson, J.A., Itskovitz-Eldor, J., Shapiro, S.S., Waknitz, M.A., Swiergiel, J.J., Marshall, V.S., and Jones, J.M., Embryonic stem cell lines derived from human blastocysts, *Science* 282, 1145–1147, 1998.

[163] Bianco, P. and Robey, P.G., Stem cells in tissue engineering, *Nature* 414, 118–121, 2001.

49

Gene Therapy and Tissue Engineering Based on Muscle-Derived Stem Cells: Potential for Musculoskeletal Tissue Regeneration and Repair

Johnny Huard
Baohong Cao
Yong Li
Hairong Peng
University of Pittsburgh

49.1 Introduction

Recent discoveries in cell biology have significantly advanced our knowledge of disease mechanisms. Newly developed techniques, coupled with advances in cell biology and polymer chemistry, are enabling the evolvement of novel tissue engineering approaches for the treatment of various disorders. Surgeons, who have traditionally used the tools of excision and reconstruction to treat patients, may now act as surgical gardeners who create microenvironments conducive to tissue regeneration. Our research team has isolated a novel population of muscle-derived stem cells (MDSCs) that display enhanced regenerative capability due to their multipotency, self-renewal ability, and immune-privileged behavior. This paper presents evidence supporting the existence of MDSCs and reviews some current MDSC-based gene therapy and tissue engineering applications designed to improve the healing of various musculoskeletal tissues, including skeletal muscle, bone, and intra-articular tissues. This review updates readers on the foundational principles and current advances in muscle-based gene therapy and tissue engineering for the musculoskeletal system.

49.1.1 Tissue Engineering

"Tissue engineering" refers to the science of creating living tissue to replace, repair, or augment diseased tissue. The engineered tissue may be created *in vitro* and subsequently implanted into the patient or the tissue may be created entirely *in vivo*. Regardless of the technique, tissue engineering requires at least three components: a growth-inducing stimulus (induction), a scaffold to support tissue formation (conduction), and responsive cells (production). The mechanical stimulation that occurs after the appropriate tissue engineering constructs have been introduced also strongly influences the remodeling of the newly regenerated tissue.

49.1.2 Growth Factors and Gene Therapy

"Growth factors" are soluble proteins that promote cell division, maturation, and differentiation. Recombinant DNA techniques have increased our understanding of the function of these proteins, which influence various tissue regeneration and repair processes. These techniques also have enabled the production of large quantities of growth factors for use in experimental investigations. Currently, a great deal of research is focused on the identification of optimal growth factors for particular applications. After identifying the ideal growth factor, scientists must determine the optimal method for delivering the growth factor within the surgical microenvironment. Direct application of a particular recombinant protein is the most straightforward means of delivering growth factors *in situ*. Research conducted during the 36 years since the discovery of bone morphogenetic proteins (BMPs) has demonstrated that one of the most important factors for *in vivo* healing is the presence of high, sustained doses of growth factors. Most growth factor proteins have half-lives of minutes and are cleared rapidly by the bloodstream. Even when the protein is bound to a collagen scaffold, its half-life is limited to several days. Although microgram doses are sufficient for *in vitro* manipulation of cells, milligram doses typically are required for *in vivo* regional regeneration. Researchers thus have turned to regional gene therapy for the sustained delivery of a growth factor to a local site *in vivo*.

One common gene therapy approach involves the transfer of a gene encoding a desired protein into cells via viral or nonviral vectors. The transduced cells subsequently secrete the desired protein into the microenvironment. Gene therapy generally assumes one of two forms: *in vivo* or *ex vivo* (indirect). The *in vivo* approach, which involves the direct injection or implantation of a gene-carrying vector into a recipient or patient, is attractive due to its technical simplicity. However, when using *in vivo* gene-therapy techniques it is impossible to perform *in vitro* safety testing on the transduced cells. In the *ex vivo* approach, cells are isolated from a tissue biopsy, expanded, and then transfected or transduced *in vitro*. Before being introduced into the recipient or patient, the genetically altered cells can be tested *in vitro* to assess the efficiency of gene transfer or to identify any abnormal behavior.

Clinical application of a particular gene therapy or tissue engineering technique requires identification of the protein required for proper tissue function, the gene that expresses this protein, and a reproducible method by which to deliver the protein to the diseased or injured tissue in sufficient quantities with adequate persistence. During the last few years, muscle cells have emerged as promising vehicles for gene therapy and tissue engineering in the musculoskeletal system. Several attributes make muscle an ideal tissue for tissue engineering such as, (1) Obtaining a muscle biopsy or tissue harvest involves a simple surgical procedure that can be repeated without compromising patients' health; (2) Muscle-derived cells tolerate *ex vivo* manipulation well and it is possible to obtain a large number of muscle-derived cells rather quickly (within 1 to 2 weeks) via expansion [1,2]; (3) After reinjection *in vivo*, these cells naturally fuse to form permanent postmitotic myotubes that allow for long-term expression of the desired protein; (4) Muscle cells can be transduced easily by a variety of viral vectors [3–6]; and (5) Muscle tissue contains a population of muscle stem cells that display an enhanced regenerative capacity when used in tissue engineering applications [1,2,7,8].

Because of the aforementioned characteristics, muscle cells have been used extensively as vehicles in gene therapy protocols for various muscle-related diseases, including Duchenne muscular dystrophy (DMD) [9–12]. Researchers also have used these cells as vehicles in many nonmuscle-related gene-therapy applications, such as the transfer and expression of factor IX for hemophilia B [13]; systemic delivery of human growth hormone for growth retardation [14]; gene delivery of human adenosine deaminase for the adenosine deaminase deficiency syndrome [15]; gene transfer of human proinsulin for diabetes mellitus [16]; expression of tyrosine hydroxylase for Parkinson's disease [17]; expression of FasL to prevent immunorejection of pancreatic islet cell transplants [18]; and injection of muscle cells into the joint (i.e., the meniscus, synovium, and ligament) for the treatment for arthritis and improvement of intra-articular tissue healing (see the sections that follow in this chapter) [19–21].

49.1.3 Isolation of Muscle-Derived Stem Cells

Muscle is composed of a heterogeneous population of cell types. Skeletal muscle contains satellite cells, which are resting, mononucleated, myogenic precursor cells capable of fusing to form postmitotic, multinucleated myotubes and myofibers. Skeletal muscle also contains stem cells. These unique cells are identifiable based on their capacity for protracted renewal; production of daughter cells, which may proceed toward lineage commitment and terminal differentiation; multipotency; and the ability to exhibit such behaviors throughout life [7]. Accordingly, muscle-derived stem cells produce populations of daughter cells that can undergo terminal differentiation into muscle cells, some of which subsequently can differentiate into myofibers while others remain undifferentiated [22]. These stem cells do not express markers of mature muscle tissue, but are capable of prolonged production of progeny and are multipotent [7,8,23–25]. Of the various cells that constitute any given postmitotic muscle sample, approximately 1% are committed satellite cells; the percentage of muscle-derived stem cells is substantially lower — roughly 1% of the number of satellite cells [7,8].

Researchers have used a variety of techniques to isolate stem cells from skeletal muscle digest. These cells can differentiate into myogenic, hematopoietic, osteogenic, adipogenic, chondrogenic, neural, and endothelial lineages [7,26–33]. Importantly, these stem cells also appear to display distinct marker profiles that distinguish them from satellite cells. Expression profiles for satellite cells vary depending on the activated state and the degree of differentiation. In our laboratory, we have used the preplate technique to isolate a novel population of highly purified MDSCs [7,8]. These cells express both early myogenic markers (e.g., desmin, c-met, MNF, and Bcl-2) and stem cell markers (e.g., Sca-1, Flk-1, and CD34) [7,8]. Because these cells can differentiate into various lineages (mesodermal, endodermal, and ectodermal) *in vitro* and *in vivo* and display an enhanced ability to regenerate various tissues, they constitute ideal cellular vehicles for gene therapy and tissue engineering applications. During the last few years, we have investigated the use of this technology to improve the healing of different components of the musculoskeletal system, including skeletal muscle, bone, and various intra-articular structures.

49.2   Skeletal Muscle

49.2.1   Muscle Disease: Duchenne Muscular Dystrophy

Patients with DMD lack the dystrophin protein in the sarcolemma of the muscle fiber; its absence disrupts the integration of the cytoskeleton with the extracellular matrix, a process normally controlled by the dystrophin associated proteins (DAPs), and consequently renders muscle fibers more susceptible to damage after contraction. Intensive efforts have been made to develop an effective cell therapy for DMD [9–12]. Although myoblast transplantation can transiently deliver dystrophin and improve the strength of injected dystrophic muscle, this approach is hindered by immune rejection, poor cellular survival rates, and limited dissemination of the injected cells. Animal and human clinical trial results have demonstrated that myoblast transplantation, although feasible, is rather inefficient [10–12]. In animal experiments, immunodeficient animals and immunosuppressive regimens, preirradiation of the injected muscle, or myonecrotic agents have been used extensively to improve the efficiency of this technique [34–43]. Although these approaches have ameliorated the restoration of dystrophin in mdx mice, success remains quite limited. More importantly, these attempts to improve myoblast transplantation in mdx mice are not applicable to human DMD patients and are therefore clinically irrelevant.

Our research team has used a modified preplate technique to isolate a novel population of MDSCs that display an improved transplantation capacity when injected into skeletal muscle [8]. These cells can be expanded *in vitro* for more than 30 passages while preserving their phenotype (Sca-1[+], CD34[low/−], c-kit[−], CD45[−]) and their ability to differentiate into various lineages both *in vitro* and *in vivo*. The transplantation of these MDSCs, in contrast to transplantation of other myogenic cells such as satellite cells, improved the efficiency of muscle regeneration and dystrophin delivery to dystrophic muscle in mice. The number of dystrophin-positive myofibers observed 90 days after injection of these MDSCs was not significantly different than the high number observed 10 days after transplantation, despite the fact that the mdx mice used as recipients in this experiment were not immunosuppressed and the injected muscles were not preirradiated or injured with a myonecrotic agent. Examination at 30 and 90 days after cell transplantation revealed that the injection of these MDSCs resulted in ten times more dystrophin-positive myofibers in the injected muscle than did the transplantation of satellite cells, although the same number of cells was injected in both groups. The ability of these MDSCs to proliferate *in vivo* for an extended period of time — combined with their strong capacity for self-renewal, their multipotency, and their immune-privileged behavior — reveals, at least in part, a basis for the benefits associated with their use in cell transplantation [8].

Although the above results show that allogeneic transplantation of normal MDSCs can restore dystrophin within dystrophic animals, autologous transplantation of MDSCs genetically engineered to express dystrophin may be more suitable for DMD patients. Our research group currently is investigating such autologous transplantation of genetically engineered MDSCs to determine the feasibility of this technology.

49.2.2   Sports-Related Muscle Injuries

Muscle injuries, particularly pulls and strains, pose a challenging problem in traumatology and are among the most common and most frequently disabling injuries to afflict athletes [44,45]. Although injured muscles can heal, such healing occurs very slowly and often results in incomplete functional recovery [44,45]. The regeneration initiated in injured muscle shortly after injury is inefficient and hindered by fibrosis, that is, scar tissue formation [44,45]. The scar tissue that often replaces the damaged myofibers is a potential contributing factor in the tendency of strains to recur.

We have identified various growth factors with the ability to enhance muscle regeneration by increasing myoblast proliferation and differentiation. The delivery of these growth factors via genetically engineered muscle cells improves the regeneration of injured muscle, but fibrosis still impedes full recovery [46–48]. The overexpression of transforming growth factor (TGF)-β1 in various injured tissues has been identified as the major cause of fibrosis in animals and humans [49]. We have observed that TGF-β1 plays a central role in skeletal muscle fibrosis [50] and, more importantly, that the use of antifibrotic agents that inactivate this molecule (e.g., decorin, suramin, γIFN, and relaxin) can reduce muscle fibrosis and consequently improve muscle healing to near-complete recovery levels [51–53].

The overall goal of our research on sports-related muscle injuries is the development of biological approaches to improve muscle healing after common muscle injuries. Because the development of muscle fibrosis has greatly hindered our attempts to improve muscle healing by enhancing muscle regeneration, the prevention of such fibrosis has become the major emphasis of our ongoing research. Although numerous studies have demonstrated the involvement of TGF-β1 in fibrosis in various tissues, very few have examined the significance of fibrosis or the role played by TGF-β1 in the scarring process in injured skeletal muscle. As described above, our recent data show that TGF-β1 plays a central role in skeletal muscle fibrosis and that the use of antifibrotic agents (e.g., decorin, suramin, γIFN, and relaxin) to inactivate this molecule can reduce muscle fibrosis and consequently improve muscle healing to near-complete recovery levels. We believe that the ultimate approach to improving muscle healing after sports-related muscle injuries may involve the transplantation of muscle cells genetically engineered to express antifibrotic agents in order to block scar tissue formation while promoting muscle regeneration.

49.3 Bone Healing

49.3.1 The Problem of Bone Healing

Fracture healing constitutes a fundamental problem in orthopaedic surgery. Although the majority of fractures heal well, difficulty in the form of delayed healing or nonunions can be devastating. Fractures in anatomically compromised locations (e.g., the talar neck or scaphoid), with inadequate fixation or infection, resulting from high-energy-type injuries with soft tissue stripping or segmental bone loss, or occurring in poor bone stock (osteoporosis) often result in delayed healing. According to a recent review, 5 to 10% of the 5.6 million fractures that occur annually in the United States exhibit delayed or impaired healing [54]. Treatment options for the orthopaedic surgeon confronted with these complex fractures, particularly fractures involving segmental bone loss, include bone autograft, vascularized bone grafting, allograft supplemented with osteogenic proteins, bone transport, or amputation [55,56]. Unfortunately, patients generally must endure a lengthy recovery period, numerous procedures, potential donor site morbidity, and, often, a less-than-satisfactory end result [57]. Similar difficulties are associated with closure of the residual bony defects in craniofacial reconstruction and oncology or trauma surgery. Consequently, research directed toward improving fracture treatment and the development of optimal bone substitutes continues to garner intense interest.

49.3.2 The Use of Muscle-Derived Cells to Improve Bone Healing

We have demonstrated that a population of MDSCs isolated from mouse skeletal muscle produced alkaline phosphatase in a dose-dependent manner after stimulation with recombinant human BMP-2 and BMP-4 [1,2,7,58,59]. After being genetically engineered to express the osteogenic proteins BMP-2 and BMP-4 and injected into skeletal muscle, these mouse muscle-derived cells induced and participated in ectopic bone formation [1,2,7,58,59]. These MDSCs were also able to differentiate toward the osteogenic lineage and consequently improve bone healing in calvarial defects in both immunodeficient mice and immunocompetent mice [1,2,7,58,59].

Although angiogenesis is integral to normal bone development, it remains largely unknown whether bone regeneration can be further improved by the use of angiogenic factors, either alone or in combination with BMPs — the most promising growth factors for inducing bone formation. To address this question, we transduced MDSCs to express human BMP-4, vascular endothelial growth factor (VEGF), or both growth factors. VEGF significantly improved the efficacy of BMP-4-elicited bone formation and regeneration by enhancing angiogenesis, but VEGF alone did not improve bone regeneration. We have also characterized the mechanism by which VEGF accelerates the bone formation mediated by genetically engineered

MDSCs expressing BMP-4. In addition to improved vasculature, we observed increased mesenchymal cell infiltration and cartilage formation, decreased cell apoptosis at the injured site, earlier cartilage resorption, and a subsequent increase in mineralized bone formation within the regenerated bone that had been treated with the combination of BMP-4 and VEGF compared to that treated with BMP-4 alone [58]. Thus VEGF appears to enhance BMP-4-induced endochondral bone formation by influencing steps before and after cartilage formation. Intriguingly, we have also demonstrated that the beneficial effect of VEGF on the bone healing elicited by BMP-4 requires proper dosing, with high doses of VEGF leading to detrimental effects on bone healing [58]. These findings open a new avenue by which to improve bone repair based on the synergistic effects of osteogenic and angiogenic factors delivered via MDSCs.

49.3.3 Can we Isolate Human Muscle-Derived Stem Cells that Display Similar Osteogenic Behavior?

To translate this research to the clinical setting, our research group is pursuing the isolation of a similar population of MDSCs from human skeletal muscle. We have recently evaluated whether muscle-derived cells isolated from the skeletal muscle of humans (~50 years of age) via the preplate technique can be used in gene therapy and tissue engineering applications to support bone regeneration and repair. We have explored the use of primary human muscle-derived cells (isolated via the preplate technique) for *ex vivo* gene therapy to deliver BMP-2 and produce bone *in vivo*. Our findings indicate that certain cells isolated from a primary cell culture taken from human skeletal muscle responded to BMP-2 by differentiating into osteogenic cells, which suggests that these cells possessed osteocompetence [60]. Using *ex vivo* gene transfer, we were able to transduce these cells to secrete BMP-2 at levels sufficient to induce radiographically detectable ectopic bone formation within skeletal muscle [60]. Histological assessment of the injected, transduced, human muscle-derived cells suggests that the cells may have responded to the secreted BMP-2 in an autocrine fashion by becoming osteoblasts, thereby contributing to the induction of bone formation [60].

We also have used adenoviral and retroviral constructs to genetically engineer these freshly isolated human skeletal muscle cells to express human BMP-2. We implanted these cells into nonhealing bone defects (skull defects) in severe combined immunodeficient (SCID) mice and monitored the closure of the defect grossly and histologically. Mice implanted with BMP-2–producing human muscle-derived cells displayed full closure of the defect by 4 to 8 weeks after transplantation [61]. Remodeling of the newly formed bone was histologically evident during the 4 to 8 week period [61]. Analysis by fluorescent *in situ* hybridization (FISH) revealed a small fraction of the injected human muscle-derived cells within the newly formed bone in the location where osteocytes normally reside [61]. These results indicate that genetically engineered human muscle-derived cells enhance bone healing primarily by delivering BMP-2, although a small fraction of the cells seems to differentiate into osteogenic cells. We are investigating whether this small fraction of human muscle cells is the human counterpart of the mouse MDSCs that display osteogenic behavior.

49.3.4 Can we Regulate the Expression of Osteogenic Proteins and the Resultant Bone Formation?

Regulated therapeutic gene expression has become increasingly important to the success of various gene therapy applications — particularly stem cell-based ones — due to the potential long-term persistence of genetically engineered cells within the body. To develop a system by which to regulate the expression of osteogenic proteins, we first investigated the use of antagonist proteins to limit bone formation. Heterotopic ossification (HO) of muscles, tendons, and ligaments is a common problem encountered by orthopaedic surgeons. We evaluated the ability of noggin, a BMP antagonist, to inhibit HO in various mouse models. First, we developed a retroviral vector carrying the gene encoding human noggin and used this vector to transduce MDSCs. MDSCs transduced with BMP-4 were implanted into both hind limbs of mice along with 100,000, 500,000, or 1,000,000 noggin-expressing MDSCs (treated limb) or with an equivalent number of nontransduced MDSCs (control limb). The mice were sacrificed and radiographed 4 weeks after implantation to look for evidence of HO. In a second set of experiments, 80 mg of human demineralized bone matrix (DBM) was implanted into the hind limbs of SCID mice along with 100,000, 500,000 or 1,000,000 noggin-expressing MDSCs (treated limb) or nontransduced MDSCs (control limb). The mice were sacrificed and radiographed 8 weeks after cell implantation. In a final set of experiments, immunocompetent mice underwent bilateral Achilles tenotomy along with the implantation of 1,000,000 noggin-expressing MDSCs (treated limb) or nontransduced MDSCs (control limb). The mice were sacrificed and radiographed 10 weeks after surgery.

Our *in vitro* results showed that the MDSCs expressed noggin at a high level (280 ng/million cells/24 h) [62]. Four weeks after implantation, we found that the BMP-4-expressing MDSCs combined with the three varying doses of noggin-expressing MDSCs had formed 53, 74, and 99% less HO in a dose-dependent manner ($p < .05$) [62]. Similarly, DBM formed 91, 99, and 99% less HO when combined with the three varying doses of noggin-expressing MDSCs ($p < .05$) [62]. Additionally, all 11 animals that underwent Achilles tenotomy developed HO at the site of injury in the control limbs, whereas the limbs treated with the noggin-expressing MDSCs exhibited 84% less HO formation; 8 of the 11 animals exhibited no radiographic evidence of HO formation ($p < .05$) [62]. These findings suggest that the delivery of noggin mediated by MDSCs can inhibit HO in three different animal models. Gene therapy to deliver noggin may consequently serve as a powerful method to inhibit HO and perhaps regulate the amount of bone formation mediated by osteogenic proteins delivered by MDSCs [62].

We have also developed a retroviral vector that appears to be suitable for regulated gene therapy to improve bone healing. To date, one of the most intensively studied inducible gene expression systems comprises the tetracycline (tet)-controlled gene and its corresponding synthetic promoter [63]; researchers have used this system for either tet-on (gene expression activated by the presence of tet) or tet-off (gene expression activated in the absence of tet) applications. Scientists have developed retroviral vectors containing tet-on- or tet-off-controlled therapeutic genes with varying degrees of success [64]. We tried to optimize the most promising design to date — the self-inactivating (SI) tet-on retroviral vector — to develop a retroviral vector suitable for regulated gene therapy to improve bone healing. After extensive investigation, we identified and optimized a retroviral vector that confers a high level of inducible transgene expression (i.e., BMP-4 expression) to transduced, muscle-derived stem cells (MDSCs) [65]. This novel retroviral vector also enables us to regulate the amount of bone formation elicited by the transduced cells after transplantation [65]. We believe that the findings generated by this study could be translated to a wide variety of other gene-therapy applications that require stringent regulation of a transgene's therapeutic effect, such as the codelivery of inducible VEGF and its specific antagonist to achieve regulated angiogenesis.

49.3.5   Is the Bone Regenerated by BMP-Producing Muscle-Derived Cells Biomechanically Relevant?

We have evaluated the ability of muscle-derived cells transduced with retroBMP4 to heal a long bone defect both structurally and functionally. Primary muscle-derived rat cells were genetically engineered to express BMP-4 and implanted into 7-mm rat femoral defects; muscle-derived cells transduced with retroLacZ were used as the control. Bone healing was monitored via radiography, histology, and biomechanical testing. Our results indicate that 78.6% of the defects treated with muscle-derived cells expressing BMP-4 formed bridging callous by 6 weeks after surgery, and 12 of the 13 femora exhibited radiographically evident union 12 weeks after implantation. Histological analysis at the 12-week time point revealed that the medullary canal of the femur was restored and the cortex was remodeled between the proximal and distal ends of each BMP-4-treated defect. In contrast, nonunions were observed at all tested time points in the defects treated with muscle-derived cells expressing β-galactosidase (a marker gene). The maximum torque-to-failure in the treatment group (BMP-4–producing cells) indicated up to 73% strength of the contralateral intact femur, while the torsional stiffness and energy-to-failure were not significantly different between the treated and the intact limbs. This study demonstrates that retroBMP4-transduced muscle-derived cells can elicit both structural and functional healing of critical sized segmental defects in rat femora [66].

49.4   Articular Disorders

Various articular disorders, including arthritis, chondral and osteochondral defects, meniscal tears, and damaged ligaments, are potential candidates for novel treatment using gene therapy and tissue engineering applications.

49.4.1   Articular Cartilage

Articular cartilage defects and progressive osteoarthritis are among the most frequent and challenging conditions encountered in orthopaedics. In contrast to bone, articular cartilage heals poorly. Current repair techniques include cartilage debridement and resurfacing [67,68], subchondral drilling [69], arthroscopic abrasion, and microfracture. Common to these techniques is the disruption of subchondral bone to allow osteochondral progenitors from the marrow to gain access to and participate in repair of the cartilage defect. The repaired cartilage, however, is structurally inferior to native cartilage and contains significantly less proteoglycan [70]. Newer strategies for cartilage repair seek to provide an alternate source of cells to stimulate healing. Strategies have included the use of autologous chondrocyte transplantation [71] and transplantation of cartilage plugs [72]. Although adult or embryonic chondrocytes may be used for transplantation, the limiting factor is chondrocyte supply. Other researchers have tried to overcome this limitation by generating chondrocytes from mesenchymal stem cells [73]. These cells then are induced to become osteochondral progenitor cells in culture before reimplantation.

Partly because muscle-derived cells are easily accessible, we have explored their capacity for repairing articular defects. The ability of muscle-derived cells to promote cartilage formation/restoration and bone formation through an endochondral pathway (see earlier sections) further justifies the evaluation of their potential use for articular cartilage repair. For these reasons, we have investigated the utilization of transplanted allogeneic muscle-derived cells embedded in collagen gels for the repair of full thickness articular cartilage defects [74]. The results were compared to chondrocyte transplantation and control (nontreated) groups. Although grafted cells were found in the defects only up to 4 weeks after transplantation, histological assessment at 12 and 24 weeks after transplantation revealed that the tissue repaired with muscle-derived cells or chondrocytes displayed comparably higher levels of healing than observed in the control groups [74]. Notably, at 24 weeks the repaired tissues in the muscle-derived cell and chondrocyte groups were composed primarily of type II collagen, indicating the presence of hyaline articular cartilage [74]. These results demonstrated that allogeneic muscle-derived cells could be used as both gene-delivery vehicles and a cell source to promote full-thickness cartilage repair. The implantation of muscle-derived cells appeared to improve the healing of the defects with an efficiency equivalent to that of chondrocyte cartilage transplantation. Muscle-derived cell transplantation is a particularly attractive option given the fact that the muscle biopsy required to obtain muscle cells is less invasive than the arthroscopy required to obtain chondrocytes [74].

49.4.2   Meniscus

Allograft meniscal transplantation is one of the few available treatment options after meniscectomy. Despite acceptable early results, considerable controversy exists due to the subsequent poor graft regeneration, shrinkage, and biomechanical failure of transplanted menisci. Meniscal injuries are promising candidates for treatment via gene therapy and tissue engineering applications. The possible *in vitro* creation of a custom, replacement meniscus by using scaffolds, cells, and gene therapy for subsequent *in vivo* implantation is intriguing. Alternatively, gene therapy could be used to genetically engineer meniscal cells in order to promote the healing of certain injuries. Meniscal cells are amenable to gene transfer of both marker genes and various growth factor genes via either direct or *ex vivo* gene therapy, with gene expression persisting for up to 6 weeks [75]. Successful *ex vivo* gene transfer to the meniscus has been accomplished using either muscle-derived cells [20] or meniscal cells [75]. Identification of the growth factors that best promote meniscal healing, techniques to improve long-term gene expression, and the optimal scaffold required to create de novo menisci is the focus of ongoing research.

We have recently investigated the feasibility of using gene transfer in meniscal allografts in rabbits to eventually deliver specific growth factor genes that may improve the regeneration of meniscal allograft [76]. Four different viral vectors encoding marker genes, including LacZ, luciferase, and green fluorescence protein, were used to investigate viral transduction in 50 lapine menisci for 4 weeks *in vitro*. Subsequently, 16 unilateral meniscus replacements were performed with *ex vivo* retrovirally transduced meniscal allografts; the expression of the LacZ gene was examined histologically at 2, 4, 6, and 8 weeks after transplantation. Gene expression in the superficial cell layers of the menisci was detected for up to 4 weeks *in vitro*, but the level of gene transfer declined over time [76]. The retrovirally transduced cells displayed more persistent transgene expression and penetrated the menisci more deeply after implantation [76]. *In vivo*, declining numbers of β-galactosidase-positive cells were detected in the retrovirally transduced allografts for up to 8 weeks. Transduced cells consistently were found at the meniscosynovial junction of the transplants and in deeper layers of the menisci. There was no evidence of cellular immune response in the transduced transplants. This investigation demonstrates the promise of growth factor delivery in auto- and allografts. We will conduct additional experiments to assess the potential of vectors expressing therapeutic proteins (e.g., growth factors) to improve remodeling and healing of meniscal allografts [76].

49.4.3 Ligaments

Researchers also are investigating the use of gene-therapy techniques for treatment of injured ligaments. LacZ gene transfer to ligaments via either direct or *ex vivo* adenoviral or retroviral approaches has proven feasible in animal models. *Ex vivo* gene transfer to ligaments has been achieved using either ligament fibroblasts or skeletal muscle-derived cells [21]. Many growth factors, such as basic fibroblast growth factor (bFGF), platelet-derived growth factor (PDGF), VEGF, insulin-like growth factor (IGF)-1 and -2, TGF-β, and BMP-12, are believed to possibly play roles in ligament healing. Data suggest that PDGF stimulates cell division and migration, whereas TGF-β and the IGFs promote extracellular matrix synthesis [77]. Use of a viral-liposome conjugate vector for the direct gene transfer of PDGF-β into rat patellar ligaments was found to initially improve angiogenesis and subsequently enhance extracellular matrix synthesis [78].

The integration of tendon grafts typically used for anterior cruciate ligament replacement continues to be unsatisfactory and may be associated with postoperative anterior–posterior laxity. We have evaluated whether BMP-2 gene transfer can improve the integration of semitendinosus tendon grafts at the tendon–bone interface after anterior cruciate ligament reconstruction in rabbits [79]. Anterior cruciate ligament reconstruction using autologous double-bundle semitendinosus tendon grafts was performed in 46 adult rabbits. The semitendinosus tendon grafts were genetically engineered *in vitro* with adenovirus–luciferase, adenovirus–LacZ (AdLacZ), or adenovirus–BMP-2 (AdBMP-2); untreated grafts served as controls. The anterior cruciate ligament grafts were examined histologically 2, 4, 6, and 8 weeks after surgery. In an additional series of experiments, the structural properties of the femur–anterior cruciate ligament graft–tibia complexes were investigated in 10 untreated controls and 10 specimens with AdBMP-2-transduced semitendinosus tendon grafts. The animals were sacrificed 8 weeks after anterior cruciate ligament surgery, and the femur–anterior cruciate ligament graft–tibia complexes were tested under uniaxial tension. The stiffness (N/mm) and ultimate load at failure (N) were determined from load-elongation curves.

Our results indicate that genetically engineered semitendinosus tendon grafts expressed reporter genes and BMP-2 *in vitro* [79]. The AdLacZ-infected anterior cruciate ligament grafts showed two different histological patterns of transduction. Intra-articular, infected cells were mostly aligned along the surface and decreased in number during the 6 weeks after surgery. In the intra-tunnel portions of the anterior cruciate ligament grafts, the number of infected cells did not decrease during the observation period. Moreover, we observed a high number of transduced cells in the deeper layers of the tendons. In the control group, granulation-type tissue at the tendon–bone interface showed progressive reorganization into a dense connective tissue, and subsequent establishment of fibers resembling Sharpey's fibers.

In the specimens receiving AdBMP-2-infected anterior cruciate ligament grafts, a broad zone of newly formed matrix resembling chondro-osteoid was observed at the tendon–bone interface 4 weeks after surgery. This area had increased by 6 weeks after surgery, showing a transition from bone to mineralized and nonmineralized cartilage. In addition, in the BMP-2-treated specimens, the tendon–bone interface in the osseous tunnel was similar to that of a normal anterior cruciate ligament insertion. The stiffness (29.0 ± 7.1 vs. 16.7 ± 8.3 N/mm) and the ultimate load at failure (108.8 ± 50.8 vs. 45.0 ± 18.0 N) were significantly enhanced in the specimens with BMP-2-transduced anterior cruciate ligament grafts when compared with controls. This study demonstrated that BMP-2 gene transfer significantly improves the integration of semitendinosus tendon grafts in the tunnels after anterior cruciate ligament reconstruction in rabbits [79]. Before introducing gene transfer as a therapeutic method in orthopaedics, however, researchers must answer questions regarding safety and regulatory issues.

49.5 Summary

This paper summarizes the current knowledge and most recent achievements in gene therapy and tissue engineering for the musculoskeletal system; many of these advances are attributable to or strongly influenced by the research findings of our laboratory. Although this review focuses on a population of muscle-derived stem cells isolated by our research team, we are not excluding the possible use of alternative cell populations, including stem cells from various sources (e.g., hematopoietic cells, mesenchymal stem cells, or fat-derived cells) for future applications. Bringing tissue engineering technology to clinical fruition, however, will require multidisciplinary collaboration to identify and optimize the appropriate cell type, growth factor, and scaffold construct for each application. Future investigations should elaborate upon the utility of stem cells derived from various adult tissues in autologous, allogeneic, or perhaps xenogeneic settings. Details regarding these cells' proliferative potential, susceptibility to genetic engineering, and immunogenic potential remain to be characterized. Furthermore, researchers must learn to combine stem cells with growth factors in a viable spatiotemporal relationship in order to re-create the *in situ* microenvironment. Much work remains before the regeneration of tissue for healing the musculoskeletal system — a complicated endeavor with vast potential applicability — becomes a clinical reality.

Acknowledgments

The authors wish to thank Marcelle Pellerin, James Cummins, and Brian Gearhart (Children's Hospital of Pittsburgh, Pittsburgh, PA) for technical support and Ryan Sauder (University of Pittsburgh, Pittsburgh, PA) for editorial assistance with the manuscript. This work was supported by grants to Dr. Johnny Huard from the Muscular Dystrophy Association (USA), the National Institutes of Health (NIH P01 AR 45925-01, R01 AR 49684-01, R01 AR 47973-01, R01 DE 13420-01A2), the Orris C. Hirtzel and Beatrice Dewey Hirtzel Memorial Foundation and the William F. and Jean W. Donaldson Chair at Children's Hospital of Pittsburgh, and the Henry J. Mankin Endowed Chair at the University of Pittsburgh.

The authors also want to thank the clinical fellows Chan Y.S., Fukushima K., Shen H.C., Adachi N., and Martinek V. for their contribution to this work.

References

[1] Bosch, P. et al., Osteoprogenitor cells within skeletal muscle. *J. Orthop. Res.* 2000; 18: 933–944.

[2] Musgrave, D.S. et al., *Ex vivo* gene therapy to produce bone using different cell types. *Clin. Orthop.* 2000: 290–305.

[3] Booth, D.K. et al., Myoblast-mediated *ex vivo* gene transfer to mature muscle. *Tissue Eng.* 1997; 3: 125.

[4] Floyd, S.S. Jr. et al., *Ex vivo* gene transfer using adenovirus-mediated full-length dystrophin delivery to dystrophic muscles. *Gene Ther.* 1998; 5: 19–30.

[5] van Deutekom, J.C. et al., Implications of maturation for viral gene delivery to skeletal muscle. *Neuromuscul. Disord.* 1998; 8: 135–148.

[6] van Deutekom, J.C., Hoffman, E.P., and Huard, J., Muscle maturation: implications for gene therapy. *Mol. Med. Today* 1998; 4: 214–220.

[7] Lee, J.Y. et al., Clonal isolation of muscle-derived cells capable of enhancing muscle regeneration and bone healing. *J. Cell Biol.* 2000; 150: 1085–1100.

[8] Qu-Petersen, Z. et al., Identification of a novel population of muscle stem cells in mice: potential for muscle regeneration. *J. Cell Biol.* 2002; 157: 851–864.

[9] Huard, J. et al., Dystrophin expression in myotubes formed by the fusion of normal and dystrophic myoblasts. *Muscle Nerve* 1991; 14: 178–182.

[10] Karpati, G. et al., Dystrophin is expressed in mdx skeletal muscle fibers after normal myoblast implantation. *Am. J. Pathol.* 1989; 135: 27–32.

[11] Partridge, T.A., Invited review: myoblast transfer: a possible therapy for inherited myopathies? *Muscle Nerve* 1991; 14: 197–212.

[12] Tremblay, J.P. et al., Results of a triple blind clinical study of myoblast transplantations without immunosuppressive treatment in young boys with Duchenne muscular dystrophy. *Cell Transplant* 1993; 2: 99–112.

[13] Dai, Y., Roman, M., Naviaux, R.K., and Verma, I.M., Gene therapy via primary myoblasts: long-term expression of factor IX protein following transplantation *in vivo*. *Proc. Natl Acad. Sci. USA* 1992; 89: 10892–10895.

[14] Dhawan, J. et al., Systemic delivery of human growth hormone by injection of genetically engineered myoblasts. *Science* 1991; 254: 1509–1512.

[15] Lynch, C.M. et al., Long-term expression of human adenosine deaminase in vascular smooth muscle cells of rats: a model for gene therapy. *Proc. Natl Acad. Sci. USA* 1992; 89: 1138–1142.

[16] Simonson, G.D., Groskreutz, D.J., Gorman, C.M., and MacDonald, M.J., Synthesis and processing of genetically modified human proinsulin by rat myoblast primary cultures. *Hum. Gene Ther.* 1996; 7: 71–78.

[17] Jiao, S., Gurevich, V., and Wolff, J.A., Long-term correction of rat model of Parkinson's disease by gene therapy. *Nature* 1993; 362: 450–453.

[18] Lau, H.T., Yu, M., Fontana, A., Stoeckert, C.J. Jr., Prevention of islet allograft rejection with engineered myoblasts expressing FasL in mice. *Science* 1996; 273: 109–112.

[19] Day, C.S. et al., Myoblast-mediated gene transfer to the joint. *J. Orthop. Res.* 1997; 15: 894–903.

[20] Kasemkijwattana, C. et al., The use of growth factors, gene therapy and tissue engineering to improve meniscal healing. *Mater. Sci. Eng.* 2000; 13: 19–28.

[21] Menetrey, J. et al., Direct-, fibroblast- and myoblast-mediated gene transfer to the anterior cruciate ligament. *Tissue Eng.* 1999; 5: 435–442.

[22] Baroffio, A. et al., Identification of self-renewing myoblasts in the progeny of single human muscle satellite cells. *Differentiation* 1996; 60: 47–57.

[23] Miller, J.B., Schaefer, L., and Dominov, J.A., Seeking muscle stem cells. *Curr. Top. Dev. Biol.* 1999; 43: 191–219.

[24] Nicolas, J.F., Mathis, L., Bonnerot, C., and Saurin, W., Evidence in the mouse for self-renewing stem cells in the formation of a segmented longitudinal structure, the myotome. *Development* 1996; 122: 2933–2946.

[25] Slack, J.M.W., *From Egg to Embryo*. 2nd ed. New York: Cambridge University Press, 1991.

[26] Cao, B. et al., Muscle stem cells differentiate into haematopoietic lineages but retain myogenic potential. *Nat. Cell Biol.* 2003; 5: 640–646.

[27] Gussoni, E. et al., Dystrophin expression in the mdx mouse restored by stem cell transplantation. *Nature* 1999; 401: 390–394.

[28] Kawada, H. and Ogawa, M., Bone marrow origin of hematopoietic progenitors and stem cells in murine muscle. *Blood* 2001; 98: 2008–2013.

[29] McKinney-Freeman, S.L. et al., Muscle-derived hematopoietic stem cells are hematopoietic in origin. *Proc. Natl Acad. Sci. USA* 2002; 99: 1341–1346.

[30] Torrente, Y. et al., Intraarterial injection of muscle-derived CD34(+)Sca-1(+) stem cells restores dystrophin in mdx mice. *J. Cell Biol.* 2001; 152: 335–348.

[31] Williams, J.T. et al., Cells isolated from adult human skeletal muscle capable of differentiating into multiple mesodermal phenotypes. *Am. Surg.* 1999; 65: 22–26.

[32] Young, H.E. et al., Pluripotent mesenchymal stem cells reside within avian connective tissue matrices. *In Vitro Cell Dev. Biol. Anim.* 1993; 29A: 723–736.

[33] Young, H.E. et al., Human reserve pluripotent mesenchymal stem cells are present in the connective tissues of skeletal muscle and dermis derived from fetal, adult, and geriatric donors. *Anat. Rec.* 2001; 264: 51–62.

[34] Beauchamp, J.R., Morgan, J.E., Pagel, C.N., and Partridge, T.A., Dynamics of myoblast transplantation reveal a discrete minority of precursors with stem cell-like properties as the myogenic source. *J. Cell Biol.* 1999; 144: 1113–1122.

[35] Fan, Y., Maley, M., Beilharz, M., and Grounds, M., Rapid death of injected myoblasts in myoblast transfer therapy. *Muscle Nerve* 1996; 19: 853–860.

[36] Guerette, B. et al., Control of inflammatory damage by anti-LFA-1: increase success of myoblast transplantation. *Cell Transplant* 1997; 6: 101–107.

[37] Huard, J. et al., Gene transfer into skeletal muscles by isogenic myoblasts. *Hum. Gene Ther.* 1994; 5: 949–958.

[38] Huard, J. et al., High efficiency of muscle regeneration after human myoblast clone transplantation in SCID mice. *J. Clin. Invest.* 1994; 93: 586–599.

[39] Kinoshita, I. et al., Very efficient myoblast allotransplantation in mice under FK506 immunosuppression. *Muscle Nerve* 1994; 17: 1407–1415.

[40] Morgan, J.E., Pagel, C.N., Sherratt, T., and Partridge, T.A., Long-term persistence and migration of myogenic cells injected into pre-irradiated muscles of mdx mice. *J. Neurol. Sci.* 1993; 115: 191–200.

[41] Petersen, Z.Q. and Huard, J., The influence of muscle fiber type in myoblast-mediated gene transfer to skeletal muscles. *Cell Transplant* 2000; 9: 503–517.

[42] Qu, Z. et al., Development of approaches to improve cell survival in myoblast transfer therapy. *J. Cell Biol.* 1998; 142: 1257–1267.

[43] Qu, Z. and Huard, J., Matching host muscle and donor myoblasts for myosin heavy chain improves myoblast transfer therapy. *Gene Ther.* 2000; 7: 428–437.

[44] Huard, J., Li, Y., and Fu, F.H., Muscle injuries and repair: current trends in research. *J. Bone Joint Surg. Am.* 2002; 84-A: 822–832.

[45] Li, Y., Cummins, J., and Huard, J., Muscle injury and repair. *Curr. Opin. Orthop.* 2001; 12: 409–415.

[46] Kasemkijwattana, C. et al., Use of growth factors to improve muscle healing after strain injury. *Clin. Orthop.* 2000: 272–285.

[47] Kasemkijwattana, C., Menetrey, J., Day, C.S., and Huard, J., Biologic intervention in muscle healing and regeneration. *Sports Med. Arthrosc. Rev.* 1998; 6: 95–102.

[48] Menetrey, J. et al., Growth factors improve muscle healing *in vivo*. *J. Bone Joint Surg. Br.* 2000; 82: 131–137.

[49] Border, W.A. and Noble, N.A., Transforming growth factor beta in tissue fibrosis. *N. Engl. J. Med.* 1994; 331: 1286–1292.

[50] Li, Y. and Huard, J., Differentiation of muscle-derived cells into myofibroblasts in injured skeletal muscle. *Am. J. Pathol.* 2002; 161: 895–907.

[51] Chan, Y.S. et al., Antifibrotic effects of suramin in injured skeletal muscle after laceration. *J. Appl. Physiol.* 2003; 95: 771–780.

[52] Foster, W. et al., Gamma interferon as an antifibrosis agent in skeletal muscle. *J. Orthop. Res.* 2003; 21: 798–804.

[53] Fukushima, K. et al., The use of an antifibrosis agent to improve muscle recovery after laceration. *Am. J. Sports Med.* 2001; 29: 394–402.

[54] Einhorn, T.A., Enhancement of fracture-healing. *J. Bone Joint Surg. Am.* 1995; 77: 940–956.

[55] Fiebel, R.J. et al., Simultaneous free-tissue transfer and Ilizarov distraction osteosynthesis in lower extremity salvage: case report and review of the literature. *J. Trauma* 1994; 37: 322–327.

[56] Prokuski, L.J. and Marsh, J.L., Segmental bone deficiency after acute trauma. The role of bone transport. *Orthop. Clin. North Am.* 1994; 25: 753–763.

[57] De Oliveira, J.C., Bone grafts and chronic osteomyelitis. *J. Bone Joint Surg. Br.* 1971; 53: 672–683.

[58] Peng, H. et al., Synergistic enhancement of bone formation and healing by stem cell-expressed VEGF and bone morphogenetic protein-4. *J. Clin. Invest.* 2002; 110: 751–759.

[59] Wright, V. et al., BMP4-expressing muscle-derived stem cells differentiate into osteogenic lineage and improve bone healing in immunocompetent mice. *Mol. Ther.* 2002; 6: 169–178.

[60] Musgrave, D.S. et al., Human skeletal muscle cells in *ex vivo* gene therapy to deliver bone morphogenetic protein-2. *J. Bone Joint Surg. Br.* 2002; 84: 120–127.

[61] Lee, J.Y. et al., Enhancement of bone healing based on *ex vivo* gene therapy using human muscle-derived cells expressing bone morphogenetic protein 2. *Hum. Gene Ther.* 2002; 13: 1201–1211.

[62] Hannallah, D. et al., Retroviral delivery of Noggin inhibits the formation of heterotopic ossification induced by BMP-4, demineralized bone matrix, and trauma in an animal model. *J. Bone Joint Surg. Am.* 2004; 86-A: 80–91.

[63] Gossen, M. and Bujard, H., Tight control of gene expression in mammalian cells by tetracycline-responsive promoters. *Proc. Natl Acad. Sci. USA* 1992; 89: 5547–5551.

[64] Iida, A., Chen, S.T., Friedmann, T., and Yee, J.K., Inducible gene expression by retrovirus-mediated transfer of a modified tetracycline-regulated system. *J. Virol.* 1996; 70: 6054–6059.

[65] Peng, H. et al., Converse relationship between *in vitro* osteogenic differentiation and *in vivo* bone healing elicited by different populations of muscle-derived cells genetically engineered to express BMP4. *J. Bone Miner. Res.* 2004; 19: 630–641.

[66] Shen, H.C. et al., Structural and functional healing of critical-size segmental bone defects by transduced muscle-derived cells expressing BMP4. *J. Gene Med.* 2004; 6: 984–991

[67] Insall, J., The Pridie debridement operation for osteoarthritis of the knee. *Clin. Orthop.* 1974; 101: 61–67.

[68] Pridie, K., A method of resurfacing osteoarthritic knee joints. *J. Bone Joint Surg. Br.* 1959; 41: 618–619.

[69] Mitchell, N. and Shepard, N., The resurfacing of adult rabbit articular cartilage by multiple perforations through the subchondral bone. *J. Bone Joint Surg. Am.* 1976; 58: 230–233.

[70] Shapiro, F., Koide, S., and Glimcher, M.J., Cell origin and differentiation in the repair of full-thickness defects of articular cartilage. *J. Bone Joint Surg. Am.* 1993; 75: 532–553.

[71] Brittberg, M. et al., Treatment of deep cartilage defects in the knee with autologous chondrocyte transplantation. *N. Engl. J. Med.* 1994; 331: 889–895.

[72] Hangody, L. et al., Mosaicplasty for the treatment of articular cartilage defects: application in clinical practice. *Orthopedics* 1998; 21: 751–756.

[73] Wakitani, S. et al., Repair of rabbit articular surfaces with allograft chondrocytes embedded in collagen gel. *J. Bone Joint Surg. Br.* 1989; 71: 74–80.

[74] Adachi, N. et al., Muscle derived, cell based *ex vivo* gene therapy for treatment of full thickness articular cartilage defects. *J. Rheumatol.* 2002; 29: 1920–1930.

[75] Goto, H. et al., Transfer of lacZ marker gene to the meniscus. *J. Bone Joint Surg. Am.* 1999; 81: 918–925.

[76] Martinek, V. et al., Genetic engineering of meniscal allografts. *Tissue Eng.* 2002; 8: 107–117.

[77] Evans, C.H., Cytokines and the role they play in the healing of ligaments and tendons. *Sports Med.* 1999; 28: 71–76.

[78] Nakamura, N. et al., Early biological effect of *in vivo* gene transfer of platelet-derived growth factor (PDGF)-B into healing patellar ligament. *Gene Ther.* 1998; 5: 1165–1170.

[79] Martinek, V. et al., Enhancement of tendon–bone integration of anterior cruciate ligament grafts with bone morphogenetic protein-2 gene transfer: a histological and biomechanical study. *J. Bone Joint Surg. Am.* 2002; 84-A: 1123–1131.

50

Tissue Engineering Applications — Bone

Ayse B. Celil
Scott Guelcher
Jeffrey O. Hollinger
Carnegie Mellon University

Michael Miller
University of Texas

50.1 Biology of the Bone

Bone is a complex living tissue that provides internal support for all higher vertebrates. It develops by osteogenesis, the process of ossification, starting out as a highly specialized form of connective tissue. Two major players in the formation of bone are the bone cells called osteoblasts (bone-forming) and the osteoclasts (bone-resorbing). During the process of ossification, osteoblasts secrete type I collagen, in addition to many noncollagenous proteins such as osteocalcin, bone sialoprotein, and osteopontin. Osteoblast-secreted extracellular matrix may initially be amorphous and noncrystalline, but it gradually transforms into more crystalline forms [1]. Mineralization is a process of bone formation promoted by osteoblasts and is thought to be initiated by the matrix vesicles that bud from the plasma membrane [2] of osteoblasts to create an environment for the concentration of calcium and phosphate, allowing crystallization. Collagen serves as a template and may also initiate and propagate mineralization independent of the matrix vesicles [3,4]. Eventually, some osteoblasts are surrounded by the bone matrix that they help to form and are called osteocytes. Despite their location, osteocytes are not metabolically inactive; they dissolve and resorb some bone mineral though osteolysis [5]. Bone resorption is in fact the primary function of another bone cell, the osteoclast, which can also digest calcified cartilage and is then called the chondroclast. Formation by the osteoblasts and resorption by the osteoclasts maintains bone in constant renewal as a dynamic tissue.

Bone formation in the developing embryo occurs by two developmental processes: intramembranous and endochondral ossification. Intramembranous ossification is the direct differentiation of osteoblasts from mesenchymal cells. Several craniofacial bones and parts of the mandible and clavicle develop by intramembranous ossification [6]. Most other bones are formed by endochondral ossification. In this process of bone formation, mesenchymal cells condense and differentiate into cartilage. The cartilage anlage matures, undergoes hypertrophy, mineralizes, and subsequently becomes invaded by blood vessels as well as osteoprogenitor cells [7,8].

Woven and lamellar bone are the two types of bone observed at the microscopic level. Woven bone is a disoriented arrangement of collagen fibers [9] and is the first bone formed in the embryo. After birth, woven bone is gradually replaced by lamellar bone except in a few places (e.g., tooth sockets). Lamellar bone is highly organized and has collagen bundles oriented in the same direction [9]. Structural organization of woven and lamellar bone is in two categories:

1. Trabecular bone (spongy, cancellous)
2. Cortical bone (compact)

The inherent architecture of bone is influenced by the mechanical stresses. The structure–function relationship of bone was described in 1892 by Wolff's law [10], which states that mechanical stress is responsible for the architecture of the bone. Bone undergoes adaptive changes in response to the demands of mechanical stress from the environment [5]. It has been shown that bone formation is upregulated in response to increased load application [11,12] and that bone tissue is removed from the skeleton in response to reduced loading as in microgravity [13,14]. The mechanical signals to the osteoprogenitor cells of the bone are also important in determining the formation of the tissue that forms during development and healing [14]. Several noninvasive techniques are currently used to evaluate bone mechanical properties in the clinic such as quantitative computer tomography (QCT), magnetic resonance imaging (MRI), ultrasound, and dual-energy x-ray absorptiometry (DEXA) [15–17]. In a laboratory setting several bone marker genes are used to evaluate differentiation into the osteoblast phenotype and formation of bone. Among these marker genes are: alkaline phosphatase (alp), type I collagen (type I col), osteopontin (opn), osteocalcin (ocn) and bone sialoprotein (bsp). Alp and type I col are induced earlier in differentiation, whereas ocn and bsp are considered to be late markers. Techniques such as conventional and quantitative real-time PCR and northern blot allow the detection of these genes at the RNA level. For genome wide analysis microarray technology can be used for the analysis of a large sample population.

Alkaline phosphatase (Alp) is an enzyme that catalyzes the hydrolysis of phosphate esters at an alkaline pH. It has several different isoforms: tissue nonspecific, placental, and intestinal [18]. Three isoforms exist for the tissue nonspecific isoenzyme including bone, liver, and kidney. The skeletal isoform is a glycoprotein on the cell membrane of osteoblasts [19]. Alp is important in bone matrix mineralization and its activity is recognized as an indicator of osteoblast function.

Type I collagen (type I col) is the major organic component of bone matrix. Collagen has a basic structure of repeating primary amino acid sequence of -gly-X-Y. Osteoblasts synthesize type I collagen molecules to form fibrils, which give the characteristic cross-banding pattern. Collagen secretion by osteoblasts promotes their differentiation into a more mature phenotype [20].

Osteopontin (Opn) is a noncollagenous, acidic, sialic acid-rich phosphorylated glycoprotein; it binds to hydroxyapatite and is abundant in the mineral matrix of bones [21].

Osteocalcin (Ocn) is the most abundant noncollagenous protein in bone, comprising approximately 2% of total protein in the human body. It is important in bone metabolism and its recently revealed structure indicates a negatively charged protein surface that places calcium ions in positions complementary to those in hydroxyapatite. Ocn could potentially modulate the crystal morphology and growth of hydroxyapatite [22].

Bone sialoprotein (Bsp) is a noncollagenous protein that promotes RGD (ARG-GLY-ASP) dependent cell attachment via integrins. Bsp is thought to be involved in the nucleation of hydroxyapatite for mineralization of bone [23].

The restoration of skeletal tissue to its normal state and function, also known as fracture repair, is dependent on the careful arrangement of the action of several factors. A number of growth factors, cytokines, and their receptors are present around the fracture site to start the repair process. Whereas many of these components are expressed in the skeletal tissue at all times, several other molecules are released from the inflammatory cells at the site of injury. Fracture repair has been discussed in several reviews and some of the factors and signaling pathways involved in this process are illustrated in Figure 50.1 [24,25]. In Section 50.2 we will overview some of the signaling molecules in bone formation and repair.

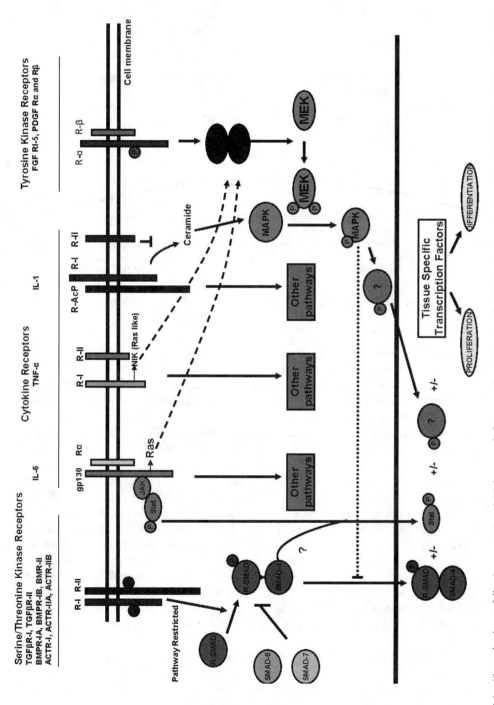

FIGURE 50.1 (See color insert following page **20**-14.) Major growth factors and cytokines involved in fracture repair. Reproduced from *J. Bone Miner. Res.* 1999, 14:1808 with permission of the American Society for Bone and Mineral Research.

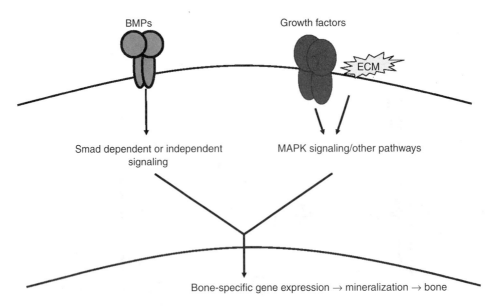

FIGURE 50.2   Growth factors, ECM proteins, BMPs exert their effects on cells to promote osteoblastic differentiation and bone formation.

50.2 Signaling Molecules for Bone

50.2.1 Growth Factors

Bone formation and development is the arrangement of the actions of a wide variety of signaling molecules (Figure 50.2). These signaling molecules include growth factors, hormones, vitamins, and cytokines. Hormones may be several categories including amino acid derivatives, peptides, steroids and fatty acid derivatives. Growth factors are peptide hormones, which induce cellular proliferation. Cytokines, which are also peptide-based can affect inflammatory and immune responses of the metabolism. The orchestration of these factors regulates mitogenesis, cell shape, movement, differentiation, and apoptosis.

Growth factor effects are concentration-dependent and are exerted through their receptors on the cell surface. A secreted growth factor may bind to matrix molecules, carrier molecules, or binding proteins to regulate its activity and stabilization [26]. Growth factors can associate with specific binding proteins that limit access to their receptors to control the bioavailability of the growth factor (e.g., IGF-I, IGF-II, TGFβ, BMPs) [27–29]. The conversion of a growth factor to a bioactive state requires an activation event. Using IGF-I as an example, greater than 99% are bound by IGFBPs (IGF binding proteins) in fluid and solid phase [26,30] and requires protease activation to release IGF-I. This mechanism of sequestration allows temporal and spatial regulation. For tissue engineering applications it is crucial to control the concentration and physical placement and sequestration of a growth factor. Several methods are available for controlling the physical placement of a growth factor including, but not limited to microfluidics, microencapsulation, entrapment and release from polymeric systems, and nonspecific adsorption to matrices [26,31]. Growth factors can also be immobilized to engineered matrices to localize delivery [32], but spatial patterning remains a challenge.

The design of a tissue engineering application requires an appreciation of the mechanism by which a factor elicits its signal and the downstream effect originating from this signal. In this section we will briefly overview some of the factors involved in bone formation and regulation.

50.2.1.1 Insulin-Like Growth Factors

The putative functions of insulin-like growth factors (IGF-I and IGF-II) include embryonic and natal growth, bone matrix mineralization, cartilage development and homeostasis [33,34]. IGFs can stimulate collagen production and prevent collagen degradation by reducing collagenase synthesis [35]. IGF-I is known to activate osteocalcin expression [36] inside the cell. It has been reported to be important for maintaining bone mass and promoting longitudinal bone growth [37].

The IGFs transduce their signals via two different receptors known as IGF-I and IGF-II receptors [38]. IGF-II mediates its signal through the type II IGF receptor although it can tissue-specifically activate the type I IGF receptor. IGF-I is a single chain peptide with a structure similar to proinsulin, but consisting of four domains (insulin contains three domains) [39]. During posttranslational modification of the molecule, one of the peptide domains is cleaved from the rest of the domains and the rest are joined to one another by forming disulfide bonds [39,40]. Growth hormone induces IGF-I synthesis [41]. The kidney, muscle, and bone also contribute to the circulating IGF-I levels [41].

IGF-II has 60% homology to IGF-I and acts independent of growth hormone [41,42]. It appears to be more important during fetal growth than in postnatal growth [43,44]. In a study where it was systemically administered to rats, IGF-II was found to be less potent than IGF-I in stimulating skeletal growth [45]. A study on chimeric mice carrying one inactivated IGF-II allele indicated that these mice were smaller than their wild type littermates [46] indicating the significance of IGF-II on the skeleton during early stages of growth. More studies have been conducted on IGF-I than IGF-II for tissue engineering applications. Studies in rats suggest that IGF-I increases intramembranous ossification [47], improves the effects of age-related osteopenia [48,49], and accelerates functional recovery from Achilles tendon injury [50]. IGF-I has also been used for spinal fusion application in sheep, giving a successful outcome when delivered via poly-(D, L-lactide) (PDLLA)-coated titanium [51]. In another study, IGF-I was delivered via polyacetate (PLLA) microspheres to metacarpal defects in calves of pigs and showed enhancement of bone formation [52].

50.2.1.2 Fibroblast Growth Factors

Fibroblast growth factors FGF-1 and -2, also known as acidic and basic FGF, respectively, belong to a family of growth factors with heparin binding domains. FGFs regulate mitogenesis, differentiation, protease production, receptor modulation, and cell maintenance [53]. FGF-2 (also called basic FGF or bFGF) is produced by the osteoblasts and stored in skeletal tissues [54]. FGF-1 has been associated with chondrocyte proliferation [55].

The FGF-1 and FGF-2 systemically and locally administered to ovariectomized rats increased new bone formation and bone density [56,57]. Systemic delivery of FGF-1 appeared to be effective in restoring the microarchitecture of bone and preventing bone loss associated with estrogen withdrawal [56]. In a rabbit ulcer model, FGF-1 delivery within a modified fibrin matrix stimulated angiogenic and fibroblastic responses in addition to an increased epithelialization rate [57]. Several studies indicated that scaffold mediated delivery rather than direct injection of FGF-2 was more effective in improving bone healing in rats [58], rabbits [59], and dogs [49,60]. Local infusion of recombinant FGF-2 increased bone ingrowth in a rabbit tibia model in the presence of polyethylene particles [61].

50.2.1.3 Vascular Endothelial Growth Factors

Vascular endothelial growth factors, of which there are six different isoforms [62], are vascular cytokines that promote angiogenesis, increased vascular permeability, and vasodilation [62]. Prosthetic vascular grafts that were coated with VEGF supported endothelial cell proliferation and migration [63]. Several studies indicated increased capillary density and vasodilator-induced blood flow in response to VEGF treatment [64–66]. Synergistic effects of VEGF and FGF-2 have also been demonstrated in the production of new blood vessels [67]. Macroporous scaffolds with poly(lactide-co-glycolide) which were designed to release VEGF increased the generation of mineralized tissue due to an increase in vascularization, but did not increase osteoid formation [68]. VEGF is a crucial factor for tissue engineering due to its role in angiogenesis; it is the main provider of nutrients and growth factors to the wound repair site.

50.2.1.4 Transforming Growth Factor-ß

Transforming growth factor-ß family consists of five members, bone morphogenetic proteins (BMP), growth and differentiation factors (GDF), activins, inhibins, and Mullerian substance [69]. Osteoblasts and chondrocytes express TGFß receptors [70,71]. Mainly found in bone, platelets, and cartilage TGFß triggers growth, differentiation, and extracellular matrix synthesis [72]. TGFß is thought to be a coupler between bone formation and resorption. Studies on the use of TGFß as a therapeutic reagent have been difficult to assess due to the use of different isoforms and superphysiological doses of TGFß.

50.2.1.5 Bone Morphogenetic Proteins

Bone morphogenetic proteins are members of the TGFß superfamily. These proteins are highly conserved with sequence homology across species. BMPs play a critical role in embryonic development and regulate a wide range of cellular activities including cell proliferation, differentiation, cell determination, and apoptosis. At the cellular level BMPs bind to their transmembrane receptors and initiate a cascade of phosphorylation events which transduces the signal to upregulate downstream genes. BMPs elicit their signals through phosphorylation of Smad molecules, which translocate to the nucleus when activated and regulate the transcription of specific target genes. Recently Hassel et al. [73] have demonstrated that a Smad independent pathway is activated if the BMP-2 signaling pathway is initiated via BMP-2 induced signaling receptor complexes instead of preformed receptor complexes (see Figure 50.3). Several studies on animals have demonstrated the osteoinductive (inducing bone formation) properties of BMPs in healing nonunions and enhancing spinal fusion. Recombinant human BMP-2 protein delivered to diaphyseal defects in dogs was able to achieve union (heal a fracture) [74]. A similar study in dogs also showed promising results using BMP-7 [75]. BMP-7 has been shown to enhance spinal fusion in rabbits [76] and sheep [77]. Recombinant human BMP-2 successfully healed critical-sized defects in sheep [78], rabbit [79], and rat [80].

Since their discovery by Dr. Marshall Urist, BMPs have been used in a number of human clinical trials as well. BMP-7 was effective in healing critical sized defects in the fibula [81] whereas BMP-2 promoted lumbar interbody fusion [82]. Transgenic BMP-2 produced by human mesenchymal stem cells was effective in bone regeneration [83]. Currently, only BMP-2 is available for clinical use. BMP-7 (rhOP-1) may be approved to treat long bone nonunions secondary to trauma. BMP-2 is approved for tibial nonunions and in a spinal fusion construct which consists of a spinal fusion cage and rhBMP-2 on a type I collagen scaffold [84].

50.2.1.6 Platelet Derived Growth Factors

Platelet derived growth factor (PDGF) is composed of two polypeptide chains that may exist as a homodimer (PDGF-AA, PDGF-BB) or heterodimer (PDGF-AB) [85]. Several reports have indicated that PDGF-AA and PDGF-BB can enhance wound repair [86], support angiogenesis [87–90], and stimulate cell proliferation in the fetal rat calvarial system and in cultures of osteoblast-like cells derived from adult human bone explants [91,92]. The PDGF A and B genes act as regulators of cell growth and have been shown to be chemotactic [88,89,91]. PDGF-BB has been reported to be the most potent PDGF isoform in skeletal and nonskeletal cells [93]. As a consequence of its role in cell growth, PDGF may exert its effect by increasing the number of collagen synthesizing cells, although it does not increase collagen synthesis on a cellular basis [93]. The role of PDGF in osteoblast differentiation may be to increase the number of cells that can progress into osteoblastic lineage and express the osteoblast phenotype [93]. PDGF expression at fracture sites in addition to its mitogenic effects indicates a role for PDGF in wound healing and fracture repair. Systemic administration of PDGF in an osteoporotic animal model demonstrated that it could stimulate bone formation and improve mechanical strength in long bones and vertebrae [94]. Howes and colleagues showed that subcutaneously implanted demineralized bone matrix augmented with PDGF could enhance bone healing in a rat model [95]. Locally administered recombinant human PDGF-BB (rhPDGF-BB) delivered with an injectable collagen gel to rabbit tibial osteotomies enhanced fracture repair and stimulated osteogenesis [96]. Currently, PDGF-BB is approved by FDA for soft tissue

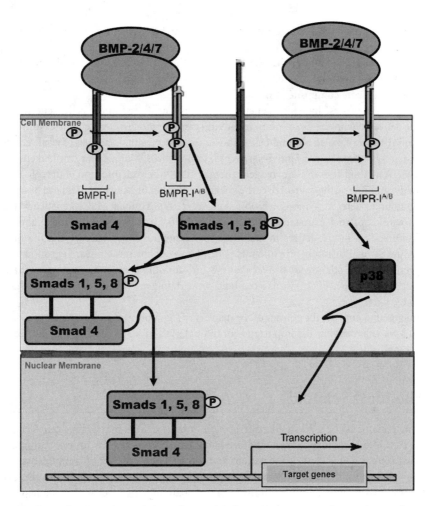

FIGURE 50.3 (See color insert.) Smad dependent and independent BMP signaling pathways. "Reprinted from Schmitt J.M., Hwang K., Winn S.R., and Hollinger J.O. 1999. *J. Orthop. Res.* 17: 269–278. With permission from the Orthopedic Research Society."

healing and remains as a compelling agent for tissue engineering applications especially in the treatment of osteoporotic fractures.

Despite the indispensable roles of these factors in osteoblast differentiation and bone formation, there are a number of concerns about their use in human patients. For instance, one concern with the injection of a growth factor like IGF-I is hypoglycemia, as reported in a study [97]. Another concern has been the use of superphysiological doses of these factors in order to trigger a response from the host. In the case of BMP-2, milligram doses (1.7 to 3.4 mg/dl) have to be used in patients due to diffusion from the wound site and instability *in vivo* [98,99]. Another reason for the rapid degradation of BMPs may be the presence of its natural inhibitors such as noggin and chordin at the fracture site [100,101]. Excessive bone formation remains a concern due to the risk of bony overgrowth leading to inadvertent fusion of adjacent levels or compression of the neural elements [102]. The potential side effects also need to be studied in longer time course experiments and trials for a fair assessment of the outcome.

50.2.2 Stem Cells and Gene Therapy

Mesenchymal stem cells (MSCs) are a population of self-renewing, undifferentiated cells. They can progress into a number of different cell fates, for example, adipocytic, osteogenic, chondrogenic, fibroblastic.

Stem cells can be harvested from fat, muscle, and bone marrow and can be genetically engineered to express bone signaling molecules [103–105]. Bruder et al. [106] implanted human bone marrow MSCs seeded on a ceramic carrier into the critical-sized defects of the femora of adult athymic rats and observed evidence for bone formation within 8 weeks. Parietal bone defects in adult sheep were repaired with MSCs added to a calcium alginate composite [107].

Gene therapy is the process by which genetic material is transferred into a cell's genome. A gene of interest can be delivered with the use of nonviral or viral carriers into targeted cell lines. Nonviral delivery methods include the use of naked plasmid DNA, liposomes, or gene gun. Examples of viral vectors include adenovirus, adeno-associated virus, lentivirus, herpes simplex virus, Moloney murine leukemia virus and retrovirus [108]. A method known as *ex vivo* gene therapy allows the viral infection of the cells to take place outside the body, thus increasing control over the system. A number of *ex vivo* studies have been performed to treat various bone defects in mouse, rabbit, and rat [109]. Human MSCs genetically engineered with an adenoviral construct expressing BMP-2 were able to form bone and cartilage and regenerate nonunion fractures in a mouse radius model [53]. An adenoviral construct carrying the BMP-2 gene was able to achieve spinal fusion in athymic rats [110]. However, the same research group also reported an immune response with adenoviral BMP-2 delivery into immunocompetent rats rather than athymic rats [111,112]. Furthermore, FDA has placed a hold on certain gene therapy applications due to safety concerns.

One method used to improve the efficacy of the delivery of signaling molecules is to use matrix scaffolds. In Section 50.3 we will overview the importance of biomaterials in tissue engineering and some current developments in this field.

50.3   The Ideal Scaffold

Autograft bone remains as the gold standard treatment of bone defects in the clinic due to its capability of providing cells, differentiative factors, and a reliable matrix required for fusion. Autograft bone is usually isolated from the iliac crest of the patient and can lead to a number of complications including chronic pain, infection, and fracture. One other option is to use allograft bone in the clinic; however, in this case immune response and disease transmission remain major concerns. The inadequacies of the current treatment methods have generated a need for alternative therapeutics for the treatment of bone defects.

Delivery of an osteoblast-specific gene or a signaling molecule remains a desirable option, but the therapeutic molecule requires an osteoconductive scaffold for its delivery. The ideal scaffold should encourage cell attachment, promote and support vascularization, and resist soft tissue forces [113]. The scaffold needs to be osteoinductive, osteoconductive, and biodegradable; this means that it needs to have the ability to induce bone formation at a nonbony site, the ability to provide a scaffold for new bone formation at the delivered site, and the ability to decompose without any toxic components to the cells and tissues, respectively.

Biomaterials for scaffold design can be classified under two major groups: acellular and cellular systems. Absorbable filter materials that can promote bone formation without a cellular component are called acellular systems. Cellular systems have cells embedded in the matrix to guide bone development [112].

Naturally derived matrices are derived from primary components of bone matrix and have natural affinity to growth factors as well as other osteoinductive factors; however they are difficult to sterilize and can trigger immune response from the host. Examples include hyaluronic acid, chitosan, and collagen matrices [69,113,114–117]. Inorganic materials include hydroxyapatite, porous coralline, calcium phosphate cements, and calcium sulfate. Their major advantage is the resemblance to bone structure, they can be resorbable or nonresorbable, but they are difficult to mold and are brittle [115,118–121]. Synthetic polymers are easy to manufacture and sterilize and they can be designed with controlled release parameters; however, they may degrade into toxic components and may be difficult to get recognized by the cells. Examples of synthetic polymers include poly (α-hydroxy acids), polypropylene fumarate, polyanhidrides, polyphosphazenes, polyethylene glycol, and poloxamers [115,122–128]. Ceramics such as tri-calcium phosphate and hydroxyapatite are biocompatible and display osteoconductivity [129–132]; however, resorption and porosity remain as concerns in these types of matrices. Oxidized cellulose and oxidized cellulose esters are also biocompatible polymers and have application in surgically implantable materials [133,134].

New biomaterial composites are being created to overcome the limitations of the different types of scaffolds mentioned above. Tsuchiya et al. [135] reported that they achieved osteogenesis with the design of a web-like structured biodegradable hybrid sheet composed of PLGA sheets containing collagen microsponges in their openings when seeded with bone marrow stem cells. These biodegradable hybrid sheets could be laminated or rolled into any shape. Photoencapsulation of hydrogels in different layers may help to mimic zonal organization of tissues which may be crucial in tissue engineering of the cartilage [136]. Recent fabrication techniques allow the synthesis of biomaterials that contain signal recognition ligands such as RGD domains to enable molecular and cellular responses.

Biocompatible and biodegradable polyurethane scaffolds have also been prepared for bone tissue engineering applications [137–144]. Polyurethanes are prepared by reacting diisocyanates with diols, whereas polyureas are the reaction product of diisocyanates with diamines (Figure 50.4). To be useful as resorbable scaffolds, conventional diisocyanates, such as methylene bis diphenylisocyanate (MDI) and toluene diisocyanate (TDI), which degrade to carcinogenic and mutagenic compounds [145], cannot be used. To avoid the toxicity problems associated with aromatic diisocyanates, aliphatic diisocyanates, such as lysine ethyl ester diisocyanate (LDI), and 1, 4-diisocyanatobutane (BDI), have been reacted with polyether and polyester polyols to synthesize resorbable polyurethanes [139,146–148].

Diisocyanates react with water to form a disubstituted urea and carbon dioxide gas, which acts as blowing agent [149]. The water reaction is exploited commercially to manufacture flexible and rigid polyurethane foams. Zhang et al. [139,140] have prepared porous scaffolds by adding water to an isocyanate-terminated prepolymer (i.e., the low molecular weight reaction product of a diisocyanate with a polyol). By varying the concentration of water added, the pore size distribution was controlled to support the growth and proliferation of rabbit bone marrow stromal cells. Porous scaffolds for the knee-joint meniscus have also been prepared by the solvent casting/salt leaching technique [150,151].

Bioactive molecules can be incorporated into polyurethanes through the reaction of diisocyanate with primary amine and hydroxyl groups. Following this approach, Zhang et al. [141] have recently synthesized a bioactive polyurethane scaffold from lysine ethyl ester diisocyanate (LDI), glycerol, polyethylene glycol (PEG), water, and ascorbic acid [142]. As the polyurethane degraded, ascorbic acid was released to the extracellular matrix and stimulated both cell proliferation and type I col and Alp synthesis *in vitro*. Other degradation products included lysine and PEG, which are biocompatible. Polyurethanes are potentially useful biomaterials for preparing bioactive porous scaffolds from both high (e.g., proteins) and low (e.g., signal recognition ligands) molecular weight bioactive molecules.

In the previous sections, we overviewed some of the required components for bone tissue regeneration: signaling molecules, cells, and scaffolds. In Section 50.4, we will summarize applications for reconstructive medicine in a clinical setting. We will review some of the current techniques applied to augment bone deficits.

50.4 Clinical Reconstruction of Bone Defects

Physical deformities caused by missing or defective tissues affect people of all ages. Most often they are due to cancer, trauma, or congenital abnormalities. Each year over 500,000 reconstructive procedures to correct these deformities are performed by plastic surgeons in the United States [152]. There are two fundamental types of deformities. One is when all tissue elements are present but not according to normal anatomy. An example is a fracture that heals with bone segments in improper orientations (i.e., fracture malunion). The second type is when the tissues are significantly impaired or absent altogether.

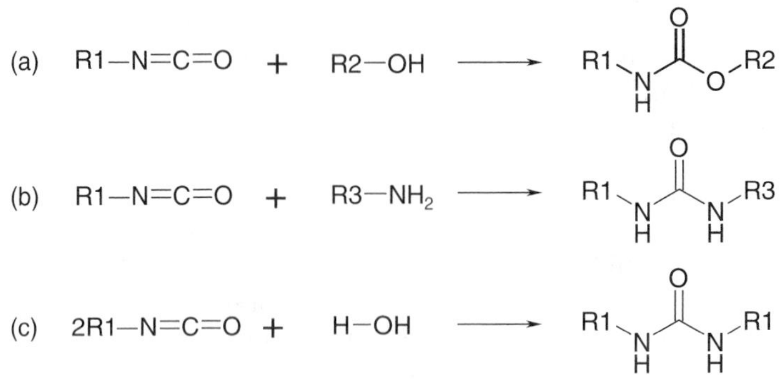

(a)   R1—N=C=O   +   R2—OH $\longrightarrow$ R1—N(H)—C(=O)—O—R2

(b)   R1—N=C=O   +   R3—NH$_2$ $\longrightarrow$ R1—N(H)—C(=O)—N(H)—R3

(c)   2R1—N=C=O   +   H—OH $\longrightarrow$ R1—N(H)—C(=O)—N(H)—R1

FIGURE 50.4   Reactions of isocyanates with (a) alcohols to form urethane groups, (b) amines to form urea groups, and (c) water to form disubstituted ureas.

An example is damage caused by cancer radiotherapy (i.e., osteoradionecrosis) or massive trauma (e.g., a shotgun blast). When a deformity contains all essential elements, repair is possible by rearranging or augmenting the local tissues. On the other hand, when useful tissues are absent then new tissue must be supplied. Ideally, tissue replacements should be readily available, easily implanted, reliably incorporated into the surrounding normal tissues. This is the goal of tissue engineering for reconstructive surgery.

It is important to understand current clinical techniques of reconstructive surgery in order to develop practical new methods. Repairing every deformity involves similar steps of planning, tissue manipulation, and patient care. During the planning phase, the clinician will assess the defect to determine the exact form and amount of the deficient tissue. Conventional radiographs and computed tomography (CT) scanning are the most useful diagnostic tools for the osseous component. Magnetic resonance imaging (MRI) best demonstrates the soft tissue component. It is important to always consider both elements. A bone defect due to trauma may have the same anatomic appearance as one caused by cancer, but the best reconstructive method may be different in each case because of the health and stability of the surrounding soft tissues. After characterizing the defect, the next step is to select a source of replacement tissue. The clinician must balance the tissue requirements with the potential morbidity related to harvest. After considering all of these issues, the clinician and patient discuss them and agree upon a plan for surgery.

Repairing deformities by tissue replacement is a two-step process that first involves tissue transfer followed by tissue modification [153]. In the transfer step, tissue is harvested from an uninjured location (i.e., tissue donor site) and moved into the defect (i.e., recipient site). It is important to understand the principles that govern this manipulation in natural tissues because they also apply to engineered tissues. Living tissue may be transferred either as a surgical graft or a surgical flap. Grafts derive a blood supply from the tissues that surround them in the new location. Except for cartilage and thin pieces of skin, only small amounts of tissue can be transferred as grafts because survival of the cellular elements by simple diffusion of oxygen and nutrients is limited to volumes of less than 0.3 cm^3 [154,155]. Success depends on the potential for angiogenesis and specialized tissue formation that exists in the tissues surrounding the graft in the new location. During the initial 48 h after transfer, the graft must survive by diffusion alone [156]. Afterward, blood vessels arising from the tissues surrounding graft begin to align with and make connections to remnants of blood vessels found in the graft [157]. It takes up to 5 days for revascularization to occur, depending on the grafted tissue and condition of the tissue bed into which it is placed. This far exceeds the time during which most whole tissues can survive without a blood supply. Skeletal muscle tissue, for example, undergoes degeneration within 4 h after being deprived of blood supply. As new vessels penetrate the graft there is cell-mediated destruction of the degenerating muscle fibers. The basal laminae and some of the satellite cells appear to be the only elements of the muscle tissue persists [158]. Bone grafts are unique, however. They essentially are porous, calcified, degradable scaffolds that guide tissue formation (i.e., osteoconduction) and deliver a set of bioactive molecules to induce new bone formation (i.e., osteoinduction). Only a limited number of cellular elements survive and contribute to healing because of diffusion limitations [159,160]. The surviving cells are mostly located on the surfaces of the calcified matrix and appear to consist mainly of endosteal lining cells and marrow stromal cells [161,162]. Even though most cellular components do not survive transfer, bone grafts still contribute to bone healing because they supply the other essential components of tissue repair. Bone grafts must be completely replaced over time in order to achieve healing. This can require up to 2 years. They have limited utility for defects greater than 6 cm in length and are avoided when there is significant local tissue impairment due to significant bacterial contamination, poor vascularity, unstable soft tissues, or radiation injury in the area of the defect [163]. Tissue engineered bone created without a capillary system *ex vivo* in a bioreactor can be expected to perform clinically in a way analogous to a bone graft.

In contrast to grafts, surgical flaps are tissues transferred with a blood supply independent of the tissues surrounding the defect. They are called flaps because originally they were actual flaps of skin elevated with an attachment at the base and rotated into an adjacent area. Over time the definition broadened to include any unit of skin, muscle, fat, bone, or viscera (e.g., small intestine) that has a discreet vascular source permitting surgical isolation from the donor site and transfer to a distant recipient site. The most advanced method of transfer is by detaching the flap completely and reestablishing the blood supply by suturing the blood vessels of the flap to vessels adjacent to the defect. This is called microvascular surgery because it involves operating on blood vessels less than 5 mm in diameter using an operating microscope. Bone transferred in this way allows survival of all tissue elements and yields the most reliable healing. Bone flaps incorporate more rapidly than grafts and do not require resorption and replacement before achieving full strength [161]. They are the treatment of choice in circumstances with large defects, significant soft tissue deficits, or impaired local tissues due to severe trauma, infection, or exposure to radiation [163–166]. The ultimate goal of bone tissue engineering for reconstructive surgery is to fabricate surgical bone flaps.

After transfer, the tissue must then be modified to simulate the missing parts. Bones have a complex three-dimensional shape and must tolerate powerful deforming forces. The relative importance of shape and load bearing differs based on the anatomic site. The long bones of the extremities function primarily as load bearing members. Minor shape discrepancies are tolerable as long as there is no significant loss of strength. On the other hand, craniofacial bones have a limited load bearing function. Their shape is critical to support and protect the complex and delicate soft tissue structures of the head and neck. They also determine human facial appearance and play a major role in psychosocial health [168,169]. Therefore, bone replacements in the craniofacial skeleton must maintain a durable shape. In addition, craniofacial bones have thin soft tissue coverage, and they are located in close proximity to heavily bacteria-contaminated surfaces of oral and nasal cavities. The oral cavity is one of the most heavily contaminated areas of the body with numerous bacterial species present including aerobes, anaerobes, fungi, viruses, and protozoa [170]. The paranasal sinuses are normally not sterile, although the bacterial load appears much less [171]. It is impossible to perform tissue implantation surgery in this area without a high probability of bacterial contamination. Therefore, the tissue replacement must be compatible with the thin soft tissues to avoid erosion and have an intrinsic resistance to infection. These features of the craniofacial skeleton make fabricating replacements by tissue engineering particularly challenging.

After the surgery is complete, the patient requires special care to recover. The reconstructed areas must be protected from disruption and infection. Grafted tissues must be stably fixed to prevent shearing motion at the interface with the tissue bed, which slows the process of revascularization. Flaps must be closely monitored to rapidly detect thrombosis and occlusion of the blood vessels that supply the tissues. After complete healing and tissue incorporation, the final step is often a period of rehabilitation to ensure maximum restoration of function. Finally, additional surgery may be required to make revisions and improve minor deficiencies that are not able to be avoided during the primary reconstruction or which may have appeared later due to scar contracture, for example. The entire process can require many months to completely restore the patient (Figure 50.5a,b and Figure 50.6a–d).

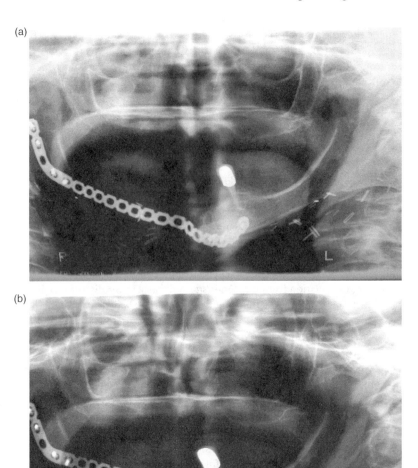

FIGURE 50.5 Panoramic radiographs of a patient after right mandible reconstruction with only a titanium reconstruction plate showing appearance after surgery (a) and appearance several months later after fracture of the plate due to metal fatigue (b).

50.5 Conclusion

Tissue engineering may offer a new dimension of therapeutic care for patients. The design and development of the tissue engineered therapeutics must be guided by basic, fundamental biological pathways targeting specific clinical applications. Targeted clinical performance standards for the tissue engineered therapeutic must be achieved in the design, validated by the appropriate standardized characterization protocols (e.g., ASTM, ISO 10993), preclinical and clinical phase I–III studies. To fulfill stringent clinical requirements for a tissue engineered bone therapeutic, specific clinical targets must be identified. Is the target a nonload bearing or load bearing bone? Is the target a fracture in the tibia of a healthy, young male? Or is the clinical target a distal radius fracture in a postmenopausal osteoporotic?

In this chapter, we have briefly reviewed the pathways of bone formation and some of the key signaling molecules cuing discrete outcome events. Tissue engineered products must integrate into their design fundamental biological elements consistent with bone formation pathways. Many of the key temporal

(a)

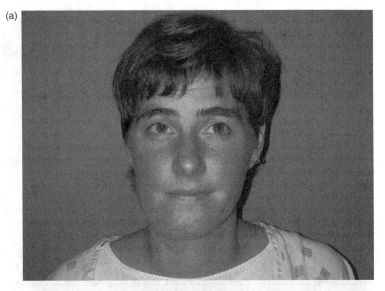

(b)

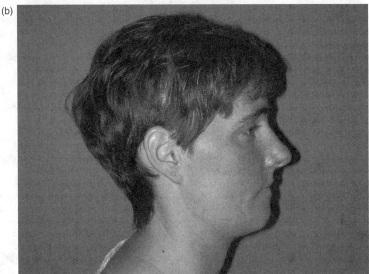

FIGURE 50.6 Appearance of a young woman treated with surgery for a tumor involving the right mandible. The entire mandible on the right was removed and replaced using a bone flap harvested from the fibula. Appearance before surgery (a),(b) and 1 year after surgery (c),(d). Although surgery resulted in a durable reconstruction, note the changes in appearance due to the difference in the shape of the fibula and native mandible.

and spatial aspects of bone formation (developmental, homeostatic, healing) remain a mystery. Unless these key aspects are elucidated, rational, effective tissue engineered therapeutics will not develop.

A broad understanding by tissue engineers of the complex anatomical and physiological issues challenging surgeons and patients will provide tissue engineers with an important foundational head start for robust design options that may include uniquely engineered compositions of cells, genes, and biomimetic extracellular matrices (e.g., bioactive matrices). The biomimetic extracellular matrix was especially emphasized in this chapter to stress the importance of spatially and temporally directing the process of tissue regeneration. Matrix design is the pivotal tissue engineering challenge.

We provided some clinical examples where bone tissue engineering will benefit craniofacial reconstruction. The craniofacial surgeon faces different clinical challenges than the orthopedic surgeon. Tissue

(c)

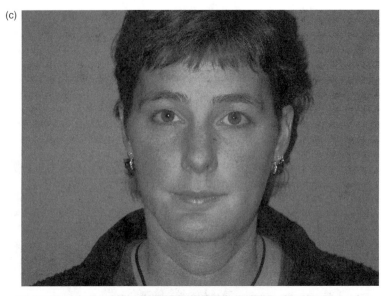

(d)

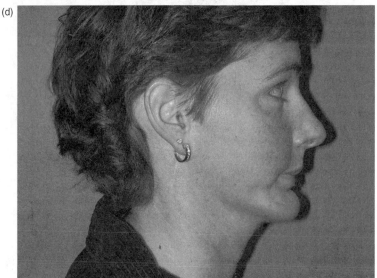

FIGURE 50.6   Continued.

engineering must emphasize a regional-anatomic and physiological approach to design and development. A single platform treatment for a tibial diaphyseal fracture in the healthy adult male may be inadequate for the patient with an avulsive bone wound of the oral–antral complex.

There are significant opportunities for the tissue engineer to improve the quality of patient care. The bedrock underscoring tissue engineering is basic biology, clinical performance standards, and patient application focus.

References

[1] Boskey A.L. 2003. Biomineralization: an overview. *Connect Tissue Res.* 44: 5.

[2] Barckhaus R.H. and Hohling H.J. 1978. Electron microprobe analysis of freeze dried and unstained mineralized epiphyseal cartilage. *Cell Tissue Res.* 18693: 541–549.

[3] Marks S.C. and Odgreen P.R. 2002. Structure and development of the skeleton. In J.P. Bilezikian, L.G. Raisz, and G.A. Rodan (Eds.), *Principles of Bone Biology*, Vol. 1, pp. 3–14, New York, Academic Press.

[4] Gay C.V., Donahue H.J., Siedlecki C.A., and Vogler E. 2004. Cellular elements of the skeleton: osteoblasts, osteocytes, osteoclasts, bone marrow stromal cells. In J.O. Hollinger, T.A. Einhorn, and B.A. Doll (Eds.), *Bone Tissue Engineering*, Chapter 3, Boca Raton, FL, CRC Press.

[5] Olsson S.E. and Ekman S. 2002. Morphology and physiology of the growth cartilage under normal and pathologic conditions. In G.E. Fackelman (Ed.), *Bone in Clinical Orthopedics*, p. 117, Stuttgart, Germany, AO Publishing.

[6] Scott, C.K. and Hightower J.A. 1991. The matrix of endochondral bone differs from the matrix of intramembranous bone. *Calcif. Tissue Int.* 49: 349–354.

[7] Sandberg M.M. 1991. Matrix in cartilage and bone development: current views on the function and regulation of the major organic components. *Ann. Med.* 23: 207–217.

[8] Tuan R.S. 1994. Developmental skeletogenesis. In C.T. Brighton, G. Friedlaender, and J.M. Lane (Eds.), *Bone Formation and Repair*, pp. 13, Rosemont, IL, AAOS.

[9] Doll, B.A. 2004. Developmental biology of the skeletal system. In J.O. Hollinger, T.A. Einhorn, and B.A. Doll (Eds.), *Bone Tissue Engineering*, Chapter 1, Boca Raton, FL, CRC Press.

[10] Wolff J. 1892. *The Law of Bone Remodelling*. Translated by Maquet P. and Furlong R. 1986. New York, NY, Springer-Verlag.

[11] Mikuni-Takagaki Y. 1999. Mechanical responses and signal transduction pathways in stretched osteocytes. *J. Bone Miner. Metab.* 17: 57–60.

[12] Dehority W., Halloran B.P., Bikle D.D., Curren T., Kostenuik P.J., Wronski T.J., Shen Y., Rabkin B., Bouraoui A., and Morey-Holton E. 1999. Bone and hormonal changes induced by skeletal unloading in the mature male rat. *Am. J. Physiol.* 276: E62–E69.

[13] Montufar-Solis D., Duke P.J., and Morey-Holton E. 2001. The Spacelab 3 stimulation: basis for a model of growth plate response in microgravity in the rat. *J. Gravit. Physiol.* 8: 67–76.

[14] Cullinane D.M. and Salisbury K.T. 2004. Biomechanics. In J.O. Hollinger, T.A. Einhorn, and B.A. Doll (Eds.), *Bone Tissue Engineering*, Chapter 10, Boca Raton, FL, CRC Press.

[15] Ferretti J.L., Capozza R.F., and Zanchetta J.R. 1996. Mechanical validation of a tomographic QCT index for noninvasive estimation of rat femur bending strength. *Bone* 18: 97–102.

[16] Beck T.J., Mourtada F.A., Ruff C.B., Scott W.W., and Kao G. 1998. Experimental testing of a DEXA-derived curved beam model of the proximal femur. *J. Orthop. Res.* 16: 394–398.

[17] Toyras J., Nieminen M.T., Kroger H., and Jurvelin J.S. 2002. Bone mineral density, ultrasound velocity, and broadband attention predict mechanical properties of trabecular bone differently. *Bone* 31: 503–507.

[18] Stigbrand T. 1984. *Present Status and Future Trends of Human Alkaline Phosphatases*, pp. 3–14, New York, NY, Alan R. Liss.

[19] Cole D.E. and Cohen M.M. 1990. Mutations affecting bone forming cells. In B.K. Hall (Ed.), *Bone: The Osteoblast and the Osteocyte*, pp. 442–452, New Jersey, The Telford Press.

[20] Risteli L. and Risteli J. 1993. Biochemical markers of bone metabolism. *Ann. Med.* 25: 385–393.

[21] Butler W.T. 1989. The nature and significance of osteopontin. *Connect Tissue Res.* 23: 123–136.

[22] Hoang Q.Q., Sicheri F., Howard A.J., and YANG D.S.C. 2003. Bone recognition mechanism of porcine osteocalcin from crystal structure. *Nature* 425: 977–980.

[23] Hunter G.K. and Goldberg H.A. 1993. Nucleation of hydroxyapatite by bone sialoprotein. *Proc. Natl Acad. Sci. USA* 90: 8562–8565.

[24] Barnes G.L., Kostenuik P.J., Gerstenfeld L.C., and Einhorn T.A. 1999. Growth factor regulation of fracture repair. *J. Bone Miner. Res.* 14: 1805–1815.

[25] Learnmoth I.D. 2004. The management of periprosthetic fractures around the femoral stem. *J. Bone Joint Surg. Br.* 86: 13–19.

[26] Sfeir C., Jadlowiec J.J., Koch H., and Campbell P.G. 2004. Signaling molecules for tissue engineering. In J.O. Hollinger, T.A. Einhorn, and B.A. Doll (Eds.), *Bone Tissue Engineering*, Chapter 5, Boca Raton, FL, CRC Press.

[27] Mohan S. and Baylink D.J. 2002. IGF-binding proteins are multifunctional and act via IGF-dependent and -independent mechanisms. *J. Endocrinol.* 175: 19–31.

[28] Nunes I., Gleizes P.E., Metz C.N., and Rifkin D.B. 1997. Latent transforming growth factor-beta binding protein domains involved in activation and transglutaminase-dependent cross-linking of latent transforming growth factor-beta. *J. Cell Biol.* 136: 1151–1163.

[29] Balemans W. and Hul W.V. 2002. Extracellular regulation of BMP signaling in vertebrates: a cocktail of modulators. *Dev. Biol.* 250: 231–250.

[30] Baxter, R.C. 2000. Insulin-like growth factor (IGF)-binding proteins: interactions with IGFs and intrinsic bioactivities. *Am. J. Physiol. Endocrinol. Metab.* 278: E967–E976.

[31] Saltzman W.M. and Olbreicht W.L. 2002. Building drug delivery into tissue engineering. *Nat. Rev.: Drug Dis.* 1: 177–186.

[32] Richardson T.P., Peters M.C., Ennett A.B., and Mooney D.J. 2001. Polymeric system for dual growth factor delivery. *Nat. Biotechnol.* 19: 1029–1034.

[33] Nixon A.J., Brower-Toland B.D., Bent S.J., Saxer R.A., Wilke M.J., Robbins P.D., and Evans C.H. 2000. Insulin-like growth factor-I gene therapy applications for cartilage repair. *Clin. Orthop.* 379: S201–1113.

[34] Zhang M., Xuan S., Bouxsein M.L., von Stechow D., Akeno N., and Fougere M.C. et al. 2002. Osteoblast-specific knockout of the IGF receptor gene reveals an essential role of IGF signaling in bone matrix mineralization. *J. Biol. Chem.* 277: 44005–44012.

[35] McCarthy T.L., Centrella M., and Canalis E. 1989. Regulatory effects of insulin-like growth factors I and II on bone collagen synthesis in rat calvarial cultures. *Endocrinology* 124: 301–309.

[36] Ogata N., Chikazu D., Kubota N., Terauchi Y., and Tobe K. et al. 2000. Insulin receptor substrate-1 in osteoblast is indispensable for maintaining bone turnover. *J. Clin. Invest.* 105: 935–943.

[37] Zhang M., Faugere M.C., Malluche H., Rosen C.J., Chernausek S.D., and Clemens T.L. 2003. Paracrine overexpression of IGFBP-4 in osteoblasts of transgenic mice decreases bone turnover and causes global growth retardation. *J. Bone Miner. Res.* 18: 836–843.

[38] Raile K., Hoflich A., Hessler U., Yang Y., Pfuender M., Blum W.F., Kolb H., Schwartz H.B., and Kiess W. 1994. Human osteosarcoma (U-2 OS) cells express both insulin-like growth factor-I (IFG-I) receptors and insulin-like growth factor-II/mannose-6-phosphate (IGF-II/M6P) receptors and synthesize IGF-II: autocrine growth stimulation by IGF-II via the IGF-I receptor. *J. Cell Physiol.* 159: 531–541.

[39] Rosenfeld R.G. and Roberts C.T. 1999. *The IGF System: Molecular Biology, Physiology and Clinical Applications*, p. 19, NJ, Homana Press.

[40] Chan S.J., Magamatsu S., Cao Q.-P., and Steiner D.F. 1992. Structure and evolution of insulin and insulin-like growth factors in chordates. *Prog. Brain Res.* 1992: 15–24.

[41] Mohan S. and Baylink D.J. 1996. The I.G.Fs as Potential therapy for metabolic bone diseases. In J.P. Bilezikian, L.G. Raisz, and G.A. Rodan (Eds.), *Principles of Bone Biology*, pp. 1100–1107, New York, Academic Press.

[42] Gray A., Tam A., Dull W., Hayflick T.J., Pintar J., Cavenee W.K., Koufos A., and Ulrich A. 1987. Tissue-specific and developmentally-regulated transcription of the IGF 2 gene. *DNA* 6: 283–295.

[43] Trippel, S.B. 1994. Biologic regulation of bone growth. In C.T. Brighton, G. Friedlaender, and J.M. Lane (Eds.), *Bone Formation and Repair*, p. 43, Rosemont, IL, AAOS.

[44] Underwood L.E. and Van Wyk J.J. 1992. Normal and aberrant growth. In J.D. Wilson and D.W. Foster (Eds.), *Williams Textbook of Endocrinology*, pp. 1079–1138, Philadelphia, PA, WB Saunders.

[45] Schoenle E., Zapf J., Hauri C. et al. 1985. Comparison of *in vivo* effects of insulin-like growth factors I and II and of growth hormone in hypophysectomized rats. *Acta Endocrinol.* 108: 167–174.

[46] DeChiara T.M., Efstratiadis A., and Robertson E.J. 1990. A growth factor deficiency phenotype in heterozygous mice carrying an insulin-like growth factor II gene disrupted by targeting. *Nature.* 345: 78–80.

[47] Thaler S.R., Dart A., and Tesluk H. 1993. The effect of insulin-like growth factor-I on critical sized calvarial defects in Sprague-Dawley rats. *Ann. Plast. Surg.* 31: 429–433.

[48] Tanaka H., Quarto R., Williams S., Barnes J., and Liang C.T. 1994. *In vivo* and *in vitro* effects of insulin-like growth factor-I (IGF-I) on femoral mRNA expression in old rats. *Bone* 15: 647–653.

[49] Jadlowiec J.J., Celil A.B., and Hollinger J.O. 2003. Bone tissue engineering: recent advances and promising therapeutic agents. *Exp. Opin. Biol. Ther.* 3: 409–423.

[50] Kurtz C.A., Loebig T.G., Anderson D.D., Demeo P.J., and Campbell P.G. 1999. Insulin-like growth factor I accelerates functional recovery from Achilles tendon injury in a rat model. *Am. J. Sports Med.* 27: 363–369.

[51] Kandziora F., Schmidmaier G., Schollmeier G. et al. 2002. IGF-I and TGF-beta application by a poly-(D,L-lactide)-coated cage promotes intervertebral bone matrix formation in the sheep cervical spine. *Spine* 27: 1710–1723.

[52] Illi O.E. and Feldmann C.P. 1998. Stimulation of fracture healing by local application of humoral factors integrated in biodegradable implants. *Eur. J. Pediatr. Surg.* 8: 251–255.

[53] Trippel S.B., Whelan M.C., Klagsbrun M. et al. 1992. Interaction of basic fibroblast growth factor with bovine growth plate chondrocytes. *J. Orthop. Res.* 10: 638–646.

[54] Canalis E., McCarthy T.L., and Centrella M. 1989. Effects of platelet-derived growth factor on bone formation *in vitro. J. Cell Physiol.* 140: 530–537.

[55] Jingushi S., Heydemann A., Kana S.R., Macey L.R., and Bolander M.E. 1990. Acidic fibroblast growth factor (aFGF) injection stimulates cartilage enlargement and inhibits cartilage gene expression in rat fracture healing. *J. Orthop. Res.* 8: 364–371.

[56] Dunstan C.R., Boyce R., Boyce B.F. et al. 1999. Systemic administration of acidic fibroblast growth factor (FGF-1) prevents bone loss and increases new bone formation in ovariectomized rats. *J. Bone Miner. Res.* 14: 953–959.

[57] Pandit A.S., Feldman D.S., Caulfield J. et al. 1998. Stimulation of angiogenesis by FGF-1 delivered through a modified fibrin scaffold. *Growth factors* 15: 113–123.

[58] Kimoto T., Hosokawa R., Kubo T., Maeda M., Sano A., and Akagawa Y. 1998. Continuous administration of basic fibroblast growth factor (FGF-2) accelerates bone induction on rat calvaria — an application of a new drug delivery system. *J. Dent. Res.* 77: 1965–1969.

[59] Inui K., Maeda M., Sano A. et al. 1998. Local application of basic fibroblast growth factor minipellet induces the healing of segmental bony defects in rabbits. *Calcif. Tissue Int.* 63: 490–495.

[60] Hosokawa R., Kikuzaki K., Kimoto T. et al. 2000. Controlled local application of basic fibroblast growth factor (FGF-2) accelerates the healing of GBR. An experimental study in beagle dogs. *Clin. Oral Implants Res.* 11: 345–353.

[61] Goodman S.B., Song Y., Yoo J.Y., Fox N., Trindale M.C., Kajiyama G., Ma T., Regula D., Brown J., and Smith R.l. 2003. Local infusion of FGF-2 enhances bone ingrowth in rabbit chambers in the presence of polyethylene particles. *J. Biomed. Res.* A: 454–461.

[62] Bates D.O., Lodwick D., and Williams B. 1999. Vascular endothelial growth factor and microvascular permeability. *Microcirculation* 6: 83–96.

[63] Stone D., Phaneuf M., Sivamurthy N. et al. 2002. A biologically active VEGF construct *in vitro*: implications for bioengineering-improved prosthetic vascular grafts. *J. Biomed. Mater. Res.* 59: 160–165.

[64] Bauters C., Asahara T., Zheng L.P. et al. 1995. Recovery of disturbed endothelium-dependent flow in the collateral-perfused rabbit ischemic hindlimb after administration of vascular endothelial growth factor. *Circulation* 91: 2802–2809.

[65] Takeshita S., Pu L.Q., Stein L.A. et al. 1994. Intramuscular administration of vascular endothelial growth factor induces dose-dependent collateral artery augmentation in a rabbit model of chronic limb ischemia. *Circulation* 90: II228–II234.

[66] Takeshita S., Tsurumi Y., Couffinahl T. et al. 1996. Gene transfer of naked DNA encoding for three isoforms of vascular endothelial growth factor stimulates collateral development *in vitro*. *Lab. Invest.* 75: 487–501.

[67] Pepper M.S., Ferrara N., Orci L. et al. 1992. Potent synergism between vascular endothelial growth factor and basic fibroblast growth factor in the induction of angiogenesis *in vitro*. *Biochem. Biophys. Res. Commun.* 189: 824–831.

[68] Murphy W.L., Simmons C.A., Kaigler D., and Mooney D.J. 2004. Bone regeneration via a mineral substrate and induced angiogenesis. *J. Dent. Res.* 83: 204–210.

[69] Massague J. and Wotton D. 2000. Transcriptional control by the TGF-beta/Smad signaling system. *EMBO J.* 19: 1745–1754.

[70] Bourque W.T., Gross M., and Hall B.K. 1993. Expression of four growth factors during fracture repair. *Int. J. Dev. Biol.* 37: 573–579.

[71] Robey P.G., Young M.F., Flanders K.C. et al. 1987. Osteoblasts synthesize and respond to transforming growth factor type beta (TGF-beta) *in vitro*. *J. Cell Biol.* 105: 457–463.

[72] Abe N., Lee Y.P., Sato M. et al. 2002. Enhancement of bone repair with a helper-dependent adenoviral transfer of bone morphogenetic protein-2. *Biochem. Biophys. Res. Commun.* 297: 523–527.

[73] Hassel S., Schmitt S., Hartung A. et al. 2003. Initiation of Smad-dependent and Smad independent signaling via distinct BMP-receptor complexes. *J. Bone Joint Surg. Am.* 85: 44–51.

[74] Sciadini M.F. and Johnson K.D. 2000. Evaluation of recombinant human bone morphogenetic protein-2 as a bone graft substitute in a canine segmental defect model. *J. Orthop. Res.* 18: 289–302.

[75] Salkeld S.L., Parton L.P., Barrack R.L., and Cook S.D. The effect of osteogenic protein-1 on the healing of segmental bone defects treated with autograft or allograft bone. *JBJS Am.* 2001: 83–1: 803–816.

[76] Grauer J.N., Patel T.C., Erulkar J.S., Troiano N.W., Panjabi M.M., and Friedlaender G.E. 2001. Young Investigator research award winner: evaluation of OP-1 as a graft substitute for intertransverse process lumbar fusion. *Spine* 26: 127–133.

[77] Magin M.N. and Delling G. 2001. Improved lumbar vertebral interbody fusion using rhOP-1: a comparison of autogenous bone graft, bovine hydroxyapatite and BMP-7 in sheep. *Spine* 26: 469–478.

[78] Gerhart T.N., Kirker-Head C.A., Kriz M.J. et al. 1993. Healing segmental defects in sheep using recombinant human bone morphogenetic protein. *Clin. Orthop.* 293: 317–326.

[79] Bostrom M., Lane J.M., Tomin E. et al. 1996. Use of bone morphogenetic protein-2 in the rabbit ulnar nonunion model. *Clin. Orthop.* 327: 272–282.

[80] Yasko A.W., Lane J.M., Fellinger E.J., Rosen V., Wozney J.M., and Wang E.A. 1992. The healing of segmental defects, induced by human bone morphogenetic protein (rhBMP-2). A radiographic, histological, and biomechanical study in rats. *J. Bone Joint Surg. Am.* 74: 659–670.

[81] Geesink R.G., Hoefnagels N.H., and Bulstra S.K. 1999. Osteogenic activity of OP-1 bone morphogenetic protein (BMP-7) in a human fibular defect. *J. Bone Joint Surg. Br.* 81: 710–718.

[82] Boden S.D., Zdeblick T.A., Sandhu H.S., and Heim S.E. 2000. The use of rhBMP-2 in interbody fusion cages: definitive evidence of osteoinduction in human — a preliminary report. *Spine* 25: 376–381.

[83] Turgeman G., Pittman D.D., Muller R. et al. 2001. Engineered human mesenchymal stem cells: a novel platform for skeletal cell mediated gene therapy. *J. Gene Med.* 3: 240–251.

[84] Issack P.S. and DiCesare P.E. 2003. Recent advances toward the clinical application of bone morphogenetic proteins in bone and cartilage repair. *Am. J. Orthop.* 32: 429–436.

[85] Westermark B. and Heldin C.H. 1993. Platelet-derived growth factor. *Acta Oncol.* 32: 101–105.

[86] Pierce G.F. and Musote T.A. 1995. Pharmacologic enhancement of wound healing. *Annu. Rev. Med.* 46: 467–481.

[87] Centrella M., McCarthy T., Kusik W., and Canalis E. 1992. Isoform specific regulation of platelet derived growth factor activity and binding in osteoblast-enriched cultures from fetal rat bone. *J. Clin. Invest.* 89: 1076–1084.

[88] Rodan S.B. and Rodan G.A. 1992. Fibroblast growth factor and platelet derived growth factor. In Gowan M. (Ed.), *Cytokines and Bone Metabolism*, pp. 116–140, Boca Raton, FL, CRC Press.

[89] Andrew J.J., Hoyland J., Freemont A., and Marsh D. 1995. Platelet derived growth factor expression in normally healing human fractures. *Bone* 16: 455–460.

[90] Gruber R., Varga F., Fishcer M., and Watzek G. 2002. Platelets stimulate proliferation of bone cells: involvement of platelet derived growth factors, microparticles and membranes. *Clin. Oral Implant. Res.* 3: 529–535.

[91] Lynch, S.E., Colvin R.B., and Antoinades H.N. 1989. Growth factors in wound healing: single and synergistic effects on partial thickness porcine skin wounds. *J. Clin. Invest.* 84: 640–646.

[92] Pierce G.F., Mustoe T.A., Altrock B.W., Deuel T.F., and Thomason A. 1991. Role of platelet derived growth factor in wound healing. *J. Cell Biochem.* 10: 131–138.

[93] Canalis E. and Rydziel S. 1996. Platelet-derived growth factor and the skeleton. In J.P. Bilezikian, L.G. Raisz, and G.A. Rodan (Eds.), *Principles of Bone Biology*, p. 621, New York, Academic Press.

[94] Mitlak B., Finkelman R., Hill E., Li J., Martin B., Smith T., D'Andrea M., Antoniades H., and Lynch S. 1996. The effect of systemically administered PDGF-BB on the rodent skeleton. *J. Bone Miner. Res.* 11: 238–247.

[95] Howes R., Bowness J., Grotendorst G., Martin G., and Reddi A. 1988. Platelet derived growth factor enhances demineralized bone matrix-induced cartilage and bone formation. *Calcif. Tissue Int.* 42: 34–38.

[96] Nash T., Howlett C., Martin C., Steele J., Johnson K., and Hicklin D. 1994. Effect of platelet derived growth factor on tibial osteotomies in rabbit. *Bone* 15: 203–208.

[97] Guler H.P., Zapf J., and Froesch E.R. 1987. Short-term metabolic effects of recombinant human insulin-like growth factor I in healthy adults. *N. Engl. J. Med.* 317: 137–140.

[98] Boden S.D., Zdeblick T.A., Sandhu H.S., and Heim S.E. 2002. Use of recombinant human bone morphogenetic protein-2 to achieve postrolateral lumbar spine fusion in humans: a prospective, randomized clinical pilot trial. *Spine* 27: 2661–2673.

[99] Boyne P.J., Marx R.E., Nevins M. et al. 1997. A feasibility study evaluating rhBMP-2/absorbable collagen sponge for maxillary sinus floor augmentation. *Int. J. Periodont. Restorat. Dent.* 17: 11–25.

[100] Abe E., Yamamoto M., Taguchi Y. et al. 2000. Essential requirement of BMPs-2/4 for both osteoblast and osteoclast formation in murine bone marrow cultures from adult mice: antagonism by noggin. *J. Bone Miner. Res.* 15: 663–673.

[101] Aspenberg P., Jeppson C., and Economides A.N. 2001. The bone morphogenetic proteins antagonist Noggin inhibits membranous ossification. *J. Bone Miner. Res.* 3: 15.

[102] Poynton A.R. and Lane J.M. 2002. Safety profile for the clinical use of bone morphogenetic proteins in the spine. *Spine* 27: S40–S48.

[103] Morizono K., De Ugarte D.A., Zhu M. et al. 2003. Multilineage cells from adipose tissue as gene delivery vehicles. *Hum. Gene Ther.* 14: 59–66.

[104] Jankowski R.J., Deasy B.M., and Huard J. 2002. Muscle-derived stem cells. *Gene Ther.* 9: 642–647.

[105] Lee J.Y., Peng H., Usas A. et al. 2002. Enhancement of bone healing based on *ex vivo* gene therapy using human muscle-derived cells expressing bone morphogenetic protein-2. *Hum. Gene Ther.* 13: 1201–1211.

[106] Bruder S.P., Kurth A.A., Shea M., Hayes W.C., Jaiswal N., and Kadiyala S. 1998. Bone regeneration by implantation of purified, culture-expanded human mesenchymal stem cells. *J. Orthop. Res.* 16: 155–162.

[107] Shang Q., Wang Z., Liu W., Shi Y., Cui L., and Cao Y. 2001. Tissue engineered bone repair of sheep cranial defects with autologous bone marrow stromal cells. *J. Craniofac. Surg.* 12: 586–593.

[108] Hannallah D., Peterson B., Lieberman J.R., Fu F.H., and Huard J. 2003. Gene therapy in orthopedic surgery. *Inst. Course Lect.* 52: 753–768.

[109] Gamradt S.C. and Lieberman J.R. 2004. Genetic modification of stem cells to enhance bone repair. *Ann. Biomed. Eng.* 32: 136–147.

[110] Alden T.D., Pittman D.D., Beres E.J. et al. 1999. Percutaneous spinal fusion using bone morphogenetic protein-2 gene therapy. *J. Neurosurg.* 90: 109–114.

[111] Alden T.D., Pittman D.D., Hankins G.R., Beres E.J. et al. 1999. *In vivo* endochondral bone formation using a bone morphogenetic protein-2 adenoviral vector. *Hum. Gene Ther.* 10: 2245–2253.

[112] Kakar S. and Einhorn T.A. 2004. Tissue engineering of bone. In J.O. Hollinger, T.A. Einhorn, and B.A. Doll (Eds.), *Bone Tissue Engineering*, Chapter 11, Boca Raton, FL, CRC Press.

[113] Hutmacher D.W. 2000. Scaffolds in tissue engineering bone and cartilage. *Biomaterials* 21: 2529–2543.

[114] Gerhart T.N., Kirker-Head C.A., Kriz M.J. et al. 1993. Healing segmental femoral defects in sheep using recombinant human bone morphogenetic protein. *Clin. Orthop.* 293: 317–326.

[115] Li R.H. and Wozney J.M. 2001. Delivering on the promise of bone morphogenetic proteins. *Trends Biotechnol.* 19: 255–265.

[116] Radomsky M.L., Aufdemorte T.B., Swain L.D. et al. 1999. Novel formulation of fibroblast growth factor-2 in a hyaluronan gel accelerates fracture healing in nonhuman primates. *J. Orthop. Res.* 17: 607–614.

[117] Sellers R.S., Zhang R., Glasson S.S. et al. 2000. Repair of articular cartilage defects one year after treatment with recombinant human bone morphogenetic protein-2 (rhBMP-2). *J. Bone Joint Surg. Am.* 82: 151–160.

[118] Boden S.D. 1999. Bioactive factors for bone tissue engineering. *Clin. Orthop.* 367: S84–S94.

[119] Wang S. 2000. Study on the mechanism of bone formation of bioactive materials BMP/Beta-TCP restoring bone defects by using quantitative analysis methods. Society for Biomaterials, *6th World Biomaterials Conference*, Hawaii, USA.

[120] Jin Q.M., Takita H., Kohgo T. et al. 2000. Effects of geometry of hydroxyapatite as a cell substratum in BMP-induced ectopic bone formation. *J. Biomed. Mater. Res.* 51: 491–499.

[121] Ijiri S., Nakamura T., Fujisawa Y. et al. 1997. Ectopic bone induction in porous apatite-woolastonite-containing glass ceramic combined with bone morphogenetic protein. *J. Biomed. Mater. Res.* 35: 421–432.

[122] Winn S.R., Uludag H., and Hollinger J.O. 1999. Carrier systems for bone morphogenetic proteins. *Clin. Orthop.* 3679: S95–S106.

[123] Whang K., Goldstick T.K., and Healy K.E. 2000. A biodegradable polymer scaffold for delivery of osteotropic factors. *Biomaterials* 21: 2545–2551.

[124] Lee S.C., Shea M., Battle M.A. et al. 1994. Healing of large segmental defects in rat femurs is aided by rhBMP-2 in PLGA matrix. *J. Biomed. Mater. Res.* 28: 1149–1156.

[125] Hollinger J.O. and Leong K. 1996. Poly(alpha-hydroxy acids): carriers for bone morphogenetic proteins. *Biomaterials* 17: 187–194.

[126] Lucas P.A., Laurencin C., Syftestad G.T. et al. 1990. Ectopic induction of cartilage and bone by water soluble proteins from bovine bone using a polyanhydride delivery vehicle. *J. Biomed. Mater. Res.* 24: 901–911.

[127] Clokie C.M. and Urist M.R. 2000. Bone morphogenetic protein excipients: comparative observations on poloxamer. *Plast. Reconstr. Surg.* 105: 628–637.

[128] Saito N., Okada T., Toba S. et al. 1999. New synthetic absorbable polymers as BMP carriers: plastic properties of poly-D,L-lactic acid-polyethylene glycol block copolymers. *J. Biomed. Mater. Res.* 47: 104–110.

[129] Kenley R., Marden L., Turek T. et al. 1994. Osseous regeneration in the rat calvarium using novel delivery systems for recombinant human bone morphogenetic protein-2 (rhBMP-2). *J. Biomed. Mater. Res.* 28: 1139–1147.

[130] Gao T., Lindholm T.S., Marttinen A. et al. 1996. Composite of bone morphogenetic protein (BMP) and Type I. V. collagen, coral-derived coral hydroxyapatite, and tricalcium phosphate ceramics. *Int. Orthop.* 20: 321–325.

[131] Higuchi T., Kinoshita A., Takahashi K. et al. 1999. Bone regeneration by recombinant human bone morphogenetic protein-2 in rat mandibular defects. An experimental model of defect filling. *J. Periodontol.* 70: 1026–1031.

[132] Ripamonti U. 1996. Osteoinduction in porous hydroxyapatite implanted in heterotropic sites of different animal models. *Biomaterials* 17: 31.

[133] Galgut P.N. 1994. A technique for treatment of extensive periodontal defects: a case study. *J. Oral Rehabil.* 21: 27–32

[134] Askar I., Gultan S.M., Erden E., and Yormuk E. 2003. Effects of polyglycolic acid bioabsorbable membrane and oxidized cellulose on the osteogenesis in bone defects: an experimental study. *Acta Chir. Plast.* 45: 131–138.

[135] Tsuchiya K., Mori T., Chen G., Ushida T., Tateishi T., Matsuno T., Sakamoto M., and Umezawa A. 2004. Custom shaping system for bone regeneration by seeding marrow stromal cells onto a web-like biodegradable hybrid sheet. *Cell Tissue Res.* 316: 141–153.

[136] Sharma B. and Elisseeff J.H. 2004. Engineering structurally organized cartilage and bone tissues. *Ann. Biomed. Eng.* 32: 148–159.

[137] Aurell C.J. and Flodin P. 2002. *New Linear Block Polymer.* July 11, 2002.

[138] Aurell C.J. and Flodin P. 2003. *A Method for Preparing an Open Porous Polymer Material and an Open Porous Polymer Material.* EP1353982.

[139] Zhang J.Y., Beckman E.J., Hu J., Yuang G.G., Agarwal S., and Hollinger J.O. 2002. Synthesis, biodegradability, and biocompatibility of lysine diisocyanate-glucose polymers. *Tissue Eng.* 8: 771–785.

[140] Zhang J.Y., Beckman E.J., Piesco N.J., and Agarwal S. 2002. A new peptide-based urethane polymer: synthesis, biodegradation, and potential to support cell growth *in vitro*. *Biomaterials* 21: 1247–1258.

[141] Zhang J.Y., Doll B.A., Beckman E.J., and Hollinger J.O. 2003. Three-dimensional biocompatible ascorbic acid-containing scaffold for bone tissue engineering. *Tissue Eng.* 9: 1143–1157.

[142] Doll B.A., Beckman E.J., and Hollinger J.O. 2003. A biodegradable polyurethane–ascorbic acid scaffold for bone tissue engineering. *J. Biomed. Mater. Res.* 67A: 389–400.

[143] De Groot J.H., Kuijper H.W., and Pennings A.J. 1997. A novel method for fabrication of biodegradable scaffolds with high compression moduli. *J. Mater. Sci.: Mater. Med.* 8: 707–712.

[144] De Groot J.H., de Vrijer R., Pennings A.J., Klompmaker J., Veth R. P.H., and Jansen H.W.B. 1996. Use of porous polyurethanes for meniscal reconstruction and meniscal prosthesis. *Biomaterials* 17: 163–174.

[145] Szycher M. Biostability of polyurethane elastomers: a critical review. 1988. *J. Biomater. Appl.* 3: 297–402.

[146] Spaans C.J., De Groot J.H., Van der Molen L.M., and Pennings A.J. 2001. New biodegradable polyurethane-ureas, polyurethane and polyurethane-amide for *in-vivo* tissue engineering: structure–properties relationships. *Polym. Mater. Sci. Eng.* 85: 61–62.

[147] Spaans C.J., De Groot J.H., Belgraver V.W., and Pennings A.J. 1988. A new biomedical polyurethane with a high modulus based on 1,4-butanediisocyanate and e-caprolactone. *J. Mater. Sci.: Mater. Med.* 9: 675–678.

[148] Skarja G.A. and Woodhouse K.A. 2000. Structure–property relationships of degradable polyurethane elastomers containing an amino acid-based chain extender. *J. Appl. Polym. Sci.* 75: 1522–1534.

[149] Oertel G. *Polyurethane Handbook.* 1994. 2nd ed., Berlin, Germany, Hanser Gardner Publications.

[150] Spaans C.J., Belgraver V.W., Rienstra O., De Groot J.H., Veth R.P.H., and Pennings A.J. 2000. Solvent-free fabrication of micro-porous polyurethane-amide and polyurethane-urea scaffolds for repair and replacement of the knee-joint meniscus. *Biomaterials* 21: 2453–2460.

[151] Spaans C.J., De Groot J.H., Dekens F.G., Veth R.P.H., and Pennings A.J. 1999. Development of new polyurethanes for repair and replacement of the knee joint meniscus. *Polym. Preprints* 40: 589–590.

[152] Surgeons, A.S.O.P., *Procedural Statistics*. 2004.

[153] Miller M.J. and Patrick C.W. 2003. Tissue engineering. *Clin. Plast. Surg.* 30: 91–103, vii.

[154] Folkman J. and Hochberg M.M. 1973. Self-regulation of growth in three dimensions. *J. Exp. Med.* 138: 745.

[155] Vacanti J.P. et al. 1988. Selective cell transplantation using bioabsorbable artificial polymers as matrices. *J. Pediatr. Surg.*, 23: 3.

[156] Smahel J. 1971. Biology of the stage of plasmatic imbibition. *Br. J. Plast. Surg.* 24: 140–143.

[157] Converse J.M. et al. 1975. Inosculation of vessels of skin graft and host bed: a fortuitous encounter. *Br. J. Plast. Surg.* 28: 274–282.

[158] Hansen-Smith F.M. and Carlson B.M. 1979. Cellular responses to free grafting of the extensor digitorum longus muscle of the rat. *J. Neurol. Sci.* 41: 149–173.

[159] Heslop B.F., Zeiss I.M., and Nisbet N.W. 1960. Studies on transference of bone: I. A comparison of autologous and homologous implants with reference to osteocyte survival, osteogenesis, and host reaction. *Br. J. Exp. Pathol.* 41: 269.

[160] DeLeu J. and Trueta J. 1965. Vascularization of bone grafts in the anterior chamber of the eye. *J. Bone Joint Surg.* 47B: 319.

[161] Gray J.C. and Elves M.W. 1979. Early osteogenesis in compact bone isografts: a quantitative study of contributions of the different graft cells. *Calcif. Tissue Int.* 29: 225–37.

[162] Dell P.C., Burchardt H., and Glowczewskie F.P. 1985. A roentgenographic, biomechanical, and histological evaluation of vascularized and non-vascularized segmental fibular canine autografts. *J. Bone Joint Surg. Am.* 67: 105–112.

[163] Finkemeier C.G. 2002. Bone-grafting and bone-graft substitutes. *J. Bone Joint Surg. Am.* 84-A: 454–464.

[164] Han C.S. et al. 1992. Vascularized bone transfer. *J. Bone Joint Surg. Am.* 74: 1441–1449.

[165] Pogrel M.A. et al. 1997. A comparison of vascularized and nonvascularized bone grafts for reconstruction of mandibular continuity defects. *J. Oral Maxillofac. Surg.* 55: 1200–1206.

[166] Chang D.W. et al. 2001. Management of advanced mandibular osteoradionecrosis with free flap reconstruction. *Head Neck* 23: 830–835.

[167] Ang E. et al., 2003. Reconstructive options in the treatment of osteoradionecrosis of the craniomaxillofacial skeleton. *Br. J. Plast. Surg.* 56: 92–99.

[168] Pertschuk M.J. and Whitaker L.A. 1985. Psychosocial adjustment and craniofacial malformations in childhood. *Plast. Reconstr. Surg.* 75: 177–184.

[169] Pruzinsky T. 1992. Social and psychological effects of major craniofacial deformity. *Cleft Palate-Craniofacial J.* 29: 578–584; discussion 570.

[170] Schuster G.S. 1999. Oral flora and pathogenic organisms. *Infect. Dis. Clin. North Am.* 13: 757–774, v.

[171] Jiang R.S. et al. 1999. Bacteriology of endoscopically normal maxillary sinuses. *J. Laryngol. Otol.* 113: 825–828.

51

Cartilage Tissue Engineering

Fan Yang
Jennifer H. Elisseeff
Johns Hopkins University

51.1 Introduction

This chapter provides a review of important developments in the field of cartilage tissue engineering, with an emphasis on articular cartilage. Clinical significance of cartilage repair is discussed and the necessity of using tissue engineering approach to solve this problem is presented. Structure, function, and biochemical components of cartilage are described. This chapter will compare and contrast the various options available for cartilage tissue engineering. Four major components of tissue engineering in relation to cartilage are discussed including cells, scaffolds, growth factors, and mechanical stimuli.

Cartilage is a highly specialized connective tissue consisting of dispersed chondrocytes embedded in a rich extracellular matrix [1]. The matrix, primarily composed of proteoglycans, collagen, and water, is directly responsible for the unique functional properties of cartilage and provides shape, resilience, and resistance against compression and shear [2,3]. Despite the relatively simple structure, cartilage has little capacity for repair and regeneration due to many factors such as lack of vascularity and progenitor cells, a sparse and highly differentiated cell population, and a slow matrix turnover [4–6].

There are three types of cartilage: hyaline cartilage, fibrocartilage, and elastic cartilage. Each type of cartilage has different functional properties and hence different biochemical contents. Hyaline cartilage is rich in Type II collagen and proteoglycans and is found mainly on the articular surface of joints where it serves as a shock absorber. Elastic cartilage consists of elastic fibers, not exclusively collagen. The elastic fibers give this type of cartilage the ability to be deformed and return to shape. Examples of elastic cartilage include external ear, epiglottis, and upper portion of larynx. Fibrocartilage is rich in Type I collagen and is found in tissues that are subject to tensile forces such as the intervertebral disk.

More than 1 million surgical procedures in the United States involve cartilage replacement. Conventional therapies include drilling and debriding, autologous cartilage transplantation, and implantation of artificial polymers or metal prostheses [7]. Drilling and debriding may provide immediate relief of symptoms but usually result in the production of a fibrocartilaginous tissue with poor long-term outcome. Transplantation can be an effective treatment for patients with small cartilage defects, but its application is limited due to insufficient donor tissue supply, donor site morbidity, and technical difficulties to shape host cartilage into desired, delicate three-dimensional shapes. Artificial prostheses can be a source of infection, unwanted protein deposition, and immune responses without being able to adapt to environmental stresses.

51.1.1 Prospects for Tissue Engineering

Given the clinical significance of cartilage injury and the poor outcomes of the conventional therapies outlined above, investigators have been motivated to seek other approaches for improving cartilage treatment. One possible solution is to create new cartilage using tissue engineering strategies. Tissue engineering is an interdisciplinary area that combines biology, material sciences, and clinical medicine to regenerate or restore tissue structure and function that is lost due to trauma, disease, or congenital abnormalities. Cartilage contains only one cell type and has no blood supply. This relatively simple cartilage structure has allowed significant progress in the area of cartilage tissue engineering [8,9].

51.2 Cells

Cells are the building blocks of tissues and the fundamental source of extracellular matrix that forms tissues. Identification and creation of a suitable cell population is the first critical step toward cartilage tissue engineering and often requires a large number of cells. Numerous cell types have been explored including chondrocytes [10,11], bone-marrow derived mesenchymal stem cells (MSCs) [12,13], stem cells isolated from adipose tissue [14], from muscle [15], and embryonic stem cells [16,17]. All these cell types have been shown to exhibit a chondrogenic potential under appropriate culture conditions. When choosing the optimal cell type, it is important to consider the cell proliferative capacity, phenotype stability, and immunogenicity.

51.2.1 Chondrocytes

Chondrocytes, the major cell type that is present in differentiated cartilage, is the most obvious cell option for cartilage tissue engineering. Thus far, autologous chondrocyte transplantation (ACT) is the only Food and Drug Administration (FDA) approved cartilage repair product in the United States. This procedure uses *in vitro* expanded autologous chondrocytes, harvested from a biopsy, combined with a periosteal membrane to repair a cartilage defect (Figure 51.1).

The ACT was first used in humans in 1987 and results of the first pilot study was published in 1994 [10]. Since then more than 950 patients have been treated with this technique with 2 to 10 years follow-up [11]. Histology of the repair tissue shows that this technique gives stable long-term results with a higher success rate in femoral condyle (84 to 90%) than in other locations (average 74%). Despite the encouraging results that ACT has shown, several problems remain with the approach. First, the age or disease state of the patient may limit the availability and function of desired chondrocytes. *In vitro* expansion is also limited due to replicative senescence that chondrocytes exhibit. More importantly, once removed from their extracellular environment and expanded in monolayer, chondrocytes would rapidly lose their differentiated phenotype, characterized by transforming into a fibroblastic morphology, decreasing expression of Type II Collagen and aggrecan with an increase in Type I Collagen expression [18,19]. Studies have shown that chondrocyte phenotype can be retained or reexpressed by suspending

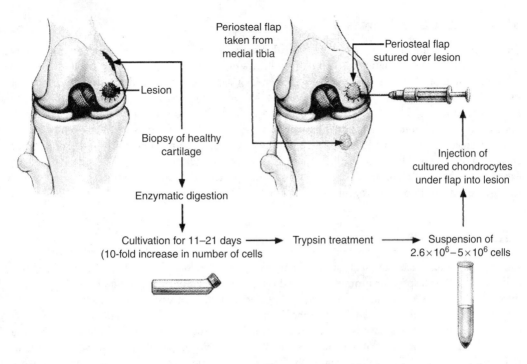

FIGURE 51.1   Flow diagram for ACT articular chondrocyte harvest and implantation. (From Brittberg, M., Lindahl, A., Nilsson, A., Ohlsson, C., Isaksson, O., and Peterson, L. *N. Engl. J. Med.* 1994; 331: 889–895. With permission.)

chondrocytes in a three-dimensional environment such as agarose gel [20], alginate beads [21], and collagen gel [22]. Optimal combinations of monolayer and three-dimensional cultures for cartilage tissue engineering are currently being investigated [23]. Challenges remain for patients who do not have healthy cartilage where autologous cell transplantation cannot be used and alternate cell sources need to be explored.

51.2.2 Mesenchymal Stem Cells

Mesenchymal stem cells are multipotent progenitor cells that have the capacity to differentiate into a variety of connective tissue cells including bone [24], cartilage [25], and adipose tissue [12] both *in vitro* and *in vivo*. MSCs are present in various tissue types during human development and are prevalent in adult bone marrow. As a readily available source, MSCs can be isolated, expanded in culture, and differentiated into chondrogenic cells under appropriated tissue conditions. Numerous studies have shown that transforming growth factor-beta (TGF-β) plays an important role in inducing undifferentiated MSCs into the chondrogenic pathway. In the presence of TGF-β, MSCs will gradually transform from a fibroblastic morphology to a mature chondrocyte morphology, accompanied by a production of cartilage-specific extracellular matrix proteins including Type II collagen, glycoaminoglycan, and proteoglycans. Unlike osteogenesis, which can be induced in monolayer culture, chondrogenesis of MSCs can only be achieved in micromass pellet culture [25] or high density suspension in a three-dimensional environment [26]. This close cell–cell contact requirement resembles the natural environment of embryonic cartilage development, which suggests that MSCs are undergoing a similar pathway. These results indicate that successful tissue-engineered cartilage repair based on MSCs can be achieved by recapitulating aspects of embryonic tissue formation. Studies so far demonstrated the great potential of using MSCs for cartilage regeneration as an alternate resource, which may eliminate the need harvest cartilage from the patient. More *in vivo* studies on cartilage regeneration using MSCs will occur as they reach clinical application.

51.2.3 Other Cell Sources

The discovery of human embryonic stem cells (hESCs) capable of indefinite replication and the ability to differentiate into all somatic cells of the body brings optimism that great progress will be made to cell transplantation therapies [27,28]. Theoretically, hESCs can be used to generate any desired cell or tissue for the treatment of degenerative diseases. So far, very few studies have been performed inducing hESCs into chondrogenic lineage [16,17]. Challenges with hESCs include potential of undesired growth, difficulty to achieve homogeneous differentiation *in vivo*, and related ethics issues. Other potential cell sources were found by Mizuno [29], who demonstrated that human dermal fibroblasts seeded onto Type I collagen sponges containing demineralizd bone matrix can be stimulated to produce a cartilaginous tissue expressing Type II collagen. Also, Lorenz [30] recently reported that human adipose tissue derived cells can also be induced into chondrogenic pathway *in vitro*.

51.3 Scaffolds

Although some approaches to cartilage tissue engineering use cells alone (i.e., ACT), most studies indicate that the scaffold is helpful for promoting desired cell phenotypes and regeneration of cartilage. Ideally, the scaffold serves as a structural support for cells at the early stage of tissue development and degrades into nontoxic products at a rate related to the formation of a functional extracellular matrix. Numerous scaffolds and matrices have been explored for cartilage tissue engineering including both natural and synthetic polymers. Natural polymers are usually porous, biocompatible, and can degrade without immunogenicity. Problems related to naturally derived scaffolds include batch-to-batch quality variance and weak structural properties. By contrast, synthetic polymers provide a more consistent quality and more control over the material properties such as degradation rate, mechanical properties, and surface biology. When choosing a scaffold, tissue engineers must decide which genre of materials, or combination, is more appropriate depending on the specific purpose and location of use.

51.3.1 Natural Polymers

As a major component of cartilage extracellular matrix, collagen was the first natural material explored as scaffold for cartilage tissue engineering. Collagen can be easily extracted from tissues such as tendon and can be readily processed into multiple forms including sponges or meshes. Collagen is liquid at 4°C and can be polymerized by raising the temperature. Further crosslinking after gelation introduces extended degradation times and greater mechanical strength [31]. Chondrocytes have been shown to maintain their morphology and phenotype when seeded in collagen gels [32–34]. Grande et al. [35] showed that collagen sponges stimulate collagen synthesis while bioabsorbable polymer such as polyglycolic acid (PGA) enhanced proteoglycan synthesis.

Hyaluronan comprises 1 to 10% of the cartilage glycosaminoglycan (GAG) and plays an important role in many biological processes such as cell attachment, hydration, and matrix synthesis. HYAFF® 11 (Fidia Advanced Biopolymers, Abano Terme, Italy) is a semisynthetic derivative of Hyaluronan by esterification of carboxyl groups of the glucuronic acid with benzyl alcohol. This processing greatly improves the originally poor ductility of hyaluronan, enabling HYAFF® 11 to be processed into multiple forms such as fibers, membranes, or microspheres. HYAFF and ACP, two hyaluronan-based biomaterials with different degradation profiles, were tested as chondrogenic delivery vehicles for rabbit MSCs and compared with a well-characterized porous calcium phosphate ceramic delivery vehicle [36]. Results showed that HYAFF 11 sponges incorporated twice as many cells and produced a 30% increase in the relative amount of bone and cartilage per unit area.

Agarose and alginate are examples of natural materials that are based on linear polysaccharide polymers that are extracted from seaweed [37]. These polymers are highly water-soluble due to a large number of hydroxyl groups. Agarose gels can be easily formed by pouring a warm liquid solution of the polymer into a mold, which gels as the solution cools to room temperature. Benya et al. [38] demonstrated that dedifferentiated rabbit articular chondrocytes can survive and redifferentiate during suspension culture in firm agarose gels. Recently, it has also been shown that dynamic pressure transmission through agarose gel was complete and immediate, which validates the use of agarose gels in studies employing dynamic pressurization in cartilage tissue engineering [39].

Alginate is a block copolymer of alternating residues of M (D-mannuronic acid) and G (L-guluronic acid). Alginate forms a gel in the presence of divalent ions such as calcium or magnesium. Alginate has been widely used as scaffold in cartilage tissue engineering because its solubility, gelation rate, and mechanical properties can be adjusted by the G/M ratio in the polymer backbone. Hauselmann showed that human chondrocytes cultured in alginate formed a similar matrix to native human articular cartilage [40]. When exposed to reduced oxygen tension (5%), chondrocytes encapsulated in an alginate gel has been shown to upregulate aggrecan and Type II collagen gene expression while downregulating Type I collagen expression [41].

51.3.2 Synthetic Polymers

No single existing polymer can meet the demands of all tissue-engineering applications, given the unique biochemical and mechanical requirements for different tissues or sites of implantation. Poly(lactic acid, PLA), PGA, and poly(lactic-co-glycolic acid, PLGA) are among the earliest synthetic polymers that were investigated for cartilage tissue engineering [7]. Originally designed for use as biodegradable surgical sutures, these polyesters can form highly porous lattice structures that allow cell encapsulation and proliferation with effective nutrient and waste transfer. A number of cell types, such as chondrocytes and bone-marrow derived MSCs have been seeded [42,43] in these polyester materials and cartilage matrix production have been achieved both *in vitro* and *in vivo*. Most studies involve implantation of cell-seeded polymer constructs into subcutaneous pockets in nude mice. Grande has shown neocartilage formation when implanted a chondrocyte-PGA construct into the rabbit knee defects [44]. PGA and PLA scaffolds are also biodegradable via nonspecific hydrolytic cleavage at the ester linkage site. Although polyester scaffolds have been widely used, they too have drawbacks such as poor cell attachment, difficulty in molding, and mild inflammatory reaction once implanted *in vivo*.

Injectable hydrogels are a genre of scaffolds that can be administered to fill defects of any shape and polymerize *in situ* with precise temporal and spatial control in a minimally invasive manner. Sims initially investigated the utilization of polyethylene oxide, a linear polyether-$(CH_2CH_2O)_n$ as encapsulating polymer scaffolds for delivering large numbers of isolated chondrocytes via injection [45]. New cartilage formation was observed as early as 6 weeks, with specimens exhibiting a white opalescence and histological characteristics consistent with those of hyaline cartilage.

Moreover, polyethylene oxide gels can be modified by adding acrylate end group that can potentially allow the transformation from a liquid to a solid with a defined structure in the presence of ultraviolet light. Elisseeff demonstrated that this transdermal photopolymerization technique can be used to implant the chondrocyte-seeded scaffolds, allowing simple exposure of the skin surface to light to induce gelation of scaffolds injected subcutaneously in nude mice [46,47] (see Figure 51.2). Williams et al. [26] has further shown the feasibility of applying photopolymerizing poly(ethylene glycol)-based hydrogels for chondrogenesis of adult goat MSCs, in the presence of growth factors. Pluronics is a commercially available copolymer of poly-(ethylene oxide) and poly-(propylene oxide) (Pluronics; BASF Corporation; Mount Olive, NJ). Pluronics forms a gel through physical crosslinks by hydrophobic group association at body temperature [48]. The main limitation of hydrogels for cartilage tissue engineering is the relatively weak mechanical properties when compared to other solid fibrous scaffolds. Mechanical properties of hydrogels may be improved by creating composite materials that incorporate a solid and hydrogel.

Ideally, polymers used in tissue engineering should be not only biocompatible, but also bioresponsive and biodegradable. The common feature of early polymers in biomedical applications was their biological inertness. Research in the past decade has been focusing more on the development of bioresponsive polymers that can respond to the local biological and physical microenvironment and elicit a controlled action and reaction. To enhance the interaction between the scaffold and the encapsulated cells, various

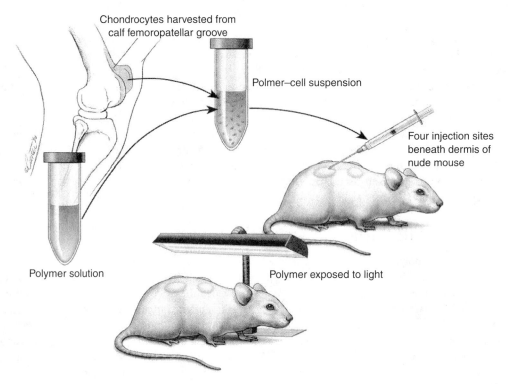

FIGURE 51.2 Schematic of procedure for cartilage tissue engineering by using transdermal photopolymerization depicting (1) isolation of bovine chondrocytes from the femoropatellar groove and combination with polymer (10 to 20% poly[ethylene oxide]-dimethacrylate) to form (2) a polymer/chondrocyte suspension. The polymer/chondrocyte suspension is subsequently (3) injected subcutaneously on the dorsal surface of a nude mouse, and (4) photopolymerized by placement of the mouse under an ultraviolet A lamp for 3 min. (From Elisseeff, J., Anseth, K., Sims, D., McIntosch, W. et al. *Plast. Reconstr. Surg.* 1999; 104: 1014–1022. With permission.)

biological signals such as cell adhesion peptides (i.e., RGD — arginine–glycine–aspartic acid), and growth factors have been incorporated into scaffolds. Enhanced cell attachment and extracellular deposition was achieved using scaffolds with biological activity [49–52]. As tissue mass increases and more extracellular matrix is deposited, it is also very important for the scaffold to degrade in a similar rate to allow effective diffusion and space for the newly formed tissue. Also, biodegradable scaffolds can play an important role as delivery vehicles for sustained growth factor release [53].

51.4   Mechanical Stimuli

Cartilage, especially articular cartilage, is a tissue that is accustomed to mechanical stimulation. During joint loading, articular cartilage undergoes compression and a plowing motion, and chondrocytes imbedded in the cartilage thus experience direct compressive deformation, shear, and hydrostatic pressure [54]. To understand the mechanotransduction pathway, various bioreactors have been designed to mimic the conditions necessary for functional cartilage tissue engineering. Freed and Vunjak-Novakovic [55] have demonstrated that dynamic stimuli is critical for cartilage matrix production by chondrocytes seeded on a PGA scaffold. Under static conditions, cell growth rates on the PGA scaffolds decreased due to limited diffusion caused by increased cell mass and new matrix deposition. Therefore, to engineer cartilage tissue that is clinically useful in size, it is essential to improve the *in vitro* culture conditions [42,56,57]. Carver and Heath [58] examined the effect of intermittent pressure on chondrocytes seeded on PGA scaffolds using a semiperfusion bioreactor. It was found that intermittent pressure increased the GAG content to native levels but the compressive modulus of the construct, though increased, did not reach the native level. This suggested that although ECM synthesis has been increased, matrix organization may be incomplete. Therefore, a current challenge in engineering functional cartilage tissue using bioreactor approach includes not only upregulation of ECM synthesis, but also its retention in the matrix and reorganization to restore the native-level mechanical function. More work is still needed to determine the type of mechanical forces, amplitude, and duty cycle that would induce the chosen cell type to form a functional cartilage tissue.

51.5 Growth Factors

Research advances in the fields of embryonic development, molecular and cellular biology have identified a variety of proteins that can affect cell chondrogenic differentiation and phenotypic expression, including transforming growth factor TGF-βs, insulin-like growth factor (IGF-1), bone morphogenetic proteins (BMPs), fibroblast growth factors (FGFs), and epidermal growth factor (EGF) [59]. These molecules have a broad range of activities, including proliferation induction, increasing the synthesis and deposition of cartilage extracellular matrix by chondrocytes, and inducing chondrogenesis by MSCs. Transforming growth factor (TGF-β) superfamily, including TGF-βs 1–3 and insulin-like growth factor-1 (IGF-1), stimulate GAG synthesis while chondrocyte synthesis of collagen II is strongly stimulated by IGF-1. It has also been demonstrated that MSC cultures exposed to TGF-βs show increased cell density, nodule formation, GAG, and Type II collagen synthesis [26,60].

The majority growth factor studies have been *in vitro* and focused on simply adding a soluble growth factor to the medium [26]. However, for clinical application, a continuous and stable effect of growth factors is a challenge. This challenge may be overcome by several possible approaches. Growth factors can be tethered to the scaffold by chemical modification and being released as the scaffold degrades [51]. They can also be encapsulated in polymer microspheres to achieve a sustained release [61]. The major limitation of both the above methods is that growth factors are proteins that can easily denature and it is challenging to retain biological activities during relative harsh chemical synthesis or microsphere suspension process.

Advances in gene transfer technology provide another novel alternative to achieve sustained and localized presentation of growth factors or gene products [62]. A variety of cDNAs have been cloned to stimulate biological processes that could promote chondrogenesis. Direct injection of a vector or genetically modified cells into the defect is conceptually the simplest approach to gene transfer. Besides the growth factors mentioned above, this method can also be applied to deliver chondrogenesis-related transcriptional factors such as Sox-9, signal transduction molecules such as SMADS [63]. Since these molecules function intracellularly and cannot be delivered to cells in a soluble form, gene transfer is a unique method for translation of these technologies in a clinical setting.

51.6 Zonal Organization

Articular cartilage is comprised of three zones that exhibit significant differences in their metabolic rate, matrix synthesis, and response to mechanical stimuli [54]. As opposed to current tissue engineering strategies where chondrocytes from all zones are seeded homogeneously, isolation of chondrocyte subpopulations from specific cartilage zones and their organization into a scaffold to mimic the native organization may provide engineered cartilage with enhanced structure and functional properties [64]. The superficial zone has a relatively low glycoaminoglycan content and compressive modulus, which facilitates the conformation of superficial zone to the opposing interface and allows stress distribution under compressive conditions. Klein isolated chondrocytes from the superficial and middle zones of immature bovine cartilage and cultured in alginate for 1 to 2 weeks. Analysis indicated that chondrocyte subpopulations play an important role in determining the structure, composition, metabolism, and mechanical function of tissue-engineered cartilage constructs [65]. Sharma has demonstrated the feasibility of using multilayered photopolymerizing hydrogel to recreate the zonal organization of articular cartilage [66].

Chondrocytes from the upper, middle, and lower zones of bovine articular cartilage were isolated and photoencapsulated in a trilayered poly(ethylene oxide)-diacrylate, PEODA, hydrogel. Cell tracking and viability assay showed that cells remained in their respective polymerized layer and cell viability was comparable throughout all three layers. Biochemical analysis further demonstrated that distinct metabolic characteristics are maintained when the chondrocytes are cultured in the layers, suggesting that this multilayer culture system may provide a native tissue mimicking environment that promotes regulatory signal molecules exchange.

51.7 Conclusion

Advances in tissue-engineering research provided an alternative possible therapeutic approach to restore lost tissue and function. Many researchers have focused on cartilage tissue engineering with encouraging results that will continue to motivate research efforts to engineer cartilage tissue with biological and mechanical properties similar to native tissue. The zonal organization of cartilage can be recreated using layered scaffolds, allowing a better mimic of the native cartilage tissue. Further development of cartilage tissue engineering is also closely related to the advances in polymer science to synthesize bioactive and biodegradable polymer with suitable biocompatibility. More research is required to achieve a sustained delivery of biological signals such as growth factors and transcriptional factors to promote tissue development *in vivo*. Identifying and providing suitable mechanical stimuli may also help engineering tissue to produce cartilage-specific biochemical compositions in an organized manner and hence acquire the mechanical properties that would meet the physiological needs of clinical application.

References

[1] Moss, M.L. and Moss-Salentijn, L. Vertebrate cartilages. In: Hall, B.K. (Ed.), *Cartilage: Structure, Function and Biochemistry*. Academic Press, New York, 1983; pp. 1–24.

[2] Heinegard, D., Bayliss, M., and Lorenzo, P. Biochemistry and metabolism of normal and osteoarthritis cartilage. In: Brandt, K.D., Doherty, M., and Lohmander, L.S. (Eds.), *Osteoarthritis*. Oxford University Press, Oxford, 1998; pp. 74–84.

[3] Mow, V.C. and Setton, L.A. Mechanical properties of normal and osteoarthritic articular cartilage. In: Brandt, K.D., Doherty, M., and Lohmander, L.S. (Eds.), *Osteoarthritis*. Oxford University Press, Oxford, 1998; pp. 108–122.

[4] Mankins, H.J. Currents concepts review: the response of articular cartilage to mechanical injury. *J. Bone Joint Surg.* 1982; 64A: 460–466.

[5] Silver, F.H. and Glasgold, A.I. Cartilage wound healing: an overview. *Otolaryngol. Clin. North Am.* 1995; 28: 847–864.

[6] Hunziker, E.B. Articular cartilage repair: problems and prospectives. *Biorheology* 2000; 37: 163–164.

[7] Langer, R. and Vacanti, J.P. Tissue engineering, *Science* 1993; 260: 920–926.

[8] Vacanti, C.A. and Upton, J. Tissue-engineered morphogenesis of cartilage and bone by means of cell transplantion using synthetic biodegradable polymer matrices [review]. *Clin. Plas. Surg.* 1994; 21: 445–462.

[9] Vacanti, C.A. and Vacanti, J.P. Bone and cartilage reconstruction with tissue engineering approaches [review]. *Otolaryngol. Clin. North Am.* 1994; 27: 263–276.

[10] Brittberg, M., Lindahl, A., Nilsson, A., Ohlsson, C., Isaksson, O., and Peterson, L. Treatment of deep cartilage defects in the knee with autologous chondrocyte transplantation. *N. Engl. J. Med.* 1994 331: 889–895.

[11] Brittberg, M., Tallheden, T., Sjogren-Jansson, B., Lindahl, A., and Peterson, L. Autologous chondrocytes used for articular cartilage repair: an update. *Clin. Orthop.* 2001; (391 Suppl.): S337–S348.

[12] Pittenger, M.F. et al. Multilineage potential of adult human mesenchymal stem cells. *Science* 1999; 284: 143–147.

[13] Jiang Y. et al. Pluripotency of mesenchymal stem cells derived from adult marrow. *Nature* 2002; 418: 41–49.

[14] Wickham, M.Q., Erickson, G.R., Gimble, J.M., Vail, T.P., and Guilak, F. Multipotent stromal cells derived from the infrapatellar fat pad of the knee. *Clin. Orthop.* 2003; (412): 196–212.

[15] Deasy, B.M. and Huard, J. Gene therapy and tissue engineering based on muscle-derived stem cells. *Curr. Opin. Mol. Ther.* 2002; 4: 382–389.

[16] Kramer, J. et al. Embryonic stem cell-derived chondrogenic differentiation *in vitro*: Activation by BMP-2 and BMP-4. *Mech. Dev.* 2000; 92: 193–205.

[17] Nakayama, N. et al. Macroscopic cartilage formation with embryonic-stem-cell-derived meso-dermal progenitor cells. *J. Cell Sci.* 2003; 116: 2015–2028.

[18] Schnabel, M. et al. Dedifferentiation-associated changes in morphology and gene expression in primary human articular chondrocytes in cell culture. *Osteoarthr. Cartil.* 2002; 10: 62–70.

[19] Benya, P.D., Padilla, S.R., and Nimni, M.E. Independent regulation of collagen types by chondrocytes during the loss of differentiated function in culture. *Cell* 1978; 15: 1313–1321.

[20] Benya, P.D. and Shaffer, J.D. Dedifferentiated chondrocytes reexpress the differentiated collagen phenotype when cultured in agarose gels. *Cell* 1982; 30: 215–224.

[21] Bonaventure, J. et al. Reexpression of cartilage-specific genes by dedifferentiated human articular chondrocytes cultured in alginate beads. *Exp. Cell Res.* 1994; 212: 97–104.

[22] Gibson, G.J. et al. Effects of matrix molecules on chondrocyte expression: synthesis of a low molecular weight collagen species by cells cultured within collagen gels. *J. Cell Biol.* 1982; 93: 767–774.

[23] Kuriwaka, M. et al. Optimum combination of monolayer and three-dimensional cultures for cartilage-like tissue engineering. *Tissue Eng.* 2003; 9: 41–49.

[24] Jaiswal, N., Haynesworth, S.E., Caplan, A.I., and Bruder, S.P. Osteogenic differentiation of purified, culture-expanded human mesenchymal stem cells *in vitro*. *J. Cell Biochem.* 1997; 64: 295–312.

[25] Barry, F., Boynton, R.E., Liu, B., and Murphy, J.M. Chondrogenic differentiation of mesenchymal stem cells from bone marrow: differentiation-dependent gene expression of matrix components. *Exp. Cell Res.* 2001; 268: 189–200.

[26] Williams, C.G., Kim, T.K., Taboas, A., Malik, A., Manson, P., and Elisseeff, J. *In vitro* chondrogenesis of bone marrow-derived mesenchymal stem cells in a photopolymerizing hydrogel. *Tissue Eng.* 2003; 9: 679–688.

[27] Thomson, J.A., Itskovitz-Eldor, J., Shapiro, S.S. et al. Embryonic stem cell lines derived from human blastocysts. *Science* 1998; 282: 1145–1147.

[28] Amit, M., Carpenter, M.K., Inokuma, M.S. et al. Clonally derived human embryonic stem cell lines maintain pluripotency and proliferative potential for prolonged periods of culture. *Dev. Biol.* 2000; 227: 271–278.

[29] Mizuno, S. and Glowacki, J. Three-dimensional composite of demineralized bone powder and collagen for *in vitro* analysis of chondroinduction of human dermal fibroblasts. *Biomaterials* 1996; 17: 1819–1825.

[30] Zuk, P.A., Zhu, M., Mizuno, H., Huang, J., Futrell, J.W., Katz, A.J. et al. Multilineage cells from human adipose tissue: implications for cell-based therapies. *Tissue Eng.* 2001; 7: 211–228.

[31] Bell, E. Deterministic models for tissue engineering. *Mol. Eng.* 1995; 1: 28–34; Campoccia, D., Doherty, P., Radice, M., Brun, P., Abatangelo, G., and Williams, D.F. Semisynthetic resorbable matrices from hyaluronan esterification. *Biomaterials* 1998; 19: 2101–2127.

[32] Weiser, L., Bhargava, M., Attia, E., and Torzilli, P.A. Effect of serum and platelet-derived growth factor on chondrocyte growth in collagen gels. *Tissue Eng.* 1999; 5: 533–544.

[33] Ochi, M., Uchio, Y., Tobita, M., and Kuriwaka, M. Current concepts in tissue engineering techniques for repair of cartilage defect. *Artif. Organs* 2001; 25: 172–179.

[34] Yamamoto, T., Katoh, M., Fukushima,R., Kurushima, T., and Ochi, M. Effect of glycosaminoglycan production on hardness of cultured cartilage fabricated by the collagen-gel embedding method. *Tissue Eng.* 2002; 8: 119–129.

[35] Grande, D.A., Halberstadt, C., Naughton, G., Schwartz, R., and Manji, R. Evaluation of matrix scaffolds for tissue engineering of articular cartilage grafts. *J. Biomed. Mater. Res.* 1997; 34: 211–220.

[36] Solchaga, L.A., Dennis, J.E., Goldberg, V.M., and Caplan, A.I. Hyaluronic acid-based polymers as cell carriers for tissue-engineered repair of bone and cartilage. *J. Orthop. Res.* 1999; 17: 205–213.

[37] Paige, K.T., Cima, L.G., Yaremchuk, M.J., Vacanti, J.P., and Vacanti, C.A. Injectable Cartilage. *Plast. Reconstr. Surg.* 1995; 96: 168–178.

[38] Benya, P.D. and Shaffer, J.D. Dedifferentiated chondrocytes reexpress the differentiated collagen phenotype when cultured in agarose gels. *Cell* 1982; 30: 215–224.

[39] Saris, D.B., Mukherjee, N., Berglund, L.J., Schultz, F.M., An, K.N., and O'Driscoll, S.W. Dynamic pressure transmission through agarose gels. *Tissue Eng.* 2000; 6: 531–537.

[40] Hauselmann, H.J. et al Adult human chondrocytes cultured in alginate form a matrix similar to native human articular cartilage. *Am. J. Physiol.* 1996; 271: C742–C752.

[41] Murphy, C.L. and Sambanis, A. Effect of oxygen tension and alginate encapsulation on restoration of the differentiated phenotype of passaged chondrocytes. *Tissue Eng.* 2001; 7: 791–803.

[42] Agrawal, C.M. and Ray, B. Biodegradable polymeric scaffolds for musculoskeletal tissue engineering. *J. Biomed. Mater. Res.* 2001; 55: 141–150.

[43] Martin, I. et al. Selective differentiation of mammalian bone marrow stromal cells cultured on three-dimensional polymer foams. *J. Biomed. Mater. Res.* 2001; 55: 229–235.

[44] Grande, D.A., Pitman, M.I., Peterson, L., Menche, D., and Klein, M. The repair of experimentally produced defects in rabbit articular cartilage by autologous chondrocyte transplantation. *J. Orthop. Res.* 1989; 7: 208–218.

[45] Sims, C.D., Butler, P.E., Casanova, R., Lee, B.T., Randolph, M.A., Lee, W.P. et al. Injectable cartilage using poly-ethylene oxide polymer substrates. *Plast. Reconstr. Surg.* 1996; 98: 843–850.

[46] Elisseeff, J., Anseth, K., Sims, D., McIntosh, W., Randolph, M., Yaremchuk, M. et al. Transdermal photopolymerization of poly(ethylene oxide)-based injectable hydrogels for tissue-engineered cartilage. *Plast. Reconstr. Surg.* 1999; 104: 1014–1022.

[47] Elisseeff, J., Anseth, K., Sims, D., McIntosh, W., Randolph, M., and Langer, R. Transdermal photopolymerization for minimally invasive implantation. *Proc. Natl Acad. Sci. USA* 1999; 96: 3104–3107.

[48] Cao, Y., Rodriguez, A., Vacanti, M., Ibarra, C., Arevalo, C., and Vacanti, C.A. Comparative study of the use of poly(glycolic acid), calcium alginate and pluronics in the engineering of autologous porcine cartilage. *J. Biomater. Sci. Polym. Ed.* 1998; 9: 475–487.

[49] Hern, D.L. and Hubbell, J.A. Incorporation of adhesion peptides into nonadhesive hydrogels useful for tissue resurfacing. *J. Biomed. Mater. Res.* 1998; 39: 266–276.

[50] Mann, B.K. et al. Modification of surfaces wit cell adhesion peptides alters extracellular matrix deposition. *Biomaterials* 1999; 20: 2281–2286.

[51] Mann, B.K., Schmedlen, R.H., and West, J.L. Tethered TGF-beta increases extracellular matrix production of vascular smooth muscle cells. *Biomaterials* 2001; 22: 439–444.

[52] Rowley, J.A. and Mooney, D.J. Alginate type and RGD density control myoblast phenotype. *J. Biomed. Mater. Res.* 2002; 60: 217–223.

[53] Holland, T.A., Tessmar, J.K., Tabata, Y., and Mikos, A.G. Transforming growth factor-beta1 release from oligo(poly(ethylene glycol) fumarate) hydrogels in conditions that model the cartilage wound healing environment. *J. Controll. Release* 2004; 94: 101–114.

[54] Mow, V.C. and Guo, X.E. Mechano-electrochemical properties of articular cartilage: their inhomogeneities and anisotropies. *Annu. Rev. Biomed. Eng.* 2002; 4: 175–209. Epub 2002, March 22.

[55] Freed, L.E., Hollander, A.P., Martin, I., Barry, J.R., Langer, R., and Vunjak-Novakovic, G. Chondrogenesis in a cell-polymer-bioreactor system. *Exp. Cell Res.* 1998; 240: 58–65.

[56] Vunjak-Novakovic, G., Martin, I., Obradovic, B., Treppo, S., Grodzinsky, A.J., Langer, R., and Freed, L.E. Bioreactor cultivation conditions modulate the composition and mechanical properties of tissue-engineering cartilage. *J. Orthop. Res.* 1999; 17: 130–138.

[57] Freed, L.E., Vunjak-Novakovic, G., and Langer, P. Cultivation of cell-polymer cartilage implants in bioreactors. *J. Cell Biochem.* 1993; 51: 257–264.

[58] Carver, S.E. and Heath, C.A. 1999. Influence of intermittent pressure, fluid flow, and mixing on the regenerative properties of articular chondrocytes. *Biotechnol. Bioeng.* 1999; 65: 274–281.

[59] Trippel, S.B. Growth factor actions on articular cartilage. *J. Rheumatol. Suppl.* 1995; 43: 129–132.

[60] Worster, A.A., Nixon, A.J., Brower-Toland, B.D., and Williams, J. Effect of transforming growth factor beta1 on chondrogenic differentiation of cultured equine mesenchymal stem cells. *Am. J. Vet. Res.* 2000; 61: 1003–1010.

[61] Elisseeff, J., McIntosh, W., Fu, K., Blunk, T., and Langer, R. Controlled Released IGF-I and TGF-beta on Bovine Chondrocytes Encapsulated in a Photopolymerizing Hydrogel. *J. Orthop. Res.* 2001; 19: 1098–1104 .

[62] Trippel, S.B., Ghivizzani, S.C., and Nixon, A.J. Gene-based approaches for the repair of articular cartilage. *Gene Ther.* 2004; 11, 351–359.

[63] Tsuchiya, H., Kitoh, H., Sugiura, F., and Ishiguro, N. Chondrogenesis enhanced by overexpression of sox9 gene in mouse bone marrow-derived mesenchymal stem cells. *Biochem. Biophys. Res. Commun.* 2003; 301: 338–343.

[64] Schinagl, R.M., Gurskis, D., Chen, A.C., and Sah, R.L. Depth-dependent confined compression modulus of full-thickness bovine articular cartilage. *J. Orthop. Res.* 1997; 15: 499–506.

[65] Klein, T.J., Schumacher, B.L., Schmidt T.A., and Sah, R.L. Tissue engineering of stratified articular cartilage from chondrocyte subpopulations. *Osteoarth. Cartil.* 2003; 11: 595–602.

[66] Sharma, B. and Elisseeff, J. Engineering structurally organized cartilage and bone tissues. *Ann. Biomed. Eng.* 2004; 32: 148–159.

52

Tissue Engineering of the Temporomandibular Joint

Mark E.K. Wong
Kyriacos A. Athanasiou
University of Texas Dental Branch
Rice University

Kyle D. Allen
University of Texas Dental Branch

52.1 Introduction

Tissue engineering of the temporomandibular joint (TMJ) is very much in its infancy. Similar to efforts directed at the replacement of other diseased joints, tissue engineering of the TMJ requires a detailed understanding of anatomy, normal joint activity and various pathologies. The body of knowledge available for the TMJ is relatively incomplete compared to other joints, which accounts for many of the problems encountered in previous reconstructive attempts. To date, very little is known about the manner in which the joint functions and the environment most conducive to its physiology. Even less is known about the impact of skeletal morphology and the presence or absence of a dentition. However, it is believed that both these parameters affect the type and range of motion as well as the forces created during joint function. The manner by which disease affects the TMJ has been derived largely from orthopedic and rheumatology studies of other diarthrodial joints. As various investigators attempt to apply basic tissue engineering techniques to produce replacement components for the TMJ, aggressive efforts are also underway to characterize its normal and abnormal behavior. These studies will provide an essential basis for the development of successful and lasting tissue engineering techniques for the reconstruction of the TMJ.

52.2   Gross Anatomy and Function of the TMJ

Movement of the lower jaw, or mandible, can occur through three planes of space as the result of *rotation* around a transcranial axis (vertical opening and closure), *translation* relative to the skull base (protrusion, retrusion, and side-to-side motion), or a combination of the two actions. These movements are possible, because of the presence of paired joints that separate the lower jaw from the skull base on either side of the cranium. The joints are named for the two bones that provide the articulating surfaces, namely the temporal bone (*temporo*) which houses the superior articulation in an area known as the glenoid fossa and articular eminence, and the mandible (*mandibular*), whose condylar processes provide the inferior portion of the articulation.

The TMJs are diarthrodial structures, which is to say that within the joint, a complete interpositional disc creates separate superior and inferior joint spaces. While this nomenclature suggests that the disc is isolated from its superior and inferior relationships by true "spaces," under normal functional conditions, the separations are extremely small and filled with synovial fluid. Conceptually, it would be more accurate to characterize these areas as *potential* spaces, with superior and inferior volumes approximating 1.0 and 0.5 ml, respectively [1]. This arrangement allows the fibrocartilaginous disc to fill the void between the condylar head and the glenoid fossa, promoting congruity between two dissimilarly shaped and sized structures [2] (Figure 52.1). Alterations in discal properties as a result of disease, improper position, or perforation are common precursors to degeneration of the articular surfaces of the joint, as mechanisms for the dissipation of normal physiological loads are lost. These degenerative conditions provide ample reasons for employing tissue engineering techniques to fabricate replacements for damaged discs [3] as well as condylar and fossa surfaces.

The disc sits astride the condylar head and together with its peripheral attachments and surrounding joint capsule, produces a closed space separating intra- and extra-articular environments. Three morphological zones have been described for the disc [4] and these are best appreciated in a sagittal view of the joint (Figure 52.1). The thickest region of the disc is the posterior band, followed by the anterior band. The intermediate zone represents the thinnest portion of the disc. The junctions between the zones are indistinct by gross examination and appear to blend with each other. In sagittal section, the disc has been described as a biconcave structure (Figure 52.1), but this is not a true depiction of its morphology. Instead, the disc resembles a cap attached along its entire peripheral margin to both the condylar neck and the skull base through a variety of different connective tissues. The superior attachments are less tenuous and allow the condylar head to slide forwards and from side to side in relation to the fossa during *translatory* movements of the joint. These attachments are composed of reflections of the superior surface of the disc, in association with the synovial membrane anteriorly and the superior laminar of the retrodiscal tissue (*bilaminar zone*) posteriorly. The synovial membrane in turn attaches to the skull base anterior to the articular eminence while the superior laminar of the retrodiscal tissue inserts into the petrous portion of the temporal bone. Medially and laterally, the superior surface of the disc turns inferiorly, blending with fibers of the capsule producing medial and lateral gutters. The inferior surface of the disc is more closely adapted to the condylar head, especially in its medial and lateral aspects. This relationship promotes *rotary* movements of the condyle in relation to the disc and glenoid fossa. Anteriorly, inferior reflections of the disc are interspersed with tendinous insertions of the superior head of the lateral pterygoid muscle, which attach to a concavity in the condylar head termed the *pterygoid fovea*. Posteriorly, the disc attaches to the inferior lamina of the retrodiscal tissue, which contains elastic fibers and blood vessels (Figure 52.2). As a result of these attachments, rotation occurs in the inferior space while translation of the joint occurs primarily involves the superior joint space. The different movements of the jaw rely upon the contraction of the lateral pterygoid muscle and its angle of attachment to the mandibular condyle (Figure 52.3).

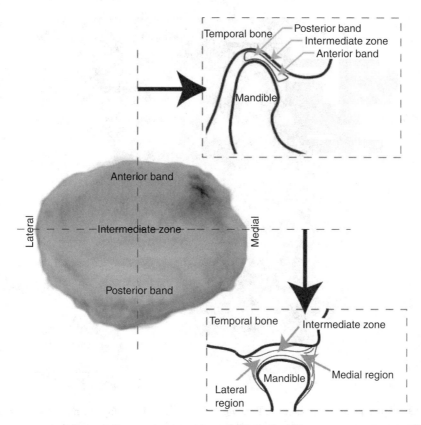

FIGURE 52.1 Superior, sagittal, and coronal views of the TMJ disc. The TMJ disc divides the joint into superior and inferior spaces. From a superior view, the disc displays an ellipsoidal shape, being thicker in the mediolateral dimension than anteroposteriorly. In a sagittal view of the disc, thicker anterior and posterior bands and a substantially thinner intermediate zone (central regions of the disc) can be appreciated. In coronal sections, the disc presents a similar biconcave shape, with thicker medial and lateral regions compared with the intermediate zone. However, regional variations in thickness are less obvious in the coronal plane.

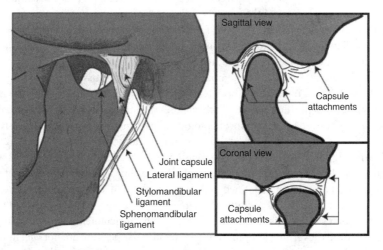

FIGURE 52.2 Ligament and capsule attachments in the TMJ. The TMJ capsule and various mandibular ligaments serve to guide and constrain mandibular movement. The capsule also separates intra- and extra-articular environments and produces a closed space containing synovial fluid, which serves both metabolic and lubricative functions. Various specialized neural elements within the capsule provide sensory input to guide joint position and movement.

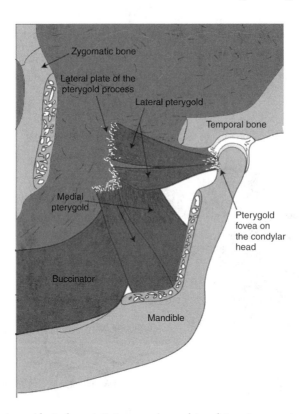

FIGURE 52.3 Lateral pterygoid attachment. Rotary opening and translatory movements of the mandible are the result of contraction of the superior and inferior bellies of the lateral pterygoid muscle. This muscle originates from the lateral surface of the lateral pterygoid plate and inserts into the pterygoid fovea, a depression in the anterior surface of the condylar head.

While the mouth is capable of opening widely, an interincisal opening of greater than 40 mm is the result of condylar rotation and translation. Most physiological opening movements are the result of smaller rotations of the condylar head. Under normal conditions, these movements produce complex compressive loads between the anterior surface of the condyle and the posterior slope of the articular eminence [5]. In the presence of a normally positioned disc, forces in this region are reduced and dissipated by the interposed intermediate zone of the disc along with the lubricating actions of synovial fluid. Only with excessive opening are shear forces generated at the interface of the superior surface of the disc and the glenoid fossa–eminence complex. The temporomandibular joints' tissues, particularly the TMJ disc, appear to have been designed to distribute both tensile and compressive forces during jaw movement.

The TMJ is enclosed by a fibrous capsule, which encloses the joint on its medial and lateral aspects. Laterally, the capsule is reinforced by the temporomandibular ligament. As described previously, attachments between the capsule and disc produce closed superior and inferior joint spaces (Figure 52.2). The capsule and ligament are highly innervated structures, containing a significant number of receptors which are capable of detecting stretch and pressure. Pacinian corpuscles, Ruffini nerve endings, Golgi tendon bodies, and free nerve endings have all been identified in the joint capsule [6]. These receptors provide important proprioceptive signals that guide the position of the mandible through neural relays with the muscles of mastication. While joint sensation is commonly ascribed to the auriculotemporal nerve, the role of other neurological mechanisms governing joint motion and mandibular position are not well understood. This lack of characterization contributes to the morbidity associated with reconstructive procedures.

The inner surfaces of the capsule are lined by the synovial membrane, a specialized structure containing cells and vessels responsible for both the phagocytosis of foreign particles and potentially pathological organisms and the production of synovial fluid. Synovial fluid serves two principal functions within a joint. As a lubricating fluid, synovial fluid is extremely effective exhibiting a coefficient of friction of approximately 0.00001. The lubricating action of synovial fluid is complex in itself and involves the interaction of multiple proteins [7]. Synovial fluid also acts a medium for the transmission of nutrients and the removal of metabolic waste from the cells present within the joint. As a dialysate of plasma, it contains all the components of plasma with the exception of large coagulation proteins. This composition suggests that synovial fluid is capable of performing most of the physiological functions of blood and is essential to the viability of joint structures. Tissue engineering products aimed at reconstruction of the TMJ or its components must be coupled with efforts to restore the functions of the synovium.

Potential movement of the mandible through three planes of space has already been described. Of interest is the considerably larger bulk of musculature responsible for closing movements as opposed to opening and excursive actions. Closure of the mandible is under the influence of the masseter, temporalis, and medial pterygoid muscles. These muscles form a robust sling around and above the mandible that generate a considerable amount of force. In contrast, opening movements are produced through the relatively small contractions of the superior head of the lateral pterygoid and (possibly) suprahyoid muscles (Figure 52.4). This muscular arrangement suggests that under normal conditions, opening movements constitute relatively passive actions through smaller ranges, while closure of the mandible invokes a power stroke to resist loads imposed by gravity and the presence of a bolus of food between the teeth. Consideration of the functional loads imposed upon the TMJ is critical in the design of tissue-engineered constructs [3]. Constructs must survive joint loading conditions, especially if protective neuromuscular controls are compromised by disease or surgical reconstructive procedures.

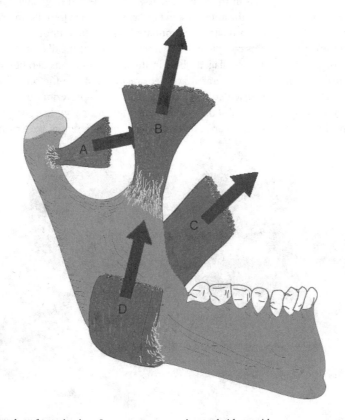

FIGURE 52.4   Muscles of mastication. In contrast to opening and side-to-side movements, mandibular closure is produced by contraction of three large muscles: the temporalis muscle (B), masseter muscle (C), and medial pterygoid muscle (D). These muscles, along with the lateral pterygoid (A), are collectively referred to as muscles of mastication since their principal activity is associated with eating.

52.3 Microscopic Anatomy of the TMJ Disc

Extensive histological studies of the TMJ utilizing light and scanning electron microscopy have been conducted in both human [8,9] and animal specimens [10,11]. Unlike most diarthrodial joints, the articular surfaces of the TMJ appear to be formed by nonvascularized and noninnervated fibrous connective tissue instead of hyaline cartilage, but these structures have not been completely characterized. The interpositional disc, on the other hand, is the subject of considerable interest in both human and animal models and these studies confirm that the disc is composed of fibrocartilage with an organic matrix composed primarily of collagen fibers enclosing a mixed fibroblastic and chondrocytic cell population [12–14]. In studies using porcine disc specimens, the ratio of fibroblasts to fibrochondrocytes is approximately 7 : 3 [14]. The presence of true chondrocytes, which are characteristic of hyaline cartilage, is debatable and indicative of the difficulty in phenotyping cells on the basis of their light microscopic appearance, especially when artifactual errors are taken into consideration. Using collagen typing, which provides strong evidence of the type of cell present based on its secretory product, a predominance of type I collagen in the TMJ disc [12,13,15] implies that the major cellular constituent is derived from a fibroblastic lineage. Trace amounts of type II collagen and a procollagen precursor have also been detected in human discs near the superior and inferior surfaces [16]. The cellular population of the disc appears to vary with age and also with the animal model studied. This is not surprising considering the different functional loads applied by various dietary patterns present in old and young ruminants and carnivores alike, and suggests that discal cells possess the ability to differentiate (or dedifferentiate) according to function. In general, higher cell numbers have been identified in the anterior and posterior bands relative to the intermediate zone [14]. The population of cells in the intermediate zone, subjected to greater compressive forces, appears to be more chondrocytic than the anterior and posterior bands [14]. In the anterior and posterior attachment regions, fibroblasts and fibrocytes predominate [14]. Smaller amounts of elastin fibers and other noncollagenous matrix proteins complete the organic structure of the disc [17].

The histological organization of the collagen fibers in the disc shows considerable regional variation between the intermediate zone and peripheral attachment regions [18]. In the central area of the intermediate zone, the collagen fibers are oriented primarily in an anterior–posterior direction. In areas where the disc attaches to the condylar neck and skull base, the fibers assume a ring-like structure (Figure 52.5). The distribution of the elastin fibers also appears to follow a circumferential pattern [17] with smaller

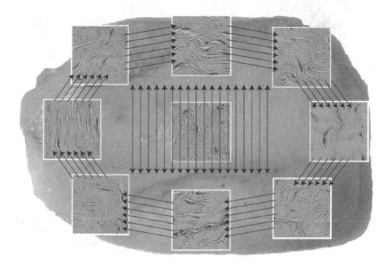

FIGURE 52.5 Collagen fiber alignment in the TMJ disc. The collagen fibers of the TMJ disc are arranged in a ring-like structure around the periphery of the disc. In the intermediate zone, the fibers are predominantly aligned in an anterior-posterior direction. In transition regions between the intermediate zone and the anterior and posterior bands, the collagen fibers curve medially, laterally, inferiorly, and superiorly.

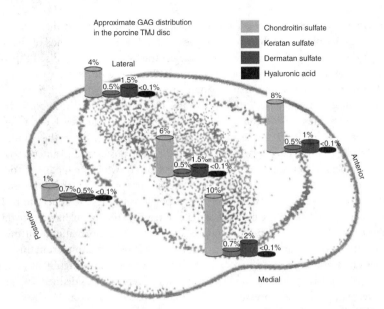

FIGURE 52.6 GAG content and distribution in the TMJ disc. Chondroitin sulfate is the predominant GAG in the TMJ disc, followed by dermatan sulfate. Keratan sulfate and hyaluronic acid GAGs are also found in the TMJ disc. Regionally, the medial portion of the disc appears to possess the largest concentration of GAGs followed by the anterior region. (Data from Detamore, M.S., et al. [2004] *Matrix Biol.* 24, 45–57. With permission.)

amounts of elastin present near the center of the disc and larger numbers of fibers in the posterior band [19]. By characterizing the disc according to the orientation of fibers, a different functional view of the disc is derived. Instead of dividing the disc into the intermediate zone and anterior and posterior bands, the disc can be regarded as possessing a central zone surrounded by peripheral attachment regions.

The collagen fibers also vary in appearance between the superior and inferior surfaces of the disc. Fibers within the inferior surface of the disc exhibit a more wavy appearance than those closer to the superior surface. This arrangement supports the need to dissipate larger compressive forces within the inferior joint space as opposed to tensile forces in the superior joint space.

At the molecular level, the presence, type, and distribution of glycosaminoglycans (GAGs) helps determine the response of articular tissue to function. The literature is not entirely in agreement regarding the total amount of GAGs present, the type and relative proportion of GAG, and the zonal distribution of each GAG [10,20–24]. The variable observations may be the result of differences in the animal model selected as well as different analytical techniques, which have included inhibition ELISA assays, ion exchange chromatography, electrophoresis, high-performance liquid chromatography, and colorimetric analysis [10,20–24].

Most studies suggest that GAGs represent between 0.5 and 10% of the dry weight of the TMJ disc [10,20–25]. The predominant GAG appears to be either chondroitin sulfate or dermatan sulfate, with small amounts of keratan sulfate and hyaluronic acid also detected [22,26]. Similar to the knee meniscus, water content of the disc is high, approximately 70% [27]. Antero-posteriorly, the highest concentration of chondroitin sulfate and keratan sulfate is found in the intermediate zone [10]. Medio-laterally, a higher concentration of GAGs is found in the medial regions [10]. The approximate values of GAG content in the TMJ disc are presented in Figure 52.6.

52.4 Biomechanical Behavior and Failure of the Disc

The TMJ disc under tension and compression exhibits significant anisotropy [28–31]. This behavior is believed to be directly related to the heterogeneous structure and organization of its cellular and molecular components. Furthermore, the disc appears to have much more tensile integrity than compressive; tensile moduli are 100- to 1000-fold larger than compressive moduli [28,29]. The bands of the disc also show a larger capacity to resist compressive loading than the central portions of the disc [28]. While the disc experiences both tensile and compressive loading, its role in the joint appears to be primarily compressive, yet its material properties under compressive loading are much smaller than other compressive tissues such as articular cartilage. The material properties of the TMJ disc support the hypothesis that the TMJ disc operates in a "trampoline-like" fashion. As the disc experiences increased levels of tensile deformation, the mesh-like collagen fiber network increases its resistance to deformations from the mandibular condyle.

The TMJ disc's material properties vary regionally [28–31]. The posterior and anterior bands appear to possess the largest resistance to instantaneous compressive loading, while the medial portions of the disc exhibits a significant relaxed resistance [28]. Under antero–posterior loading, the TMJ disc demonstrates considerable stiffness in all regions, however, the lateral portions of the disc appear to be less stiff than the central and medial portions [29]. Under medio-lateral tension, the disc behaves very differently. The anterior and posterior bands each display large resistance to tensile deformation, but the intermediate zone appears to be much weaker and consequently, more prone to deformation. From this account, we see strong correlations between a disc's tensile properties and its collagen fiber alignment [29]. Correlations between the disc's compressive properties and its matrix constituents are less defined. While GAG content is believed to increase the hydrostatic pressure within a matrix, and thus its compressive stiffness, the GAG content of the TMJ disc may not be large enough to account for significant variations throughout the tissue. Other factors, such as the specific type of GAGs or the size of collagen fibers present, account for the regional variations [28].

52.5   Common Conditions Affecting the TMJ

Within the context of clinical disease, four categories of pathology have been recognized to affect the TMJ to the extent that treatment is required. *Internal derangement of the TMJ* is a condition characterized by incoordinate movements of the disc relative to the condyle. It is believed to be the result of several inter-related pathological processes, including softening (*chondromalacia*) which produces either a deformed or malpositioned disc (most commonly in an anteromedial direction), disc *perforation* as a result of functional loads applied to diseased tissue, intra-articular reparative processes which limit joint and disc motion (*adhesions or scar bands*), and an alteration of synovial fluid properties which affect lubrication and metabolism (*synovitis*). When a disc is displaced from its normal position, a variety of responses occur depending on the extent and duration of the displacement. Minimally displaced discs that are capable of reduction often provoke adaptive responses within a joint, consisting of remodeling of the articular surfaces and discal tissue. However, if the disc is displaced significantly for a prolonged period, degeneration occurs as the result of unfavorable loading forces and the consequences of reduced mobility [32].

Degenerative joint disease represents a different state where catabolic loss of articular tissue exceeds anabolic attempts to restore joint structure. Various etiologies are capable of producing degeneration and these include excessive and repetitive loading patterns (*osteoarthritis*) and autoimmune conditions, where inflammatory antibodies against joint matrix proteins destroy the structural organization of the joint (*rheumatoid and psoriatic arthritis*). The etiology of osteoarthritis is unknown, but the interaction of several factors such as heredity, prolonged loading, trauma to a joint, immobility, obesity, joint instability, and advanced age appear to affect the normal mechanism by which cartilage cells replenish matrix macromolecules responsible for cartilage integrity [33]. The capacity for internal remodeling of both the discal and articular cartilage diminishes as a result of changes in matrix composition, biosynthetic activity of cartilage cells, and responsiveness of these cells to stimulation.

The cause of rheumatoid arthritis is also unknown, and while a strong genetic predisposition has been suggested by the presence of the HLA-DR4/DR1 epitope in over 90% of patients, the concordance of disease in monozygotic twins is between 15 and 20%, suggesting the significant influence of nongenetic factors. Macroscopic hallmarks of disease include synovial proliferation (*rheumatoid pannus*) and uncontrolled inflammation, reflected on a microscopic level by synovial cell hyperplasia and endothelial cell proliferation. The inflammatory process is also associated with activation of various cells of the reticulo-endothelial system, including CD_4 T lymphocytes, B cells, phagocytes, and neutrophils. Fibroblast and osteoclast activation result in both cartilage and bone resorption and thickening of the periarticular tissue.

Both internal derangement of the TMJ and degenerative joint disease can produce a reduction in the range of motion of a TMJ. These conditions may also be associated with significant pain. The origins of pain remain controversial, often because of the difficulty in localizing the sources of pain. Activation of nerve endings by inflammatory mediators and stimulation of neural elements present within the capsule, TMJ ligament, synovial membrane, and retrodiscal tissue by distortion or compression have been implicated. In addition, compromised joint function is capable of altering the normal behavior of the mandibular musculature. This sequela of joint disease produces reactive muscular responses and the phenomenon has been characterized as *myofascial pain dysfunction* (MPD), a condition which includes myospasm and muscle fatigue. The combination of pain derived from multifactorial origins and reduction in joint mobility produces the principal signs and symptoms associated with *temporomandibular dysfunction* (TMD), a clinical syndrome associated with pain and an inability to achieve normal mandibular motion.

The third category of TMJ disease differs from the preceding conditions, because it reflects a disorder of bone metabolism, rather than cartilage. Here, the local intra- and extra-articular environment favors the formation of heterotopic bone. When the dystrophic bone bridges the joint space (temporal–condyle interphase), complete immobility of the joint (and mandible) occurs. This condition is referred to as *ankylosis* of the TMJ.

The last category of conditions affecting the TMJ consists of different neoplasms or cysts that affect the mandible. These diseases rarely affect the joint without involvement of the adjacent mandibular bone and as such, will not be considered in this discussion on tissue engineering of the TMJ, because the defect requiring reconstruction usually extends beyond the confines of the joint.

The successful application of tissue engineering strategies to reconstruct either individual joint components or the entire joint mandates a full appreciation of the pathological condition(s) responsible for the destruction of the joint in the primary instance. Ignoring the etiology of joint disease may result in a diminished capacity for successful implementation of an engineered construct and an inability of tissue engineering to fulfill its promise as a reconstructive modality.

52.6 Current Methods for TMJ Reconstruction

Reconstruction of the TMJ can involve the replacement of a disc, reconstruction of the superior articulation (*hemi-arthroplasty*), or replacement of the superior and inferior articulating surfaces (*total joint reconstruction*). A variety of autogenous and alloplastic materials have been used for joint reconstruction with varying and conflicting results. It is beyond the scope of this chapter to discuss comparative outcomes from these procedures. Analyzing the relative success and failure of each technique or material is complicated by an inability to fully appreciate the normal function of a particular patient's joint, which has lead to difficulty in gauging outcomes. Criteria used to evaluate treatment of patients with TMJ pathology usually include a comparison between the mandibular range of motion and pain levels before and after surgery, which are imprecise measurements fraught with subjective error.

Removal of a diseased or severely displaced disc (*discectomy or meniscectomy*) is a procedure employed when repositioning maneuvers of the malposed disc fail or are not possible because of advanced degeneration of the disc. Following removal, treatment alternatives include leaving the joint empty, replacement of the disc with an autogenous fat, fascia (e.g., fascia lata), cartilage (e.g., auricular cartilage), dermal graft, or rotating a fascia flap (e.g., temporalis fascia) into the defect. Whichever modality is selected, it appears that the formation of an interarticular scar band either through a *de novo* process or metaplastic transformation of grafts and flaps into fibrous tissue provides a common endpoint.

Experiences with different alloplastic materials for discal replacement have been characterized by a number of significant failures resulting in severe joint resorption, alteration of mandibular skeletal relationships, compromised motion, pain, and allegations of systemic immune compromise. These surgical disasters and the resultant lawsuits have unfortunately tainted all forms of TMJ surgery and discouraged many surgeons from seeking alternative methods to reconstruct the joint. Before the controversy surrounding the implantation of medical-grade silicone developed, silicone (*Silastic*) interpositional implants were available for disc replacement. As permanent replacements, these devices were capable of fragmentation, but when used as a temporary interpositional implant ("pull-out" technique), they were observed to provoke the formation of a dense fibrous tissue capsule, which served as an interarticular cushion. Their relatively successful use following discectomy might be attributed to this reaction.

One of the most litigious experiences associated with the alloplastic replacement of a disc occurred with the use of a Teflon–Proplast implant in the late 1980s and early 1990s. Produced by the Vitek® Corporation, fragmentation of the implant under functional and parafunctional loads was associated with an exuberant foreign body giant cell response and significant osteoclastic activity, resulting in the resorption of condylar and fossa surfaces and severe local inflammatory events. The lessons learned from this experience are essential, and include the significance of characterizing the loading patterns within a joint, and the importance of recognizing the effects of degradation products upon the local joint environment.

The TMJ hemi-arthroplasty was a procedure popularized by Christensen and Morgan in the 1960s, in which the superior articulation of the joint was replaced with an implant fabricated out of chrome–cobalt alloy. The Christensen implant reconstructed both the fossa and articular eminence while the Morgan implant covered the eminence only. Concerns over accelerated degeneration of the natural condyle articulating against a less-deformable surface eventually resulted in the replacement of the hemi-arthroplasty with total joint reconstructive procedures utilizing both prosthetic fossa and condylar components. Several systems are currently licensed by the Food and Drug Administration (FDA) (ca. 2004) for implantation into patients, though limitations have been imposed on surgeons wishing to use these devices and the selection of patient candidates. Stringent follow-up of patients treated with these implants form the basis of various clinical trials designed to test not only the ability of the procedure to improve a patient's condition, but also the integrity of the devices over time.

As an alternative to prosthetic devices, autogenous grafting techniques are available. Reconstruction of the TMJ with autogenous tissue involves the harvesting of a costochondral graft (fourth to sixth rib) and attaching the graft to the remaining mandibular ramus following removal of the diseased joint. The rib is usually placed on the lateral surface of the ramus and fixated with multiple transcortical screws or a bone plate (Figure 52.7). The rib may also be placed on the posterior border of the ramus so that its widest dimension occupies the fossa, but fixation with either bone plates or screws becomes a little more difficult. When the disc is removed along with the condyle, alternatives for discal reconstruction are similar to those following discectomy and range from leaving the interarticular space empty to using some form of autogenous soft tissue to fill the void.

In general, reconstruction following joint removal for neoplastic or cystic disease enjoys a higher rate of success than similar procedures performed in patients with temporomandibular dysfunction. Several reasons have been proposed for this dichotomy, including persistence of parafunctional loading of the articulation, excessive scarring from multiple operations, the physical and psychological consequences of chronic illness, and degenerative disease states which are directed against bone and cartilage.

The principal indications for considering an alloplastic total joint over an autogenous costochondral graft include the treatment of joints where heterotopic bone formation is a concern (e.g., ankylosis of the TMJ), joints affected by a resorptive inflammatory process (e.g., rheumatoid arthritis or joints affected by a foreign body response to previously implanted alloplasts), and multiply operated patients where the soft tissue bed is excessively scarred and relatively avascular. Under these adverse conditions, autogenous grafts may be compromised by further disease or conditions which do not favor graft survival. The ability to customize an alloplastic device is also useful for correcting a skeletal discrepancy that may occur in

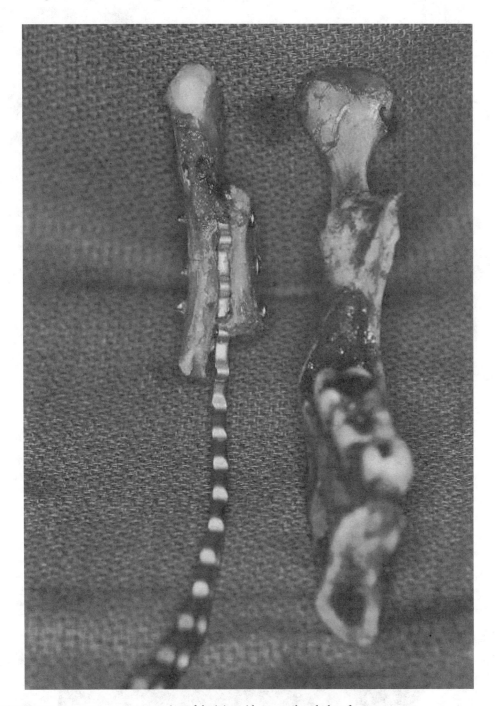

FIGURE 52.7 Autogenous reconstruction of the joint with a costochondral graft.

patients with severe degenerative joint disease, where retrusion and rotation of the mandible is the result of decreased posterior vertical support (Figure 52.8a,b).

Customized prosthetic devices involve complex surgical techniques. In order to accurately reproduce the skeletal bases to which the devices will be attached, two separate surgeries are ideally required. During the first procedure, the diseased joint (or failed implant) is removed and the area derided. A temporary alloplastic space maintaining implant is used to reduce the amount of soft tissue in-growth into the

(a)

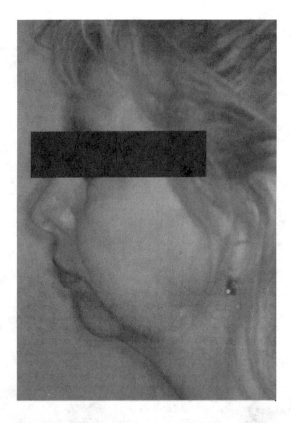

(b)

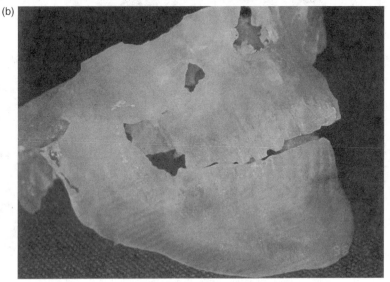

FIGURE 52.8 Mandibular retrusion secondary to bilateral condylar resorption. (a) Profile view of patient with severe, bilateral rheumatoid degeneration of the mandibular condyles. Retrusion of the mandible can be appreciated from the posterior position of the chin; (b) stereolithographic model of the same patient demonstrating the resulting malocclusion created by loss of condylar height. Correction of mandibular skeletal position with bilateral alloplastic total joint reconstruction. (c) Patient with bilateral degenerative rheumatoid disease of the mandibular condyles following surgical reconstruction of the joints with alloplastic total joint prosthesis. Note restoration of mandibular projection; and (d) Postero-anterior (PA) skull radiograph demonstrating bilateral alloplastic total joints.

(c)

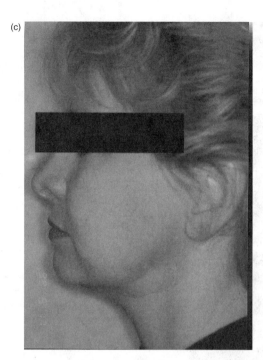

(d)

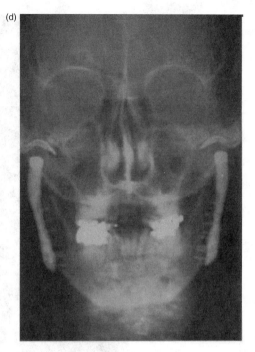

FIGURE 52.8 *Continued.*

resulting space. Following this surgery, a thin-cut Computerized Tomography (CT) scan is obtained using a protocol devised by companies specializing in the fabrication of stereolithographic models. The anatomically accurate model is sent to a joint fabrication company where CAD–CAM technology is used to produce a prototype of the final device. Each device is composed of a prosthetic fossa and eminence as well as a condylar head attached to a ramus component. The prototype is returned to the surgeon who confirms that the surgical defect has been correctly reconstructed. At this time, minor modifications to the skeletal defect may be proposed to better accommodate and fit the implant. Once the customized implant has been completed, the patient undergoes a second surgery during which time, the surgical sites are adjusted to match the defect created on the stereolithographic model before the prosthetic fossa and condyle are attached to their bony bases. The entire process is time-consuming and expensive, but justification for its use lies in the magnitude of the problem requiring correction (Figure 52.8c,d).

Single surgery reconstruction of a joint is also possible with custom devices. In this procedure, a stereolithographic model of the diseased joint is prepared. If an alloplastic device is already in place, digital subtraction technology is employed to artificially remove the prosthesis. Otherwise, the surgeon creates the anticipated surgical defect on the model and the device is fabricated. Minor adjustments to the skeletal remnants can be made at the time of implantation to promote a close adaptation of the device to the defect.

The Christensen total joint system has been available since 1965, though the current device, which employs a Vitallium fossa articulating against a chrome–cobalt condylar head, is significantly modified from the original design which used a metallic fossa matched with a condylar head composed of polymethylmethacrylate (PMMA) (Figure 52.9a). Concerns over the development of a giant cell mediated foreign body response to particulate PMMA prompted this change. Both the fossa and condylar prosthesis are fixated to the temporal bone and mandibular ramus, respectively, with screws (Figure 52.9b). Both patient-specific implants, customized according to computerized tomographic data, as well as stock devices with different sizes and shapes for the fossa and condyle are available.

Another system currently available is offered by TMJ Concepts® (Figure 52.10). This system utilizes a chromium–cobalt–molybdenum condylar head attached to a ramus framework made out of titanium alloy

(a)

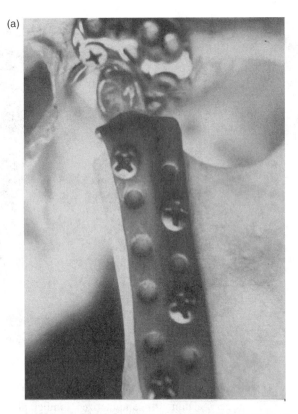

(b)

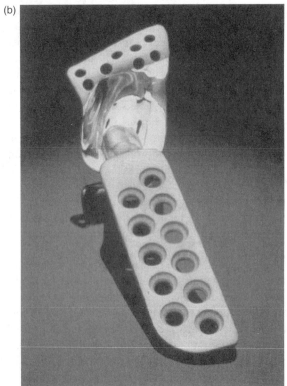

FIGURE 52.9   Christensen® total joint prosthesis with (a) acrylic condyle and (b) metal condyle.

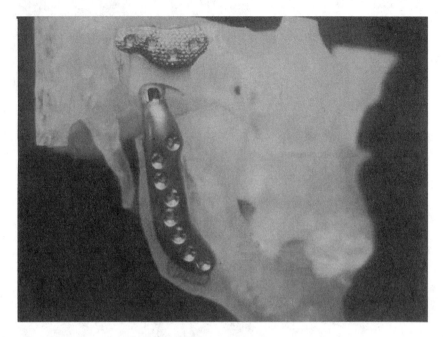

FIGURE 52.10 TMJ Concepts® total joint prosthesis.

(6AL–4V) and a fossa component composed of ultra-high molecular weight polyethylene (UHMWPE) with a nonalloy titanium mesh backing. The respective components are customized to the individual patient's anatomical defect and are produced with advanced CAD–CAM technology. After fabrication, the condyle and fossa are attached to their respective skeletal components with multiple screws (titanium alloy) placed in a nonlinear fashion to promote maximum stability. There are no stock components available for this system.

The third device is currently available only to surgeons who are formally registered to participate in an FDA-sanctioned clinical trial for the Lorenz-Biomet prosthetic total joint. The fossa consists of a UHMWPE articular surface mounted on a metallic base which is used to secure the prosthesis with screws to the lateral margins of the glenoid fossa. Since this is a stock device available in three sizes, the patient's anatomy requires preparation to conform with the prosthetic contours. This is achieved in part by removing most of the articular eminence and if indicated, filling the space between the fossa and device with orthopedic cement (e.g., Simplex P). A significant difference between the design of this fossa prosthesis and those used in the Christensen or TMJ Concepts systems is the thickness of the articular surface. The Lorenz-Biomet total joint system attempts to shift the center of rotation of the reconstructed joint inferiorly to simulate translatory movements by increasing the thickness of the UHMWPE to a minimum of 4 mm. The condylar portion of this device is composed of a cobalt–chromium–molybdenum alloy and is available in 45, 50, and 55 mm lengths to accommodate various ramus heights. Several design features have also been incorporated including augmenting the peripheral margin of the fossa prosthesis to reduce the likelihood of re-ankylosis and the in-setting of the condylar head so that it articulates against the middle of the fossa instead of the lateral aspect.

52.7 Tissue Engineering Strategies for TMJ Reconstruction

52.7.1 Tissue Engineering Motivation and Philosophy

The motivations for tissue engineering in the TMJ are abundant [3,34]. While surgical removal of diseased articular surfaces or a pathologically affected disc with or without reconstruction remains a viable treatment option, the resulting articulation is left without the benefit of physiologically adaptive tissues. Tissue

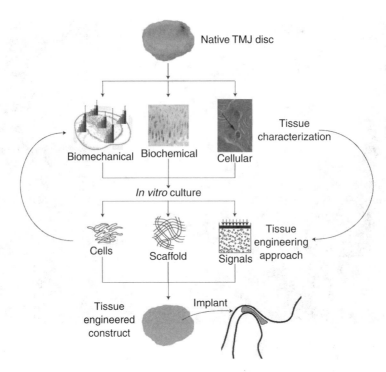

FIGURE 52.11 Developmental approach toward tissue engineering. The combination of cells, scaffolding, and signals provide the foundations for the creation of a tissue engineered construct. However, before designing such an implant, the material characteristics of the native tissue should be fully characterized and incorporated into the design.

engineering offers the potential to replace tissues that have been destroyed and removed [3]. Laboratory fabricated biological constructs would be capable of immediate structural reconstruction, reproducing normal joint physiology, and reducing the need for multiple surgical procedures. Current tissue engineering efforts in the TMJ are focused on the replacement of bony, cartilage, and fibrocartilage structures as separate components. There are currently no documented efforts to reconstruct the capsule or synovium, which places the field at a considerable distance from the engineering of a true total joint system.

The tissue engineering approach to articular reconstruction combines cells, a scaffold, and biological agents that control the formation and maintenance of tissue with properties comparable to native structures [3]. Several variations to this general approach include the use of different cell lineages [35], various scaffold materials and shapes [36], and the methods by which biological signals are applied [37]. In order for engineered constructs to succeed, characterization of the native tissue properties (cellular, biochemical, and mechanical) must first be conducted, such that tissue engineering efforts may be designed to create constructs which emulate the native tissues' functions [18]. Figure 52.11 summarizes the progression and philosophy associated with tissue engineering efforts. Each level of tissue characterization, as well as general efforts to engineer joint components, is the focus of active research. A comprehensive understanding of the challenges in these research areas will lead to the development of viable, implantable tissue engineered construct for TMJ reconstruction.

52.7.2 Cellular Issues

Cells are the factories responsible for the formation and maintenance of replacement tissues. Through the action of proteins responsible for creating or degrading the surrounding extracellular matrix, cells produce and remodel tissue structure to comply with functional requirements. Cells for TMJ tissue engineered constructs are derived from one of three sources: native cells isolated from healthy mature tissue, undifferentiated progenitor cells isolated from a variety of autogenous sites, and cells which infiltrate a noncellular, implanted scaffold from the surrounding tissue *in vivo*. Each cell source is associated with distinct advantages balanced against phenotypical limitations. The selection of an appropriate cell source is therefore based upon the requirements of a particular tissue engineering application.

Several issues govern the selection of cells for tissue engineering in the TMJ. For example, the presence of a healthy native cell source may be impossible due to joint pathologies. Also, these mature cells may have fewer propensities to produce ECM proteins. For these reasons, the promotion of an undifferentiated cellular phenotype has been suggested as a possible cell source for diseased joints. However, this promotion may be unnecessary if healthy, native cells which have retained their phenotype are available.

Further complicating the selection of the cell source is a tissue's phenotypic nature. In the case of the TMJ disc, a heterogeneous group of cells are found throughout the disc, thus native cell harvesting techniques may yield the best approximation of the disc's cellular constituency. Mature cells could have a reduced ability to produce extracellular matrix proteins, but these effects may be a result of other factors such as passaging effects. In addition to these issues are the multiple phenotypic origins which may assist in TMJ development. Cell populations in the TMJ have been shown to possess origins associated with mesenchymal and neural crest derivatives. These lineages may play very different and interrelated roles in TMJ development [38].

When a reconstruction aims to replace the entire TMJ and not the disc alone, multiple cell lines, scaffolds, and molecular factors have to be considered. In the most extensive form of joint reconstruction, it may be necessary to replace bone, cartilage, fibrocartilage, capsule, and synovium simultaneously. The concurrent regeneration of these different tissues in a single scaffold with multiple cell lines and specialized molecular signals may prove extremely difficult. An alternative approach would attempt to engineer components of the joint separately and to combine these elements after they have been formed, in a process similar to the use of current alloplastic devices.

To complete the reconstruction, an implantable construct may require the incorporation of a neural network capable of mediating joint neuromuscular responses as well as a vascular supply to support various metabolic requirements of the reconstructed joint. Current tissue engineering studies are not sufficiently developed to handle this level of complexity and ultimately, this effort might prove unnecessary if the capsule, synovium, and temporomandibular ligament are preserved and re-attached after the implantation of the construct. Currently, the focus of TMJ tissue engineering is the separate regeneration of the major tissue constituents of the joint, namely bone, cartilage, or fibrocartilage, but success in this area does not necessarily translate into a successful reconstruction of the total joint.

52.7.3 Scaffold Issues

The scaffold is used to support cells while they produce a three-dimensional biological matrix. The choice of material for the scaffold is based upon how the construct will be utilized. Important considerations include the characteristics of the tissue being regenerated, the mechanical environment to which the scaffold is subjected, interactions between cells and the scaffolding material, the biocompatibility of the scaffold and its degradation products, and the ability of a scaffold to convey various biological signals. The scaffold should also elicit a minimal immunogenic response to reduce rejection and facilitate the formation of biological tissue. Current TMJ tissue engineering efforts have focused on scaffolds composed of hydrogels and meshes fabricated from different natural and synthetic materials [39].

Hydrogels are scaffolds used in current tissue engineering applications for bone, cartilage, and fibrocartilage regeneration. Some of the advantages of hydrogels include controlled rates of degradation, the ability to be injected, photopolymerization capabilities, and the assembly of protein sequences conducive to cell attachment [40,41]. Specific hydrogels such as oligo(poly(ethyleneglycol)fumarate) (OPF) have shown promise in the regeneration of bone and might prove effective in the promotion of cartilage regeneration [35]. Alginate hydrogels have also been used in the regeneration of the TMJ disc using porcine TMJ disc fibrochondrocytes [39]. However, the cellular population of the construct was not stable and observed to decrease with time [39]. The importance of a scaffold to the production of bone and cartilage from cells has been well documented. When cells remain unattached, tissue formation is absent, while suspension in hydrogels can promote both bone and cartilage formation [42].

Meshes can be made from degradable or nondegradable synthetic materials. Natural porous meshes, such as coral hydroxyapatite have also been utilized as scaffolds [43]. Nonwoven meshes of polyglycolic acid (PGA) and polylactic acid (PLA), used alone or as copolymers, are popular in tissue engineering, because they have already received approval from the FDA for medical implantation into humans [39]. These materials can be formed into complex shapes by polymerizing or fashioning the material within anatomic molds. The rate of degradation of the copolymeric scaffolds can also be adjusted by changing the ratio of the copolymers. While complete hydrolysis of many polymeric meshes will occur, acidic degradation products may incite an inflammatory response which can adversely affect the formation of bone or cartilage. Nonwoven meshes have already demonstrated their ability to support TMJ disc fibrochondrocytes [39], osteoblast-like cells [44], and chondrocytes [45] *in vitro*. These studies demonstrate the promise of these materials for the reconstruction of an interpositional disc and articular cartilage.

52.7.4 Signals and Stimulation Issues

Molecular signals and nonbiological stimuli may be used to induce positive and negative gene expression, and thus biosynthetic responses, in cells. These modulators can take a variety of forms such as growth factor application, mechanical stimulation, the use of adhesion peptides, and the generation of oxygen gradients, electrical currents, and sonic stimulation. The effects of these agents can be direct or synergistic and may produce single or inter-related responses. By varying parameters, such as the bioactivity of growth factors and proteins, the size and frequency of mechanical and sonic stimulations, the length of stimulations, and dosage and saturation effects, the regeneration of tissue can be optimized.

Several studies have investigated the effect of growth factors, mechanical stimulation, and oxygen on tissue engineered constructs. Each stimulant, acting through the modulation of the local environment, is capable of producing tissue-like ECM proteins. However, the formation of an organized, three-dimensional tissue array with biochemical and biomechanical properties similar to native tissue will probably require a combination of signals. One method for creating a multisignal environment employs bioreactors to supply mechanical stimulation, such as hydrostatic pressure, in combination with a variety of other signals such as growth factors. Bioreactors capable of perfusion are also able to deliver molecular signals more efficiently by dispersing the biochemical agent throughout the tissue engineered construct.

52.7.5 Specific Issues Related to Joint Reconstruction

Since a tissue engineered construct is composed of biological tissue, consideration must be given to the original disease process or joint loading patterns that initially produced a dysfunctional joint. If parafunctional forces exist, strategies to decrease joint loading must be employed. These include the use of dental orthotic devices, which reduce forces generated by the muscles of mastication and provide protective responses through neuromuscular afferent signals from the periodontium surrounding the teeth.

Another challenge is the maintenance of construct viability following implantation. In order to survive, cells require nutrients diffusing from the surrounding vasculature and a method to remove metabolic waste. Establishing a vascular supply in a tissue engineered construct is critical, especially for vascular tissues like bones. Fortunately, fibrocartilage has even lower metabolic requirements, an advantage where TMJ reconstruction is concerned. A separate concern involves the creation and connection of the nervous system in a tissue engineered construct to guide the complex movements of the joint and provide proprioceptive input to the neuromuscular system. Meeting this requirement is important for the return of normal function to the reconstructed joint. It may be possible to utilize native tissue for these two functions, if efforts are made at the time of joint or disc removal to preserve the capsule, synovium, and vascular supply from the bony resection margins. When these structures are compromised, such as the case with multiply operated patients, the success of any reconstruction diminishes. Avoidance of multiple surgeries should therefore be part of the overall strategy for using tissue engineering to provide improved results compared to current modalities.

There are also concerns with the immunogenicity of tissue engineered constructs if nonautologous cells and a synthetic matrix are used for the construct. This is especially significant if xenogeneic sources are employed. Possible sources for TMJ cells include the contralateral joint, provided that it is not also diseased. Alternatively, fibroblasts and fibrochondrocytes, the lineages found in TMJ tissue, may be harvested from another fibrocartilaginous joint such as the sternoclavicular joint. It should be kept in mind that biological tissue is capable of varying degrees of adaptation according to the local environment. While this tenet has not been explored in tissue engineering reconstruction of the TMJ, it would not be unreasonable to expect that an engineered construct composed of cells from other diarthrodial joints or cartilaginous structures are capable of phenotypical transformation into cells more closely resembling those of the native TMJ. The successful use of such unrelated tissues as scar bands, fascia, auricular cartilage, costochondral cartilage, dermis, and fat support this contention.

The time required to create a viable tissue engineered construct for the reconstruction of a disc or total joint must also be considered. At this stage, an estimation of the period necessary for the population of an implant with sufficient cells of the desired lineage with properties suitable for handling, surgical implantation and attachment, is unknown. While TMJ reconstruction is generally an elective procedure, it would be unreasonable to consider tissue engineering techniques requiring more than several months as viable alternatives to current modalities.

Another important concern focuses on the ability to stabilize a construct within the joint. Even after the successful creation of replacement tissue, the implant must be anchored to existing structures. To facilitate this process, the implant must possess sufficient bulk, surface area, strength, and tenacity to attach it to the remaining skeleton. Current methods for repositioning a disc include the use of sutures threaded through holes made in the adjacent bone or attaching it to bone anchors such as the Mitek® device inserted into the condylar head. Single point attachment of structures which usually require circumferential fixation for positional anchorage are inherently unstable. Methods for providing multiple attachments of a disc replacement need to be developed for successful function to be restored. This is especially true when the zonal differences and functional properties of each zone are considered. Attachment of a condylar or fossa engineered implant is a little easier, provided that the construct possesses sufficient bulk and strength. Bone plates and screws are currently available for the fixation of skeletal structures and these could be used for a tissue engineered construct.

With the reconstruction of a joint, lubrication of the articulating surfaces must be considered. This function is normally performed by the synovial fluid, but the effects of disease or surgery may compromise the normal secretion and composition of the fluid available. Synthetic adjuvants, such as hyaluronic acid substitutes, may be used in conjunction with joint replacement procedures to protect the implant from unwanted forces, while the synovium heals.

The last issue concerning the successful application of tissue engineering techniques for the reconstruction of TMJ components concerns the unavoidable consequences of any surgical maneuver, specifically the development of intra-articular scars. Steroid injections can help reduce this natural consequence of surgery, but perhaps the most effective results are seen through the fastidious employment of postoperative physical therapy exercises. These maneuvers promote the formation of long vs. short, scars. They also encourage the necessary plasmatic diffusion of fluids responsible for joint nutrition and metabolism.

52.7.6 The Future of Tissue Engineering in the TMJ

The challenges associated with tissue engineering are immense, but the benefit of utilizing tailored biological constructs without the morbidity of an autogenous donor site, are obvious. Tissue engineered initiatives for the reconstruction of the TMJ and disc avoids the problems associated with the implantation of prosthetic devices or tissues dissimilar from natural joint components. Efforts toward tissue engineering in the TMJ are relatively new, however, emergent technologies and studies add promise to the goal of tissue engineering TMJ replacement tissues. Along the way, characteristics about TMJ tissues are revealed and our comprehension of this complex joint's function and structure increases. Solutions for several challenges facing biomedical engineers will be developed with each progressive study. Currently, TMJ tissue engineering is in its formative years. Only four original studies on tissue engineering of the TMJ disc had been published at the date of this article's submission. However, the future promises new knowledge and innovative technologies which may yet allow for the creation of viable, implantable tissue engineered constructs.

References

[1] Dolwick, M.F. (1983) The temporomandibular joint: normal and abnormal anatomy. In *Internal Derangements of the Temporomandibular Joint* (Helms, C.A. et al., eds.), pp. 1–14, Radiology Research and Education Foundation.

[2] Gillbe, G.V. (1975) The function of the disc of the temporomandibular joint. *J. Prosthet. Dent.* 33, 196–204.

[3] Detamore, M.S. and Athanasiou, K.A. (2003) Motivation, characterization, and strategy for tissue engineering the temporomandibular joint disc. *Tissue Eng.* 9, 1065–1087.

[4] Rees, L.A. (1954) The structure and function of the mandibular joint. *Br. Dent. J.* 96, 125–133.

[5] Gallo, L.M. et al. (2000) Stress-field translation in the healthy human temporomandibular joint. *J. Dent. Res.* 79, 1740–1746.

[6] Zimny, M.L. (1988) Mechanoreceptors in articular tissues. *Am. J. Anat.* 182, 16–32.

[7] Hills, B.A. and Monds, M.K. (1998) Enzymatic identification of the load-bearing boundary lubricant in the joint. *Br. J. Rheumatol.* 37, 137–142.

[8] Minarelli, A.M. et al. (1997) The structure of the human temporomandibular joint disc: a scanning electron microscopy study. *J Orofac. Pain* 11, 95–100.

[9] Minarelli, A.M. and Liberti, E.A. (1997) A microscopic survey of the human temporomandibular joint disc. *J. Oral Rehabil.* 24, 835–840.

[10] Detamore, M.S. et al. (2004) Quantitive analysis and comparative regional investigation of the extracellular matrix of the porcine temporomandibular joint disc. *Matrix Biol.* 24, 45–57.

[11] Berkovitz, B.K. and Pacy, J. (2000) Age changes in the cells of the intra-articular disc of the temporomandibular joints of rats and marmosets. *Arch. Oral Biol.* 45, 987–995.

[12] Mills, D.K. et al. (1994) Morphologic, microscopic, and immunohistochemical investigations into the function of the primate TMJ disc. *J. Orofac Pain.* 8, 136–154.

[13] Landesberg, R. et al. (1996) Cellular, biochemical and molecular characterization of the bovine temporomandibular joint disc. *Arch. Oral Biol.* 41, 761–767.

[14] Detamore, M.S. et al. (2003) Cell type and distribution in the porcine temporomandibular joint disc. *J. Oral Maxillofac. Surg.* Accepted.

[15] Milam, S.B. et al. (1991) Characterization of the extracellular matrix of the primate temporomandibular joint. *J. Oral Maxillofac. Surg.* 49, 381–391.

[16] Kondoh, T. et al. (1998) Prevalence of morphological changes in the surfaces of the temporomandibular joint disc associated with internal derangement. *J. Oral Maxillofac Surg.* 56, 339–343; discussion 343–334.

[17] Keith, D.A. (1979) Elastin in the bovine mandibular joint. *Arch. Oral Biol.* 24, 211–215.

[18] Detamore, M.S. et al. (2003) Structure and function of the temporomandibular joint disc: implications for tissue engineering. *J. Oral Maxillofac. Surg.: Offic. J. Am. Assoc. Oral Maxillofac. Surg.* 61, 494–506.

[19] Gross, A. et al. (1999) Elastic fibers in the human temporo-mandibular joint disc. *Int. J. Oral Maxillofac. Surg.* 28, 464–468.

[20] Almarza, A.J. et al. (2005) Biochemical content and distribution in the porcine temporomandibular joint disc. *Br. J. Oral Maxillofac. Surg.*

[21] Nakano, T. and Scott, P.G. (1989) A quantitative chemical study of glycosaminoglycans in the articular disc of the bovine temporomandibular joint. *Arch. Oral Biol.* 34, 749–757.

[22] Nakano, T. and Scott, P.G. (1989) Proteoglycans of the articular disc of the bovine temporomandibular joint. I. High molecular weight chondroitin sulphate proteoglycan. *Matrix* 9, 277–283.

[23] Sindelar, B.J. et al. (2000) Effects of intraoral splint wear on proteoglycans in the temporomandibular joint disc. *Arch. Biochem. Biophys.* 379, 64–70.

[24] Axelsson, S. et al. (1992) Glycosaminoglycans in normal and osteoarthrotic human temporomandibular joint disks. *Acta Odontol. Scand.* 50, 113–119.

[25] Scott, P.G. et al. (1989) Proteoglycans of the articular disc of the bovine temporomandibular joint. II. Low molecular weight dermatan sulphate proteoglycan. *Matrix* 9, 284–292.

[26] Nakano, T. and Scott, P.G. (1996) Changes in the chemical composition of the bovine temporomandibular joint disc with age. *Arch. Oral Biol.* 41, 845–853.

[27] Gage, J.P. et al. (1995) Collagen type in dysfunctional temporomandibular joint disks. *J. Prosthet. Dent.* 74, 517–520.

[28] Allen, K.D. and Athanasiou, K.A. (2005) A surface-regional and freeze-thaw characterization of the porcine temporomandibular joint disc. *Ann. Biomed. Eng.* 33, 859–897.

[29] Detamore, M.S. et al. (2003) Tensile properties of the porcine temporomandibular joint disc. *J. Biomech. Eng.* 125, 558–565.

[30] del Pozo, R. et al. (2002) The regional difference of viscoelastic property of bovine temporomandibular joint disc in compressive stress-relaxation. *Med. Eng. Phys.* 24, 165–171.

[31] Kim, K.W. et al. (2003) Biomechanical characterization of the superior joint space of the porcine temporomandibular joint. *Ann. Biomed. Eng.* 31, 924–930.

[32] Berteretche, M.V. et al. (2001) Histologic changes associated with experimental partial anterior disc displacement in the rabbit temporomandibular joint. *J. Orofac. Pain* 15, 306–319.

[33] Hinton, R. et al. (2002) Osteoarthritis: diagnosis and Therapeutic Considerations. *Am. Family Phys.* 65, 841–847.

[34] Feinberg, S.E. et al. (2001) Image-based biomimetic approach to reconstruction of the temporomandibular joint. *Cells Tissues Organs* 169, 309–321.

[35] Temenoff, J.S. et al. (2004) Thermally cross-linked oligo(poly(ethylene glycol) fumarate) hydrogels support osteogenic differentiation of encapsulated marrow stromal cells *in vitro*. *Biomacromolecules* 5, 5–10.

[36] Fisher, J.P. et al. (2004) Effect of biomaterial properties on bone healing in a rabbit tooth extraction socket model. *J. Biomed. Mater. Res.* 68A, 428–438.

[37] Holland, T.A. et al. (2004) Transforming growth factor-beta1 release from oligo(poly(ethylene glycol) fumarate) hydrogels in conditions that model the cartilage wound healing environment. *J. Controll. Release: Offic. J. Control. Release Soc.* 94, 101–114.

[38] Chai, Y. et al. (2000) Fate of the mammalian cranial neural crest during tooth and mandibular morphogenesis. *Development* 127, 1671–1679.

[39] Almarza, A.J. and Athanasiou, K. (2004) Seeding techniques and scaffolding choice for the tissue engineering of the temporomandibular joint disc. *Tissue Eng.* 10, 1787–1795.

[40] Poshusta, A.K. and Anseth, K.S. (2001) Photopolymerized biomaterials for application in the temporomandibular joint. *Cells Tissues Organs* 169, 272–278.

[41] Behravesh, E. et al. (2003) Three-dimensional culture of differentiating marrow stromal osteoblasts in biomimetic poly(propylene fumarate-co-ethylene glycol)-based macroporous hydrogels. *J. Biomed. Mater. Res.* 66A, 698–706.

[42] Weng, Y. et al. (2001) Tissue-engineered composites of bone and cartilage for mandible condylar reconstruction. *J. Oral Maxillofac. Surg.: Offic. J. Am. Assoc. Oral Maxillofac. Surg.* 59, 185–190.

[43] Roux, F.X. et al. (1988) Madreporic coral: a new bone graft substitute for cranial surgery. *J. Neurosurg.* 69, 510–513.

[44] Lu, H.H. et al. (2003) Three-dimensional, bioactive, biodegradable, polymer-bioactive glass composite scaffolds with improved mechanical properties support collagen synthesis and mineralization of human osteoblast-like cells *in vitro*. *J. Biomed. Mater. Res.* 64A, 465–474.

[45] Ma, P.X. and Langer, R. (1999) Morphology and mechanical function of long-term *in vitro* engineered cartilage. *J. Biomed. Mater. Res.* 44, 217–221.

53

Engineering Smooth Muscle

Yu Ching Yung
University of Michigan

David J. Mooney
University of Michigan
Harvard University

53.1 Introduction

Tissue engineering has emerged over the past two decades to address the growing need for biological substitutes to restore or replace damaged tissues and organs [1]. Current approaches to organ repair rely primarily on transplantation of whole or partial organs and tissues from autogeneic, allogeneic, and less frequently, xenogeneic sources. The imbalance of need versus availability of organs poses as a significant and inherent limitation to this method [2]. Tissue engineering promises an alternative via rebuilding tissues or organs from targeted cell populations, often with the participation of matrices that guide tissue regeneration while providing specific instructions with signaling molecules.

Diseases related to the malfunction of cardiovascular, gastrointestinal and urinary tissues account for millions of deaths annually [1], and smooth muscle (SM) tissue has a critical role in the structure and function of a number of these tissues. In blood vessels of the cardiovascular system, the smooth muscle cell (SMC) component (medial layer) provides mechanical strength and elasticity. SM tissue plays a key role in the gastrointestinal system through its ability to drive the transport of solids and liquids, and malfunction of these tissues typically result in malnutrition. The SM in the intestinal tract, in contrast to SM tissue in blood vessels, is organized in two layers of opposing orientation, and provides for propulsive movements of food through peristalsis. The SM of the bladder also regulates the reservoir function of this tissue, as it controls the storage and release of urine. In all of these tissues, the SMCs contain a highly organized structure of actin and myosin filaments that allow the cells to efficiently modulate and respond to a mechanically dynamic environment and regulate the operation of the organ. A functional smooth muscle component will be critical to the success of engineered tissues intended to replace any of these tissues or organs.

53.2 Cell Source

A critical question in the engineering of smooth muscle tissues is the appropriate source of the SMCs that will comprise the tissue. The majority of research to date has utilized smooth muscle procured from the tissue of interest. However, the isolation of smooth muscle progenitors may allow for a less invasive and destructive approach. In addition, it may be possible to directly recruit SMCs to the site at which one wants a tissue to form.

53.2.1 Differentiated SMCs

The most direct approach to form smooth muscle tissues is to utilize SMCs obtained from the tissue that one desires to engineer. In this approach, smooth muscle containing tissue is typically explanted and dissociated into individual cells. The cells are then directly transplanted or expanded in culture, and subsequently transplanted (Figure 53.1a,b). Direct transplantation may be advantageous as it bypasses *in vitro* culturing, which can alter the contractile phenotype of SMCs. In contrast, culture of SMCs prior to transplantation may lead to phenotypic changes [3,4], but this approach allows one to greatly expand the cell population. This may allow a relatively small explant to ultimately yield sufficient cells to engineer a large tissue. The phenotypic changes noted in SMCs, as they revert to a synthetic phenotype [5] may be reversed or prevented through appropriate culture conditions (i.e., cyclic mechanical loading) [6].

Although smooth muscle tissues characteristically contain contractile apparatus and form the muscular components of visceral structures, there are differences between SM in various tissues [7]. These likely relate to the specific microenvironment and physiology of each tissue type. For this reason, SM biopsies are typically procured for the specific type of tissue being engineered. The artery is the most commonly excised tissue for vascular regeneration [8–11] primarily because it is the largest blood vessel, and hence contains the thickest medial layer. Current methods for bladder replacement require a biopsy to obtain

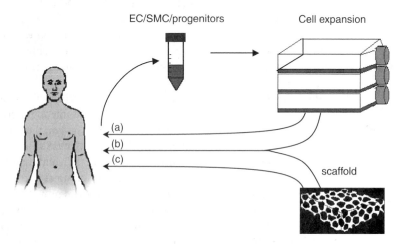

FIGURE 53.1 Scheme of approaches to engineer SM tissue. (a) The direct cell transplantation approach first involves the procurement of the appropriate cell types for the tissue of interest (e.g., EC, SM, or progenitor cells). The cells are typically expanded in culture, and induced to differentiate into SMCs before implantation if necessary. (b) Alternatively, the expanded cells may be seeded onto a scaffold, and subsequently implanted as a cell–matrix construct. (c) Third, acellular matrices may be implanted without seeded cells, and in this situation one relies on the recruitment of neighboring SMCs or progenitors to infiltrate scaffold and form the new SM tissue.

a small specimen of the donor or host bladder tissue, which is then used to expand separate cultures of urothelial and SMCs [12]. Ureter or renal pelvis cells can be similarly harvested. Regeneration of gastrointestinal organs, specifically the stomach and the intestine, has most commonly utilized organoid units which contain SM precursors [13,14].

Differentiated SMCs have shown tremendous utility for the successful regeneration of SM tissues. However the invasive nature of this cell procurement, the inherent limited proliferation capability of primary cells, and maintenance of smooth muscle phenotype are all limitations to this cell source.

53.2.2 Smooth Muscle Progenitor Cells

Smooth muscle progenitors may potentially be isolated using minimally invasive techniques, and subsequently induced to differentiate down a smooth muscle lineage. Cells isolated from bone marrow are termed bone marrow stromal cells (BMSCs), or mesenchymal stem cells (MSCs) depending on the mode of cell purification selection *in vitro*.

Bone marrow can be obtained easily from the medullary canals of long bones or the cancellous cavities [15], and the resultant BMSC can be readily expanded in culture. BMSCs have demonstrated the ability to differentiate into multiple mesenchymal cell lineages, and offer an alternative source of SMCs [7,16–23]. Recent studies have shown that BMSCs are inducible down a smooth muscle pathway, and this process is regulated by an interplay between stimulatory molecules [24,25], with TGF-β and PDGF as the main modulators [24]. Mechanical stimulation has also been shown to effect differentiation of bone marrow stromal cells [26]. However, the mechanism of this effect is still unclear. SM progenitors can also be derived from embryonic stem cells [27,28], circulating blood [29,30], bone marrow [31,32], and other tissues [33].

53.2.3 Recruitment of SMCs

The recruitment of SMCs or progenitors from a surrounding tissue to an engineered tissue provides an alternative to SM transplantation (Figure 53.1c). Signaling molecules such as PDGF and TGF-β have chemotactic effects on SMCs [34], and growth factors (Figure 53.2) released by endothelial cells (ECs) can also induce the migration of MSCs and their subsequent differentiation into SM like cells [35,36]. Similarly, myoblast recruitment can be modulated by a gradient of a chemotactic agent [37]. This recruitment approach greatly simplifies the process of SM tissue engineering, as it eliminates the isolation and expansion of cells *in vitro*. In addition, this approach could have utility in applications such as blood

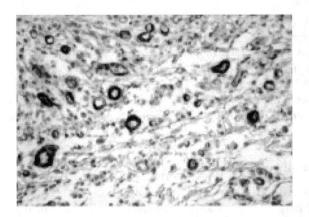

FIGURE 53.2 Sustained and localized delivery of PDGF can lead to the recruitment of SMCs to nascent blood vessels. Photomicrograph of tissue section stained using standard immunohistochemical techniques to detect (brown stain) cells containing α-SMA (SMCs) associating with blood vessels. (Photomicrograph was taken from Richardson, T.P. et al., *Nat. Biotechnol.*, 2001, **19**: 1029–1034 used with permission from the Nature Publishing Group.)

vessel repair where direct placement of smooth cells in the lumen could cause a thrombogenic effect. The use of signaling molecules to recruit circulating progenitor cells may provide a useful alternative in this situation.

53.3 Extracellular Signaling

The extracellular environment plays a pivotal role in SM tissue engineering by providing instructions to the SMCs. Both signaling molecules and mechanical stimuli similar to that found in the native extracellular environment of SM tissues may be used to induce specific SM responses.

Mitogenic factors that have shown to possess a significant effect on SMCs in culture include platelet derived growth factor (PDGF), TGF-β, angiopoietin, and to a lesser extent, heparin-binding epidermal growth factor (HB-EGF) and fibroblast growth factor-2 (FGF-2) [38,39]. PDGF has been shown to have potent effects on proliferation, migration, and matrix production by SMCs [27,28,34,35,37,40–42] and potentially has a significant role in cell transplantation where SMC proliferation is necessary. An increase in the synthesis of SM extracellular proteins is stimulated by TGF-β and these matrix components provide mechanical integrity to engineered SM tissues [34,36,43–48]. Particularly in strategies where SM recruitment is important, angiopoietin and HB–EGF have both shown to mediate EC and SMC interactions [39,49–51]. However, SM tissue engineering strategies that utilize growth factors must consider the mode of delivery. Polymeric encapsulation of growth factors is a common approach to deliver the molecules to the developing SM tissues in a controlled and sustained manner [52].

Mechanical signals modulate the phenotype of SMCs [40,53,54] and enhance the development and function of engineered tissues [55–57]. Cyclic mechanical strain of engineered SM tissues [53,56] result in an increase of matrix production and increased mechanical strength. These mechanical signals are transmitted intracellularly though various signaling pathways that initiate at the transmembrane receptors known as integrins [58], which link the extracellular matrix to the cytoskeleton [59,60]. Integrins activate mitogen activated protein kinase (MAPK) cascades via signaling through extracellular signal-regulated kinase (ERK) [60–63], either through focal adhesion kinases (FAKs) or through coactivation of growth factor receptors (GFRs). Cyclic mechanical strain increases levels of focal contact components [64], which may increase integrin clustering [61], and provide a potential mechanism for the role of mechanical signals in activation of FAKs. It is currently unclear whether these pathways act synergistically with growth factor stimulation, but optimal development and function of engineered SM tissues will likely require appropriate chemical and mechanical signals.

53.4 Synthetic Extracellular Matrix

Tissue engineering utilizes synthetic extracellular matrices (ECMs) to provide an infrastructure for the formation of tissues by providing a predefined space to localize tissue growth and the mechanical support necessary to facilitate this growth. Synthetic ECMs may also provide specific signals to the SMCs. Two general designs of synthetic ECMs for SM tissue regeneration are being pursued, one involving a biological approach where the matrix is assembled by the resident cells and the other utilizing predefined polymeric structures.

53.4.1 Self-Assembly

SMCs maintained for extended times in culture will synthesize, secrete, and assemble an ECM with sufficient mechanical integrity to allow a sheet of confluent SMCs to be manipulated and formed into a three-dimensional tissue [65]. This technique is attractive for tissue engineering because it eliminates the need for exogenous biomaterials, and thereby eradicates any potential inflammatory issues related to the material [66,67]. Self-assembly approaches have focused on engineering vascular grafts by individually culturing cellular sheets to model the defined layers of the blood vessel. A sheet of SMCs is used to form the medial layer, which is subsequently wrapped with a sheet composed of fibroblasts to form the adventitial layer, and finally seeded with endothelial cells to create the lumen. Initial studies on tissues formed utilizing this approach reported poor mechanical strength [68,69], which is indicative of a deficient medial and, or adventitial layers. A revised approach increased the mechanical strength of tissues formed with this approach [65]. However, a limitation to this approach is the extensive time required to form the cellular sheets.

53.4.2 Polymer Scaffolds: Synthetic and Naturally Derived

Most approaches to engineer SM tissues have utilized three-dimensional, biodegradable polymeric scaffolds. Polymeric scaffolds formed from exogenous biomaterials provide mechanical stability and can deliver signaling molecules or adhesion peptides to induce appropriate tissue development. These polymeric biomaterials are fabricated from either synthetic or naturally derived materials. Synthetic polymers typically used for engineering SM tissues include several forms of polyesters, elastomeric polymers, and hydrogels. The most common used naturally derived polymer used to engineer SMC is type I collagen.

53.4.2.1 Synthetic Polymers

The most prevalent synthetic polymers used to engineer smooth muscle tissues are the polyesters poly(glycolic acid) (PGA) (Figure 53.3a), poly(L-lactic acid) (PLLA), and poly (lactic-co-glycolic acid) (PLGA). Advantageous features of these polymers include their reproducible and readily altered mechanical properties and degradation rates [70,71]. These polymer scaffolds provide temporary mechanical support [72] sufficient to resist cellular contractile forces *in vitro* [73–76], and scaffolds exhibiting partial elastic properties under cyclic strain enabled induction of a more contractile, differentiated smooth muscle phenotype from attached SMCs [56]. In addition to structural stability, appropriate signals may be required to guide the development of smooth muscle tissues. Synthetic polymers can be modified to incorporate signals to alter cellular function, including cell adhesion molecules [77–79] and growth factors [80,81].

Hydrogel forming polymers have also been investigated for engineering SM tissues. Polyethylene glycol (PEG) hydrogels intrinsically resist protein adsorption and cell adhesion [82] and this characteristic

(a) 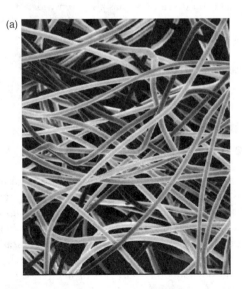 (b)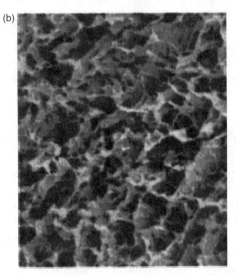

FIGURE 53.3 Scanning electron photomicrographs of typical polymeric scaffolds utilized for engineering SM tissue. (a) PGA fiber based scaffold, and (b) type I collagen scaffold. (Photomicrograph was taken from Kim, B.S. and D.J. Mooney, *J. Biomech. Eng.*, 2000, **122**: 210–215; Kim, B.S. and D.J. Mooney, *J. Biomed. Mater. Res.*, 1998, **41**: 322–332, and used with permission from John Wiley & Sons and ASME, respectively.)

offers advantages for studying the effects of specific bioactive ligands or peptides presented from the scaffold [83,84]. Studies utilizing surface modified PEGs have demonstrated that a number of cellular functions, including adhesion [83], migration [85], and matrix production [46] can be regulated by ligand presentation. In general, hydrogels are an appealing scaffold material because they are structurally similar to the highly hydrated ECM of many tissues [86]. However, the use of hydrogels is often constrained by their limited range of mechanical properties.

The elasticity provided by elastin in SM tissues has motivated the development of elastomeric scaffolds that can similarly provide this property to engineered SM. Elastomeric polymers can recover from extensive deformation [87–89] and are designed to resemble the incompressible nature of the ECM [90]. This property of biomaterials may be ideal to engineer functional SM tissues that require transduction of mechanical signals from the extracellular environment in order to elicit and activate key cellular functions [40,53,54]. This type of biomaterial resolves the limitations of lack of pliancy that limits many synthetic polymer scaffolds (i.e., poly[lactic acid] [PLA]).

53.4.2.2 Naturally Derived Biomaterials

Type I collagen (Figure 53.3b) has been frequently used to create polymer scaffolds for engineering SM tissues [56,73,91,92]. Naturally derived collagen is an attractive biologic material because collagen is the primary constituent of the ECM [58], and contains adhesion ligands that facilitate cell attachment. Although type I collagen does not require additional surface modification to promote tissue formation, glycosaminoglycans (GAGs) [93] and growth factors [45] can be incorporated to improve mechanical properties and to induce specific cellular functions. Type I collagen matrices used to engineer SM tissues have demonstrated partial elasticity and are capable of withstanding cyclic stain [56]. The high tensile strength of type I collagen can be attributed to its molecular structure, while the elasticity is conferred by the intermolecular cross-linking. The degradation of type I collagen scaffolds is dependent on the extent of cross-linking, pore structure and the apparent density, which are variables that can be readily altered to meet a desired target. Although type I collagen is typically extracted from xenogeneic sources, it is considered biocompatible and exhibits low immunogenic responses, likely due to the similarity of this molecule between species [94]. However, naturally derived materials may suffer from batch to batch variations.

Another collagen based biomaterial, small intestinal submucosa (SIS), has also been widely used in tissue engineering research [95–97]. This xenogeneic matrix is harvested from the submucosal layer of the intestine. SIS may provide functional growth factors [98]. that contribute to SM tissue formation. In addition, SIS matrices maintain elasticity and high strength [99]. SIS has typically been obtained from porcine sources, but isolation from rats [100] and canines [101] has also been attempted. SIS has been used to promote regeneration of several SM tissues, in the blood vessels [102,103] and in the bladder [99,101,104].

53.5 Engineered Smooth Muscle Tissues

A number of studies to date have utilized a combination of scaffolding technologies and cells to reconstruct the smooth muscle component of cardiovascular, gastrointestinal, and urinary tissues. The two primary tissue-engineering approaches used to regenerate tissues are cell transplantation and cell recruitment from surrounding tissue. Cell transplantation requires an initial step of procuring cells, often via biopsy from the host, followed by dissociation and expansion *in vitro*. The cells are then seeded onto a scaffold and implanted as a cell–matrix construct. Alternatively, an implanted acellular matrix may be implanted to promote the recruitment of neighboring SMCs and possibly other cell types of interest (e.g., ECs, urothelial cells). Work to date in engineering SM tissues is briefly summarized in this section.

A great deal of research has been performed with the goal of developing blood vessel substitutes, due to the large impact this advance would have on the millions of patients that annually suffer from diseases of blood vessels [105]. Strategies to engineer blood vessel must provide adequate mechanical properties,

(a) 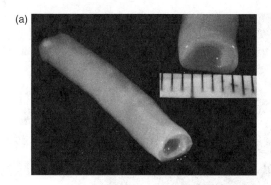   (b)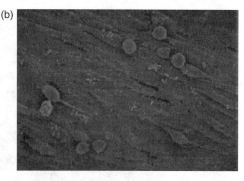

FIGURE 53.4 Engineered blood vessel substitutes. (a) Self-assembly approach to blood vessel formation relies on the ability of sheets of cells to form their own ECM, and multiple cells sheets can subsequently be combined to form tissues (b) Cyclic mechanical strain can play a prominent role in the development of engineered vascular tissues, as it can lead to alignment of cells, as shown in this photomicrograph, and also leads to an increase in tissue mechanical properties. (Photomicrograph was taken from Kim, B.S. et al., *Nat. Biotechnol.*, 1999, **17**: 979–983; L'Heureux, N. et al., *FASEB J.*, 1998, **12**: 47–56, and used with permission from FASEB and the Nature Publishing Group, respectively.)

to avoid catastrophic failure in this mechanically demanding site, and appropriate cellular components to form the complex vascular wall. An early approach to engineer the blood vessels involved the culture of different vascular cell populations in collagen gels to form three distinct layers, resembling the three layers of native blood vessel [68]. However, this model did not lead to tissues with adequate mechanical strength. A later approach exploited the ability of fibroblasts and SM cells to synthesize and secrete their own ECM and form self assembled sheets. These sheets were subsequently wrapped around a mandrel to form distinct layers of the native vessels [65] (Figure 53.4a). This method led to tissues with much greater mechanical strength, comparable to that of human vessels [69]. The increased mechanical strength of these tissues my be partially attributed to paracrine effects between ECs and SMCs [35,39,51] that contribute to the stability of nascent blood vessels by increasing matrix production. Also, implantation of a decellularized SIS with additional type I bovine collagen into a rabbit artery led to the formation of a blood vessel characterized by reasonable burst strength, cell and matrix organization [102].

Several groups have utilized externally applied mechanical stimulation to improve the mechanical integrity of engineered SM tissues (Figure 53.4b). Blood vessel substitutes formed from allogeneic vascular SMCs and ECs cultured on biodegradable PGA scaffolds were maintained under pulsatile stress, and this resulted in an increased matrix production [57]. These engineered constructs were subsequently implanted into swine for seven weeks and the explanted vessels exhibited adequate burst pressures and histology. Several studies document that one can improve the properties of constructs engineered using collagen through the use of mechanical stimulation [55,106]. The significance of mechanical stimulation was also demonstrated by studies where synthetic SMCs cultured with ECs on collagen gels were found to undergo a phenotypic reversion under contractile forces [5,107].

Currently, a common approach to replace or repair bladder tissue utilizes gastrointestinal segments, but this method can result in mucus production, stone formation, and other abnormalities that may be attributed to the different physiologic role of each tissue type. These complications have motivated investigation into new methods for bladder replacement utilizing tissue engineering techniques. One common acellular approach to engineer bladder tissue utilizes SIS membranes, as SIS membranes grafted during partial cystectomy of canines have displayed development of all three layers of the bladder (urothelium, SM, and serosa) [95]. Additionally, these regenerated tissues demonstrated contractile nerve regeneration. Acellular biomaterial extracted from rat bladder also resulted in a well integrated construct when implanted, but one that developed a compromised SM layer [108]. While these studies utilizing acellular scaffold implantation resulted in bladder regeneration, but function of the resultant tissues was not reported. In contrast to this approach, PGA–PLGA scaffolds seeded with autologous canine cells led to formation of a new tissue (Figure 53.5) that regained bladder function [12].

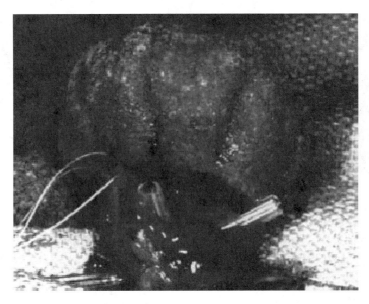

FIGURE 53.5 Engineered bladder formed from autologous cells cultured on polymeric scaffolds *in vitro*. The neo-bladders can be implanted to replace lost bladder tissue. (Photomicrograph was taken from Oberpenning, F. et al., *Nat. Biotechnol.*, 1999, **17**: 149–155, and used with permission from the Nature Publishing Group.)

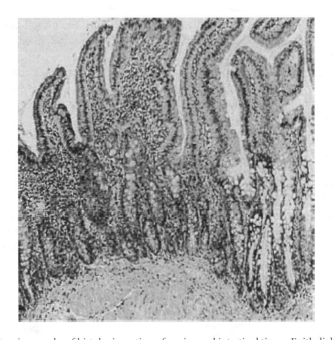

FIGURE 53.6 Photomicrographs of histologic section of engineered intestinal tissue. Epithelial organoid units were isolated, seeded onto polymeric scaffolds, and implanted. Ultimately, the transplanted cells differentiate and form new tissue. (Photomicrograph was taken from Vacanti, J.P., *J. Gastrointest. Surg.*, 2003, **7**: 831–835., and used with permission from Elsevier Inc.)

A number of studies suggest it may be feasible to engineer functional gastrointestinal tissues. Isolated crypt cells implanted on PGA tubes formed epithelial-lined tubular structures lacking in a SM component [109] (Figure 53.6). The transplantation of intestinal organoid units, in place of individual cells on PLGA scaffolds led to the development of a neomucosa layer [14] and SM layers [109]. However, the neomucosa may have been lacking in its ability to control nutrient. SIS patch implantation, without cells, into canines led to formation of both the epithelial and SM layer. However, a large percentage of animals died and a large number of inflammatory cells were found in explanted SIS patches. One study utilized transplantation of precursor cells derived from bone marrow in the place of differentiated SMCs [110], but the engineered tissues did not regenerate a functional muscle layer, potentially due to a lack of appropriate extracellular signals to induce the differentiation of the mesenchymal stem cells into SMCs.

53.6   Conclusion/Future Directions

Impressive progress has been made to date in SM engineering, and these tissues may have significant clinical impact and provide models to study basic biological processes. However our current understanding of the complex interplay of factors that modulate the SM function are far from comprehensive, and advances in this knowledge will likely translate to improved systems for engineering functional SM tissues. One important issue yet to be addressed is whether approaches that successfully regenerate one type of SM tissue will necessarily be successful for other organ systems. Physiologically, there are distinct differences between the SM in cardiovascular, gastrointestinal, and urinary tissues. Similar approaches have been utilized to date in most SM engineering approaches. However, inherent differences exist in the microenvironment of different SM tissues that may have a significant effect on the developing SM tissue. The substratum to which SMCs adhere also plays an important role in the presentation of paracrine signals and that may regulate SMC phenotype [35,37,111]. An ideal cell source is also currently lacking, but stem cells may fill this need. BMSCs contain a population of SM progenitors, but the difficulties in reproducibly isolating and regulating the differentiation of these cell populations pose as an obstacle to their use. Embryonic stem cells may provide a more homogeneous population of pluripotential cells, but these cells have not yet been demonstrated to form functional SM tissue. In addition, for engineered SM tissues to be truly functional, they must also be innervated and vascularized. Current research in the therapeutic angiogenesis field may provide methods to induce formation of vascular networks [81]. However, development of fully functional SM tissues will also require a means to transduce neural signals critical for blood vessel vasoactivity.

References

[1]   Langer, R. and J.P. Vacanti, Tissue engineering. *Science*, 1993, **260**: 920–926.
[2]   Gridelli, B. and G. Remuzzi, Strategies for making more organs available for transplantation. *N. Engl. J. Med.*, 2000, **343**: 404–410.
[3]   Owens, G.K., Regulation of differentiation of vascular smooth muscle cells. *Physiol. Rev.*, 1995, **75**: 487–517.
[4]   Campbell, J.H. and G.R. Campbell, *Vascular Smooth Muscle in Culture*. Boca Raton, FL: CRC Press, 2 vol, 1987.
[5]   Kanda, K., H. Miwa, and T. Matsuda, Phenotypic reversion of smooth muscle cells in hybrid vascular prostheses. *Cell Transplant.*, 1995, **4**: 587–595.
[6]   Nikolovski, J., B.S. Kim, and D.J. Mooney, Cyclic strain inhibits switching of smooth muscle cells to an osteoblast-like phenotype. *FASEB J.*, 2003, **17**: 455–457.
[7]   Young, B. et al., *Wheater's Functional Histology: A Text and Colour Atlas*. Churchill Livingstone: Edinburgh; New York, 2000.
[8]   Stegemann, J.P. and R.M. Nerem, Altered response of vascular smooth muscle cells to exogenous biochemical stimulation in two- and three-dimensional culture. *Exp. Cell Res.*, 2003, **283**: 146–155.
[9]   McKee, J.A. et al., Human arteries engineered *in vitro*. *EMBO Rep.*, 2003, **4**: 633–638.
[10] Stock, U.A. et al., Tissue engineering of heart valves — current aspects. *Thorac. Cardiovasc. Surg.*, 2002, **50**: 184–193.
[11] Shinoka, T. et al., Creation of viable pulmonary artery autografts through tissue engineering. *J. Thorac. Cardiovasc. Surg.*, 1998, **115**: 536–545; discussion 545–546.

[12] Oberpenning, F. et al., *De novo* reconstitution of a functional mammalian urinary bladder by tissue engineering. *Nat. Biotechnol.*, 1999, **17**: 149–155.

[13] Maemura, T. et al., A tissue-engineered stomach as a replacement of the native stomach. *Transplantation*, 2003, **76**: 61–65.

[14] Kaihara, S. et al., Long-term follow-up of tissue-engineered intestine after anastomosis to native small bowel. *Transplantation*, 2000, **69**: 1927–1932.

[15] Junqueira, L.C.U. and J. Carneiro, Basic Histology: Text & Atlas. 10th ed. 2003, New York: Lange Medical Books McGraw-Hill Medical Pub. Division, p. viii, 515.

[16] Pittenger, M.F. et al., Multilineage potential of adult human mesenchymal stem cells. *Science*, 1999, **284**: 143–147.

[17] Bianco, P. and P.G. Robey, Stem cells in tissue engineering. *Nature*, 2001, **414**: 118–121.

[18] Bianco, P. et al., Bone marrow stromal stem cells: nature, biology, and potential applications. *Stem Cells*, 2001, **19**: 180–192.

[19] Krebsbach, P.H. et al., Bone marrow stromal cells: characterization and clinical application. *Crit. Rev. Oral Biol. Med.*, 1999, **10**: 165–181.

[20] Ferrari, G. et al., Muscle regeneration by bone marrow-derived myogenic progenitors. *Science*, 1998, **279**: 1528–1530.

[21] Ferrari, G. and F. Mavilio, Myogenic stem cells from the bone marrow: a therapeutic alternative for muscular dystrophy? *Neuromuscul. Disord.*, 2002, **12**(Suppl 1): S7–S10.

[22] Hirschi, K.K. and M.A. Goodell, Hematopoietic, vascular and cardiac fates of bone marrow-derived stem cells. *Gene Ther.*, 2002, **9**: 648–652.

[23] Kadner, A. et al., A new source for cardiovascular tissue engineering: human bone marrow stromal cells. *Eur. J. Cardiothorac. Surg.*, 2002, **21**: 1055–1060.

[24] Dennis, J.E. and P. Charbord, Origin and differentiation of human and murine stroma. *Stem Cells*, 2002, **20**: 205–214.

[25] Kinner, B., J.M. Zaleskas, and M. Spector, Regulation of smooth muscle actin expression and contraction in adult human mesenchymal stem cells. *Exp. Cell Res.*, 2002, **278**: 72–83.

[26] Altman, G.H. et al., Cell differentiation by mechanical stress. *FASEB J.*, 2002, **16**: 270–272.

[27] Yamashita, J. et al., Flk1-positive cells derived from embryonic stem cells serve as vascular progenitors. *Nature*, 2000, **408**: 92–96.

[28] Koike, N. et al., Tissue engineering: creation of long-lasting blood vessels. *Nature*, 2004, **428**: 138–139.

[29] Han, C.I., G.R. Campbell, and J.H. Campbell, Circulating bone marrow cells can contribute to neointimal formation. *J. Vasc. Res.*, 2001, **38**: 113–119.

[30] Simper, D. et al., Smooth muscle progenitor cells in human blood. *Circulation*, 2002, **106**: 1199–1204.

[31] Sata, M. et al., Hematopoietic stem cells differentiate into vascular cells that participate in the pathogenesis of atherosclerosis. *Nat. Med.*, 2002, **8**: 403–409.

[32] Shimizu, K. et al., Host bone-marrow cells are a source of donor intimal smooth-muscle-like cells in murine aortic transplant arteriopathy. *Nat. Med.*, 2001, **7**: 738–741.

[33] Majka, S.M. et al., Distinct progenitor populations in skeletal muscle are bone marrow derived and exhibit different cell fates during vascular regeneration. *J. Clin. Invest.*, 2003, **111**: 71–79.

[34] Hirschi, K.K., S.A. Rohovsky, and P.A. D'Amore, PDGF, TGF-beta, and heterotypic cell–cell interactions mediate endothelial cell-induced recruitment of 10T1/2 cells and their differentiation to a smooth muscle fate. *J. Cell Biol.*, 1998, **141**: 805–814.

[35] Hirschi, K.K. et al., Endothelial cells modulate the proliferation of mural cell precursors via platelet-derived growth factor-BB and heterotypic cell contact. *Circ. Res.*, 1999, **84**: 298–305.

[36] Darland, D.C. and P.A. D'Amore, TGF beta is required for the formation of capillary-like structures in three-dimensional cocultures of 10T1/2 and endothelial cells. *Angiogenesis*, 2001, **4**: 11–20.

[37] Corti, S. et al., Chemotactic factors enhance myogenic cell migration across an endothelial monolayer. *Exp. Cell Res.*, 2001, **268**: 36–44.

[38] Adam, R.M. et al., Signaling through PI3K/Akt mediates stretch and PDGF-BB-dependent DNA synthesis in bladder smooth muscle cells. *J. Urol.*, 2003, **169**: 2388–2393.

[39] Iivanainen, E. et al., Angiopoietin-regulated recruitment of vascular smooth muscle cells by endothelial-derived heparin binding EGF-like growth factor. *FASEB J.*, 2003, **17**: 1609–1621.

[40] Stegemann, J.P. and R.M. Nerem, Phenotype modulation in vascular tissue engineering using biochemical and mechanical stimulation. *Ann. Biomed. Eng.*, 2003, **31**: 391–402.

[41] Hellstrom, M. et al., Role of PDGF-B and PDGFR-beta in recruitment of vascular smooth muscle cells and pericytes during embryonic blood vessel formation in the mouse. *Development*, 1999, **126**: 3047–3055.

[42] Stringa, E. et al., Collagen degradation and platelet-derived growth factor stimulate the migration of vascular smooth muscle cells. *J. Cell Sci.*, 2000, **113**(Pt 11): 2055–2064.

[43] Wrenn, R.W. et al., Transforming growth factor-beta: signal transduction via protein kinase C in cultured embryonic vascular smooth muscle cells. *In Vitro Cell Dev. Biol.*, 1993, **29A**: 73–78.

[44] Desmouliere, A. et al., Transforming growth factor-beta 1 induces alpha-smooth muscle actin expression in granulation tissue myofibroblasts and in quiescent and growing cultured fibroblasts. *J. Cell Biol.*, 1993, **122**: 103–111.

[45] Vaughan, M.B., E.W. Howard, and J.J. Tomasek, Transforming growth factor-beta1 promotes the morphological and functional differentiation of the myofibroblast. *Exp. Cell Res.*, 2000, **257**: 180–189.

[46] Mann, B.K., R.H. Schmedlen, and J.L. West, Tethered-TGF-beta increases extracellular matrix production of vascular smooth muscle cells. *Biomaterials*, 2001, **22**: 439–444.

[47] Hirschi, K.K. et al., Transforming growth factor-beta induction of smooth muscle cell phenotpye requires transcriptional and post-transcriptional control of serum response factor. *J. Biol. Chem.*, 2002, **277**: 6287–6295.

[48] Cutroneo, K.R., Gene therapy for tissue regeneration. *J. Cell Biochem.*, 2003, **88**: 418–425.

[49] Lobov, I.B., P.C. Brooks, and R.A. Lang, Angiopoietin-2 displays VEGF-dependent modulation of capillary structure and endothelial cell survival *in vivo*. *Proc. Natl Acad. Sci. USA*, 2002, **99**: 11205–11210.

[50] Du, L. et al., Signaling molecules in nonfamilial pulmonary hypertension. *N. Engl. J. Med.*, 2003, **348**: 500–509.

[51] Nishishita, T. and P.C. Lin, Angiopoietin 1, PDGF-B, and TGF-beta gene regulation in endothelial cell and smooth muscle cell interaction. *J. Cell Biochem.*, 2004, **91**: 584–593.

[52] Holland, T.A. et al., Transforming growth factor-beta1 release from oligo(poly(ethylene glycol) fumarate) hydrogels in conditions that model the cartilage wound healing environment. *J. Control. Release*, 2004, **94**: 101–114.

[53] Kim, B.S. et al., Cyclic mechanical strain regulates the development of engineered smooth muscle tissue. *Nat. Biotechnol.*, 1999, **17**: 979–983.

[54] Owens, G.K., Role of mechanical strain in regulation of differentiation of vascular smooth muscle cells. *Circ. Res.*, 1996, **79**: 1054–1055.

[55] Seliktar, D. et al., Dynamic mechanical conditioning of collagen-gel blood vessel constructs induces remodeling *in vitro*. *Ann. Biomed. Eng.*, 2000, **28**: 351–362.

[56] Kim, B.S. and D.J. Mooney, Scaffolds for engineering smooth muscle under cyclic mechanical strain conditions. *J. Biomech. Eng.*, 2000, **122**: 210–215.

[57] Niklason, L.E. et al., Functional arteries grown *in vitro*. *Science*, 1999, **284**: 489–493.

[58] Alberts, B., *Molecular Biology of the Cell*. 4th ed. New York: Garland Science, 2002.

[59] Davis, M.J. et al., Integrins and mechanotransduction of the vascular myogenic response. *Am. J. Physiol. Heart Circ. Physiol.*, 2001, **280**: H1427–H1433.

[60] Assoian, R.K. and M.A. Schwartz, Coordinate signaling by integrins and receptor tyrosine kinases in the regulation of G1 phase cell-cycle progression. *Curr. Opin. Genet. Dev.*, 2001, **11**: 48–53.

[61] Giancotti, F.G. and E. Ruoslahti, Integrin signaling. *Science*, 1999, **285**: 1028–1032.

[62] Schwartz, M.A. and M.H. Ginsberg, Networks and crosstalk: integrin signalling spreads. *Nat. Cell Biol.*, 2002, **4**: E65–E68.

[63] Howe, A.K., A.E. Aplin, and R.L. Juliano, Anchorage-dependent ERK signaling–mechanisms and consequences. *Curr. Opin. Genet. Dev.*, 2002, **12**: 30–35.

[64] Cunningham, J.J., J.J. Linderman, and D.J. Mooney, Externally applied cyclic strain regulates localization of focal contact components in cultured smooth muscle cells. *Ann. Biomed. Eng.*, 2002, **30**: 927–935.

[65] L'Heureux, N. et al., A completely biological tissue-engineered human blood vessel. *FASEB J.*, 1998, **12**: 47–56.

[66] Shin, H. et al., *In vivo* bone and soft tissue response to injectable, biodegradable oligo(poly(ethylene glycol) fumarate) hydrogels. *Biomaterials*, 2003, **24**: 3201–3211.

[67] Cao, Y. et al., Comparative study of the use of poly(glycolic acid), calcium alginate and pluronics in the engineering of autologous porcine cartilage. *J. Biomater. Sci. Polym. Ed.*, 1998, **9**: 475–487.

[68] Weinberg, C.B. and E. Bell, A blood vessel model constructed from collagen and cultured vascular cells. *Science*, 1986, **231**: 397–400.

[69] L'Heureux, N. et al., *In vitro* construction of a human blood vessel from cultured vascular cells: a morphologic study. *J. Vasc. Surg.*, 1993, **17**: 499–509.

[70] Thomson, R.C. et al., Fabrication of biodegradable polymer scaffolds to engineer trabecular bone. *J. Biomater. Sci. Polym. Ed.*, 1995, **7**: 23–38.

[71] Wong, W. and D. Mooney, Synthesis and properties of biodegradable polymers used in synthetic matrices for tissue engineering, In Atala, M.D., Ed., *Synthetic Biodegradable Polymer Scaffolds*, Birkhäuser: Boston. pp. 51–84, 1997.

[72] Mikos, A.G. et al., Laminated three-dimensional biodegradable foams for use in tissue engineering. *Biomaterials*, 1993, **14**: 323–330.

[73] Kim, B.S. and D.J. Mooney, Engineering smooth muscle tissue with a predefined structure. *J. Biomed. Mater. Res.*, 1998, **41**: 322–332.

[74] Peter, S.J. et al., Polymer concepts in tissue engineering. *J. Biomed. Mater. Res.*, 1998, **43**: 422–427.

[75] Niklason, L.E. and R.S. Langer, Advances in tissue engineering of blood vessels and other tissues. *Transpl. Immunol.*, 1997, **5**: 303–306.

[76] Mooney, D.J. et al., Stabilized polyglycolic acid fibre-based tubes for tissue engineering. *Biomaterials*, 1996, **17**: 115–124.

[77] Nikolovski, J. and D.J. Mooney, Smooth muscle cell adhesion to tissue engineering scaffolds. *Biomaterials*, 2000, **21**: 2025–2032.

[78] Mann, B.K. et al., Modification of surfaces with cell adhesion peptides alters extracellular matrix deposition. *Biomaterials*, 1999, **20**: 2281–2286.

[79] Gao, J., L. Niklason, and R. Langer, Surface hydrolysis of poly(glycolic acid) meshes increases the seeding density of vascular smooth muscle cells. *J. Biomed. Mater. Res.*, 1998, **42**: 417–424.

[80] Mooney, D.J. et al., Novel approach to fabricate porous sponges of poly(D,L-lactic-co-glycolic acid) without the use of organic solvents. *Biomaterials*, 1996, **17**: 1417–1422.

[81] Richardson, T.P. et al., Polymeric system for dual growth factor delivery. *Nat. Biotechnol.*, 2001, **19**: 1029–1034.

[82] Gombotz, W.R. et al., Protein adsorption to poly(ethylene oxide) surfaces. *J. Biomed. Mater. Res.*, 1991, **25**: 1547–1562.

[83] Mann, B.K. and J.L. West, Cell adhesion peptides alter smooth muscle cell adhesion, proliferation, migration, and matrix protein synthesis on modified surfaces and in polymer scaffolds. *J. Biomed. Mater. Res.*, 2002, **60**: 86–93.

[84] Tulis, D.A. et al., YC-1-mediated vascular protection through inhibition of smooth muscle cell proliferation and platelet function. *Biochem. Biophys. Res. Commun.*, 2002, **291**: 1014–1021.

[85] Gobin, A.S. and J.L. West, Cell migration through defined, synthetic ECM analogs. *FASEB J.*, 2002, **16**: 751–753.

[86] Drury, J.L. and D.J. Mooney, Hydrogels for tissue engineering: scaffold design variables and applications. *Biomaterials*, 2003, **24**: 4337–4351.

[87] Guan, J. et al., Synthesis, characterization, and cytocompatibility of elastomeric, biodegradable poly(ester-urethane)ureas based on poly(caprolactone) and putrescine. *J. Biomed. Mater. Res.*, 2002, **61**: 493–503.

[88] Lee, S.H. et al., Elastic biodegradable poly(glycolide-co-caprolactone) scaffold for tissue engineering. *J. Biomed. Mater. Res.*, 2003, **66A**: 29–37.

[89] Fromstein, J.D. and K.A. Woodhouse, Elastomeric biodegradable polyurethane blends for soft tissue applications. *J. Biomater. Sci. Polym. Ed.*, 2002, **13**: 391–406.

[90] Wang, Y. et al., A tough biodegradable elastomer. *Nat. Biotechnol.*, 2002, **20**: 602–6.

[91] Nakanishi, Y. et al., Tissue-engineered urinary bladder wall using PLGA mesh-collagen hybrid scaffolds: a comparison study of collagen sponge and gel as a scaffold. *J. Pediatr. Surg.*, 2003, **38**: 1781–1784.

[92] Pariente, J.L., B.S. Kim, and A. Atala, *In vitro* biocompatibility evaluation of naturally derived and synthetic biomaterials using normal human bladder smooth muscle cells. *J. Urol.*, 2002, **167**: 1867–1871.

[93] Cavallaro, J.F., P.D. Kemp, and K.H. Kraus, Collagen fabrics as biomaterials. *Biotechnol. Bioeng.*, 1994, **43**: 781–791.

[94] Li, S.T., Biologic biomaterials: tissue-derived biomaterials (collagen). In Brozino, J.D., Ed. *The Biomedical Engineering Handbook*. Boca Raton, FL: CRC Press, pp. 627–647, 1995.

[95] Kropp, B.P. et al., Regenerative urinary bladder augmentation using small intestinal submucosa: urodynamic and histopathologic assessment in long-term canine bladder augmentations. *J. Urol.*, 1996, **155**: 2098–2104.

[96] Badylak, S.F. et al., Comparison of the resistance to infection of intestinal submucosa arterial autografts versus polytetrafluoroethylene arterial prostheses in a dog model. *J. Vasc. Surg.*, 1994, **19**: 465–472.

[97] Zhang, Y. et al., Coculture of bladder urothelial and smooth muscle cells on small intestinal submucosa: potential applications for tissue engineering technology. *J. Urol.*, 2000, **164**: 928–934; discussion 934–935.

[98] Voytik-Harbin, S.L. et al., Identification of extractable growth factors from small intestinal submucosa. *J. Cell Biochem.*, 1997, **67**: 478–491.

[99] Chen, M.K. and S.F. Badylak, Small bowel tissue engineering using small intestinal submucosa as a scaffold. *J. Surg. Res.*, 2001, **99**: 352–358.

[100] Wang, Z.Q., Y. Watanabe, and A. Toki, Experimental assessment of small intestinal submucosa as a small bowel graft in a rat model. *J. Pediatr. Surg.*, 2003, **38**: 1596–1601.

[101] Yoo, J.J. et al., Bladder augmentation using allogenic bladder submucosa seeded with cells. *Urology*, 1998, **51**: 221–225.

[102] Huynh, T. et al., Remodeling of an acellular collagen graft into a physiologically responsive neovessel. *Nat. Biotechnol.*, 1999, **17**: 1083–6.

[103] Badylak, S.F. et al., Small intestinal submucosa as a large diameter vascular graft in the dog. *J. Surg. Res.*, 1989, **47**: 74–80.

[104] Falke, G., J. Caffaratti, and A. Atala, Tissue engineering of the bladder. *World J. Urol.*, 2000, **18**: 36–43.

[105] Tu, J.V. et al., Use of cardiac procedures and outcomes in elderly patients with myocardial infarction in the United States and Canada. *N. Engl. J. Med.*, 1997, **336**: 1500–1505.

[106] Seliktar, D., R.M. Nerem, and Z.S. Galis, Mechanical strain-stimulated remodeling of tissue-engineered blood vessel constructs. *Tissue Eng.*, 2003, **9**: 657–666.

[107] Reusch, P. et al., Mechanical strain increases smooth muscle and decreases nonmuscle myosin expression in rat vascular smooth muscle cells. *Circ. Res.*, 1996, **79**: 1046–1053.

[108] Probst, M. et al., Reproduction of functional smooth muscle tissue and partial bladder replacement. *Br. J. Urol.*, 1997, **79**: 505–515.

[109] Choi, R.S. and J.P. Vacanti, Preliminary studies of tissue-engineered intestine using isolated epithelial organoid units on tubular synthetic biodegradable scaffolds. *Transplant Proc.*, 1997, **29**: 848–851.

[110] Hori, Y. et al., Experimental study on tissue engineering of the small intestine by mesenchymal stem cell seeding. *J. Surg. Res.*, 2002, **102**: 156–160.

[111] Master, V.A. et al., Urothlelium facilitates the recruitment and trans-differentiation of fibroblasts into smooth muscle in acellular matrix. *J. Urol.*, 2003, **170**: 1628–1632.

[112] Vacanti, J.P., Tissue and organ engineering: can we build intestine and vital organs? *J. Gastrointest. Surg.*, 2003, **7**: 831–835.

54

Esophagus: A Tissue Engineering Challenge

B.D. Ratner
B.L. Beckstead
University of Washington

K.S. Chian
A.C. Ritchie
Nanyang Technological University

54.1 Medical Need/Clinical Problem

The esophagus, a muscular/mucosal tube connecting the mouth and pharynx to the stomach, is critical for life (and good quality of life) (Figure 54.1). This seemingly simple organ is surgically challenging to repair or replace. There are a number of conditions where surgical repair of the esophagus is indicated. These include accident and trauma, congenital defects such as esophageal atresia (incomplete formation of the esophagus) and tracheoesophageal fistulas and cancer. In 2003, roughly 14,000 people in the United States were diagnosed with esophageal cancer. The prevalence of esophageal cancer in the general population can be 10 to 100 times higher in Iran, China, Singapore, India, and South Africa. Worldwide, cancer of the esophagus is the seventh leading cause of cancer death.

Surgical removal of a section of the esophagus and reconnection with the stomach, the most common strategy for more advanced cancers, leads to complication rates as high as 40%. Strictures, dilation, leakage, and infection are often observed. Attempts to use synthetics such as polyethylene, polypropylene, teflon, or elastomers have also met with very limited success, problems being stenosis, leakage, infection, scarring,

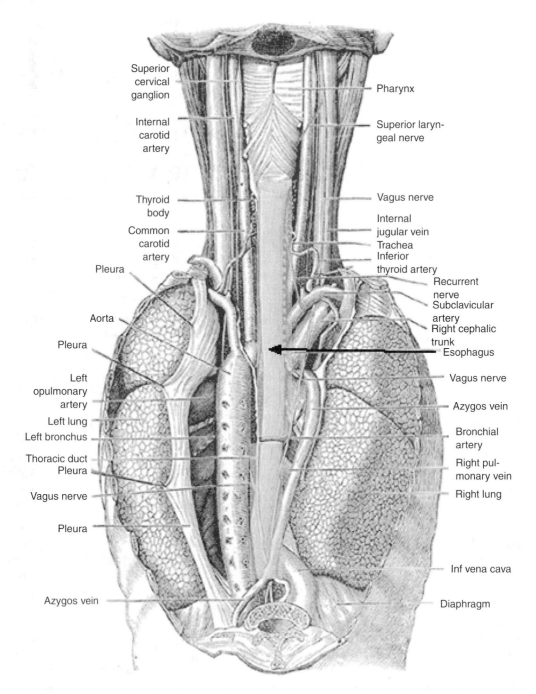

FIGURE 54.1 Diagram illustrating the anatomical location of the esophagus (from Gray's Anatomy).

ulceration, and migration [Leininger et al., 1970; Watanabe and Mark, 1971; Sato et al., 1997; Ure et al., 1998; Fuchs et al., 2001]. A living, nonimmunologic esophageal replacement could make a significant contribution to medical practice and patient treatment.

Tissue engineering, using healthy cells supplied by the patient, offers the possibility of a normal esophageal reconstruction after surgery, trauma, or for congenital repair. In recent years, the tissue engineering approach has been investigated as an alternative treatment of esophageal diseases [Natsume et al., 1993; Miki et al., 1999; Badylak et al., 2000; Yamamoto et al., 2000; Kajitani et al., 2001].

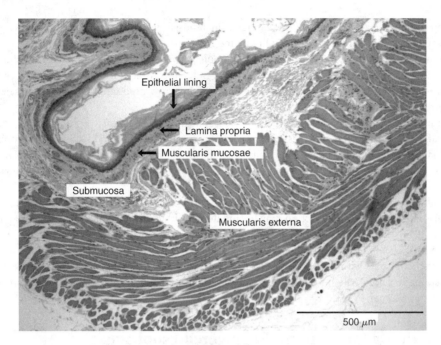

FIGURE 54.2 A cross-sectional histological section of the esophagus.

54.2 Anatomy and Physiology of the Esophagus

The esophagus is a thick-walled muscular tube extending from the pharynx to the stomach. It descends through the posterior mediasternum, passes through the diaphragm at the esophageal hiatus, and joins the stomach at the T9 level [Kumar, 1993]. Its length in adults is typically between 9 and 10 in. (225 to 250 mm). It consists of three main layers, the mucosa, submucosa, and muscularis. The esophagus has no serosa [Gray, 1995; Goyal and Sivarao, 1999; Ergun and Kahrilas, 1997; Wood, 1994].

Innervation: Sensory and motor function is supplied by branches of cranial nerves V, VII, IX, X, XI, and XII [Wood, 1994; Ergun and Kahrilas, 1997; Goyal and Sivarao, 1999]. Neural networks lie between the longitudinal and circular muscle layers (Auerbach's or myenteric plexus) and the circular muscle and submucosa (Meissner's or submucosal plexus) [Wood, 1994; Ergun and Kahrilas, 1997]. Swallowing and esophageal peristalsis come under the control of both the somatic and enteric nervous systems, with signal conduction primarily through the vagus nerve.

Vasculature: Blood supply to the esophagus is via shared vasculature. Along its length, branches of larger vessels including the thyroid artery, esophageal aortic arteries, and left gastric and splenic arteries supply blood to the arterial network around the esophageal lumen [Gershon et al., 1994; Ergun and Kahrilas, 1997]. Capillaries within the tissues drain into deep intrinsic and adventitial veins. Blood is transported back to the heart via the extrinsic serosal and periesophageal veins, which drain into the left gastric veins and azygos vein [Ergun and Kahrilas, 1997].

Structure: A cross-sectional diagram of a rat esophagus is shown in Figure 54.2. The layer closest to the lumen is typically composed of stratified squamous epithelium [Burkitt et al., 1993]. Acid reflux may cause Barrett's esophagus, where the stratified squamous epithelium is transformed into columnar epithelium [Goyal and Sivarao, 1999]. Lying beneath this layer is a thin lamina propria and a thin layer of smooth muscle, the muscularis mucosa [Burkitt et al., 1993].

The submucosa is a layer of highly vascularized and relatively loose connective tissue, which allows distension. Within the submucosa are small mucous glands for lubrication [Burkitt et al., 1993].

The muscularis layer is normally classified as two sublayers according to the orientation of the muscle cells. Closest to the submucosa is the circular muscle layer, where the myocytes are aligned tangentially to the esophageal lumen. The next layer is the longitudinal muscle, where the myocytes are aligned parallel to the esophageal axis [Burkitt et al., 1993; Ergun and Kahrilas, 1997].

The muscle type varies along the length of the esophagus. In the cervical esophagus, the muscularis layer is made up, almost exclusively, of skeletal muscle, and in the distal third (closest to the stomach), the muscularis layer consists of smooth muscle. The middle third is composed of a mixture of skeletal and smooth muscle.

Contraction of the skeletal muscle in the cervical esophagus may be initiated voluntarily or reflexively. The initial stage of swallowing occurs as the tongue pushes a bolus of masticated food into the oropharynx. This initiates the involuntary pharyngeal stage of swallowing, as the bolus of food stimulates receptors in the oropharynx, which then sends impulses to the deglutition center of the medulla oblongata and lower pons [Ergun and Kahrilas, 1997].

The bolus of masticated food is then pushed through the esophagus by peristaltic contraction of the muscularis layer. Peristaltic contraction may be initiated by either extrinsic or intrinsic neural pathways [Wingate, 1993]. Longitudinal muscles ahead of the bolus contract to widen the esophagus while the circular muscles behind the bolus of food contract to push it toward the stomach. Food normally passes through the esophagus within 10 sec [Ergun and Kahrilas, 1997]. The junction between the esophagus and the stomach is not a true sphincter and in certain conditions, matter may pass from the stomach into the esophagus [Kumar, 1993].

54.3 Criteria for a Tissue-Engineered Esophagus

Based upon the above anatomical description, and from an engineering and biology standpoint, what are the criteria that must be met before a practical and functional surgical alternative through tissue engineering is in place? The following demands challenge us in the development of a tissue-engineered living prosthesis:

Radially elastic/longitudinally rigid: The normal biomechanical behavior of the esophagus must be duplicated in a surgical replacement. First, this mechanically strong and compliant tube must expand radially to permit ingestion of a bolus of food or liquid, yet it should exhibit relatively little elasticity longitudinally. The organization of collagen and elastin within the structure, along with its convoluted luminal cross section can account for these mechanical properties.

Muscular: The esophagus is a highly muscular organ. Smooth muscle cells and skeletal muscle cells are present with proportions varying along the length of the tube. Muscle laminae in the walls of the esophagus are organized orthogonally to one another. The act of swallowing produces a peristaltic pulse along the esophagus to drive contents to the stomach. This peristaltic process must be replicated in a tissue-engineered construct.

Mucosal lining: The epithelial cell lining of the lumen of the esophagus generates a mucosal exterior layer that lubricates and also protects the air–tissue interface. This lining enables the esophagus able to deal with the range of "chemicals" and insults it must tolerate including hot foods, strong alcoholic beverages, abrasive foods, and acidic foods.

Innervation: A nerve network in the esophagus coordinates the peristaltic action.

Angiogenesis: The esophageal wall is a relatively thick tissue (>1 mm) and requires its own blood vessel network to sustain the core muscle tissue and remove cell wastes.

Cell sources: Since we do not know how to deal with the immunological issues associated with allogeneic cell sources, a practical surgical prosthesis will probably be comprised of autologous cells. Cell harvesting from a biopsy should not be a problem. However, sterility issues, cell separation, expansion, and seeding on a scaffold are all challenges to address.

Scaffolds: A scaffold will be used to give anatomical shape and biological signals to the growing cells forming the new tissue. The criteria for scaffolds are many. Of course, it should be nontoxic (nominally "biocompatible"). The esophageal scaffold should have a shape and form similar to the organ to be replaced (including the puckered or invaginated form of the lumen). It should separate epithelial and muscular lamina, but allow biological communication between them. It should give cells the proper signals for attachment, growth, and orientation. This scaffold should be elastomeric as opposed to stiff. It should allow or even encourage angiogenesis and integration into the anatomical site. Finally, it should biodegrade without a trace after the living tissue has gained sufficient strength to support itself and function anatomically.

Bioreactor issues: The seeded cells will be cultured *in vitro* until the evolving tissue is adequate for transplantation into the patient. A bioreactor must sustain the cells with oxygen and nutrients, remove wastes, provide an appropriate mechanical environment to condition the cells, provide a sterile environment, and also create the air–tissue interface necessary for proper development of the epithelial cell–mucosal layer.

Surgical issues: Finally, the growing tissue engineered construct must be taken from the bioreactor and implanted. What is the optimal period of *in vitro* development before *in vivo* implantation? How should it be sutured? How should it be implanted to optimize angiogenesis? What patient management issues are needed pre and post surgery?

The following sections illustrate research efforts underway at the Nanyang Technological University and the University of Washington to take an engineering systems approach to the esophageal replacement problem and address the demanding criteria for a tissue-engineered esophagus.

54.4 Scaffold Possibilities

54.4.1 Background

Currently two main approaches to tissue/organ regeneration are *in vivo* and *in vitro* tissue engineering. *In vivo* tissue engineering uses noncell-seeded biomaterials, which include decellularized tissues such as the acellular small intestinal submucosa, amniotic membranes, and pig-heart valves [Badylak et al., 1995; Khan et al., 2001]. In contrast, *in vitro* approaches involve the manipulation of cells on biomaterial scaffolds *in vitro* prior to implantation. Despite these obvious differences, both approaches involve the use of biomaterial scaffold and rely on the body's ability to regenerate.

The scaffold plays a crucial role in tissue engineering of the esophagus. The growth of the anchorage-dependant esophageal cells requires a suitable scaffold for attachment in order to proliferate and function. These scaffolds are three-dimensional biodegradable structures that provide spatial cellular signaling environment necessary for the regenerative processes. These signaling processes are responsible for triggering the expression or repression of genes that regulate cell division, production of extracellular matrix (ECM), differentiation, proliferation, migration, and even apoptosis [Peters and Mooney, 1997; Bottaro and Heidaran, 2001]. In essence, a scaffold is a temporary biodegradable structure containing the appropriate cells that, through various biological remodeling processes, will eventually form vital tissues/organs.

A suitable tissue engineered scaffold for esophageal replacement must closely mimic the host tissue it replaces with respect to mechanical, surface, structural, and biological properties. Some of these considerations necessary for esophageal tissue engineering include (i) materials selection, (ii) scaffold design, and (iii) choice of fabrication techniques.

54.4.2 Materials Selection

The esophagus is a highly elastic and muscular organ, and one of the main considerations is to identify materials that are mechanically compatible. This criterion limits the choice to only polymeric biomaterials. These polymers must be biocompatible, biodegradable, mechanically compliant, and have suitable surface chemistry. In addition, the polymers must be amenable to fabrication and sterilization techniques without altering their biocompatibility and properties. Some of these biodegradable polymers used in tissue engineering applications have been comprehensively reviewed elsewhere [Pachence and Kohn, 2000; Langer and Tirrell, 2004].

The three groups of polymeric biomaterials commonly used in tissue engineering applications include (1) naturally derived polymers, that is, alginates, chitosan, hyaluronic acid; (2) biologically derived materials such as the decellularized tissues, that is, collagens, small intestinal submucosa, urinary bladder matrix, and amniotic membranes; and (3) synthetic polymers, that is, poly(lactic acid), poly(glycolic acid), and poly(lactic-co-glycolic acid), poly(hydroxybutyrate-valerate). Some of the recent developments in biomaterials for tissue engineering applications include self-assembly nanofibers [Huang et al., 2000; Hartgerink et al., 2002], and elastic protein-based polymer systems [Urry et al., 1991; McMillan and Conticello, 2000].

Many materials have been evaluated for esophagus repair and reconstruction. These include collagens [Natsume et al., 1993], poly(glycolic acid) [Shinhar et al., 1998, Miki et al., 1999], urinary bladder matrix [Badylak, et al. 2000]; elastin biomaterials obtained from porcine aorta [Kajitani et al., 2001], and Alloderm®[Isch et al., 2001]. All the above materials showed promise, especially the collagen and acellular matrices, but the problem of stenosis remained. The acellular matrices appear to show better cell–matrix interactions than synthetic ones. This may be due to the fact that these acellular matrices, being the ECM materials, contain a complex mixture of structural and functional proteins, glycoproteins, and proteoglycans arranged in a unique, tissue-specific three-dimensional ultrastructure [Badylak, 2002]. However, cell adhesion to degradable synthetic polymers can be improved by modifying the surfaces with RGD peptide for cell surface adhesion receptors [Glass et al., 1994; Cook et al., 1997; Schmedlen et al., 2002].

Our research group is currently evaluating the interactions between the esophageal epithelial and smooth muscle cells on various materials including chitosan, various blends of biodegradable polymers with chitosan, collagens; and decellularized porcine matrices such as urinary bladder matrix, small intestinal submucosa, and esophagus.

54.4.3 Scaffold Design

With the exception of the acellular matrices, all other scaffolds using synthetic polymers or pure collagen must be fabricated. As such, important structural features of the scaffold design must be considered. The ideal scaffold should direct the biological process of tissue formation and regeneration. One of the principal objectives in tissue engineering is to mimic the ECM in terms of their surface chemistry, mechanical properties and structure. In addition to the choice of biomaterials, to provide suitable surfaces for cell attachment and recognition, the physical structure of the scaffold plays an equally important role. The effects of pore size, morphology, microgeometry, and scaffold thickness are known to influence cellular adhesion, tissue organization, angiogenesis, and matrix deposition [Wake et al., 1994; Brauker et al., 1995; Zeltinger et al., 2001; Ward et al., 2002; Rosengren and Bjursten, 2003].

Pore size and total porosity, for example, are also known to influence fibrovascular tissue invasion and extent of fibrosis [Mikos et al., 1993]. In the case of the esophagus, fibrosis reaction must be minimized in order to maintain its mechanical performance. Conceptually, the scaffold for esophageal tissue should have a range of pore sizes. On the outer surface of the scaffold, the pore size should be large (ranging from 50 to 200 μm) to facilitate cell seeding, and transport of nutrients and waste. There should also be smaller pores (ranging from 35 to 70 μm) necessary to promote angiogenesis [Marshall et al., 2004]. The luminal surface, in order to mimic the basal membrane in the esophagus, should be dense (in the range of several microns in size). This barrier layer is to facilitate diffusion of signaling molecules and nutrients but prevents cell migration across the surface. An example of such a scaffold structure with varying pore sizes is shown in Figure 54.3a,b [Chian, 2003].

Another important aspect of the esophageal scaffold is the need for pores with specific orientation. The muscularis mucosa of the esophagus consists of a single layer of longitudinally oriented smooth muscle fibers, whereas the muscularis externa has an inner circular and outer longitudinal muscle layers. It is therefore advantageous to have channels in the scaffold that can provide directional guidance for these muscular tissues. Examples of such scaffolds with porous channels are shown in Figures 54.4a,b [Chian, 2003]. Our research effort is currently underway to study if these channels in the scaffold are effective in guiding these smooth muscle cells in culture.

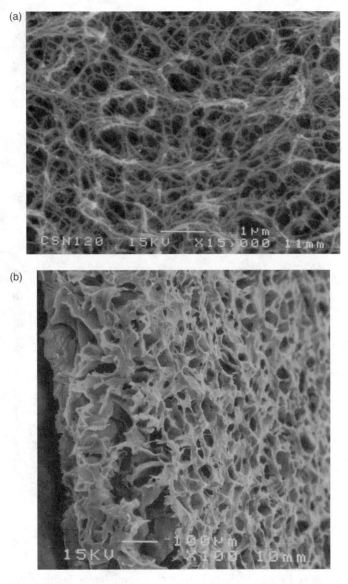

FIGURE 54.3 Chitosan scaffold showing a graded pore structure that may be suitable for replicating features found in the natural esophagus (a) Scaffold showing a dense basement membrane-like surface. (b) Scaffold showing highly interconnecting porous structure.

However, it must be noted that the features designed into the scaffold are only important in the initial stages of cell attachment and proliferation. As these scaffolds are biodegradable, the porous features and mechanical strengths are only transient. In an ideal situation, it is hoped that as the implanted cells interact suitably with the scaffold material, ECM produced by the cells will be laid down to replace the scaffold materials as they degrade. Therefore it is very important to select a suitable biomaterial as scaffold material that has a degradation timescale similar to the tissue forming process, which ranges from seconds to weeks.

54.5 Fabrication Processes

The methods of producing porous scaffolds for tissue engineering are well reviewed elsewhere [Thomson et al., 2000; Atala and Lanza, 2002]. Many of these processes used in scaffold fabrication are adapted from

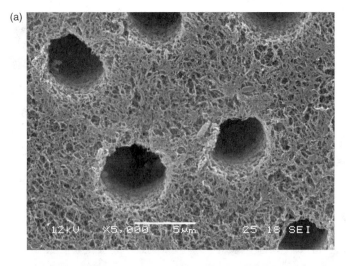

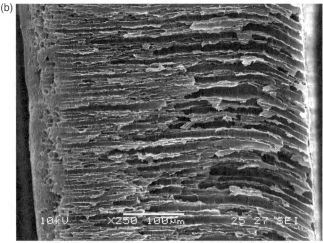

FIGURE 54.4 Examples of chitosan scaffolds with channel structures that may be useful for aligning muscle cells. (a) Porous surface of scaffold. (b) Cross section of a chitosan scaffold.

textile [Summanasinghe and King, 2003] and membrane technologies. Some of the common scaffold fabrication process that have been widely evaluated and reviewed [Sachlos and Czernuszka, 2003] include the following: Fiber bonding [Mooney et al., 1996], solvent casting and particulate leaching [Mikos et al., 1994; Wake et al., 1996], membrane lamination [Mikos et al., 1993], melt molding [Thomson et al., 1995], extrusion [Widmer et al., 1998], solid free-form methods [Giordano et al., 1996; Park et al., 1998], gas forming [Mooney et al., 1996], freeze drying [Whang et al., 1995], and phase inversion [Lo et al., 1995].

In this chapter, we will highlight some of the newer methods that are currently being explored for fabricating tissue engineering of tubular scaffolds. These include (i) electrostatic spinning, (ii) cryogenic molding, and (iii) rapid freeze prototyping.

54.5.1 Electrostatic spinning

Electrostatic spinning is a well-established method for producing porous materials [Formhals, 1934; Amato, 1972; Bornat, 1982]. More recently, this technique has been adapted for producing biodegradable scaffolds from a range of polymers and collagens [Stitzel et al. 2000; Bowland et al., 2001; Matthews et al., 2002; Li et al., 2002; Wnek et al., 2003; Chu et al., 2004]. In an electrostatic spinning process, a high-voltage

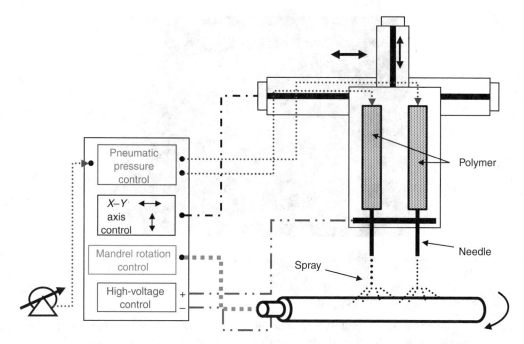

FIGURE 54.5   An electrostatic spinning system (a) apparatus for electrostatic spinning. (b) Porous nanofibers of PLA.

field is created between the polymer solution/melt and a collector. The polymer solution/melt is usually contained in a syringe and the needle is connected to an electrode. The oppositely charged electrode is connected to a collector, which can be either a stationary plate or a rotating mandrel. Typically, a high-voltage source of up to 30 kV is required for this process. Figure 54.5a shows a schematic diagram of a typical electrostatic spinning system. In order to form the electrostatic spray, the electric field between the end of the needle and the collector must increase until the mutual charge repulsion overcomes the surface tension of the polymer solution [Doshi and Reneker, 1995]. Increasing the electric field results in a charged stream of polymer fluid ejecting from the tip of the Taylor cone [Yarin et al., 2001]. The ejecting solution undergoes a whipping process [Shin et al., 2001], wherein the solvent evaporates leaving a charged polymer fiber randomly laid onto the grounded collector. The electrostatic spinning system offers many advantages over conventional methods of scaffold manufacture, and these include (i) the ability to produce varying fiber size, from nanometer to micron size, (ii) fabricating composite scaffolds, (iii) good porosity control, and (iv) the process is amenable to a wide range of synthetic and biological polymers. Figure 54.5b shows this use of this technique to produce nanofibers of polylactic acid with porous surfaces [Leong et al., 2004]. We are exploring further the potential of this method to fabricate scaffolds with various biodegradable polymers.

54.5.2   Cryogenic molding

Another method for forming the esophageal scaffold that we are currently evaluating is the cryogenic molding process. In this process, the polymer solution is injected into a metal mould and allowed to freeze completely. The mould is then opened and the frozen polymer removed for freeze-drying or coagulated immediately. We have used this method successfully to produce a tubular scaffold made from chitosan solution. Figure 54.6 shows esophageal scaffolds that were made using this cryogenic molding process. This process offers the advantages of (i) reproducible scaffolds, (ii) it is amenable to a wide range of polymers, (iii) low cost, and (iv) it provides good porosity control, comparable to other phase separation methods commonly used in forming tissue engineering scaffolds.

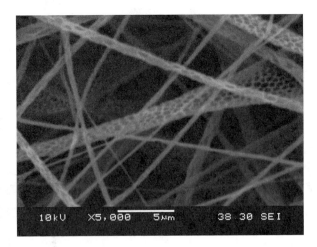

FIGURE 54.6   A cryogenically molded tubular chitosan scaffold.

54.5.3 Rapid freeze prototyping

The various forms of rapid prototyping techniques have been successfully used in producing three-dimensional scaffolds for hard tissue implants [Giordano et al., 1996; Levy et al., 1997; Matsuda and Mizutani, 2002]. Attempts to produce scaffolds using the rapid prototyping technique for soft tissue engineering applications from agar hydrogels [Landers et al., 2002], fibrin hydrogels [Landers et al., 2002], chitosan, or chitosan-hydroxyapatite [Ang et al., 2002] have also been reported.

A new method was recently developed by our research group for producing scaffolds for soft tissue engineering application that is suitable for a wide range of polymers and biological materials. The method is adapted from the rapid freeze prototyping process that uses water to build ice prototypes. This process is capable of and has been successfully used to generate three-dimensional ice objects by depositing and rapidly freezing water layer by layer [Zhang et al., 2001; Chao et al., 2002]. However, in our adapted system, we used a robotic dispensing system to dispense chitosan solution onto a cold stage where it is allowed to freeze. The layers are built by repeatedly dispensing chitosan solution onto the previously frozen structure. When the required frozen structure is formed, it can be either freeze-dried or coagulated in alkaline solution to form the porous scaffold. Figure 54.7 shows samples of chitosan scaffolds fabricated using the adapted rapid freeze prototyping process.

The challenges in scaffold technology are many. The combination of selecting or developing a suitable material and utilizing a suitable fabrication method is often difficult. As cells have specific interactions with a substrate, a synthetic scaffold may eventually need to be a structure made from different materials, and with different pore size and surface chemistry. As we learn more about cell–material interactions, the closer we get to understanding, and enhancing our ability to mimic, the complex scaffold structure that nature can provide so readily. More research needs to be done in understanding the biological processes involved in tissue regeneration, and to develop novel and ingenious methods for fabricating scaffolds that replicate nature's ECM structures.

54.6 Cell Possibilities

54.6.1 Epithelial Characteristics

The epithelial lining of the esophagus is composed of stratified, squamous epithelial cells. In the human esophagus, these cells are nonkeratinizing, whereas in the rat they form a stratum corneum (see Figure 54.8) [Leeson and Leeson, 1981]. This epithelium is organized into distinct cellular layers, distinguished by appearance and protein expression. As the epithelial cells advance from the basal layer to the lumen, their

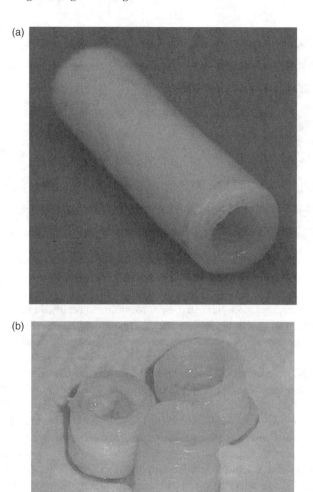

FIGURE 54.7 Samples of chitosan scaffolds fabricated using the rapid freeze prototyping process.

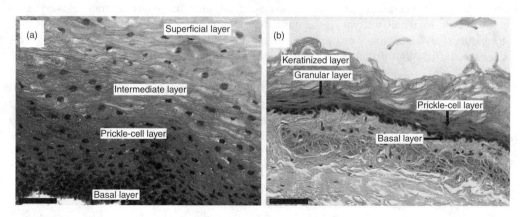

FIGURE 54.8 Esophageal epithelial morphology. (a) Nonkeratinizing human esophageal epithelium. (b) Keratinizing rat esophageal epithelium (H&E, bar = 50 μm).

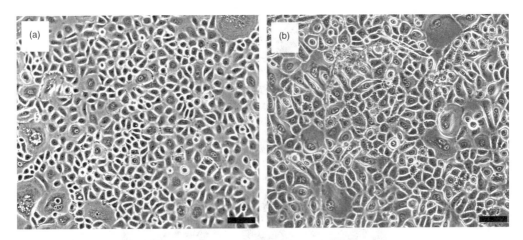

FIGURE 54.9 Esophageal epithelial cells in serum-free culture. (a) Human esophageal epithelial cells. (b) Rat esophageal epithelial cells (bar = 100 μm).

appearance becomes flatter and more elongated. In nonkeratinizing epithelium, the various layers consist of the basal layer, prickle-cell layer, intermediate layer, and superficial layer (see Figure 54.8a) [Squier et al., 1976]. A keratinized esophagus shows a slightly different morphology and the epithelial layers are termed basal, prickle-cell, granular, and keratinized (see Figure 54.8b) [Squier et al., 1976]. As the cells progress toward the lumen, they become more differentiated and lose proliferative potential. In this manner, there is constant turnover and shedding of the epithelial cells. The turnover time for the epithelial lining is relatively short: 21 days in humans [Squier and Kremer, 2001] and 7 days in mice [Eastwood, 1977].

Epithelial stem cells reside in the basal layer of the esophagus and serve to replenish the lining [Seery and Watt, 2000]. Upon division of the stem cell, the daughter cells can either remain in their primitive state or enter the differentiation pathway [Seery and Watt, 2000]. This entrance into differentiation results in the development of a so-called transit-amplifying cell that is capable of further division, but quickly loses proliferative potential and becomes terminally differentiated [Seery and Watt, 2000]. The option between differentiation and proliferation has shown to be influenced by various factors, including calcium, phorbol esters, retinoic acid, vitamin A, air–liquid interface, and vitamin D3 [Fuchs and Green, 1981; Watt, 1984; Asselineau et al., 1985, 1989; Dotto, 1999]. The state of differentiation is spatially defined within the esophagus: cells residing in the basal layer are in a more primitive state, whereas differentiation progresses as the cell moves toward the lumen [Squier and Kremer, 2001]. Cytokeratin (intermediate cytoskeletal filaments) expression also varies spatially and provides a means to monitor differentiation of the epithelial cells. For example, within the human esophageal epithelial lining, cytokeratin 14 is expressed exclusively in the basal cells, whereas cytokeratin 13 is expressed in suprabasal cells [Takahasi et al., 1995]. Cytokeratin expression is closely tied to function and abnormal cytokeratin expression in other tissues has been associated with carcinomas and genetic diseases, such as epidermolysis bullosa [Takahasi et al. 1995; Fuchs, 1996].

The *in vitro* culture of esophageal epithelial cells has been well established [Compton et al., 1998; Oda et al., 1998; Okumura et al., 2003]. The majority of isolations involve an enzymatic digestion to allow for easy separation of the epithelium and underlying lamina propria. The epithelium is then trypsin-treated to obtain a single cell suspension. These cells can either be grown using a 3T3 feeder layer [Rheinwald and Green, 1975; Compton et al., 1998] or in a serum-free keratinocyte growth medium [Oda et al., 1998; Miki et al., 1999; Okumura et al., 2003], and propagated in culture for multiple passages (see Figure 54.9).

54.6.2 Epithelial Cell Source for Tissue Engineering

Attempts at engineering a replacement esophagus have exclusively employed the use of esophageal epithelial cells, rather than epithelial cells isolated from other tissues. Most likely, this stems from ease of isolation and physiological relevance. The most extensive research has been done by Kitajima and associates [Sato et al., 1993, 1994, 1997; Miki et al., 1999]. Originally, their work focused on seeding human esophageal epithelial cells on a collagen gel or poly(glycolic) acid (PGA) mesh embedded within a collagen gel. Using these scaffolds, they were able to obtain two to five layers of epithelial cells prior to implantation in the latissimus dorsi of a rat or mouse [Sato et al., 1993, 1994]. *In vivo*, the number of cell layers did increase and after 2 weeks, the epithelium was comparable to normal esophagus [Sato et al., 1993, 1994]. More recent studies have investigated the effect on epithelial cells of fibroblasts embedded in the collagen gels [Miki et al., 1999]. These fibroblasts serve a similar function as a 3T3 feeder layer used in monolayer culture. They reported a positive correlation between the number of dermal fibroblasts embedded in the collagen and the number of epithelial cell layers. At 8×10^5 fibroblasts/ml, the authors were able to obtain greater than 18 epithelial cell layers after 21 days of *in vitro* culture [Miki et al., 1999]. For *in vivo* studies, they seeded human esophageal epithelial cells with human esophageal fibroblasts in a collagen gel embedded within a PGA matrix. After implantation in the latissimus dorsi of a rat for 2 weeks, they observed approximately 20 layers of epithelial cells, with morphology similar to native esophagus [Miki et al., 1999]. However, no immunocytochemical staining was done to evaluate differentiation or cytokeratin expression of the epithelial lining and this construct has yet to be implanted in either a partial or a full circumferential esophageal defect.

The Vacanti research group has also reported creation of a tissue-engineered esophagus [Grikscheit et al., 2003]. For their epithelial cell source, they created "organoid units" (OUs), which are mesenchymal cells surrounded by epithelium. To create the OUs, a rat esophagus was harvested and digested using a dispase/collagenase type I solution. The suspension was washed, resuspended in culture media, and seeded immediately onto a PGA mesh for implantation. For *in vivo* implantation, the rat's omentum was wrapped around the construct before securing it in the peritoneum. After 4 weeks, the engineered construct was removed from the peritoneum and either used for histological analysis, implantation as an esophageal patch, or as an interposition graft. The epithelial lining of these grafts was similar to native rat esophagus with a stratified squamous keratinizing epithelium. The authors reported that the esophageal patch showed good integration and no stenosis, unlike the interposition graft, which showed stenosis at the upper anastomosis and dilation at the lower anastomosis [Grikscheit et al., 2003].

Our research group has also employed esophageal epithelial cells for use in esophageal tissue engineering. Both human and rat epithelial cells have been successfully isolated and cultured using previous published techniques [Oda et al., 1998]. We are currently investigating epithelial interactions with various synthetic and natural matrices.

54.6.3 Muscle Component of the Esophagus

In addition to the epithelial cells, another critical cellular component of a tissue-engineered esophagus is the muscle layers. The esophagus has two muscle layers: the muscularis mucosa and the muscularis externa [Leeson and Leeson, 1981]. The muscularis mucosa lies between the lamina propria and the submucosa. Its main function appears to be a support for the luminal lining during contraction of the muscularis externa [Squier and Kremer, 2001]. The muscularis externa is the outermost layer of the esophagus and serves to push the food down the esophagus through peristalsis [Leeson and Leeson, 1981]. In humans, the composition of the muscularis externa has traditionally been reported as striated muscle in the upper third of the esophagus, smooth muscle in the lower third, and mixed in the middle third [Leeson and Leeson, 1981]. However, this reported composition has been modified by other investigators. Meyer and Castell report that the inner circular layer of the muscularis externa is approximately 4% striated muscle, 35% mixed, and 62% smooth muscle [Meyer and Castell, 1983]. The outer longitudinal layer of the muscularis externa, follows similar trends with approximately 6% striated, 41% mixed, and 54% smooth muscle [Meyer and Castell, 1983]. In the rat esophagus, the compositions of the muscularis mucosa and externa are more defined. The muscularis mucosa is strictly smooth muscle, whereas the muscularis externa is striated muscle [Linnes, 2004].

54.6.4 Engineering the Muscularis Mucosa and Externa

The muscle layer of the esophagus has surprisingly received little attention in attempts to engineer a replacement esophagus. As stated above, Miki et al. [1999] attempted to improve epithelial differentiation through a coculture with fibroblasts. For *in vivo* studies, human esophageal fibroblasts were isolated from subepithelial tissues by mincing and enzymatic digestion [Miki et al., 1999]. Besides staining with an antihuman fibroblast antibody after implant harvest, no characterization of the cells was reported. It is unknown whether these cells can serve as an appropriate source for the muscularis mucosa or if they will populate the lamina propria or submucosa. For *in vivo* studies, the engineered tubes were implanted in the muscle flaps of the latissimus dorsi, which could theoretically serve to generate a muscularis externa [Miki et al., 1999]. However, no in-depth histological analysis of the muscularis mucosa or muscularis externa of these constructs has been reported.

Within the esophageal organoid units created by the Vacanti group are mesenchymal cells, which could serve as a smooth muscle cell source [Grikscheit et al., 2003]. As stated above, these organoid units were seeded onto a PGA mesh and wrapped with the omentum before suturing into the peritoneum. After 4 weeks, the construct was harvested and analyzed for alpha-smooth muscle actin expression [Grikscheit et al., 2003]. The staining did appear in the expected site of the muscularis mucosa, but was sparse and discontinuous. No mention of a muscularis externa was made. Thus, it is unclear whether the OU approach can lead to a morphological and functional equivalent to either muscle layer.

Clearly, engineering of the esophageal muscle layers is an area that requires increased attention. Since the muscle layer's composition varies from species to species, animal models will need to anticipate this variation. Studies investigating potential cell sources, matrix production, mechanical strength, and cellular alignment are needed to thoughtfully engineer the esophagus.

54.6.5 Esophageal Regeneration

As an alternative to the *in vitro* construction of a tissue-engineered esophagus, much research has been aimed at developing methods to stimulate *in vivo* regeneration. One widely employed approach has been to use a collagen-coated silicone tube to promote regeneration [Ike et al., 1989; Natsume et al., 1990, 1993; Takimoto et al., 1993, 1998; Yamamoto et al., 1999a, b, 2000; Hori et al., 2003]. In this approach, a silicone stent is coated with collagen types I and III, and the collagen is freeze-dried and lightly cross-linked around the stent. Both layers serve distinct purposes in the regeneration. The collagen provides a matrix for cell infiltration and tissue regeneration; the silicone stent provides mechanical integrity and protection from displacement, leakage, and infection [Natsume et al., 1990]. At the desired time after implantation, the silicone stent is dislodged endoscopically, leaving behind the neo-esophageal tissue. In one study, a 5-cm long prosthesis was implanted in the cervical esophagus of a canine animal model [Takimoto et al., 1998]. If the silicone stent was removed at 2 or 3 weeks, the neo-esophagus constricted rendering the dogs unable to swallow. However, if the stent was removed at 4 weeks, the regenerated tissue showed remarkable similarity to native esophagus. The regenerated tissue showed a stratified epithelium (8 to 10 layers) and both inner circular and outer longitudinal muscle layers [Takimoto et al., 1998]. The esophagus remained patent even after 12 months. Variations on this stent design have included preseeding with oral mucosal cells [Natsume et al., 1990], omental-pedicle wrapping [Yamamoto et al., 2000], and delivery of basic fibroblast growth factor from the collagen [Hori et al., 2003].

Extracellular matrix materials have also been studied as scaffolds for esophageal regeneration. Acellular human skin (AlloDerm®, LifeCell, Branchburg, NJ) was used as an esophageal patch by Isch and associates [Isch et al., 2001]. In this study, a section of canine esophagus was removed (2 × 1 cm) and replaced with AlloDerm®. While epithelial coverage was incomplete at 1 month, by 2 months, coverage was complete and vascularization was evident. However, elastin staining indicated that the AlloDerm® was still present in the wound site at 3 months. Also, there was no indication of smooth muscle cell repopulation [Isch et al., 2001].

Small intestinal submucosa (SIS) has also found use in esophageal repair. Badylak et al. reported using SIS for both partial (3 × 5 cm) and complete (5-cm length) circumferential defect repair in canines [Badylak et al., 2000]. By 35 days, epithelialization was complete and the repair site showed indications of striated muscle infiltration from adjacent esophagus. While remnants of the SIS could be seen at 35 days, by 50 days, the SIS appears to have been completely degraded. Stenosis was seen in the complete circumferential defect repair site, with an approximate 50% decrease in circumference. The authors hypothesize that this narrowing is caused by the lack of intraluminal pressure [Badylak et al., 2000].

Finally, Kajitani et al. [2001] employed acellular porcine aorta as an esophageal patch. A small half-circle defect (2-cm diameter) was made in the distal esophagus of a pig and the acellular aorta was used to repair the site. Complete epithelial coverage and evidence of muscle regeneration was seen in the defect site by 7 weeks. However, residual elastin fibers indicated incomplete degradation of the acellular patch [Kajitani et al., 2001].

Thus, the initial results for esophageal regeneration are promising. To repair circumferential defects, the collagen–silicone stent has shown the ability to form a neo-esophagus with morphological similarities to native esophagus [Takimoto et al., 1998]. For patch defects, use of ECM materials has resulted in esophageal regeneration, but these materials have yet to be successful as full circumferential replacements [Badylak, et al., 2000; Isch et al., 2001; Kajitani et al., 2001]. In addition, further studies must be performed to evaluate the effect of the residual ECM material that remains in the wound site after regeneration appears to be complete.

54.7 Bioreactors for Esophageal Tissue Engineering

54.7.1 Mechanical Conditioning of Smooth Muscle Tissue Constructs

The outcome of culture of cells on a scaffold has shown to be influenced by the underlying substrate in addition to the biochemical and biomechanical environment [Kanda et al., 1992; Kim and Mooney, 2000]. The effect of mechanical stimulation on vascular smooth muscle cells has been much studied as part of the ongoing research focus to develop bioartificial vascular prostheses [Nerem and Seliktar, 2001]. There is less data available in the literature on mechanical stimulation of visceral smooth muscle but the general principles and effects of mechanical stimulation are similar for the two myocyte types [Karim et al., 1992; Gooch and Tennant, 1997]. Mechanical stimulation of smooth muscle cells has been shown to have the following effects:

Cells align perpendicular to the stress direction in one-dimensional stress and exhibit morphological changes [Kanda et al., 1992; Gooch and Tennant, 1997]. Cyclic stretching significantly increases elastin production and promotes expression of contractile phenotype. Cells subjected to cyclic strain display prominent bundles of myofilaments while control cells (no strain) exhibited no such bundles, but conversely displayed significant amounts of rough endoplasmic reticulum (synthetic phenotype) [Kim and Mooney, 2000]. Mechanical stress causes elevated protein synthesis and gene expression in cells [Nerem and Seliktar, 2001], and has a favorable effect on cell proliferation [Stegemann and Nerem, 2001] and DNA synthesis [Gooch and Tennant, 1997; Karim et al., 1992].

In developing the bioartificial esophagus, the relationship between magnitude and frequency of stimulation and the optimal function of the smooth muscle cells has been examined *in vitro* using the apparatus shown schematically in Figure 54.10a. This apparatus is based on one-dimensional mechanical stimulators reported in the literature [Kanda et al., 1992; Kim and Mooney, 2000]. Apparatus for the conditioning of tissue constructs consists of a reservoir of culture medium, and a means for applying the mechanical stimulus, as shown schematically in Figure 54.10a,b. Simulation may be by means of a slider-crank mechanism [Kim and Mooney, 2000], lead screw [Kanda et al., 1992], or linear motor, as in the bioreactor in Figure 54.10b. One-dimensional stimulation as shown in Figure 54.10a,b has shown to influence the alignment of smooth muscle cells, so that they align perpendicular to the direction of principal strain [Kanda et al., 1992]. If this effect is not desired, a bioreactor as shown in Figure 54.11a may be used to subject the construct to a two-dimensional stress state [Gooch and Tennant, 1997]. The pressure difference

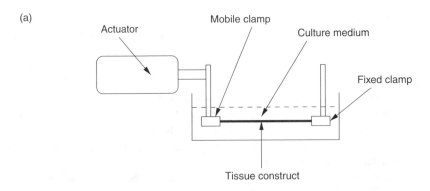

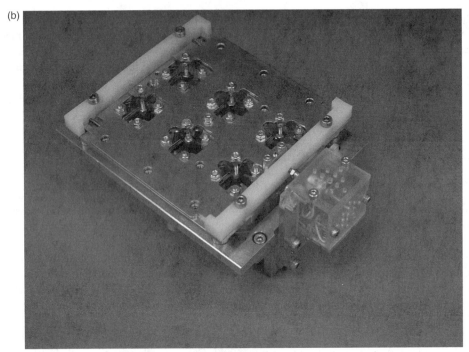

FIGURE 54.10   (a) Schematic of apparatus for tissue engineering. (b) Bioreactor developed at Nanyang Technological University for one-dimensional stimulation of smooth muscle and endothelial cells.

between the two chambers causes the scaffold to stretch, resulting in the bi-axial stress state as shown in Figure 54.11b. The culture chamber is maintained at atmospheric pressure (P1), while a pressure controller varies the pressure in the lower chamber [Gooch and Tennant, 1997]. Bioreactors based on this principle are available commercially, an example being the Flexcell Stage Flexer (Flexcell International Corp., Hillsborough, NC, USA).

Thicker tissue constructs have been fabricated from sheets incorporating a single layer of cells by rolling a matured, conditioned flat construct into a tubular structure [Nerem and Seliktar, 2001]. Alternatively, the tubular construct may also be mechanically conditioned, as shown in Figure 54.12. The construct is mounted between two tubular clamps and pressurized intermittently to provide radial and circumferential stress. This approach finds particular application in the tissue engineering of blood vessels although it also has application in the development of the bioartificial esophagus [Niklason et al., 1999; Nerem and Seliktar, 2001]. Mechanical conditioning has been found to significantly increase the burst strength of tissue-engineered blood vessels and may be expected to have a similar effect on the strength of an esophageal construct.

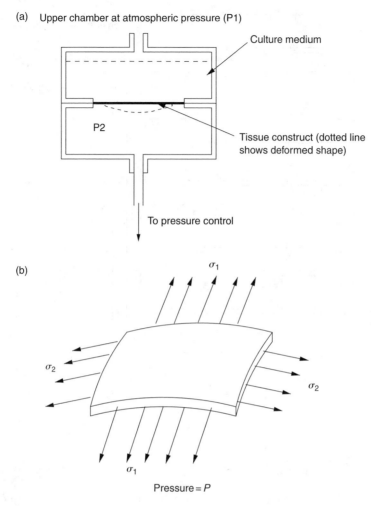

FIGURE 54.11 (a) Bioreactor for two-dimensional stress stimulation of cells. (b) Two-dimensional stress state in tissue construct.

As the esophagus is a thick-walled structure, necrosis of cells due to insufficient nutrition becomes a major issue. Myocytes are highly metabolically active and do not tolerate hypoxia well [Carrier et al., 1999; Radisic et al., 2003], and insufficient nutrition may result in necrosis of cells, particularly toward the center of the construct [Bethiaume and Yarmush, 2000]. A novel approach to this problem has been proposed [Kofidis et al., 2003] in which a section of native artery is used to provide a central vessel in a thick construct. The authors report viable cells in vascular constructs up to 8 mm in thickness, with a central vessel of mean diameter 2 mm.

The esophagus presents novel bioreactor challenges, and while much of the science generated in the development of bioartificial vascular constructs will influence application in other tissue types, a bioreactor must be developed to provide an analog of developmental conditions in the esophagus. A baby is able to swallow at birth: the neonatal esophagus is fully developed. We must therefore provide a means to replicate neonatal conditions *in vitro*. The final phase of development will be to build the bioreactor shown in Figure 54.13. It incorporates a tubular cell/scaffold construct with culture medium supplied to the outer jacket. The central canal of the esophagus can be drained from the bottom to provide the air/endothelium interface found in the esophagus. The central canal also incorporates a stimulator, consisting of a series of expandable chambers, which may be inflated in sequence by compressed air to simulate the passage of a bolus of masticated food through the esophagus.

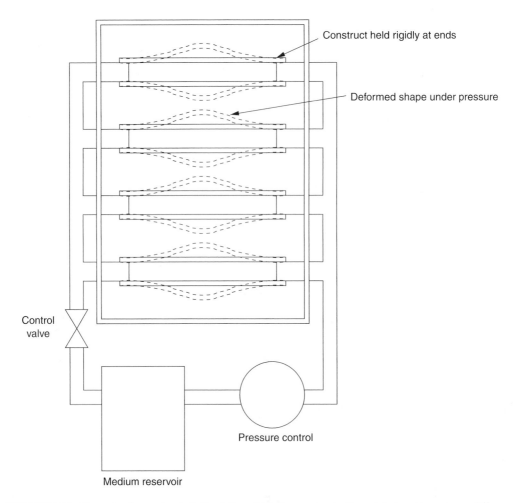

FIGURE 54.12 Bioreactor for mechanical stimulation of tubular constructs. Stress is induced by pressure difference between the inside of the construct and surroundings.

54.8 Conclusions and Prognostications

The potential to have significant impact on medicine and to make a positive contribution to the quality of life for esophagus surgery patients exists in the tissue engineering of esophagus. When this technology/biology triumph is realized, tissue engineering of other epithelial tissues such as stomach and colon will quickly follow.

The innovations that will make esophageal tissue engineering a routine procedure will come from interdisciplinary team efforts and an engineering systems approach. There are still many issues with regard to science and technology that must be resolved to develop the system for esophageal replacement. It is more than cell growth. It is more than surgery. It is more than chemistry. No one discipline can marshal all of the needed skills to make this happen. The engineered systems concept charts a path from science discoveries to products and generates a roadmap with needed team players, economic issues, milestones, and alternate strategies.

There are still significant technical challenges, challenges without clear solutions at this time. How we will go from an *in vitro* seeded cell construct to a vascularized, integrated tissue before hypoxic cell death occurs is not clear. How we will ultimately use allogeneic cells allowing an "off-the-shelf" surgical replacement challenges our understanding of cell-induced immune response. Matching (or exceeding) the mechanical properties of the natural tissue remains challenging. Many other sizable challenges remain.

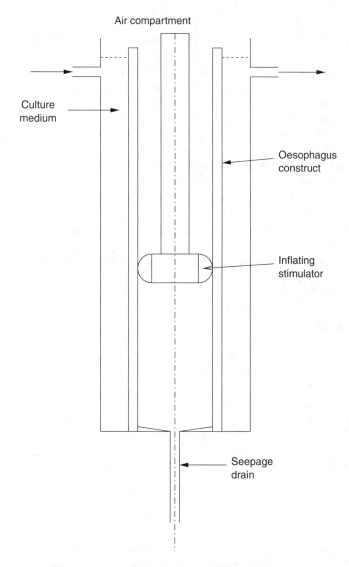

FIGURE 54.13 Schematic of bioreactor for environmental conditioning of constructs.

Acknowledgments

The authors acknowledge the generous support of the Singapore Agency for Science, Technology and Research (A*Star) to the Singapore-University of Washington Alliance (SUWA), and NSF support to the University of Washington Engineered Biomaterials (UWEB) program. SUWA is a close collaboration between UWEB and the Nanyang Technological University Biomedical Engineering Research Centre (BMERC).

References

Amato R. 1972. Textile machine. US Patent no. 3665695.

Ang T., Sultana F., Hutmacher D., Wong Y., Fuh J., Mo X., Loh H., Burdet E., and Teoh S. 2002. Fabrication of 3-d chitosan-hydroxyapatite scaffolds using a robotic dispensing system. *Mater. Sci. Eng.*, C20: 35.

Asselineau D., Bernard B., Bailly C., and Darmon M. 1989. Retinoic acid improves epidermal morphogenesis. *Dev. Biol.*, 133: 322–335.

Asselineau D., Bernhard B., Bailly C., and Darmon M. 1985. Epidermal morphogenesis and induction of the 67 kd keratin polypeptide by culture of human keratinocytes at the liquid–air interface. *Exp. Cell Res.*, 159: 536.

Atala A. and Lanza R. 2002. *Methods of Tissue Engineering.*, Academic Press, USA.

Badylak S. 2002. The extracellular matrix as a scaffold for tissue reconstruction. *Cell Dev. Biol.*, 13: 377.

Badylak S., Meurling S., Chen M., Spievack A., and Simmons-Byrd A. 2000. Resorbable bioscaffold for esophageal repair in a dog model. *J. Pediatr. Surg.*, 35: 1097.

Badylak S., Tullius R., Kokini K., Shelbourne K., Klootwyck T., Voytik S., Kraine M., and Simmons C. 1995. The use of xenographic small intestinal submucosa as a biomaterial for achilles tendon repair in a dog model. *J. Biomed. Mater. Res.*, 29: 977–985.

Bethiaume F. and Yarmush M. 2000. Tissue engineering. In: *The Biomedical Engineering Handbook*, Bronzino J., Ed., 2nd ed. CRC Press, Boca Raton, FL.

Bornat A. 1982. Electrostatic spinning of tubular products. US Patent no. 4323525.

Bottaro D. and Heidaran M. 2001. Engineered extracellular matrices: a biological solution for tissue repair, regeneration, and replacement. *e-Biomed*, 2: 9–12.

Bowland E., Wnek G., Simpson D., Pawlowski K., and Bowlin G. 2001. Tailoring tissue engineering scaffolds by employing electrostatic processing techniques: A study of poly(glycolic acid). *J. Macromol. Sci.*, 31: 1231–1243.

Brauker J., Carr-Brendel V., Martinson L., Crudele J., Johnston W., and Johnson R. 1995. Neovascularisation of synthetic membranes directed by membrane microarchitecture. *J. Biomed. Mater. Res.*, 29: 1517.

Burkitt H., Young B., and Heath J. 1993. *Wheater's Functional Histology.* 3rd ed. Longman, London.

Carrier R., Papadaki M., Rupnick M., Schoen F., Bursac N., Langer R., Freed L., and Vunjak-Novakovic G. 1999. Cardiac tissue engineering: cell seeding, cultivation parameters, and tissue construct characterization. *Biotechnol. Bioeng.*, 64: 580.

Chao F., Yan Y., and Zhang R. 2002. Comparison and analysis of continuously jetting and discretely jetting method in rapid ice prototype forming. *Mater. Des.*, 23: 77.

Chian K.S. 2003. Unpublished data. Nanyang Technological University.

Chu B., Hsiao B., Fang D., and Braithwaite C. 2004. Biodegradable and/or bioabsorbable fibrous articles and methods for using the article for medical applications. US Patent no. 6685956.

Compton C., Warland G., Nakagawa H., Opitz O., and Rustgi A. 1998. Cellular characterization and successful transfection of serially subcultured normal human esophageal keratinocytes. *J. Cell Physiol.*, 177: 274.

Cook A., Hrkach J., Gao N., Johnson I., Pajvani U., Cannizzaro S., and Langer R. 1997. Characterisation and development of rgd-peptide modified poly(lactic acid-co-lysine) as an interactive, resorbable biomaterial. *J. Biomed. Mater. Res.*, 35: 513.

Doshi J. and Reneker D. 1995. Electrospinning process and applications of electrospun fibers. *J. Electrostat.*, 35: 151.

Dotto G. 1999. Signal transduction pathways controlling the switch between keratinocyte growth and differentiation. *Crit. Rev. Oral Biol. Med.*, 10: 442.

Eastwood G. 1977. Gastrointestinal epithelial renewal. *Gastroenterology*, 72: 962.

Ergun G, and Kahrilas P. 1997. Esophageal anatomy and physiology. In: *Gastroenterology and Hepatology*, Orlando R, Ed., 3rd ed. Churchill Livingstone, Philadelphia.

Formhals A. 1934. Process and apparatus for preparing artificial threads. US Patent no. 1975504.

Fuchs E. 1996. The cytoskeleton and disease: genetic disorders of intermediate filaments. *Annu. Rev. Genet.*, 30: 197.

Fuchs E. and Green H. 1981. Regulation of terminal differentiation of cultured human keratinocytes by vitamin A. *Cell*, 25: 617.

Fuchs J., Nasseri B., and Vacanti J. 2001. Tissue engineering: a 21st century solution to surgical reconstruction. *Ann. Thorac. Surg.*, 72: 577.

Gershon M., Kirchgessner A., and Wade P. 1994. Functional anatomy of enteric nervous system. In: *Physiology of the Gastrointestinal Tract*, Johnson L., Ed., 3rd ed. Raven Press, New York.

Giordano R., Wu B., Borland S., Cima L., Sachs E., and Cima M. 1996. Mechanical properties of dense polylactic acid structures fabricated by three dimensional printing. *J. Biomat. Sci. Polym. Ed.*, 8: 63.

Glass J., Blevitt J., Dickerson K., Pierschbacher M., and Craig W. 1994. Cell attachment and motility on materials modified by surface-active rgd-containing peptides. *Ann. NY Acad. Sci.*, 745: 177.

Gooch K. and Tennant C. 1997. *Mechanical Forces: Their Effects on Cells and Tissues.* Spinger-Verlag and Landes Bioscience, Berlin.

Goyal R. and Sivarao D. 1999. Functional anatomy and physiology of swallowing and esophageal motility. In: *The Esophagus*, Castell D. and Richter J. Eds., 3rd ed. Lippincott Williams and Wilkins, Philadelphia.

Gray H. 1995. *Gray's Anatomy: The Anatomical Basis of Medicine and Surgery.* Churchill Livingstone, New York.

Grikscheit T., Ochoa E., Srinivasan A., Gaissert H., and Vacanti J. 2003. Tissue-engineered esophagus: experimental substitution by onlay patch or interposition. *J. Thorac. Cardiovasc. Surg.*, 126: 537.

Hartgerink J., Beniash E., and Stupp S. 2002. Peptide-amphiphile nanofibers: A versatile scaffold for the preparation of self-assembling materials. *Proc. Natl Acad. Sci. USA*, 99: 5133.

Hori Y., Nakamura T., Kimura D., Kaino K., Kurokawa Y., Satomi S., and Shimizu Y. 2003. Effect of basic fibroblast growth factor on vascularization in esophagus tissue engineering. *Int. J. Artif. Organs*, 26: 241.

Huang L., McMillan R., Apkarian R., Pourdeyhimi B., Conticello V., and Chaikof E. 2000. Generation of synthetic elastin-mimetic small diameter fibers and fiber networks. *Macromolecules*, 33: 2989.

Ike O., Shimizu Y., Okada T., Natsume T., Watanabe S., Ikada Y., and Hitomi S. 1989. Experimental studies on an artificial esophagus for the purpose of neoesophageal epithelization using a collagen-coated silicone tube. *ASAIO Trans.*, 35: 226.

Isch J., Engum S., Ruble C., Davis M., and Grosfeld J. 2001. Patch esophagoplasty using alloderm as a tissue scaffold. *J. Pediatr. Surg.*, 36: 266.

Kajitani M., Wadia Y., Hinds M., Teach J., Swartz K., and Gregory K. 2001. Successful repair of esophageal injury using an elastin based biomaterial patch. *J. Am. Soc. Artific. Internal Organs*, 47: 342.

Kanda K., Matsuda T., and Oka T. 1992. Two dimensional orientational response of smooth muscle cells to cyclic stretching. *J. Am. Soc. Artific. Internal Organs*, 38: M382.

Karim O., Pienta K., Seki N., and Mostwin J. 1992. Stretch-mediated visceral smooth muscle growth *in vitro*. *Am. J. Physiol.*, 262: R895–R992.

Khan S., Trento A., DeRoberts M., Kass R., Sandhu M., Czer L., Blanche C., Raissi S., Fontana G., Cheng W., Chaux A., and Matloff J. 2001. Twenty-year comparison of tissue and mechanical valve replacement. *J. Thorac. Cardiovasc. Surg.*, 122: 257–269.

Kim B., and Mooney D. 2000. Scaffolds for engineering smooth muscle under cyclic mechanical strain conditions. *Transac. ASME J. Biomech. Eng.*, 122: 210.

Kofidis T., Lenz A., Boublik J., Akhyari P., Wachsmann B., Stahl K., Haverich A., and Leyh R. 2003. Bioartificial grafts for transmural myocardial restoration: a new cardiovascular tissue culture concept. *Eur. J. Cardio-Thorac. Surg.*, 24: 906.

Kumar D. 1993. Morphology of the gastrointestinal motor system - gross morphology. In: *Gastrointestinal Motility*, Kumar D. and Wingate D., Eds., 2nd ed. Churchill Livingstone, Edinburgh.

Landers R., Pfister A., Hubner U., John H., Schmelzeisen R., and Mulhaupt R. 2002. Fabrication of soft tissue engineering scaffolds by means of rapid prototyping techniques. *J. Mater. Sci.*, 37: 3107.

Langer R. and Tirrell D. 2004. Designing materials for biology and medicine. *Nature*, 428: 487.

Leeson T. and Leeson C. 1981. *Histology.* 4th ed. W.B. Sauders, Philadelphia.

Leininger B., Peacock H., and Neville W. 1970. Esophageal mucosal regeneration following experimental prosthetic replacement of the esophagus. *Surgery*, 67: 468.

Leong M.F., Chian K.S., and Ritchie A.C. 2004. Unpublished data. Nanyang Technological University.

Levy R., Chu T., Halloran J., Feinberg S., and Hollister S. 1997. CT generated porous hydroxyapatite orbital floor prosthesis on a prototype bioimplant. *Am. J. Neuroradiol.*, 18: 1522.

Li W., Laurencin C., Caterson E., Tuan R., and Ko F. 2002. Electrospun nanofibrous structure: a novel scaffold for tissue engineering. *J. Biomed. Mater. Res.*, 60: 613.

Linnes M. 2004. Unpublished data. University of Washington.

Lo H., Ponticiello M., and Leong K. 1995. Fabrication of controlled release biodegradable foams by phase separation. *Tissue Eng.*, 1: 15.

Marshall A., Barker T., Sage E., Hauch K., and Ratner B. 2004. Pore size controls angiogenesis in subcutaneously implanted porous matrices. *Proceedings of the 7th World Biomaterials Congress in Sydney, Australia.*

Matsuda T., and Mizutani M. 2002. Liquid acrylate-endcapped biodegradable poly(e-caprolactone-co-trimethylene carbonate). ii. computer aided stereolithographic microarchitectural surface photoconstructs. *J. Biomed. Mater. Res.*, 62: 395.

Matthews J., Wnek G., Thomson D., and Bowlin G. 2002. Electrospinning of collagen nanofibers. *Biomolecules*, 3: 232.

McMillan R. and Conticello V. 2000. Synthesis and characterization of elastin-mimetic protein gels derived from a well-defined polypeptide precursor. *Macromolecules*, 33: 4809.

Meyer G. and Castell D. 1983. Anatomy and physiology of the esophageal body. In: *Esophageal Function in Health and Disease*, Castell D. and Johnson L., Eds., Elsevier Biomedical, New York.

Miki H., Ando N., Ozawa S., Sato M., Hayashi K., and Kitajima M. 1999. An artificial esophagus constructed of cultured human esophageal epithelial cells, fibroblasts, polyglycolic acid mesh and collagen. *J. Am. Soc. Artific. Internal Organs*, 45: 502.

Mikos A., Bao Y., Cima L., Ingber D., Vacanti J., and Langer R. 1993. Preparation of poly(glycolic acid) bonded fiber structures for cell attachment and transplantation. *J. Biomed. Mater. Res.*, 27: 183.

Mikos A., Lyman M., Freed L., and Langer R. 1994. Wetting of poly(l-lactic acid) and poly(dl-lactic-co-glycolic) foams for tissue culture. *Biomaterials*, 15: 55.

Mooney D., Baldwin D., Suh N., Vacanti J., and Langer R. 1996. Novel approach to fabricate porous sponges of poly(d,l-lactic-co-glycolic) without the use of organic solvents. *Biomaterials*, 17: 1417.

Natsume T., Ike O., Okada T., Shimizu Y., Ikada Y., and Tamura K. 1990. Experimental studies of a hybrid artificial esophagus combined with autologous mucosal cells. *ASAIO Trans.*, 36: M435.

Natsume T., Ike O., Okada T., Takimoto N., Shimizu Y., and Ikada Y. 1993. Porous collagen sponge for esophageal replacement. *J. Biomed. Mater. Res.*, 27: 867.

Nerem R. and Seliktar D. 2001. Vascular tissue engineering. *Annu. Rev. Biomed. Eng.*, 3: 225.

Niklason L., Gao J., Abbott W., Hirschi K., Houser S., Marini R., and Langer R. 1999. Functional arteries grown *in vitro*. *Science*, 284: 489.

Oda D., Savard C., Eng L., Sekijima J., Haigh G., and Lee S. 1998. Reconstituted human oral and esophageal mucosa in culture. *In vitro Cell Dev. Biol. Anim.*, 34: 46.

Okumura T., Shimada Y., Imamura M., and Yasumoto S. 2003. Neurotrophin receptor p75(ntr) characterizes human esophageal keratinocyte stem cells *in vitro*. *Oncogene*, 22: 4017.

Pachence J. and Kohn J. 2000. Biodegradable polymers. In: *Principles of Tissue Engineering*, Lanza R., Langer R., and Vacanti J., Eds., 2nd ed. Academic Press, New York.

Park A., Wu B., and Griffith L. 1998. Integration of surface modification and 3-d fabrication techniques to prepare patterned poly(l-lactide) substrates allowing regionally selective cell adhesion. *J. Biomater. Sci., Polym. Ed.*, 9: 89.

Peters M. and Mooney D. 1997. Synthetic extracellular matrices for cell transplantation. In: *Porous Materials for Tissue Engineering.*, Liu D. and Dixit V., Eds., volume 250 of *Materials Science Forum*. Trans Tech Publications, Enfield, pp. 43–52.

Radisic M., Euloth M., Yang L., Langer R., Freed L., and Vunjak-Novakovic G. 2003. High density seeding of myocyte cells for cardiac tissue engineering. *Biotechnol. Bioeng.*, 82: 403.

Rheinwald J. and Green H. 1975. Serial cultivation of strains of human epidermal keratinocytes: the formation of keratinizing colonies from single cells. *Cell*, 6: 331.

Rosengren A. and Bjursten L. 2003. Pore size in implanted polypropylene filters is critical for tissue organization. *J. Biomed. Mater. Res.*, 67A: 918.

Sachlos E. and Czernuszka J. 2003. Making tissue engineering scaffolds work. review on the application of solid freeform fabrication technology to the production of tissue engineering scaffolds. *Europ. Cells Mater.*, 5: 29.

Sato M., Ando N., Ozawa S., Miki H., Hayashi K., and Kitajima M. 1997. Artificial esophagus. In: *Porous Materials for Tissue Engineering.*, Liu D. and Dixit V., Eds., volume 250 of *Materials Science Forum.* Trans Tech Publications, Enfield.

Sato M., Ando N., Ozawa S., Miki H., and Kitajima M. 1994. An artificial esophagus consisting of cultured human esophageal epithelial cells, polyglycolic acid mesh, and collagen. *J. Am. Soc. Artific. Internal Organs*, 40: M389.

Sato M., Ando N., Ozawa S., Nagashima A., and Kitajima M. 1993. A hybrid artificial esophagus using cultured human esophageal epithelial cells. *J. Am. Soc. Artific. Internal Organs*, 39: M554.

Schmedlen R., Masters K., and West J. 2002. Photocrosslinkable polyvinyl alcohol hydrogels that can be modified with cell adhesion peptides for use in tissue engineering. *Biomaterials*, 23: 4325.

Seery J. and Watt F. 2000. Asymmetric stem-cell divisions define the architecture of human oesophageal epithelium. *Curr. Biol.*, 10: 1447.

Shin M., Hohman M., and Brenner M. 2001. Experimental characterization of electrospinning: the electrically forced jet and instabilities. *Polymer*, 42.

Shinhar D., Finaly R., Niska A., and Mares A. 1998. The use of collagen-coated vicryl mesh for reconstruction of the canine cervical esophagus. *Pediatr. Surg. Int.*, 13: 84.

Squier C., Johnson N., and Hopps R. 1976. *Human Oral Mucosa: Development, Structure, and Function.* Blackwell Scientific Publications, Oxford.

Squier C. and Kremer M. 2001. Biology of oral mucosa and esophagus. *J. Natl Cancer Inst. Monogr.*, 29: 7.

Stegemann J. and Nerem R. 2001. Effect of mechanical stimulation on smooth muscle cell proliferation and phenotype. *ASME Bioeng. Conf.*, BED 50: 609.

Stitzel J., Bowlin G., Mansfield K., Wnek G., and Simpson D. 2000. Electrospraying and electrospinning of polymers for biomedical applications: poly(lactic-co-glycolic acid) and poly(ethylene-co-vinyl acetate). In: *Proceedings of the 32nd Annual SAMPE Meeting.*

Summanasinghe R. and King M. 2003. New trends in biotextile — the challenges of tissue engineering. *J. Textile and Apparel, Technol. and Manag.*, 3: 1.

Takahashi H., Shikata N., Senzaki H., Shintaku M., and Tsubura A. 1995. Immunohistochemical staining patterns of keratins in normal oesophageal epithelium and carcinoma of the oesophagus. *Histopathology*, 26: 45.

Takimoto Y., Nakamura T., Yamamoto Y., Kiyotani T., Teramachi M., and Shimizu Y. 1998. The experimental replacement of a cervical esophageal segment with an artificial prosthesis with the use of collagen matrix and a silicone stent. *J. Thorac. Cardiovasc. Surg.*, 116: 98.

Takimoto Y., Okumura N., Nakamura T., Natsume T., and Shimizu Y. 1993. Long-term follow-up of the experimental replacement of the esophagus with a collagen–silicone composite tube. *J. Am. Soc. Artific. Internal Organs*, 39: M736.

Thomson R., Shung A., Yaszemski M., and Mikos A. 2000. Polymer scaffold processing. In: *Principles of Tissue Engineering*, Lanza R., Langer R., and Vacanti J., Eds., 2nd ed. Academic Press, New York.

Thomson R., Yaszemski M., Powers J., and Mikos A. 1995. Fabrication of biodegradable polymer scaffolds to engineer trabecular bone. *J. Biomater. Sci. Polymer Ed.*, 7: 23.

Ure B., Slany E., Eypasch E., Weiler K., Troidl H., and Holschneider A. 1998. Quality of life more than 20 years after repair of esophageal atresia. *J. Paediatr. Surg.*, 33: 511.

Urry D., Parker T., Reid M., and Gowda D. 1991. Biocompatibility of the bioelastic material poly(gvgvp) and its γ-irradiation crosslinked matrix. *J. Bioact. Compat. Polym.*, 3: 263.

Wake M., Gupta P., and Mikos A. 1996. Fabrication of pliable biodegradable polymer foams to engineer soft tissues. *Cell Transplant.*, 5: 465.

Wake M., Patrick C., and Mikos A. 1994. Pore morphology effects on the fribovascular tissue growth in porous polymer substrates. *Cell Transplant.*, 3: 339.

Ward W., Slobodzian E., Tiekotter K., and Wood M. 2002. The effect of microgeometry, implant thickness and polyurethane chemistry on the foreign body response to subcutaneous implants. *Biomaterials*, 23: 4185.

Watanabe K. and Mark J. 1971. Segmental replacement of the thoracic esophagus with silastic prosthesis. *Am. J. Surg.*, 121: 238.

Watt F. 1984. Selective migration of terminally differentiating cells from the basal layer of cultured human epidermis. *J. Cell Biol.*, 98: 16.

Whang K., Thomas H., and Healy K. 1995. A novel method to fabricate biodegradable scaffolds. *Polymer*, 36: 837.

Widmer M., Gupta P., Lu L., Meszlenyi R., Evans G., Brandt K., Savel T., Gurlek A., Patrick C., and Mikos A. 1998. Manufacture of porous biodegradable polymer conduits by an extrusion process for guided tissue regeneration. *Biomaterials*, 19: 1945.

Wingate D. 1993. Regulation of gastrointestinal motility — intrinsic and extrinsic neural control. In: *Gastrointestinal Motility*, Kumar D. and Wingate D., Eds., 2nd ed. Churchill Livingstone, Edinburgh.

Wnek G., Carr M., Simpson D., and Bowlin G. 2003. Electrospinning of nanofibrous fibrinogen structures. *Nano Lett.*, 3: 213.

Wood J. 1994. Physiology of enteric nervous system. In: *Physiology of the Gastrointestinal Tract*, Johnson L., Ed., 3rd ed. Raven Press, New York.

Yamamoto Y., Nakamura T., Shimizu Y., Matsumoto K., Takimoto Y., Kiyotani T., Sekine T., Ueda H., Liu Y., and Tamura N. 1999a. Intrathoracic esophageal replacement in the dog with the use of an artificial esophagus composed of a collagen sponge with a double-layered silicone tube. *J. Thorac. Cardiovasc. Surg.*, 118: 276.

Yamamoto Y., Nakamura T., Shimizu Y., Takimoto Y., Matsumoto K., Kiyotani T., Yu L., Ueda H., Sekine T., and Tamura N. 1999b. Experimental replacement of the thoracic esophagus with a bioabsorbable collagen sponge scaffold supported by a silicone stent in dogs. *J. Am. Soc. Artific. Internal Organs*, 45: 311.

Yamamoto Y., Nakamura T., Shimizu Y., Matsumoto K., Takimoto Y., Liu Y., Ueda H., Sekine T., and Tamura N. 2000. Intrathoracic esophageal replacement with a collagen sponge-silicone double layer tube: evaluation of omental-pedicle wrapping and prolonged placement of an inner stent. *J. Am. Soc. Artific. Internal Organs*, 46: 734.

Yarin A., Koombhongse S., and Reneker D. 2001. Taylor cone and jetting from liquid droplets in electrospinning of nanofibers. *J. Appl. Phys.*, 90: 4836–4846.

Zeltinger J., Sherwood J., Graham D., Meuller R., and Griffith L. 2001. Effect of pore size and void fraction on cellular adhesion, proliferation, and matrix deposition. *Tissue Eng.*, 7: 557.

Zhang W., Leu M., Ji Z., and Yan Y. 2001. Method and apparatus for rapid freeze prototyping. US Patent no. 6253116.

55

Tissue Engineered Vascular Grafts

Rachael H. Schmedlen
Wafa M. Elbjeirami
Andrea S. Gobin
Jennifer L. West
Rice University

55.1 Introduction

Cardiovascular disease remains the leading cause of death in the United States, claiming more lives each year than the next five leading causes of death combined (American Heart Association National Center for Health Statistics). Coronary heart disease caused more than 1 in every 5 American deaths in 2000 and required approximately 500,000 coronary artery bypass graft surgeries (CABGs) that year. Bypass grafting is also used in the treatment of aneurysmal disease or trauma. At present, surgeons use autologous tissue and synthetic biomaterials as vascular grafts. Transplantation of autologous tissue has the best outcome in small diameter applications such as CABG because synthetic grafts lack long-term patency for small diameter applications (<6 mm). However, autologous tissue is limited in supply. Recent advances in tissue engineering provide hope that new blood vessel substitutes may one day be fabricated for small diameter applications, such as CABG, where treatment options are often severely limited.

55.1.1 Current Vascular Grafts

Currently, occluded vessels with diameters <6 mm are bypassed with autologous native blood vessels such as the saphenous vein as a treatment. Autologous blood vessels were first employed in the beginning of the 20th century when Goyanes reported the use of a graft to replace an excised segment of artery by bridging the defect with the patient's own popliteal vein [Goyanes, 1906]. Since then, venous grafts have retained the best long-term patency rate, although limitations such as deterioration when exposed to increased flow and pressure still remain [Crawford et al., 1981; Szilagyi et al., 1973]. More recently, the internal mammary artery from the chest has shown to be a superior conduit to the saphenous vein with better long-term patency and has gained increasing use [Kock et al., 1996]. These native vessels generally display 50 to 70% graft patency over 10 years (VA study). Moreover, the superior patency of native vessels is attributed to their compliant natural tissue characteristics and to their antithrombogenic luminal endothelial lining [Richardson et al., 1980]. Unfortunately, ~60% of patients who require vascular bypass surgery do not have a suitable vessel for grafting [Moneta and Porter, 1995], either due to earlier procedures or advanced peripheral vascular disease. As a result, alternative conduits constructed with synthetic materials have been investigated.

The use of synthetic vascular prostheses for replacement of natural blood vessels has been explored since the 1950s [Vorhees et al., 1952]. The most widely employed materials include Dacron™ (polyethylene terepthalate; PET), Gore-Tex™ (expanded polytetrafluoroethylene; ePTFE), and compliant polyurethanes. A strong, yet flexible polymer, PET may be fabricated in woven, velour, or knitted fiber configurations [Coury et al., 1996]. ePTFE possesses a smooth surface and exhibits good durability and biocompatibility. Polyurethane has been increasingly studied because it has been developed to more closely match the compliance of native vessels than Gore-Tex™ or Dacron, which may reduce some clinical complications [Giudiceandrea et al., 1998]. These materials are readily available, relatively inexpensive, and have seen success clinically in applications with vessel diameters greater than 6 mm. However, synthetic grafts with a small diameter (<6 mm, e.g., coronary artery bypass and femoral-crural bypass) exhibit unsatisfactory long-term patency due to graft thrombogencity and neointima formation.

Platelet adhesion and aggregation on the graft surface often results in reocclusion of the vessel. This is caused by the adsorption of proteins that mediate platelet adhesion and coagulation processes on the relatively hydrophobic polymeric materials. The need for a nonthrombogenic surface has lead to the investigation of endothelial cell (EC) seeding on the lumen of the graft. Although EC seeding improves synthetic graft patency, EC retention under physiological shear conditions remains problematic [Thompson et al., 1994; Deutsch et al., 1999]. Furthermore, differences in elasticity between a synthetic material and the adjacent tissue create discrepancies in strain at the anastomoses, referred to as compliance mismatch, contributing to intimal hyperplasia [Geary et al., 1993; Greisler et al., 1993]. Moreover, synthetic grafts have been shown to carry an increased risk of infection [Clowes, 1993], further limiting their clinical efficacy.

55.1.2 Tissue Engineering

Most tissue engineering strategies attempt to create small caliber vascular grafts by closely mimicking the structure, function, and physiologic environment of native vessels. Normal arteries possess three distinct tissue layers (Figure 55.1): the intima, media, and adventitia. The intima consists of an EC

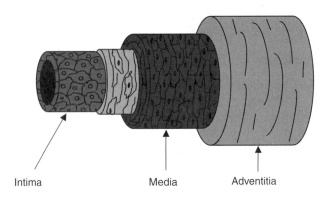

Intima   Media   Adventitia

FIGURE 55.1 The arterial wall is composed of three distinct layers: the intima, media, and adventitia. The intima, composed of endothelial cells, provides a nonthrombogenic surface. In the medial layer, smooth muscle cells and elastin fibers align circumferentially and provide mechanical integrity and contractility. The outer adventitia is a supportive connective tissue.

monolayer, which prevents platelet aggregation and regulates vessel permeability, vascular smooth muscle cell behavior, and homeostasis. Within the medial layer, smooth muscle cells (SMCs) and elastin fibers are aligned circumferentially, contributing the majority of the vessel's mechanical strength [Wight, 1996]. Dilation and constriction of the vessel are due to medial SMCs' response to external stimuli. Finally, the adventitial layer contains fibroblasts, connective tissue, the microvascular supply, and a neural network that regulates the vasotone of the blood vessel. The recreation of some or all of the vessel layers and their properties may result in the development of a patent, functional vascular graft. In all likelihood, an intima and media will be required to achieve any degree of success.

The general concept for creating a tissue-engineered vascular graft (TEVG) usually involves the harvest of desired cells, cell expansion in culture, cell seeding onto a scaffold, construct culture in an environment that induces tissue formation, and implantation of the construct back into the patient. Many options exist at each step of this process and each must be carefully considered. First, cell source and culture conditions must be determined. Due to concerns regarding immunogenicity, autologous cells are likely to be required, but these may be differentiated SMCs and ECs or a variety of types of vascular progenitors. Expansion *in vitro* is usually necessary, but *in vitro* culture time must also be minimized to avoid cell dedifferentiation. Genetic modification of cells may also be a means to improve TEVG performance. In addition to the cellular component, some type of material, or scaffolding, is generally required to provide mechanical support and integrity. Many varieties of scaffolds are used in tissue engineering, primarily composed of extracellular matrix (ECM) proteins and synthetic polymeric materials. Once cells are seeded onto scaffolds, another *in vitro* culture period is usually needed to allow for new tissue formation and development of appropriate mechanical and functional characteristics. During the culture period, the construct should receive appropriate chemical and mechanical signals for cells to synthesize proteins, remodel the tissue, and organize their environment such that the construct will develop into a functional graft with mechanical properties similar to native vessels. Therefore, a tissue-engineered construct may require several weeks of preparation before it can be implanted into the patient.

While efforts to create TEVGs remain in an early developmental stage, several problems potentially exist. Graft patency is still threatened by thrombosis, in all likelihood due to issues with retention of ECs after implantation or with alterations in EC function after culture *in vitro*. Also, the possibility of burst failure after implantation in the physiological flow environment raises concern since the consequences would be catastrophic. Mechanical properties of TEVGs are generally observed to be lower than those of native arteries, and thus a number of approaches have begun to address these issues. All of the strategies discussed above — cell source, genetic modification, scaffold materials, and culture conditions — will likely impact the fabrication of an optimal, clinically useful TEVG.

55.2 Cell Sources for Vascular Tissue Engineering

The development of a functional TEVG is likely to require the construction of an intima and media composed of ECs and SMCs. Limitations imposed by immunogenicity will probably require the use of autologous cells, so the majority of studies to date have utilized differentiated SMCs and ECs isolated from harvested blood vessels. Issues with donor site morbidity and the performance of these cells types in the engineered tissues have led to the consideration of alternative cell sources. Recent advances in stem cell biology offer hope for suitable progenitors that can be effectively differentiated into ECs and SMCs for use in vascular tissue engineering.

Circulating endothelial progenitor cells [Wijelath et al., 2004; Griese et al., 2003; He et al., 2003; Shirota et al., 2003] and smooth muscle progenitor cells [Simper et al., 2002] can be isolated from blood, offering a potential source of autologous cells for tissue engineering if they can be appropriately expanded in culture. Blood-derived endothelial progenitors have already been utilized as linings on synthetic vascular grafts in several studies [He et al., 2003; Shirota et al., 2003]. Grafts lined with these endothelial progenitors have been implanted in a canine carotid model, and after more than 30 days, 11 out of 12 grafts remained patent, and cells lining the surface appeared to be ECs [He et al., 2003]. Umbilical cord blood [Murga et al., 2004] and bone marrow [Hamilton et al., 2004] may be additional sources of autologous vascular progenitor cells.

55.3   Genetic Modification of Vascular Cells

The leading cause of vascular graft failure has been attributed to thrombosis. Genetic engineering of vascular cells *ex vivo* may provide an effective strategy to improve graft properties for tissue engineering applications. Investigators have reported transduction of vascular cells such as ECs [Wilson et al., 1989; Dunn et al., 1996], fibroblasts [Scharfmann et al., 1991], and SMCs [Lynch et al., 1992]. The seeding of small-diameter vascular graft constructs with either ECs or SMCs genetically engineered to secrete anti-thrombotic factors exists as a potential method of improving graft patency rates. As an example, baboon ECs have been genetically modified with a retroviral vector encoding antithrombotic factors, namely tissue plasminogen activator (tPA) and glycosylphosphatidylinositol-anchored urokinase-plasminogen activator (uPA) [Dichek et al., 1996]. The modified cells were seeded on the luminal surface of collagen-coated Dacron surfaces and introduced in arteriovenous shunts in baboons. A significant reduction in platelet and fibrin accumulation was observed in grafts containing modified ECs expressing either tPA or uPA. In another approach, the use of a platelet aggregation inhibitor, nitric oxide (NO), has shown to be promising. Using an *ex vivo* approach, bovine SMCs liposomally transfected with nitric oxide synthase III (NOS III) and GTP cyclohydrolase, which produces a cofactor essential for NOS activity, were grown as monolayers on plastic slides or biomaterials of interest and then placed in a parallel-plate flow chamber. Whole blood was introduced into the flow chamber to assess platelet adherence to the cell monolayers. The number of platelets that adhered to the NOS-transduced SMCs was significantly lower than those bound to mock-transduced SMCs and similar to the numbers adhered to cultured ECs. Moreover, the NOS-expressing SMCs exhibited decreased proliferative activity, which may reduce the incidence of intimal hyperplasia [Scott-Burden et al., 1996]. These studies demonstrated that an *ex vivo* genetic engineering approach may be useful for altering thrombogenicity of TEVG surfaces.

An alternative gene therapy approach to reducing the thrombogenicity of TEVG surfaces would utilize transfected VEGF. VEGF has shown to be mitogenic for ECs *in vitro* and stimulates angiogenesis *in vivo* [reviewed in Ahrendt et al., 1998]. More importantly, the mitogenic response associated with VEGF is restricted to ECs, which allows VEGF to be administered without concerns of SMC intimal hyperplasia. VEGF production in the TEVG may encourage proliferation of ECs seeded on the lumenal surface as well as stimulate endogenous host EC migration from the anastomoses. Transfecting SMCs with VEGF may allow for localized and prolonged treatment. Additionally, VEGF-producing SMCs have been found to promote EC proliferation and migration using *in vitro* models [Elbjeirami et al., 2004].

Improving the mechanical properties of TEVGs has also been a goal of numerous research efforts, and genetic modification of cells used to seed the TEVG may prove beneficial. The mechanical properties of a TEVG will be related in large part to the ECM that forms, both its composition and structure. ECM crosslinking can result from the enzymatic activity of lysyl oxidase (LO) or tissue transglutaminase [Aeschlimann et al., 1991] and may be a means to improve the mechanical properties of the TEVG. LO, a copper-dependent amine oxidase, forms lysine-derived crosslinks in connective tissue, particularly in collagen and elastin [Rucker et al., 1998]. Desmosine is produced in LO-mediated crosslinking of elastin and is commonly used as a biochemical marker of ECM crosslinking [Venturi et al., 1996]. The LO-catalyzed crosslinks are present in various connective tissues within the body including bone, cartilage, skin, and lung and are believed to be a major source of mechanical strength in tissues. Additionally, the LO-mediated enzymatic reaction renders crosslinked fibers less susceptible to proteolytic degradation [Vater et al., 1979]. A gene therapy strategy has demonstrated the enhancement of mechanical properties of tissue-engineered collagen constructs using vascular SMCs transfected with LO [Elbjeirami et al., 2003]. The elastic modulus and ultimate tensile strength of collagen gels seeded with LO-transfected SMCs nearly doubled as compared to gels seeded with mock-transfected SMCs. These enhanced mechanical properties resulted from increased ECM crosslinking rather than increased amounts of ECM, changes in the ECM composition, or increased cellularity. LO-mediated crosslinking, tissue transglutaminase, or glycation, may potentially be used in combination with mechanical conditioning, or biochemical factors, such as TGF-β, that increase the synthesis of ECM proteins to achieve synergistic effects. This strategy may ultimately enhance mechanical characteristics of TEVGs and minimize *in vitro* culture times prior to implantation.

Another effort in the use of genetic modification of vascular cells to improve TEVG performance has focused on regulation of SMC phenotype [Stegemann et al., 2004]. SMCs that were stably transfected with the gene for cyclic guanosine monophosphate-dependent protein kinase (PKG) were seeded into type I collagen constructs. PKG is an important regulator of SMC phenotype, and PKG-transfected cells showed substantially increased expression of smooth muscle α-actin, indicating a reduction in dedifferentiation during culture. Thus, TEVGs formed with such genetically modified cells may function more similarly to native tissues.

55.4   Scaffolds for Vascular Tissue Engineering

55.4.1   Natural Scaffold Materials

55.4.1.1   Collagen

One of the first TEVGs developed was based on a natural collagen type I scaffold supported by knitted Dacron [Weinberg and Bell, 1986]. This study provided early evidence of the feasibility of tissue engineering a blood vessel substitute by creating layers similar to those of a blood vessel using ECM components and vascular cells. Cultured bovine ECs, SMCs, and fibroblasts embedded within denatured bovine collagen were used to construct a multilayered vascular graft. Endothelium formation was confirmed by production of biosynthetic markers such as prostacylcin and von Willebrand's factor. The burst strength of the engineered tissue was proportional to the collagen content and cell density. However, the resultant engineered graft did not achieve sufficient mechanical strength to withstand physiological conditions unless a supporting Dacron mesh sleeve was added. In fact, maximum burst strengths seen in this model ($\approx$325 mmHg) were significantly lower than that of native coronary artery ($\approx$ 5000 mmHg) or saphenous vein ($\approx$2000 mmHg).

Glycation, the nonenzymatic crosslinking of ECM proteins by reducing sugars, has been proposed as a strategy to enhance the stiffness and strength of collagen gel constructs seeded with SMCs [Girton et al., 1999, 2000]. These constructs were cultured for 10 weeks under high concentrations of glucose or ribose and then assessed for mechanical properties. The circumferential tensile stiffness of constructs incubated in medium containing 30 mM ribose showed a 16-fold increase over normally cultured constructs while tensile strength increased by 4-fold. Although the compliance of the construct compared favorably, the tensile strength and burst pressure still fell significantly below that of arteries.

Expanding upon work with collagen scaffolds, others have further explored the potential utility of collagen scaffolds by evaluating decellularized collagen matrices from porcine tissue [Hiles et al., 1993; Huynh et al., 1999]. Small intestine submucosa (SIS) has been isolated and chemically treated to remove the cellular component, leaving an intact matrix containing mainly collagen. The mechanical properties and remodeling ability of SIS have been previously investigated for numerous tissue-engineering applications [Sacks et al., 1999; Gloeckner et al., 2000]. For vascular grafts, SIS possesses acceptable mechanical properties and exhibits better compliance than currently employed vein grafts [Roeder et al., 1999]. In one effort, Huynh et al. prepared SIS tubes and minimally chemically crosslinked the collagen layers to provide mechanical strength while maintaining biocompatibility. The inner surface of the grafts were additionally treated with a heparin complex to inhibit thrombosis and then implanted into rabbits. For time periods up to 13 weeks, grafts remained patent, and SMCs and ECs were found to have migrated into the graft from the surrounding tissue.

55.4.1.2 Decellularized Vascular matrix

Xenogenic acellular matrix conduits have also been investigated for the development of TEVG. In this approach, vessels are treated with reagents such as trypsin and EDTA [Bader et al., 2000] or sodium dodecyl sulfate [Schaner et al., 2004] to remove the cells, leaving an intact matrix that can be used as a scaffold. Decellularized porcine arteries have been seeded with human ECs and SMCs isolated from the saphenous vein [Teebken et al., 2000]. After exposure to pulsatile flow, the cell-seeded porcine matrix developed an endothelial monolayer. This study demonstrated the feasibility of generating vascular grafts *in vitro* from acellular, animal-derived, vascular matrices and human cells. Attempts to improve biocompatibility of xenograft matrices have included proteolysis of bovine or porcine carotid arteries [Moazami et al., 1998; Teebken et al., 2000]. This decellularized form provided an ECM with properly arranged collagen and elastin fibers that had minimal immune or inflammatory response [Teebken et al., 2000]. However, fibrosis eventually rendered these grafts unsuccessful.

55.4.1.3 Cell Sheets

L'Heureux and his collegues have applied a unique approach in the fabrication of a TEVG using biological materials, essentially using cells to generate the scaffold for the tissue-engineering construct [L'Heureux et al., 1998]. Umbilical vein SMCs and human skin fibroblasts were cultured for 5 weeks to form sheets containing superconfluent cells and cell-synthesized ECM. The cell sheets were sequentially rolled around a mandrel to form first the medial layer, then the adventitial layer. For 8 weeks, the construct was cultured in a bioreactor designed to provide perfusion of the culture medium and mechanical support. Following culture, the mandrel was removed, and the lumen was seeded with ECs, thus forming the three layers representative of a native artery. The burst strength of these grafts well exceeded that of native veins. Based on histological analysis, it appeared that SMCs were aligned circumferentially and produced a significant amount of new ECM. When implanted *in vivo*, these vascular substitutes had a 50% patency rate at one week after implantation. The construct consists entirely of human cells and human ECM proteins while exhibiting impressive mechanical strength, which makes this strategy attractive. However, much of the constructs' strength was attributed to the adventitial layer instead of the medial layer, as is normally observed in blood vessels. Some thrombus formation was also observed at the graft site following implantation. Furthermore, a 12-week time span was required to prepare a construct.

55.4.2 Synthetic Polymer Scaffolds

While the natural scaffold materials discussed above have achieved some success, concerns with disease transmission, difficulties with material processing, and often poor mechanical properties have led some groups to concentrate on the development of synthetic biomaterials as scaffolds. Bioabsorbable synthetic polymers may be designed to provide a transitional environment by providing a supporting structure to developing tissue. The degradation rate of these constructs may often be tailored to match the rate at which new tissue is formed, so that space is created for cell growth and matrix deposition. These materials serve as guides for tissue regeneration in three dimensions and offer the possibility to control structural variables and scaffold properties, such as the molecular structure, molecular weight, degradation properties, porosity, and mechanical properties [Ma et al., 1995].

55.4.2.1 Polyester Scaffolds

Polyglycolic acid (PGA), a biodegradable polyester, has demonstrated relatively good biocompatibility and has been extensively studied for numerous tissue-engineering applications [Freed et al., 1993; Kim et al., 1998; Mooney et al., 1996]. These well-characterized materials have been the first to illustrate the feasibility of polymeric scaffolds in vascular tissue engineering [Niklason et al., 1999]. TEVGs were fabricated using PGA mesh scaffolds, seeded with bovine aortic SMCs, then cultured in pulsatile flow bioreactors. After 8 weeks, these cultured vessels exhibited increased concentrations of collagen and enhanced mechanical properties. Burst pressure of these grafts compared well to that of typical vein grafts (human saphenous vein = 1680 ± 307 mmHg vs. PGA graft = 2150 ± 700 mmHg). When these grafts were seeded with autologous ECs on their luminal surface, continuously perfused for 3 days, and then implanted into pigs, they remained patent for up to 4 weeks.

55.4.2.2 Hydrogel Scaffolds

Derivatives of polyethylene glycol (PEG) currently are being studied as hydrogel scaffolds for blood vessel substitutes. These materials are hydrophilic, biocompatible, and intrinsically resistant to protein adsorption and cell adhesion [Merrill et al., 1983; Gombotz et al., 1991]. Thus, PEG essentially provides a "blank slate," devoid of biological interactions, upon which the desired biofunctionality can be built. Aqueous solutions of acrylated PEG can be rapidly photopolymerized in direct contact with cells and tissues [Sawhney et al., 1994; Hill-West et al., 1994]. Furthermore, PEG-based materials can be rendered bioactive by inclusion of proteolytically degradable peptides into the polymer backbone [West et al., 1999] and by grafting adhesion peptides [Hern et al., 1998] or growth factors [Mann et al., 2001a] into the hydrogel network during the photopolymerization process. Recently, PEG hydrogels that largely mimic the properties of collagen have been developed. PEG hydrogels grafted with a synthetic adhesive peptide RGDS and the collagenase-sensitive peptide sequence GGGLGPAGGK permitted cell migration [Gobin and West 2002; Mann et al., 2001b]. Following 7 days of incubation, approximately 70% as many cells migrated through collagenase-sensitive hydrogels as through collagen gels, with no statistically significant difference between the two groups. The elastin-derived peptide VAPG has shown to be specific for SMC adhesion, and PEG hydrogels modified with this adhesive peptide rather than RGDS supported adhesion and growth of vascular SMCs but not fibroblasts or platelets [Gobin et al., 2003]. Moreover, bioactive molecules like TGF-β may be covalently incorporated into scaffolds to induce protein synthesis by vascular SMCs. TGF-β has been reported to stimulate expression of several matrix components, including elastin, collagen, fibronectin, and proteoglycans [Amento et al., 1991; Lawrence et al., 1994; Tajima, 1996]. TGF-β covalently immobilized to PEG-based hydrogels significantly increased collagen production of vascular SMCs seeded within these scaffold materials [Mann et al., 2001]. Mechanical testing of these engineered tissues also determined that the elastic modulus was higher in TGF-β-tethered PEG scaffolds than PEG scaffolds without TGF-β, indicating that material properties for TEVGs may be improved using this technology. A cell-seeded graft formed from this biomimetic hydrogel scaffold is shown in Figure 55.2. These types of bioactive materials may allow one to capture the advantages of a natural scaffold, such as specific cell–material interactions and proteolytic remodeling in response to tissue formation, while also having the benefits of a synthetic material, namely the ease of processing and the ability to manipulate mechanical properties.

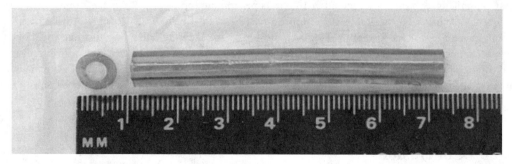

FIGURE 55.2 A PEG-based scaffold seeded with smooth muscle cells and endothelial cells ready for insertion into a bioreactor for *in vitro* culture of a TEVG (left, standing upright; right, laying on side). The cell-seeded scaffold is formed via photopolymerization, so the dimensions are easily tailored for a given application and cells are homogeneously seeded throughout the material. The scaffold is designed to degrade in response to cellular proteolytic activity during tissue formation.

55.5 Bioreactors for Mechanical Conditioning

In vivo, the pulsatile nature of blood flow imposes radial pressure upon the vessel wall, which subjects SMCs within the medial layer to cyclic strain. Thus, a great deal of research has examined SMC behavior in response to cyclic stretch and found such stimuli important in the fabrication of vascular tissue, particularly with respect to ECM synthesis and tissue organization. For example, SMCs seeded on purified elastin membranes and exposed to 2 days of cyclic stretching (10% beyond the resting length) have been shown to incorporate hydroxyproline into protein three to five times more rapidly than stationary controls, indicating increased collagen synthesis in response to strain [Leung et al., 1976]. Cyclic strain also increased the synthesis of collagen types I and III and chondroitin-6-sulfate without stimulating DNA synthesis. Another study also detected enhanced matrix production in collagen constructs seeded with rat aortic SMCs and subjected to 7% cyclic strain [Kim et al., 1999]. Over 20 weeks of culture under cyclic strain, SMCs upregulated expression of elastin and collagen type I. Elastin content from these SMCs increased 49% over unstretched controls. Furthermore, organization of the tissue was observed, as evidenced by perpendicular alignment of SMCs to the direction of the applied strain.

Similar results have been obtained in three-dimensional constructs. Tubular collagen constructs seeded with SMCs were cultured over thin-walled silicone sleeves and subsequently exposed to regulated intraluminal pressures to stretch the vessel in a repeatable fashion for up to 8 days. The 10% cyclic distension in diameter caused the scaffolds to contract, SMCs and bundles of collagen fibers to align circumferentially around the vessel, and improvement of the scaffold's mechanical properties [Seliktar et al., 2000]. Moreover, this model system was employed to investigate the remodeling capacity of these constructs via the activity of matrix metalloproteinases (MMPs) known to cleave solubilized type I collagen fragments [Seliktar et al., 2001]. Constructs mechanically conditioned for 4 days contained five times higher amounts of MMP-2 compared to static controls and increased MMP-2 activity. The increases in MMP-2 levels correlated favorably with improvements in mechanical strength and material modulus as a result of cyclic strain. When a nonspecific inhibitor of MMP-2 was added to the culture media, MMP-2 levels decreased and mechanical properties were reduced, negating the benefits of mechanical conditioning. These studies indicate that strain-mediated remodeling of collagen scaffolds is essential for improved construct of mechanical properties.

Because of the profound effects of cyclic strain on SMC orientation, ECM production, and tissue organization, preculture of vascular graft constructs in a pulsatile flow bioreactor system may help recreate the natural structure of native vessels and allow one to better achieve the mechanical properties required of the construct. A schematic of a typical pulsatile flow bioreactor system is shown in Figure 55.3. The mechanical stimuli from pulsatile flow could generate the cyclic strain necessary to alter ECM production, thereby creating a histologically organized, functional construct with satisfactory mechanical characteristics for implantation. To develop a blood vessel substitute, Niklason et al. [1999], cultured PGA constructs in a pulsatile blow bioreactor generating 165 beats per minute (bpm) and 5% radial strain. The pulse frequency of this system was chosen to mimic a fetal heart rate, believed to possibly provide optimal conditions for new tissue formation. However, most mechanical conditioning investigations mentioned above conducted strain studies at 60 bpm, more representative of an adult heart rate, with promising outcomes. Therefore, the optimal bioreactor culture conditions for the development of a TEVG remain to be elucidated. Nevertheless, such a system shows promise for the production of a blood vessel substitute with the necessary mechanical and biochemical components.

55.6 Conclusions

In the past couple of decades, a great deal of progress on TEVGs has been made. Still, many challenges remain and are currently being addressed, particularly with regard to the prevention of thrombosis and the improvement of graft mechanical properties. In order to develop a patent TEVG that grossly resembles native tissue, required culture times in most studies exceed 8 weeks. Even with further advances in the

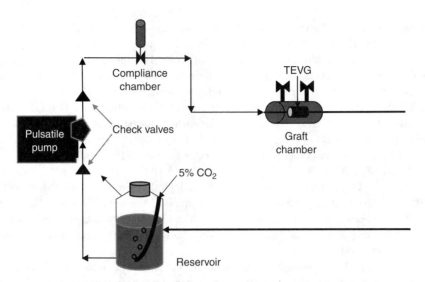

FIGURE 55.3 Diagram of a typical pulsatile flow bioreactor for culture of TEVGs.

field, TEVGs will likely not be used in emergency situations because of the time necessary to allow for cell expansion, ECM production and organization, and attainment of desired mechanical strength. Furthermore, TEVGs will probably require the use of autologous tissue to prevent an immunogenic response, unless advances in immune acceptance render allogenic and xenogenic tissue use feasible. TEVGs have not yet been subjected to clinical trials, which will determine the efficacy of such grafts in the long term. Finally, off the shelf availability and cost will become the biggest hurdles in the development of a feasible TEVG product.

Although many obstacles still exist in the effort to develop a small-diameter TEVG, the potential benefits of such an achievement are exciting. In the near future, a nonthrombogenic TEVG with sufficient mechanical strength may be developed for clinical trials. Such a graft will have the minimum characteristics of biological tissue necessary to remain patent over a time period comparable to current vein graft therapies. As science and technology advance, TEVGs may evolve into complex blood vessel substitutes. TEVGs may become living grafts, capable of growing, remodeling, and responding to mechanical and biochemical stimuli in the surrounding environment. These blood vessel substitutes will closely resemble native vessels in almost every way, including structure, composition, mechanical properties, and function. They will possess vasoactive properties, able to dilate and constrict in response to stimuli. Close mimicry of native blood vessels may ultimately aid in the engineering of other tissues dependent upon vasculature to sustain function. With further understanding of the factors involved in cardiovascular development and function combined with the foundation of knowledge already in place, the development of TEVGs should one day lead to improved quality of life for those with vascular diseases and other life threatening conditions.

References

Aeschlimann, D. and Paulsson, M. Cross-linking of laminin-nidogen complexes by tissue transglutaminase. A novel mechanism for basement membrane stabilization. *J. Biol. Chem.* 1991; **266**: 15308–15317.

Ahrendt, G., Chickering, D.E., and Ranieri, J.P. Angiogenic growth factors: a review for tissue engineering. *Tissue Eng.* 1998; **4**: 117–130.

Amento, E.P., Ehsani, N., Palmer, H., and Libby, P. Cytokines and growth factors positively and negatively regulate interstitial collagen gene expression in human vascular smooth muscle cells. *Arterioscler. Thromb.* 1991; **11**: 1223–1230.

American Heart Association. Heart Disease and Stroke Statistics — 2003 Update. http://www.americanheart.org/presenter.jhtml?identifier=4439

Anderson, J.M., Cima, L.G., Eskin, S.G., Graham, L.M., Greisler, H., Hubbell, J., Levy, R.J., Naughton, G., Northup, S.J., Ratner, B.D., Scott-Burden, T., Termin, P., and Didisheim, P. Tissue engineering in cardiovascular disease: a report. *J. Biomed. Mater. Res.* 1995; **29**:1473–1475.

Bader, A., Steinhoff, G., Strobl, K., Schilling, T., Brandes, G., Mertsching, H., Tsikas, D., Froelich, J., and Haverich, A. Engineering of human vascular aortic tissue based on a xenogenic starter matrix. *Transplantation* 2000; **70**: 7–14.

Clowes, A.W. Intimal hyperplasia and graft failure. *Cardiovasc. Pathol.* 1993; **2**: 179S-186S.

Coury, A.J., Levy, R.J., McMillin, C.R., Pathak, Y., Ratner, B.D., Schoen, F.J., Williams, D.F., and Williams, R. L. Degradation of materials in the biological environment. In *Biomaterials Science.* Ratner, B.D., Hoffman, A.S., Schoen, F.J., Lemons, J.E., Eds. Academic Press: San Diego, 1996.

Crawford, E.S., Bomberger, R.A., Glaeser, D.H., Saleh, S.A., and Russell, W.L. Aortoiliac occlusive disease: factors influencing survival and function following reconstructive operation over a twenty-five year period. *Surgery* 1981; **90**: 1055–1067.

Deutsch, M., Meinhart, J., Fischlein, T., Preiss, P., and Zilla, P. Clinical autologous *in vitro* endothelialization of infrainguinal ePTFE grafts in 100 patients: a 9-year experience. *Surgery* 1999; **126**: 847–855.

Dichek, D.A., Anderson, J., Kelly, A.B., Hanson, S.R., and Harker, L.A. Enhanced *in vivo* antithrombotic effects of endothelial cells expressing recombinant plasminogen activators transduced with retroviral vectors. *Circulation* 1996; **93**: 301–309.

Dunn, P.F., Newman, K.D., Jones, M., Yamada, I., Shayani, V., Virmani, R., and Dichek, D.A. Seeding of vascular grafts with genetically modified endothelial cells. *Circulation* 1996; **93**: 1439–1446.

Elbjeirami, W.M., Yonter, E.O., Starcher, B.C., and West, J.L. Enhancing mechanical properties of tissue engineered constructs via lysyl oxidase crosslinking activity. *J. Biomed. Mater. Res.* 2003; **66A**: 513–521.

Freed, L.E., Marquis, J.C., Nohia, A., Emmanual, J., Mikos, A.G., and Langer, R. Neocartilage formation *in vitro* and *in vivo* using cells cultured on synthetic biodegradable polymers. *J. Biomed. Mater. Res.* 1993; **27**: 11–23.

Geary, R.L, Kohler, T.R., Vergel, S., Kirkman, T.R., and Clowes, A.W. Time course of flow-induced smooth muscle cell proliferation and intimal thickening in endothelialized baboon vascular grafts. *Circulation Res.* 1993; **74**: 14–23.

Girton, T.S., Oegema, T.R., and Tranquillo, R.T. Exploiting glycation to stiffen and strengthen tissue equivalents for tissue engineering. *J. Biomed. Mater. Res.* 1999; **46**: 87–92.

Girton, T.S., Oegema, T.R., Grassel, E.D., Isenberg, B.C., and Tranquillo, R.T. Mechanisms of stiffening and strengthening in media-equivalents fabricated using glycation. *J. Biomech. Eng.* 2000; **122**: 216–223.

Giudiceandrea, A., Seifalian, A.M., Krijgsman, B., and Hamilton, G. Effect of prolonged pulsatile shear stress *in vitro* on endothelial cell seeded PTFE and compliant polyurethane vascular grafts. *Eur. J. Vasc. Endovasc. Surg.* 1998; **15**: 147–154.

Gloeckner, D.C., Sacks, M.S., Billiar, K.L., and Bachrach, N. Mechanical evaluation and design of a multilayered collagenous repair biomaterial. *J. Biomed. Mater. Res.* 2000; **52**: 365–373.

Gobin, A.S. and West, J.L. Cell migration through defined, synthetic extracellular matrix analogues. *FASEB J.* 2002.

Gobin, A.S. and West, J.L. Val-ala-pro-gly, an elastin-derived non-integrin ligand: smooth muscle cell adhesion and specificity, *J. Biomed. Mater. Res.* 2003; **67A**: 255–259.

Gombotz, W.R., Guanghui, W., Horbett, T.A., and Hoffman, A.S. Protein adsorption to poly(ethylene oxide) surfaces. *J. Biomed. Mater. Res.* 1991; **25**: 1547–1562.

Goyanes, J. Nuevos trabajos de cirugia vascular, substitucion plastica de les arterias por las venas or arterioplasia venosa, applicada, como nuevo metodo, al tratamiento de la aneurismas. *Siglo Med.* 1906; **53**: 546–549.

Griese, D.P., Ehsan, A., Melo, L.G., Kong, D, Zhang, L, Mann, M.J., Pratt, R.E., Mulligan, R.C., and Dzau, V.J. Isolation and transplantation of autologous circulating endothelial cell into denuded vessels and prosthetic grafts: implications for cell-based vascular therapy. *Circulation* 2003; **108**: 2710–2715.

Hamilton, D.W., Maul, T.M., and Vorp, D.A. Characterization of the response of bone marrow-derived progenitor cells to cyclic strain: implications for vascular tissue engineering applications. *Tissue Eng.* 2004; **10**: 361–369.

He, H., Shirota, T., and Matsuda, T. Canine endothelial progenitor cell-lined hybrid vascular graft with nonthrombogenic potential. *J. Thorac. Cardiovasc. Surg.* 2003; **126**: 455–464.

Hern, D.L. and Hubbell, J.A. Incorporation of adhesion peptides into nonadhesive hydrogels useful for tissue resurfacing. *J. Biomed. Mater. Res.* 1998; **39**: 266–276.

Hiles, M.C., Badylak, S.F., Geddes, L.A., Kokini, K., and Morff, R.J. Porosity of porcine small-intestinal submucosa for use as a vascular graft. *J. Biomed. Mater. Res.* 1993; **27**: 139–144.

Hill-West, J.L., Chowdhury, S.M., Sawhney, A.S., Pathak, C.P., Dunn, R.C., and Hubbell, J.A. Prevention of postoperative adhesions in the rat by *in situ* photopolymerization of bioresorbable hydrogel barriers. *Obstet. Gynecol.* 1994; **83**: 59–64.

Huynh, T., Abraham, G., Murray, J., Brockbank, K., Hagen, P.O., and Sullivan, S. Remodeling of an acellular collagen graft into a physiologically responsive neovessel. *Nat. Biotechnol.* 1999; **17**: 1083–1086.

Kim, B.S. and Mooney, D.J. Engineering smooth muscle tissue with a predefined structure. *J. Biomed. Mater. Res.* 1998; **41**: 322–332.

Kim, B.S., Nikolovski, J., Bonadio, J., and Mooney, D.J. Cyclic mechanical strain regulates the development of engineered smooth muscle tissue. *Nat. Biotech.* 1999; **17**: 979–983.

Kock, G., Gutschi, S., Pascher, O., Fruhwirth, J., and Hauser, H. Zur problematik des femoropoplitealen Gefassersatzes: vene ePTFE oder ovines Kollagen? *Zentralbl Chir* 1996; **121**: 761–767.

L'Heureux, N., Paquet, S., Labbe, R., Germain, L., and Auger, F.A. A completely biological tissue-engineered human blood vessel. *FASEB J.* 1998; **12**: 47–56.

Lawrence, R., Hartmann, D.J., and Sonenshein, G.E. Transforming growth factor β1 stimulates type V collagen expression in bovine vascular smooth muscle cells. *J. Biol. Chem.* 1994; **269**: 9603–9609.

Leung, D.Y.M., Glagov, S., and Mathews, M.B. Cyclic stretching stimulates synthesis of matrix components by arterial smooth muscle cells *in vitro*. *Science* 1976; **191**: 475–477.

Lynch, C.M., Clowes, M.M., Osborne, W.R.A., Clowes, A.W., and Miller, A.D. Long-term expression of human adenosine deaminase in vascular smooth muscle cells of rats: a model for gene therapy. *Proc. Natl Acad. Sci. USA* 1992; **89**: 1138–1142.

Ma, P.X. and Langer, R. Degradation, structure and properties of fibrous nonwoven poly(glycolic acid) scaffolds for tissue engineering. *Mat. Res. Soc. Symp. Proc.* 1995; **394**: 99–104.

Mann, B.K., Schmedlen, R.H., and West, J.L. Tethered-TGF-β increases extracellular matrix production of vascular smooth muscle cells. *Biomaterials* 2001; **22**: 439–444.

Mann, B.K., Gobin, A.S., Tsai, A.T., Schmedlen, R.H., and West, J.L. Smooth muscle cell growth in photopolymerized hydrogels with cell adhesive and proteolytically degradable domains: synthetic ECM analogs for tissue engineering. *Biomaterials* 2001; **22**: 3045–3051.

Merrill, E.A. and Salzman, E.W. Polyethylene oxide as a biomaterial. *ASAIO J.* 1983; **6**: 60–64.

Moazami, N., Argenziano, M., Williams, M., Cabreriza, S.B., Oz, M.C., and Nowygrod, R. Photo-oxidized bovine arterial grafts: short-term results. *ASAIO J.* 1998; **44**: 89–93.

Moneta, G.L. and Porter, J.M. Arterial substitutes in peripheral vascular surgery: a review. *J. Long-Term Effects Med. Implants* 1995; **5**: 47–67.

Mooney, D.J., Mazzoni, C.L., Breuer, C., McNamara, K., Hern, D., Vacanti, J.P., and Langer, R. Stabilized polyglycolic acid fibre-based tubes for tissue engineering. *Biomaterials* 1996; **17**: 115–124.

Murga, M., Yao, L., and Tosato, G. Derivation of endothelial cells from CD34-umbilical cord blood. *Stem Cells* 2004; **22**: 385–395.

Niklason, L.E., Gao, J., Abbott, W.M., Hirschi, K.K., Houser, S., Marini, R., and Langer, R. Functional arteries grown in *vitro*. *Science* 1999; **284**: 489–493.

Richardson, J.V., Wright, C.B., and Hiratzka, L.F. The role of endothelium in the patency of small venous substitutes. *J. Surg. Res.* 1980; **28**: 556–562.

Roeder, R., Wolfe, J., Lianakis, N., Hinson, T., Geddes, L.A., and Obermiller, J. Compliance, elasitic modulus, and burst pressure of small-intestine submucosa (SIS), small-diameter vascular grafts. *J. Biomed. Mater. Res.* 1999; **47**: 65–70.

Rucker, R.B., Kosonen, T., Clegg, M.S., Mitchell, A.E., Rucker, B.R., Uriu-Hare, J.Y., and Keen, C.L. Copper, lysyl oxidase, and extracellular matrix protein cross-linking. *Am. J. Clin. Nutri.* 1998; **67** Suppl: 996S–1002S.

Sacks, M.S. and Gloeckner, D.C. Quantification of the fiber architecture and biaxial mechanical behavior of porcine intestinal submucosa. *J. Biomed. Mater. Res.* 1999; **46**: 1–10.

Sawhney, A.S., Pathak, C.P., and Hubbell, J.A. Bioerodible hydrogels based on photopolymerized poly(ethylene glycol)-*co*-poly(α-hydroxy acid) diacrylate macromers. *Macromolecules* 1993; **26**: 581–587.

Schaner, P.J., Martin, N.D., Tulenko, T.N., Shapiro, I.M., Tarola, N.A., Leichter, R.F., Carabasi, R.A., and Dimuzio, P.J. Decellularized vein as a potential scaffold for vascular tissue engineering. *J. Vasc. Surg.* 2004; **40**: 146–153.

Scharfmann, R., Axelrod, J.H., and Verma, I.M. Long-term expression of retrovirus-mediated gene transfer in mouse fibroblast implants. *Proc. Natl Acad. Sci. USA* 1991; **88**: 4626–4630.

Scott-Burden, T., Tock, C.L., Schwarz, J.J., Casscells, S.W., and Engler, D.A. Genetically engineered smooth muscle cells as linings to improve the biocompatibility of cardiovascular prostheses. *Circulation* 1996; **94**[Suppl II]: II235–II238.

Seliktar, D., Black, R.A., Vito, R.P., and Nerem, R.M. Dynamic mechanical conditioning of collagen-gel blood vessel constructs induces remodeling *in vitro*. *Ann. Biomed. Eng.* 2000; **28**: 351–362.

Seliktar, D., Nerem, R.M., and Galis, Z.S. The role of matrix metalloproteinase-2 in the remodeling of cell-seeded vascular constructs subjected to cyclic strain. *Ann. Biomed. Eng.* 2001; **29**: 923–934.

Shirota, T., He, H., and Matsuda, T. Human endothelial progenitor cell-seeded hybrid graft: proliferative and antithrombogenic potentials *in vitro* and fabrication processing. *Tissue Eng.* 2003; **9**: 127–136.

Simper, D., Stalboerger, P.G., Panetta, C.J., Wang, S., and Caplice, N.M. Smooth muscle progenitor cells in human blood. *Circulation* 2002; **106**: 1199–1204.

Sinnaeve, P., Varenne, O., Collen, D., and Janssens, S. Gene therapy in the cardiovascular system: an update. *Cardiovasc. Res.* 1999; **44**: 498–506.

Stegemann, J.P., Dey, N.B., Lincoln, T.M., and Nerem, R.M. Genetic modification of smooth muscle cells to control phenotype and function in vascular tissue engineering. *Tissue Eng.* **10**: 189–199.

Szilagyi, D.E., Elliott, J.P., and Hageman, J.H. Biological fate of autologous implants as arterial substitutes: clinical angiographic and histopathological observations in femoropopliteal opertations for atherosclerosis. *Ann. Surg.* 1973; **178**: 232–246.

Tajima, S. Modulation of elastin expression and cell proliferation in vascular smooth muscle cells *in vitro*. *Keio J. Med.* 1996; **45**: 58–62.

Teebken, O.E., Bader, A., Steinhoff, G., and Haverich, A. Tissue engineering of vascular grafts: human cell seeding of decellularized porcine matrix. *Eur. J. Vasc. Endovasc. Surg.* 2000; **19**: 381–386.

Thompson, M.M., Budd, J.S., Eady, S.L., James, R.F.L., and Bell, P.R.F. Effect of pulsatile shear stress on endothelial attachment to native vascular surfaces. *Br. J. Surg.* 1994; **81**: 1121–1127.

VA Coronary Artery Bypass Surgery Cooperative Study Group. Eighteen-year follow-up in the veterans affairs cooperative study of coronary artery bypass surgery for stable angina. *Circulation* 1992; **86**: 121–130.

Vater, C.A., Harris, E.D., and Siegel, R.C. Native cross-links in collagen fibrils induce resistance to human synovial collagenase. *Biochem. J.* 1979; **181**: 639–645.

Venturi, M., Bonavina, L., Annoni, F., Colombo, L., Butera, C., Peracchia, A., and Mussini, E. Biochemical assay of collagen and elastin in the normal and varicose vein wall. *J. Surg. Res.* 1996; **60**: 245–248.

Vorhees, A.B., Jaretski, A., and Blakeore, A.H. Use of tubes constructed from vinyon "n" cloth in bridging arterial deficits. *Ann. Surg.* 1952; **135**: 332–338.

Weinberg, C.B. and Bell, E. A blood vessel model constructed from collagen and cultured vascular cells. *Science* 1986; **231**: 397–400.

West, J.L. and Hubbell, J.A. Polymeric biomaterials with degradation sites for proteases involved in cell migration. *Macromolecules* 1999; **32**: 241–244.

Wight, T.N. Arterial wall. In: *Extracellular Matrix*, Vol. 1. Howard Academic Publishers: Netherlands, 1996, pp. 175–202.

Wijelath, E.S., Rahman, S., Murray, J., Patel, Y., Savidge, G., and Sobel, M. Fibronectin promotes VEGF-induced CD34 cell differentiation into endothelial cells. *J. Vasc. Surg.* 2004; **39**: 655–660.

Wilson, J.M., Birinyi, L.K., Salomon, R.N., Libby, P., Callow, A.D., and Mulligan, R.C. Implantation of vascular grafts lined with genetically modified endothelial cells. *Science* 1989; **244**: 1344–1346.

56

Cardiac Tissue Engineering: Matching Native Architecture and Function to Develop Safe and Efficient Therapy

Nenad Bursac
Duke University

56.1 Introduction

After an acute myocardial infarction, lost cardiomyocytes are replaced by a noncontractile fibrous tissue. Although it is suggested that heart has a small regenerative potential via cell proliferation [1], or stem cell recruitment [2], the rate of renewal is insufficient to compensate for myocyte loss. As a result, altered workload of a surviving myocardium may ultimately lead to deterioration in contractile function and congestive heart failure (CHF). Besides traditional pharmacological therapies (diuretics, β-blockers, angiotensine, and aldosterone inhibitors) [3] or heart transplant [4], investigators are evaluating innovative approaches for treatment of CHF including mechanical assist devices [5], dynamic cardiomyoplasty [6], transmyocardial laser revascularization [7], and artificial heart [8]. Nevertheless, in end stage disease, heart transplant remains the only option with good long-term results [4]. However, inadequate availability of donor organs (~10% of current needs [9]) requires new strategies for treatment of increasing number of heart failure patients.

One promising approach is augmentation of the number of functional myocytes in the diseased heart using methodologies for cardiomyocyte cell cycle activation [10], adult stem cell mobilization [11], or cellular transplantation [12]. Cellular transplantation at the site of injury in the heart can be accomplished either by injecting isolated cells ("cellular cardiomyoplasty") [13], or by implanting a cardiac tissue patch engineered *in vitro* ("tissue cardiomyoplasty") [14].

56.1.1 Cellular Cardiomyoplasty

More than 10 years ago, pioneering studies in the laboratory of Lauren Field have shown feasibility of cell transplantation in the heart [15,16]. Since then, different investigators have used cardiac [15] or skeletal myoblast cell lines [16], fetal [17,18], neonatal [19], and adult [20] cardiac myocytes, autologous [21,22] and syngeneic [23] skeletal myoblasts, smooth muscle cells [24], endothelial cells [25], native [26] or genetically altered fibroblasts [27], embryonic [28], bone marrow [29], mesenchymal [30], or heart derived [31] stem cells, as potential donor cells. As a result, treated hearts have shown improvement in diastolic function, almost independent of transplanted cell type [26]. The improvement in the systolic function (generation of active force) on the other hand required use of cells with the myogenic (contractile) potential [26,32]. The possible therapeutic benefit of cellular cardiomyoplasty stems from structural remodeling of scar region [33], enhancement of myocardial revascularization [12], and direct structural and functional integration of donor cells with the host myocardium [18]. Presently, clinical studies in the United States, Europe, and Asia are under way to investigate feasibility and safety in using autologous bone marrow derived stem cells and skeletal myoblasts in treatment of postinfarction left ventricular disfunction [13,34,35]. Initial results are promising, but reveal risk for ventricular arrhythmias [34], limiting in some studies the pool of patients to only those that already have internal defibrillators. Since no systematic studies have been performed to assess the electrical performance of the heart postcardiomyoplasty, and little data exists on electrical interaction between donor and host cells *in vivo* or *in vitro* [36], the causes of the postoperative electrical instability are not known. Plausible explanations include inflammatory response and subsequent fibrosis at implantation site [35], possible electrical coupling in conjunction with different electrophysiology between implanted cells and cardiomyocytes [18,34], and possible stimulation of sympathetic nerve sprouting and overexpression of neurotransmitters after the cell transplantation [37].

56.1.2 Tissue Cardiomyoplasty

Some of the major hurdles in restoring heart function by cellular cardiomyoplasty include limited survival of injected cells in the region of scar tissue, and no architectural repair of the infarcted area. An alternative approach is tissue cardiomyoplasty, which involves *in vitro* cultivation of compact three-dimensional (3D) cardiac tissue patch, and subsequent implantation over or instead of the infracted scar tissue. Although surgically more challenging compared to cellular cardiomyoplasty, this methodology has a potential to improve efficiency and localization of tissue repair in larger size cardiac injury such as infarction of major coronary vessels, or congenital heart defects [38]. Ideally, based on the location, shape, and size of injury and architecture of surrounding tissue (assessed by ultrasound, MRI, or other noninvasive technique [39]), functional cardiac patch with needed geometry and 3D structure is engineered *in vitro* starting from selected cell type, natural or synthetic scaffold, and appropriate culturing vessel (bioreactor). Inside the bioreactor, cells attach to biocompatible (and possibly degradable) scaffold, interconnect, and assemble in three dimensions to reconstitute an *in vivo*-like cardiac tissue equivalent (construct). The combination of biochemical and physical stimuli during culture is designed to best mimic physiological state of tissue, and to support cell differentiation or transdifferentiation and desired 3D tissue architecture. At a proper time point, tissue construct is removed from the bioreactor and surgically implanted in the site of injury in order to restore or improve electrical and mechanical function of diseased heart.

In reality, however, the successful reconstitution of cardiac-like tissue patch *in vitro* starting from single cells is an extremely challenging problem due to limited proliferation potential and high metabolic demand of cardiac cells, as well as complex anisotropic architecture and electro-mechanical function of native cardiac tissue. While recent reviews on cardiac tissue engineering [14,40] have focused on scaffold biomaterials, bioreactors, and cultivation conditions, this chapter will provide emphasis on the electrophysiological considerations and role of tissue architecture in the development of functional cardiac patch. It is this author's view, that these factors will play an important role in the design of efficient and safe therapies, despite the fact that they are frequently neglected in current *in vitro* and *in vivo* studies.

56.2 Cardiac Architecture and Function

The crucial architectural and functional feature of cardiac muscle tissue (Figure 56.1) is anisotropy, that is, anatomically and biophysically, properties of cardiac muscle vary in different directions [41]. Microscopic structural anisotropy in cardiac tissue results from the spatial alignment of elongated cardiac myocytes (Figure 56.1a), and the preferential location of intercellular junctions (e.g., fascia adherence, gap junctions, desmosomes) in end-to-end vs. side-to-side cell connections [42]. Macroscopic anisotropy is a result of the presence of aligned cardiac muscle fibers and sheets that transmurally rotate inside the heart wall (180° rotation from endo- to epicardium) [43]. The unique anisotropic architecture of cardiac tissue enables an orderly sequence of electrical and mechanical activity, and efficient pumping of blood from the heart. Beside architecture, electrical membrane properties of cardiac myocytes also vary substantially depending on the location in the heart with distinct differences between atria and ventricles, endo- and epicardial regions, left and right heart, base and apex, etc. [44–46]. Moreover, the heart contains a large variety of nonmyocytes (e.g., fibroblasts, endothelial cells, smooth muscle cells, neural cells, leukocytes) with specific roles in the cardiac function that are still not fully elucidated.

Structural anisotropy and intercellular continuity of the excitable cardiac substrate have profound effect on electrical and mechanical functioning of the heart. For example, anatomical anisotropy in heart tissue causes a larger intracellular resistance per unit length in the transverse (across fiber) than longitudinal (along fiber) direction, resulting in smaller velocity but larger maximum slope of action potential upstroke and safer electrical propagation in the transverse direction [47,48]. As a consequence, electrical stimulation of a small region in the heart tissue results in development of elliptical rather than circular propagating wavefront [49] (Figure 56.1b). Directly related to anisotropy is evidence that cardiac impulse conduction at the microscopic level is discontinuous at sites of gap junctions, and even stochastic due to small local variations in ion channel function, gap junction distribution, and adjoining tissue architecture [50,51]. In contrast to these small physiological variations, larger variations of electrical properties (e.g., action potential duration, intercellular coupling, electrical load) at the cellular and tissue level may result in increased susceptibility to propagation slowing and conduction block [46,51]. Slow propagation velocity and unidirectional block are some of the main prerequisites for the initiation of reentrant cardiac arrhythmias [51,52].

The degree of anatomical and functional anisotropy depends on location in the heart and age of the individual, with main determinants being cell size and geometry, type, amount, and distribution of cell junctions in membrane, and macroscopic tissue architecture [53–55]. Electrical anisotropy changes in certain cardiac pathologies such as ischemia, infarction, and heart failure [56,57]. This change is a consequence of the altered gap junction distribution and expression, as well as formation of longitudinal collagenous septa between the cardiac fibers which result in discontinuous transverse propagation ("nonuniform anisotropy") and increased susceptibility to reentrant arrhythmias [58]. In particular, in canine hearts, "border zone" between infracted and normal tissue exhibits disarray of cardiac cells and gross change in anisotropy, resulting in conduction slowing, block, and reentrant "figure of eight" circuits

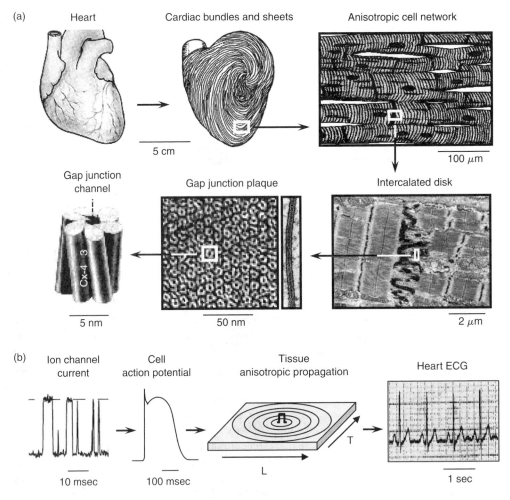

FIGURE 56.1   Levels of anatomical and electrophysiological organization in cardiac muscle. (a) Intercalated disk is specialized end-to-end connection between cardiac cells. Gap junction plaque is shown in cross-section and en face. Cx-43 is gap junction protein connexin-43. Note that structural complexity in heart spans many orders of magnitude from nanometer-size scale in single channels to centimeter-size scale in the heart. (b) Time constants of electrophysiological function in cardiac muscle range from nanoseconds for a single channel gating to seconds for heart beats. L and T denote longitudinal and transverse direction, respectively. Pulse sign denotes site of stimulus.

in the heart [59]. In addition, presence of noncontractile scar in heart milieu can cause locally increased stress gradients, which through mechano-electric feedback may yield in stretch-induced arrhythmias [60].

56.3   Current State of Cardiac Tissue Engineering

Over the last several years different strategies have been developed to design engineered cardiac tissues that could be used for pharmacological, genetic, and functional studies *in vitro* and possible implantation *in vivo*, as outlined in Table 56.1. These studies have shown that structure and function of cardiac tissue constructs depend on the animal species used for the cell dissociation [61–63], composition of seeded cells [14,64], initial cell seeding density [62,63,65,66], scaffold characteristics [40,67–70], composition of culture medium [69], type of bioreactor [63,65,69], and applied physical forces [61,71]. Most of these results are based on the evaluation of general histology, and assessment of cellular properties including cell

TABLE 56.1 Cardiac Tissue Engineering *In Vitro* and *In Vivo*

		In vitro		
Cell source	Scaffold	Bioreactor	Assessment	References
Neonatal rat ventricle	Microcarrier beads	HARV	Immunohistology, ultrastructure, pharmacology	[77,78]
Embryonic chick ventricle	Planar collagen gel with supplements	Static petri dish attachment to velcro	Immunohistology, pharmacology, ultrastructure, gene manipulation, mechanical contractile force	[79]
Neonatal rat ventricle	planar collagen gel with supplements	Static petri dish attachment to velcro	Immunohistology, pharmacology, ultrastructure, contractile force	[62]
Neonatal rat ventricle	Collagen gel ring with supplements	Static petri dish and cyclic stretch	Immunohistology, pharmacology, ultrastructure, contractile force	[72]
Rat smooth muscle, skin fibroblasts, fetal ventricle, human atria and ventricle	Rectangular gelatin mesh	Static petri dish	Histology, cell proliferation	[86]
Young human ventricle	Rectangular gelatin mesh	Cyclic stretch in dish	Histology, proliferation, mechanical	[71]
Neonatal rat ventricle	Rectangular collagen scaffold ("tissue fleece")	Static petri dish	RT-PCR, pharmacology, ultrastructure, mechanical	[73,87]
Neonatal rat ventricle	Fibrin glue and thick collagen gel around aorta	Unperfused and perfused through aorta	FDG-PET, Immunohistology	[88]
Neonatal rat ventricle	Cross-linked collagen mesh	HARV	Immunohistology, ultrastructure	[89]
Fetal and neonatal rat ventricle	Electrospun tubular collagen scaffold	HARV	Immunohistology, ultrastructure mechanical stress–strain curves	[74,90]
Neonatal rat ventricle	No scaffold	Static petri dish	Immunohistology, ultrastructure, electrical connectivity, mechanical, subcutaneous implantation	[75,92]
Embryonic chick and neonatal rat ventricle	Fibrous PGA disk	Static petri dish, spinner flask, HARV	Viability, metabolic activity, immunohistology, ultrastructure	[63]
Neonatal rat ventricle	Fibrous PGA disk	Spinner flask	Viability, metabolic activity, immunohistology, ultrastructure, tissue scale electrophysiology	[64]
Neonatal rat ventricle	Fibrous PGA disk	Perfusion cartridge	Viability, metabolic activity, immunohistology, ultrastructure	[94,95]
Neonatal rat ventricle C2C12 myoblasts	collagen sponge disk with matrigel	Orbitally mixed dish, Perfusion cartridge	Viability, metabolic activity, immunohistology, pharmacology, excitation threshold, capture rates	[65,96]
Neonatal rat ventricle	Surface hydrolyzed, laminin-coated PGA disk	Spinner flask, 3D gyrator, HARV	Immunohistology, immunoblotting, ultrastructure, viability, metabolic activity, tissue electrophysiology	[69]

Continued

TABLE 56.1   Continued

<table>
<tr><td colspan="5" align="center">*In vitro*</td></tr>
<tr><td>Cell source</td><td>Scaffold</td><td>Bioreactor</td><td>Assessment</td><td>References</td></tr>
<tr>
<td>Neonatal rat ventricle</td>
<td>Surface hydrolyzed, laminin-coated PGA disk</td>
<td>HARV</td>
<td>Immunohistology, immunoblotting, pharmacology, cell electrophysiology</td>
<td>[76]</td>
</tr>
<tr>
<td>Neonatal rat ventricle</td>
<td>Fibronectin coated PLGA disk</td>
<td>HARV</td>
<td>Histology, ultrastructure, optical mapping of action potentials</td>
<td>[121,122]</td>
</tr>
<tr>
<td>Fetal rat ventricle</td>
<td>Alginate disk</td>
<td>Static petri dish</td>
<td>Viability, metabolic activity, histology</td>
<td>[66]</td>
</tr>
</table>

<table>
<tr><td colspan="5" align="center">*In vivo* implantation in heart</td></tr>
<tr><td>Cell source</td><td>Scaffold</td><td>Site of implantation</td><td>Postoperative assessment</td><td>References</td></tr>
<tr>
<td>Fetal rat ventricle</td>
<td>Gelatin mesh cube</td>
<td>Infarct in cryoinjured left rat ventricle</td>
<td>Histology, ultrastructure, ventricular pressure in Langendorf preparation</td>
<td>[97]</td>
</tr>
<tr>
<td>Rat aortic smooth muscle</td>
<td>Gelatin mesh, PTFE patch, PGA, and PCLA sponge</td>
<td>Defect in right outflow ventricular tract in rat</td>
<td>Immunostaining, cell proliferation, morphometry</td>
<td>[67,98]</td>
</tr>
<tr>
<td>Rat aortic smooth muscle</td>
<td>PCLA sponge</td>
<td>Postinfarct aneurysm in rat left ventricular</td>
<td>Immunohistology, echocardiography, ventricular pressure</td>
<td>[99]</td>
</tr>
<tr>
<td>Fetal rat ventricle</td>
<td>Alginate disk</td>
<td>Rat coronary occlusion site</td>
<td>Immunohistology, echocardiography</td>
<td>[100]</td>
</tr>
<tr>
<td>Neonatal rat ventricle</td>
<td>Collagen gel ring with supplements</td>
<td>Perimeter of healthy rat ventricle</td>
<td>Immunohistology, ultrastructure, pharmacology, echocardiography</td>
<td>[85]</td>
</tr>
</table>

HARV — high-aspect-ratio-vessel, HFDG-PET — Fluor-Deoxy-Glucose-Positron-Emission-Tomography, PLGA — poly(lactic-co-glycolic) acid, PTFE — polytetrafluoroethylene, PCLA — ε-caprolactone-co-L-lactide reinforced with knitted poly-L-lactide fabric.

number, viability, metabolic activity, expression of cardiac-specific proteins, and ultrastructural features. Few groups also focused on measurements of contractile force at tissue scale [62,72–75], while only one group has studied in detail microscopic and macroscopic electrical properties of tissue constructs [64,69,76]. The following paragraphs will give an overview of existing *in vitro* and *in vivo* efforts in the emerging field of cardiac tissue engineering.

56.3.1 Cardiogenesis *In Vitro*

Akins et al. [77,78] have shown that neonatal rat ventricular myocytes can form multilayered interconnected structures when cultivated on fibronectin-coated polystyrene beads or collagen fibers inside high-aspect-ratio-vessel (HARV) bioreactors. After 6 days in culture, cardiac cells formed small, several layers thick clusters in the regions between the beads, exhibited presence of sarcomeres and gap junctions, and rhythmically contracted at rates that were slower in the presence of propranolol. The nonmyocytes were distributed throughout the tissue clusters, with most of the endothelial cells lining on the interface between the cluster and culture medium.

Group of Eschenhagen has done some of the most comprehensive work in the field, using mixtures of embryonic chick [79] or neonatal rat cardiac cells [62,72] and gels made of collagen type I supplemented with matrigel, chick embryo extract, and horse serum. Their initial work was based on Vandenburgh's approach for engineering of skeletal muscle [80], where cell–gel mixture was cast in the thin planar geometry between two parallel Velcro-coated glass tubes. Firm attachment to Velcro-imposed static stress on free edges of the gel resulting in thin biconcave tissue construct ($8 \times 15 \times 0.18$ mm^3) with loose, aligned cardiac cell network formed mostly along the construct edges [79]. The alignment and density of this network was improved by use of the chronic cyclic stretch during cultivation [61]. In their current approach [72], cardiac constructs termed engineered heart tissues (EHTs) are made by embedding neonatal rat ventricular cells in circularly molded collagen gels, which are subsequently cultivated in static conditions for 7 days and subjected to chronic cyclic stretch (10%, 2 Hz) for additional 7 days. Resulting submillimeter thick rings of tissue contain aligned cardiomyocytes organized in loose but uniform tissue-like network with frequently forming 20 to 50 μm thick cardiac fibers [72]. Myocytes in this network spontaneously contract at steady rates of ~2 Hz, and exhibit differentiated cardiac-specific ultrastructure including parallel sarcomeres, T-tubules, SR vesicles, formed dyads, and basement membrane [72]. The initial seeding of unpurified cell mixture (no differential preplating) result in the presence of microphages and abundant fibroblasts, scattered throughout the EHT, as well as endothelial and smooth muscle cells, packed more densely in the outer compared to inner region. When electrically and pharmacologically stimulated, EHTs exhibit cardiac-specific mechanical properties including Frank–Starling behavior, a positive inotropic response to extracellular calcium and isoprenaline, and negative inotropic effect to carbachol. Although recorded twitch amplitudes of 1 to 2 mN/mm^2 are an order of magnitude lower than those found in native cardiac tissues [81], the twitch to resting tension ratio is larger than 1, similar to native muscle. The use of rat cells, horse serum, chick embryo extract, matrigel, and unpurified cell seeding mixture are all found to increase the maximum developed force and mechanical integrity of EHTs, while increase in collagen content seems to decrease twitch tension [14,70]. Up to now, EHTs have been used for studying the effect of genetic and pharmacological manipulations on cardiac contractile function [62,82–84], and were also implanted *in vivo* (see work by Zimmermann et al. [85]).

Group of Li [86] seeded biodegradable gelatin meshes with different cell types including stomach smooth muscle cells, skin fibroblasts and fetal ventricular myocytes from rat, and adult atrial and ventricular myocytes from humans. Rat cells and human atrial, but not ventricular, cells proliferated over 3 to 4 weeks in culture. All cells migrated in a 300 to 500 μm thick outside layer of gelatin scaffold, which slowly degraded with the highest degradation rate found in the presence of fibroblasts. In separate *in vitro* study [71], the same group showed that 2 weeks of cyclic mechanical stretch improved cell proliferation, distribution, and mechanical strength of tissue constructs made using gelatin scaffolds and heart cells isolated from children who underwent repair of Tetralogy of Fallot.

Kofidis et al. [73,87], used $20 \times 15 \times 2$ mm^3 commercially available collagen-based scaffolds ("tissue fleece") that were inoculated with neonatal rat cardiac cells and cultured in petri dishes. The randomly distributed cells formed sparse synchronously contractile networks, and exhibited cardiac specific mechanical responses to stretch, extracellular calcium, and epinephrine. In an attempt to increase the thickness of the engineered cardiac tissue, the same group recently embedded a rat aorta in the 8.5 mm thick mixture of collagen gel and cardiac cells, and used pulsatile flow through the aorta for 2 weeks as a vehicle for nutrition and oxygen delivery [88]. The aorta remained patent throughout the culture and viability was increased compared to unperfused controls.

van Luyn et al. [89] have also used neonatal rat cells and commercially available cross-linked collagen I bovine matrices, and cultured them in HARV bioreactors for up to 3 weeks. Spatially scattered cells exhibited immature sarcomeres, gap junctions, and stained for troponin-T.

In recent studies, Evans et al. [90] and Yost et al. [74] cultured embryonic and neonatal rat cardiac cells on fibronectin coated aligned tubular scaffolds (15 mm long, 4 mm inner, 5 mm outer diameter) made from extruded collagen I fibers [91]. After 3 to 6 weeks in HARV bioreactors, cardiac cells aligned, contracted spontaneously, formed few interconnected cell layers (with total thickness of ~20 μm) on the inside and outside lumen of the tube, and exhibited registered sarcomeres and randomly distributed gap junctions. Tubular collagen scaffolds exhibited viscoelastic properties qualitatively resembling those of native papillary muscle [74] only when seeded with cardiac cells, as inferred from the shape of the stress–strain hysteresis loops.

Very elegant studies by Shimizu et al. [75,92,93] have demonstrated that cardiac cells can form 3D multilayer tissue-like structures without the use of any type of scaffold. Isotropic monolayers of purified cardiac cells were cultured to confluence on the surfaces made of temperature responsive polymer poly(N-isopropylacrylamide). This polymer is slightly hydrophobic and cell adhesive at 37°C and becomes hydrophilic and cell repellent when cooled below 32°C. After 4 days, up to four cardiac sheets were detached (together with secreted extracellular matrix) from polymer surface by cooling to 20°C and overlaid using pipette or polyethylene mesh. Overlaid sheets exhibited uniform gap junction distribution, connected electrically, and formed compact multilayered spontaneously contractile cardiac constructs with area of 1 cm^2 and thickness of up to 50 μm. After subcutaneous implantation, cardiac constructs survived up to 12 weeks, spontaneously contracted, appeared vascularized and at 3 weeks exhibited twitch tension of 1.2 mN [75].

Group of Freed and Vunjak-Novakovic has utilized various approaches to engineering of cardiac tissue based on the use of biodegradable polymer scaffolds and different tissue culture bioreactors. Initial studies of Bursac et al. [64], and Carrier et al. [63] have demonstrated that cardiac cells formed tissue-like constructs when seeded on 5 mm diameter × 2 mm thick fibrous poly(glycolic) acid (PGA) disks inside spinner flask bioreactors. Cells in the outer 50 to 70 μm thick region were randomly oriented and connected in the relatively dense multilayer network. These cells expressed cardiac specific proteins (α-sarcomeric actin and troponin-T), end ultrastructural features characteristic of cardiac myocytes (parallel sarcomeres, all types of specialized junctions, dense mitochondria, glycogen granules). The cells in the interior of these tissue constructs were sparsely distributed and often necrotic. Spontaneous macroscopic contractions were observed at days 2 to 4 of culture and generally ceased thereafter, with occasional activity at rates of less then 1 Hz on culture day 7. Action potential propagation and electrical excitability were studied using linear array of eight metal microelectrodes with 500 μm spatial resolution (Figure 56.2a). Constructs were electrically excitable and exhibited isotropic, macroscopically continuous electrical propagation with velocities as high as 60% of those found in native ventricles [64]. Use of purified cell mixture (after differential preplating) for seeding resulted in superior electrophysiological properties including higher velocity of propagation, increased maximum rates of tissue capture and lower excitation threshold compared with use of unpurified (no preplating) cell mixture. In addition, use of neonatal vs. chick cardiac cells, dynamic seeding and cultivation in bioreactors vs. static petri dishes, and increase in the number of seeded cells up to 8 × 10^6 cells per scaffold have all improved cell packing density, metabolic activity, and electrophysiological properties of constructs [63,64]. In further studies, Carrier et al. [94] looked in the use of perfusion through tissue construct as means to improve the cellularity and tissue architecture, and studied effect of oxygen deprivation on engineered cardiac muscle [95]. In the most recent studies from the same group, Radisic et al. [65,96] used cell–matrigel mixture to densely inoculate cardiac cells inside collagen sponge scaffolds, and employed similar perfusion bioreactor for construct cultivation. The viability, metabolic activity, and cellular density through ~1 mm thick region were higher than in constructs cultured in orbital shakers and those from studies by Carrier et al. In a different study, Papadaki et al. [69] have shown significant improvements in structure and function of cardiac constructs when PGA scaffolds were hydrophilized and coated with laminin, percentage of serum in culture medium reduced after 2 days of cultivation, constructs seeded with concentrated cell suspension in rotating gyrators, and cultivation performed in HARV bioreactors. Compared to previous studies, tissue constructs exhibited better cell viability yielding thicker (120 to 160 μm) cardiac-like outer region, and higher cellular expression of differentiation marker proteins including creatine kinase-MM (involved in metabolism), sarcomeric myosin heavy chain (involved in contractile function), and gap junction protein Connexin-43. Tissue scale electrical properties approached those found in native muscle with conduction velocity at basic stimulation rate of 1 Hz and maximum capture rate reaching 90 and 70% of those found in donor neonatal ventricles, respectively (Figure 56.2a). Macroscopic electrical propagation was effectively isotropic due to random cell orientation and uniform gap junction distribution. Further electrophysiological and pharmacological studies at microscopic scale by Bursac et al. [76] demonstrated that action potentials in cardiac cells from 7-day constructs were comparable to those in 2-day old donor ventricles with respect to depolarization upstroke, amplitude, and resting potential. The major difference was prolonged action potential duration

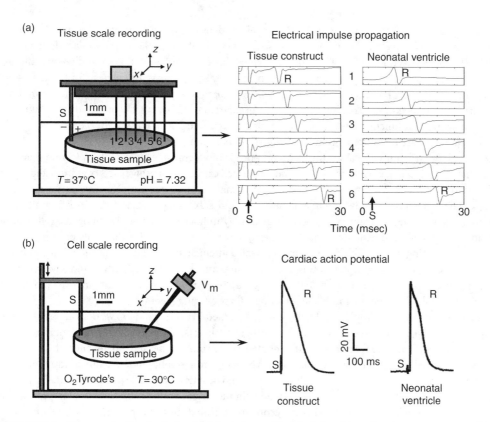

FIGURE 56.2   Tissue and cell scale electrophysiological recordings in 7-day old cardiac tissue constructs and 2-day old neonatal ventricles. (a) Custom-built linear array of two stimulating and eight recording microelectrodes (only six are shown) was used for assessment of macroscopic impulse propagation. S and R in two tracings denote stimulus artifact and responses, respectively. Note relatively smooth biphasic shapes of recorded extracellular waveforms in constructs and ventricles. The response amplitude in constructs is an order of magnitude lower than in ventricles due to smaller number of cardiac cell layers present. Propagation velocities in constructs and ventricles are comparable (i.e., times for propagation from electrode 1 to 6 are similar). (b) Glass capillary microelectrodes are used for action potential recordings from single cells in the tissue sample. Note fast upstroke and similar resting potential, but longer action potential in constructs than in ventricles. S and R denote stimulus artifact and response, respectively.

(Figure 56.2b) and absence of early repolarization notch due to downregulation of transient outward potassium current. In addition, cardiac cells cultured in 3D tissue constructs maintained more differentiated phenotype (higher expression of marker proteins) and more *in-vivo* like action potential features compared to those cultured in 2D monolayers under similar cultivation conditions.

56.3.2   *In Vivo* Implantation for Cardiac Repair

By April 2004, *in vivo* implantation of engineered cardiac tissue in infracted heart was attempted by only three groups.

Li et al. [97] cultured fetal rat myocytes on biodegradable gelatin meshes ($15 \times 15 \times 5$ mm^3) for 7 days and implanted cardiac constructs over the scar area in cryoinjured syngeneic rat hearts. Cells populated sparse interstices of gelatin meshes (see *in vitro* work by Li's group) and continued to proliferate and spontaneously contract *in vitro* for at least 26 days. Epicardially implanted grafts survived for 5 weeks, exhibited increased cellularity, slight degradation, and moderate degree of vascularization. Left ventricular developed pressure, showed no improvement over the control animals. In other studies [67,98], the same group evaluated use of various scaffold materials seeded with aortic smooth muscle cells (used to presumably increase elasticity of the patch) for repair of defect in the right ventricular outflow tract in syngeneic rats. Eight weeks postimplantation constructs made of ε-caprolactone-co-L-lactide reinforced with knitted poly-L-lactide fabric (PCLA) outperformed those made of gelatin, PGA, and polytetrafluoro-ethylene (PTFE) with respect to cellularity, elastin content, and preserved thickness. In the next study [99], grafts made of PCLA and smooth muscle cells were used to repair left ventricular aneurysm in the rat hearts after transmural infraction. Cell-seeded grafts reduced abnormal chamber distensibility and improved ventricular function compared with implanted cell-free grafts, as assessed by echocardiography and constant pressure measurements in Langendorff preparation.

Leor et al. [100] cultured fetal rat myocytes on porous biodegradable alginate disks (6 mm diameter, 1 mm thick) inside 96-well plates for 4 days, and implanted cardiac tissue constructs over infracted region in rat hearts 7 days after permanent occlusion of left main coronary artery. Nine weeks postimplant-ation, cardiac constructs survived, while alginate scaffold substantially degraded. Cardiac grafts were neovascularized, contained infiltrated macrophages and lymphocytes due to use of allogenic cells and no immunosuppression, and exhibited small number of sparsely distributed cardiac cells presumably due to low initial seeding density. Echocardiography revealed attenuated left ventricular dilatation and main-tained contractile function, although it was not clear if implanted cell-free scaffolds would have produced similar results. Further *in vitro* study from the same group [66] focused on methods to increase cell density in alginate scaffolds by applying moderate centrifugal forces during seeding.

Zimmermann et al. [85] implanted 12-day old ring-shaped EHTs (see *in vitro* work from Eschehagen's group) around the circumference of healthy syngeneic rat hearts. Two weeks after implantation, EHTs were vascularized, innervated, expressed differentiated cardiac phenotype, and did not alter left ventricular function compared to preoperative state, as assessed by echocardiography. Spontaneous contractions were preserved *in vivo*, but no intercellular coupling of EHTs and host tissue could be demonstrated. Despite the syngeneic approach, EHTs were completely degraded in the absence of immunosuppression, presumably due to presence of allogenic components in reconstitution mixture (e.g., matrigel, horse serum, chick embryo extract).

In all of the described *in vivo* attempts no electrophysiological studies of engineered patch were done pre- or postimplantation.

56.4 Design Considerations

Ultimate success of cardiac tissue repair with an implanted cardiac patch depends on thorough under-standing of the key parameters of tissue design *in vitro*, and careful definition of the desired tissue engineering outcomes.

56.4.1 Cell Source and Immunology

One of the crucial aspects for successful engineering of cardiac tissue is a choice of implanted cells. Experiences from cellular cardiomyoplasty show that for the improvement of heart systolic function implanted cells need to be (or be capable of becoming) contractile [26]. Although fetal and neonatal cardiac cells are clearly shown to functionally incorporate in the myocardium [17–19], they are not cells of choice due to limited proliferation potential, immunological, and ethical issues. For this reason, their use will probably stay limited to *in vitro* model systems and proof-of-concept *in vivo* studies. Possible "ideal" cell source may be human embryonic or adult stem cells. Although human embryonic stem cells are shown to differentiate into cardiac myocytes [101,102], their immunogenic and tumorogenic nature, and low efficiency and specificity of differentiation (<1% of cells differentiate into mixture of atrial, ventricular, and nodal cells), as well as ethical issues, may finally preclude their clinical use. Some hope lies in the nuclear transfer technology ("therapeutic cloning") [103], and genetic knock-out of major histocompatibility complexes [104], which may offer strategies for preventing immune rejection. Autologous adult stem cells from skeletal muscle, peripheral blood, or bone marrow appear as better choice for cell transplantation than embryonic stem cells. For example, autologous skeletal myoblasts are easy to proliferate *in vitro* and implant *in vivo* and cause no immune response, which currently makes them one of the cell types used in clinical trials [33]. Unfortunately, they do not express gap junction proteins and are still not shown to functionally couple with host cardiac tissue when implanted [105,106], although this may be resolved with stable transgene expression of connexin molecules [107]. Mesenchymal or hematopoietic stem cells derived from bone marrow may represent an ideal cell source [29,108]. However, the efficiency of their transdifferentiation into cardiac myocytes remains controversial in light of recent findings that question techniques used to quantify the number of transdifferentated cells in heart [109,110]. Still their beneficial effect may come from induced neovascularization in implantation sites. Current research efforts are focused on increase in percentage of embryonic or adult stem cells that commit to cardiac phenotype by use of different growth factors or media compositions, introduction of early cardiac genes in undifferentiated stem cells *in vitro*, or coculture of stem cells with differentiated cardiac myocytes. Another promising alternative is *in vitro* genetic reprogramming of differentiated somatic cells (for review see Reference 111).

56.4.2 Cellular Composition

The heart is composed of different types of cells. Engineering of functional tissue patch requires selection of the appropriate composition of seeded cell mixture. For example, if an implant were to be localized in the ventricle, cardiac myocytes that comprise a main fraction of seeded cells should be of ventricular origin or with ventricular characteristics. The percentage of nonmyocytes in the seeding mixture is a parameter that can be varied. Eschenhagen's group found that it was necessary to use higher percentage of nonmyocytes (no preplating after cell isolation) to improve mechanical integrity and twitch tension of EHTs [14]. In contrast, scaffold-free constructs by Shimizu et al. [75] developed similar twitch tensions despite the fact that they were made of purified cardiac cell mixture. This suggests that the percentage of "needed" nonmyocytes may actually depend on the presence and type of scaffold. It is possible that in EHTs, higher number of fibroblasts contributed initial contraction of collagen gel [112], which in turn increased the proximity and intercellular connectivity between myocytes, yielding increased contractile force. In addition, Bursac et al. [64] have shown that use of unpurified cardiac cell mixture decreased propagation velocity and compromised electrical properties in cardiac constructs. Therefore, for a given type of scaffold, the percentage of seeded nonmyocytes should be selected to optimize for both mechanical and electrical function of cardiac constructs.

56.4.3 Tissue Architecture

The anisotropic architecture and dense cell packing of native cardiac tissue impose important design rules in engineering of functional cardiac patch. For instance, velocity of electrical propagation and mechanical stiffness in healthy adult human ventricles are on average 2 to 3 times larger in longitudinal (fiber) than in transverse (cross-fiber) direction [113,114]. This can vary widely with location in the heart, age of individual, and heart disease. Therefore, only a cardiac patch with dense 3D network of elongated and aligned cardiac myocytes that mimic architecture of native tissue can generate desirable spatio-temporal distribution of electrical and mechanical activity, and result in efficient and safe therapy. Aligned growth of cardiac cells can be induced by static or dynamic stretch [61,115,116], presence of free tissue boundaries [117], or by cell guidance with oriented surface topography [49,118,119] and anisotropic distribution of chemical cues for cell attachment [49,120]. Eschenhagen's group applied cyclic stretch and ring geometry creating a sparse network of oriented cardiac cells in the form of a thin (submillimeter diameter) cardiac cable. Repair of larger injured area in the heart will, however, require engineering of an anisotropic slab of 3D cardiac-like tissue with controllable shape, size, and geometry.

Bursac et al. [49] have recently shown that anisotropic monolayers of cardiac cells (that mimic longitudinal sections of native cardiac tissue) can be designed with highly controllable architecture using surface microabrasion or micropatterning of extracellular matrix proteins (e.g., fibronectin) (Figure 56.3b). These

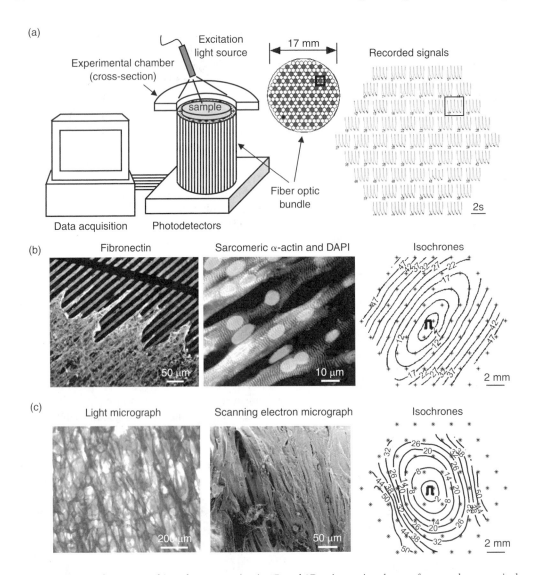

FIGURE 56.3 Architecture and impulse propagation in 2D and 3D anisotropic cultures of neonatal rat ventricular cells. (a) Optical mapping setup. Tissue samples stained with voltage sensitive dye were positioned over 61 hexagonally arranged fibers and transilluminated with excitation light. Two seconds of optically recorded action potentials from a cardiac cell monolayer are shown on the right. Gray circles denote active fibers. Square denotes a recording site in the bundle and corresponding voltage trace (for details see Reference 49). (b) Anisotropic monolayer of cardiac cells. Cells were cultured on micropatterned lines of fibronectin. On the left, culture is deliberately scratched to expose patterned lines and cell-deposited fibronectin. Aligned cells exhibit prominent sarcomeres and elongated nuclei (middle). Elliptical isochrones demonstrate anisotropic propagation (right). * denotes recording sites. Pulse symbol denotes site of stimulus. The degree of anisotropy can be systematically varied by controlling the amount of intercellular clefts and cell co-alignment [49]. (c) Anisotropic tissue construct. Oriented fibrous architecture in PLGA scaffolds (left) was accomplished by leaching sucrose from a polymer-coated template made of aligned sucrose fibers [121]. Cardiac cells were aligned in numerous regions along the direction of PLGA fibers (middle). Macroscopic propagation was anisotropic (albeit moderately), as assessed by optical mapping of transmembrane voltage (right) [122].

methodologies enabled systematic control over the degree of anisotropy (longitudinal-to-transverse velocity anisotropy ratios from 1 to 5.6), fiber direction, and amount of longitudinal intercellular clefts in the 2D cardiac monolayers. Optically recorded action potentials with voltage sensitive dye RH237 (at 61 sites over 2 cm^2 area) were used to map propagation of electrical activity and degree of functional anisotropy (Figure 56.3a). It would be ideal if techniques for 3D cardiac tissue culture could be developed with a similar level of architectural control as those used for 2D cell culture. In most recent studies Bursac et al. [121,122] extruded and baked sucrose to form 3D aligned fibrous templates in an attempt to induce anisotropic architecture in poly(lactic-co-glycolic) acid (PLGA) scaffold disks (Figure 56.3c). After 2 weeks of culture in HARV bioreactors, 12 mm diameter, 0.7 mm thick cardiac constructs exhibited regions with aligned cells, and moderate degrees of functional anisotropy (i.e., longitudinal-to-transverse velocity ratio of up to 2), as assessed by optical mapping of electrical propagation (Figure 56.3c). Using similar techniques to align elastomeric polymers [123] instead of PLGA in conjunction with chronic mechanical stimulation may yield 3D cardiac patches with physiological degrees of structural and functional anisotropy. An alternative approach is the use of electrospun scaffolds [74,91,124] providing that obtained degrees of porosity can support deeper cell penetration during seeding than achievable by current methodologies.

56.4.4 Tissue Thickness

Another important parameter in the design of a functional cardiac patch is thickness of the tissue construct. Compared to other cells in the body, cardiac myocytes require high oxygen and nutrient supply due to continuous contractile activity. High metabolic demand in myocardium is sustained by dense vascularization with average arterial intercapillary distances that range from 15 to 50 μm depending on the size of the heart and basal heart rate [125,126]. Absence of vasculature in tissue constructs is a limiting factor for engineering thicker (>200 to 300 μm) cardiac patches with physiological cell packing densities. Nonetheless, high cell density is necessary for establishment of proper intercellular communication, which in turn enables efficient generation of mechanical force and fast, electrically safe impulse propagation. Mixing and perfusion of culture medium, and/or cyclic mechanical stimulation are some of the methods that can alleviate diffusional limits of oxygen and nutrient supply, but only to a certain extent. Nevertheless, thin but dense engineered cardiac tissue is still a good *in vitro* approximation of a viable portion of explanted ventricular slice after several hours of superfusion [127], and thus could be used for different tissue-scale functional studies *in vitro*. These studies would be more versatile and technically easier than studies in monolayer cultures (e.g., they would enable variety of force measurements, and yield substantially higher signal-to-noise ratio during extracellular and optical recordings of electrical propagation). Moreover, implantation of even 10 to 20 well-coupled anisotropic cardiomyocyte layers over the infracted area may still have a significant therapeutic value regarding the facts that after epicardial infarction only several disarrayed cell layers may survive above the scar, and that increased thickness of survived layers is directly correlated with decreased incidence of arrhythmias [128]. This is one of the reasons why approach by Shimizu et al. [75] with scaffold-free cardiac multilayers deserves close attention. On the other hand, engineering of thicker cardiac slices will depend upon the development of externally perfusable, patent microcapillary-like networks inside the tissue constructs. Recent work by Vacanti's group [129] represents an interesting approach to this problem.

56.4.5 Electrical Function and Safety

One of the most important criteria for successful design of cardiac patch is the issue of electrical and mechanical safety. It is important to understand that haphazardly adding donor cells or transplanting a poorly designed tissue patch into an already compromised heart may only increase the likelihood for aneurisms, tissue rupture, or arrhythmias. In general, the injection of donor cells or implantation of a tissue patch introduces structural and functional heterogeneity in the cardiac milieu that depends on (1) electromechanical characteristics of donor cells, (2) the density, coupling, and geometrical arrangement of donor cells within the implant, (3) the degree of interaction between the donor and host cells, and

(4) architectural differences and relative position between implant and host tissue. Understanding how normal functioning of the cardiac cell network changes with the presence of different types of cellular, structural, and functional heterogeneities is a necessary step in the design of safer and more efficient cell and tissue transplantation therapies.

For example, it is already known from computational and experimental studies that contact between two cells with different resting potentials (e.g., injured and healthy cell [130]) or action potential durations (e.g., purkinje and ventricular cell [131], epicardial and M cell [132]), may trigger afterdepolarizations or create conduction block depending on the degree of their electrical coupling. It is also known that partial decoupling between the cells may actually increase the safety of propagation [133,134] as is the case in transverse vs. longitudinal propagation in healthy cardiac muscle [47]. On the other hand, excessive gap junction decoupling [134], presence of fibrotic regions [135], geometrical expansions [136], and repetitive tissue branching [137] (e.g., sparse cardiac network in ischemic or infarcted area [138]) can yield extreme slowing of impulse propagation and occurence of conduction block and introduce the susceptibility of cardiac tissue to formation of micro- or macroreentrant circuits. In the ideal world, the safest and most efficient therapy would be to engineer a cardiac patch that exactly mimics the geometry, architecture, and function of the "missing region" in the heart, and to perfectly couple it to the host tissue, as "a piece of the jigsaw puzzle." In the "semi-real" world, even if one is to produce a patch with perfect anisotropic architecture, its optimal orientation relative to host tissue when implanted may change depending on the electrical differences between the donor and host cells, or capability of patch to couple with the host tissue. In the real world, things are very complex due to interplay of many factors. For example, the use of skeletal myoblasts or stem cell-derived cardiomyocytes may demand different patch design and different implantation strategy as determined by the functional differences between these cell types (e.g., shorter vs. longer action potential, different resting potentials, none vs. significant expression of gap junctions, etc.). The simulation may be further complicated by the presence of a fibrous capsule at the implantation site.

Due to the complexity of the problem, carefully designed studies on possible implantation scenarios will be crucial as a prescreening tool before the actual implantation. The author's view is that there are at least two simplified settings that could be used to systematically and reproducibly study the factors affecting the likelihood of arrhythmia arising from cell and tissue cardiomyoplasty. One is the use of micropatterned cocultures [139,140] of host cardiomyocytes and different types of donor cells or mixtures of donor cells, with the possibility for well-controlled studies based on (1) simplified cellular composition and tissue architecture compared to the 3D heart, (2) precise control of the cell microenvironment, cellular geometry and distribution, and geometry of cellular interactions between donor, host, and donor and host cells, and (3) the possibility to optically assess and exactly correlate electrical/mechanical activity and underlying tissue architecture at microscopic and macroscopic spatial scales. Optical mapping of transmembrane potentials and intracellular calcium [141] are well-suited not only for these studies, but also for electrophysiological evaluation of engineered cardiac patch pre and postimplantation *ex vivo*. The other setting is the use of computer models that incorporate cell-specific membrane properties, cell geometry, distribution of intercellular connections, and discrete tissue microarchitecture. With increase in computing efficiency, these detailed models could be used as counterparts to different *in vitro* or *in vivo* implantation scenarios to help interpretation and design of experiments, and eventually yield safe and efficient therapies.

56.4.6 Spontaneous Activity

Another electrophysiological parameter for consideration is a somewhat misinterpreted presence of spontaneous contractile activity in cardiac cell cultures. It is important to understand that although spontaneous contractions in cardiac cultures represent convenient way to visually identify cardiac cells, they are by no means a physiologically normal state for adult or neonatal ventricular muscle (which is most often the source tissue for cell dissociation). While early embryonic ventricular cells still spontaneously depolarize and contract [142], their resting potential hyperpolarizes with maturation such that neonatal ventricular cells already exhibit steady resting potentials (less than -70 mV), fast action potential upstroke (more than 100 V/sec), and no spontaneous activity [76,142,143]. Rather, spontaneous activity of cardiac cells observed *in vitro* is an artifact of the cell culture possibly caused by (1) membrane depolarization due to cell injury during or after dissociation, (2) dedifferentiation of cultured cells to more embryonic state due to presence of high serum and inadequate media formulation, (3) large presence of nodal or other pacemaking cells due to unselective cell dissociation, and/or (4) decreased intercellular coupling compared to native tissue due to 2D or sparse 3D arrangement of ventricular cells. The first three causes can be alleviated with time in culture, proper cultivation conditions, and careful cell dissociation. However, the sparse cardiac network, if present, will always result in less electrotonic load "seen" by a cell and facilitate propagation from single or small group of pacemaking cells into the quiescent tissue, favoring spontaneous activity [144,145]. Our observations that spontaneous contractions in cardiac constructs can be more readily observed when cells are less coupled (e.g., at lower seeding density, in the beginning of cultivation, or on the perturbing polymer fibers at the edges of the tissue construct) are in agreement with this reasoning. After 5 to 7 days in culture, tissue constructs in our studies usually become quiescent, presumably due to increased packing density and connectivity of cardiac cells. The low percentage of nonmyocytes in tissue constructs as assessed by immunostaining, and increase in conduction velocity between culture days 4 and 7, exclude fibroblast overgrowth as a possible cause of cardiac cells quiescence.

Although reported spontaneous beating rates in cardiac constructs are usually lower than regular heart rate, presence of paracrine chronotropic factors (e.g., epinephrine, adrenaline) after implantation in the heart may result in faster activity and possible arrhythmogenic hazard. For electrical safety reasons, a nonstimulated ventricular cardiac patch should be electrically quiescent, but readily excitable and fast conducting, similar to native ventricular muscle. Moreover, a quiescent avascular patch may have lower metabolic demand and increased chance for survival after implantation compared to a spontaneously contractile patch. However, persistent contractions and presence of mechanical load are essential for maintenance of ventricular mass *in vivo* [146], and for cell hypertrophy [147], spreading to confluence [148], and establishment of cell contacts *in vitro* [149,150]. (Our experience is that if cardiac cell culture is noncontracting for more than 3 days, cells start to atrophy and loose cell contacts.) Therefore, spontaneously quiescent engineered cardiac constructs still need to be maintained mechanically active in culture either by use of electrical, mechanical, or chemical (e.g., small concentrations of epinephrine) stimulation [150], or by coculture with spatially distinct population of pacemaking cells, which can be easily dissected before the implantation in the ventricle.

In any case, thorough evaluation of electrical properties and susceptibility to conduction block and arrhythmic behavior should be routinely done in cultured cardiac constructs and used as one of the tissue design criteria. From our experience, it is important to assess the properties of engineered tissue in challenging regimes such as fast or premature stimulation, similar to standard clinical pacing protocols for testing the susceptibility to arrhythmias [151]. For example, a tissue construct can support macroscopically continuous and relatively fast electrical propagation at low pacing rates, but yield conduction blocks and high incidence of reentrant arrhythmias [122] when paced rapidly (Figure 56.4) due to large spatial dispersion of refractoriness, or abundance of microscopic anatomic heterogeneities.

56.5 Future Work

The crucial technical aspect of this and all other cell-based therapies will be a choice of appropriate cell source, which is to be primarily determined by developmental biologists, geneticists, and immunologists. Engineering of a functional cardiac tissue patch using embryonic or adult stem cells and subsequent implantation studies are still to be done. Simultaneous efforts on design of appropriate scaffolds and control over the cellular connectivity and tissue architecture in three dimensions will be essential to the development of functional cardiac patch for use in laboratory and clinics. Systematic *in vitro* and *in vivo* studies on the role of heterogeneities on structure and function of cardiac tissue will help in designing more efficient and safer therapies. Possible engineering of the patent capillary- and microcapillary-like networks inside the tissue constructs may enable culture of thick tissue slices, and facilitate immediate perfusion

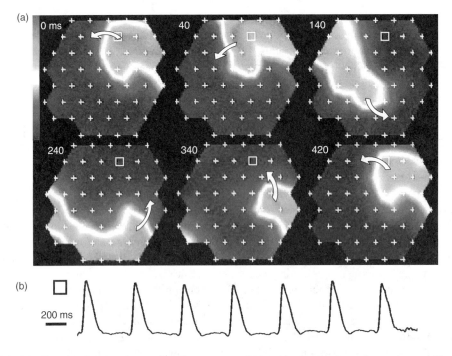

FIGURE 56.4 Functional reentry in a cardiac tissue construct induced by rapid point pacing, and assessed by optical mapping of transmembrane potential. (a) Single rotation of a counterclockwise reentrant wave shown through a series of voltage snapshots in time. Frames progress left to right, top to bottom. Time in milliseconds is marked at the top left corner of each frame. Arrows denote the direction of wave front. + denotes 2-mm spaced recording sites. Gray scale bar next to the first frame corresponds to a normalized transmembrane voltage with bottom and top denoting rest and peak of an action potential, respectively. (b) Recording of transmembrane voltage from the site marked by a white square in the frames of panel A. Reentrant activity appears stationary and periodic.

during implantation by attachment to one of the host arteries. The success will only be accomplished by a profound understanding of a number of complex topics, and achieved through a joint effort among basic scientists, engineers, and clinicians.

56.6 Conclusions

Cardiac tissue engineering is a new and exciting field with many obstacles to be surmounted before start of clinical trials. With technical aspects resolved, the main advantage of implanted cardiac tissue patch over the injected cells will be a structural and functional repair of large tissue defects. Given that implantation of cardiac patch will repair a centimeter-size tissue region, inference about the quality of tissue construct sprior to implantation should be based not only upon different assessments at cellular or subcellular level, but also upon detailed evaluation of both electrical and mechanical function at centimeter-size scale (i.e., measurements of impulse propagation and contractile force in constructs relative to those in native cardiac muscle). Similarly, only systematic micro- and macroscopic assessments of heart structure and electromechanical function postimplantation will provide necessary selectivity towards the design of safe and efficient clinical therapies.

Acknowledgment

The author would like to thank P. Bursac and K. Cahill for reviewing the manuscript. This manuscript was submitted for press on May 1, 2004. Due to rapid developments in the field, some of the most contemporary work will not be reviewed, and certain statements may be outdated at the time of press. Author apologizes in advance if this is the case.

References

[1] Anversa P. and Kajstura J. Ventricular myocytes are not terminally differentiated in the adult mammalian heart. *Circ. Res.* 1998; 83: 1–14.

[2] Laflamme M.A., Myerson D., Saffitz J.E., and Murry C.E. Evidence for cardiomyocyte repopulation by extracardiac progenitors in transplanted human hearts. *Circ. Res.* 2002; 90: 634–640.

[3] Guyatt G.H. and Devereaux P.J. A review of heart failure treatment. *Mt. Sinai. J. Med.* 2004;71: 47–54.

[4] Miniati D.N. and Robbinson R.C. Heart transplantation: a thirty year perspective. *Annu. Rev. Med.* 2002; 53: 189–205.

[5] Boehmer J.P. Device therapy for heart failure. *Am. J. Cardiol.* 2003; 91: 53D–59D.

[6] Moreira L.F. and Stolf N.A. Dynamic cardiomyoplasty as a therapeutic alternative: current status. *Heart Fail. Rev.* 2001; 6: 201–212.

[7] Szatkowski A., Ndubuka-Irobunda C., Oesterle S.N., and Burkhoff D. Transmyocardial laser revascularization: a review of basic and clinical aspects. *Am. J. Cardiovasc. Drugs* 2002; 2: 255–266.

[8] Sorelle R. Cardiovascular news: totally contained AbioCor artificial heart implanted July 3, 2001. *Circulation* 2001; 104: E9005–E9006.

[9] Association A.H. *2000 Heart and Stroke Statistical Update.* Dallas, TX: American Heart Association, 1999.

[10] Pasumarthi K.B.S. and Field L.J. Cardiomyocyte cell cycle regulation. *Circ. Res.* 2002; 90: 1044–1054.

[11] Orlic D., Kajstura J., Chimenti S., Limana F., Jakoniuk I., Quaini F., Nadal-Ginard B., Bodine D.M., Leri A., and Anversa P. Mobilized bone marrow cells repair the infarcted heart, improving function and survival. *Proc. Natl Acad. Sci. USA* 2001; 98: 10344–10349.

[12] Dowell J.D., Rubart M., Pasumarthi K.B., Soonpaa M.H., and Field L.J. Myocyte and myogenic stem cell transplantation in the heart. *Cardiovasc. Res.* 2003; 58: 336–350.

[13] Chachques J.C., Acar C., Herreros J., Trainini J.C., Prosper F., D'Attellis N., Fabiani J.N., and Carpentier A.F. Cellular cardiomyoplasty: clinical application. *Ann. Thorac. Surg.* 2004; 77: 1121–1130.

[14] Zimmermann W.H. and Eschenhagen T. Cardiac tissue engineering for replacement therapy. *Heart Fail. Rev.* 2003; 8: 259–269.

[15] Koh G., Soonpaa M., Klug M., and Field L. Long-term survival of AT-1 cardyomyocyte grafts in syngeneic myocardium. *Am. J. Physiol.* 1993; 264: H1727–H1733.

[16] Koh G., Klug M., Soonpaa M., and Field L. Differentiation and long term survival of C2C12 myoblasts graft in heart. *J. Clin. Invest.* 1993; 92: 1548–1554.

[17] Soonpa M.H., Koh G.Y., Klug M.G., and Field L.J. Formation of nascent intercalated disks between grafted fetal cardiomyocytes and host myocardium. *Science* 1994; 264: 98–101.

[18] Rubart M., Pasumarthi K.B., Nakajima H., Soonpaa M.H., Nakajima H.O., and Field L.J. Physiological coupling of donor and host cardiomyocytes after cellular transplantation. *Circ. Res.* 2003; 92: 1217–1224.

[19] Reinecke H., Zhang M., Bartosek T., and Murry C.E. Survival, integration, and differentiation of cardiomyocyte grafts: a study in normal and injured rat hearts. *Circulation* 1999; 100: 193–202.

[20] Sakai T., Li R.K., Weisel R.D., Mickle D.A., Kim E.J., Tomita S., Jia Z.Q., and Yau T.M. Autologous heart cell transplantation improves cardiac function after myocardial injury. *Ann. Thorac. Surg.* 1999; 68: 2074–2080; discussion 2080–2081.

[21] Taylor D., Atkins B., Hungspreugs P., Jones T., Reedy M., Hutcheson K., Glower D., and Kraus W. Regenerating functional myocardium: improved performance after skeletal myoblast transplantation. *Nat. Med.* 1998; 4: 929–933.

[22] Kessler P.D. and Byrne B.J. Myoblast cell grafting into heart muscle: cellular biology and potential applications. *Annu. Rev. Physiol.* 1999; 61: 219–242.

[23] Murry C., Wiseman R., Schwartz S., and Hauschka S. Skeletal myoblast transplantation for repair of myocardial necrosis. *J. Clin. Invest.* 1996; 98: 2512–2523.

[24] Li G., Ouyang Q., Petrov V.V., and Swinney H.L. Transition from simple rotating chemical spirals to meandering and traveling spirals. *Phys. Rev. Lett.* 1996; 77: 2105–2108.

[25] Kim E.J., Li R.K., Weisel R.D., Mickle D.A., Jia Z.Q., Tomita S., Sakai T., and Yau T.M. Angiogenesis by endothelial cell transplantation. *J. Thorac. Cardiovasc. Surg.* 2001; 122: 963–971.

[26] Hutcheson K.A., Atkins B.Z., Hueman M.T., Hopkins M.B., Glower D.D., and Taylor D.A. Comparison of benefits on myocardial performance of cellular cardiomyoplasty with skeletal myoblasts and fibroblasts. *Cell Transplant.* 2000; 9: 359–368.

[27] Etzion S., Barbash I.M., Feinberg M.S., Zarin P., Miller L., Guetta E., Holbova R., Kloner R.A., Kedes L.H., and Leor J. Cellular cardiomyoplasty of cardiac fibroblasts by adenoviral delivery of MyoD *ex vivo*: an unlimited source of cells for myocardial repair. *Circulation* 2002; 106: I125–I130.

[28] Klug M.G., Soonpaa M.H., Koh G.Y., and Field L.J. Genetically selected cardiomyocytes from differentiating embronic stem cells form stable intracardiac grafts. *J. Clin. Invest.* 1996; 98: 216–224.

[29] Orlic D., Kajstura J., Chimenti S., Jakoniuk I., Anderson S.M., Li B., Pickel J., McKay R., Nadal-Ginard B., Bodine D.M., Leri A., and Anversa P. Bone marrow cells regenerate infarcted myocardium. *Nature* 2001; 410: 701–705.

[30] Vulliet P.R., Greeley M., Halloran S.M., MacDonald K.A., and Kittleson M.D. Intra-coronary arterial injection of mesenchymal stromal cells and microinfarction in dogs. *Lancet* 2004; 363: 783–784.

[31] Beltrami A.P., Barlucchi L., Torella D., Baker M., Limana F., Chimenti S., Kasahara H., Rota M., Musso E., Urbanek K., Leri A., Kajstura J., Nadal-Ginard B., and Anversa P. Adult cardiac stem cells are multipotent and support myocardial regeneration. *Cell* 2003; 114: 763–776.

[32] Sakai T., Li R.K., Weisel R.D., Mickle D.A., Jia Z.Q., Tomita S., Kim E.J., and Yau T.M. Fetal cell transplantation: a comparison of three cell types. *J. Thorac. Cardiovasc. Surg.* 1999; 118: 715–724.

[33] Menasche P. Myoblast-based cell transplantation. *Heart Fail. Rev.* 2003; 8: 221–227.

[34] Menasche P., Hagege A.A., Vilquin J.T., Desnos M., Abergel E., Pouzet B., Bel A., Sarateanu S., Scorsin M., Schwartz K., Bruneval P., Benbunan M., Marolleau J.P., and Duboc D. Autologous skeletal myoblast transplantation for severe postinfarction left ventricular dysfunction. *J. Am. Coll. Cardiol.* 2003; 41: 1078–1083.

[35] Menasche P. Cellular transplantation: hurdles remaining before widespread clinical use. *Curr. Opin. Cardiol.* 2004; 19: 154–161.

[36] Reinecke H., MacDonald G.H., Hauschka S.D., and Murry C.E. Electromechanical coupling between skeletal and cardiac muscle. Implications for infarct repair. *J. Cell Biol.* 2000; 149: 731–740.

[37] Pak H.N., Qayyum M., Kim D.T., Hamabe A., Miyauchi Y., Lill M.C., Frantzen M., Takizawa K., Chen L.S., Fishbein M.C., Sharifi B.G., Chen P.S., and Makkar R. Mesenchymal stem cell injection induces cardiac nerve sprouting and increased tenascin expression in a Swine model of myocardial infarction. *J. Cardiovasc. Electrophysiol.* 2003; 14: 841–848.

[38] Hoffman J.I., Kaplan S., and Liberthson R.R. Prevalence of congenital heart disease. *Am. Heart J.* 2004; 147: 425–439.

[39] O'Dell W.G. and McCulloch A.D. Imaging three-dimensional cardiac function. *Annu. Rev. Biomed. Eng.* 2000; 2: 431–456.

[40] Shachar M. and Cohen S. Cardiac tissue engineering, *ex-vivo*: design principles in biomaterials and bioreactors. *Heart Fail. Rev.* 2003; 8: 271–276.

[41] Spach M. Anisotropy of cardiac tissue: a major determinant of conduction. *J. Cardiovasc. Electrophysiol.* 1999; 10: 887–890.

[42] Saffitz J., Kanter H., Green K., Tolley T., and Beyer E. Tissue-specific determinants of anisotropic conduction velocity in canine atrial and ventricular myocardium. *Circ. Res.* 1994; 74: 1065–1070.

[43] Arts T., Costa K.D., Covell J.W., and McCulloch A.D. Relating myocardial laminar architecture to shear strain and muscle fiber orientation. *Am. J. Physiol. Heart Circ. Physiol.* 2001; 280: H2222–H2229.

[44] Antzelevitch C., Yan G.-X., Shimizu W., and Burashnikov A. Electrical heterogeneity, the ECG, and cardiac arrhythmias. In Zipes D.P. and Jalife J., Eds. *Cardiac Electrophysiology — From Cell to Bedside.* 3rd ed. Philadelphia, PA: W. B. Saunders Co., 2000, pp. 222–238.

[45] de Bakker J.M. and OptHof T. Is the apico-basal gradient larger than the transmural gradient? *J. Cardiovasc. Pharmacol.* 2002; 39: 328–331.

[46] Wolk R., Cobbe S.M., Hicks M.N., and Kane K.A. Functional, structural, and dynamic basis of electrical heterogeneity in healthy and diseased cardiac muscle: implications for arrhythmogenesis and anti-arrhythmic drug therapy. *Pharmacol. Ther.* 1999; 84: 207–231.

[47] Spach M.S., Dolber P.C., Heidlage J.F., Kootsey J.M., and Johnson E.A. Propagating depolarization in anisotropic human and canine cardiac muscle: apparent directional differences in membrane capacitance. A simplified model for selective directional effects of modifying the sodium conductance on Vmax, tau foot, and the propagation safety factor. *Circ. Res.* 1987; 60: 206–219.

[48] Roberge F.A. and Leon L.J. Propagation of activation in cardiac muscle. *J. Electrocardiol.* 1992; 25 Suppl: 69–79.

[49] Bursac N., Parker K.K., Iravanian S., and Tung L. Cardiomyocyte cultures with controlled macroscopic anisotropy. A model for functional electrophysiological studies of cardiac muscle. *Circ. Res.* 2002; 91: e45–e54.

[50] Spach M.S. and Heidlage J.F. The stochastic nature of cardiac propagation at a microscopic level. Electrical description of myocardial architecture and its application to conduction. *Circ. Res.* 1995; 76: 366–380.

[51] Kleber A.G. and Rudy Y. Basic mechanisms of cardiac impulse propagation and associated arrhythmias. *Physiol. Rev.* 2004; 84: 431–488.

[52] Antzelevitch C. Basic mechanisms of reentrant arrhythmias. *Curr. Opin. Cardiol.* 2001; 16: 1–7.

[53] Spach M.S. and Dolber P.C. Relating extracellular potentials and their derivatives to anisotropic propagation at a microscopic level in human cardiac muscle. Evidence for electrical uncoupling of side-to-side fiber connections with increasing age. *Circ. Res.* 1986; 58: 356–371.

[54] Koura T., Hara M., Takeuchi S., Ota K., Okada Y., Miyoshi S., Watanabe A., Shiraiwa K., Mitamura H., Kodama I., and Ogawa S. Anisotropic conduction properties in canine atria analyzed by high-resolution optical mapping: preferential direction of conduction block changes from longitudinal to transverse with increasing age. *Circulation* 2002; 105: 2092–2098.

[55] McCulloch A., Bassingthwaighte J., Hunter P., and Noble D. Computational biology of the heart: from structure to function. *Prog. Biophys. Mol. Biol.* 1998; 69: 153–155.

[56] de Bakker J.M., van Capelle F.J., Janse M.J., Tasseron S., Vermeulen J.T., de Jonge N., and Lahpor J.R. Fractionated electrograms in dilated cardiomyopathy: origin and relation to abnormal conduction. *J. Am. Coll. Cardiol.* 1996; 27: 1071–1078.

[57] De Bakker J.M.T and Janse M.J. Pathophysiological correlates of ventricular tachycardia in hearts with a healed infarct. In Zipes D.P. and Jalife J., Eds. *Cardiac Electrophysiology — From Cell to Bedside.* 3rd ed. Philadelphia, PA: W.B. Saunders Co., 2000, pp. 415–422.

[58] Spach M.S. and Josephson M.E. Initiating reentry: the role of nonuniform anisotropy in small circuits. *J. Cardiovasc. Electrophysiol.* 1994; 5: 182–209.

[59] Wit A.L., Dillon S.M., and Coromilas J. Anisotropic reentry as a cause of ventricular tachyarrhythmias in myocardial infarction. In Zipes D.P. and Jalife J., Eds. *Cardiac Electrophysiology — From Cell to Bedside.* Philadelphia, PA: W.B. Saunders Co., 1995, pp. 511–526.

[60] Ravens U. Mechano-electric feedback and arrhythmias. *Prog. Biophys. Mol. Biol.* 2003; 82: 255–266.

[61] Fink C., Ergun S., Kralisch D., Remmers U., Weil J., and Eschenhagen T. Chronic stretch of engineered heart tissue induces hypertrophy and functional improvement. *FASEB J.* 2000; 14: 669–679.

[62] Zimmermann W., Fink C., Kralisch D., Remmers U., Weil J., and Eschenhagen T. Three-dimensional engineered heart tissue from neonatal rat cardiac cells. *Biotechnol. Bioeng.* 2000; 68: 106–114.

[63] Carrier R., Papadaki M., Rupnick M., Schoen F., Bursac N., Langer R., Freed L., and Vunjak-Novakovic G. Development of a model system for cardiac tissue engineering: investigation of key parameters. *Biotechnol. Bioeng.* 1999; 64: 580–589.

[64] Bursac N., Papadaki M., Cohen R., Schoen F., Eisenberg S., Carrier R., Vunjak-Novakovic G., and Freed L. Cardiac muscle tissue engineering: towards an *in vitro* model for electrophysiological studies. *Am. J. Physiol. (Heart Circ. Physiol. 46)* 1999; 277: H433–H444.

[65] Radisic M., Euloth M., Yang L., Langer R., Freed L.E., and Vunjak-Novakovic G. High-density seeding of myocyte cells for cardiac tissue engineering. *Biotechnol. Bioeng.* 2003; 82: 403–414.

[66] Dar A., Shachar M., Leor J., and Cohen S. Optimization of cardiac cell seeding and distribution in 3D porous alginate scaffolds. *Biotechnol. Bioeng.* 2002; 80: 305–312.

[67] Ozawa T., Mickle D.A., Weisel R.D., Koyama N., Ozawa S., and Li R.K. Optimal biomaterial for creation of autologous cardiac grafts. *Circulation* 2002; 106: I176–I182.

[68] Pego A.P., Poot A.A., Grijpma D.W., and Feijen J. Biodegradable elastomeric scaffolds for soft tissue engineering. *J. Control. Release* 2003; 87: 69–79.

[69] Papadaki M., Bursac N., Langer R., Merok J., Vunjak-Novakovic G., and Freed L. Tissue engineering of functional cardiac muscle: molecular, structural and electrophysiological studies. *Am. J. Physiol. (Heart Circ. Physiol.)* 2001; 280: H168–H178.

[70] Zimmermann W.H., Melnychenko I., and Eschenhagen T. Engineered heart tissue for regeneration of diseased hearts. *Biomaterials* 2004; 25: 1639–1647.

[71] Akhyari P., Fedak P.W., Weisel R.D., Lee T.Y., Verma S., Mickle D.A., and Li R.K. Mechanical stretch regimen enhances the formation of bioengineered autologous cardiac muscle grafts. *Circulation* 2002; 106: I137–I142.

[72] Zimmermann W., Schneiderbanger K., Schubert P., Didie M., Munzel F., Heubach J., Kostin S., Nehuber W., and Eschenhagen T. Tissue engineering of a differentiated cardiac muscle construct. *Circ. Res.* 2002; 90: 223–230.

[73] Kofidis T., Akhyari P., Wachsmann B., Mueller-Stahl K., Boublik J., Ruhparwar A., Mertsching H., Balsam L., Robbins R., and Haverich A. Clinically established hemostatic scaffold (tissue fleece) as biomatrix in tissue- and organ-engineering research. *Tissue Eng.* 2003; 9: 517–523.

[74] Yost M.J., Baicu C.F., Stonerock C.E., Goodwin R.L., Price R.L., Davis J.M., Evans H., Watson P.D., Gore C.M., Sweet J., Creech L., Zile M.R., and Terracio L. A novel tubular scaffold for cardiovascular tissue engineering. *Tissue Eng.* 2004; 10: 273–284.

[75] Shimizu T., Yamato M., Isoi Y., Akutsu T., Setomaru T., Abe K., Kikuchi A., Umezu M., and Okano T. Fabrication of pulsatile cardiac tissue grafts using a novel 3-dimensional cell sheet manipulation technique and temperature-responsive cell culture surfaces. *Circ. Res.* 2002; 90: e40.

[76] Bursac N., Papadaki M., White J.A., Eisenberg S.R., Vunjak-Novakovic G., and Freed L.E. Cultivation in rotating bioreactors promotes maintenance of cardiac myocyte electrophysiology and molecular properties. *Tissue Eng.* 2003; 9: 1243–1253.

[77] Akins R.E., Schroedl N.A., Gonda S.R., and Hartzell C.R. Neonatal rat heart cells cultured in simulated microgravity. *In Vitro Cell Dev. Biol.* 1997; 337–343.

[78] Akins R.E., Boyce R.A., Madonna M.L., Schroedl N.A., Gonda S.R., McLaughlin T.A., and Hartzell C.R. Cardiac organogenesis in vitro: reestablishment of three-dimensional tissue architecture by dissociated neonatal rat ventricular cells. *Tissue Eng.* 1999; 5: 103–118.

[79] Eschenhagen T., Fink C., Remmers U., Scholz H., Wattchow J., Weil J., Zimmerman W., Dohmen H., Schafer H., Bishopric N., Wakatsuki T., and Elson E. Three-dimensional reconstitution of embryonic cardimyocytes in a collagen matrix: a new heart muscle model system. *FASEB J.* 1997; 11: 683–694.

[80] Vandenburgh H., Del Tatto M, Shansky J., Lemaire J., Chang A., Payumo F., Lee P., Goodyear A., and Raven L. Tissue-engineered skeletal muscle organoids for reversible gene therapy. *Hum. Gene Ther.* 1996; 7: 2195–2200.

[81] Holubarsch C., Ruf T., Goldstein D.J., Ashton R.C., Nickl W., Pieske B., Pioch K., Ludemann J., Wiesner S., Hasenfuss G., Posival H., Just H., and Burkhoff D. Existence of the Frank–Starling mechanism in the failing human heart. Investigations on the organ, tissue, and sarcomere levels. *Circulation* 1996; 94: 683–689.

[82] Rau T., Nose M., Remmers U., Weil J., Weissmuller A., Davia K., Harding S., Peppel K., Koch W.J., and Eschenhagen T. Overexpression of wild-type Galpha(i)-2 suppresses beta-adrenergic signaling in cardiac myocytes. *FASEB J.* 2003; 17: 523–525.

[83] El-Armouche A., Rau T., Zolk O., Ditz D., Pamminger T., Zimmermann W.H., Jackel E., Harding S.E., Boknik P., Neumann J., and Eschenhagen T. Evidence for protein phosphatase inhibitor-1 playing an amplifier role in beta-adrenergic signaling in cardiac myocytes. *FASEB J.* 2003; 17: 437–439.

[84] Zolk O., Munzel F., and Eschenhagen T. Effects of chronic endothelin-1 stimulation on cardiac myocyte contractile function. *Am. J. Physiol. Heart Circ. Physiol.* 2004; 286: H1248–H1257.

[85] Zimmermann W.H., Didie M., Wasmeier G.H., Nixdorff U., Hess A., Melnychenko I., Boy O., Neuhuber W.L., Weyand M., and Eschenhagen T. Cardiac grafting of engineered heart tissue in syngenic rats. *Circulation* 2002; 106: I151–I157.

[86] Li R.K., Yau T.M., Weisel R.D., Mickle D.A., Sakai T., Choi A., and Jia Z.Q. Construction of a bioengineered cardiac graft. *J. Thorac. Cardiovasc. Surg.* 2000; 119: 368–375.

[87] Kofidis T., Akhyari P., Wachsmann B., Boublik J., Mueller-Stahl K., Leyh R., Fischer S., and Haverich A. A novel bioartificial myocardial tissue and its prospective use in cardiac surgery. *Eur. J. Cardiothorac. Surg.* 2002; 22: 238–243.

[88] Kofidis T., Lenz A., Boublik J., Akhyari P., Wachsmann B., Mueller-Stahl K., Hofmann M., and Haverich A. Pulsatile perfusion and cardiomyocyte viability in a solid three-dimensional matrix. *Biomaterials* 2003; 24: 5009–5014.

[89] van Luyn M.J., Tio R.A., Gallego y van Seijen X.J., Plantinga J.A., de Leij L.F., DeJongste M.J., and van Wachem P.B. Cardiac tissue engineering: characteristics of in unison contracting two- and three-dimensional neonatal rat ventricle cell (co)-cultures. *Biomaterials* 2002; 23: 4793–4801.

[90] Evans H.J., Sweet J.K., Price R.L., Yost M., and Goodwin R.L. Novel 3D culture system for study of cardiac myocyte development. *Am J. Physiol. Heart Circ. Physiol.* 2003; 285: H570–H578.

[91] Matthews J.A., Wnek G.E., Simpson D.G., and Bowlin G.L. Electrospinning of collagen nanofibers. *Biomacromolecules* 2002; 3: 232–238.

[92] Shimizu T., Yamato M., Akihiko K., and Okano T. Two-dimensional manipulation of cardiac myocyte sheets utilizing temperature-responsive culture dishes augments pulsatile amplitude. *Tissue Eng.* 2001; 7: 141–151.

[93] Shimizu T., Yamato M., Akutsu T., Shibata T., Isoi Y., Kikuchi A., Umezu M., and Okano T. Electrically communicating three-dimensional cardiac tissue mimic fabricated by layered cultured cardiomyocyte sheets. *J. Biomed. Mater. Res.* 2002; 60: 110–117.

[94] Carrier R.L., Rupnick M., Langer R., Schoen F.J., Freed L.E., and Vunjak-Novakovic G. Perfusion improves tissue architecture of engineered cardiac muscle. *Tissue Eng.* 2002; 8: 175–188.

[95] Carrier R.L., Rupnick M., Langer R., Schoen F.J., Freed L.E., and Vunjak-Novakovic G. Effects of oxygen on engineered cardiac muscle. *Biotechnol. Bioeng.* 2002; 78: 617–625.

[96] Radisic M., Yang L., Boublik J., Cohen R.J., Langer R., Freed L.E., and Vunjak-Novakovic G. Medium perfusion enables engineering of compact and contractile cardiac tissue. *Am. J. Physiol. Heart Circ. Physiol.* 2004; 286: H507–H516.

[97] Li R.K., Jia Z.Q., Weisel R.D., Mickle D.A., Choi A., and Yau T.M. Survival and function of bioengineered cardiac grafts. *Circulation* 1999; 100: II63–II69.

[98] Ozawa T., Mickle D.A., Weisel R.D., Koyama N., Wong H., Ozawa S., and Li R.K. Histologic changes of nonbiodegradable and biodegradable biomaterials used to repair right ventricular heart defects in rats. *J. Thorac. Cardiovasc. Surg.* 2002; 124: 1157–1164.

[99] Matsubayashi K., Fedak P.W., Mickle D.A., Weisel R.D., Ozawa T., and Li R.K. Improved left ventricular aneurysm repair with bioengineered vascular smooth muscle grafts. *Circulation* 2003; 108 Suppl 1: II219–II225.

[100] Leor J., Aboulafia-Etzion S., Dar A., Shapiro L., Barbash I., Battler A., Granot Y., and Cohen S. Bioengineered cardiac grafts: a new approach to repair the infarcted myocardium? *Circulation* 2000; 102: III56–III61.

[101] Kehat I., Kenyagin-Karsenti D., Snir M., Segev H., Amit M., Gepstein A., Livne E., Binah O., Itskovitz-Eldor J., and Gepstein L. Human embryonic stem cells can differentiate into myocytes with structural and functional properties of cardiomyocytes. *J. Clin. Invest.* 2001; 108: 407–414.

[102] Xu C., Police S., Rao N., and Carpenter M.K. Characterization and enrichment of cardiomyocytes derived from human embryonic stem cells. *Circ. Res.* 2002; 91: 501–508.

[103] Lanza R., Moore M.A., Wakayama T., Perry A.C., Shieh J.H., Hendrikx J., Leri A., Chimenti S., Monsen A., Nurzynska D., West M.D., Kajstura J., and Anversa P. Regeneration of the infarcted heart with stem cells derived by nuclear transplantation. *Circ. Res.* 2004; 94: 820–827.

[104] Grusby M.J., Auchincloss H., Jr., Lee R., Johnson R.S., Spencer J.P., Zijlstra M., Jaenisch R., Papaioannou V.E., and Glimcher L.H. Mice lacking major histocompatibility complex class I and class II molecules. *Proc. Natl Acad. Sci. USA* 1993; 90: 3913–3917.

[105] Leobon B., Garcin I., Menasche P., Vilquin J.T., Audinat E., and Charpak S. Myoblasts transplanted into rat infarcted myocardium are functionally isolated from their host. *Proc. Natl Acad. Sci. USA* 2003; 100: 7808–7811.

[106] Reinecke H., Poppa V., and Murry C.E. Skeletal muscle stem cells do not transdifferentiate into cardiomyocytes after cardiac grafting. *J. Mol. Cell Cardiol.* 2002; 34: 241–249.

[107] Suzuki K., Brand N.J., Allen S., Khan M.A., Farrell A.O., Murtuza B., Oakley R.E., and Yacoub M.H. Overexpression of connexin 43 in skeletal myoblasts: relevance to cell transplantation to the heart. *J. Thorac. Cardiovasc. Surg.* 2001; 122: 759–766.

[108] Thompson R.B., Emani S.M., Davis B.H., van den Bos E.J., Morimoto Y., Craig D., Glower D., and Taylor D.A. Comparison of intracardiac cell transplantation: autologous skeletal myoblasts versus bone marrow cells. *Circulation* 2003; 108 Suppl 1: II264–II271.

[109] Murry C.E., Soonpaa M.H., Reinecke H., Nakajima H., Nakajima H.O., Rubart M., Pasumarthi K.B., Virag J.I., Bartelmez S.H., Poppa V., Bradford G., Dowell J.D., Williams D.A., and Field L.J. Haematopoietic stem cells do not transdifferentiate into cardiac myocytes in myocardial infarcts. *Nature* 2004; 428: 664–668.

[110] Balsam L.B., Wagers A.J., Christensen J.L., Kofidis T., Weissman I.L., and Robbins R.C. Haematopoietic stem cells adopt mature haematopoietic fates in ischaemic myocardium. *Nature* 2004; 428: 668–673.

[111] Leor J., Battler A., Kloner R.A., and Etzion S. Reprogramming cells for transplantation. *Heart Fail. Rev.* 2003; 8: 285–292.

[112] Lijnen P., Petrov V. and Fagard R. *In vitro* assay of collagen gel contraction by cardiac fibroblasts in serum-free conditions. *Meth. Find. Exp. Clin. Pharmacol.* 2001; 23: 377–382.

[113] Taggart P., Sutton P.M., Opthof T., Coronel R., Trimlett R., Pugsley W., and Kallis P. Inhomogeneous transmural conduction during early ischaemia in patients with coronary artery disease. *J. Mol. Cell Cardiol.* 2000; 32: 621–630.

[114] Hunter P.J., McCulloch A.D., and ter Keurs H.E. Modelling the mechanical properties of cardiac muscle. *Prog. Biophys. Mol. Biol.* 1998; 69: 289–331.

[115] Terracio L., Miller B., and Borg T.K. Effects of cyclic mechanical stimulation of the cellular components of the heart: *in vitro*. *In Vitro Cell Dev. Biol.* 1988; 24: 53–58.

[116] Simpson D., Majeski M., Borg T., and Terracio L. Regulation of cardiac myocyte protein turnover and myofibrillar structure *in vitro* by specific directions of stretch. *Circ. Res.* 1999; 85: e59–e69.

[117] Costa K.D., Lee E.J., and Holmes J.W. Creating alignment and anisotropy in engineered heart tissue: role of boundary conditions in a model three-dimensional culture system. *Tissue Eng.* 2003; 9: 567–577.

[118] Simpson D., Terracio L., Terracio M., Price R., Turner D., and Borg T. Modulation of cardiac myocyte phenotype *in vitro* by the composition and orientation of the extracellular matrix. *J. Cell Physiol.* 1994; 161: 89–105.

[119] Bien H., Yin L., and Entcheva E. Cardiac cell networks on elastic microgrooved scaffolds. *IEEE Eng. Med. Biol. Mag.* 2003; 22: 108–112.

[120] McDevitt T., Angello J., Whitney M., Reinecke H., Hauschka S., Murry C., and Stayton P. *In vitro* generation of differentiated cardiac myofibers on micropatterned laminin surfaces. *J. Biomed. Mater. Res.* 2002; 60: 472–479.

[121] Bursac N., Loo Y., Irby M.E., Leong K., and Tung L. Polymer scaffolds for anisotropic growth of engineered cardiac tissue. In Vossoughi J., Ed. *Southern Biomedical Engineering Conference.* Washington, DC: 2002, pp. 141–142.

[122] Bursac N., Loo Y., Irby M.E., Leong K., and Tung L. Electrophysiological studies in anisotropic 3D cardiac cultures. In Pace, Ed. *NASPE.* Washington, DC: Futura, 2003, p. 1045.

[123] Pego A.P., Siebum B., Van Luyn M.J., Gallego y Van Seijen X.J., Poot A.A., Grijpma D.W., and Feijen J. Preparation of degradable porous structures based on 1,3-trimethylene carbonate and D,L-lactide (co)polymers for heart tissue engineering. *Tissue Eng.* 2003; 9: 981–994.

[124] Li W.J., Laurencin C.T., Caterson E.J., Tuan R.S., and Ko F.K. Electrospun nanofibrous structure: a novel scaffold for tissue engineering. *J. Biomed. Mater. Res.* 2002; 60: 613–621.

[125] Stoker M.E., Gerdes A.M., and May J.F. Regional differences in capillary density and myocyte size in the normal human heart. *Anat. Rec.* 1982; 202: 187–191.

[126] Xie Z., Gao M., Batra S., and Koyama T. The capillarity of left ventricular tissue of rats subjected to coronary artery occlusion. *Cardiovasc. Res.* 1997; 33: 671–676.

[127] Spach M., Dolber P., and Heidlage J. Properties of discontinuous anisotropic propagation at a microscopic level. *Ann. N Y Acad. Sci.* 1990; 591: 62–74.

[128] Peters N.S., Coromilas J., Severs N.J., and Wit A.L. Disturbed connexin43 gap junction distribution correlates with the location of reentrant circuits in the epicardial border zone of healing canine infarcts that cause ventricular tachycardia. *Circulation* 1997; 95: 988–996.

[129] Kaihara S., Borenstein J., Koka R., Lalan S., Ochoa E.R., Ravens M., Pien H., Cunningham B., and Vacanti J.P. Silicon micromachining to tissue engineer branched vascular channels for liver fabrication. *Tissue Eng.* 2000; 6: 105–117.

[130] Arutunyan A., Swift L.M., and Sarvazyan N. Initiation and propagation of ectopic waves: insights from an in vitro model of ischemia-reperfusion injury. *Am. J. Physiol. Heart Circ. Physiol.* 2002; 283: H741–H749.

[131] Huelsing D.J., Spitzer K.W., Cordeiro J.M., and Pollard A.E. Conduction between isolated rabbit Purkinje and ventricular myocytes coupled by a variable resistance. *Am. J. Physiol.* 1998; 274: H1163–H1173.

[132] Antzelevitch C., Shimizu W., Yan G.X., Sicouri S., Weissenburger J., Nesterenko V.V., Burashnikov A., Di Diego J., Saffitz J., and Thomas G.P. The M cell: its contribution to the ECG and to normal and abnormal electrical function of the heart. *J. Cardiovasc. Electrophysiol.* 1999; 10: 1124–1152.

[133] Rohr S., Kucera J., Fast V., and Kleber A. Paradoxical improvement of impulse conduction in cardiac tissue by partial cellular uncoupling. *Science* 1997; 275: 841–844.

[134] Shaw R. and Rudy Y. Ionic mechanisms of propagation in cardiac tissue. roles of the sodium and L-type calcium currents during reduced excitability and decreased gap junctional coupling. *Circ. Res.* 1997; 81: 727–741.

[135] Gaudesius G., Miragoli M., Thomas S.P., and Rohr S. Coupling of cardiac electrical activity over extended distances by fibroblasts of cardiac origin. *Circ. Res.* 2003; 93: 421–428.

[136] Rohr S. and Salzberg B. Characterization of impulse propagation at the microscopic level across geometrically defined expansions of excitable tissue: multiple site optical recording of transmembrane voltage (MSORTV) in patterned growth heart cell cultures. *J. Gen. Physiol.* 1994; 104: 287–309.

[137] Kucera J., Kleber A., and Rohr S. Slow conduction in cardiac tissue, II. Effects of branching tissue geometry. *Circ. Res.* 1998; 83: 795–805.

[138] de Bakker J.M., van Capelle F.J., Janse M.J., Tasseron S., Vermeulen J.T., de Jonge N., and Lahpor J.R. Slow conduction in the infarcted human heart. 'Zigzag' course of activation. *Circulation* 1993; 88: 915–926.

[139] Folch A. and Toner M. Microengineering of cellular interactions. *Annu. Rev. Biomed. Eng.* 2000; 2: 227–256.

[140] Khademhosseini A., Suh K.Y., Yang J.M., Eng G., Yeh J., Levenberg S., and Langer R. Layer-by-layer deposition of hyaluronic acid and poly-L-lysine for patterned cell co-cultures. *Biomaterials* 2004; 25: 3583–3592.

[141] Fast V.G. and Ideker R.E. Simultaneous optical mapping of transmembrane potential and intracellular calcium in myocyte cultures. *J. Cardiovasc. Electrophysiol.* 2000; 11: 547–556.

[142] Sperelakis N. and Haddad G. Developmental changes in membrane electrical properties of the heart. In Sperelakis N., Ed. *Physiology and the Pathophysiology of the Heart.* 3rd ed. Norwell, MA: Kluwer Academic Publishers, 1995, pp. 669–700.

[143] Athias P., Frelin C., Groz B., Dumas J., Klepping J., and Padieu P. Myocardial electophysiology: intracellular studies on heart cell cultures from newborn rats. *Path. Biol.* 1979; 27: 13–19.

[144] Joyner R. Interactions between spontaneously pacing and quiescent but excitable heart cells. *Can. J. Cardiol.* 1997; 13: 1085–1092.

[145] Wagner M., Golod D., Wilders R., Verheijck E., Joyner R., Kumar R., Jonsma H., Van Ginneken A., and Goolsby W. Modulation of propagation from an ectopic focus by electrical load and by extracellular potassium. *Am. J. Physiol. (Heart Circ. Physiol.)* 1997; 272: H1759–H1769.

[146] Antonutto G. and di Prampero P.E. Cardiovascular deconditioning in microgravity: some possible countermeasures. *Eur. J. Appl. Physiol.* 2003; 90: 283–291.

[147] Decker M.L., Simpson D.G., Behnke M., Cook M.G., and Decker R.S. Morphological analysis of contracting and quiescent adult rabbit cardiac myocytes in long-term culture. *Anat. Rec.* 1990; 227: 285–299.

[148] Clark W.A., Decker M.L., Behnke-Barclay M., Janes D.M., and Decker R.S. Cell contact as an independent factor modulating cardiac myocyte hypertrophy and survival in long-term primary culture. *J. Mol. Cell. Cardiol.* 1998; 30: 139–155.

[149] Simpson D.G., Decker M.L., Clark W.A., and Decker R.S. Contractile activity and cell–cell contact regulate myofibrillar organization in cultured cardiac myocytes. *J. Cell Biol.* 1993; 123: 323–336.

[150] Clark W.A., Rudnick S.J., LaPres J.J., Andersen L.C., and LaPointe M.C. Regulation of hypertrophy and atrophy in cultured adult heart cells. *Circ. Res.* 1993; 73: 1163–1176.

[151] Ferrick K.J., Maher M., Roth J.A., Kim S.G., and Fisher J.D. Reproducibility of electrophysiological testing during antiarrhythmic therapy for ventricular arrhythmias unrelated to coronary artery disease. *Pacing Clin. Electrophysiol.* 1995; 18: 1395–1400.

57

Tissue Engineering of Heart Valves

K. Jane Grande-Allen
Rice University

Heart valves are essential to the normal function of the heart and cardiovascular/cardiopulmonary systems. When functioning properly, the heart valves allow unrestricted, unidirectional blood flow through the heart for subsequent distribution throughout the body. Consequently, valve disease or dysfunction can result in significant harm, as the reduction in the forward flow of blood limits the oxygenation of the tissues and can induce cardiac, cardiovascular, or cardiopulmonary compensation. Valve disease is prevalent in our society, with valve replacement or repair in approximately 90,000 people in the United States in 2001 [1] (275,000 worldwide [2]). Moreover, valve disease can be either congenital or acquired. For example, approximately 9 to 14 of every 10,000 children born are affected with the **Tetralogy of Fallot** [3,4], a congenital heart disorder characterized by a narrowing of the pulmonary valve among other anomalies. Acquired valve disease can affect people of all ages and may be due to an infectious agent (rheumatic heart disease, endocarditis), systemic diseases (lupus, carcinoid syndrome), other cardiac disease, trauma, pharmacologic agents, aging-related changes, or many other causes, some of which remain unknown [5].

The majority of current treatments for heart valve disease involve elective surgical replacement of the valve with a mechanical, bioprosthetic, or cryopreserved allograft (homograft) valve. The allograft is the treatment of choice for children, because bioprosthetic valves will calcify rapidly in children and mechanical valves cannot grow with the child [6]. Aortic and pulmonary allografts have also been used very successfully in adults, with the pulmonary conduit having a 90% freedom from replacement at 20 years [7], but the vascular remnant of these allografts eventually calcifies. Unfortunately, allografts, much like other donated organs, are in scarce supply. Moreover, allografts needs to be matched to the recipient tissue type to prevent immunological rejection [7], which narrows the diminishing pool of donated organs even further. Alternative options such as mechanical or bioprosthetic heart valves can be used in many situations, and are widely available, but have their own limitations [5]. Mechanical heart valves require anticoagulation therapy, which some patients cannot tolerate. Bioprosthetic valves do not require any anticoagulation, but do not contain any living tissues, and they undergo stiffening, calcification, and structural deterioration *in vivo* as a result of their glutaraldehyde fixation during manufacturing [8]. Bioprosthetic valves demonstrate a freedom from structural deterioration of 49% at 10 years and only 32% at 15 years, [9] and eventually require another surgical replacement. Overall, there is great need for a living, unfixed tissue-engineered heart valve (TEHV) or valved conduit in adults who require valve replacements. A TEHV with the potential for growth would also provide pediatric patients with a superior alternative for the treatment of valve defects.

57.1 The Native Heart Valve as a Design Goal

57.1.1 Anatomy and Terminology

The aortic valve is one of four valves in the heart, but it is replaced most frequently, and therefore will be discussed in greater detail. The aortic valve consists of three pieces of connective tissue (the right, left, and noncoronary leaflets) that are attached to the aorta at one edge, and are free to move at the other edge. These free edges meet centrally to close the valve and keep the blood from reentering the left ventricle. The valve is located in the bulbous base of the aorta, which is known as the aortic root (an anatomic recreation for a TEHV is shown in Figure 57.1). There are several distinct anatomic regions of the valve leaflet itself (Figure 57.2). The leaflet attachment edge inserts into the aortic root wall at the crown-shaped annulus [10]. The common region where two leaflets insert into the root wall is their commissure. The leaflet belly, or body, is the main portion of the leaflet (0.4 mm thick in humans [11]), and bears the majority of the pressure load when the valve is closed [12]. The **coaptation** area is the 0.5 to 0.6 mm thick [11] region of the leaflet that is in contact with the two other leaflets when the valve is closed. The free margin is the unattached edge of the leaflet, and suspends the leaflet between the tops of the commissures, much like cables of a suspension bridge [10,13]. Finally, the central portion of the edge of the valve leaflet is the Nodule of Arantius, a thickened area (0.95 to 1.2 mm [11]) that helps maintain valve closure [14].

The pulmonary valve (the other "**semilunar**" valve) is located in the pulmonary root between the right ventricle and pulmonary artery, and is thinner and more delicate than but otherwise almost identical to the aortic valve. The semilunar valves are quite different structurally from the "**atrioventricular**" valves. The mitral valve consists of two differently shaped leaflets attached at their outer border to the junction between the left atrium and left ventricle. The free edges and ventricular surfaces of the leaflets are connected to the papillary muscles of the left ventricle by numerous chordae tendineae. Likewise, the tricuspid valve is located between the right atrium and right ventricle. The tricuspid valve also contains chordae, but has three differently shaped leaflets as opposed to two. The tricuspid leaflets and chordae are thinner, shorter, and more delicate than those in the mitral valve.

57.1.2 Microstructure and Material Behavior

The semilunar valve leaflets consist of three histologically defined layers: the ventricularis forms the lower surface, the fibrosa forms the upper surface, and the spongiosa layer lies in between [15] (Figure 57.3 and Figure 57.4). The ventricularis contains a meshwork of elastic fibers along with loosely scattered collagen fibers [15]. The predominant elastic makeup allows this layer to expand in response to tension in the closed state of the valve, and then retract when the valve opens in response to ventricular ejection [15]. The fibrosa contains collagen fibers (predominantly type I), which are aligned largely circumferentially, although radially aligned fibers are found near the root-valve annulus [15]. The collagen fiber bundles in the fibrosa serve as the main source of strength for the diastolic pressure. The ridged appearance of the fibrosa is attributed to a corrugation of that tissue layer, in addition to the collagen bundles [16]. The spongiosa is a gelatinous layer containing loose connective tissue that is rich in proteoglycans

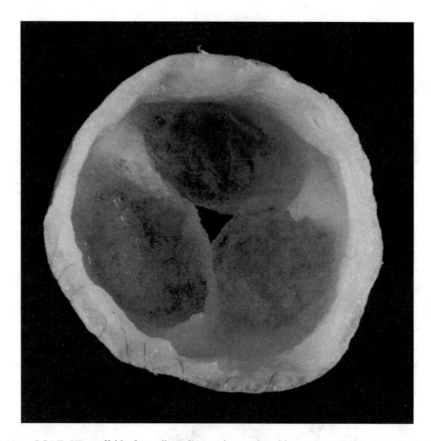

FIGURE 57.1 PGA/P4HB scaffold after cell seeding and 2 weeks of bioreactor conditioning. (Reprinted from Hoerstrup, S.P., Sodian, R., Daebritz, S., Wang, J., Bacha, E.A., Martin, D.P., Moran, A.M., Guleserian, K.J., Sperling, J. S., Kaushal, S., Vacanti, J.P., Schoen, F.J., Mayer, J.E., *Circulation*, 102, III-46, Copyright 2000, with permission from Lippincott Williams & Wilkins.)

(PGs), and serves as a mechanism for compressive resistance [17] and shear between the fibrosa and ventricularis [16].

The mitral and tricuspid valves have a similar laminated structure, except the respective outer layers are "upside down" from the arrangement shown in Figure 57.3. In these valves, the thick, heavily collagenous layer is located on the ventricular side, whereas the thin, predominantly elastic layer is found on the atrial side; these layers are also separated by a spongiosa. These similarities, which may be beneficial in future tissue engineering of atrioventricular valves, end with the chordae tendineae, which are not found in semilunar valves. The chordae are strong, thin, cable-like structures that contain a core of highly aligned collagen inside a thin outer sheath of elastic fibers and endothelial cells.

The interaction between the extracellular matrix (ECM) constituents within the valve microstructure allows distensibility, strength, elastic recovery, viscoelasticity, and an even distribution of deformation over a wide range of loading [18]. Like many other biological soft tissues, the stress–strain and load elongation curves of heart valve tissues are characterized by a low pretransition elastic modulus at initial strain (due to elastic fibers), followed by a transition zone to a higher posttransition elastic modulus at higher strains (due to the uncrimped collagen) [18]. The unique collagen and elastic fiber arrangements in the different layers, however, bestow the leaflet with anisotropic behavior (Figure 57.5). The greater circumferential stiffness (due to collagen) contributes to normal aortic valve function by restricting downward leaflet motion, while the lower radial stiffness permits the inward motion toward leaflet coaptation. This properly closing aortic valve will allow blood flow from the left ventricle into the ascending aorta, and prevent reverse flow. During this functional cycle, the leaflets interact with complex patterns of blood flow [5], and are

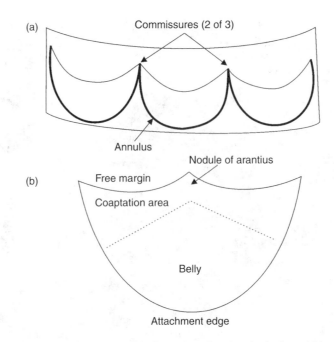

FIGURE 57.2   Semilunar valve leaflet anatomy. (a) Illustration of aortic valve leaflets within an opened aortic root. (b) Single valve leaflet.

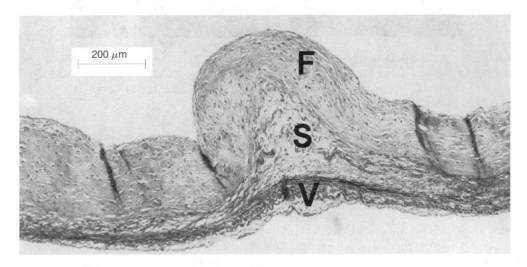

FIGURE 57.3   The histological layers of the aortic valve leaflet. Movat's Pentachrome stain. F, fibrosa; S, spongiosa; V, ventricularis.

subjected to transvalvular pressures as high as 120 mmHg [19] and shear stresses as high as 7.9 Pa [20]. These magnitudes of load are lower in the pulmonary circulation, where the transvalvular pressure across the pulmonary valve is only 25 mmHg [19].

57.1.3   Valvular Cells

Heart valves contain both endothelial and interstitial cells [21–23]. The valvular endothelial cells (VECs) populate the outer surfaces of the valves, whereas "interstitial cells" are all the cells that populate the inside

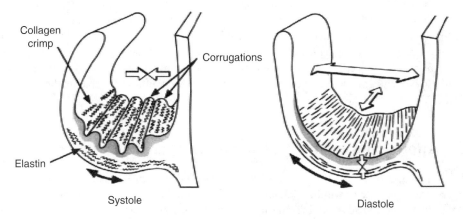

FIGURE 57.4 Illustration of the histological layers of the valve during systole and diastole. (Reprinted from Schoen, F. J., *J. Heart Valve Dis.*, 6, 2, Copyright 1997, with permission from ICR Publishers).

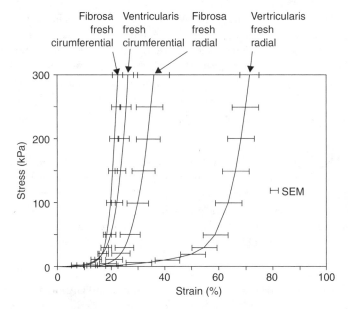

FIGURE 57.5 Radial and circumferential stress–strain curves of the ventricularis and fibrosa of aortic valve leaflets. (Reprinted from Vesely, I. and Noseworthy, R., Micromechanics of the fibrosa and the ventricularis in aortic valve leaflets, *J. Biomech.*, 25, 107, Copyright 1992, with permission from Elsevier.)

of the leaflets. Although it is presumed that the VECs provide the tissue with a nonthrombogenic surface, their functions otherwise are only beginning to be explored [23,24]. The **valvular interstitial cells** (VICs), which are only slightly better understood, are responsible for the synthesis of extracellular matrix components, including collagen, elastin, proteoglycans, and hyaluronan (for reviews see References 25 and 26). A key characteristic of VICs is that this group of cells exhibits a mixed phenotype of both fibroblastic and smooth muscle cell characteristics and are yet uniquely different from both these cell types [21,22,27,28]. It remains unclear whether this dual phenotype is caused by a single population of cells that express both features simultaneously [22,27], a single population of cells that can switch between these two phenotypes [21], or a population of several types of cells [29,30]. The different phenotypes of VICs are typically distinguished by their morphological appearance and immunohistochemical staining [21,27,28]. The fibroblastic phenotype is marked by elongated cells that contain numerous organelles for matrix synthesis, and stain for prolyl-4-hydroxlyase. The smooth muscle cell phenotype is denoted by cobblestone cells that stain for smooth muscle α-actin and stress fibers. VICs display this dual phenotype consistently throughout passaging [22,27]. Although in native valves these different cell phenotypes are slightly segregated [29,30], cells harvested from different regions of the valve had a consistent dual phenotypic appearance and growth characteristics [22]. It has also been difficult to separate these phenotypes in culture [28].

57.2 Approaches to the Tissue Engineered Heart Valve

The basic approach to constructing a TEHV, as with many other engineered tissues, is first to seed an appropriate cell type onto or within a suitable scaffold, and then to have a period of incubation during which the cells remodel or otherwise become integrated with the scaffold, and form a neotissue. This definition is intentionally ambiguous because a wide range of cells, scaffolds, and incubation environments have been used. All of the proposed TEHVs, however, have been designed to have as many of the ideal features of a heart valve substitute as possible [31,32] (i) maintain normal structural and biological function over the patient's lifetime, (ii) not elicit any inflammatory, foreign body, or immunologic responses, (iii) have antithrombotic surfaces and the potential for growth and self-repair, (iv) manufactured for each individual, (v) easy to implant with little technical variability, and (vi) available in an unlimited supply [31,32]. The majority of research of TEHVs has focused upon the structural, antithrombotic, immunologic, and availability aspects of this lofty goal. Although the studies described here do not represent an exhaustive discussion of TEHVs, several reviews provide more thorough detail [2,26,33].

57.2.1 Biodegradable Polymeric Scaffolds

Almost half of the proposed designs for TEHVs involve seeding cells on or within a polymeric biodegradable scaffold. The purpose in using a biodegradable scaffold is to anchor the seeded cells within an environment that is originally strong enough to withstand the *in vivo* mechanical forces, yet will subsequently degrade slowly, thereby transferring the function of load-bearing to the nascent ECM produced by the cells. Ideally, scaffold degradation rate and cellular synthesis rate should be balanced so that the scaffold has been completely degraded when the seeded cells have generated an amount of ECM comparable to native heart valves. The scaffold should also have initial material properties that are comparable to native valves.

The first such scaffold used to generate a TEHV was a woven mesh of 90% poly(glycolic acid) (PGA)/10% poly(lactic acid) (PLA) sandwiched between nonwoven PGA mesh, which was seeded with ovine vascular myofibroblasts and endothelial cells and used to replace the right leaflet of the pulmonary valve in a lamb model [34]. Although the resulting pulmonary valve was functional in the short term (3 weeks), this scaffold was found to be too stiff and thick for long-term use [35,36]. Conversely, seeding cells in PGA mesh alone produced a neotissue that was too delicate to handle [37], although the high porosity of this scaffold (95%) encouraged high seeding efficiencies and subsequent ECM production [35].

To avoid the mechanical limitations of the previous scaffolds, Sodian et al. [38] developed a new TEHV scaffold using poly(hydroxyalkanoate) (PHA), a thermoplastic, easily moldable polymer. The polymer was cast into a valved-conduit-shaped mold, made porous through a salt leaching process, and seeded with **autologous** ovine vascular myofibroblasts and endothelial cells. Although this valved conduit functioned normally in a sheep model for up to 17 weeks, the PHA scaffold material did not degrade fully by that time, and the developing neotissue did not contain any histologically detectable elastin or have an endothelial cell coating [38]. Moreover, PHA has a high echocardiographic density, which prevented the TEHV performance from being evaluated by Doppler echocardiography.

Because the PHA did not degrade rapidly enough, valved conduits were next assembled from nonwoven PGA mesh coated with a thin layer of poly-4-hydroxybutyrate (P4HB), a biodegradable thermoplastic moldable polymer that provided the nonwoven PGA with additional strength [39]. After seeding with

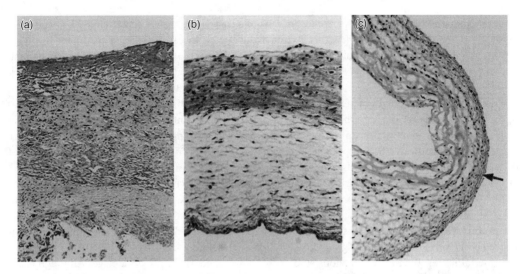

FIGURE 57.6   After 6 weeks *in vivo* (a), the TEHV from Figure 57.5 demonstrates preliminary organization (50×). After 16 weeks (b) and 20 weeks (c), the TEHV leaflet demonstrates organized, dense collagen on the outflow surface, elastic fibers on the inflow surface (arrow), and spongy organization within (both 100×). (Reprinted from Hoerstrup, S. P., Sodian, R., Daebritz, S., Wang, J., Bacha, E.A., Martin, D.P., Moran, A.M., Guleserian, K.J., Sperling, J. S., Kaushal, S., Vacanti, J.P., Schoen, F.J., Mayer, J.E., *Circulation*, 102, III-48, Copyright 2000, with permission from Lippincott Williams & Wilkins.)

autologous ovine vascular cells and 2 weeks of dynamic conditioning in a bioreactor (Figure 57.1), these TEHVs were implanted in the pulmonary position of sheep for 20 weeks. These TEHVs functioned well, with only mild to moderate pulmonary regurgitation at 16 and 20 weeks. Upon explant, the TEHV leaflets were found to have the normal three-layered structure of native heart valves (Figure 57.6), although their biochemically measured concentrations of collagen, elastin, and GAGs, as well as their ultimate tensile strength, were significantly higher than normal native pulmonary leaflets. Overall, the PGA/P4HB has been considered a very successful scaffold for TEHV development and is still being investigated [40,41]. Other biodegradable scaffolds that have been explored include biodegradable polyurethane, which was found to have not degraded completely at 6 weeks [42]. Finally, new classes of biodegradable scaffolds are being designed, such as a combination of poly(vinyl alcohol) (PVA) with brush groups of modified PLA [43]. This novel scaffold should combine the advantages of PVA, a high water content hydrogel with high elasticity and the ability to incorporate biologically active molecules on its hydroxyl groups, with the features of PLA, which is biodegradable, can be crosslinked, and is hydrophobically attractive to cells.

57.2.2 Decellularized Leaflet Scaffolds

Although polymeric biodegradable scaffolds have a long history in TEHV designs, another early approach that is still in active development today is the use of decellularized semilunar valve leaflets as a scaffold, with the rationale that they would provide the requisite strength [44], and already contain ECM in the correct microstructural arrangement [45]. Unlike polymeric designs, there is no need to fabricate or mold these scaffolds. Moreover, removing the cells would presumably eliminate the most antigenic elements, thereby avoiding any immunological response in the recipient. This reasoning has enabled the development of decellularized scaffolds from not only human heart valves (from donated allograft organs [45–47] or cadavers [48]), but also porcine heart valves. The predominant matrix element in these scaffolds, collagen, is highly conserved between species and is thus considered minimally antigenic [49,50], although there are concerns about the potential for transmission of **xenogenic** diseases [51].

A major area of research in the development of this scaffold is determining the best method to remove the cells from the original valve leaflet. Several different methods, involving ionic and nonionic detergents, solutions that are hypotonic or hypertonic, and enzyme treatments, have been attempted, abandoned, debated, and revisited, with only few direct comparisons [52]. In early studies, a treatment involving hypotonic saline to lyse the cells followed by two washes with the nonionic detergent Triton X-100 and one enzymatic soak in DNAse and RNAse was effective in the removal of all cells and cell debris [44,53]. This method preserved the majority of the thermal, physical, and material properties with the exception of a slight swelling and a slight increase in the stress relaxation of the tissue. This successful treatment was in contrast to their previous experimentation with the ionic detergent sodium dodecyl sulfate (SDS), in which the leaflet matrix swelled up to three times and had significant thermal denaturation [53]. On a single wash basis, however, SDS appears to remove more cells than Triton X-100 [54]. A combination of 0.5% trypsin and 0.2% EDTA was also successful in removing cells from human and porcine valves [48,55], as was a solution of 1% deoxycholic acid [56]. A solution of 0.1% N-cetylpyridinium chloride was shown to remove cells effectively and to preserve the tissue's microstructure and mechanics but this treatment induced calcification when the decellularized leaflet was tested in a rat subcutaneous dermal model [57]. Booth et al. [52] found that solutions of 0.03 to 0.1% SDS and 0.5% Na deoxycholate in hypotonic solutions worked best (with SDS causing a slight increase in tissue extensibility [58]), which they attribute to better protease inhibition than in the previous studies that implicated SDS in fiber damage. Although a few studies reported using protease inhibitors [48,53,55], such as phenylmethyl sulfonyl fluoride (PMSF) and EDTA, to block the endogenous lysosomal proteases released during cell lysis and to prevent degradation of the matrix scaffold, certain protease inhibitors (including PMSF) are short-lived in aqueous solutions and a more stable compound such as aprotinin may be preferable [52]. Many studies did not report any use of protease inhibitors, which could result in partial degradation of the collagen and elastic matrix components of the scaffold. The partial degradation of elastin in these scaffolds is considered particularly risky given that decellularized aortic wall, found to contain an abundance of partially degraded elastin, was prone to calcification in a rat subcutaneous dermal model [59].

Once prepared, the decellularized leaflet scaffold is almost always reseeded with autologous cells derived from the same host animal to be used in the TEHV study. Several of these scaffolds have been reseeded with endothelial cells only [56,60]. The main intent of this seeding is to form an antithrombotic coating around the bare collagen [60], and is an especially important consideration in planning for human TEHV use, because humans may have a more difficult time endothelizing structures than do the sheep models used in most of these studies [61]. Many other decellularized scaffolds, however, have also received a preliminary reseeding with vascular myofibroblasts in attempts to accelerate the eventual remodeling of the matrix [51,55,62–64]. Despite the preliminary seeding of the decellularized scaffolds, dispersing the cells within the existing matrix has proven difficult, with some tendency for the cells to remain on the surface or to merely line the largest pores [65]. In addition, Steinhoff et al. [62] found that the seeded cells tended to make new matrix on top of as opposed to within the existing scaffold matrix.

The Synergraft™ valve (Cryolife, Inc., Kennesaw, Georgia) consists of a decellularized porcine pulmonary root or composite aortic root (constructed from three noncoronary root-valve segments); decellularized human allografts are also available [46,66]. In contrast to the other approaches, the Synergraft valved conduits were not reseeded with any cells before implantation in sheep models, but became entirely repopulated with host cells and were completely functional for one year [45]. Although these scaffolds were developed with many techniques similar to those used for other TEHVs, they are not universally considered tissue-engineered structures because they are not reseeded with cells before implantation.

57.2.3 Cell Seeding

The methods used to seed the cells on and within the polymeric biodegradable scaffolds and the decellularized valve leaflets tend to be very straightforward: a concentrated solution containing the cells is dripped onto the scaffold surface and the cells disperse by gravity [67,68]. This seeding dispersion was encouraged by gentle agitation in some studies [30], but there was no report of any improved seeding efficiency due to this method. Many TEHVs have been developed by seeding first with myofibroblasts (several million cells), incubating 10 to 14 days, and then seeding with endothelial cells [34,37,38,62,69–72]. In preparation for this staged seeding process, a mixed population of vascular cells can separated into endothelial and nonendothelial cells using fluorescence-activated cell sorting (FACS)-based binding to acetylated low-density lipoprotein (positive binding in endothelial cells [73]). Staged seeding is not necessarily required [74]; mixed vascular cells seeded onto PGA/PLA–PGA sandwich scaffolds tended to segregate during incubation and *in vivo* implantation, forming neotissue with endothelial cells (staining for Factor XIII) on the outside and myofibroblasts (negative for Factor XIII) within. Other factors shown to improve seeding efficiency include 24 or 36 h seeding intervals (as opposed to 2 or 12 h intervals [68]), using polymeric scaffolds with high porosity such in PGA [67,68], mixing soluble collagen into the cell seeding solution [70], and coating the scaffold with Matrigel before seeding [75].

57.2.4 Natural Materials

Although the majority of TEHVs to date have been constructed from either biodegradable polymeric or decellularized leaflet scaffolds, there are a number of alternative scaffolds that have been developed using natural polymers such as collagen. The rationale behind using these natural materials is that the synthetic biodegradable polymers may have cytotoxic degradation products such as lactic acid, which can lower the pH of the culture medium [76]. A very early approach, reported by Carpentier et al. [77], was to inject solubilized collagen into a leaflet shaped mold. The resulting valve was implanted in sheep in the tricuspid or mitral position and functioned for up to 10 months without incompetence. Upon explant, fibroblasts were found within the collagen leaflets, but the leaflets were determined to have thickened slightly *in vivo*. More recently, valvular interstitial cells seeded within collagen sponge scaffolds were found to demonstrate phenotypic characteristics very similar to cells within intact valve leaflets [78]. Rothenburger et al. [71,75] grew human and porcine vascular and valvular cells within a freeze-dried porous type I collagen matrix *in vitro* and found that the cells produced the large hydrating proteoglycan (PG) versican, the small collagen-binding PG decorin, fibronectin, thrombospondin, and a medium-sized heparan sulfate PG (possibly perlecan or syndecan). The production of these PGs and glycoproteins indicate that the cells were interacting with and organizing the nascent ECM. Another natural material, fibrin, is being explored as a natural scaffold because fibrin gels can be made autologously from a patient's own blood and thereby prevent an immunologic reaction [67,68,76]. Fibrin gel components can also be coupled with exogenous biologically functional groups, such as growth factors, for improved neotissue formation. In addition, the use of injection molding to cast a cell-seeded fibrin gel ensures that the cells will be evenly distributed throughout the TEHV. This initial even distribution of cells is an advantage over the seeding of fibrous or sponge structures, where seeding dispersion is due to gravity and barely 50% of cells attach [67]. The disadvantage with fibrin gels is their initial weakness, which needs to be improved before *in vivo* studies can be performed. Yet another natural polymer that has been proposed is chitosan, a polysaccharide derivative that has been used for other tissue engineering applications [23]. Although three-dimensional chitosan scaffolds have yet to be tested in a TEHV, monolayer cultures of VECs adhered better to chitosan surfaces — and chitosan/collagen IV combinations in particular — than to PHA surfaces.

57.2.5 Building Block Approach

Almost without exception, the approach to TEHV development has been to use scaffolds that are destined for degradation or remodeling by the cells that will populate these constructs. The exception to this paradigm is the approach by Vesely et al. [79], in which the different ECM structural components are derived and then assembled into an approximation of the native aortic valve microstructure *in vitro*. The collagen bundles that provide the leaflet strength are replicated by neonatal rat aortic smooth muscle cells (NRASMCs) seeded within a type I collagen gel and anchored to promote uniaxial or branched contraction. The lubricating glycosaminoglycan component will be represented by cross-linked hyaluronan (also seeded with NRASMCs), and the network and sheets of elastic fibers are synthesized by the NRASMCs atop the crosslinked hyaluronan and around the collagen bundles. The final valve structure will be assembled by stacking alternating layers of hyaluronan/elastic sheets with layers of collagen bundles/elastic sheaths that are oriented as they would be in the native aortic valve (predominantly circumferential). This novel approach is still in the *in vitro* developmental stages, but it is envisaged that the multiple layers would compact, and the embedded cells would synthesize additional ECM, during a period of *in vitro* dynamic conditioning.

57.2.6 Cell Origin

It is generally agreed that the source of cells for a TEHV should be autologously derived from the intended valve recipient. This is particularly feasible given that most valve surgeries are elective, with criteria for the decisions of surgical timing being continuously reevaluated [5,80]. Autologous cells may perform best in pediatric cases, given that adult cells may have diminished proliferative ability (cell sources are discussed extensively in Reference 2). The anatomic source of these autologous cells, however, has not been firmly established. Shinoka et al. [74] determined that arterial myofibroblasts were superior to dermal fibroblasts in generating a strong, collagen-rich, and organized neotissue; Schnell et al. [42] found that venous cells were better yet. Given that saphenous veins are more easily harvested than arteries, the use of venous cells was therefore considered a promising alternative to arterial cells for seeding a TEHV scaffold. Although many studies continue to explore the use of cells derived from vascular sources, there were two recent reports that used either the stromal cells [40] or mesenchymal stem cells [81] from bone marrow. In the first case, human bone marrow stromal cells (obtained from the sternum) were seeded on a PGA/P4HB valved conduit, then conditioned in a bioreactor. After 14 days, the cells showed phenotypic characteristics of myofibroblasts (smooth muscle α-actin and vimentin), but did not show markers for muscle, osteogenic, or endothelial differentiation. In the second case, ovine bone marrow mesenchymal stem cells were seeded on the same type of valved conduit, then conditioned in bioreactor. Although the differentiation characteristics such as cell phenotype were not reported, the cells were able to form a functional neotissue *in vitro*.

Very few research groups have actually attempted to use VECs and VICs in the design of TEHVs [30,75,78]. It appears to have been assumed, if not often explicitly postulated, that whatever cell type is seeded within the TEHV will soon differentiate and begin to express the phenotypic characteristics of valvular cells. With rare exception [82], this assumption has not been tested in any depth, even though recent gene expression work has shown that VECs have many transcriptional differences from vascular endothelial cells [24]. VECs were also four times more proliferative in culture than were vascular endothelial cells [24], which may explain why vascular endothelial cells have frequently failed to form a continuous endothelial coating of the TEHV scaffolds *in vitro* [71] or *in vivo* [38,44,63]. VICs seeded in decellularized porcine leaflets differentiated and segregated into regionally specific myofibroblasts, fibroblasts, endothelial cells, and smooth muscle cells after 15 days *in vitro* [30]. After seeding in porous collagen sponge-like structures, VICs demonstrated phenotypic similarity to cells in native valve leaflets [78] and produced many of the PGs normally found in valves [75] A potential source for autologous valvular cells was proposed by Maish et al. [83], who found that valvular cells could be harvested from an ovine tricuspid valve without compromising the function of the tricuspid valve in the donor animal. This option may be important if the restoration of the VIC and VEC phenotype proves necessary and cannot be accomplished using an alternative cell source.

57.2.7 Bioreactors for Conditioning and Proof of Concept

Bioreactors have been widely used to provide the developing TEHV with strength-building mechanical stimulation prior to implantation within the animal model. Compared with static controls, bioreactor-conditioned TEHVs have demonstrated greater production of collagen, greater cell densities, improved mechanical strength, and more compact matrix organization [39,40,55]. It has also been proposed that bioreactor conditioning maintains the synthesis of ECM and DNA at levels normally found in the valve leaflets [84]. Bioreactors can also accelerate the turnover of the biodegradable matrix. Incubation in

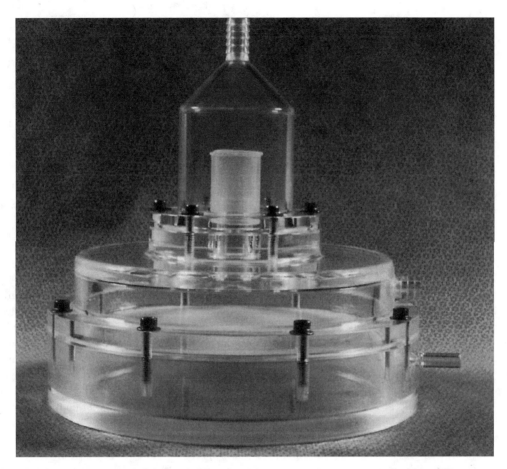

FIGURE 57.7   This bioreactor design creates pulsatile flow by cyclically pumping air beneath the silicone diaphragm separating the medium and air chambers. This action draws medium from a reservoir and propels it through the TEHV fixed to the silicone tubing above. (Reprinted from Hoerstrup, S.P., Sodian R., Sperling, J.S., Vacanti, J.P., Mayer J. E., *Tissue Eng.*, 6, 1, Copyright 2000, with permission from Mary Ann Liebert, Inc.)

a dynamic flexure bioreactor also augmented the bulk degradation of PGA/P4HB and PGA/PLA/P4HB scaffolds, resulting in significantly less flexural stiffness at 3 weeks compared to unflexed controls [41]. The types of bioreactors developed for TEHV studies can be generally classified into one of two categories. The first category, which has a continuously circulating supply of tissue culture medium, is predominantly used for the conditioning of intact TEHV and valved conduits. These bioreactors generally consist of a medium reservoir, a chamber to hold the TEHV, a pressure source, ports for gas exchange, optional pressure and flow transducers, and often have components to mimic vascular compliance and resistance [85,86] (Figure 57.7 and Figure 57.8). A similar setup was used in a study of the synthesis of collagen, GAGs, and DNA by valvular cells [84]. Because these bioreactor systems are capable of producing pulsatile flows ranging from 50 to 2000 ml/min [85] or even 20 l/min [84], and transvalvular pressures of 10 to 240 mmHg, they can easily be tailored to the conditioning or testing of aortic or pulmonary TEHVs. Feedback-driven tensioning systems have also been incorporated into these bioreactors [87]. The second category of bioreactor tends to be smaller and scalable, and is used more for proof of concept studies that examine how mechanical stimulation can improve the TEHV characteristics. An example of this was developed by Engelmayr et al. [41], in which scaffolds identical to those used in certain TEHVs were subjected to flexural conditioning, but were not bathed in circulating medium.

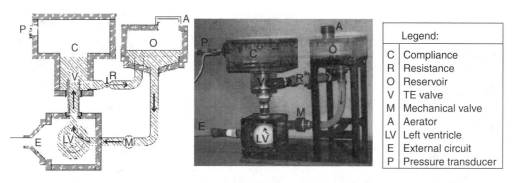

FIGURE 57.8 A bioreactor flow loop that includes components for variable compliance, resistance, and pressure measurements. (Reprinted from Dumont, K., Yperman, J., Verbeken, E., Segers, P., Mauris, B., Vandenberghe, S., Flameng, W., Verdonck, P.R., *Artif. Organs*, 26, 711, Copyright 2002, with permission from Blackwell Publishing.)

57.2.8 *In Vivo* Testing in Animal Models

Although many potential TEHV designs have been successfully compared using *in vitro* and bioreactor analyses, evaluation of the inflammatory, immunologic, and calcific responses requires an *in vivo* model. Canines have been used at least twice [44,88], but the majority of TEHVs have been tested *in vivo* in the widely accepted ovine models (either lamb or mature sheep) [33]. TEHVs have been implanted into the atrioventricular position in the past [77], and a **heterotopic** implantation in the abdominal aorta was recently reported [88], but most are tested in the pulmonary position, either as an **orthotopic** replacement of the pulmonary valve [38,39,45,51,56,72] or heterotopically interposed between the main and left pulmonary artery [44]. Single [34,69] and double [36] leaflet replacements within the pulmonary valve have been attempted with more success in the single leaflet replacement. The double leaflet replacement involved two identical PGA/PLA–PGA sandwich scaffolds: one seeded TEHV leaflet and one unseeded control. Unfortunately, this otherwise ingenious approach did not work because the stiff, thick scaffolds were unable to coapt normally and cause pulmonary insufficiency [36]. More recent TEHV designs are often tested using a valved conduit, containing all three leaflets, in the orthotopic pulmonary position.

These *in vivo* studies have often demonstrated an early but very mild inflammatory response to the TEHV [47], although this response was stronger when **allogeneic** as opposed to autologous cells were seeded [34]. A late inflammatory response (9 to 12 weeks) was reported with a reseeded decellularized porcine TEHV [63]. The remnant muscular shelf of decellularized leaflets has also been shown to invoke a mild inflammatory and calcific response [62]. Otherwise, reports of calcification of the scaffolds have been with mixed; there was heavy calcification of reseeded decellularized scaffolds after 12 and 24 weeks *in vivo* [64], while a Synergraft decellularized porcine scaffold (not reseeded) showed no calcification after 21 weeks [66].

57.2.9 Clinical Experience

The majority of TEHVs have only been tested *in vitro* or in animal models; no TEHV has been approved for clinical use in the United States. The porcine and human Synergrafts, which are technically not TEHVs since they are not reseeded with cells, have been approved in the United States [46]. As of 2003, these decellularized human valved conduits have been implanted in more than 150 patients in the United States and more than 1000 patients worldwide, approximately 84% of which have been in the pulmonary position (16% aortic). The distribution of patient age in the United States has been approximately 1/3 children and 2/3 adults, with a mean follow-up time of 231 days (range 0 to 788 days). In the two cases where these pulmonary allograft conduits were explanted (due to external fibrosis at 14 months and unrelated infection at 3 months), the leaflets and conduit had been repopulated with fibroblasts and myofibroblasts and demonstrated an endothelial lining and normal leaflet architecture. Function of the pulmonary Synergraft allografts have been comparable to cryopreserved allografts [46,61], whereas the aortic Synergraft allografts have evoked humoral antibodies in 25% of patients, but have shown normal aortic valve function with only trivial regurgitation [46]. The porcine pulmonary Synergrafts have been implanted in 20 patients [46], with 3 deaths and conduit pseudoaneurysm formation in 3 patients, but 14 other patients have had satisfactory valve performance for a maximum of one year. Unfortunately, the porcine Synergraft has not been as successful in the pediatric population, with a massive inflammatory response leading to leaflet degeneration and rupture in at least seven children in Austria and Norway [61]. One Synergraft that was examined after being implanted for one year showed no host recellularization of the implant at all and the formation of a fibrous capsule around the porcine tissue, which was very different from the results in a sheep model [45], in which the entire leaflet was repopulated with cells after one year.

In Germany, decellularized human cryopreserved pulmonary allografts that were reseeded with autologous venous endothelial cells were implanted in at least 6 **Ross procedure** patients with a mean age of 44 years [60]. All patients demonstrated an improvement of **ejection fraction** at 3 months. One patient was reported to be excellent condition after 12 months, and had not demonstrated any fever during this time. This absence of fever was interpreted as an absence of any antigenic inflammatory or immunologic response.

57.3 Conclusions and Future Challenges

There are many challenges ahead for the future of TEHVs. The first challenge appears to be the recapitulation of the many aspects of valvular biology in a living TEHV, particularly in designs involving nonvalvular cells. Quite frankly, it remains to be determined if such recapitulation would even be necessary for TEHV function, even though that finding could help direct future TEHV research. Moreover, the nascent field of valvular biology lags far behind vascular biology. Regardless, future TEHV research may wish to build upon the many studies over the last several years that have examined the contractile, synthetic, signaling, interactive, and diffusion characteristics of heart valves at the tissue, cellular, and molecular level. Normal aortic valve leaflets and VICs, for example, will contract slowly in response to stimulation with vasoactive agents such as serotonin, epinephrine, and endothelin-1 [28,89], potentially to maintain a baseline resting tension in the normal aortic valve [89]. More recently, the proliferative, migratory, synthetic, signaling, and phenotypic transdifferentiation responses of VICs to members of the renin–angiotensin system (including TGF-β) and vasoactive agents have been assessed [90–92]. Furthermore, the receptors and/or mRNA for serotonin, angiotensin II, bradykinin, and angiotensin-converting enzyme have been identified in VICs [92,93]. In fact, many of the transcriptional and proliferative characteristics of valvular cells have been shown to be different from those expressed by vascular cells [24,93]. Cell–matrix interactions have been demonstrated at the molecular level by the characterization of several integrins in bovine and baboon VICs [94]. Finally, oxygen diffusion within young porcine aortic valves was recently measured [95] and it was observed that blood vessels were present in most regions of the valve thicker than 0.5 mm. This finding highlights the differences between pediatric heart valves, which are vascularized [96,97] and even innervated [98], and adult heart valves, which have far less nerves and vessels, but contain viable, synthetic cells nonetheless. Exactly how well oxygen and nutrients diffuse to these adult VICs, and likewise to the cells within a TEHV, is a fertile topic for further research.

Another challenge for the future is the development of TEHV replacements for the aortic, atrioventricular, and venous valves. The highest clinical need is for the aortic position. To meet the higher pressure and flow requirements of the systemic circulation, the current pulmonary TEHV designs will need to be adapted to produce a stronger neotissue. In a recent proof of concept study that explored this need, a PGA/P4HB scaffold seeded with human venous myofibroblasts became more than three times stiffer when the maximum cyclic strain was raised from 7 to 10% during bioreactor conditioning [99]. Given that the atrioventricular valves are more commonly repaired than replaced [5], recent TEHV work in that regard has focused on replacement components, as opposed to the entire valve. The chordae, in particular, frequently rupture in prolapsed mitral valves [80]; torn chordae are currently replaced with Gore-Tex™ sutures. Because these sutures are several times stiffer than normal chordae [100], Vesely et al. [79] have been developing tissue-engineered chordae (large collagen fiber bundles) by seeding NRASMCs in a type 1 collagen gel and allowing the cell-seeded gel to contract uniaxially. Although these tissue-engineered chordae have not yet been tested *in vivo*, and are an order of magnitude less stiff than normal native human chordae, they have approximately normal extensibility [79]. As this avenue of TEHV research is very young, these preliminary results are likely to improve substantially in the years to come. Tissue engineered venous valves have been developed in a sheep model using allogeneic decellularized jugular veins seeded with autologous venous myofibroblasts and endothelial cells; these valves were still patent at 12 weeks [101].

The final challenge, particularly given the clinical reports of failure of the Synergraft valves in pediatric patients [61], are the ethical considerations involved as these research findings are eventually translated to clinical practice [102]. Although there are no current governmental regulatory divisions that are focusing exclusively on engineered tissues, U.S. and European regulatory agencies are planning centers that will meet this need. Beyond that goal lies the problem of developing standards to which engineered tissues such as the TEHV would be held. Furthermore, we are reminded by Sutherland and Mayer in their excellent review of this topic, "compliance with standards alone carries no guarantee that a given device will be free from risk" [102]. Applying a risk management approach, with identification and severity grading of potential hazards, is an appropriate first step along this path. Hazards particularly associated with the current characteristics of the TEHV described in this chapter could be scaffold-related, such as adverse reactions to the degradation products of the biodegradable scaffolds, or the potential for transmission of porcine endogenous retrovirus from the decellularized porcine valve scaffold to the TEHV recipient [51,102]. Other hazards could be related to the cells involved, particularly if they are not autologous, or to the performance of the TEHV *in vivo*.

The field of TEHV research is growing exponentially and has demonstrated many recent advances, particularly in the development and application of bioreactor technologies. New research in valvular biology and targeted scaffold development, together with frequent reflection and review [2,26,33], are certain to drive this field ahead. Although there are many hurdles to overcome before the many promises of TEHVs become fully realized, the potential to create a living, healing, growing valve continues to inspire significant effort in this exciting field.

Defining Terms

Allogeneic: Taken from a different individual of the same species
Atrioventricular: Referring to the position between the atrium and the ventricle. The mitral and tricuspid valves are atrioventricular valves.
Autologous: Taken or derived from the same individual.
Coaptation: Referring to contact between different heart valve leaflets, or regions of the leaflets where this contact occurs when the valve is closed.
Ejection fraction: The percentage of blood pumped out of an individual's left ventricle.
Heterotopic: Referring to a region of the body where a structure is not normally located.
Incompetence and insufficiency: Inability of the heart valve to close property.
Orthotopic: Referring to a region of the body where a structure is normallt located.
Ross Procedure: Surgical replacement of a patient's deficient aortic valve with a pulmonary autograft, followed by implantation of a cryopreserved pulmonary allograft in the pulmonary position.
Semilunar: Referring to the half-moon shape of the leaflets of the pulmonary and aortic valves.
Tetralogy of Fallot: A congenital heart defect with four predominant symptoms (ventricular septal defect, pulmonary valve stenosis, right ventricular hypertrophy, and malposition of the aorta over both ventricles.

Valvular interstitial cells: An all-encompassing term for the nonendothelial cells that are contained within the heart valve leaflets. This definition includes cells of variable phenotype.

Xenogenic: Taken from a different species.

References

[1] American Heart Association, *Heart Disease and Stroke Statistics — 2004 Update*, American Heart Association, Dallas, 2004.

[2] Rabkin, E. and Schoen, F.J., Cardiovascular tissue engineering, *Cardiovasc. Pathol.* 11, 305, 2002.

[3] American Heart Association, *Youth and Cardiovascular Diseases — Statistical Fact Sheet*, American Heart Association, Dallas, 2004.

[4] Topol, E.J., *Cleveland Clinic Heart Book*, Hyperion, New York, 2000.

[5] Otto, C.M., *Valvuar Heart Disease*, 2nd ed., Saunders, Philadephia, 2004.

[6] Mayer, J.E. Jr., In search of the ideal valve replacement device, *J. Thorac. Cardiovasc. Surg.* 122, 8, 2001.

[7] Ross, D.N., Options for right ventricular outflow tract reconstruction, *J. Cardiovasc. Surg.* 13, 186, 1998.

[8] Vesely, I., Barber, J.E., and Ratliff, N.B., Tissue damage and calcification may be independent mechanisms of bioprosthetic heart valve failure, *J. Heart Valve Dis.* 10, 471, 2001.

[9] Fann, J.I. et al., Twenty-year clinical experience with porcine bioprostheses, *Ann. Thorac. Surg.* 62, 1301, 1996.

[10] Mercer, L., Benedicty, M., and Bahnson, H., The geometry and construction of the aortic leaflet, *J. Thorac. Cardiovasc. Surg.* 65, 511, 1973.

[11] Sahasakul, Y. et al., Age-related changes in aortic and mitral valve thickness: implications for two-dimensional echocardiography based on an autopsy study of 200 normal human hearts, *Am. J. Cardiol.* 62, 424, 1988.

[12] Christie, G.W. and Stephenson, R.A., Modelling the mechanical role of the fibrosa and the ventricularis in the porcine bioprosthesis, in *Surgery for Heart Valve Disease*, Bodnar, E., Ed., Heart Valve Diseases, London, 1989, p. 815.

[13] Sutton, J.P. 3rd, Ho, S.Y., and Anderson, R.H., The forgotten interleaflet triangles: a review of the surgical anatomy of the aortic valve, *Ann. Thorac. Surg.* 59, 419, 1995.

[14] Clark, R.E. and Finke, E.H., Scanning and light microscopy of human aortic leaflets in stressed and relaxed states, *J. Thorac. Cardiovasc. Surg.* 67, 792, 1974.

[15] Sauren, A.A. et al., Aortic valve histology and its relation with mechanics — preliminary report, *J. Biomech.* 13, 97, 1980.

[16] Vesely, I. and Noseworthy, R., Micromechanics of the fibrosa and the ventricularis in aortic valve leaflets, *J. Biomech.* 25, 101, 1992.

[17] Grande-Allen, K.J. et al., Glycosaminoglycans and proteoglycans in normal mitral valve leaflets and chordae: association with regions of tensile and compressive loading, *Glycobiology* 14, 621, 2004.

[18] Sauren, A.A. et al., The mechanical properties of porcine aortic valve tissues, *J. Biomech.* 16, 327, 1983.

[19] Patton, H.D. et al., *Textbook of Physiology. Circulation, Respiration, Body Fluids, Metabolism, and Endocrinology*, W.B. Saunders, Philadelphia, 1989.

[20] Weston, M.W., LaBorde, D.V., and Yoganathan, A.P., Estimation of the shear stress on the surface of an aortic valve leaflet, *Ann. Biomed. Eng.* 27, 572, 1999.

[21] Taylor, P., Allen, S., and Yacoub, M., Phenotypic and functional characterization of interstitial cells from human heart valves, pericardium and skin, *J. Heart Valve Dis.* 9, 150, 2000.

[22] Johnson, C.M., Hanson, M.N., and Helgeson, S.C., Porcine cardiac valvular subendothelial cells in culture: cell isolation and growth characteristics, *J. Mol. Cell. Cardiol.* 19, 1185, 1987.

[23] Cuy, J.L. et al., Adhesive protein interactions with chitosan: consequences for valve endothelial cell growth on tissue-engineering materials, *J. Biomed. Mater. Res.* 67A, 538, 2003.

[24] Farivar, R.S. et al., Transcriptional profiling and growth kinetics of endothelium reveals differences between cells derived from porcine aorta versus aortic valve, *Eur. J. Cardiothorac. Surg.* 24, 527, 2003.

[25] Taylor, P.M. et al., The cardiac valve interstitial cell, *Int. J. Biochem. Cell. Biol.* 35, 113, 2003.

[26] Flanagan, T.C. and Pandit, A., Living artificial heart valve alternatives: a review, *Eur. Cell. Mater.* 6, 28, 2003.

[27] Lester, W.M. and Gotlieb, A.I., *In vitro* repair of the wounded porcine mitral valve, *Circ. Res.* 62, 833, 1988.

[28] Messier, R.H. et al., Dual structural and functional phenotypes of the porcine aortic valve interstitial population: characteristics of the leaflet myofibroblast, *J. Surg. Res.* 57, 1, 1994.

[29] Della Rocca, F. et al., Cell comparison of the human pulmonary valve: a comparison study with the aortic valve — the VESALIO project, *Ann. Thorac. Surg.* 70, 1594, 2000.

[30] Bertipaglia, B. et al., Cell characterization of porcine aortic valve and decellularized leaflets repopulated with aortic valve interstitial cells: the VESALIO project (Vitalitate Exornatum Succedaneum Aorticum Labore Ingenioso Obtenibitur), *Ann. Thorac. Surg.* 75, 1274, 2003.

[31] Cohn, L.H. and Lipson, W., Selection and complications of cardiac valvular prostheses, in *Glenn's Thoracic and Cardiovascular Surgery*, Baue, A.E. et al., Eds., Appleton & Lange, Stamford, CT, 1996, p. 2043.

[32] Harken, D.E. and Curtis, L.E., Heart surgery — legend and a long look, *Am. J. Cardiol.* 19, 393, 1967.

[33] Stock, U.A. et al., Tissue engineering of heart valves — current aspects, *Thorac. Cardiovasc. Surg.* 50, 184, 2002.

[34] Shinoka, T. et al., Tissue engineering heart valves: valve leaflet replacement study in a lamb model, *Ann. Thorac. Surg.* 60, S513, 1995.

[35] Sodian, R. et al., Evaluation of biodegradable, three-dimensional matrices for tissue engineering of heart valves, *ASAIO J.* 46, 107, 2000.

[36] Kim, W.G. et al., Tissue-engineered heart valve leaflets: an animal study, *Int. J. Artif. Organs* 24, 642, 2001.

[37] Zund, G. et al., The *in vitro* construction of a tissue engineered bioprosthetic heart valve, *Eur. J. Cardiothorac. Surg.* 11, 493, 1997.

[38] Sodian, R. et al., Early *in vivo* experience with tissue-engineered trileaflet heart valves, *Circulation* 102, III22, 2000.

[39] Hoerstrup, S.P. et al., Functional living trileaflet heart valves grown *in vitro*, *Circulation* 102, III44, 2000.

[40] Hoerstrup, S.P. et al., Tissue engineering of functional trileaflet heart valves from human marrow stromal cells, *Circulation* 106, I143, 2002.

[41] Engelmayr, G.C. Jr. et al., A novel bioreactor for the dynamic flexural stimulation of tissue engineered heart valve biomaterials, *Biomaterials* 24, 2523, 2003.

[42] Schnell, A.M. et al., Optimal cell source for cardiovascular tissue engineering: venous vs. aortic human myofibroblasts, *Thorac. Cardiovasc. Surg.* 49, 221, 2001.

[43] Nuttelman, C.R., Henry, S.M., and Anseth, K.S., Synthesis and characterization of photocrosslinkable, degradable poly(vinyl alcohol)-based tissue engineering scaffolds, *Biomaterials* 23, 3617, 2002.

[44] Wilson, G.J. et al., Acellular matrix: a biomaterials approach for coronary artery bypass and heart valve replacement, *Ann. Thorac. Surg.* 60, S353, 1995.

[45] Goldstein, S. et al., Transpecies heart valve transplant: advanced studies of a bioengineered xeno-autograft, *Ann. Thorac. Surg.* 70, 1962, 2000.

[46] Elkins, R.C., Is tissue-engineered heart valve replacement clinically applicable? *Curr. Cardiol. Rep.* 5, 125, 2003.

[47] Elkins, R.C. et al., Decellularized human valve allografts, *Ann. Thorac. Surg.* 71, S428, 2001.

[48] Cebotari, S. et al., Construction of autologous human heart valves based on an acellular allograft matrix, *Circulation* 106, I63, 2002.

[49] Yannas, I.V., Natural materials, in *Biomaterials Science. An Introduction to Materials in Medicine*, Ratner, B.D. et al., Eds., Academic Press, San Diego, 1996, p. 84.

[50] Miller, E.J., Chemistry of the collagens and their distribution, in *Extracellular Matrix Biochemistry*, Piez, K.A. and Reddi, A.H., Eds., Elsevier, New York, 1984, p. 41.

[51] Leyh, R.G. et al., Acellularized porcine heart valve scaffolds for heart valve tissue engineering and the risk of cross-species transmission of porcine endogenous retrovirus, *J. Thorac. Cardiovasc. Surg.* 126, 1000, 2003.

[52] Booth, C. et al., Tissue engineering of cardiac valve prostheses I: development and histological characterization of an acellular porcine scaffold, *J. Heart Valve Dis.* 11, 457, 2002.

[53] Courtman, D.W. et al., Development of a pericardial acellular matrix biomaterial: biochemical and mechanical effects of cell extraction, *J. Biomed. Mater. Res.* 28, 655, 1994.

[54] Kim, W.G., Park, J.K., and Lee, W.Y., Tissue-engineered heart valve leaflets: an effective method of obtaining acellularized valve xenografts, *Int. J. Artif. Organs* 25, 791, 2002.

[55] Schenke-Layland, K. et al., Complete dynamic repopulation of decellularized heart valves by application of defined physical signals — an *in vitro* study, *Cardiovasc. Res.* 60, 497, 2003.

[56] Dohmen, P.M. et al., Ross operation with a tissue-engineered heart valve, *Ann. Thorac. Surg.* 74, 1438, 2002.

[57] Spina, M. et al., Isolation of intact aortic valve scaffolds for heart-valve bioprostheses: extracellular matrix structure, prevention from calcification, and cell repopulation features, *J. Biomed. Mater. Res.* 67A, 1338, 2003.

[58] Korossis, S.A., Fisher, J., and Ingham, E., Cardiac valve replacement: a bioengineering approach, *Biomed. Mater. Eng.* 10, 83, 2000.

[59] Bailey, M.T. et al., Role of elastin in pathologic calcification of xenograft heart valves, *J. Biomed. Mater. Res.* 66A, 93, 2003.

[60] Dohmen, P.M. et al., Tissue engineering of an auto-xenograft pulmonary heart valve, *Asian Cardiovasc. Thorac. Ann.* 10, 25, 2002.

[61] Simon, P. et al., Early failure of the tissue engineered porcine heart valve SYNERGRAFT in pediatric patients, *Eur. J. Cardiothorac. Surg.* 23, 1002, 2003.

[62] Steinhoff, G. et al., Tissue engineering of pulmonary heart valves on allogenic acellular matrix conduits: *in vivo* restoration of valve tissue, *Circulation* 102, III50, 2000.

[63] Wilhelmi, M.H. et al., Role of inflammation and ischemia after implantation of xenogeneic pulmonary valve conduits: histological evaluation after 6 to 12 months in sheep, *Int. J. Artif. Organs* 26, 411, 2003.

[64] Leyh, R.G. et al., *In vivo* repopulation of xenogeneic and allogeneic acellular valve matrix conduits in the pulmonary circulation, *Ann. Thorac. Surg.* 75, 1457, 2003.

[65] Curtil, A., Pegg, D.E., and Wilson, A., Repopulation of freeze-dried porcine valves with human fibroblasts and endothelial cells, *J. Heart Valve Dis.* 6, 296, 1997.

[66] O'Brien, M.F. et al., The SynerGraft valve: a new acellular (nonglutaraldehyde-fixed) tissue heart valve for autologous recellularization first experimental studies before clinical implantation, *Semin. Thorac. Cardiovasc. Surg.* 11, 194, 1999.

[67] Ye, Q. et al., Scaffold precoating with human autologous extracellular matrix for improved cell attachment in cardiovascular tissue engineering, *ASAIO J.* 46, 730, 2000.

[68] Zund, G. et al., Tissue engineering in cardiovascular surgery: MTT, a rapid and reliable quantitative method to assess the optimal human cell seeding on polymeric meshes, *Eur. J. Cardiothorac. Surg.* 15, 519, 1999.

[69] Shinoka, T. et al., Tissue-engineered heart valves. Autologous valve leaflet replacement study in a lamb model, *Circulation* 94, II164, 1996.

[70] Kim, W.G. et al., Tissue-engineered heart valve leaflets: an effective method for seeding autologous cells on scaffolds, *Int. J. Artif. Organs* 23, 624, 2000.

[71] Rothenburger, M. et al., *In vitro* modelling of tissue using isolated vascular cells on a synthetic collagen matrix as a substitute for heart valves, *Thorac. Cardiovasc. Surg.* 49, 204, 2001.

[72] Stock, U.A. et al., Tissue-engineered valved conduits in the pulmonary circulation, *J. Thorac. Cardiovasc. Surg.* 119, 732, 2000.

[73] Hoerstrup, S.P. et al., Fluorescence activated cell sorting: a reliable method in tissue engineering of a bioprosthetic heart valve, *Ann. Thorac. Surg.* 66, 1653, 1998.

[74] Shinoka, T. et al., Tissue-engineered heart valve leaflets: does cell origin affect outcome? *Circulation* 96, II, 1997.

[75] Rothenburger, M. et al., Tissue engineering of heart valves: formation of a three-dimensional tissue using porcine heart valve cells, *ASAIO J.* 48, 586, 2002.

[76] Jockenhoevel, S. et al., Fibrin gel — advantages of a new scaffold in cardiovascular tissue engineering, *Eur. J. Cardiothorac. Surg.* 19, 424, 2001.

[77] Carpentier, A. et al., Collagen-derived heart valves: concept and experimental results, *J. Thorac. Cardiovasc. Surg.* 62, 707, 1971.

[78] Taylor, P.M. et al., Human cardiac valve interstitial cells in collagen sponge: a biological three-dimensional matrix for tissue engineering, *J. Heart Valve Dis.* 11, 298, 2002.

[79] Shi, Y., Ramamurthi, A., and Vesely, I., Towards tissue engineering of a composite aortic valve, *Biomed. Sci. Instrum.* 38, 35, 2002.

[80] Cosgrove, D.M. and Stewart, W.J., Mitral valvuloplasty, *Curr. Probl. Cardiol.* 14, 359, 1989.

[81] Perry, T.E. et al., Thoracic Surgery Directors Association Award. Bone marrow as a cell source for tissue engineering heart valves, *Ann. Thorac. Surg.* 75, 761, 2003.

[82] Narine, K. et al., Transforming growth factor-beta-induced transition of fibroblasts: a model for myofibroblast procurement in tissue valve engineering, *J. Heart Valve Dis.* 13, 281, 2004.

[83] Maish, M.S. et al., Tricuspid valve biopsy: a potential source of cardiac myofibroblast cells for tissue-engineered cardiac valves, *J. Heart Valve Dis.* 12, 264, 2003.

[84] Weston, M.W. and Yoganathan, A.P., Biosynthetic activity in heart valve leaflets in response to *in vitro* flow environments, *Ann. Biomed. Eng.* 29, 752, 2001.

[85] Hoerstrup, S.P. et al., New pulsatile bioreactor for *in vitro* formation of tissue engineered heart valves, *Tissue Eng.* 6, 75, 2000.

[86] Dumont, K. et al., Design of a new pulsatile bioreactor for tissue engineered aortic heart valve formation, *Artif. Organs* 26, 710, 2002.

[87] Sarraf, C.E. et al., Heart valve and arterial tissue engineering, *Cell. Prolif.* 36, 241, 2003.

[88] Zhao, D.E. et al., Tissue-engineered heart valve on acellular aortic valve scaffold: *in-vivo* study, *Asian Cardiovasc. Thorac. Ann.* 11, 153, 2003.

[89] Chester, A.H., Misfeld, M., and Yacoub, M.H., Receptor-mediated contraction of aortic valve leaflets, *J. Heart Valve Dis.* 9, 250, 2000.

[90] Hafizi, S. et al., Mitogenic and secretory responses of human valve interstitial cells to vasoactive agents, *J. Heart Valve Dis.* 9, 454, 2000.

[91] Jian, B. et al., Serotonin mechanisms in heart valve disease I: serotonin-induced up-regulation of transforming growth factor-beta1 via G-protein signal transduction in aortic valve interstitial cells, *Am. J. Pathol.* 161, 2111, 2002.

[92] Katwa, L.C. et al., Angiotensin converting enzyme and kininase-II-like activities in cultured valvular interstitial cells of the rat heart, *Cardiovasc. Res.* 29, 57, 1995.

[93] Roy, A., Brand, N.J., and Yacoub, M.H., Expression of 5-hydroxytryptamine receptor subtype messenger RNA in interstitial cells from human heart valves, *J. Heart Valve Dis.* 9, 256, 2000.

[94] Wiester, L.M. and Giachelli, C.M., Expression and function of the integrin alpha9beta1 in bovine aortic valve interstitial cells, *J. Heart Valve Dis.* 12, 605, 2003.

[95] Weind, K.L. et al., Oxygen diffusion and consumption of aortic valve cusps, *Am. J. Physiol. Heart Circ. Physiol.* 281, H2604, 2001.

[96] Weind, K.L., Ellis, C.G., and Boughner, D.R., Aortic valve cusp vessel density: relationship with tissue thickness, *J. Thorac. Cardiovasc. Surg.* 123, 333, 2002.

[97] Duran, C.M. and Gunning, A.J., The vascularization of the heart valves: a comparative study, *Cardiovasc. Res.* 2, 290, 1968.

[98] Marron, K. et al., Innervation of human atrioventricular and arterial valves, *Circulation* 94, 368, 1996.

[99] Mol, A. et al., The relevance of large strains in functional tissue engineering of heart valves, *Thorac. Cardiovasc. Surg.* 51, 78, 2003.

[100] Cochran, R.P. and Kunzelman, K.S., Comparison of viscoelastic properties of suture versus porcine mitral valve chordae tendineae, *J. Cardiovasc. Surg.* 6, 508, 1991.

[101] Teebken, O.E. et al., Tissue-engineered bioprosthetic venous valve: a long-term study in sheep, *Eur. J. Vasc. Endovasc. Surg.* 25, 305, 2003.

[102] Sutherland, F.W. and Mayer, J.E. Jr., Ethical and regulatory issues concerning engineered tissues for congenital heart repair, *Semin. Thorac. Cardiovasc. Surg. Pediatr. Card. Surg. Annu.* 6, 152, 2003.

58

Tissue Engineering, Stem Cells and Cloning for the Regeneration of Urologic Organs

J. Daniell Rackley
Anthony Atala
*Wake Forest University
Baptist Medical Center*

The genitourinary system is exposed to a variety of possible injuries from the time the fetus develops. Aside from congenital abnormalities, individuals may also suffer from other disorders such as cancer, trauma, infection, inflammation, iatrogenic injuries, or other conditions that may lead to genitourinary organ damage or loss, requiring eventual reconstruction. The type of tissue chosen for replacement depends on which organ requires reconstruction. Bladder and ureteral reconstruction may be performed with gastrointestinal tissues. Urethral reconstruction is performed with skin, mucosal grafts from the bladder, rectum, or oral cavity. Vaginas can be reconstructed with skin, small bowel, sigmoid colon, and rectum. However, a shortage of donor tissue may limit these types of reconstructions and there is a degree of morbidity associated with the harvest procedure. In addition, these approaches rarely replace the entire function of the original organ. The tissues used for reconstruction may lead to complications due to their inherently different functional parameters. In most cases, the replacement of lost or deficient tissues with functionally equivalent tissues would improve the outcome for these patients. This goal may be attainable with the use of tissue engineering techniques.

58.1 Cell Growth

One of the initial limitations of applying cell-based tissue engineering techniques to urologic organs had been the previously encountered inherent difficulty of growing genitourinary associated cells in large quantities. In the past, it was believed that urothelial cells had a natural senescence, which was hard to overcome. Normal urothelial cells could be grown in the laboratory setting, but with limited expansion. Several protocols were developed over the last two decades which improved urothelial growth and expansion [1–4]. A system of urothelial cell harvest was developed, which does not use any enzymes or serum and has a large expansion potential. Using these methods of cell culture, it is possible to expand a urothelial strain from a single specimen, which initially covers a surface area of 1 cm^2 to one covering a surface area of 4202 m^2 (the equivalent area of one football field) within 8 weeks [1]. These studies indicated that it should be possible to collect autologous urothelial cells from human patients, expand them in culture, and return them to the human donor in sufficient quantities for reconstructive purposes. Bladder, ureter, and renal pelvis cells can be equally harvested, cultured, and expanded in a similar fashion. Normal human bladder epithelial and muscle cells can be efficiently harvested from surgical material, extensively expanded in culture, and their differentiation characteristics, growth requirements, and other biological properties studied [1,3–13].

58.2 Biomaterials for Genitourinary Tissue Engineering

Biomaterials provide a cell–adhesion substrate and can be used to achieve cell delivery with high loading and efficiency to specific sites in the body. The configuration of the biomaterials can guide the structure of an engineered tissue. The biomaterials provide mechanical support against *in vivo* forces, thus maintaining a predefined structure during the process of tissue development. The biomaterials can be loaded with bioactive signals, such as cell–adhesion peptides and growth factors, which can regulate cellular function. The design and selection of the biomaterial is critical in the development of engineered genitourinary tissues. The biomaterial must be capable of controlling the structure and function of the engineered tissue in a predesigned manner by interacting with transplanted cells or the host cells. Generally, the ideal biomaterial should be biocompatible, promote cellular interaction and tissue development, and possess proper mechanical and physical properties.

The selected biomaterial should be biodegradable and bioresorbable to support the reconstruction of a completely normal tissue without inflammation. The degradation products should not provoke inflammation or toxicity and must be removed from the body via metabolic pathways. The degradation rate and the concentration of degradation products in the tissues surrounding the implant must be at a tolerable level [14]. The mechanical support of the biomaterials should be maintained until the engineered tissue has sufficient mechanical integrity to support itself [15].

This can be potentially achieved by an appropriate choice of mechanical and degradative properties of the biomaterials [16].

58.2.1 Types of Biomaterials

Generally, three classes of biomaterials have been utilized for engineering genitourinary tissues: naturally derived materials (e.g., collagen and alginate), acellular tissue matrices (e.g., bladder submucosa and small intestinal submucosa), and synthetic polymers (e.g., polyglycolic acid (PGA), polylactic acid (PLA), and poly(lactic-co-glycolic acid) (PLGA). These classes of biomaterials have been tested in respect to their biocompatibility with primary human urothelial and bladder muscle cells [17,18]. Naturally derived materials and acellular tissue matrices have the potential advantage of biological recognition. Synthetic polymers can be produced reproducibly on a large scale with controlled properties of their strength, degradation rate, and microstructure.

Collagen is the most abundant and ubiquitous structural protein in the body, and may be readily purified from both animal and human tissues with an enzyme treatment and salt/acid extraction [19]. Collagen implants degrade through a sequential attack by lysosomal enzymes. The *in vivo* resorption rate can be regulated by controlling the density of the implant and the extent of intermolecular crosslinking. The lower the density, the greater the interstitial space and generally the larger the pores for cell infiltration, leading to a higher rate of implant degradation. Collagen contains cell-adhesion domain sequences (e.g., RGD), which exhibit specific cellular interactions. This may assist in retaining the phenotype and activity of many types of cells, including fibroblasts [20] and chondrocytes [21].

Alginate, a polysaccharide isolated from sea weed, has been used as an injectable cell delivery vehicle [22] and a cell immobilization matrix [23] owing to its gentle gelling properties in the presence of divalent ions such as calcium. Alginate is relatively biocompatible and approved by the FDA for human use as wound dressing material. Alginate is a family of copolymers of D-mannuronate and L-guluronate. The physical and mechanical properties of alginate gel are strongly correlated with the proportion and length of polyguluronate block in the alginate chains [22].

Acellular tissue matrices are collagen-rich matrices prepared by removing cellular components from tissues. The matrices are often prepared by mechanical and chemical manipulation of a segment of tissue [24–27]. The matrices slowly degrade upon implantation, and are replaced and remodeled by ECM proteins synthesized and secreted by transplanted or ingrowing cells.

Polyesters of naturally occurring α-hydroxy acids, including PGA, PLA, and PLGA, are widely used in tissue engineering. These polymers have gained FDA approval for human use in a variety of applications, including sutures [28]. The ester bonds in these polymers are hydrolytically labile, and these polymers degrade by nonenzymatic hydrolysis. The degradation products of PGA, PLA, and PLGA are nontoxic, natural metabolites and are eventually eliminated from the body in the form of carbon dioxide and water [28]. The degradation rate of these polymers can be tailored from several weeks to several years by altering crystallinity, initial molecular weight, and the copolymer ratio of lactic to glycolic acid. Since these polymers are thermoplastics, they can be easily formed into a three-dimensional scaffold with a desired microstructure, gross shape and dimension by various techniques, including molding, extrusion [29], solvent casting [30], phase separation techniques, and gas foaming techniques [31]. Many applications in genitourinary tissue engineering often require a scaffold with high porosity and ratio of surface area to volume. Other biodegradable synthetic polymers, including poly(anhydrides) and poly(ortho-esters), can also be used to fabricate scaffolds for genitourinary tissue engineering with controlled properties [32].

58.3 Tissue Engineering of Urologic Structures

58.3.1 Urethra

Various biomaterials without cells have been used experimentally (in animal models) for the regeneration of urethral tissue, including PGA, and acellular collagen based matrices from small intestine, bladder, and skin [27,33–37]. Some of these biomaterials, like acellular collagen matrices derived from bladder submucosa, have also been seeded with autologous cells for urethral reconstruction. Our laboratory has been able to replace tubularized urethral segments with cell-seeded collagen matrices.

A cellular collagen matrices derived from bladder submucosa by our laboratory have been used experimentally and clinically. In animal studies, segments of the urethra were resected and replaced with acellular matrix grafts in an onlay fashion. Histological examination showed complete epithelialization and progressive vessel and muscle infiltration. The animals were able to void through the neourethras [27]. These results were confirmed clinically in a series of patients with hypospadias and urethral stricture disease [38,39]. Cadaveric bladders were microdissected and the submucosal layers were isolated. The submucosa was washed and decellularized. The matrix was used for urethral repair in patients with stricture disease

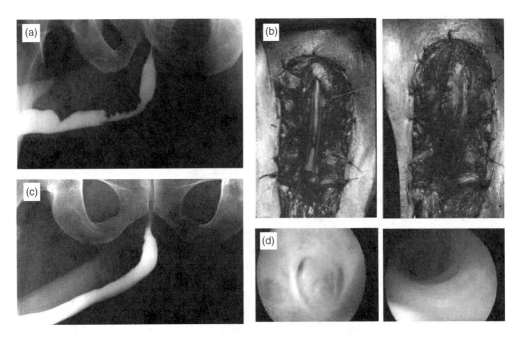

FIGURE 58.1 Representative case of a patient with a bulbar stricture repaired with a collagen matrix. (a) Preoperative urethrogram. (b) Urethral repair. Structured tissue is excised, preserving urethral plate on left side and matrix is anastomosed to urethral plate in an onlay fashion on right side. (c) Urethrogram 6 months after repair. (d) Cystoscopic view of urethra preoperatively on left side and 4 months after repair on right side.

($n = 33$; 28 adults, 5 children) and hypospadias ($n = 7$ children). The matrices were trimmed to size and the neourethras were created by anastomosing the matrix in an onlay fashion to the urethral plate. The size of the neourethras ranged from 2 to 16 cm. Voiding histories, physical examination, retrograde urethrography, uroflowmetry, and cystoscopies were performed serially, pre- and postoperatively, with up to a 7-year follow-up. After a 4- to 7-year follow-up, 34 of the 40 patients had a successful outcome. Six patients with a urethral stricture had a recurrence, and one patient with hypospadias developed a fistula. The mean maximum urine flow rate significantly increased postoperatively. Cystoscopic studies showed adequate caliber conduits. Histologic examination of the biopsies showed the typical urethral epithelium. The use of an off-the-shelf matrix appears to be beneficial for patients with abnormal urethral conditions, and obviates the need for obtaining autologous grafts, thus decreasing operative time and eliminating donor site morbidity (Figure 58.1).

Unfortunately, the above techniques are not applicable for tubularized urethral repairs. The collagen matrices are able to replace urethral segments when used in an onlay fashion. However, if a tubularized repair is needed, the collagen matrices need to be seeded with autologous cells [40,41]. Autologous bladder epithelial and smooth muscle cells from male rabbits were grown and seeded onto preconfigured tubular matrices. The entire anterior urethra was resected and urethroplasties were performed with tubularized collagen matrices seeded with cells in nine animals, and without cells in six animals. Serial urethrograms showed a wide urethral caliber without strictures in the animals implanted with the cell seeded matrices, and collapsed urethral segments with strictures within the unseeded scaffolds. Gross examination of the urethral implants seeded with cells showed normal appearing tissue without any evidence of fibrosis. Histologically, a transitional cell layer surrounded by muscle cell fiber bundles with increasing cellular organization over time were observed on the cell seeded constructs. The epithelial and muscle phenotypes were confirmed with pAE1/AE3 and smooth muscle specific alpha actin antibodies. A transitional cell layer with scant unorganized muscle fiber bundles and large areas of fibrosis were present at the anastomotic sites on the unseeded constructs. Therefore, tubularized collagen matrices seeded with autologous cells can be used successfully for total penile urethra replacement; whereas, tubularized collagen matrices without cells lead to poor tissue development and stricture formation. The cell seeded collagen matrices form new tissue which is histologically similar to native urethra. This technology may be applicable to patients requiring tubularized urethral repair.

58.3.2 Bladder

Currently, gastrointestinal segments are commonly used as tissues for bladder replacement or repair. However, gastrointestinal tissues are designed to absorb specific solutes, whereas bladder tissue is designed for the excretion of solutes. Due to the problems encountered with the use of gastrointestinal segments, numerous investigators have attempted alternative materials and tissues for bladder replacement or repair.

Over the last few decades, several bladder wall substitutes have been attempted with both synthetic and organic materials. The first application of a free tissue graft for bladder replacement was reported by Neuhoff in 1917, when fascia was used to augment bladders in dogs [42]. Since that first report, multiple other free graft materials have been used experimentally and clinically, including bladder allografts, SIS, pericardium, dura, and placenta [24,25,43–50]. In multiple studies using different materials as an acellular graft for cystoplasty, the urothelial layer was able to regenerate normally, but the muscle layer, although present, was not fully developed [24,48,51,52]. When using cell-free collagen matrices, scarring and graft contracture may occur over time [53–58]. Synthetic materials, which have been tried previously in experimental and clinical settings, include polyvinyl sponge, tetrafluoroethylene (Teflon), collagen matrices, vicryl matrices, and silicone [59–62]. Most of the above attempts have usually failed due to either mechanical, structural, functional, or biocompatibility problems. Usually, permanent synthetic materials used for bladder reconstruction succumb to mechanical failure and urinary stone formation and degradable materials lead to fibroblast deposition, scarring, graft contracture, and a reduced reservoir volume over time.

Engineering tissue using selective cell transplantation may provide a means to create functional new bladder segments [63]. The success of using cell transplantation strategies for bladder reconstruction depends on the ability to use donor tissue efficiently and to provide the right conditions for long-term survival, differentiation, and growth. Urothelial and muscle cells can be expanded *in vitro*, seeded onto the polymer scaffold, and allowed to attach and form sheets of cells. The cell-polymer scaffold can then be implanted *in vivo*. A series of *in vivo* urologic associated cell-polymer experiments were performed. Histologic analysis of human urothelial, bladder muscle, and composite urothelial and bladder muscle-polymer scaffolds, implanted in athymic mice and retrieved at different time points, indicated that viable cells were evident in all three experimental groups [64]. Implanted cells oriented themselves spatially along the polymer surfaces. The cell populations appeared to expand from one layer to several layers of thickness with progressive cell organization with extended implantation times. Cell-polymer composite implants of urothelial and muscle cells, retrieved at extended times (50 days), showed extensive formation of multilayered sheet-like structures and well-defined muscle layers. Polymers seeded with cells and manipulated into a tubular configuration showed layers of muscle cells lining the multilayered epithelial sheets. Cellular debris appeared reproducibly in the luminal spaces, suggesting that epithelial cells lining the lumina are sloughed into the luminal space. Cell polymers implanted with human bladder muscle cells alone showed almost complete replacement of the polymer with sheets of smooth muscle at 50 days. This experiment demonstrated, for the first time, that composite tissue engineered structures could be created *de novo*. Prior to this study, only single cell type tissue engineered structures had been created.

58.3.2.1 Formation of Bladder Tissue *Ex-Situ*

In order to determine the effects of implanting engineered tissues in continuity with the urinary tract, an animal model of bladder augmentation was utilized [24]. Partial cystectomies, which involved removing approximately 50% of the native bladders, were performed in 10 beagles. In five, the retrieved bladder tissue was microdissected and the mucosal and muscular layers separated. The bladder urothelial and muscle cells were cultured using the techniques described above. Both urothelial and smooth muscle cells were harvested and expanded separately. A collagen-based matrix, derived from allogeneic bladder submucosa, was used for cell delivery. This material was chosen for these experiments due to its native elasticity. Within 6 weeks, the expanded urothelial cells were collected as a pellet. The cells were seeded on the luminal surface of the allogeneic bladder submucosa and incubated in serum-free keratinocyte growth medium for 5 days. Muscle cells were seeded on the opposite side of the bladder submucosa and subsequently placed in DMEM supplemented with 10% fetal calf serum for an additional 5 days. The seeding density on the allogeneic bladder submucosa was approximately 1×10^7 cells/cm^2.

Preoperative fluoroscopic cystography and urodynamic studies were performed in all animals. Augmentation cystoplasty was performed with the matrix with cells in one group, and with the matrix without cells in the second group. The augmented bladders were covered with omentum in order to facilitate angiogenesis to the implant. Cystostomy catheters were used for urinary diversion for 10 to 14 days. Urodynamic studies and fluoroscopic cystography were performed at 1, 2, and 3 months postoperatively. Augmented bladders were retrieved 2 ($n = 6$) and 3 ($n = 4$) months after surgery and examined grossly, histologically, and immunocytochemically.

Bladders augmented with the matrix seeded with cells showed a 99% increase in capacity compared to bladders augmented with the cell-free matrix, which showed only a 30% increase in capacity. Functionally, all animals showed a normal bladder compliance as evidenced by urodynamic studies, however, the remaining native bladder tissue may have accounted for these results. Histologically, the retrieved engineered bladders contained a cellular organization consisting of a urothelial lined lumen surrounded by submucosal tissue and smooth muscle. However, the muscular layer was markedly more prominent in the cell reconstituted scaffold [24].

Most of the free grafts (without cells) utilized for bladder replacement in the past have been able to show adequate histology in terms of a well-developed urothelial layer, however they have been associated with an abnormal muscular layer that varies in terms of its full development [15,65]. It has been well established for decades that the bladder is able to regenerate generously over free grafts. Urothelium is associated with a high reparative capacity [66]. Bladder muscle tissue is less likely to regenerate in a normal fashion. Both urothelial and muscle ingrowth are believed to be initiated from the edges of the normal bladder toward the region of the free graft [67,68]. Usually, however, contracture or resorption of the graft has been evident. The inflammatory response toward the matrix may contribute to the resorption of the free graft.

It was hypothesized that building the three-dimensional structure constructs *in vitro*, prior to implantation, would facilitate the eventual terminal differentiation of the cells after implantation *in vivo*, and would minimize the inflammatory response towards the matrix, thus avoiding graft contracture and shrinkage. This study demonstrated that there was a major difference evident between matrices used with autologous cells (tissue engineered) and matrices used without cells [24]. Matrices implanted with cells for bladder augmentation retained most of their implanted diameter, as opposed to matrices implanted without cells for bladder augmentation, wherein graft contraction and shrinkage occurred. The histomorphology demonstrated a marked paucity of muscle cells and a more aggressive inflammatory reaction in the matrices implanted without cells. Of interest is that the urothelial cell layers appeared normal, even though their underlying matrix was significantly inflamed. It was further hypothesized, that having an adequate urothelial layer from the outset would limit the amount of urine contact with the matrix, and would therefore decrease the inflammatory response, and that the muscle cells were also necessary for bioengineering, being that native muscle cells are less likely to regenerate over the free grafts. Further studies confirmed this hypothesis [69]. Thus, it appears that the presence of both urothelial and muscle cells on the matrices used for bladder replacement appear to be important for successful tissue bioengineering.

58.3.2.2 Bladder Replacement Using Tissue Engineering

The results of initial studies showed that the creation of artificial bladders may be achieved *in vivo*, however, it could not be determined whether the functional parameters noted were due to the augmented segment or the intact native bladder tissue. In order to better address the functional parameters of tissue engineered bladders, an animal model was designed, which required a subtotal cystectomy with subsequent replacement by a tissue engineered organ [69].

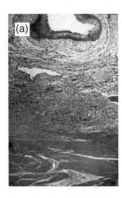 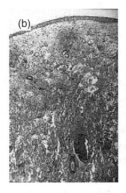 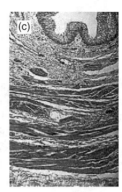

FIGURE 58.2 Hematoxylin and Eosin histological results 6 months after surgery (original magnification: ×250). (a) Normal canine bladder. (b) The bladder dome of the cell-free polymer reconstructed bladder consists of a thickened layer of collagen and fibrotic tissue. (c) The tissue engineered neo-organ shows a histo-morphologically normal appearance. A trilayered architecture consisting of urothelium, submucosa, and smooth muscle is evident.

A total of 14 beagle dogs underwent a trigone-sparing cystectomy. The animals were randomly assigned to one of three groups. Group A ($n = 2$) underwent closure of the trigone without a reconstructive procedure. Group B ($n = 6$) underwent reconstruction with a cell-free bladder shaped biodegradable polymer. Group C ($n = 6$) underwent reconstruction using a bladder shaped biodegradable polymer that delivered autologous urothelial cells and smooth muscle cells. The cell populations had been separately expanded from a previously harvested autologous bladder biopsy. Preoperative and postoperative urodynamic and radiographic studies were performed serially. Animals were sacrificed at 1, 2, 3, 4, 6, and 11 months postoperatively. Gross, histological, and immunocytochemical analyses were performed [69].

Cystectomy only controls and polymer only grafts maintained average capacities of 22 and 46% of preoperative values, respectively. An average bladder capacity of 95% of the original precystectomy volume was achieved in the tissue engineered bladder replacements. These findings were confirmed radiographically. The subtotal cystectomy reservoirs, which were not reconstructed and polymer only reconstructed bladders showed a marked decrease in bladder compliance (10 and 42%). The compliance of the tissue engineered bladders showed almost no difference from preoperative values that were measured when the native bladder was present (106%). Histologically, the polymer only bladders presented a pattern of normal urothelial cells with a thickened fibrotic submucosa and a thin layer of muscle fibers. The retrieved tissue engineered bladders showed a normal cellular organization, consisting of a trilayer of urothelium, submucosa, and muscle (Figure 58.2). Immunocytochemical analyses for desmin, alpha actin, cytokeratin 7, pancytokeratins AE1/AE3 and uroplakin III confirmed the muscle and urothelial phenotype. S-100 staining indicated the presence of neural structures. The results from this study showed that it is possible to tissue engineer bladders, which are anatomically and functionally normal [69]. Clinical trials for the application of this technology are currently being arranged.

58.3.3 Genital Tissues

Reconstructive surgery is required for a wide variety of pathologic penile conditions, such as penile carcinoma, trauma, severe erectile dysfunction, and congenital conditions like ambiguous genitalia, hypospadias, and epispadias. One of the major limitations of phallic reconstructive surgery is the availability of sufficient autologous tissue. Phallic reconstruction using autologous tissue, derived from the patient's own cells, may be preferable in selected cases.

58.3.4 Reconstruction of Corporal Tissues

One of the major components of the phallus is corporal smooth muscle. The creation of autologous functional and structural corporal tissue *de novo* would be beneficial.

Initial experiments were performed in order to determine the feasibility of creating corporal tissue *in vivo* using cultured human corporal smooth muscle cells seeded onto biodegradable polymers [70]. Primary normal human corpus cavernosal smooth muscle cells were isolated from normal young adult patients after informed consent during routine penile surgery. Muscle cells were maintained in culture, seeded onto biodegradable polymer scaffolds, and implanted subcutaneously in athymic mice. Implants were retrieved at 7, 14, and 24 days after surgery for analyses. Corporal smooth muscle tissue was identified grossly and histologically. Intact smooth muscle cell multilayers were observed growing along the surface of the polymers throughout all time points. Early vascular ingrowth at the periphery of the implants was evident by 7 days. By 24 days, there was evidence of polymer degradation. Smooth muscle phenotype was confirmed immunocytochemically and by Western blot analyses with antibodies to alpha smooth muscle actin.

In order to engineer functional corpus cavernosum, both smooth muscle and sinusoidal endothelial cells are essential. However, penile sinusoidal endothelial cells had not been extensively cultured in the past, and had not been fully characterized. A method of isolation and expansion of sinusoidal endothelial cells from corpora cavernosa was devised, and cell function and gene expression were characterized.

When grown on collagen, corporal cavernosal endothelial cells formed capillary structures, which created a complex three-dimensional capillary network. The possibility of developing human corporal tissue *in vivo* by combining smooth muscle and endothelial cells was investigated [71]. Primary normal human corpus cavernosal smooth muscle cells and ECV 304 human endothelial cells were seeded on biodegradable polymers and implanted in the subcutaneous space of athymic mice. At retrieval all polymer scaffolds seeded with cells had formed distinct tissue structures and maintained their preimplantation size. The control scaffolds without cells had decreased in size with increasing time. Histologically, all of the retrieved polymers seeded with corporal smooth muscle and endothelial cells showed the survival of the implanted cells. The presence of penetrating native vasculature was observed 5 days after implantation. The formation of multilayered strips of smooth muscle adjacent to endothelium was evident by 7 days after implantation. Increased smooth muscle organization and accumulation of endothelium lining the luminal structures were evident 14 days after implantation. A well-organized construct, consisting of muscle and endothelial cells, was noted at 28 and 42 days after implantation. A marked degradation of the polymer fibers was observed by 28 days. There was no evidence of tissue formation in the controls (polymers without cells). The results of these studies suggested that the creation of well-vascularized autologous corporal-like tissue, consisting of smooth muscle and endothelial cells, may be possible.

The aim of phallic reconstruction is to achieve structurally and functionally normal genitalia. It had been shown that human cavernosal smooth muscle and endothelial cells seeded on polymers would form tissue composed of corporal cells when implanted *in vivo*. However, corporal tissue structurally identical to the native corpus cavernosum was not achieved, due to the type of polymers used. Therefore, a naturally derived acellular corporal tissue matrix that possesses the same architecture as native corpora was developed. The feasibility of developing corporal tissue, consisting of human cavernosal smooth muscle and endothelial cells *in vivo*, using an acellular corporal tissue matrix as a cell delivery vehicle was explored [72]. Acellular collagen matrices were derived from processed donor rabbit corpora using cell lysis techniques. Human corpus cavernosal muscle and endothelial cells were derived from donor penile tissue, the cells were expanded *in vitro*, seeded on the acellular matrices, and implanted subcutaneously in athymic mice. Western blot analysis detected alpha actin, myosin and tropomyosin proteins from human corporal smooth muscle cells. Expression of muscarinic acetylcholine receptor (mAChR) subtype m4 mRNA was demonstrated by RT-PCR from corporal muscle cells 8 weeks prior to and after seeding. The implanted matrices showed neovascularity into the sinusoidal spaces by 1 week after implantation. Increasing organization of smooth muscle and endothelial cells lining the sinusoidal walls was observed at 2 weeks and continued with time. The matrices were covered with the appropriate cell architecture 4 weeks after implantation. The matrices showed a stable collagen concentration over 8 weeks, as determined by hydroxy-proline quantification. Immunocytochemical studies using alpha actin and Factor VIII antibodies confirmed the presence of corporal smooth muscle and endothelial cells, both *in vitro* and *in vivo*, at all time points. There was no evidence of cellular organization in the control matrices.

In another study, we attempted to replace entire crossectional segments of both corporal bodies of penis *in vivo* by interposing engineered tissue in rabbits and investigated their structural and functional integrity [73]. Autologous cavernosal smooth muscle and endothelial cells were harvested, expanded, and seeded on acellular collagen matrices. The entire cross section of the protruding rabbit phallus (~0.7 cm long; 1/3 of penile shaft) was excised, leaving the urethra intact. Matrices with and without cells were interposed into the excised corporal space. Additional rabbits, without surgical intervention, served as controls. The experimental corporal bodies demonstrated adequate structural and functional integrity by cavernosography and cavernosometry. Mating activity in the animals with the engineered corpora normalized by 3 months. The presence of sperm was confirmed during mating, and was present in all the rabbits with the engineered corpora. Grossly, the corporal implants with cells showed continuous integration of the graft into native tissue. Histologically, sinusoidal spaces and walls, lined with endothelium and smooth muscle, were observed in the engineered grafts. Grafts without cells contained fibrotic tissue and calcifications with sparse corporal elements. Each cell type was identified immunohistochemically and by Western blot analyses. These studies demonstrate that it is possible to engineer autologous functional penile tissue. Our laboratory is currently working on increasing the size of the engineered constructs.

58.4   Engineered Penile Prostheses

Although silicone is an accepted biomaterial for penile prostheses, biocompatibility is a concern [74,75]. The use of a natural prosthesis composed of autologous cells may be advantageous. A feasibility study for creating natural penile prostheses made of cartilage was performed initially [76].

Cartilages, harvested from the articular surface of calf shoulders, were isolated, grown, and expanded in culture. The cells were seeded onto preformed cylindrical polyglycolic acid polymer rods (1 cm in diameter and 3 cm in length). The cell-polymer scaffolds were implanted in the subcutaneous space of 20 athymic mice. Each animal had two implantation sites consisting of a polymer scaffold seeded with chondrocytes and a control (polymer alone). The rods were retrieved at 1, 2, 4, and 6 months postimplantation. Biomechanical properties, including compression, tension, and bending were measured on the retrieved structures. Histological analyses were performed to confirm the cellular composition. At retrieval, all of the polymer scaffolds seeded with cells formed milky-white rod-shaped solid cartilaginous structures, maintaining their preimplantation size and shape. The control scaffolds without cells failed to form cartilage. There was no evidence of erosion, inflammation, or infection in any of the implanted cartilage rods.

The compression, tension, and bending studies showed that the cartilage structures were readily elastic and could withstand high degrees of pressure. Biomechanical analyses showed that the engineered cartilage rods possessed the mechanical properties required to maintain penile rigidity. The compression studies showed that the cartilage rods were able to withstand high degrees of pressure. A ramp compression speed of 200 μm/sec, applied to each cartilage rod up to 2000 μm in distance, resulted in 3.8 kg of resistance. The tension relaxation studies demonstrated that the retrieved cartilage rods were able to withstand stress and were able to return to their initial state while maintaining their biomechanical properties. A ramp tension speed of 200 μm/sec applied to each cartilage rod created a tensile strength of 2.2 kg, which physically lengthened the rods an average of 0.48 cm. Relaxation of tension at the same speed resulted in retraction of the cartilage rods to their initial state. The bending studies performed at two different speeds showed that the engineered cartilage rods were durable, malleable, and were able to retain their mechanical properties. Cyclic compression, performed at rates of 500 and 20,000 μm/sec, demonstrated that the cartilage rods could withstand up to 3.5 kg of pressure at a predetermined distance of 5000 μm. The relaxation phase of the cyclic compression studies showed that the engineered rods were able to maintain their tensile strength. None of the rods were ruptured during the biomechanical stress relaxation studies.

Histological examination with hematoxylin and eosin showed the presence of mature and well-formed cartilage in all the chondrocyte-polymer implants. The polymer fibers were progressively replaced by cartilage with time progression. Undegraded polymer fibers were observed at 1 and 2 months after implantation. However, remnants of polymer scaffolds were not present in the cartilage rods at 6 months. Aldehyde fuschin-alcian blue and toluidine blue staining demonstrated the presence of highly sulfated mucopolysaccharides, which are differentiated products of chondrocytes. There was no evidence of cartilage formation in the controls.

In a subsequent study using an autologous system, the feasibility of applying the engineered cartilage rods *in situ* was investigated [77]. Autologous chondrocytes harvested from rabbit ear were grown and expanded in culture. The cells were seeded onto biodegradable poly-L-lactic acid coated polyglycolic acid polymer rods at a concentration of 50×10^6 chondrocytes/cm^3. Eighteen chondrocyte-polymer scaffolds were implanted into the corporal spaces of 10 rabbits. As controls, two corpora, one each in 2 rabbits, were not implanted. The animals were sacrificed at 1, 2, 3, and 6 months after implantation. Histological analyses were performed with hematoxylin and eosin, aldehyde fuschin-alcian blue, and toluidine blue staining. All animals tolerated the implants for the duration of the study without any complications. Gross examination at retrieval showed the presence of well-formed milky-white cartilage structures within the corpora at 1 month. All polymers were fully degraded by 2 months. There was no evidence of erosion or infection in any of the implant sites. Histological analyses with alcian blue and toluidine blue staining demonstrated the presence of mature and well-formed chondrocytes in the retrieved implants. Subsequent studies were performed assessing the functionality of the cartilage penile rods *in vivo* long term. To date, the animals have done well, and can copulate and impregnate their female partners without problems. Further functional studies need to be completed before applying this technology to the clinical setting.

58.5 Other Applications of Genitourinary Tissue Engineering

58.5.1 Injectable Therapies

Both urinary incontinence and vesicoureteral reflux are common conditions affecting the genitourinary system, wherein injectable bulking agents can be used for treatment. There are definite advantages in treating urinary incontinence and vesicoureteral reflux endoscopically. The method is simple and can be completed in less than 15 min, it has a low morbidity and it can be performed on an outpatient basis. The goal of several investigators has been to find alternate implant materials, which would be safe for human use [78].

The ideal substance for the endoscopic treatment of reflux and incontinence should be injectable, nonantigenic, nonmigratory, volume stable, and safe for human use. Toward this goal long-term studies were conducted to determine the effect of injectable chondrocytes *in vivo* [79]. It was initially determined that alginate, a liquid solution of gluronic and mannuronic acid, embedded with chondrocytes, could serve as a synthetic substrate for the injectable delivery and maintenance of cartilage architecture *in vivo*. Alginate undergoes hydrolytic biodegradation and its degradation time can be varied depending on the concentration of each of the polysaccharides. The use of autologous cartilage for the treatment of vesicoureteral reflux in humans would satisfy all the requirements of an ideal injectable substance. A biopsy of the ear could be easily and quickly performed, followed by chondrocyte processing and endoscopic injection of the autologous chondrocyte suspension for the treatment reflux.

Chondrocytes can be readily grown and expanded in culture. Neocartilage formation can be achieved *in vitro* and *in vivo* using chondrocytes cultured on synthetic biodegradable polymers [79]. In these experiments, the cartilage matrix replaced the alginate as the polysaccharide polymer underwent biodegradation. This system was adapted for the treatment of vesicoureteral reflux in a porcine model [80].

Six mini swine underwent bilateral creation of reflux. All six were found to have bilateral reflux without evidence of obstruction at 3 months following the procedure. Chondrocytes were harvested from the left auricular surface of each mini swine and expanded with a final concentration of $50-150 \times 10^6$ viable cells per animal. The animals underwent endoscopic repair of reflux with the injectable autologous chondrocyte solution on the right side only. Serial cystograms showed no evidence of reflux on the treated side and persistent reflux in the uncorrected control ureter in all animals. All animals had a successful cure of reflux in the repaired ureter without evidence of hydronephrosis on excretory urography. The harvested ears had evidence of cartilage regrowth within 1 month of chondrocyte retrieval.

At the time of sacrifice, gross examination of the bladder injection site showed a well-defined rubbery to hard cartilage structure in the subureteral region. Histologic examination of these specimens showed evidence of normal cartilage formation. The polymer gels were progressively replaced by cartilage with increasing time. Aldehyde fuschin-alcian blue staining suggested the presence of chondroitin sulfate. Microscopic analyses of the tissues surrounding the injection site showed no inflammation. Tissue sections from the bladder, ureters, lymph nodes, kidneys, lungs, liver, and spleen showed no evidence of chondrocyte or alginate migration, or granuloma formation. These studies showed that chondrocytes can be easily harvested and combined with alginate *in vitro*, the suspension can be easily injected cystoscopically and the elastic cartilage tissue formed is able to correct vesicoureteral reflux without any evidence of obstruction [80].

Two multicenter clinical trials were conducrted using the above engineered chondrocyte technology. Patients with vesicoureteral reflux were treated at 10 centers throughout the United States. The patients had a similar success rate as with other injectable substances in terms of cure (Figure 58.3). Chondrocyte formation was not noted in patients who had treatment failure. The patients who were cured would supposedly have a biocompatible region of engineered autologous tissue present, rather than a foreign material [81]. Patients with urinary incontinence were also treated endoscopically with injected chondrocytes at three different medical centers. Phase 1 trials showed an approximate success rate of 80% at both 3 and 12 months postoperatively [82].

The potential use of injectable, cultured myoblasts for the treatment of stress urinary incontinence has been investigated [83,84]. Primary myoblasts obtained from mouse skeletal muscle were transduced *in vitro* to carry the β-galactosidase reporter gene and were then incubated with fluorescent microspheres, which would serve as markers for the original cell population. Cells were then directly injected into the proximal urethra and lateral bladder walls of nude mice with a micro-syringe in an open surgical procedure. Tissue was harvested up to 35 days postinjection, analyzed histologically, and assayed for β-galactosidase expression. Myoblasts expressing B-galactosidase and containing fluorescent microspheres were found at each of the retrieved time points. In addition, regenerative myofibers expressing β-galactosidase were identified within the bladder wall. By 35 days postinjection, some of the injected cells expressed the contractile filament α-smooth muscle actin, suggesting the possibility of myoblastic differentiation into smooth muscle. The authors reported that a significant portion of the injected myoblast population persisted *in vivo*. Similar techniques of sphincteric derived muscle cells have been used for the treatment of urinary incontinence. Strasser from Innsbuck, Austria harvested muscle samples from pigs, dissociated the cells, and injected autologous pure clones of myoblasts into the urethral wall of pigs under sonographic visualization. Postoperatively maximal urethral closure pressures were increased markedly in most pigs and the zone of higher urethral closure pressure was lengthened compared to preoperative measurements [85]. The fact that myoblasts can be transfected, survive after injection, and begin the process of myogenic differentiation, further supports the feasibility of using cultured cells of muscular origin as an injectable bioimplant.

58.6   Stem Cells for Tissue Engineering

Most current strategies for engineering urologic tissues involve harvesting of autologous cells from the host diseased organ. However, in situations wherein extensive end stage organ failure is present, a tissue biopsy may not yield enough normal cells for expansion. Under these circumstances, the availability of pluripotent stem cells may be beneficial. Pluripotent embryonic stem cells are known to form teratomas *in vivo*, which are composed of a variety of differentiated cells. However, these cells are immunocompetent, and would require immunosuppression if used clinically.

The possibility of deriving stem cells from postnatal mesenchymal tissue from the same host, and inducing their differentiation *in vitro* and *in vivo*, was investigasted. Stem cells were isolated from human

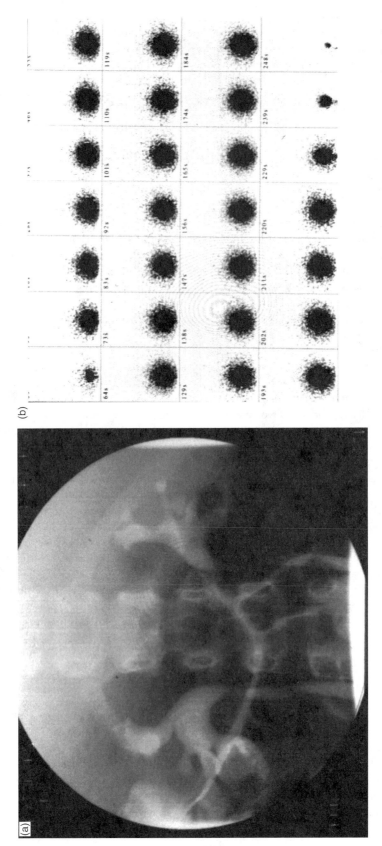

FIGURE 58.3 (a) Preoperative voiding cystourethrogram of a patient showing bilateral reflux; (b) Postoperative radionuclide cystogram of the same patient 6 months after the injection of autologous chondrocytes.

foreskin derived fibroblasts. Stem cell derived chondrocytes were obtained through a chondrogenic lineage process. The cells were grown, expanded, seeded onto biodegradable scaffolds, and implanted *in vivo*, where they formed mature cartilage structures. This was the first demonstration that stem cells can be derived from postnatal connective tissue and can be used for engineering tissues *in vivo ex situ* [86].

A second approach which has been pursued for stem lineage isolation involves the isolation of stem cells from individual organs. For example, daily female hormone supplementation is used widely, most commonly in postmenopausal women. A continuous and unlimited hormonal supply produced from ovarian granulosa cells would be an attractive alternative. The feasibility of isolating functional human ovarian granulosa stem cells, which, unlike primary cells, may have the ability to proliferate and function indefinitely, was investigated.

Granulosa stem cells were selectively isolated from postmenopausal human ovaries and their phenotype was confirmed with the stem cell marker antibodies, CD 34, CD 105, and CD 90. The granulosa stem cells in culture showed steady state progesterone (5 to 7 ng/ml) and estradiol (2500 to 3000 pg/ml) production either with or without hCG stimulation [87].

58.7 Therapeutic Cloning

Nuclear transplantation ("therapeutic cloning") could theoretically provide a limitless source of cells for regenerative therapy. According to data from the Centers for Disease Control, as many as 3000 Americans die every day from diseases that in the future may be treatable with embryonic stem (ES)-derived tissues [88]. In addition to generating functional replacement cells such as cardiomyocytes and neurons, there is also the possibility that these cells could be used to reconstitute more complex tissues and organs, including kidneys [89–91]. Somatic cell nuclear transfer (SCNT) has the potential to eliminate immune responses associated with the transplantation of these various tissues, and thus the requirement for immunosuppressive drugs or immunomodulatory protocols that carry the risk of a wide variety of serious and potentially life-threatening complications (Figure 58.4) [92].

Although the goal of "therapeutic" cloning is to generate replacement cells and tissues that are genetically identical with the donor, numerous studies have shown that animals produced by the SCNT technique

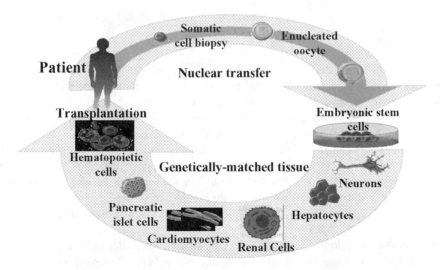

FIGURE 58.4 Therapeutic cloning strategy and its application to the engineering of tissues and organs.

inherit their mitochondria entirely or in part from the recipient oocyte and not the donor cell [93–95]. This raises the question of whether nonself mitochondrial proteins in cells could lead to immunogenicity after transplantation and defeat the main objective of the procedure.

We tested the histocompatibility of nuclear-transfer-generated cells and engineered tissues in a large animal model, the cow (*Bos taurus*). Cloned muscle cell implants were not rejected, and they remained viable after being transplanted back into the nuclear donor animal despite expressing a different mtDNA haplotype. We also showed that nuclear transplantation can be used to generate functional renal structures. Owing to its complex structure and function [95], the kidney is one of the most challenging organs to reconstruct in the body. Previous efforts at tissue engineering the kidney have been directed toward development of an extracorporeal renal support system comprising both biologic and synthetic components [97–99]. This approach was first described by Aebischer et al. [100,101] and is being focused toward the treatment of acute rather than chronic renal failure. Humes et al. [97] have shown that the combination of hemofiltration and a renal-assist device containing tubule cells can replace certain physiologic functions of the kidney when they are connected in an extravascular perfusion circuit in uremic dogs. Heat exchangers, flow and pressure monitors, and multiple pumps are required for optimal functioning of this device [102,103]. Although *ex vivo* organ substitution therapy would be life-sustaining, there would be obvious benefits for patients if such devices could be implanted long term without the need for an extracorporeal perfusion circuit or immunosuppressive drugs or immune modulatory protocols. While synthetic, selectively permeable barriers can be used *ex vivo* to separate transplanted cells from the immune system of the body, the implantation of such immunoisolation systems would pose significant difficulties in both the long and short term [104–107]. We demonstrated that it may be feasible to use therapeutic cloning to generate functional immune-compatible renal tissues [108].

Dermal fibroblasts were isolated from adult Holstein steers by ear notch. Bovine oocytes were obtained from abattoir-derived ovaries. The oocytes were mechanically enucleated at 18 to 22 h postmaturation, and complete enucleation of the metaphase plate was confirmed with *bis*Benzimide dye under fluorescence microscopy. A suspension of actively dividing cells was prepared immediately prior to nuclear transfer. Single donor cells were selected and transferred into the perivitelline space of the enucleated oocytes. Fusion of the cell–oocyte complexes was accomplished by applying a single pulse of 2.4 kV/cm for 15 μsec. Nuclear transfer embryos were activated with exposure to Ionomycin. The resulting blastocysts were nonsurgically transferred into progestrin-synchronized recipients. The cloned renal and muscle cells were isolated and expanded *in vitro* after 12 weeks. The expanded cloned renal cells were successfully seeded onto renal units, and implanted back into the nuclear donor organism without immune destruction. The cells organized into glomeruli- and tubule-like structures with the ability to excrete toxic metabolic waste products through a urine-like fluid.

58.7.1 Muscle

Tissue engineered constructs containing bovine muscle cells seeded onto PGA matrices were transplanted subcutaneously and retrieved 6 weeks after implantation. After retrieval of the first-set implants, a second set of constructs from the same donor were transplanted for a further 12 weeks. On a histological level, the cloned muscle tissue appeared intact, and showed a well-organized cellular orientation with spindle-shaped nuclei. Immunohistochemical analysis identified muscle fibers within the implanted constructs. In contrast to the cloned implants, the allogeneic, control cell implants failed to form muscle bundles, and showed an increased number of inflammatory cells, fibrosis, and necrotic debris consistent with acute rejection. Semiquantitative RT-PCR and Western blot analysis confirmed the expression of muscle specific mRNA and proteins in the retrieved tissues despite the presence of allogeneic mitochondria. In contrast, expression intensities were significantly lower or absent in constructs generated from genetically unrelated cattle.

Immunocytochemical analysis using CD4- and CD8-specific antibodies identified an approximately twofold increase in CD4+ and CD8+ T cells within the explanted first and second set control vs. cloned constructs. Importantly, first and second set cloned constructs exhibited comparable levels of CD4 and

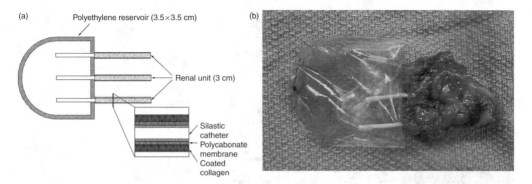

FIGURE 58.5   Tissue-engineered renal units. Illustration of renal unit (a) and unit seeded with cloned cells, showing the accumulation of urinelike fluid, retrieved 3 months after implantation (b).

CD8 expression, arguing against the presence of an enhanced second set reaction as would be expected if mtDNA-encoded minor antigen differences were present. Western blot analysis of the first-set explants indicated an approximately sixfold increase in expression intensity of CD4 in the control vs. cloned constructs at 6 weeks, confirming a primary immune response to the control grafts. There was also a significant increase in the mean expression intensities of CD8 in the control vs. cloned constructs at 6 weeks. Twelve weeks after second-set implantation, mean expression intensities of CD4 and CD8 continued to remain significantly elevated in the control vs. cloned constructs.

58.7.2 Kidney

The renal cells obtained through nuclear transfer demonstrated immunochemically the expression of renal specific proteins, including synaptopodin (produced by podocytes), aquaporin 1 (AQP1, produced by proximal tubules and the descending limb of the loop of Henle), aquaporin 2 (AQP2, produced by collecting ducts), Tamm–Horsfall protein (produced by the ascending limb of the loop of Henle), and factor VIII (produced by endothelial cells). Synaptopodin and AQP1 & 2 expressing cells exhibited circular and linear patterns in two-dimensional culture, respectively. After expansion, the renal cells were shown to produce both erythropoietin and 1,25-dihydroxyvitamin D_3, a key endocrinologic metabolite. The cloned cells produced erythropoietin and were responsive to hypoxic stimulation.

The cloned renal cells were seeded onto collagen-coated cylindrical polycarbonate membranes. Renal devices with collecting systems were constructed by connecting the ends of three membranes with catheters that terminated in a reservoir (Figure 58.5). Thirty-one units ($n = 19$ with cloned cells, $n = 6$ without cells, and $n = 6$ with cells from an allogeneic control fetus) were transplanted subcutaneously and retrieved 12 weeks after implantation back into the nuclear donor animal.

On gross examination, the explanted units appeared intact, and straw-yellow colored fluid could be observed in the reservoirs of the cloned group. There was a sixfold increase in volume in the experimental group vs. the control groups. Chemical analysis of the fluid suggested unidirectional secretion and concentration of urea nitrogen and creatinine.

Physiological function of the implanted units was further evidenced by analysis of the electrolyte levels in the collected fluid as well as specific gravity and glucose concentrations. The electrolyte levels detected in the fluid of the experimental group were significantly different from plasma or the controls. These findings indicate that the implanted renal cells possess filtration, reabsorption, and secretory functions. Urine specific gravity is an indicator of kidney function and reflects the action of the tubules and collecting ducts on the glomerular filtrate by furnishing an estimate of the number of particles dissolved in the urine. The urine-specific gravity of cattle is reported as approximately 1.025 (vs. 1.027 ± 0.001 for the fluid that was produced by the cloned renal units), and normally ranges from 1.020 to 1.040 (vs. approximately 1.010 in normal bovine serum) [16,17]. The normal range of urine pH for adult herbivores is alkaline, with values

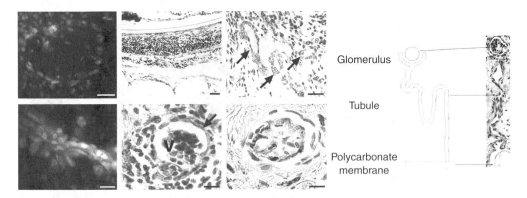

FIGURE 58.6   Characterization of renal explants. Cloned cells stained positively with synaptopodin antibody (a) and AQP1 antibody (b). The allogeneic controls displayed a foreign body reaction with necrosis (c). Cloned explant shows organized glomeruli (d) and tubule-like structures (e). H&E, reduced from 400×. Immunohistochemical analysis using factor VIII antibodies identifies vascular structure within d (f). Reduced from ×400. There was a clear unidirectional continuity between the mature glomeruli, their tubules, and the polycarbonate membrane (g).

ranging from 7.0 to 9.0 [17] (the pH of the fluid from the cloned renal units was 8.1±0.20). Glucose is reabsorbed in the proximal tubules, and is seldom present in the urine of cattle. Glucose was undetectable ($<$10 mg/dl) in the cloned renal fluid (vs. blood glucose concentrations of 76.6 $\pm$ 0.04 mg/dl).

The retrieved implants demonstrated extensive vascularization, and had self-assembled into glomeruli and tubule-like structures. The latter were lined with cuboid epithelial cells with large, spherical, and pale-stained nuclei, whereas the glomeruli structures exhibited a variety of cell types with abundant red blood cells. There was a clear continuity between the mature glomeruli, their tubules, and the polycarbonate membrane. The renal tissues were integrally connected in a unidirectional manner to the reservoirs, resulting in the excretion of dilute urine into the collecting systems.

Immunohistochemical analysis confirmed expression of renal specific proteins, including AQP1, AQP2, synaptopodin, and factor VIII. Antibodies for AQP1, AQP2, and synaptopodin identified tubular, collecting tubule, and glomerular segments within the constructs, respectively. In contrast, the allogeneic controls displayed a foreign body reaction with necrosis, consistent with the finding of acute rejection. RT-PCR analysis confirmed the transcription of AQP1, AQP2, synaptopodin, and Tamm–Horsfall genes exclusively in the cloned group. Cultured and cloned cells also expressed high protein levels of AQP1, AQP2, synaptopodin, and Tamm–Horsfall protein as determined by Western blot analysis. Expression intensity of CD4 and CD8, markers for inflammation and rejection, were also significantly higher in the control vs. cloned group (Figure 58.6).

58.7.2.1 Mitochondrial DNA analysis

Previous studies showed that bovine clones harbor the oocyte mtDNA [93–95,109]. Differences in mtDNA-encoded proteins expressed by clone cells could stimulate a T cell response specific for mtDNA-encoded minor histocompatibility antigens (miHA) [110] when clone cells are transplanted back to the original nuclear donor. The most straightforward approach to resolve the question of miHA involvement is the identification of potential antigens by nucleotide sequencing of the mtDNA genomes of the clone and fibroblast nuclear donor. The contiguous segments of mtDNA that encode 13 mitochondrial proteins and tRNAs were amplified by PCR from total cell DNA in five overlapping segments. These amplicons were directly sequenced on one strand with a panel of sequencing primers spaced at 500 bp intervals.

The resulting nucleotide sequences (13,210 bp) revealed nine nucleotide substitutions for the first donor : recipient combination (muscle constructs). One substitution was in the tRNA-Gly segment and five substitutions were synonymous. The sixth substitution, in the ND1 gene, was heteroplasmic in the nuclear donor where one of the two alternative nucleotides was shared with the clone. A Leu or Arg would be translated at this position in ND1. The eighth and ninth substitutions resulted in amino acid (AA) interchanges of Asn > Ser and Val > Ala in the ATPase6 and ND4L genes, respectively. For the second donor : recipient combination (renal constructs), we obtained 12,785 bp from both the clone and nuclear donor animal. The resulting sequences revealed six nucleotide substitutions. One substitution was in the tRNA-Arg segment and three substitutions were synonymous. The fifth and sixth substitutions resulted in AA interchanges of Ile>Thr and Thr>Ile in the ND2 and ND5 genes, respectively. The identification of two AA substitutions that distinguish the clone and the nuclear donor confirm that a maximum of only two miHA peptides could be defined by the second donor : recipient combination. Given the lack of knowledge concerning peptide binding motifs for bovine MHC class I molecules, there is no reliable method to predict the impact of these AA substitutions on the ability of mtDNA-encoded peptides to either bind to bovine class I molecules or activate CD8+CTLs.

Although the cloned renal cells derived their nuclear genome from the original fibroblast donor, their *mt*DNA was derived from the original recipient oocyte. A relatively limited number of *mt*DNA polymorphisms have been shown to define maternally transmitted miHA in mice [110]. This class of miHA has been shown to stimulate both skin allograft rejection *in vivo* and expansion of cytotoxic T lymphocytes (CTL) *in vitro* [110], and could constitute a barrier to successful clinical use of such cloned devices as hypothesized for chronic rejection of MHC-matched human renal transplants [111,112]. We chose to investigate a possible anti-miHA T cell response to the cloned renal devices through both delayed-type hypersensitivity (DTH) testing *in vivo* and Elispot analysis of IFNg-secreting T cells *in vitro*. An *in vivo* assay of anti-miHA immunity was chosen based on the ability skin allograft rejection to detect a wide range of miHA in mice with survival times exceeding 10 weeks [113] and the relative insensitivity of *in vitro* assays in detecting miHA incompatibility, highlighted by the requirement for *in vivo* priming to generate CTL [114]. We were unable to discern an immunological response directed against the cloned cells by DTH testing *in vivo*. Cloned and control allogeneic cells were intradermally injected back into the nuclear donor animal 80 days after the initial transplantation. A positive DTH response was observed after 48 h for the allogeneic control cells but not the cloned cells.

The results of DTH analysis were mirrored by Elispot-derived estimates of the frequencies of T cells that secreted IFN-gamma following *in vitro* stimulation. PBLs were harvested from the transplanted recipient 1 month after retrieval of the devices. These PBLs were stimulated in primary mixed lymphocyte cultures (MLCs) with allogeneic renal cells, cloned renal cells, and nuclear donor fibroblasts. Surviving T cells were restimulated in anti-IFN-gamma-coated wells with either nuclear donor fibroblasts (autologous control) or the respective stimulators used in the primary MLCs. Elispot analysis revealed a relatively strong T cell response to allogeneic renal stimulator cells relative to the responses to either cloned renal cells or nuclear donor fibroblasts. These results corroborate both the relative CD4 and CD8 expression in Western blots as well as the results of *in vivo* DTH testing to support the conclusion that there was no detectable rejection response that was specific for cloned renal cells following either primary or secondary challenge. Our results suggest that cloned cells and tissues can be grafted back into the nuclear donor organism without immune destruction. These were the first proof-of-principle studies to demonstrate that therapeutic cloning is feasible.

58.8   Conclusion

Tissue engineering efforts are currently being undertaken for every type of tissue and organ within the urinary system. Most of the effort expended to engineer genitourinary tissues has occurred within the last decade. Tissue engineering techniques require a cell culture, facility designed for human application. Personnel who have mastered the techniques of cell harvest, culture, and expansion as well as polymer design are essential for the successful application of this technology. Various engineered genitourinary tissues are at different stages of development, with some already being used clinically, a few in preclinical trials, and some in the discovery stage. Recent progress suggests that engineered urologic tissues may have an expanded clinical applicability in the future.

References

[1] Cilento, B.G., Freeman, M.R., Schneck, F.X., Retik, A.B., and Atala, A. Phenotypic and cytogenetic characterization of human bladder urothelia expanded *in vitro*. *J. Urol.* 1994; 152: 655.

[2] Scriven, S.D., Booth, C., Thomas, D.F., Trejdosiewicz, L.K., and Southgate, J. Reconstitution of human urothelium from monolayer cultures. *J. Urol.* 1997; 158: 1147–52.

[3] Liebert, M., Hubbel, A., Chung, M., Wedemeyer, G., Lomax, M.I., Hegeman, A., Yuan, T.Y., Brozovich, M., Wheelock, M.J., and Grossman, H.B. Expression of mal is associated with urothelial differentiation in vitro: identification by differential display reverse-transcriptase polymerase chain reaction. *Differentiation* 1997; 61: 177–85.

[4] Puthenveettil, J.A., Burger, M.S., and Reznikoff, C.A. Replicative senescence in human uroepithelial cells. *Adv. Exp. Med. Biol.* 1999; 462: 83–91.

[5] Fauza, D.O., Fishman, S., Mehegan, K., and Atala, A. Videofetoscopically assisted fetal tissue engineering: bladder augmentation. *J. Ped. Surg.* 1998; 33: 7–12.

[6] Liebert, M., Wedemeyer, G., Abruzzo, L.V., Kunkel, S.L., Hammerberg, C., Cooper, K.D., and Grossman, H.B. Stimulated urothelial cells produce cytokines and express an activated cell surface antigenic phenotype. *Semin. Urol.* 1991; 9: 124–30.

[7] Tobin, M.S., Freeman, M.R., and Atala, A. Maturational response of normal human urothelial cells in culture is dependent on extracellular matrix and serum additives. *Surgical Forum* 1994; 45: 786.

[8] Freeman, M.R., Yoo, J.J., Raab, G., Soker, S., Adam, R.M., Schneck, F.X., Renshaw, A.A., Klagsbrun, M., and Atala, A. Heparin-binding EGF-like growth factor is an autocrine factor for human urothelial cells and is synthesized by epithelial and smooth muscle cells in the human bladder. *J. Clin. Invest.* 1997; 99: 1028.

[9] Nguyen, H.T., Park, J.M., Peters, C.A., Adam, R.A., Orsola, A., Atala, A., and Freeman, M.R. Cell-specific activation of the HB-EGF and ErbB1 genes by stretch in primary human bladder cells. *In Vitro Cell Dev. Biol.* 1999; 35: 371–375.

[10] Harriss, D.R. Smooth muscle cell culture: a new approach to the study of human detrusor physiology and pathophysiology. *Br. J. Urol.* 1995; 75(Suppl 1): 18–26.

[11] Solomon, L.Z., Jennings, A.M., Sharpe, P., Cooper, A.J., and Malone, P.S. Effects of short-chain fatty acids on primary urothelial cells in culture: implications for intravesical use in enterocystoplasties. *J. Lab. Clin. Med.* 1998; 132: 279–83.

[12] Lobban, E.D., Smith, B.A., Hall, G.D., Harnden, P., Roberts, P., Selby, P.J., Trejdosiewicz, L.K., and Southgate, J. Uroplakin gene expression by normal and neoplastic human urothelium. *Am. J. Pathol.* 1998; 153: 1957–67.

[13] Rackley, R.R., Bandyopadhyay, S.K., Fazeli-Matin, S., Shin, M.S., and Appell, R. Immunoregulatory potential of urothelium: characterization of NF-kappaB signal transduction. *J. Urol.* 1999; 162: 1812–6.

[14] Bergsma, J.E., Rozema, F.R., Bos, R.R.M, van Rozendaal, A.W.M, de Jong, W.H., Teppema, J.S., and Joziasse, C.A.P. Biocompatibility and degradatin mechanism of predegraded and non-degraded poly(lactide) implants: an animal study. *Mater. Med.* 1995; 6: 715–24.

[15] Atala, A. Autologous cell transplantation for urologic reconstruction. *J. Urol.* 1998; 159: 2–3.

[16] Kim, B.S. and Mooney, D.J. Development of biocompatible synthetic extracellular matrices for tissue engineering. *Trend Biotechnol.* 1998; 16: 224–30.

[17] Pariente, J.L., Kim, B.S., and Atala, A. In vitro biocompatibility assessment of naturally-derived and sythetic biomaterials using normal human urothelial cells. *J. Biomed. Mater. Res.* 2001; 55: 33–39.

[18] Pariente, J.L., Kim, B.S., and Atala, A. *In vitro* biocompatibility evaluation of naturally derived and synthetic biomaterials using normal human bladder smooth muscle. *J. Urol.* 2002; 167: 1867–71.

[19] Li, S.T. Biologic biomaterials: tissue-derived biomaterials (collagen). In: Brozino, J.D., Ed. *The Biomedical Engineering Handbook*. Boca Ranton, FL: CRC Press, 1995, pp. 627–647.

[20] Silver, F.H. and Pins, G. Cell growth on collagen: a review of tissue engineering using scaffolds containing extracellular matrix. *J. Long-Term Effects Med. Implants* 1992; 2: 67–80.

[21] Sam, A.E. and Nixon, A.J. Chondrocyte-laden collagen scaffolds for resurfacing extensive articular cartilage defects. *Osteoarthritis Cartil.* 1995; 3: 47–59.

[22] Smidsrød, O. and Skjåk-Bræk, G. Alginate as an immobilization matrix for cells. *Trend Biotechnol.* 1990; 8: 71–78.

[23] Lim, F. and Sun, A.M. Microencapsulated islets as bioartificial endocrine pancreas. *Science* 1980; 210: 908–910.

[24] Yoo, J.J., Meng, J., Oberpennin, F., and Atala, A. Bladder augmentation using allogenic bladder submucosa seeded with cells. *J. Urol.* 1998; 51: 221.

[25] Piechota, H.J., Dahms, S.E., Nunes, L.S., Dahiya, R., Lue, T.F., and Tanagho, E.A. In vitro functional properties of the rat bladder regenerated by the bladder acellular matrix graft. *J. Urol.* 1998; 159: 1717–24.

[26] Dahms, S.E., Piechota, H.J., Dahiya, R., Lue, T.F., and Tanagho, E.A. Composition and biochemical properties of the bladder acellular matrix graft: comparative analysis in rat, pig and human. *Br. J. Urol.* 1998; 82: 411–19.

[27] Chen, F., Yoo, J.J., and Atala, A. Acellular collagen matrix as a possible "off the shelf" biomaterial for urethral repair. *Urology* 1999; 54: 407–10.

[28] Gilding, D.K. Biodegradable polymers. In: Williams, D.F., Ed. *Biocompatibility of Clinical Implant Materials*. Boca Raton, FL: CRC Press, 1981, pp. 209–32.

[29] Freed, L.E., Vunjak-Novakovic, G., Biron, R.J., Eagles, D.B., Lesnoy, D.C., Barlow, S.K., and Langer, R. Biodegradable polymer scaffolds for tissue engineering. *BioTechnology* 1994; 12: 689–93.

[30] Mikos, A.G., Thorsen, A.J., Czerwonka, L.A., Bao, Y., Langer, R., Winslow, D.N., and Vacanti, J.P. Preparation and characterization of poly(L-lactic acid) foams. *Polymer* 1994; 35: 1068–77.

[31] Harris, L.D., Kim, B.S., and Mooney, D.J. Open pore biodegradable matrices formed with gas foaming. *J. Biomed. Mater. Res.* 1998; 42: 396–402.

[32] Peppas, N.A. and Langer, R. New challenges in biomaterials. *Science* 1994; 263: 1715–20.

[33] Bazeed, M.A., Thüroff, J.W., Schmidt, R.A., and Tanagho, E.A. New treatment for urethral strictures. *Urology* 1983; 21: 53–57.

[34] Atala, A., Vacanti, J.P., Peters, C.A., Mandell, J., Retik, A.B., and Freeman, M.R. Formation of urothelial structures in vivo from dissociated cells attached to biodegradable polymer scaffolds *in vitro*. *J. Urol.* 1992; 148: 658.

[35] Olsen, L., Bowald, S., Busch, C. et al. Urethral reconstruction with a new synthetic absorbable device. *Scan. J. Urol. Nephrol.* 1992; 26: 323–6.

[36] Kropp, B.P., Ludlow, J.K., Spicer, D., Rippy, M.K., Badylak, S.F., Adams, M.C., Keating, M.A., Rink, R.C., Birhle, R., and Thor, K.B. Rabbit urethral regeneration using small intestinal submucosa onlay grafts. *Urology* 1998; 52: 138–42.

[37] Sievert, K.D., Bakircioglu, M.E., Nunes, L., Tu, R., Dahiya, R., and Tanagho, E.A. Homologous acellular matrix graft for urethral reconstruction in the rabbit: histological and functional evaluation. *J. Urol.* 2000; 163: 1958–65.

[38] Atala, A. Future perspectives in reconstructive surgery using tissue engineering. *Urol. Clin.* 1999; 26: 157–65.

[39] ElKassaby, A.W., Retik, A.B., Yoo, J.J., and Atala, A. Urethral stricture repair with an "off the shelf" collagen matrix. *J. Urol.* 2003; 169.

[40] DeFilippo, R.E., Yoo, J.J., Chen, F., and Atala, A. Urethral replacement using cell-seeded tubularized collagen matrices. *J. Urol.* 2002; 168: 1789–93.

[41] DeFilippo, R.E., Pohl, H.G., Yoo, J.J., and Atala, A. Total penile urethra replacement with autologous cell-seeded collagen matrices [abstract]. *J. Urol.* 2002; 167(Suppl): 152–3.

[42] Neuhof, H. Fascial transplantation into visceral defects: An experimental and clinical study. *Surg. Gynecol Obstet.* 1917; 25: 383.

[43] Tsuji, I., Ishida, H., and Fujieda, J. Experimental cystoplasty using preserved bladder graft. *J. Urol.* 1961; 85: 42.

[44] Kambic, H., Kay, R., Chen, J.F., Matsushita, M., Harasaki, H., and Zilber, S. Biodegradable pericardial implants for bladder augmentation: a 2.5-year study in dogs. *J. Urol.* 1992; 148: 53943.

[45] Kelami, A., Ludtke-Handjery, A., Korb, G., Roll, J., Schnell, J., and Danigel, K.H. Alloplastic replacement of the urinary bladder wall with lyophilized human dura. *Eur. Surg. Res.* 1970; 2: 195.

[46] Fishman, I.J., Flores, F.N., Scott, B., Spjut, H.J., and Morrow, B. Use of fresh placental membranes for bladder reconstruction. *J. Urol.* 1987; 138: 1291.

[47] Probst, M., Dahiya, R., Carrier, S., and Tanagho, E.A. Reproduction of functional smooth muscle tissue and partial bladder replacement. *Br. J. Urol.* 1997; 79: 505.

[48] Sutherland, R.S., Baskin, L.S., Hayward, S.W., and Cunha, G.R. Regeneration of bladder urothelium, smooth muscle, blood vessels, and nerves into an acellular tissue matrix. *J. Urol.* 1996; 156: 571–7.

[49] Kropp, B.P., Sawyer, B.D., Shannon, H.E., Rippy, M.K., Badylak, S.F., Adams, M.C., Keating, M.A., Rink, R.C., and Thor, K.B. Characterization of using small intestine submucosa regenerated canine detrusor: assessment of reinnervaation, in vitro compliance and contractility. *J. Urol.* 1996; 156: 599–607.

[50] Vaught, J.D., Kroop, B.P., Sawyer, B.D., Rippy, M.K., Badylak, S.F., Shannon, H.E., and Thor, K.B. Detrusor regeneration in the rat using porcine small intestine submucosal grafts: functional innervation and receptor expression. *J. Urol.* 1996; 155: 374–8.

[51] Probst, M., Dahiya, R., Carrier, S., and Tanagho, E.A. Reproduction of functional smooth muscle tissue and partial bladder replacement. *Br. J. Urol.* 1997; 79: 505–15.

[52] Kropp, B.P., Rippy, M.K., Badylak, S.F., Adams, M.C., Keating, M.A., Rink, R.C., and Thor, K.B. Small intestinal submucosa: urodynamic and histopahtologic evaluation in long term canine bladder augmentations. *J. Urol.* 1996; 155: 2098–2104.

[53] Lai, J.Y., Yoo, J.J., Wulf, T., and Atala, A. Bladder augmentation using small intestinal submucosa seeded with cells. [abstract]. *J. Urol.* 2002; 167(Suppl): 257.

[54] Brown, A.L., Farhat, W., Merguerian, P.A., Wilson, G.J., Khoury, A.E., and Woodhouse, K.A. 22 week assessment of bladder accellular matrix as a bladder augmentation material in a porcine model. *Biomaterials* 2002; 23: 2179–90.

[55] Reddy, P.P., Barrieras, D.J., Wilson, G., Bagli, D.J., McLorie, G.A., Khoury, A.E., and Merguerian, P.A. Regeneration of functional bladder substitutes using large segment acellular matrix allografts in a porcine model. *J. Urol.* 2000; 164: 936–41.

[56] Merguerian, P.A., Reddy, P.P., Barrieras, D.J., Wilson, G.J., Woodhouse, K., Bagli, D.J., McLorie, G.A., and Khoury, A.E. Acellular bladder matrix allografts in the regeneration of functional bladders: evaluation of large-segment (>24 cm) substitution in a porcine model. *BJU Int.* 2000; 85: 894–8.

[57] Portis, A.J., Elbahnasy, A.M., Shalhav, A.L., Brewer, A., Humphrey, P., McDougall, E.M., and Clayman, R.V. Laparascopic augmentation cystoplasty with different biodegradable grafts in an animal model. *J. Urol.* 2000; 164: 1405–11.

[58] Portis, A.J., Elbahnasy, A.M., Shalhav, A.L., Brewer, A.V., Olweny, E., Humphrey, P.A., McDougall, E.M., and Clayman, R.V. Laparoscopic midsagittal hemicystectomy and replacement of bladder wall with small intestinal submucosa and reimplantation of ureter into graft. *J. Endourol.* 2000; 14: 203–11.

[59] Gleeson, M.J. and Griffith, D.P. The use of aloplastic biomaterials in bladder substitution. *J. Urol.* 1992; 148: 1377.

[60] Bona, A.V. and De Gresti, A. Partial substitution of urinary bladder with Teflon prothesis. *Minerva Urol.* 1966; 18: 43.

[61] Monsour, M.J., Mohammed, R., Gorham, S.D., French, D.A., and Scott, R. An assessment of a collagen/vicryl composite memebrane to repair defects of the urinary bladder in rabbits. *Urology* 1987; 15: 235.

[62] Rohrmann, D., Albrecht, D., Hannappel, J., Gerlach, R., Schwarzkopp, G., and Lutzeyer, W. Alloplastic replacement of the urinary bladder. *J. Urol.* 1996; 156: 2094.

Atala, A. Tissue engineering in the genitourinary system. In: Atala, Moone, D. (Eds.) *Tissue Engineering* Boston: Birkhouser Press, 1997, p. 149.

[63] Atala, A., Freeman, M.R., Vacanti, J.P., Shepard, J., and Retik, A.B. Implantation *in vivo* and retrieval of artificial structures consisting of rabbit and human urothelium and human bladder muscle. *J. Urol.* 1993; 150: 608–12.

[64] Atala, A. Commentary on the replacement of urologic associated mucosa. *J. Urol.* 1995; 156: 338.

[65] De Boer, W.I., Schuller, A.G., Vermay, M., and van der Kwast, T.H. Expression of growth factors and receptors during specific phases in regenerating urothelium after acute injury *in vivo. Am. J. Pathol.* 1994; 145: 1199.

[66] Baker, R., Kelly, T., Tehan, T., Putman, C., and Beaugard, E. Subtotal cystectomy and total bladder regeneration in treatment of bladder cancer. *J. Am. Med. Assoc.* 1955; 168: 1178.

[67] Gorham, S.D., French, D.A., Shivas, A.A., and Scott, R. Some observations on the regeneration of smooth muscle in the repaired urinary bladder of the rabbit. *Eur. Urol.* 1989; 16: 440.

[68] Oberpenning, F.O., Meng, J., Yoo, J., and Atala, A. *De novo* reconstitution of a functional urinary bladder by tissue engineering. *Nat. Biotechnol.* 1999; 17: 2.

[69] Kershen, R.T., Yoo, J.J., Moreland, R.B., Krane, R.J., and Atala, A. Novel system for the formation of human corpus cavernosum smooth muscle tissue *in vivo. J. Urol.* 1998; 159(Suppl): 156.

[70] Park, H.J., Kershen, R., Yoo, J., and Atala, A. Reconstitution of human corporal smooth muscle and endothelial cells *in vivo. J. Urol.* 1999; 162: 1106–9.

[71] Falke, G., Yoo, J., Machado, M., Moreland, R., and Atala, A. Formation of corporal tissue *in vivo* using human cavernosal muscle and endothelium cells seeded on collagen matrices. *Tissue Eng.* 2003; 9: 871–9.

[72] Kwon, T.G., Yoo, J.J., and Atala, A. Autologous penile corpora cavernosa replacement using tissue engineering techniques. *J. Urol.* 2002; 168: 1754–58.

[73] Nukui, F., Okamoto, S., Nagata, M., Kurokawa, J., and Fukui, J. Complications and reimplantation of penile implants. *Int. J. Urol.* 1997; 4: 52.

[74] Thomalla, J.V., Thompson, S.T., Rowland, R.G., and Mulcahy, J.J. Infectious complications of penile prosthetic implants. *J. Urol.* 1987; 138: 65–7.

[75] Yoo, J.J., Lee, I., and Atala, A. Cartilage rods as a potential material for penile reconstruction. *J. Urol.* 1998; 160: 1164.

[76] Yoo, J.J., Park, H., Lee, I., and Atala, A. Autologous engineered cartilage rods for penile reconstruction. *J. Urol.* 1999; 162: 1119–21.

[77] Kershen, R.T. and Atala, A. Advances in injectable therapies for the treatment of incontinence and vesicoureteral reflux. *Urol. Clin.* 1999; 26: 81–94.

[78] Atala, A., Cima, L.G., Kim, W., Paige, K.T., Vacanti, J.P., Retik, A.B., and Vacanti, C.A. Injectable alginate seeded with chondrocytes as a potential treatment for vesicoureteral reflux. *J. Urol.* 1993; 150: 745–5.

[79] Atala, A., Kim, W., Paige, K.T., Vacanti, C.A., and Retik, A.B. Endoscopic treatment of vesicoureteral reflux with chondrocyte-alginate suspension. *J. Urol.* 1994; 152: 641.

[80] Diamond, D.A., and Caldamone, A.A. Endoscopic correction of vesicoureteral reflux in children using autologous chondrocytes: preliminary results. *J. Urol.* 1999; 162: 1185.

[81] Bent, A., Tutrone, R., McLennan, M., Lloyd, K., Kennelly, M., and Badlani, G. Treatment of intrinsic sphincter deficiency using autologous ear chondrocytes as a bulking agent. *Neurourol. Urodynam* 2001; 20: 157–65.

[82] Yokoyama, T., Chancellor, M.B., Watanabe, T., Ozawa, H., Yoshimura, N., de Groat, W.C., Qu, Z., and Huard, J. Primary myoblasts injection into the urethra and bladder as a potential treatment of stress urinary incontinence and impaired detrusor contractility ; long term survival without significant cytotoxicity. *J. Urol.* 1999; 161: 307.

[83] Chancellor, M.B., Yokoyama, T., Tirney, S., Mattes, C.E., Ozawa, H., Yoshimura, N., de Groat, W.C., and Huard, J. Preliminary results of myoblast injection into the urethra and bladder wall: a possible method for the treatment of stree urinary incontinence and impaired detrusor contractility. *Neurourol. Urodyn.* 2000; 19: 279–87.

[84] Strasser, H., Marksteiner, R., Eva, M., Stanislav, B., Guenther, K., Helga, F. et al. Transurethral Ultrasound Guided Injection of Clonally Cultured Autologous Myoblasts and Fibroblasts: Experimental Results. In: *Proceedings of the 2003 International Bladder Symposium*, 2003 March 6–9; Arlington, VA. Ridgefield, CT: National Bladder Foundation, 2003, p. 6.

[85] Bartsch, G., Yoo, J., Kim, B., and Atala, A. Stem cells in tissue engineering applications for incontinence. *J. Urol.* 2000; 1009S: 227.

[86] Raya-Rivera, A., Yoo, J., and Atala, A. Hormone producing granulosa stem cells for intersex disorders [abstract 29]. American Academy of Pediatrics Meeting, Urology section, Chicago, 2000.

[87] Lanza, R.P. et al. The ethical reasons for stem cell research. *Science* 2001; 293: 1299.

[88] Machluf, M. and Atala, A. Emerging concepts for tissue and organ transplantation. *Graft* 1998; 1: 31. .

[89] Atala, A. and Lanza, R.P. *Methods of Tissue Engineering.* San Diego, CA: Academic Press, 2001.

[90] Atala, A. and Mooney, D. *Synthetic Biodegradable Polymer Scaffolds.* Boston, MA: Birkhaüser, 1997.

[91] Lanza, R.P., Cibelli, J.B., and West, M.D. Prospects for the use of nuclear transfer in human transplantation. *Nat. Biotechnol.* 1999; 17: 1171–4.

[92] Evans, M.J. et al. Mitochondrial, DNA genotypes in nuclear transfer-derived cloned sheep. *Nat. Genet.* 1999; 23: 90–3.

[93] Hiendleder, S., Schmutz, S.M., Erhardt, G., Green, R.D., and Plante, Y. Transmitochondrial differences and varying levels of heteroplasmy in nuclear transfer cloned cattle. *Mol. Reprod. Dev.* 1999; 54: 24–31.

[94] Steinborn, R., et al. Mitochondrial DNA heteroplasmy in cloned cattle produced by fetal and adult cell cloning. *Nat. Genet.* 2000; 25: 255–7.

[95] Amiel, G.E. and Atala, A. Current and future modalities for functional renal replacement. *Urol. Clin.* 1999; 26.

[96] Humes, H.D., Buffington, D.A., MacKay, S.M., Funke, A.J., and Weitzel, W.F. Replacement of renal function in uremic animals with a tissue-engineered kidney. *Nat. Biotechnol.* 1999; 17: 451455.

[97] Cieslinsk, D.A. and Humes, H.D. Tissue engineering of a bioartificial kidney. *Biotechnol. Bioeng.* 1994; 43: 781–91.

[98] MacKay, S.M., Kunke, A.J., Buffington, D.A., and Humes, H.D. Tissue engineering of a bioartificial renal tubule *ASAIO J.* 1998; 44: 179–83.

[99] Aebischer, P., Ip, T.K., Panol, G., and Galletti, P.M. The bioartificial kidney: progress towards an ultrafiltration device with renal epithelial cells processing. *Life Support Syst.* 1987; 5: 159–68.

[100] Ip, T., Aebischer, P., and Galletti, P.M. Cellular control of membrane permeability. Implications for a bioartificial renal tubule. *ASAIO Trans.* 1988; 34: 351–55.

[101] Humes, H.D. Renal replacement devices. In: Lanza, R.P., Langer, R., and Vacanti, J. Eds. *Principles of Tissue Engineering*, 2nd ed. San Diego: Academic Press, 2000, pp. 645–653.

[102] Amiel, A., Yoo, J., and Atala, A. Renal therapy using tissue engineered constructs and gene delivery. *J. Urol.* 2000; 18: 71–9.

[103] Lanz, R.P., Hayes, J.L., and Chick, W.L. Encapsulated cell technology. *Nat. Biotechol.* 1996; 14: 1107–11.

[104] Kuhtreiber, W.M., Lanza, R.P., and Chick, W.L. (Eds). *Cell Encapsulation Technology and Therapeutics.* Boston: Birkhauser, 1998.

[105] Lanza, R.P. and Chick, W.L. (Eds.) *Immunoisolation of Pancreatic Islets.* Austin, TX: R.G. Landes, 1994.

[106] Joki, T., Machluf, M., Atala, A., Zhu, J., Seyfried, N.T., Dunn, I.F., Abe, T., Carroll, R.S., and Black, P.M. Continuous release of endostatin from microencapsuled engineered cells for tumor therapy. *Nat. Biotechnol.* 2001; 19: 35–9.

[107] Lanza, R.P., Chung, H.Y., Yoo, J.J., Wettstein, P., Blackwell, C., Atala, A. et al. Generation of histocompatible tissues using nuclear transplantation. *Nat. Biotechnol.* 2002; 20: 689.

[108] Lanza, R.P. et al. Cloning of an endangered species (Bos gaurus) using interspecies nuclear transfer. *Cloning* 2000; 2: 79–90.

[109] Fischer Lindahl, K., Hermel, E., Loveland, B.E., and Wang, C.R. Maternally transmitted antigen of mice. *Ann. Rev. Immunol.* 1991; 9: 351–72.

[110] Hadley, G.A., Linders, B., and Mohanakumar, T. Immunogenicity of MHC class I alloantigens expressed on parenchymal cells in the human kidney. *Transplantation* 1992; 54: 537–42.

[111] Yard, B.A. et al. Analysis of T cell lines from rejecting renal allografts. *Kidney Int.* 1993; 43: S133–8.

[112] Bailey, D.W. Genetics of histocompatibility in mice. I. New loci and congenic lines. *Immunogenetics* 1975; 2: 249–56.

[113] Mohanakumar, T. The role of MHC and non-MHC antigens in allograft immunity. Austin, TX: R.G. Landes Company, 1994, pp. 1–115.

59

Hepatic Tissue Engineering for Adjunct and Temporary Liver Support

François Berthiaume
Arno W. Tilles
Mehmet Toner
Martin L. Yarmush
Harvard Medical School
Shriners Hospital for Children

Christina Chan
Harvard Medical School
Shriners Hospital for Children
Michigan State University

59.1 Introduction

Approximately 30,000 patients die each year from end-stage liver disease in the United States. About 80% of these patients have decompensated chronic liver disease, typically caused by alcoholism or chronic hepatitic C infection, and less commonly by a genetic — hepatocellular or anatomic — defect of liver function, or cancer. The other 20% die of acute liver failure (without preexisting chronic liver disease), which has various etiologies, including ischemia–reperfusion injury during liver surgery, acetaminophen poisoning, viral hepatitis, severe sepsis, idiosyncratic drug reactions, etc. Acute liver failure symptoms develop over a period of 6 weeks to 6 months and lead to death in over 80% of the cases, usually from cerebral edema, complications due to coagulopathy, and renal dysfunction. A more severe form of acute liver failure — fulminant hepatic failure — is characterized by a more rapid evolution (2 to 6 weeks).

Orthotopic liver transplantation (OLT) is the only clinically proven effective treatment for patients with end-stage liver disease. The majority of donor livers are obtained from brain-dead cadavers that still possess respiratory and circulatory functions at the time of organ retrieval. Expansion of the donor pool to include living donors, marginal and domino livers, as well as using split livers has been a major focus of transplant surgeons in the past few years. Although this may alleviate the donor organ shortage, there still remains a great potential benefit to developing alternatives that could be more cost-effective and less invasive, such as adjunct and temporary liver support. These approaches may find applications in the treatment of acute liver failure by allowing endogenous liver regeneration, as well as in chronic liver failure by ameliorating complications arising from the disease. Temporary liver support may also serve as a bridge to OLT by allowing more time to find a better match between donor and recipient or stabilize the patient prior to surgery.

59.2 Adjunct Internal Liver Support

A situation in which the native liver retains some functional capabilities is most amenable to adjunct liver support. The concept of adjunct liver support has been validated by the success of auxiliary partial liver transplantation [1,2]. However, primary nonfunction and vascular complications, for example, portal vein thrombosis, are more frequent with auxiliary partial liver transplantation than with whole liver transplantation. On the other hand, in certain situations, for example, fulminant hepatic failure (FHF), the native liver recovered and the patients could be safely removed from immunosuppressive drug therapy. Hepatocyte transplantation and hepatocyte-based implantable devices are an appealing alternative to auxiliary partial liver transplantation for several reasons (a) several patients could be treated with one single donor liver; (b) the implantation procedure could be performed using less invasive surgery; (c) isolated liver cells can be cryopreserved for long times; and (d) the liver cells could be genetically engineered *in vitro* to upregulate specific functions.

59.2.1 Hepatocyte Transplantation

Hepatocyte transplantation is the simplest form of adjunct internal liver support and has been investigated for over 25 years. In general, the efficiency of engraftment has been found to be quite low and a lag time, which may be as much as 48 h, is necessary before any clinical benefit occurs [3]. Thus, this approach offers an attractive prospect for correcting mostly nonemergency conditions such as inherited metabolic defects of the liver [4]. In early studies the choice of the transplantation site was dictated by accessibility and ease of procedure, as well as by spatial considerations: the pulmonary vascular bed, dorsal and inguinal fat pads, and peritoneal cavity. However, expression of liver-specific functions by transplanted hepatocytes could not be achieved in most of these ectopic sites. A microenvironment resembling that of liver, including a basement substrate to promote hepatocyte anchorage and a venous blood supply mimicking the mechanical and biochemical environment of the hepatic sinusoid is required [5]. The splenic pulp and the host liver itself are now the preferred sites for transplantation of hepatocytes [6]. When implanted into the spleen, hepatocytes may engraft locally or migrate into the liver. Some of the successes with hepatocyte transplantation in experimental animals, although often not very dramatic, have prompted clinical studies. The best results have been obtained in the treatment of specific metabolic disorders; however, except for one case with Crigler–Najjar syndrome type I, there was no detectable long-term function of transplanted human hepatocytes [7].

59.2.2 Implantable Devices

To improve the survival and function of implanted hepatocytes, the latter have been incorporated into biocompatible support materials, effectively constituting an implantable device. There are two major types of implantables devices (a) hepatocytes in open matrices that allow tissue — especially blood vessels — ingrowth from the host, thus leading to integration with the surrounding tissue, and (b) hepatocytes isolated from the surrounding environment in the host by a selective membrane barrier.

In early studies, isolated hepatocytes attached to collagen-coated dextran microcarriers were transplanted by intraperitoneal injection in two rat models of liver dysfunction (a) the Nagase analbuminemic rat, and (b) the Gunn rat, which has and inherited deficiency of bilirubin–uridine disphosphate glucuronosyltransferase activity causing a lack of conjugated bilirubin in the bile [8]. In both models, microcarriers promoted cell attachment, survival, and function of the transplanted hepatocytes.

Prevascularizing the cell polymer devices in combination with hepatotrophic stimulation have been used to encourage liver tissue regeneration around the implant [9]. Furthermore, materials that biodegrade at controlled rates *in vivo* (such as collagen and poly-lactic-glycolic co-polymers) can be used [10,11], and novel techniques, such as solid freeform fabrication can be used to reproducibly manufacture three-dimensional porous materials of well-defined pore size, distribution and interconnectivity [12,13]. Recently, novel biomaterials that are bioactive as well as resorbable have been developed [14]. For example, biomaterials are being designed to stimulate tissue repair through the release of factors that elicit specific cellular responses, such as cell proliferation, differentiation, and synthesis of extracellular matrix. Thus far, one of the more common approaches is to incorporate growth factors into tissue-engineering scaffolds [15,16]. There is also an interest in using "smart" materials consisting of stimuli-responsive polymers that change their properties in response to changes in the external environment [17].

59.2.3 Encapsulated Hepatocytes

A limitation of hepatocyte-based devices using open matrices is the need to use the host's own cells or at the very least an allogeneic cell source, both of which are very difficult to obtain, which seriously limits the usefulness of these devices. To circumvent this problem, there is great interest in using hepatocytes from xenogeneic sources. Since there is no immunosuppressive regimen that currently exists to prevent rejection of xenografts, hepatocytes have been encapsulated into small microspheres as well as into hollow fibers. In theory, encapsulating with a synthetic, permeable membrane provides a physical separation which protects the cells from the immune system of the host by excluding high molecular weight immunocompetent proteins (e.g., antibodies and complement) as well as leukocytes, while allowing free exchange of nutrients and oxygen. Nevertheless, if the microcapsule causes complement activation after implantation, the breakdown complement products could be small enough to enter the microcapsules and damage the transplanted cells. Initial applications of semipermeable microcapsules contained hemoglobin as blood substitute, enzymes to treat inborn errors of metabolism or absorbents to treat drug overdoses [18]. With advances in genetically engineered cells, microencapsulated cells have been used to remove ammonia in liver failure and amino acids such as phenylalanine in phenylketonuria [19]. Numerous studies have been performed with encapsulated hepatocytes without immunosuppressive drugs. Transplantation of microencapsulated xenogeneic hepatocytes into Gunn rats without immunosuppression reduced serum bilirubin levels for up to 9 weeks before returning to control rat levels, possibly due to the deterioration of the biomaterial [20]. The viability and function of encapsulated hepatocytes is highly dependent on the composition of the hollow fiber material [21]. Better results may be possible if angiogenesis near the capsule surface can be promoted [22], and the formation of a fibrotic layer around the capsule can be avoided [23].

59.3 Extracorporeal Temporary Liver Support

Extracorporeal temporary liver support systems are life-support systems that are analogous in concept to kidney dialysis machines, but specifically designed for liver failure patients. Since the liver has the ability to regenerate, temporary liver support may be sufficient to prevent patient death during the most severe phase of the illness, and allow regeneration of the host liver. The other main purpose of liver support systems is to provide a bridge to transplantation while awaiting a suitable donor. Table 59.1 provides a listing of the various techniques and systems currently being tested in a clinical setting.

59.3.1 Extracorporeal Whole Liver Perfusion

This technique was first used in humans in 1964 [24]. Xenogeneic (pig) livers were used for the first time in human studies in 1965 [25]. Although it fell out of favor due to the development of OLT, extracorporeal

TABLE 59.1   Clinical Trials for Temporary Extracorporeal Liver Support

Device[a]	Configuration	Cell mass and source	Perfusate and treatment protocol	Trial phase	Refs.
Whole liver perfusion					
Whole pig, baboon, or human liver			Whole blood, 5 h median perfusion time, most patients received 1 or 2 perfusions	I/II	[26,36]
Dialysis and filtration systems					
MARS (Teraklin AG, Rostock, Germany)	Albumin-loaded hemofilter, 60-kDa cut-off	None	Whole blood, 12–132 h	I/II	[123,124]
Liver Dialysis Unit (HemoCleanse Technologies, West Lafayette, IN)	Hemodiabsorption across 5-kDa cut-off cellulosic membranes	None	Whole blood, 6 h/day; up to 5 days	FDA approved	[38,39]
Prometheus (Fresenius Medical Care AG, Bad Homburg, Germany)	Hemofilter, 250-kD a cut-off, connected to two adsorber cartridges, in series with conventional dialyser	None	Whole blood, up to 12 h divided into 2 treatments over 2 days	I	[40,125]
Bioartificial livers					
HepatAssist (Circe Biomedical, Lexington, MA)	Hollow-fiber, polysulphone, 0.15–0.20 μm pore size	50 g cryopreserved primary porcine hepatocytes on microcarrier beads[b]	Plasma, 6 h/session; up to 14 sessions	II/III	[126–128]
BLSS (Excorp Medical, Oakdale, MN)	Hollow-fiber, cellulose acetate, 100-kDa cut-off	70–100 g primary porcine hepatocytes	Whole blood, 12 h/session; up to 2 sessions	I/II	[129,130]
MELS (Charité Virchow, Berlin, Germany)	Hollow-fiber (Interwoven, multi-compartment)	250–500 g primary porcine or human hepatocytes	Plasma, continuous up to 3 days	I/II	[131]
ELAD (Vital Therapies, La Jolla, CA)	Hollow-fiber, cellulose acetate, 120-kDa cut-off	100 g human hepatoblastoma C3A cells per cartridge, up to 4 cartridges/device	Plasma, continuous up to 107 h	II (due to resume in 2004)	[132]
AMC-BAL (Hep-Art Medical Devices, B.V., Amsterdam, The Netherlands)	Spirally wound, nonwoven polyester matrix, no membrane	70–150 g[b] primary porcine hepatocytes	Plasma, up to 18 h/session; up to 2 sessions	I	[99,133]
Radial-flow bioreactor (Sant'Anna University Hospital, Italy)	Radial-flow bioreactor	230 g primary porcine hepatocytes	Plasma, 6–24 h treatments, mostly in one session	I/II	[134]
LiverX-2000 (Algenix, Inc., Minneapolis, MN)	Cells embedded in collagen matrix within hollow-fibers	40 g primary porcine hepatocytes per cartridge, 2 cartridges/device	Blood	I/II	[135][c]
Hybrid bioartificial liver (Hepatobiliary Institute of Nanjing University, China)	Polysulfone hollow-fiber cartridge with 100-kDa cut-off combined with adsorption column	100 g primary porcine hepatocytes[b]	Plasma, one 6 h treatment, except one patient with 2 × 6 h treatments	I	[136]

[a] ELAD, Extracorporeal liver assist device; BLSS, bioartificial liver support system; MELS, modular extracorporeal liver system; AMC-BAL, Amsterdam bioartificial liver system; MARS, molecular adsorbent recycling system; FDA, Food and Drug Administration.

[b] Based on 10^8 hepatocytes/g liver tissue.

[c] Clinical data not yet published, reference describes device design.

whole liver perfusion has experienced renewed interest in recent years. Pascher et al. [26] analyzed data from nearly 200 patients from studies conducted from 1964 to 2000, and overall the study concluded that extracorporeal whole liver perfusion was not superior to conventional intensive care treatment approaches.

Early on, a major challenge of this technique was the relatively poor and unstable function of the extracorporeal liver and hemodynamic instability of the patient, which have been improved by using dual vessel (hepatic artery and portal vein) perfusion [27]. Studies in the period ranging from 1990 to 2000 have shown that patients treated with an extracorporeal liver and that survived all eventually received OLT; thus, the extracorporeal liver was potentially effective as a bridge to transplantation, but not as a substitute.

The shortage of human donors provides a strong motivation for the use of xenogeneic livers. Transgenic pigs and immunoabsorption techniques have been used to reduce the effects of hyperacute rejection [28–30]. Given that immune function is severely depressed in acute liver failure patients, this may not be necessary for perfusions lasting 24 to 36 h [31–33]. Borie et al. [34] described an alternative approach to isolate the xenogeneic liver from the host whereby a pig liver is perfused with pig blood in a secondary circuit which is separated from the host's blood by a microporous membrane. Although it appears that immune incompatibilities could be addressed, some of the data suggest that baboon and human livers may be more effective than livers from other species, suggesting an important role for proper matching of the metabolic and physiological activities of the extracorporeal liver and host [35,36].

59.3.2 Dialysis and Filtration Systems

The first attempts at developing devices for temporary and adjunct liver support consisted of nonbiological devices incorporating hemodialysis, hemofiltration, and/or plasma exchange units aimed at removing toxins accumulating in the patient's blood. Charcoal perfusion, the most extensively characterized nonbiological method, showed benefits in various animal models, but no survival benefit was reported in the only one reported randomized clinical trial [37]. Recently, there has been renewed interest in further refining these approaches, with three different systems at various stages of clinical assessment.

The Liver Dialysis Unit (Hemocleanse Technologies, West Lafayette, IN), an approved device in the United States since 1996, is a modified dialysis machine wherein blood is dialyzed against a solution that is continuously recycled through a mixture of sorbents including activated charcoal and an ion-exchange resin. In several small randomized prospectively controlled trials carried out from 1992 to 1998, patients were treated 6 h/day for 1 to 5 days, and the results showed a better outcome with patients with acute on chronic liver failure, although there was no benefit for patients with FHF [38]. The lack of benefit in FHF patients was attributed to the inability to clear strongly protein- or lipid-bound toxins, including bilirubin, endotoxin, and inflammatory cytokines, that are too big to go across the 5 kDa molecular weight cut-off of the dialysis module. A modified version of the device includes a plasma filter module wherein plasma interacts directly with the sorbent particles, thus eliminating this barrier. In preliminary clinical studies, including the plasma filter module resulted in decreases in bilirubin, aromatic amino acids, ammonium, creatinine, and inflammatory mediators such as interleukin-1β [39], but not enough information was available to make conclusions on the overall clinical benefit. A "second-generation" system is currently being designed as kit to convert an existing kidney dialysis into a liver dialysis system, and being touted as a more cost-effective system than its predecessor.

The Prometheus System (Fresenius Medical Care AG, Bad Homburg, Germany) is conceptually very similar to the competing system described above, in that it also includes of two separate modules (a) a high-flux dialyzer that removes water soluble toxins, and (b) a plasma filter module. The latter consists of a large pore (250 kDa) hollow-fiber module that enables albumin along with hydrophobic toxins bound to it to enter a closed loop circuit that contains sorbent materials that strip off the toxins and free up the binding sites on albumin before it is returned to the blood stream. A clinical study in patients with acute-on-chronic liver failure with accompanying hepatorenal syndrome shows that treatment decreased circulating levels of many toxins, such as ammonia, bilirubin, bile acids, etc. although there was no improvement in the hepatic encephalopathy score [40]. More information on clinical efficacy awaits prospective controlled studies with longer treatment periods.

The Molecular Adsorbent Recirculating System, also known as "MARS" (Teraklin, Rostock, Germany) is a device wherein the patient's blood is dialyzed against an albumin solution, the latter of which is recycled continuously over stripping columns containing various sorbent materials, including activated charcoal [41]. The dialysis membrane has a pore size of 50 kDa, which in principle allows small water-soluble toxins (such as ammonia) to escape, and a hydrophobic coating which allows albumin-bound liposoluble substances in the blood (such as bilirubin and benzodiazepines) to cross the membrane and be picked up by the albumin in the dialysate. In this design, a single module can remove both water-soluble and lipid-soluble toxins. Furthermore, the patient's blood contacts the biocompatible membrane only, and never comes into direct contact with the sorbent materials. Over 3000 patients with various etiologies of liver dysfunction have been treated with this device, and generally show neurological improvement, hemodynamic stabilization, and better hepatic and kidney functions following treatment [42,43]. The small number of controlled trials available for acute liver failure also suggest increased survival in MARS-treated patients [44–47]. Larger multicenter trials in the United States and Europe are currently under way to confirm these very encouraging, yet preliminary, findings. Evidence shows that markers of oxidative stress and systemic inflammation are also reduced after MARS treatment [48].

A meta-analysis published early in 2003 suggests that, overall, artificial liver support systems containing no cells significantly reduced mortality in acute-on-chronic liver failure, although not acute liver failure [49]. Preliminary economic evaluations of such treatments have been performed. In one study with cirrhosis patients undergoing superimposed acute liver injury, cost savings due to reduced liver-disease-related complications more than offset the additional cost of MARS treatment relative to conventional therapy [50]. In another study with patients with acute-on-chronic liver failure due to alcoholic liver disease, cumulative costs per patient in the first year were much higher in the MARS-treated group, although the main explanation appears to be an increase in mean survival time of the patients [51].

59.3.3 Bioartificial Livers

Although such devices are in principle more complex than dialysis and filtration systems, they could provide biochemical and synthetic functions that are not available in the systems containing no cells [52]. The mechanisms of liver failure are not yet well understood and the most critical hepatic functions in patients undergoing liver failure not known; therefore, it is yet unclear whether dialysis and filtration systems, which are likely to be cheaper, will supplant hepatocyte- or cell-based bioartificial livers.

59.3.3.1 Long-Term Hepatocyte Culture Systems

The availability of stable long-term liver cell culture systems that express high levels of liver-specific functions is an essential step in the development of liver-assist devices using hepatocytes. Three types of long-term culture techniques for adult hepatocytes have been used for bioartificial liver development: (a) co-culture of hepatocytes with a "feeder" cell line, such as fibroblasts, (b) three-dimensional network of collagen or other matrix, and (c) hepatocyte aggregates or spheroids. Hepatoma cell lines, which do not require specific substrate configurations, have been used as well. Some of these techniques can be combined; for example, Takezawa et al. [53,54] used thermally responsive polymer substrates to develop multicellular spheroids of fibroblasts and hepatocytes.

59.3.3.1.1 Introducing Non-Parenchymal Cells

Approximately 20 years ago, it was discovered that hepatocytes could be cultured on "feeder or supportive cells" to maintain their viability and function [55]. More recent studies showed that nonhepatic cells, even from other species, could be used. In these culture systems, cell–cell interactions among hepatocytes and cells of another type (rat liver epithelial cells, liver sinusoidal endothelial cells, or mouse embryonic fibroblasts), or "heterotypic interactions," are critical for the expression of hepatocellular functions. The disadvantages of co-culture systems include the potential variability in the cell line used, and the additional work needed to propagate that cell line in addition to attending to the isolation of hepatocytes.

It may be desirable to optimize heterotypic cell–cell interactions in order to maximize the expression of liver-specific functions of the co-cultures. Keeping in mind that cells cultured on surfaces do not usually layer onto each other (except for malignant cancer cell lines), random seeding using a low ratio of parenchymal cells to feeder cells will achieve this goal, but at the expense of using a lot of the available surface for fibroblasts, which do not provide the desired metabolic activity. On the other hand, micropatterning techniques enable the optimization of the seeding pattern of both cell types so as to ensure that each hepatocyte is near a feeder cell while minimizing the number of feeder cells [56]. As a result, metabolic function per area of culture is increased and the ultimate size of a BAL with the required functional capacity is reduced. In prior studies using circular micropatterns, function per hepatocyte increased when the hepatocyte circle diameter decreased, and function per unit area of culture increased when the space occupied by fibroblasts in-between the hepatocyte islands decreased (for a constant cell number ratio of the two cell types).

Various methods for patterning the deposition of extracellular matrix or other cell attachment factors onto surfaces have been developed [57]. Photolithography involves spin-coating a surface (typically silicon or glass) with a ~1 μm thick layer of photo-resist material, exposing the coated material to ultraviolet light through a mask which contains the pattern of interest, and treating the surface with a developer solution which dissolves the exposed regions of photo-resist only. This process leaves photo-resist in previously unexposed areas of the substrate. The exposed areas of substrate can be chemically modified for attaching proteins, etc., or treated with hydrofluoric acid to etch the material. The etching time controls the depth of the channels created. The etched surfaces produced by photolithography can be used to micromold various shapes in a polymer called poly(dimethylsiloxane) (PDMS). The PDMS cast faithfully reproduces the shape of the silicon or glass mold to the micrometer scale, and can be used in various "soft lithography" techniques, including microstamping, microfluidic patterning, and stencil patterning. An infinite number of identical PDMS casts can be generated from a single master mold, which makes the technique very inexpensive. Soft lithography methods can be used on virtually any type of surface, including curved surfaces, owing to the flexibility of PDMS.

59.3.3.1.2 *Hepatocyte Functional Heterogeneity*
In the hepatic lobule, blood flows from the periportal outer region towards the central hepatic vein. Hepatocytes in the periportal, intermediate or centrilobular, and perivenous zones exhibit different morphological and functional characteristics. Spatial heterogeneity in the hepatic lobule is clearly important for some aspects of hepatic function (Figure 59.1a). For example, urea synthesis is a process with high capacity to metabolize ammonia but low affinity for the substrate. Ammonia removal by glutamine synthesis is a high affinity process which removes traces of ammonia which cannot be metabolized by the urea cycle [58]. Co-expression of both enzyme systems would not be productive because the higher affinity process (glutamine synthesis) would be saturated under most operating conditions, leading to a reduced efficiency in ammonia extraction. On the other hand, replicating the functional heterogeneity of hepatocytes in the lobule would likely enhance the performance at the tissue level.

Functional heterogeneity also has important implications in the metabolism of hepatotoxins such as acetaminophen. Acetaminophen is normally degraded by glucuronidation and sulfation reactions which are uniformly distributed along the acinus. After acetaminophen overdose, these processes are saturated and cytochrome P450 activities primarily located in the centrilobular region metabolize significant amounts to toxic metabolites causing oxidative stress and protein cross-linking. Although these metabolites can be detoxified by glutathione-dependent reactions, centrilobular hepatocytes do not have an efficient glutathione recycling system, and as a result are the main target of acetaminophen-induced hepatotoxicity. Repeat exposure to incremental doses of acetaminophen increases the tolerance to hepatic damage by partially shifting the expression of cytochrome P450 towards the periportal region [59], which has the most active glutathione recycling metabolism in the liver [60].

The maintenance of functional heterogeneity in the liver is dependent on several factors, including gradients of hormones, substrates, oxygen, and extracellular matrix composition, although the relative importance of each one of these factors is currently unknown. In one study where hepatocytes were

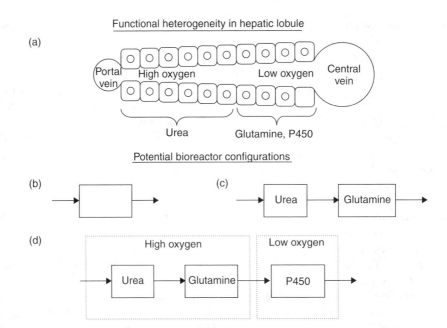

FIGURE 59.1 Potential bioreactor configurations in a bioartificial liver. (a) *In vivo* distribution of hepatocellular functions. (b) Single unit optimized to perform all functions. (c) Two subunits, the first one optimized for ammonia conversion to urea, a high capacity but low affinity process, and the second one optimized for ammonia conversion to glutamine, a high affinity process that scavenges ammonia not metabolized in the first subunit. (d) Three subunits, the first two designed to clear ammonia under high oxygen tension, and a third subunit operating at lower oxygen tension that is optimized for efficient P450 detoxification pathways.

chronically exposed to increasing oxygen tensions within the physiological range of about 5 mmHg (perivenous) to 85 mmHg (periportal), urea synthesis increased about 10 fold, while P450IA1 activity decreased slightly and albumin secretion was unchanged [61]. These data suggest that by creating environmental conditions which emulate certain parts of the liver sinusoid, it is possible to modulate hepatocyte metabolism in a way that is consistent with *in vivo* behavior. Spatial control of the layout of the cells in the device may be achieved using micropatterning and microfabrication techniques [62,63], or using separate bioreactor modules that are optimized to perform a subset of hepatocellular functions, as illustrated in Figure 59.1b–d.

It is also possible to profoundly affect the expression of liver-specific functions by hepatocytes by changing a number of environmental conditions in the bioreactor environment. For example, urea synthesis dramatically increases with increasing oxygen tension while cytochrome P450 decreases [64]. Amino acid supplementation to human plasma increases urea and albumin synthesis, as well as cytochrome P450 activities [65]. Co-culture with mouse 3T3 cells also increases albumin and urea secretion to levels which exceed *in vivo* rates severalfold [66,67]. While albumin and urea secretion decrease at higher fluid shear rates, the latter tend to increase cytochrome P450 detoxification rates, at least in the short term [68]. Sophisticated optimization techniques that can tackle the large number of adjustable environmental variables may be helpful for optimizing the bioreactor environment [69,70]. Since varying one specific environmental condition increases the expression of liver-specific functions many times, it is reasonable to assume that optimization of several such parameters simultaneously may yield an order of magnitude or more in improvement.

59.3.3.1.3 Pre-Conditioning Hepatocytes Prior to Plasma Exposure

Rat hepatocytes which are seeded and maintained in standard hepatocyte culture medium and then exposed to either rat or human plasma become severely fatty within 24 h with a concomitant reduction in

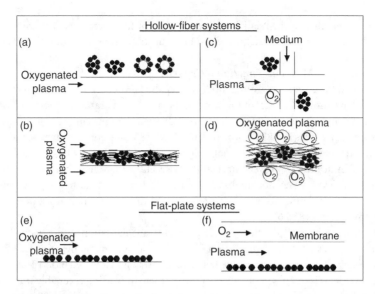

FIGURE 59.2 Most common bioreactor design for bioartificial livers. (a) Hepatocyte aggregates or seeded on microcarriers are placed on the outside of hollow fibers. Oxygenated plasma is flown through the hollow fibers. (b) Hepatocyte aggregates in a supporting matrix are inside hollow fibers and oxygenated plasma is flown outside the hollow fibers. (c) Similar to panel A, although separate hollow fibers are used to deliver hepatocyte culture medium and oxygen into the system. Circle with O_2 is a hollow fiber perpendicular to the plane of the paper. (d) Hepatocyte aggregates are in a supporting matrix next to hollow fibers that deliver oxygen. Oxygenated plasma is flown in the space outside of the hollow fibers and percolates through the matrix–hepatocyte network. (e) Hepatocytes are seeded as a monolayer on the bottom surface of a flat plate and placed within a parallel-plate flow chamber. Oxygenated plasma is flown directly above the cells. (f) System is similar to panel E, except that oxygen is delivered through a permeable membrane directly above the flow channel with the hepatocytes.

liver-specific functions. Thus, plasma appears to be a rather inhospitable environment to the hepatocytes, yet it is clear that hepatocytes must be made to tolerate it for the concept of bioartificial liver to become reality. Supplementation of human anticoagulated plasma with hormones and amino acids (to bring those metabolites to levels similar to that found in standard hepatocyte culture medium) eliminate intracellular lipid accumulation and restores albumin and urea synthesis as well as P450-dependent detoxification [71,72]. However, direct supplementation of plasma, especially with respect to the high levels of hormones used, would be very costly and pose a health risk to the patient.

In prior studies, we have shown that the culture conditions used prior to placing the hepatocytes in contact with human plasma as well as during plasma exposure, can dramatically affect hepatocellular metabolism. For example, hepatocytes cultured in standard hepatocyte culture medium containing supra-physiological levels of insulin become fatty once they are exposed to plasma, and this can be prevented by "preconditioning" the cells in a medium containing physiological levels of insulin [64]. Direct amino acid supplementation to the plasma also increased both urea and albumin secretion rates by the hepatocytes. Thus, a combination of preconditioning and plasma supplementation can be used to upregulate liver-specific functions of hepatocytes during plasma exposure.

59.3.3.2 Hepatocyte Bioreactor Designs

The most popular bioreactor designs are shown in Figure 59.2 and discussed in greater detail below. Most devices tested clinically consist of hollow fiber cartridges containing either porcine hepatocytes or human hepatoblastoma cells. In most cases, cells are loaded into the extraluminal compartment and patient plasma or blood is perfused through the fiber lumens [73–75]. Similar hollow fiber cartridges have also been used in animal studies with hepatocytes seeded inside the fibers and the plasma flowing over the outer surface of the fibers [76,77]. Because of the relatively large diameter of the fibers as well as transport limitations associated with the fiber wall, these systems are prone to substrate transport limitations [78].

59.3.3.2.1 Minimum Cell Mass and Functional Capacity

The cell mass required to support an animal model of hepatic failure has not been systematically determined. Prior studies have shown significant improvements in various parameters using as low as 2 to 3% of the normal liver mass of the animal [79,80]. Devices that have undergone clinical testing have used 6×10^9 to 1×10^{11} porcine hepatocytes [81,82] or 4×10^{10} C3A cells [83]. Recently, in an experimental pig model of hepatic failure, treatment with a bioartificial liver containing 6×10^8 pig hepatocytes (about 3 to 5% of the liver mass) significantly improved survival [84]. Recently, there have been efforts to improve cell viability in large-scale devices. Hepatocytes have been transfected with an antiapoptotic gene (nitric oxide synthase) or exposed to an antiapoptotic drug (ZVAD-fmk) to increase their resistance to what appears to be mainly hypoxic injury [85,86].

Clinical improvements have also been seen in hepatocyte transplantation studies using less than 10% of the host's liver mass. Intrasplenic transplantation of 2.5×10^7 allogeneic rat hepatocytes (about 5% of the rat liver mass) prolonged the survival, improved blood chemistry, and lowered blood TGF-β_1 (an inhibitor of hepatocyte growth) levels in anhepatic rats [87]. In another study using reversibly transformed human hepatocytes, 50×10^6 cells were injected intra-splenically into rats subjected to a 90% hepatectomy [88]. In a recent study on humans with acute liver failure, intrasplenic and intra-arterial injections of human hepatocytes (ranging from 10^9 to 4×10^{10} per patient, i.e., 1 to 10% of the total liver mass) transiently improved several blood chemistry parameters and brain function after a lag time of about 48 h, but did not improve survival [3]. The lag time before any benefit is observed may reflect the time required for the engraftment of the cells in the host liver. Better survival of the injected cells may be possible if the cells are seeded in prevascularized polymeric scaffolds [89]. The relatively low number of hepatocytes needed to effect a therapeutic benefit may be due, in part, to the fact that the exogenously supplied hepatocytes may aid the regeneration of the native liver [79].

Assuming that the minimum cell mass necessary to support a patient undergoing acute liver failure is about 5 to 10% of the total liver weight, this yields a bioartificial liver containing about 10^{10} cells. Designing this system with a priming volume not exceeding about 1 l is still a daunting challenge. Knowing which functions are most critical would help to rationally improve the efficacy of bioartificial liver systems and dramatically reduce the minimum therapeutic cell mass. For example, it is well known that hepatocytes exhibit a metabolic zonation along the acinus [61]. Periportal and centrilobular hepatocytes express high levels of urea cycle enzymes and low levels of glutamine synthetase while pericentral hepatocytes are the opposite [58]. Another example is the reduction in albumin synthesis during the acute phase response, a process which may help sustain the increased level of acute phase proteins [90].

59.3.3.2.2 Oxygen Transport Issues

In a normal liver, no hepatocyte is further than a few micrometers from circulating blood; thus, transport by diffusion only has to occur over very short distances. Although oxygen diffusivity is an order of magnitude greater that that of many other small metabolites (e.g., glucose and amino acids), it has a very low solubility in physiological fluids deprived of oxygen carriers. Thus, it is not possible to create large concentration gradients which would provide the driving force for rapid oxygen transport over long distances. This, in addition to the fact that hepatocytes have a relatively high oxygen uptake rate [91,92], makes oxygen transport the most constraining parameter in the design of BAL devices.

Oxygen transport and uptake of hepatocytes has been extensively studied in the sandwich culture configuration in order to obtain the essential oxygen uptake parameters needed in the design of bioreactor configurations [93]. The maximum oxygen uptake rate of cultured rat hepatocytes was measured to be about 13.5 pmol/sec/μg DNA, which is fairly stable after the first day in culture and for up to 2 weeks. Interestingly, the oxygen uptake was about twice in the first day after cell seeding, presumably because of the increased energy requirement for cell attachment and spreading. This may need to be taken into account when seeding hepatocytes into a BAL. Oxygen uptake was not sensitive to the oxygen tension in the vicinity of the hepatocytes up to a lower limit of about 0.5 mmHg, below which oxygen uptake decreased, suggesting that it becomes a limiting substrate for intercellular hepatocyte metabolism. Since oxygen is essential for hepatic ATP synthesis, a reasonable design criterion is that the oxygen tension should remain above ~0.5 mmHg.

Based on these parameters, it is possible to estimate oxygen concentration profiles in various bioreactor configurations based on a simple diffusion–reaction models assuming Michaelis–Menten kinetics. Generally, one can estimate that the maximum thickness of a static layer of aqueous medium on the surface of a confluent single hepatocyte layer is about 400 μm [94]. Calculations on oxygen transport through hepatocyte aggregates suggest that even a relatively low density of cells (10^7 cells/cm^3) cannot have a thickness exceeding about 300 to 500 μm. At cell densities of 10^8 cells/cm^3, which is similar to that found in normal liver, that thickness is only 100 to 200 μm.

59.3.3.2.3 Hollow-Fiber Systems

The hollow fiber system has been the most widely used type of bioreactor in BAL development [77,95]. The hollow fiber cartridge consists of a shell traversed by a large number of small diameter tubes. The cells may be placed within the fibers in the intracapillary space or on the shell side in the extracapillary space. The compartment which does not contain the cells is generally perfused with culture medium or the patient's plasma or blood. The fiber walls may provide the attaching surface for the cells and/or act as barrier against the immune system of the host. Microcarriers have also been used as a way to provide an attachment surface for anchorage-dependent cells introduced in the shell side of hollow fiber devices. There are many studies on how to determine optimal fiber dimensions, spacing, and reactor length based on oxygen transport considerations [78].

One difficulty with the hollow fiber configuration is that interfiber distances, and consequently transport properties within the shell space, are not well controlled. Thus, it may be advantageous to place cells in the lumen of small fibers because the diffusional distance between the shell (where the nutrient supply would be) and the cells is essentially equal to the fiber thickness. In one configuration, hepatocytes have been suspended in a collagen solution and injected into the lumen of fibers where the collagen is allowed to gel. Contraction of the collagen lattice by the cells even creates a void in the intraluminal space, which can theoretically be perfused with hormonal supplements, etc. to enhance the viability and function of the cells, while the patient's plasma flows on the shell side. Because of the relatively large diameter of the fibers used as well as transport limitations associated with the fiber wall, these systems have been prone to substrate transport limitations.

To improve oxygen delivery, novel designs using additional fibers which carry gaseous oxygen straight into the device have been used [96,97]. Using this approach, Gerlach et al. [82] were able to demonstrate that hepatocytes could express differentiated functions over several weeks. Using a device consisting of hepatocytes seeded onto a woven polyester substrate with integrated hollow fibers for oxygen supply, Flendrig et al. [96,98] showed that the survival time of pigs undergoing total hepatic ischemia was significantly increased over the control group; more recently, this device was successfully used to treat seven acute liver failure patients, of which six were bridged to a transplant and one spontaneously recovered [99].

59.3.3.2.4 Parallel Plate Systems

An alternative bioreactor configuration is based on a flat surface geometry [80,93,100,101] where it is easier to control the internal flow distribution and ensure that all cells are adequately perfused. Its main drawback is that it is difficult to build a system which contains a sufficient cell concentration (Figure 59.3). For example, a channel height of 1 mm would result in a 10 l reactor to support 20×10^9 hepatocytes cultured on an area of 10 m^2. For a liver failure patient who is probably hemodynamically unstable, it is generally accepted that the priming volume of the system should not exceed 1 l.

The volume of the device in the flat-plate geometry can be decreased by reducing the channel height (Figure 59.3). However, this forces the fluid to move through a smaller gap, which rapidly increases the drag force (shear stress) imparted by the flow on the cells. Recent data suggest that hepatocyte function decreases significantly at shear stresses >5 dyn/cm^2 [102]. To reduce the deleterious effects of high shear,

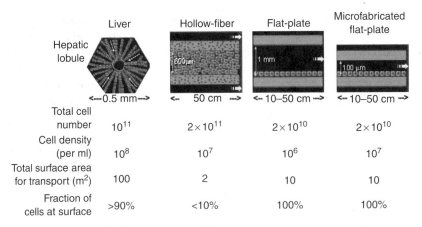

	Liver	Hollow-fiber	Flat-plate	Microfabricated flat-plate
	Hepatic lobule			
	<---0.5 mm--->	<- 50 cm ->	<- 10–50 cm ->	<- 10–50 cm ->
Total cell number	10^{11}	2×10^{11}	2×10^{10}	2×10^{10}
Cell density (per ml)	10^{8}	10^{7}	10^{6}	10^{7}
Total surface area for transport (m^2)	100	2	10	10
Fraction of cells at surface	>90%	<10%	100%	100%

FIGURE 59.3   Comparison between popular hepatocyte bioreactor configurations.

it may be possible to use grooved surfaces where cells lodge and are less exposed to the shear stress, as previously done for blood cells [103,104]. Cells lodge inside the grooves where they are less exposed to the shear stress, which allows for faster flow without causing cell damage. The grooves may on the other hand significantly increase the fluid hold-up volume [105].

In an attempt to provide to cells adequate oxygenation and protection from shear in perfused bioreactors, gas-permeable membranes as well as membranes separating cells from plasma have been incorporated into the flat-plate geometry. Recently, a flat-plate microchannel bioreactor where cells directly contact the circulating medium was developed [93]. The channel is closed by a gas-permeable membrane on one surface, which decouples oxygen transport from the flow rate in the device. Comparing this with a similar flat-plate design where a nonpermeable glass surface is substituted to the membrane, internal membrane oxygenation removed the oxygen limitations that occur at low volumetric flow rates [105]. De Bartolo et al. [80] incorporated two membranes into the flat-plate geometry. The first membrane is gas-permeable and minimizes the oxygen transport limitations in the system. The second membrane separates cells from plasma and adds a significant barrier to the transport of protein-bound toxins that need to be processed by the cells [78]. Others have reported the design of a radial flow bioreactor with an internal membrane oxygenator for the culture of hematopoietic cells [106]. Based on a theoretical analysis, the proposed design would have removed oxygen transport limitations in the bioreactor, but no experimental data were shown.

59.3.3.3   Potential Sources of Cells for Bioartificial Livers

Although several technical difficulties remain to be addressed with respect to the design of implantable and extracorporeal liver-assist devices, clearly a major hurdle for both approaches is the procurement of a sufficient number of cells that are required to achieve a therapeutic effect. Human hepatocytes appear to be the "natural" choice for hepatocyte transplantation, internal and external liver assist devices, however, they are scarce due to a competing demand of OLT. Whether adult human hepatocytes can be induced to replicate *in vitro* and the daughter cells express high levels of liver-specific functions remains to be shown. Human hepatocyte cell lines have been developed via spontaneous transformation [107], as well as via retroviral transfection of the simian virus 40 large T antigen [108]. Recently, a novel technology which uses a reversible transformation strategy with the SV40 T antigen and Cre–Lox recombination was used to grow human hepatocytes *in vitro* [88]. These cells, when transplanted into the spleen of 90% hepatectomized rats, improved biochemical and clinical parameters. In bioartificial liver devices tested so far, the only human cells used have been the cancer-derived C3A line [74,83]. However, one study suggests that C3A cells have lower levels of P450IA1 activity, ammonia removal, and amino acid metabolism that adult porcine hepatocytes [109]. Furthermore, when using immortalized human cell lines, there are concerns with the possibility of transmission of tumorigenic products into the patient. Xenogeneic hepatocytes offer no risk of transmitting malignancies to the patient, but pose other problems, including the risk of hyperacute rejection [110], transmission of zoonoses [111], and potential mismatch between xenogeneic and human liver functions. The first two could be addressed by dedicated breeding programs of transgenic animals. On the other hand, little is known about the third factor.

Although no one has achieved the goal of generating a safe, fully functional yet clonal, immortalized, or genetically engineered human cell that can be substituted for primary hepatocytes, a new promising avenue is the discovery of liver stem cells. The existence of hepatic stem cells was hypothesized over 40 years ago [112], and recent data suggest that there are stem cells present within [113–115] as well as outside the liver [116], which can differentiate into fully mature hepatocytes. *In vitro* studies suggest the presence of a subpopulation of small hepatocytes in rat liver with a high proliferative potential [117]. Three independent studies in rats, mice, and humans have shown that a major extrahepatic source is stem cells of the bone marrow which may take part in normal tissue renewal as well as in liver regeneration after severe experimentally induced hepatic injury [116,118,119].

59.3.3.4 Techniques for Preservation of Hepatocytes and Liver Cells

The development of optimal preservation protocols for hepatocytes that enable the storage and ready availability of cells for BALs, has been the subject of several studies. Hepatocytes have been cryopreserved shortly after isolation as well as after culture for several days. Compared to isolated cells, cultured hepatocytes exhibit greater resistance to high concentrations of the cryoprotective agent dimethyl sulfoxide, as evidenced by preservation of cell viability, cytoskeleton, and function. Based on experimental and theoretical studies, cooling rates between 5 and 10°C/min caused no significant decrease in albumin secretion rate compared to control, unfrozen, cultures [120,121]. There have been attempts to store hepatocyte cultures in various solutions used for cold storage of whole donor livers. One study showed that cultured hepatocytes maintained at 4°C lose significant viability after a few hours of cold storage, but that addition of polyethylene glycol significantly extends functionality and survival [122]. Interestingly, the use of the University of Wisconsin (UW) solution, currently the most widely used solution for cold organ storage, has not performed better than leaving the cells in standard hepatocyte culture medium. It is conceivable that the UW solution mediates its effect by prolonging the survival of nonparenchymal cells. It is hoped that further improvements in preservation solutions will enable the storage of BAL systems, as well as lengthen the useful cold storage time of whole livers for transplantation.

59.4 Summary

The severe donor liver shortage, high cost, and complexity of orthotopic liver transplantation have prompted the search for alternative treatment strategies for end-stage liver disease that would require less donor material, be cheaper, and less invasive. Adjunct internal liver support, which may be provided via auxiliary partial liver transplantation or hepatocyte transplantation, is most suitable for cases where the native liver retains some functional capabilities, and may be a cure for patients who suffer from specific metabolic disorders. Acute liver failure patients will benefit most from extracorporeal temporary liver support, which can be used as a bridge to transplantation, or as a means to support the patient until its own liver regenerates. Currently, there are three approaches for extracorporeal temporary liver support: extracorporeal liver perfusion, dialysis and filtration systems containing no cells, and bioartificial livers. Dialysis and filtration systems, which do not contain any living cells, are ahead with respect to clinical testing and gaining regulatory approval. A concern with such systems is that their efficacy may be limited due to the lack of metabolic and protein synthetic activities which are normally present in the liver. Bioartificial livers containing liver cells would overcome this limitation, and have passed the "proof of principle" test in preclinical and clinical studies, although tangible clinical benefits have not yet been demonstrated. Important unresolved issues for bioartificial livers and extracorporeal liver perfusion are the identification of a reliable cell/tissue source and a better understanding of metabolic and immune incompatibilities arising from the use of allogeneic and xenogeneic liver cells. Ultimately, several temporary and adjunct treatment approaches may be available, and the best choice may depend on the etiology of liver failure in each individual patient.

Acknowledgments

This work was partially supported by the NIH grant R01 DK37743 and the Shriners Hospitals for Children.

References

[1] Boudjema, K. et al., Auxiliary liver transplantation and bioartificial bridging procedures in treatment of acute liver failure, *World J. Surg.*, 26, 264, 2002.

[2] Azoulay, D. et al., Auxiliary partial orthotopic versus standard orthotopic whole liver transplantation for acute liver failure: a reappraisal from a single center by a case-control study, *Ann. Surg.*, 234, 723, 2001.

[3] Bilir, B.M. et al., Hepatocyte transplantation in acute liver failure, *Liver Transplant.*, 6, 32, 2000.

[4] Fox, I.J. et al., Treatment of the Crigler-Najjar syndrome type I with hepatocyte transplantation, *N. Engl. J. Med.*, 338, 1422, 1998.

[5] Fox, I.J. and Roy-Chowdhury, J., Hepatocyte transplantation, *J. Hepatol.*, 40, 878, 2004.

[6] Gupta, S., Bhargava, K.K., and Novikoff, P.M., Mechanisms of cell engraftment during liver repopulation with hepatocyte transplantation, *Semin. Liver Dis.*, 19, 15, 1999.

[7] Fox, I.J. and Chowdhury, J.R., Hepatocyte transplantation, *Am. J. Transpl.*, 4, 7, 2004.

[8] Demetriou, A.A. et al., Survival, organization, and function of microcarrier-attached hepatocytes transplanted in rats, *Proc. Natl Acad. Sci. USA*, 83, 7475, 1986.

[9] Fontaine, M. et al., Human hepatocyte isolation and transplantation into an athymic rat, using prevascularized cell polymer constructs, *J. Pediatr. Surg.*, 30, 56, 1995.

[10] Hasirci, V. et al., Expression of liver-specific functions by rat hepatocytes seeded in treated poly(lactic-co-glycolic) acid biodegradable foams, *Tissue Eng.*, 7, 385, 2001.

[11] Ranucci, C.S. et al., Control of hepatocyte function on collagen foams: sizing matrix pores toward selective induction of 2-D and 3-D cellular morphogenesis, *Biomaterials*, 21, 783, 2000.

[12] Sachols, E. and Czernuszka, J.T., Making tissue engineering scaffolds work. Review on the application of solid freeform fabrication technology to the production of tissue engineering scaffolds, *Eur. Cells Mater.*, 5, 29, 2003.

[13] Leong, K.F., Cheah, C.M., and Chua, C.K., Solid freeform fabrication of three-dimensional scaffolds for engineering replacement tissues and organs, *Biomaterials*, 295, 2363, 2003.

[14] Hench, L.L. and Polak, J.M., Third-generation biomedical materials, *Science*, 295, 1014, 2002.

[15] Whitaker, M.J. et al., Growth factor release from tissue engineering scaffolds, *J. Phar. Pharmacol.*, 53, 1427, 2001.

[16] Sakai, Y. et al., *In vitro* organization of biohybrid rat liver tissue incorporating growth factor- and hormone-releasing biodegradable polymer microcapsules, *Cell Transplant.*, 10, 479, 2001.

[17] Jeong, B. and Gutowska, A., Lessons from nature: stimuli-responsive polymers and their biomedical applications, *Trends Biotechnol.*, 20, 305, 2002.

[18] Chang, T.M. and Prakash, S., Therapeutic uses of microencapsulated genetically engineered cells, *Mol. Med. Today*, 4, 221, 1998.

[19] Lanza, R.P., Hayes, J.L., and Chick, W.L., Encapsulated cell technology, *Nat. Biotechnol.*, 14, 1107, 1996.

[20] Gomez, N. et al., Evidence for survival and metabolic activity of encapsulated xenogeneic hepatocytes transplanted without immunosuppression in Gunn rats, *Transplantation*, 63, 1718, 1997.

[21] Yang, M.B., Vacanti, J.P., and Ingber, D.E., Hollow fibers for hepatocyte encapsulation and transplantation: studies of survival and function in rats, *Cell Transplant.*, 3, 373, 1994.

[22] Yoon, J.J. et al., Surface immobilization of galactose onto aliphatic biodegradable polymers for hepatocyte culture, *Biotechnol. Bioeng.*, 78, 1, 2002.

[23] Granicka, L.H. et al., Polypropylene hollow fiber for cells isolation: methods for evaluation of diffusive transport and quality of cells encapsulation, *Artif. Cells Blood Substit. Immobil. Biotechnol.*, 31, 249, 2003.

[24] Sen, P.K. et al., Use of isolated perfused cadaveric liver in the management of hepatic failure, *Surgery*, 59, 774, 1966.

[25] Eiseman, B.,Liem, D.S., and Raffucci, F., Heterologous liver perfusion in treatment of hepatic failure, *Ann. Surg.*, 162, 329, 1965.

[26] Pascher, A. et al., Extracorporeal liver perfusion as hepatic assist in acute liver failure: a review of world experience, *Xenotransplantation*, 9, 309, 2002.

[27] Mora, N. et al., Single vs. dual vessel porcine extracorporeal liver perfusion, *J. Surg. Res.*, 103, 228, 2002.

[28] Pascher, A. et al., Immunopathological observations after xenogeneic liver perfusions using donor pigs transgenic for human decay-accelerating factor, *Transplantation*, 64, 384, 1997.

[29] Pascher, A. et al., Application of immunoapheresis for delaying hyperacute rejection during isolated xenogeneic pig liver perfusion, *Transplantation*, 63, 867, 1997.

[30] Pascher, A. et al., Impact of immunoadsorption on complement activation, immunopathology, and hepatic perfusion during xenogeneic pig liver perfusion, *Transplantation*, 65, 737, 1998.

[31] Tector, A.J. et al., Mechanisms of resistance to injury in pig livers perfused with blood from patients in liver failure, *Transplant. Proc.*, 29, 966, 1997.

[32] Horslen, S.P. et al., Extracorporeal liver perfusion using human and pig livers for acute liver failure, *Transplantation*, 70, 1472, 2000.

[33] Collins, B.H. et al., Immunopathology of porcine livers perfused with blood of humans with fulminant hepatic failure, *Transplant. Proc.*, 27, 280, 1995.

[34] Borie, D.C. et al., Functional metabolic characteristics of intact pig livers during prolonged extracorporeal perfusion: potential for a unique biological liver-assist device, *Transplantation*, 72, 393, 2001.

[35] Foley, D.P. et al., Bile acids in xenogeneic *ex-vivo* liver perfusion: function of xenoperfused livers and compatibility with human bile salts and porcine livers, *Transplantation*, 69, 242, 2000.

[36] Pascher, A., Sauer, I.M., and Neuhaus, P., Analysis of allogeneic versus xenogeneic auxiliary organ perfusion in liver failure reveals superior efficacy of human livers, *Int. J. Artif. Organs*, 25, 1006, 2002.

[37] O'Grady, J.G. et al., Controlled trials of charcoal haemoperfusion and prognostic factors in fulminant hepatic failure, *Gastroenterology*, 94, 1186, 1998.

[38] Ash, S.R. et al., Push-pull sorbent-based pheresis and hemodiabsorption in the treatment of hepatic failure: preliminary results of a clinical trial with the BioLogic-DTPF System, *Ther. Apher.*, 4, 218, 2000.

[39] Ash, S.R. et al., Treatment of acetaminophen-induced hepatitis and fulminant hepatic failure with extracorporeal sorbent-based devices, *Adv. Ren. Replace Ther.*, 9, 42, 2002.

[40] Rifai, K. et al., Prometheus((R)) — a new extracorporeal system for the treatment of liver failure (small star, filled), *J. Hepatol.*, 39, 984, 2003.

[41] Stange, J. et al., Molecular adsorbent recycling system (MARS): clinical results of a new membrane-based blood purification system for bioartificial liver support, *Artif. Organs*, 23, 319, 1999.

[42] Butterworth, R.F., Role of circulating neurotoxins in the pathogenesis of hepatic encephalopathy: potential for improvement following their removal by liver assist devices, *Liver Int.*, 23, 5, 2003.

[43] Mitzner, S. et al., Improvement in central nervous system functions during treatment of liver failure with albumin dialysis MARS — a review of clinical, biochemical, and electrophysiological data, *Metab. Brain Dis.*, 17, 463, 2002.

[44] Heemann, U. et al., Albumin dialysis in cirrhosis with superimposed acute liver injury: a prospective, controlled study, *Hepatology*, 36, 949, 2002.

[45] Chen, S. et al., Molecular adsorbent recirculating system: clinical experience in patients with liver failure based on hepatitis B in China, *Liver*, 22, 48, 2002.

[46] Schmidt, L.E. et al., Systemic hemodynamic effects of treatment with the molecular adsorbents recirculating system in patients with hyperacute liver failure: a prospective controlled trial, *Liver Transpl.*, 9, 290, 2003.

[47] Mitzner, S.R. et al., Improvement of hepatorenal syndrome with extracorporeal albumin dialysis MARS: results of a prospective, randomized, controlled clinical trial, *Liver Transplant.*, 6, 277, 2000.

[48] Sen, S., Jalan, R., and Williams, R., Liver failure: basis of benefit of therapy with the molecular adsorbents recirculating system, *Int. J. Biochem. Cell Biol.*, 35, 1306, 2003.

[49] Kjaergard, L.L. et al., Artificial and bioartificial support systems for acute and acute-on-chronic liver failure: a systematic review, *JAMA*, 289, 217, 2003.

[50] Hassanein, T. et al., Albumin dialysis in cirrhosis with superimposed acute liver injury: possible impact of albumin dialysis on hospitalization costs, *Liver Int.*, 23, 61, 2003.

[51] Hessel, F.P. et al., Economic evaluation and 1-year survival analysis of MARS in patients with alcoholic liver disease, *Liver Int.*, 23, 66, 2003.

[52] Chamuleau, R.A., Artificial liver support in the third millennium, *Artif. Cells Blood Substit. Immobil. Biotechnol.*, 31, 117, 2003.

[53] Takezawa, T. et al., Morphological and immuno-cytochemical characterization of a hetero-spheroid composed of fibroblasts and hepatocytes, *J. Cell Sci.*, 101, 495, 1992.

[54] Takezawa, T. et al., Characterization of morphology and cellular metabolism during the spheroid formation by fibroblasts, *Exp. Cell Res.*, 208, 430, 1993.

[55] Guguen-Guillouzo, C. et al., Maintenance and reversibility of active albumin secretion by adult rat hepatocytes co-cultured with another liver epithelial cell type, *Exp. Cell Res.*, 143, 47, 1983.

[56] Bhatia, S.N. et al., Effect of cell–cell interactions in preservation of cellular phenotype: cocultivation of hepatocytes and nonparenchymal cells, *FASEB J.*, 13, 1883, 1999.

[57] Folch, A. and Toner, M., Microengineering of cellular interactions, *Annu. Rev. Biomed. Eng.*, 2, 227, 2000.

[58] Häussinger, D., Gerok, W., and Sies, H., Regulation of flux through glutaminase and glutamine synthetase in isolated perfused rat liver, *Biochim. Biophys. Acta*, 755, 272, 1983.

[59] Shayiq, R.M. et al., Repeat exposure to incremental doses of acetaminophen provides protection against acetaminophen-induced lethality in mice: an explanation for high acetaminophen dosage in humans without hepatic injury, *Hepatology*, 29, 451, 1999.

[60] Kera, Y., Penttila, K.E., and Lindros, K.O., Glutathione replenishment capacity is lower in isolated perivenous than in periportal hepatocytes, *Biochem. J.*, 254, 411, 1988.

[61] Bhatia, S.N. et al., Zonal liver cell heterogeneity: effects of oxygen on metabolic functions of hepatocytes, *Cell Eng.*, 1, 125, 1996.

[62] Bhatia, S.N. et al., Selective adhesion of hepatocytes on patterned surfaces, *Ann. NY Acad. Sci. USA*, 745, 187, 1994.

[63] Bhatia, S.N., Yarmush, M.L., and Toner, M., Controlling cell interactions by micropatterning in co-cultures: hepatocytes and 3T3 fibroblasts, *J. Biomed. Mater. Res.*, 34, 189, 1997.

[64] Chan, C. et al., Metabolic flux analysis of hepatocyte function in hormone- and amino acid-supplemented plasma, *Metab. Eng.*, 5, 1, 2003.

[65] Washizu, J. et al., Optimization of rat hepatocyte culture in citrated human plasma, *J. Surg. Res.*, 93, 237, 2000.

[66] Bhatia, S.N. et al., Probing heterotypic cell interactions: hepatocyte function in microfabricated co-cultures, *J. Biomater. Sci. Polym. Ed.*, 9, 1137, 1998.

[67] Bhatia, S.N. et al., Microfabrication of hepatocyte/fibroblast co-cultures: role of homotypic cell interactions, *Biotechnol. Prog.*, 14, 378, 1998.

[68] Roy, P. et al., Effect of flow on the detoxification function of rat hepatocytes in a bioartificial liver reactor, *Cell Transplant.*, 10, 609, 2001.

[69] Chan, C. et al., Application of multivariate analysis to optimize function of cultured hepatocytes, *Biotechnol. Prog.*, 19, 580, 2003.

[70] Chan, C. et al., Metabolic flux analysis of cultured hepatocytes exposed to plasma, *Biotechnol. Bioeng.*, 81, 33, 2003.

[71] Washizu, J. et al., Amino acid supplementation improves cell-specific functions of the rat hepatocytes exposed to human plasma, *Tissue Eng.*, 6, 497, 2000.

[72] Washizu, J. et al., Long-term maintenance of cytochrome P450 activities by rat hepatocyte/3T3 cell co-cultures in heparinized human plasma, *Tissue Eng.*, 7, 691, 2001.

[73] Watanabe, F.D. et al., Clinical experience with a bioartificial liver in the treatment of severe liver failure. A phase I clinical trial, *Ann. Surg.*, 225, 484, 1997.

[74] Kamohara, Y.,Rozga, J., and Demetriou, A.A., Artificial liver: review and Cedars–Sinai experience, *J. Hepatobil. Pancreat. Surg.*, 5, 273, 1998.

[75] Ellis, A.J. et al., Pilot-controlled trial of the extracorporeal liver assist device in acute liver failure, *Hepatology*, 24, 1446, 1996.

[76] Hu, W.-S. et al., Development of a bioartificial liver employing xenogeneic hepatocytes, *Cytotechnology*, 23, 29, 1997.

[77] Tzanakakis, E.S. et al., Extracorporeal tissue engineered liver-assist devices, *Annu. Rev. Biomed. Eng.*, 2, 607, 2000.

[78] Catapano, G., Mass transfer limitations to the performance of membrane bioartificial liver support devices, *Int. J. Artif. Organs*, 19, 18, 1996.

[79] Eguchi, S. et al., Loss and recovery of liver regeneration in rats with fulminant hepatic failure, *J. Surg. Res.*, 72, 112, 1997.

[80] De Bartolo, L. et al., A novel full-scale flat membrane bioreactor utilizing porcine hepatocytes: cell viability and tissue-specific functions, *Biotechnol. Prog.*, 16, 102, 2000.

[81] Rozga, J. et al., Development of a hybrid bioartificial liver, *Ann. Surg.*, 217, 502, 1993.

[82] Gerlach, J.C. et al., Bioreactor for a larger scale hepatocyte *in vitro* perfusion, *Transplantation*, 58, 984, 1994.

[83] Sussman, N.L. et al., The Hepatix extracorporeal liver assist device: initial clinical experience, *Artif. Organs*, 18, 390, 1994.

[84] Cuervas-Mons, V. et al., *In vivo* efficacy of a bioartificial liver in improving spontaneous recovery from fulminant hepatic failure: a controlled study in pigs, *Transplantation*, 69, 337, 2000.

[85] Tzeng, E. et al., Adenovirus-mediated inducible nitric oxide synthase gene transfer inhibits hepatocyte apoptosis, *Surgery*, 124, 278, 1998.

[86] Nyberg, S.L. et al., Cytoprotective influence of ZVAD-fmk and glycine on gel-entrapped rat hepatocytes in a bioartificial liver, *Surgery*, 127, 447, 2000.

[87] Arkadopoulos, N. et al., Intrasplenic transplantation of allogeneic hepatocytes prolongs survival in anhepatic rats, *Hepatology*, 28, 1365, 1998.

[88] Kobayashi, N. et al., Prevention of acute liver failure in rats with reversibly immortalized human hepatocytes, *Science*, 287, 1258, 2000.

[89] Kim, S.S. et al., Survival and function of hepatocytes on a novel three-dimensional synthetic polymer scaffold with an intrinsic network of channels, *Ann. Surg.*, 228, 8, 1998.

[90] Baumann, H. and Gauldie, J., The acute phase response, *Immunol. Today*, 15, 74, 1994.

[91] Rotem, A. et al., Oxygen uptake rates in cultured hepatocytes, *Biotechnol. Bioeng.*, 40, 1286, 1992.

[92] Rotem, A. et al., Oxygen is a factor determining *in vitro* tissue assembly: effects on attachment and spreading of hepatocytes, *Biotechnol. Bioeng.*, 43, 654, 1994.

[93] Tilles, A.W. et al., Critical issues in bioartificial liver development, *Technol. Health Care*, 10, 177, 2002.

[94] Yarmush, M.L. et al., Hepatic tissue engineering. Development of critical technologies, *Ann. N. Y. Acad. Sci. USA*, 665, 238, 1992.

[95] Allen, J.W., Hassanein, T., and Bhatia, S.N., Advances in bioartificial liver devices, *Hepatology*, 34, 447, 2001.

[96] Flendrig, L.M. et al., *In vitro* evaluation of a novel bioreactor based on an integral oxygenator and a spirally wound nonwoven polyester matrix for hepatocyte culture as small aggregates, *J. Hepatol.*, 26, 1379, 1997.

[97] Sauer, I.M. et al., Development of a hybrid liver support system, *Ann. NY Acad. Sci.*, 944, 308, 2001.

[98] Flendrig, L.M. et al., Significantly improved survival time in pigs with complete liver ischemia treated with a novel bioartificial liver, *Int. J. Artif. Organs*, 22, 701, 1999.

[99] van de Kerkhove, M.P. et al., Phase I clinical trial with the AMC-bioartificial liver, *Int. J. Artif. Organs*, 25, 950, 2002.

[100] Kan, P. et al., Effects of shear stress on metabolic function of the co-culture system of hepatocyte/nonparenchymal cells for a bioartificial liver, *ASAIO J.*, 44, M441, 1998.

[101] Taguchi, K. et al., Development of a bioartificial liver with sandwiched-cultured hepatocytes between two collagen gel layers, *Artif. Organs*, 20, 178, 1996.

[102] Tilles, A.W. et al., Effects of oxygenation and flow on the viability and function of rat hepatocytes cocultured in a microchannel flat-plate bioreactor, *Biotechnol. Bioeng.*, 73, 379, 2001.

[103] Sandstrom, C.E. et al., Development of novel perfusion chamber to retain nonadherent cells and its use for comparison of human "mobilized" peripheral blood mononuclear cell cultures with and without irradiated bone marrow stroma, *Biotechnol. Bioeng.*, 50, 493, 1996.

[104] Horner, M. et al., Transport in a grooved perfusion flat-bed bioreactor for cell therapy applications, *Biotechnol. Prog.*, 14, 689, 1998.

[105] Roy, P. et al., Analysis of oxygen transport to hepatocytes in a flat-plate microchannel bioreactor, *Ann. Biomed. Eng.*, 29, 947, 2001.

[106] Peng, C.A. and Palsson, B.O., Determination of specific oxygen uptake rates in human hematopoietic cultures and implications for bioreactor design, *Ann. Biomed. Eng.*, 24, 373, 1996.

[107] Roberts, E.A. et al., Characterization of human hepatocyte lines derived from normal liver tissue, *Hepatology*, 19, 1390, 1994.

[108] Kobayashi, N. et al., Transplantation of highly differentiated immortalized human hepatocytes to treat acute liver failure, *Transplantation*, 69, 202, 2000.

[109] Wang, L. et al., Comparison of porcine hepatocytes with human hepatoma (C3A) cells for use in a bioartificial liver support system, *Cell Transplant.*, 7, 459, 1998.

[110] Butler, D., Last chance to stop and think on risks of xenotransplants, *Nature*, 391, 320, 1998.

[111] Le Tissier, P. et al., Two sets of human-tropic pig retrovirus, *Nature*, 389, 681, 1997.

[112] Wilson, J.W. and Leduc, R.H., Role of cholangioles in restoration of the liver of the mouse after dietary injury, *J. Pathol. Bacteriol.*, 76, 441, 1958.

[113] Sigal, S.H. et al., The liver as a stem cell and lineage system, *Am. J. Physiol.*, 263, G139, 1992.

[114] Thorgeirsson, S.S., Hepatic stem cells in liver regeneration, *FASEB J.*, 10, 1249, 1996.

[115] Theise, N.D. et al., The canals of Hering and hepatic stem cells in humans, *Hepatology*, 30, 1425, 1999.

[116] Theise, N.D. et al., Liver from bone marrow in humans, *Hepatology*, 32, 11, 2000.

[117] Tateno, C. et al., Heterogeneity of growth potential of adult rat hepatocytes *in vitro*, *Hepatology*, 31, 65, 2000.

[118] Theise, N.D. et al., Derivation of hepatocytes from bone marrow cells in mice after radiation-induced myeloablation, *Hepatology*, 31, 235, 2000.

[119] Petersen, B.E. et al., Bone marrow as a potential source of hepatic oval cells, *Science*, 284, 1168, 1999.

[120] Borel-Rinkes, I.H.M. et al., Nucleation and growth of ice crystals insude cultured hepatocytes during freezing in the presence of dimethylsulfoxide, *Biophys. J.*, 65, 2524, 1993.

[121] Karlsson, J.O.M. et al., Long-term functional recovery of hepatocytes after cryopreservation in a three-dimensional culture configuration, *Cell Transplant.*, 1, 281, 1992.

[122] Stefanovich, P. et al., Effects of hypothermia on the function, membrane integrity, and cytoskeletal structure of hepatocytes, *Cryobiology*, 23, 389, 1995.

[123] Stange, J. et al., The molecular adsorbents recycling system as a liver support system based on albumin dialysis: a summary of preclinical investigations, prospective, randomized, controlled clinical trial, and clinical experience from 19 centers, *Artif. Organs*, 26, 103, 2002.

[124] Chang, M.-H. et al., Albumin dialysis MARS 2003, *Liver Int.*, 23, 3, 2003.

[125] Kramer, L. et al., Successful treatment of refractory cerebral oedema in ecstasy/cocaine-induced fulminant hepatic failure using a new high-efficacy liver detoxification device (FPSA-Prometheus), *Wien. Klin. Wochenschr.*, 115, 599, 2003.

[126] Samuel, D. et al., Neurological improvement during bioartificial liver sessions in patients with acute liver failure awaiting transplantation, *Transplantation*, 73, 257, 2002.

[127] Pazzi, P. et al., Serum bile acids in patients with liver failure supported with a bioartificial liver, *Aliment. Pharmacol. Ther.*, 16, 1547, 2002.

[128] Demetriou, A.A. et al., Prospective, randomized, multicenter, controlled trial of a bioartificial liver in treating acute liver failure, *Ann. Surg.*, 239, 660, 2004.

[129] Patzer II, J. et al., Bioartificial liver assist devices in support of patients with liver failure, *Hepatobiliary Pancreat. Dis. Int.*, 1, 18, 2002.

[130] Mazariegos, G.V. et al., Safety observations in phase I clinical evaluation of the Excorp Medical Bioartificial Liver Support System after the first four patients, *ASAIO J.*, 47, 471, 2001.

[131] Sauer, I.M. et al., Clinical extracorporeal hybrid liver support — phase I study with primary porcine liver cells, *Xenotransplantation*, 10, 460, 2003.

[132] Millis, J.M. et al., Initial experience with the modified extracorporeal liver-assist device for patients with fulminant hepatic failure: system modifications and clinical impact, *Transplantation*, 74, 1735, 2002.

[133] van de Kerkhove, M.P. et al., Bridging a patient with acute liver failure to liver transplantation by the AMC-bioartificial liver phase I clinical trial with the AMC-bioartificial liver, *Cell Transplant.*, 12, 563, 2003.

[134] Morsiani, E. et al., Early experiences with a porcine hepatocyte-based bioartificial liver in acute hepatic failure patients, *Int. J. Artif. Organs*, 25, 192, 2002.

[135] Sielaff, T.D. et al., Characterization of the three-compartment gel-entrapment porcine hepatocyte bioartificial liver, *Cell Biol. Toxicol.*, 13, 357, 1997.

[136] Ding, Y.-T. et al., The development of a new bioartificial liver and its application in 12 acute liver failure patients, *World J. Gastroenterol.*, 9, 829, 2003.

60

Tissue Engineering of Renal Replacement Therapy

William H. Fissell
H. David Humes
University of Michigan

60.1 Background

The kidney is unique among body organs in that it is the first organ for which maintenance replacement therapy has become available and widespread. At the time of this writing, approximately a quarter million people in the United States receive maintenance dialysis as a lifesaving treatment for end-stage renal disease (ESRD) [1]. Despite its successes in preventing immediate death from volume overload, hyperkalemia, and uremia, one should not confuse the *ex vivo* application of a technology developed for chemical purification with complete organ replacement.

Epidemiologic data suggest that patients with chronic renal insufficiency who do not yet require renal replacement therapy have worse operative mortality than those with better renal function, suggesting that adequate clearance and metabolic function of the kidney is necessary for recovery from injury [2,3]. Wolfe, Ashby, and Port published a landmark study comparing the survival of ESRD patients on dialysis awaiting kidney transplant to the survival of recipients of a first deceased donor kidney transplant [4]. This study, the first to directly compare survival of otherwise similar groups treated with dialysis or transplant, showed an annual death rate 1.7-fold higher in patients remaining on the wait-list and receiving dialysis compared with the death rate of those receiving a renal transplant. This suggests a survival benefit associated with renal function over and above waste removal. It has been suggested that the poor outcomes seen in U.S. dialysis patients are related to underdosing of dialysis. Multiple observational studies have noted a correlation between delivered dialysis dose and patient survival, yet the data are subject to attack on several grounds: first, dialytic dosing is measured by clearance of a marker molecule, urea, which itself is not particularly toxic; second, measurement of clearance of urea is easily confounded by the volume of distribution of urea, which is related to patient body mass and obesity; and last, delivered dose of dialysis may be a surrogate for another factor, such as patient adherence or physician attentiveness. Prospective trials in ESRD and in acute renal failure (ARF) have failed to show a conclusive cause and effect relationship between dialysis dose and survival [5–7].

Given that mortality in ESRD is high (18 deaths per 100 patient-years at risk) compared with mortality in patients with a functioning kidney, it is instructive to examine the causes of death in dialysis patients. The leading cause of death is cardiovascular disease, accounting for almost half of all deaths in ESRD patients, and this affects diabetics and nondiabetics alike. The second most common cause of death is infection, and even after controlling for infections related to dialysis access, dialysis patients die from pulmonary infections at a rate 16 times that of the general population and 8 times that of the renal transplant population — a group of patients treated with immunosuppressive drugs [1,8].

The molecular mechanisms underlying accelerated cardiovascular disease and susceptibility to infection in the ESRD population remain unclear, and this is a major concern to the tissue engineer who contemplates design considerations for renal replacement therapy. Putative mechanisms of vascular disease in ESRD include the observation that chronic kidney disease before and after initiation of dialysis is associated with increased plasma markers of oxidative stress, which have in turn been proposed as accelerants of vascular disease [9–11]. Similarly, differences in serum and stimulated peripheral blood mononuclear cell cytokine levels between control subjects and subjects with acute and chronic renal failure have been identified in humans and in animal models, and that has been hypothesized to play a role in the diminished immunologic competence observed in ESRD [12,13].

60.2　Renal Physiology

With the explicit understanding that the high mortality observed in ESRD cannot yet be attributed to lack of specific physiologic processes of the native kidney, let us begin to consider the engineering of a renal replacement system. A diagram of the kidney and its functional units, nephrons, are shown in Figure 60.1. The glomerulus is a specialized tuft of capillaries which permit high-flux transudation of fluid out of the bloodstream and into a receptacle, Bowman's capsule. Bowman's capsule drains into

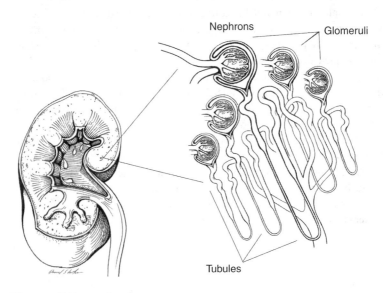

FIGURE 60.1　Diagram of kidney and nephrons.

TABLE 60.1 Renal Functions in the Native Kidney and in Hemodialysis

Function	Renal physiology	Dialysis therapy
Volume homeostasis	Direct control of filtered volume by glomerular capillaries, with passive regulation of reabsorption in the proximal tubule via glomerulo-tubular balance and active control of sodium reabsorption in the cortical collecting system	Patient is weighed at each treatment and technician enters an ultrafiltration volume into the dialysis machine
Control of blood tonicity	Generation of medullary concentration gradient by loop of Henle; ADH-regulated insertion of aquaporin channels into luminal membrane of collecting duct cells; ADH-mediated thirst	Concentration of electrolytes in dialysate prescribed by physician; water and sodium diffuse freely across dialysis membrane; ADH-mediated thirst
Toxin clearance	Bulk filtration by glomerular capillaries, with resorptive concentration of ultrafiltrate into urine, including reabsorption of important metabolites, such glutathione, glucose, amino acids	Passive diffusion of small solutes from blood into dialysate
Acid-base homeostasis	pH-dependent ammoniagenesis in the proximal tubule; active pH-dependent proton excretion in collecting duct	Bicarbonate concentration in dialysate controlled by prescription
Potassium metabolism	Potassium ion excretion by principal cells of the collecting duct under active regulation by aldosterone-mediated Na–K ATPase activity	Serum potassium measured periodically and dialysate potassium concentration adjusted
Calcium–phosphorus metabolism	Hydroxylation of 25-(OH) Vit D_3 in proximal tubule cells; PTH-regulated calcium reabsorption and phosphorus excretion	Calcium present in dialysate; dietary phosphorus absorption blocked with phosphorus binders, oral or intravenous vitamin D analogs prescribed
Regulation of red blood cell mass	Oxygen-dependent synthesis and release of erythropoetin from capillary endothelium	Erythropoetin analogs injected at time of dialysis

a multisegmented tube, the renal tubule, which progressively reabsorbs the majority of the fluid which enters it, but does not reabsorb toxins to the same degree, thus concentrating toxins in the remaining fluid, urine. An understanding of the known physiologic processes of the kidney is a first step towards outlining the task list of a hypothetical artificial kidney, and a comparison to existing dialytic therapy may be helpful.

The major filtration, excretion, and metabolic functions of the healthy kidney are contrasted with dialysis therapy in Table 60.1.

The kidney's algorithm for waste excretion is at first confusing: why does the kidney in effect discard everything and then struggle to reabsorb its losses? In contrast, the body's other major toxin clearinghouse, the liver, has evolved a complex web of enzymes to degrade and detoxify bloodborne toxins. Each normal kidney's filters produce approximately 60 ml/min of an ultrafiltrate of blood, and the kidney's tubules progressively extract salt and water from that ultrafiltrate, concentrating toxins until that ultrafiltrate is urine. A unique and underappreciated feature of the kidney's approach is that the organism has an opportunity via the kidney to excrete novel toxins for which it has not been evolutionarily prepared. The kidney has evolved a narrow set of transport proteins to scavenge from the ultrafiltrate stream the salt, water, glucose, and amino acids necessary for life, and with that toolkit, to discard all that is not needed, whether the body recognizes a particular molecule as a toxin or not. Curiously, despite a half century of research, the identities of the molecules responsible for the uremic state have proven elusive, which argues against an engineering approach that targets individual toxins. This suggests that adsorbent or catalytic systems are not the approach of choice for a tissue-engineered artifical kidney.

The kidney also employs a combination of active and passive negative feedback systems to confer redundancy in the event of failure. In advanced renal failure, when glomerular filtration has dropped to 10% of its original value, despite dilution of the medullary concentrating gradient and increased single-nephron glomerular filtration rate (GFR), the kidney can still maintain volume homeostasis, albeit over a narrower range of intake and output. A successful implantable artificial kidney will need closed-loop feedback algorithms integrating sensors of blood pressure and flow, tonicity, and potassium concentration to autonomously replace the failed organ.

It is worthwhile to include some order-of-magnitude estimates of the fluxes and volumes, and working pressures necessary for renal function. Patients with chronic renal insufficiency develop symptoms insidiously with wide variability in actual GFR at the time of clinical illness, but it is generally accepted that a GFR of 10 ml/min is enough for some patients to survive, and almost all will be manageable with a GFR of 20 ml/min. This corresponds to just under 29 l/day of blood clearance. Typical dietary consumption in the United States includes 1.5 to 2 l of fluid intake, 100 to 200 mEq of sodium, and 90 mEq of potassium, although both of the latter vary widely with dietary intake. This same diet also includes approximately 50 to 100 mM of acid. An ultrafiltrate stream of 20 ml/min thus bears some 4000 mEq of sodium and 120 mEq of potassium over 24 h. Of this 2000 to 4000 Eq of sodium filtered each day, all but 100 to 200 mEq must be returned to the blood stream, illustrating the efficient reclamation of sodium performed by the kidney. Of the 29 l of water, all but one to two l need to be reabsorbed. All of this filtration and reabsorption occur at hydrostatic pressures approximating capillary perfusion pressure of 25 mmHg, or about 0.1 PSI.

60.3   Engineering Renal Replacement

Design of an artifical kidney begins with the enumeration of a set of tasks for the proposed device. At a minimum, to replace present dialytic therapy, an engineered kidney will need to remove approximately 100 to 200 mM of sodium, 100 mM of potassium, 1 to 2 l of water, and 50 to 100 mM of acid from the bloodstream, while also providing 20 to 30 l a day of small-molecule clearance. In addition, calcium-phosphorus balance, in particular, avoidance of hyperphosphatemia, must be maintained, as well as regulation of serum tonicity.

Several of the functions of the native kidney may not need replacing in a tissue-engineered artificial kidney. Regulation of red blood cell mass, (1,25)-OH Vitamin D$_3$, and buffering of dietary acids are solved problems from an engineering viewpoint; weekly injections and well-tolerated oral medications appear sufficient to replace these metabolic and endocrine functions of the kidney. Serum tonicity is controlled by two redundant pathways in the healthy organism: vasopressin is a short peptide hormone synthesized and released by the periventricular and supraoptic nuclei of the hypothalamus in response to increased plasma tonicity. Elevated levels of vasopressin, also called antidiuretic hormone, stimulate water reabsorption in the kidney and the sensation of thirst. Hemodialysis patients appear to be able to regulate plasma tonicity solely through the latter mechanism, as well as patients with advanced renal insufficiency who have little urinary diluting or concentrating capacity. It is when these patients either imbibe excess water or are deprived of it that they lose osmoregulation. This suggests that although tight control of plasma tonicity is important, it can be achieved in the absence of a renal regulatory mechanism.

Renal potassium excretion varies with dietary input under control of a serum steroid hormone, aldosterone. Longterm success of an implantable artifical kidney will be predicated in part on sensing and responding to serum potassium levels, as it is difficult to tailor a varied diet to contain identical amounts of potassium each day. As failure of potassium control may be promptly fatal, development of online noninvasive potassium monitors is a major challenge in renal tissue engineering. However, given information regarding potassium levels, external control of potassium levels may be accomplished via oral medicines.

The single largest challenge facing renal tissue engineering is providing 30 to 50 l each day of small-molecule clearance. In present clinical practice, this clearance is provided by hemodialysis, peritoneal dialysis, or hemofiltration. Dialysis is an unattractive strategy for providing clearance in a totally implanted device, given the large volumes of electrolytically pure nonpyrogenic fluid necessary. Patients receiving peritoneal dialysis wash their peritoneal cavities with 10 to 15 l of electrolyte each day. Scarring of the peritoneal membrane, caloric load from the hypertonic glucose, and infection related to the dialysis catheter limit the effectiveness of this approach, as well as the labor of maintaining a stock of dialysate near the patient. Dialysate regeneration, wherein toxins are adsorbed or catabolized in the dialysate in essence simply transfers the clearance problem from the blood to the dialysate. In the absence of detailed knowledge of specific molecules to be cleared, selection of reagents for dialysate regeneration is problematic.

A second strategy for clearance is already used to clear excess potassium from patients with chronic hyperkalemia and block dietary phosphorus absorption from patients with hyperphosphatemia. Oral administration of binding resins with high affinity for the solute of choice (Kayexelate® Renegel®) can alter serum electrolyte levels promptly and, if used regularly, can maintain neutral balance for months to years. This strategy in essence uses the enteric epithelium to confer biocompatibility to the chemicals used to adsorb the solutes. The broader applicability of absorbent technologies hinges on the absorption of the toxins responsible for uremia. They are at present unknown and by extension not only is the design of a sorbent difficult, but the transport of such toxins into the intestinal lumen remains speculative.

A third strategy for providing clearance is high-volume ultrafiltration and selective reabsorption of that ultrafiltrate, as occurs in the native nephron. This poses the problem as a two-stage filtration problem: one filter generating an ultrafiltrate and a second reabsorbing part of the ultrafiltrate back into the feed solution of the first membrane. The remaining of the chapter will address the nature of these passive and active membranes and the forces driving mass transport across them in the nephron and present tissue-engineering constructs.

60.4 Hemofiltration

60.4.1 The Renal Glomerulus

The fundamental structure of the glomerulus, and fundamental physiologic determinants of glomerular filtration have been well described. Three distinct layers, the endothelium, the basement membrane — glomerular basement membrane (GBM), and a specialized cell junction, the podocyte slit diaphragm, comprise the filter (Figure 60.2). The glomerulus itself is a tuft of capillaries tethered by smooth muscle-like cells continuous with the arteriolar wall called mesangial cells. The outer surface of the glomerular capillary tube is covered with a mesh-like array of interdigitated epithelial cells called podocytes, and the inner surface of the capillary tube is a specialized endothelium with regular pores called fenestrae. The capillary tuft is enclosed in a small receptacle for ultrafiltrate called Bowman's space, which drains ultrafiltrate into the renal tubule. The glomerulus permits low-molecular weight substances, such as

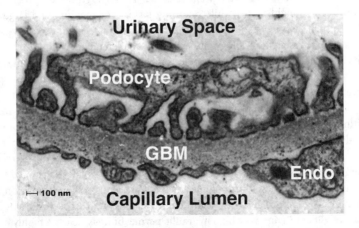

FIGURE 60.2   Transmission electron micrograph of the glomerular filtration barrier, GBM.

electrolytes, urea, creatinine, glucose, and amino acids, to pass with water as ultrafiltrate into Bowman's space for processing by the renal tubule. Larger molecules, such as proteins, which are energetically expensive for the body to synthesize, are retained in the bloodstream. The exact contribution of each component of the glomerular capillary to the filtration barrier is unknown.

The glomerular endothelium is a specialized structure featuring unusual endothelial cells with fenestrations, considered to be the loci at which water enters the glomerular basement membrane. Other vessels in the kidney subject to high-volume convective transport, such as peritubular capillaries, also have fenestrations. The individual glomerular fenestrae are not bridged by proteinaceous diaphragms, although such diaphragms are described in other fenestrated endothelia. Endothelial proteins which localize to other fenestrated endothelia in the kidney and the lung do not localize in the glomerular endothelial fenestrae [14]. Glomerular endothelial cells also form intracapillary ridges, which are thought to impair laminar flow and promote mixing at the capillary walls. The role of the fenestrae in glomerular filtration may solely lie in this mixing and in directing site of entry of fluid into the GBM.

The GBM is a 200 to 300 nm thick gel of extracellular matrix proteins, primarily collagen IV, laminin, fibronectin, and heparan sulfate proteoglycan. The GBM is composed of two separate and superimposed collagen IV networks, one of $\alpha(1,2)$ collagen IV chains adjacent to and synthesized by endothelial cells, and one of $\alpha(3,4,5)$ collagen IV chains adjacent to and synthesized by the podocytes. Laminin, fibronectin, and entactin are thought to crosslink the collagen IV molecules and add mechanical rigidity to the basement membrane. A heparan sulfate proteoglycan, perlecan, is the major proteglycan constituent of the GBM and forms a hydrated meshwork within the GBM.

The glomerular slit diaphragm is a unique intercellular junction whose fundamental ultrastructure was elucidated by Karnovsky et al. 30 years ago [15]. The protein constituents of the glomerular slit diaphragm have been the subject of intense recent study. Nephrin, a 185 D protein product of NPHS1, a gene mutated in congenital nephropathy of the Finnish type, has been localized to the glomerular slit diaphragm [16]. The slit diaphragm is a somewhat delicate structure, in that neutralization of fixed anion charges with polycations such as protamine can induce reversible podocyte rearrangement and obliteration of the slit diaphragm structure. Detailed analysis of the functional properties of the glomerular slit diaphragm have been hampered by the terminally differentiated phenotype of the glomerular podocyte. The podocyte does not easily replicate in cell culture, and has not yet been observed to form the slit diaphragm structure *in vitro*. Strategies for understanding glomerular filtration to date have centered on ultrastructural imaging and mathematical modeling of the glomerular barrier as an array of pores [15,17–21].

60.4.2 Toward a Synthetic Glomerulus

The modern hollow-fiber hemodialyzer is an excellent glomerular analog, providing passage of electrolytes, water, and low-molecular weight toxins while retarding passage of medium and large serum proteins such as albumin. As such, it provides life-saving clearance to a quarter-million dialysis patients in the United States. However, present technology poses several challenges to integration into a durable or implantable artificial organ. The first and most obvious is the fairly low hydraulic permeability of existing membranes. To achieve meaningful filtration rates in clinical practice, transmembrane pressures of 200 to 400 mmHg are applied to the membrane by peristaltic pumps. Incorporation of these technologies into an implantable or wearable organ will require either pumps, a very large membrane area, or significant advances in existing polymer technology. Second, membrane fouling presently limits service lifetime to around 100 h with present technology. Last, and possibly most significant, the glomerulus appears to have a fairly sharp cutoff for molecular weights around 60 kDa, probably attributable to the extraordinary uniformity of the glomerular slit diaphragm. Polymer filters have a normally distributed spectrum of pore sizes arising from the characteristics of the polymer melt or cast. Thus, a sharp transition from passage to retardation with increasing molecular weight is difficult to achieve in practice. A durable hemofilter with a sharp molecular weight cutoff and very high hydraulic permeability is clearly a highly desireable goal of tissue engineering an artifical kidney.

Two recent approaches are worthy of a brief introduction. If, as evidence suggests, the podocyte slit diaphragm is the locus of glomerular permselectivity, growth of the podocyte in tissue or organ culture may promise a glomerular replacement. Unfortunately, podocytes are terminally differentiated epithelial cells and resist expansion in cell or tissue culture. Cultured podocytes harvested from organs do not easily form the octopus-like structures of the podocyte foot processes. In an attempt to expand understanding of podocyte biology, Mundel and colleagues have engineered a conditionally transformed podocyte cell line using a temperature-sensitive SV40 construct [22]. This cell line appears to display many cellular proteins characteristic of differentiated podocytes, and is a promising area for tissue engineering. Live human podocytes are shed in the urine in patients with glomerular disease, and the potential to harvest, transform and expand these cells is an exciting prospect in renal tissue engineering.

Our laboratory has begun testing mechanical analogs of the glomerular slit diaphragm. Using nanofabrication technology, silicon membranes comprised of slit shaped pores 6 to 100 nm in smallest dimension have been tested for hydraulic permeability. This approach allows extremely narrow pore size dispersions, unprecedented control over pore size and shape, as well as batch fabrication using conventional silicon micromachining techniques. Silicon surfaces are easily functionalized with polymer and peptide moeities giving rise to the possibility of independent control of electrostatic and steric hindrance of molecules by selection of pore size and surface treatment. Most promising, slit-shaped pores, as are found in the glomerular slit diaphragm, potentially have higher hydraulic permeability than an equivalent area of cylindrical pores, while retaining steric hindrance to macromolecules. Initial characterization of these membranes suggests that prototype slit-pore membranes with low porosity ($\sim 10^{-3}$) have hydraulic permeabilities on a par with polymer membranes with porosities two orders of magnitude higher [23]. Further work characterizing protein permselectivity of these membranes is underway.

60.5 Reabsorption of Filtered Fluid

60.5.1 The Renal Tubule

The renal tubule affects the controlled reabsorption of salt, water, glucose, and amino acids from the ultrafiltrate stream. It permits the body to excrete a urine stream that may vary in tonicity from about 100 to about 1000 mOsm under the control of a single hormone, vasopressin. The tubule is loosely described as having, in sequence, eight segments: the proximal convoluted tubule, the descending limb of the loop of Henle, the thick and thin ascending limbs of the loop of Henle, the distal convoluted and straight tubules, and the cortical and medullary collecting ducts. Each segment is composed of one or more individual cell types, which may be interspersed, as in the principal and intercalated cells of the collecting ducts, or may transition from one type to the next along the length of the segment, as occurs in the proximal tubule. Postglomerular blood accompanies the tubule in peritubular capillaries. In concert with the spatial distribution of cell types, the anatomy of the tubule gives rise to a corticomedullary gradient in tonicity, with the renal cortex approximating systemic tonicity, and the inner medulla of the kidney approaching 1200 mOsm. It is this progressive concentration and dilution of the ultrafiltrate stream that permits the kidney to regulate serum tonicity.

A slight majority of tubular reabsorption of salt, water, electrolytes, glucose, and amino acids takes place in the proximal tubule, with the balance occurring more distally. The maximum fractional reabsorption of salt and water by the tubule remains unclear. The driving force for sodium reabsorption in all nephron segments in which it occurs is the basolateral localization of the sodium–potassium ATPase transporter. This plasma membrane protein moves three sodium ions from the interior of the cell to the exterior, while transporting two potassium ions into the cell.

Both movements are against and in fact give rise to the prevailing concentration gradient, and so require energy in the conversion of adenosine triphosphate (ATP) to adenosine diphosphate (ADP). The resulting very low intracellular sodium concentration allows passive transport of sodium into the interior of the cell from the ultrafiltrate stream via apical sodium channels. Intracellular sodium is then transported across the basolateral membrane by the Na–K ATPase, accomplishing bulk transport of sodium from ultrafiltrate to pericapillary interstitium. The transport of ions results in an increase in basolateral tonicity, and water moves from the tubular lumen to the peritubular interstitium under osmotic pressure. In the proximal tubule, this takes place by passive, unregulated paracellular means, but in more distal segments this occurs via highly regulated transcellular pathways.

Broadly speaking, there are two approaches to engineering tubular reabsorption: employing living cells to mimic the function of their native counterparts, or manufacturing a second filtration membrane which permits the passage of salt, water, glucose, and sodium bicarbonate but retards the passage of urea, creatinine, and other uremic toxins. The advantage of the former lies in the simplicity of the approach; there is no need to separately implement each of the many transporters on the apical surface of the cell; supply the cell and the cell will supply not only the transporters but in addition the driving force for reabsorption. The disadvantage of the cellular approach is that it is subject to the same supply pressures as renal transplantation: the cells need to come from somewhere. Despite these pressures, a tissue-engineered bioartificial tubule containing human cells has entered clinical trials in the United States, and the design and engineering of that device will be described.

60.5.2 Isolation and Culture of Proximal Tubule Cells

Our laboratory developed experience in the isolation and culture of porcine proximal tubule cells until we could reproducibly harvest cells and maintain them stably in culture [24,25]. In brief, Yorkshire breed pigs were sacrificed at 4 to 6 weeks of age and their kidneys harvested. The renal cortices were dissected, minced, digested with collagenase, and the resulting mixture was separated on a Percoll density gradient. Renal proximal tubule fragments were isolated and grown in a serum-free hormonally derived medium. After third passage and reaching confluence on 100 mm culture dishes, cells were mobilized with trypsin into a suspension and seeded into polysulfone single hollow-fiber bioreactors for *in vitro* assessment of cell viability and metabolic activity.

Cellular attachment, stability, and confluence on the interior lumen of the bioreactor is of paramount importance. To promote attachment of the cells, the luminal surface of the polysulfone membrane was coated with ProNectin-L, a synthetic protein sharing the intercellular attachment domains of laminin, a protein found in the renal glomerular and tubular basement membrane. Laminin and collagen type IV, key components of the tubular basement membrane, also provide an effective biomatrix for cell attachment and growth. After seeding of the hollow fiber with tubule cells, the hollow fibers were perfused with culture media. As newly seeded cells need time to attach, perfusion was initially performed via diffusion from the exterior through the polysulfone membrane, and after time for attachment, convective flow through the interior of the fiber was initiated. A graduated increase in flow (and thus shear forces) was used to condition the cells and minimize cellular detachment. Studies demonstrated confluence was reached in 7 to 10 days. After 14 days in culture the hollow fiber bioreactors were assessed for cellular confluency and viability. Light microscopy of fixed sections showed evidence of a confluent monolayer formed on the inside of the hollow fibers, and intercellular tight junction formation was verified by measuring low inulin leak rates across the monolayer [26].

60.5.3 Transport and Metabolic Characteristics of Hollow-Fiber Bioreactors

As initial experiments using the single hollow-fiber model were promising, the design was scaled up to use commercially available polysulfone hollow fiber dialysis cartridges from the manufacturers of the single hollow fibers. Single hollow-fiber measurements of transport and metabolic activity were repeated with 97 cm^2 and 0.4 m^2 surface area cartridges.

We further explored the metabolic characteristics of the cultured proximal tubule cells. We examined the transport of glucose, bicarbonate, and glutathione and expressed the data in terms of fractional reabsorption accomplished by the bioreactor. For each of the molecules listed, fractional excretion was measured in the absence and presence of a known inhibitor of an enzyme essential for the reabsorption. In each case, there was evidence of active transport and specific inhibition [26].

The synthesis and secretion of ammonia into the tubule is essential for renal excretion of an acid load, as it buffers secreted protons. Proximal tubule cells are able to increase their ammoniagenesis in response to a decline in pH, and the proximal tubule cells in the bioreactor demonstrated a stepwise increase in ammonia production with changes in pH [26].

The experiments detailed above were performed with porcine tubule cells, and our laboratory has demonstrated similar results in culture, attachment, and activity with human proximal tubule cells from cadaveric organs. The final selection of cell type for use in a renal tubule device rests not only on supply and safety of cells, but also depends on the ability of xenotransplanted cells to participate in the homeostasis of the host.

The above data suggest that our laboratory has successfully isolated and cultured renal proximal tubule cells, established stable confluent monolayers within hollow fiber bioreactors, and scaled the initial construct to a level approximating the number of proximal tubule cells in a single kidney.

60.5.4 Preclinical Characterization of the Renal Assist Device (RAD)

In keeping with its role as a metabolically active replacement for the renal proximal tubule, an extracorporeal circuit was devised that recapitulated nephron anatomy (Figure 60.3). A conventional hollow-fiber dialyser and a hollow fiber bioreactor were connected in series, so that a portion of the ultrafiltrate exiting the hemofilter was directed into the luminal spaces of the bioreactor, and thus presented to the apical aspect of the cultured proximal tubule cells. Concentrated blood exiting the hemofilter was directed to the extraluminal space (conventionally the dialysate compartment) of the bioreactor, just as post glomerular blood surrounds the renal tubules via the peritubular capillaries. In order to allow independent control of the subject's volume status and clearance parameters during experiments, the balance of the ultrafiltrate was discarded and the subject infused with a balanced electrolyte solution, as in a conventional hemofiltration circuit.

The bioartificial kidney setup consists of a filtration device (a conventional hemofilter) followed in series by the tubule RAD unit. Specifically, blood is pumped out of a large animal using a peristaltic pump. The blood then enters the fibers of a hemofilter, where ultrafiltrate is formed and delivered into the fibers of the tubule lumens within the RAD downstream to the hemofilter. Processed ultrafiltrate exiting the RAD is collected and discarded as "urine." The filtered blood exiting the hemofilter enters the RAD through the extracapillary space port and disperses among the fibers of the device. Upon exiting the RAD, the processed blood travels through a third pump and is delivered back to the animal. This additional pump is required to maintain appropriate hydraulic pressures within the RAD. Heparin is delivered continuously into the blood before entering the RAD to diminish clotting within the device. The RAD is oriented horizontally and placed into a temperature-controlled environment. The temperature of the cell compartment of the RAD must be maintained at 37°C throughout its operation to ensure optimal functionality of the cells. Maintenance of a physiologic temperature is a critical factor in the functionality of the RAD. The tubule unit is able to maintain viability because metabolic substrates and low-molecular weight growth factors are delivered to the tubule cells from the ultrafiltration unit and the blood in the extracapillary space. Furthermore, immunoprotection of the cells grown within the hollow fiber is achieved because of the impenetrability of immunoglobulins and immunologically competent cells through the hollow fibers. Rejection of the cells, therefore, does not occur. This arrangement thereby allows the filtrate to enter the internal compartments of the hollow fiber network, lined with confluent monolayers of renal tubule cells for regulated transport and metabolic function.

Large animal studies have been completed with the use of this extracorporeal circuit. Dogs were made uremic by performing bilateral nephrectomies. A double lumen catheter was placed into the internal jugular vein, extending into the heart. After 24 h of postoperative recovery, the dogs were treated either with hemofiltration and the RAD or with hemofilter and a sham control cartridge containing no cells. The blood flow rate to the hemofiltrator was maintained at 80 ml/min, with a controlled ultrafiltration rate of 5 to 7 ml/min. Dogs were treated daily for either 7 or 9 h or for 24 h continuously. The dogs in these experiments developed ARF with average blood urea nitrogen (BUN) and plasma creatinine levels of 68 and 6.6 mg/dl,

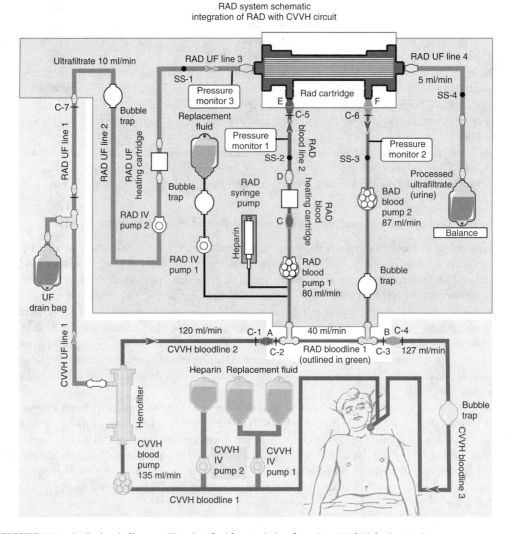

FIGURE 60.3   RAD circuit diagram. (Reprinted with permission from RenaMed Biologics, Inc.)

respectively. The RADs maintained viability and functionality when connected in series to a hemofiltration cartridge within an extracorporeal perfusion circuit in an acutely uremic animal. During a 24-h perfusion period, fewer than 10^5 cells were lost from the RAD, which contained more than 1.4×10^8 cells. Treatment with the RAD and hemofiltration maintained BUN and plasma creatinine levels similar to those of sham controls. In addition, plasma HCO_3, P_i, and K^+ levels were more readily maintained near normal values in RAD treatment than in sham treatment. The RADs were able to reabsorb 40 to 50% of ultrafiltrate volume presented to the devices. Furthermore, active transport of K^+, HCO_3, and glucose was accomplished by the RAD in this *ex vivo* situation. Metabolic activity of the RAD was also shown in these experiments. Virtually no ammonia excretion occurred in the processed ultrafiltrate of the sham control group, in contrast with an ammonia excretion level as high as 100 μM/h in the RAD-treated group. Glutathione processing by the RAD was also shown, with greater than 50% glutathione removal from the ultrafiltrate presented to the RAD. Finally, uremic animals treated with the RAD attained 1,25-$(OH)_2$-D_3 levels of 19.5 ± 0.5 pg/ml, a value no different from the normal levels of the prenephrectomy condition. In contrast, sham treatment resulted in a further fall of 4.0 ± 2.4 pg/ml from the already low plasma levels of 1,25-$(OH)_2$-D_3 in the acutely uremic animals. Thus, these experiments clearly showed that the combination of

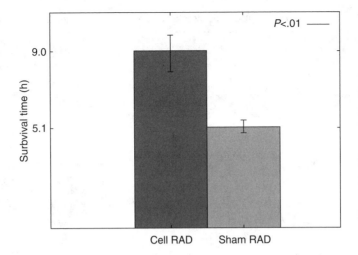

FIGURE 60.4 Survival times of RAD- and sham-treated animals. (Reprinted from Fissell and Humer, Cell therapy of renal failure, Transplantation Proceedings, 35, 2837–2842, 2003, with permission from Elsevier.)

a synthetic hemofiltration cartridge and a RAD in an extracorporeal circuit successfully replaced filtration, transport, and metabolic and endocrinologic functions of the kidney in acutely uremic dogs.

After a series of experiments demonstrating bioactivity, longevity, and systemic activity of the proximal tubule cells in a large animal model, further experiments were conducted to examine the impact of cell therapy on the course of sepsis complicated by renal failure. Septic shock with ARF was chosen as an experimental model for several reasons. First, there is no established animal model of chronic renal failure, largely due to the cost involved in maintaining a herd of animals on dialysis. Second, the time course of well-dialyzed chronic renal failure is months to years of subject survival, which would be prohibitively expensive. Lastly, animal models of septic shock have been well established and can serve as a starting point for understanding the disease physiology.

After two initial studies supported a systemic effect and hemodynamic benefit from cell therapy in large animal models of sepsis [27,28], we pursued further evidence that cell therapy with renal proximal tubule cells altered the physiologic response to sepsis. A porcine model of septic shock was developed from the previous work. It was noted in nonnephrectomized animals that in response to bacteria, the animals rapidly became oligoanuric. We hypothesized that septic shock rapidly induced tubule cell injury, and that replacement of the function of injured tubule cells would confer benefit upon the animals.

Purpose-bred pigs were anesthetized and administered an intraperitoneal dose of bacteria, causing shock and renal failure. An hour later CVVH was initiated with either cell or sham RAD. Urine output and mean arterial pressure declined within the first few hours after insult. Cell-treated animals survived 9.0 ± 0.83 h vs. 5.1 ± 0.4 h ($P < .005$) for sham-treated animals (Figure 60.4).

Serum cytokines were similar between the two groups, with the striking exception of IL-6 and IFN-γ. Treatment with the cell RAD resulted in significantly lower plasma levels of both IL-6 ($P < .04$) and IFN-γ ($P < .02$) throughout the experimental time course compared to sham RAD exposure (Figure 60.5).

This controlled trial of cell therapy of renal failure in a realistic animal model of sepsis has several findings not immediately expected from a priori assumptions regarding renal function. Heretofore, although renal failure has been strongly associated with poor outcome in hospitalized patients, and chronic renal failure is associated with specific defects in humoral and cellular immunity, a direct immunomodulatory effect of the kidney had not been accepted. In this trial, clear differences in survival and clear differences in a serum cytokine associated with mortality in sepsis were found between animals treated with cells and with sham cartridges. This hearkens back to statements made earlier in the chapter: that the increased mortality in renal failure has not been conclusively attributed to inadequate clearance, but may arise from other bioactivity of the kidney. With a series of preclinical experiments demonstrating the extracorporeal

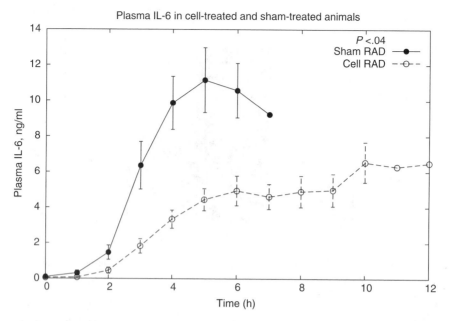

FIGURE 60.5 Serum cytokine levels in septic animals treated with a bioartificial kidney. (Reprinted with modifications from Humer, H.D., Buffington, D.A., Lou, L., Abrishami, S., Wang, M., Xia, J., and Fissell, W.H. *Critical Care Med.*, 31: 2421–2428, 2003, with permission from Lippincott Williams & Wilkins.)

circuit containing the bioreactor, the U.S. Food and Drug Administration granted Investigational New Drug approval to the bioreactor, and a multicenter Phase I/II clinical trial of the bioartificial kidney was begun.

60.6 Clinical Trials of the RAD

With the suggestive preclinical data from the canine studies, the FDA approved an investigational new drug (IND) application to study the RAD containing human cells in patients with acute tubular necrosis and multisystem organ failure who were receiving continuous renal replacement therapy. Human kidney cells were isolated from kidneys donated for cadaveric transplantation but which could not be used for this end due to anatomic or fibrotic defects.

At the time of this writing, ten human patients at two investigational centers have been treated with the RAD in this Phase I trial. The initial clinical experience with the RAD is detailed in Reference 29. The data collected to date suggests that the RAD remains functional with proximal tubules remaining viable and continuing to display differentiated functions of the proximal tubule. The cells demonstrated glutathione degradation and 25-OH Vitamin D_3 hydroxylation out to 24 h of use, the longest time tested to date. This represents an important milestone in medical therapeutics. We have shown the practicability and safety of treating an acute illness characterized by damage to and loss of function of a cell type with human cells grown in tissue culture and delivered to the patient in a bedside bioreactor.

References

[1] U.S. Renal Data System. *USRDS 2003 Annual Data Report*: Atlas of End-Stage Renal Disease in the United States. National Institutes of Health, National Institute of Diabetes and Digestive and Kidney Diseases, 2003.

[2] O'Brien, M.M., Gonzales, R., Shroyer, A.L., Grunwald, G.K., Daley, J., Henderson, W.G., Khuri, S.F., and Anderson, R.J. Modest serum creatinine elevation affects adverse outcome after general surgery. *Kidney Int.*, 62: 585–592, 2002.

[3] Anderson, R.J., O'Brien, M.M., MaWhinney, S., VillaNueva, C.B., Moritz, T.E., Sethi, G.K., Henderson, W.G., Hammermeister, K.E., Grover, F.L., and Shroyer, A.L. Renal failure predisposes patients to adverse outcome after coronary artery bypass surgery. *Kidney Int.*, 55: 1057–1062, 1999.

[4] Wolfe, R.A., Ashby, V.B., Milford, E.L., Ojo, A.O., Ettenger, R.E., Agodoa, L.Y.C., Held, P.J., and Port, F.K. Comparison of mortality in all patients on dialysis, patients on dialysis awaiting transplantation, and recipients of a first cadaveric transplant. *NEJM*, 341: 1725–1730, 1999.

[5] Schiffl, H., Lang, S.M., and Fischer, R. Daily hemodialysis and the outcome of acute renal failure. *NEJM*, 346: 305–310, 2002.

[6] Ronco, C., Bellomo, R., Homel, P., Brendolan, A., Dan, M., Piccinni, P., and La Greca, G. Effects of different doses in continuous veno-venous haemofiltration on outcomes of acute renal failure: a prospective randomised trial. *Lancet*, 356: 26–30, 2000.

[7] Eknoyan, G., Beck, G.J., Cheung, A.K., Daugirdas, J.T., Greene, T., Kusek, J.W., Allon, M., Bailey, J., Delmez, J.A., Depner, T.A., Dwyer, J.T., Levey, A.S., Levin, N.W., Milford, E., Ornt, D.B., Rocco, M.V., Schulman, G., Schwab, S.J., Teehan, B.P., Toto, R., and the Hemodialysis (HEMO) Study Group. Effect of dialysis dose and membrane flux in maintenance hemodialysis. *NEJM*, 347: 2010–2019, 2002.

[8] Sarnak, M.J. and Jaber, B.L. Mortality caused by sepsis in patients with end-stage renal disease compared to the general population. *Kidney Int.*, 58: 1758–1764, 2000.

[9] Himmelfarb, J., Stenvinkel, P., Ikizler, T.A., and Hakim, R.M. The elephant in uremia: oxidant stress as a unifying concept of cardiovascular disease in uremia. *Kidney Int.*, 62: 1524–1538, 2002.

[10] Himmelfarb, J., McMenamin, E., and McMonagle, E. Plasma aminothiol oxidation in chronic hemodialysis patients. *Kidney Int.*, 62: 705–716, 2002.

[11] Himmelfarb, J., McMonagle, E., and McMenamin, E. Plasma protein thiol oxidation and carbonyl formation in chronic renal failure. *Kidney Int.*, 58: 2571–2578, 2000.

[12] Girndt, M., Kohler, H., and Schiedhelm-Weick, E. Production of interleukin-6, tumor necrosis factor alpha and interleukin-10 *in vitro* correlates with the clinical immune defect in chronic hemodialysis patients. *Kidney Int.*, 47: 559–565, 1995.

[13] Girndt, M., Sester, U., Sester, M., Kaul, H., and Kohler, H. Impaired cellular immune function in patients with endstage renal failure. *Nephrol. Dial. Transplant.*, 14: 2807–2830, 1999.

[14] Stan, R.V., Kubitza, M., and Palade, G.E. Pv-1 is a component of the fenestral and stomatal diaphragms in fenestrated endothelia. *Proc. Natl Acad. Sci. USA*, 96: 13203–13207, 1999.

[15] Rodewald, R. and Karnovsky, M.J. Porous substructure of the glomerular slit diaphragm in the rat and the mouse. *J. Cell Biol.*, 60: 423, 1974.

[16] Holzman, L.B., St. John, P.L., Kovari, I.A., Verma, R., Holthofer, H., and Abrahamson, R. Nephrin localizes to the slit pore of the glomerular slit diaphragm. *Kidney Int.*, 56: 1481–1491, 1999.

[17] Ohlson, M., Sorensson, J., and Haraldsson, B. Glomerular size and charge selectivity in the rat as revealed by fitc-ficoll and albumin. *Am. J. Physiol.*, 279: F84–F91, 2000.

[18] Sorensson, J., Ohlson, M., and Haraldsson, B. A quantitative analysis of the glomerular charge barrier in the rat. *Am. J. Physiol. Renal Physiol.*, 280: F646–F656, 2001.

[19] Ohlson, M., Sorensson, J., and Haraldsson, B. A gel-membrane model of glomerular charge and size selectivity in series. *Am. J. Physiol. Renal Physiol.*, 280: F396–F405, 2001.

[20] Drumond, M.C. and Deen, W.M. Structural determinants of glomerular hydraulic permeability. *Am. J. Physiol. Renal Physiol.*, 266: F1–F12, 1994.

[21] Deen, W.M., Satvat, B., and Jamieson, J.M. Theoretical model for glomerular filtration of charged solutes. *Am. J. Physiol. Renal Physiol.*, 238: F126–F139, 1980.

[22] Saleem, M.A., O'Hare, M.J., Reiser, J., Coward, R.J., Inward, C.D., Farren, T., Xing, C.Y., Ni, L., Mathieson, P.W., and Mundel, P. A conditionally immortalized podocyte cell line demonstrating nephrin and podocin expression. *J. Am. Soc. Nephrol.*, 13: 630–638, 2002.

[23] Fissell, W.H., Humes, H.D., Roy, S., and Fleischman, A. Initial characterization of a nanoengineered ultrafiltration membrane. *J. Am. Soc. Nephrol.*, 13: 602A, 2002.

[24] Humes, H.D. and Cieslinski, D.A. Interaction between growth factors and retinoic acid in the induction of kidney tubulogenesis in tissue culture. *Exp. Cell Res.*, 201: 8–15, 1992.

[25] Humes, H.D., Krauss, J.C., Cieslinski, D.A., and Funke, A.J. Tubulogenesis from isolated single cells of adult mammalian kidney: clonal analysis with a recombinant retrovirus. *Am. J. Physiol.*, 271: F42–49, 1996.

[26] Humes, H.D., MacKay, S.M., Funke, A.J., and Buffington, D.A. Tissue engineering of a bioartificial renal tubule assist device: *in vitro* transport and metabolic characteristics. *Kidney Int.*, 55: 2502–2514, 1999.

[27] Fissell, W.H., Dyke, D.B., Weitzel, W.F., Buffington, D.A., Westover, A.J., Mackay, S.M., Gutierrez, J.M., and Humer, H.D., Bioartificial kidney alters cytokine response and hemodynamics in endotoxin- challenged uremic animals. Blood Purif., 20: 55–60, 2002.

[28] Fissell, W.H., Lou, L., Abrishami, S., Buffington, D.A., and Humer, H.D., Bioartificial kidney ameliorates gram-negative bacteria-induced septic shock in uremic animals. *J. Am. Soc. Nephrol.* 14: 456–461, 2003.

[29] Weitzel, W.F., Fissell, W.H., and Humes, H.D. Initial clinical experience with a human proximal tubule cell renal assist device (RAD). *J. Am. Soc. Nephrol.*, 12: 279a, 2001.

61

The Bioengineering of Dental Tissues

Rena N. D'Souza
University of Texas Health Science Center at Houston

Songtao Shi
*National Institutes of Health
National Institute of Dental and Craniofacial Research*

61.1 Introduction

The proper size, shape, color, and alignment of teeth influences the nature of our smile and determines our uniqueness as individual humans. In addition to their esthetic value, teeth are important for the mastication of food and for proper speech. Despite these critical functions, the importance and uniqueness of teeth are frequently overlooked by health professionals. The loss of dentition to common diseases like caries, periodontal disease and to trauma imposes significant emotional and financial burdens on patients and their families. Despite the overall success of osseo-integrated titanium implants, tooth forms that are bioengineered from natural tissues/cells represent the next wave of dental regenerative medicine. The calcified tooth matrices of enamel, dentin, and cementum each possesses unique biomechanical, structural and biochemical properties. When consideration is given to the bioengineering of whole tooth forms, several challenges exist that relate to the restoration of specific shapes and sizes as well as the (re)generation of these highly specialized mineralized matrices. In order to provide an appreciation for the complexity of the tooth as a whole, this chapter first discusses the components of a mature tooth and its surrounding structures. Next, the basic principles of tooth development that lend the molecular and genetic bases for modern bioengineering strategies is presented. Important contributions from mouse and human genetic studies is also briefly overviewed. Finally, recent data from successful tooth engineering initiatives involving somatic and stem cell approaches along with whole tooth organ strategies is discussed. In projecting future research directions, this chapter concludes with a brief discussion of the challenges and opportunities that exist for bioengineering one of the most complex of all vertebrate organ systems.

61.2   The Tooth and Its Supporting Structures

The crowns of teeth that are exposed in the oral cavity are covered by enamel. Under the enamel is a thick layer of dentin and a soft central core, the pulp chamber (Figure 61.1). Enamel is the hardest calcified structure as it is about 99.5% mineralized. It varies from 2 to 3 mm in thickness at the height of cusps and narrows to a knife-edge thickness at the cementoenamel junction. Enamel is deposited by ameloblasts, cells that are believed to undergo programmed cell death. Because enamel is acellular and nonvital it cannot regenerate itself. Underlying enamel is dentin, a specialized mineralized matrix that shares several biochemical characteristics with bone. In contrast to enamel, dentin is a vital tissue that harbors odontoblastic processes and some nerve endings. The formation of dentin follows the same principles that guide the formation of other hard connective tissues in the body, namely, cementum and bone.

As described by Linde and Goldberg [1] and Butler and Ritchie [2], the composition of dentin matrix and the process of dentinogenesis are highly complex. The organic phase of dentin is composed of proteins, proteoglycans, lipids, various growth factors, and water. Among the proteins, collagen is the most abundant and offers a fibrous matrix for the deposition of carbonate apatite crystals. The collagens that are found in dentin are primarily type I collagen with trace amounts of type V collagen and some type I collagen trimer. An important class of dentin matrix proteins is the noncollagenous proteins or NCPs [2]. The dentin-specific NCPs are dentin phosphoproteins (DPP) or phosphophoryns and dentin sialoprotein (DSP). After type I collagen, DPP is the most abundant of dentin matrix proteins and represents almost 50% of the dentin extracellular matrix. DPP is a polyionic macromolecule that is rich in phosphoserine and aspartic acid. Its high affinity for type I collagen as well as calcium makes it a strong candidate for the initiation of dentin mineralization. DSP accounts for 5 to 8% of the dentin matrix and has a relatively high sialic acid and carbohydrate content. Its role in dentin mineralization is unclear at the present time. For several years it was believed that DSP and DPP were two independent proteins that were encoded by individual genes. DPP and DSP are specific cleavage products of a larger precursor protein that was translated from one large transcript [3]. This single gene encoding for DSP and DPP is named dentin sialophosphoprotein or Dspp.

A second category of NCPs with Ca-binding properties are classified as mineralized tissue-specific as they are found in all the calcified connective tissues, namely, dentin, bone, and cementum. These

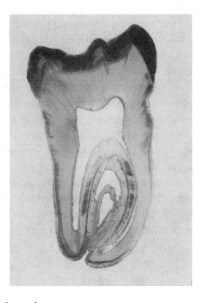

FIGURE 61.1   Component parts of a tooth.

include osteocalcin (OC) and bone sialoprotein (BSP). A serine-rich phosphoprotein called dentin matrix protein 1, Dmp-1, whose expression was first described as being restricted to odontoblasts [4], was later shown to be expressed by osteoblasts and cementoblasts [5]. Other NCPs include osteopontin (OP) and osteonectin (secreted protein, acidic, cycteine-rich; SPARC). The fourth category of dentin NCPs are not expressed in odontoblasts but are primarily synthesized in the liver and are released into the circulation. An example of a serum borne protein is α2HS-glycoprotein. Diffusible growth factors that appear to be sequestered within dentin matrix constitute the fifth group of dentin NCPs. This group includes the BMPs, IGFs, and TGF-βs [6].

The central chamber of the tooth is occupied by a soft connective tissue called the dental pulp that is comprised of a heterogeneous cell population of fibroblasts, undifferentiated mesenchymal cells, nerves, blood vessels, and lymphatics. The regenerative capacity of dental pulp is well documented in the literature and best illustrated by the formation of a layer of reparative dentin beneath a carious lesion or a cavity base. As will be discussed later, somatic stem cells from the dental pulp are capable of regenerating several tissues when transplanted *in vivo*. Cementum is another calcified tissue of mesodermal origin. The cementum covering the apical third of the root is cellular (contains cementocytes), whereas that of the remaining two-thirds is acellular. Since the fibers of the periodontal ligament are anchored within cementum, the regeneration of this complex is important when bioengineering of whole tooth structures is considered.

61.3   Genetic Control of Tooth Development

61.3.1   Stages of Tooth Development

Teeth develop in distinct stages that are easily recognizable at the microscopic level. Hence, stages in odontogenesis are described in classic terms by the histologic appearance of the tooth organ. From early to late, these stages are described as the lamina, bud, cap, and bell (early and late) stages of tooth development [7,8]. Recent advances made in the understanding of the molecular control of tooth development have led to the development of new terminology to describe tooth development as occurring in four phases: initiation, morphogenesis, cell or cyto-differentiation, and matrix apposition (Figure 61.2). The appearance of the dental lamina marks the first visible sign of tooth initiation that is seen about five weeks of human

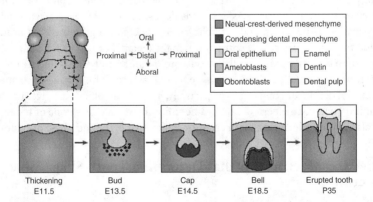

FIGURE 61.2   (See color insert following page **20**-14.) Stages of tooth development. A schematic frontal view of an embryo head at embryonic day (E)11.5 is shown with a dashed box to indicate the site where the lower (mandibular) molars will form. Below, the stages of tooth development are laid out from the first signs of thickening at E11.5 to eruption of the tooth at around 5 weeks after birth. The tooth germ is formed from the oral epithelium and neural-crest-derived mesenchyme. At the bell stage of development, the ameloblasts and odontoblasts form in adjacent layers at the site of interaction between the epithelium and mesenchyme. These layers produce the enamel and dentin of the fully formed tooth. (Reproduced from Tucker, A. and Sharpe, P. *Nat. Rev. Genet.* 5: 499–508, 2004. With permission.)

development. The inductive influence of the dental lamina to dictate the fate of the underlying ectomesenchyme has been confirmed by several researchers [9]. The table below summarizes the molecules expressed in the epithelium and mesenchyme at this inductive phase. The bud stage is characterized by the continual growth of cells of the dental lamina and ectomesenchyme. The latter is condensed and termed the dental papilla. At this stage, the inductive or tooth-forming potential is transferred from the dental epithelium to the dental papilla. The transition from the bud to the cap stage is an important step in tooth development as it marks the onset of crown formation. The tooth bud assumes the shape of a cap that is surrounded by the dental papilla. The ectodermal compartment of the tooth organ is referred to as the dental or enamel organ. The enamel organ and dental papilla become encapsulated by a sac called the dental follicle that separate the tooth organ papilla from the other connective tissues of the jaws. A cluster of cells called the enamel knot is an important organizing center within the dental organ and is important for the formation of cusps [10,11]. The enamel knot expresses a unique set of signaling molecules that influence the shape of the crown as well as the development of the dental papilla. Similar to the fate of signaling centers in other organizing tissues like the developing limb bud, the enamel knot undergoes programmed cell death or apoptosis, after cuspal patterning is completed at the onset of the early bell stage. As the dental organ assumes the shape of a bell, several layers of cells continue to divide but at differential rates. A single layer of cuboidal cells called the external or outer dental epithelium lines the periphery of the dental organ while cells that border the dental papilla and are columnar in appearance form the internal or inner dental epithelium. The latter gives rise to the ameloblasts, cells responsible for enamel formation. Cells located in the center of the dental organ produce high levels of glycosaminoglycans that are able to sequester fluids as well as growth factors that lead to its expansion. This network of star-shaped cells is named the stellate reticulum. Interposed between the stellate reticulum and the internal dental epithelium is a narrow layer of flattened cells termed the stratum intermedium that express high levels of alkaline phosphatase. The stratum intermedium is believed to influence the biomineralization of enamel. In the region of the apical end of the tooth organ, the internal and external dental epithelial layers meet at a junction called the cervical loop.

At the early bell stage, each layer of the dental organ has assumed special functions and exchanges molecular information that leads to cell differentiation at the late bell stage. The dental lamina that connects the tooth organ to the oral epithelium gradually disintegrates at the late bell stage. At the future cusp tips, cells of the internal dental epithelium stop dividing and assume a columnar shape. The most peripheral cells of the dental papilla organize along the basement membrane and differentiate into odontoblasts, the dentin-forming cells. At this time, the dental papilla is termed the dental pulp. After the first layer of predentin matrix is deposited, cells of the internal dental epithelium differentiate into ameloblasts or enamel-producing cells. As enamel is deposited over dentin matrix, ameloblasts retreat to the external surface of the crown and are believed to undergo programmed cell death. In contrast, odontoblasts line the inner surface of dentin and remain metabolically active throughout the life of a tooth. Root formation then proceeds as epithelial cells proliferate apically and influence the differentiation of odontoblasts from the dental papilla as well as cementoblasts from follicle mesenchyme. This leads to the deposition of root dentin and cementum respectively. The dental follicle that gives rise to components of the periodontium, namely the periodontal ligament fibroblasts, alveolar bone of the tooth socket and the cementum also plays a role during tooth eruption which marks the end phase of odontogenesis.

61.3.2 Molecular Mechanisms that Determine Tooth Shape, Size, and Structure

Similar to other organs like the limb bud, kidney, lung, and hair follicles, tooth development is regulated by temporally and spatially restricted interactions between epithelial and mesenchymal compartments. Molecular approaches used in expression analyses as well as functional *in vivo* and *in vitro* tooth recombinations and bead implantation assays have greatly increased our understanding about the molecular control of tooth development. In addition, the use of genetic approaches involving transgenic mice with targeted inactivation of various genes have provided a powerful means to delineate the *in vivo* functions of individual molecules [12,13].

In vivo and *in vitro* recombination studies have shown that during the formation of the epithelial bud (E12), the inductive potential shifts to the dental mesenchyme that later influences the fate of the enamel organ and its morphogenesis from the bud stage to the early bell stage (E16) [9,14–16]. Reciprocal interactions between the morphologically distinct enamel organ and papilla mesenchyme at the late bell stage (E18) then leads to the differentiation of dentin-forming odontoblasts and enamel-forming ameloblasts. As morphogenesis advances, the matrices of dentin and enamel are deposited in an organized manner and root formation begins. Interactions between the apical extension of the enamel organ (epithelial root sheath) and papilla/follicle mesenchyme lead to the patterning of roots, the differentiation of cementoblasts and the formation of cementum. Hence, during crown and root development, morphogenesis, and cytodifferentiation are controlled by epithelial-mesenchymal interactions.

As depicted in Table 61.1 [13], molecular changes in dental mesenchyme involve proteins in the bone morphogenetic protein (BMP), fibroblast growth factor (FGF) and wingless-type MMTV integration site family WNT families; *sonic hedgehog* (*Shh*) as well as transcriptional molecules like the *Msx-1, -2* homeobox genes; lymphoid enhancer-binding factor 1 (Lef-1) and Pax-9, a member of the paired-box-containing transcription factor gene family. The actions and interactions of these molecules are complex and described eloquently in recent reviews [12,17].

The BMPs are among the best-characterized signals in tooth development. In addition to directly influencing morphogenesis of the enamel organ (see discussion on enamel knot later), epithelial BMP-2 and -4 are able to induce expression of *Msx1*, *Msx2*, and *Lef-1* in dental mesenchyme as shown in bead implantation assays [18–20]. The shift in *Bmp-4* expression from epithelium to mesenchyme occurs around E12 and is coincident with the transfer of inductive potential from dental epithelium to mesenchyme [18]. In mesenchyme, *Bmp-4* in turn, requires *Msx-1* to induce its own expression [19]. The FGFs, in general, are potent stimulators of cell proliferation and division both in dental mesenchyme and epithelium. *Fgf-2, -4,-8,* and -9 expression are each restricted to dental epithelium and can stimulate *Msx-1* but not *Msx-2* expression in underlying mesenchyme. *Fgf-8* is expressed early in odontogenesis (E10.5 to E11.5), in presumptive dental epithelium, and can induce the expression of *Pax-9* in underlying mesenchyme. Interestingly, BMP-4 prevents this induction and may share an antagonistic relationship with the FGFs similar to what is observed in limb development [21]. Recent studies by Hardcastle et al., 1998, have shown that Shh in beads cannot induce *Pax9*, *Msx-1* or *Bmp-4* expression in dental mesenchyme but is able to stimulate other genes encoding the transmembrane protein *patched* (*Ptc*) and *Gli1*, a zinc finger transcription factor [22–24]. Since neither FGF-8 nor BMP-4 can stimulate *Ptc* or *Gli1*, it can be assumed at the present time that the Shh signaling pathway is independent of the BMP and FGF pathways during tooth development [24]. Several *Wnt* genes are expressed during tooth development and may be required for the formation of the tooth bud [12]. These genes are believed to play a role in activating the intracellular pathway involving frizzled receptors, β-catenin and nuclear transport of Lef-1. Other signaling molecules including the Notch genes, epidermal growth factor (EGF), hepatocyte growth factor (HGF) and, platelet derived growth factor (PDGF) families may also influence tooth development, though the exact nature of their involvement remains to be elucidated.

The enamel knot is a transient epithelial structure that appears at the onset of cusp formation. For years, it was thought that the enamel knot controlled the folding of the dental epithelium and hence cuspal morphogenesis. Recently, the morphological, cellular and molecular events leading to the formation and disappearance of the enamel knot have been described, thus linking its role as an organizing center for tooth morphogenesis [11,25,26]. Interestingly, cells of the enamel knot are the only cells within the enamel organ that stop proliferating [10] and that undergo apoptosis [27]. Another intriguing finding linked p21, a cyclin-dependent kinase inhibitor associated with terminal differentiation events, to apoptosis of the enamel knot [11].

The enamel knot cells express several signaling molecule genes including *Bmp-2, -4, -7*; *Fgf-4, -9*; *Msx-2* and *Shh* [22,25,28–30]. Although the precise function of each morphogen is not known at the present time, a model for the relationship of inductive signaling molecules involved has been proposed by integrating morphological and molecular data [11]. Since the instructive signaling influence lies with the dental mesenchyme prior to the development of the primary enamel knot, it is likely that this tissue

TABLE 61.1   Genes Expressed During Tooth Development in Mouse[a]

Stage of development	Expressed in epithelium	References	Expressed in mesenchyme	References
Up to epithelial thickening				
(E10–E11)	*Fgf8,9*	[21,60,63,64]	*Activin*	[70]
	Bmp4	[21,35,60,75]	*Pax9*	[21]
	Shh	[24,69]	*Barx1*	[60]
	Islet1	[65]	*Msx1 & Msx2*	[19,83,84]
	Pitx2	[66,67]	*Dlx1,2,3,5,6*	[61,62]
	Wnt 10b	[76]	*Ptc*	[24]
	Follistatin	[70]	*Gli1,2,3*	[24]
	Lef1	[20]	*Lhx6,7*	[63]
	Eda, Edar	[72]		
Bud stage				
(E12–E13)	*Eda, Edar*	[72]	*Runx2*	[71]
	Pitx2	[66,67]	*Bmp4*	[35,75]
			Msx1	[35]
			Lef1	[20]
			Fgf3,10	[73]
			Dlx1,2	[62]
			Lhx6,7	[63]
Cap stage				
(E14–E15)	*Enamel knot*		*Non-EK* epithelium	[74]
	p21	[11]	*FgfR*	[72]
	Shh	[24]	*Eda*	
	Edar	[72]		
	Edaradd	[68]		
	Bmp 2,4,7	[75]		
	Wnt10a	[76]		
	Msx2	[11,29]		
	Fgf3,4	[10,73]		
Bell stage				
(E16 Onward)	*Amelogenin*	[77]	*Dspp*	[78]
	Bmp5	[75]		

[a] This list indicates the expression pattern of several genes that are thought to be important in tooth development in the mouse. A more comprehensive list of genes and their expression patterns can be found at the Gene Expression in Tooth web site (http://bite-it.helsinki.fi/) [79]. *Barx*, BarH-like homeobox; *Bmp*, bone morphogenetic protein; *Dlx*, distal-less homeobox; *Dspp*, dentin sialophosphoprotein; E, embryonic stage; *Eda*, ectodysplasin-A; *Edar*, Eda receptor; *Edaradd*, EDAR (ectodysplasin-A receptor)-associated death domain; *EK*, enamel knot; *Fgf*, fibroblast growth factor; *FgfR*, fibroblast growth factor receptor; *Gli*, GLI-Kruppel family member; *Lef*, lymphoid enhancer binding factor; *Lhx*, LIM homeodomain genes; *Msx*, homeobox, msh-like; *p21* (*CDKN1A*), cyclin-dependent kinase inhibitor 1A; *Pax*, pairedbox gene; *Pitx*, paired-related homeobox gene; *Ptc*, patched; *Runx*, runt homologue; *Shh*, sonic hedgehog; *Wnt*, wingless-related protein.

Source: Reproduced from Tucker, A. and Sharpe, P. *Nat. Rev. Genet.* 5: 499–508, 2004. With permission.

influences enamel knot formation. In this regard, BMP-4 in condensing dental mesenchyme, functions as a paracrine molecule that can upregulate *Msx2* and *p21* expression within the enamel knot [11,26]. It is hypothesized that *p21* then prevents proliferation within the enamel knot allowing for the growth stimulatory *Fgf-4* to be expressed exclusively in this region [10]. FGF-4 in turn, may act singly or in concert with *Fgf-9* to influence patterning or to regulate expression of downstream genes like *Msx1* in underlying papilla mesenchyme [19,28]. Intriguingly, later in development, BMP-4 participates in the regulation of apoptosis perhaps in an autocrine fashion by involving genes like *Msx-2*.

Mice genetically engineered with targeted mutations in transcription factor genes like *Msx-1*, *Lef-1*, and *Pax9* as well as activin-βA, a member of the TGF-β superfamily, have revealed important information.

Knockouts of *Bmp-2, -4*, and *Shh* have proven less informative largely due to death that occurs *in utero* prior to the onset of tooth development. In *Msx-1, Lef*-1, *Pax9*, and activin-βA mutant strains, tooth development fails to advance beyond the bud stage. Thus, these molecules are important in directing the fate of the dental mesenchyme and its ability to influence the progress of epithelial morphogenesis to the cap stage [31–34]. Curiously, *Msx2* molars develop fully but show abnormal cuspal patterning, a poorly differentiated stellate reticulum and enamel matrix defects, suggesting that this homeobox gene is involved in the patterning and differentiation of the enamel organ [17; Maas, personal communication]. As reviewed by Tucker and Sharpe [13], molecular information on tooth development can be used to alter the shape and size of teeth. For example, when beads soaked with Bmp4 are placed on mesenchyme within the presumptive incisor region, *Msx1* expression is downregulated and expression of the transcription factor *Barx1* is upregulated. Since *Barx1* is normally restricted to the molar region, its misexpression within the incisor region results in the formation of a molar tooth organ instead of an incisor [35].

In addition to use of the mouse tooth organ model, the legacy of inheritable anomalies of human dentition involving the failure of teeth to develop offers a powerful system for studying the genetic pathways that control the development of human dentition. Familial tooth agenesis is the most common dental anomaly that affects up to 25% of the population. It is transmitted either as an autosomal-dominant, autosomal-recessive or X-linked trait, and presents in syndromic and nonsyndromic forms. Genes involved in epithelial-mesenchymal interactions as shown by studies in the mouse are strong candidates for human tooth agenesis. Until recently, mutations in two genes that encode for the key transcription factors *PAX9* and *MSX1* were associated with agenesis of molars and premolars [36]. Importantly, PAX9 and MSX1 have each been excluded in other families with autosomal dominant forms of tooth agenesis. Recently, tooth agenesis has been linked to a mutation in AXIN2, a molecule known to regulate cell homeostasis [37]. Several members of this four-generation family are affected by or are at risk for colon cancer suggesting a broader role for this molecule in cell proliferation.

Taken together, the data from mouse and human studies have provided valuable insights into the molecular and genetic control of tooth development. As illustrated later, such basic information provided the rationale for tooth bioengineering initiatives for the regeneration of dentin matrix and whole tooth forms.

61.4 Tooth Regenerative Strategies

Over the years, the research on the use of stem cells for clinical therapies has been growing, especially after researchers have found that hematopoietic stem cells, a well-characterized population of postnatal stem cells, have been successfully utilized in clinics to treat hematopoietic diseases [38] autoimmune diseases [39] and solid tumors [40]. Stem cells are defined as cells that have clonogenic and self-renewing capabilities and that differentiate into multiple-cell lineages. In general, there are two kinds of stem cells: embryonic and postnatal stem cells. Embryonic stem cells are derived from mammalian embryos in the blastocyst stage and have the ability to generate any terminally differentiated cell in the body; postnatal stem cells are part of tissue-specific cells of the postnatal organism into which they are committed to differentiate. Stem cell-based tissue regeneration has great clinical potential to regain physiological functions that have been damaged by various diseases.

61.4.1 Human Dental Pulp Stem Cells

Isolation and identification of stem cells are the first step in studying the potential of stem cell-mediated therapy. Postnatal stem cells have been isolated from a variety of tissues including but not limited to skin, liver, brain, bone marrow, and peripheral blood. Recently, dental pulp stem cells (DPSCs) have been successfully isolated from adult dental pulp in extracted human teeth [41]. Similar to the other mesenchymal stem cells, DPSCs are able to generate clonogenic cell colonies *in vitro*. The majority of the individual colonies (67%) failed to proliferate beyond 20 population doublings in the culture, suggesting that only a small portion of cells maintain high proliferation potential *in vitro* [42]. Mixed multi-colony DPSCs show a higher proliferation rate than bone marrow stromal stem cells (BMSSCs) in culture. cDNA microarray analysis demonstrated that highly expressed cyclin-dependent kinase 6 (cdk6) and IGF-2 in DPSCs might be, at least partially, responsible for the promoted progression of cells through G1 to the start of DNA synthesis [43–45], leading to an elevated replicative proliferation. Most postnatal stem cells reside in a specific niche microenvironment to maintain their stemness. To elucidate the DPSCs' niche environment, DPSCs were first found to express various markers associated with endothelial and/or smooth muscle cells such as STRO-1, 3G5, VCAM-1, MUC-18 and α-smooth muscle actin [41,46]. Then, immunohistochemical staining and magnetic beads sorting were applied to confirm that DPSCs, similar to BMSSCs, reside in a perivascular niche microenvironment [46]. Taken together with their clonogenic nature, higher proliferation rate, and specific niche microenvironment, DPSCs satisfy three criteria characteristic of human postnatal somatic stem cells.

61.4.2 Dentin Tissue Regeneration

One of the most important characteristics of DPSCs is their capability to form a dentin/pulp-like complex upon *in vivo* transplantation in conjunction with hydroxyapatite/tricalcium phosphate as a carrier (Figure 61.3). Backscatter EM analysis demonstrated that the dentin-like material formed in the

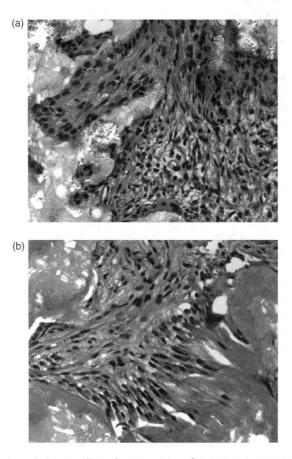

FIGURE 61.3   (See color insert.) Hematoxylin and eosin staining of representative DPSC transplants. (a) After one week posttransplantation, DPSC transplants contain connective tissue (*CT*) around HA/TCP carrier (*HA*), without any sign of dentin formation. (b) After six week posttransplantation, DPSCs differentiate into odontoblasts (arrows) that are responsible for the dentin formation on the surface of HA/TCP (*HA*). Original magnification: 40×.

transplants had a globular appearance consistent with the structure of dentin *in situ* [42]. DPSC-mediated odontogenesis is differentiable from BMSSC-mediated osteogenesis by regenerating different organ-like structures and involving different regulating molecules [47]. This implies that critical factor(s) may regulate mineralized matrix forming stem cells to generate defined mineralized tissue along with associated soft tissues. The property of multipotential differentiation of DPSCs has been demonstrated by the findings that under the proper culture conditions, DPSCs are capable of differentiating into osteo/odontogenic cells, adipocytes, and neural cells [42]. However, the assets of multipotential differentiation of DPSCs at functional levels remain to be confirmed.

The findings on DPSCs may provide a potential for utilizing them for dentin and pulp tissues regeneration. Human teeth do not undergo the type of remodeling that is seen in other mineralized tissues such as bone, which remodels to maintain organ integrity. Once a tooth has erupted, dentinal damage caused by mechanical trauma, exposure to chemicals or by infectious processes, induces the formation of reparative dentin that is even though structurally poorly organized, but serves as a protective barrier to the dental pulp with limited capacity [48–52]. It was reported that bone morphogenetic protein-7 is capable of stimulating tertiary dentin formation when applied to freshly cut dentin both *in vitro* and *in vivo* [53,54]. This probably occurs through an osteo/odontogenic induction property of BMP-7, since BMP-7 transfected human fibroblasts were able to express osteogenic characteristic and form bone tissue *in vivo* [55]. DPSCs were also capable of forming reparative dentin structure on the surfaces of regular human dentin [47]. However, it seems that DPSCs exhibit a decreased and altered *in vivo* odontogenic capacity when loaded on the surface of human dentin. Although the reason is not known, it may be associated with the microenvironment that accommodates *in vivo* differentiation of DPSCs [47]. Recently, it was demonstrated that autogenous transplantation of BMP2-treated DPSCs was able to stimulate reparative dentin formation on the amputated pulp [56]. This finding suggests that combination therapy using stem cells and growth factors may improve stem cell-mediated dentin regeneration.

61.4.3 Tooth Regeneration

Recently, whole tooth regeneration *in vivo* has become a hot topic in dental research. Tooth development involves a mutual signaling interaction between epithelial and mesenchymal cells of neural ectodermal origin. It was demonstrated that tooth crown structures including dentin, odontoblasts, pulp chamber, putative Hertwig's root sheath epithelia, putative cementoblasts, and enamel organ could be regenerated using dissociated cells from pig tooth bud tissues (Figure 61.4) [57]. Further, the same research group identified that cultured cells from rat tooth bud were also able to regenerate tooth structure when loaded on the PGA or PLGA scaffolds [58]. These studies demonstrate for the first time that mammalian tooth structure can be regenerated in a system consisting of tooth bud progenitors and the proper scaffold. Moreover, Sharpe's group conducted a promising study to demonstrate that mice embryonic oral epithelium along with nondental stem cells can induce an odontogenic response, showing the expression of odontogenic mesenchymal cell associated genes such as Msx1, Lhx7, and Pax9 [59]. After being transplanted into adult renal capsules, the recombination of embryonic oral epithelium with nondental stem cells (embryonic, neural, and bone marrow stem cells) gave rise to both tooth structure and bone tissue (Figure 61.5) [59]. Also, transplanted embryonic tooth primordial were able to maintain their tooth development potential within an adult environment [59]. This study clearly indicates that the inductive function of embryonic oral epithelium may be an important driving force for future prospects of achieving entire tooth regeneration *in vivo*.

Human DPSCs have been successfully isolated and characterized, which open the door for using these cells for potential tooth structure regeneration. In addition, stem cell-mediated whole tooth structure regeneration implies a great potential for regenerating functional entire tooth *in vivo*. However, substantial experimentation is still required for translating these technologies into clinical applications.

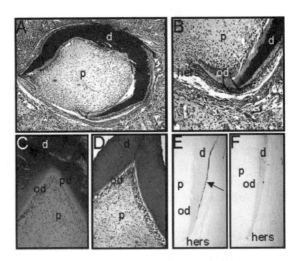

FIGURE 61.4   (See color insert.) Histology and immunohistochemistry of a 20-week implant. (a) Von Kossa stain for calcified mineralization in bioengineered tooth crown (50× magnification). Dark brown stain is positive for mineralized tissues. (b) A high-magnification (400×) photomicrograph of the Hertwig's epithelial root sheath is shown, stained by the Von Kossa method to detect calcified mineralization. (c) High-magnification (200×) photomicrograph of cuspal region in bioengineered tooth crown. The tissue was stained by the Von Kossa method. (d) Hematoxylin and eosin (H&E) stain of a positive control porcine third molar cuspal region demonstrates morphology similar to that of the bioengineered tooth structure (200×). (e) BSP immunostain of 20-week bioengineered tooth crown (100×). Positive BSP expression is indicated by the arrow. (f) Negative preimmune control immunostain for BSP in bioengineered tooth crown (100×). Abbreviations: d, dentin; od, odontoblasts; p, pulp; pd, predentin; hers, Hertwig's epithelial root sheath.

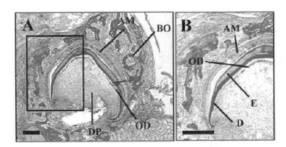

FIGURE 61.5   (See color insert.) Recombinant explant between bone-marrow-derived cells and oral epithelium following 12 days of development in a renal capsule. All the tissues visible are donor-derived, since the host kidney makes no cellular contribution to the tissue. Where epithelium in the recombinations was from GFP mice, *in situ* hybridization of sections of these tissues confirmed that all mesenchyme-derived cells were of wildtype origin (not shown). BO, bone; Am, ameloblasts; DP, dental pulp; OD, odontoblasts; E, enamel; D, dentin. Scale bar: 80 μm. (Reproduced from Ohazama, et al. *J. Dent. Res.* 83: 518–522. With permission.)

61.5   Conclusions

The last decade has witnessed an explosion of scientific and technological advances that will undoubtedly propel the field of tooth bioengineering forward. This chapter was limited in scope in as much as only a few tooth regenerative strategies were discussed. Therefore, readers should be mindful of several other dimensions of research that exist. As presented in the current literature, there is much interest in understanding the structural, biomechanical, and bioregulatory features of dentin and bone matrices as well as the complex process of enamel biomineralization and remineralization. Such basic knowledge is essential for the development of tooth-specific biological substitutes that will best restore, maintain, or improve the functions of normal dentition. The legacy of inheritable anomalies that involve tooth patterning and extracellular matrices will continue to provide a powerful means of identifying new molecular pathways that influence normal and abnormal development. Clearly, advances in the field of tooth bioengineering will depend on the clever integration of basic science knowledge from animal and human developmental and genetic studies with emerging technologies in the field of stem cell biology, autologous cell therapy, gene therapy, materials sciences, and nanotechnology. Although the clinical applications for the use of bioengineered tooth forms and matrices remain limitless, several challenges must be surmounted prior to successful therapeutic interventions. As important as the timely diagnosis, accurate prognosis and proper treatment of diseases affecting dentition will be the preparation of host sites within the oral cavity to receive bioengineered materials. In every respect, the field of tooth bioengineering encompasses broad strategies and multidisciplinary approaches directed at restoring one of the most complex organs in vertebrates.

Acknowledgments

The authors acknowledge the support of the National Institute of Dental and Craniofacial Research (NIDCR), National Institutes of Health (NIH). The research program of RDS has been funded through NIH grants DE10517; DE07252; DE12269; DE11663 and DE13368. STS is supported by the Division of Intramural Research at the NIDCR.

References

[1] Linde, A. and Goldberg, M. Dentinogenesis. *Crit. Rev. Oral. Biol. Med.* 4: 679–728, 1993.
[2] Butler, W.T. and Ritchie, H. The nature and functional significance of dentin extracellular matrix proteins. *Int. J. Dev. Biol.* 39: 169–179, 1995.
[3] MacDougall, M. et al. Dentin phosphoprotein and dentin sialoprotein are cleavage products expressed from a single transcript coded by a gene on human chromosome 4. Dentin phosphoprotein DNA sequence determination. *J. Biol. Chem.* 272: 835–842, 1997.
[4] George, A. et al. Characterization of a novel dentin matrix acidic phosphoprotein. Implications for induction of biomineralization. *J. Biol. Chem.* 268: 12624–12630, 1993.
[5] D'Souza, R.N. et al. Gene expression patterns of murine dentin matrix protein 1 (Dmp1) and dentin sialophosphoprotein (DSPP) suggest distinct developmental functions *in vivo. J. Bone Miner. Res.* 12: 2040–2049, 1997.
[6] Smith, A.J. and Lesot, H. Induction and regulation of crown dentinogenesis: embryonic events as a template for dental tissue repair? *Crit. Rev. Oral Biol. Med.* 12: 425–437, 2001.
[7] Ten Cate, A.R. *Oral Histology: Development, Structure, and Function*, 5th ed. St. Louis, MO, Mosby, Inc. 1998.
[8] Avery, J.K. *Oral Development and Histology*. Pine, J.W. (ed.) Baltimore, MD, Waverly Press, 1987.
[9] Mina, M. and Kollar, E.J. The induction of odontogenesis in non-dental mesenchyme combined with early murine mandibular arch epithelium. *Arch. Oral Biol.* 32: 123–127, 1987.
[10] Jernvall, J. et al. Evidence for the role of the enamel knot as a control center in mammalian tooth cusp formation: non-dividing cells express growth stimulating Fgf-4 gene. *Int. J. Dev. Biol.* 38: 463–469, 1994.
[11] Jernvall, J. et al. The life history of an embryonic signaling center: BMP-4 induces p21 and is associated with apoptosis in the mouse tooth enamel knot. *Development* 125: 161–169, 1998.
[12] Thesleff, I. and Sharpe, P. Signalling networks regulating dental development. *Mech. Dev.* 67: 111–123, 1997.
[13] Tucker, A. and Sharpe, P. The cutting-edge of mammalian development; how the embryo makes teeth. *Nat. Rev. Genet.* 5: 499–508, 2004.
[14] Lumsden, A.G.S. Spatial organization of the epithelium and the role of neural crest cells in the initiation of the mammalian tooth. *Development* 103: 155–169, 1988.

[15] Kollar, E.J. and Baird, G.R. The influence of the dental papilla on the development of tooth shape in embryonic mouse tooth germs. *J. Embryol. Exp. Morphol.* 21: 131–148, 1969.

[16] Kollar, E.J. and Baird, G.R. Tissue interactions in embryonic mouse tooth germs. I. Reorganization of the dental epithelium during tooth-germ reconstruction. *J. Embryol. Exp. Morphol.* 24: 159–171, 1970.

[17] Maas, R. and Bei, M. The genetic control of early tooth development. *Crit. Rev. Oral Biol. Med.* 8: 4–39, 1997.

[18] Vainio, S. et al. Identification of BMP-4 as a signal mediating secondary induction between epithelial and mesenchymal tissues during early tooth development. *Cell* 75: 45–58, 1993.

[19] Chen, Y. et al. Msx1 controls inductive signaling in mammalian tooth morphogenesis. *Development* 122: 3035–3044, 1996.

[20] Kratochwil, K. et al. Lef1 expression is activated by BMP-4 and regulates inductive tissue interactions in tooth and hair development. *Genes Dev.* 10: 1382–1394, 1996.

[21] Neubüser, A. et al. Antagonistic interactions between FGF and BMP signaling pathways: a mechanism for positioning the sites of tooth formation. *Cell* 90: 247–255, 1997.

[22] Bitgood, M.J. and McMahon, A.P. Hedgehog and Bmp genes are coexpressed at many diverse sites of cell-cell interaction in the mouse embryo. *Dev. Biol.* 172: 126–138, 1995.

[23] Koyama, E. et al. Polarizing activity, Sonic hedgehog, and tooth development in embryonic and postnatal mouse. *Dev. Dyn.* 206: 59–72, 1996.

[24] Hardcastle, Z. et al. The Shh signalling pathway in tooth development: defects in Gli2 and Gli3 mutants. *Development* 125: 2803–2811, 1998.

[25] Vaahtokari, A. et al. The enamel knot as a signaling center in the developing mouse tooth. *Mech. Dev.* 54: 39–43, 1996a.

[26] Thesleff, I. and Jernvall, J. The enamel knot: a putative signaling center regulating tooth development. *Cold spring harbour Symp. Quant. Biol.* 62: 257–267, 1997.

[27] Vaahtokari, A., Åberg, T., and Thesleff, I. Apoptosis in the developing tooth: association with an embryonic signaling center and suppression by EGF and FGF-4. *Development* 122: 121–129, 1996b.

[28] Kettunen, P. and Thesleff, I. Expression and function of FGFs-4, -8, and -9 suggest functional redundancy and repetitive use as epithelial signals during tooth morphogenesis. *Dev. Dyn.* 211: 256–268, 1998.

[29] MacKenzie, A., Ferguson, M.W., and Sharpe, P.T. Expression patterns of the homeobox gene, Hox-8, in the mouse embryo suggest a role in specifying tooth initiation and shape. *Development* 115: 403–420, 1992.

[30] Iseki, S. et al. Sonic hedgehog is expressed in epithelial cells during development of whisker, hair, and tooth. *Biochem. Biophys. Res. Commun.* 218: 688–693, 1996.

[31] Satokata, I. and Maas, R. Msx1 deficient mice exhibit cleft palate and abnormalities of craniofacial and tooth development. *Nat. Genet.* 6: 348–356, 1994.

[32] van Genderen, C. et al. Development of several organs that require inductive epithelial-mesenchymal interactions is impaired in LEF-1-deficient mice. *Genes Dev.* 8: 2691–2703, 1994.

[33] Peters, H., Neubüser, A., and Balling, R. Pax genes and organogenesis: Pax9 meets tooth development. *Eur. J. Oral Sci.* 106: 38–43, 1998.

[34] Matzuk, M.M., Kumar, T.R., and Bradley, A. Different phenotypes for mice deficient in either activins or activin receptor type II. *Nature* 374: 356–360, 1995.

[35] Tucker, A.S., Al Khamis, A., and Sharpe, P.T. Interactions between Bmp-4 and Msx-1 act to restrict gene expression to odontogenic mesenchyme. *Dev. Dyn.* 212, 533–539, 1998.

[36] Vieira, A.R. Oral clefts and syndromic forms of tooth agenesis as models for genetics of isolated tooth agenesis. *J. Dent. Res.* 82: 162–165, 2003.

[37] Lammi, L. et al. Mutations in AXIN2 cause familial tooth agenesis and predispose to colorectal cancer. *Am. J. Hum. Genet.* 74: 1043–1050, 2004. Epub 2004 Mar 23.

[38] Thomas, E.D. Bone marrow transplantation from bench to bedside. *Ann. NY Acad. Sci.* 770: 34–41, 1995.

[39] Snowden, J.A. et al. Autologous hemopoietic stem cell transplantation in severe RA: a report from the EBMT and ABMTR. *J. Rheumatol.* 31: 482–488, 2004.

[40] Rini, B.I. et al. Allogeneic stem-cell transplantation of renal cell cancer after nonmyeloablative chemotherapy: feasibility, engraftment, and clinical results. *J. Clin. Oncol.* 20: 2017–2024, 2002.

[41] Gronthos, S. et al. Postnatal human dental pulp stem cells (DPSCs) *in vitro* and *in vivo. Proc. Natl Acad. Sci. USA* 97: 13625–30136, 2000.

[42] Gronthos, S. et al. Stem cell properties of human dental pulp stem cells. *J. Dental. Res.* 81: 531–535, 2002.

[43] Shi, S., Robey, P.G., and Gronthos, S. Comparison of gene expression profiles for human, dental pulp and bone marrow stromal stem cells by cDNA microarray analysis. *Bone* 29: 532–539, 2001.

[44] Ekholm, S.V. and Reed, S.I. Regulation of G(1) cyclin-dependent kinases in the mammalian cell cycle. *Curr. Opin. Cell Biol.* 12: 676–684, 2000.

[45] Grossel, M.J., Baker, G.L., and Hinds, P.W. cdk6 can shorten G(1) phase dependent upon the N-terminal INK4 interaction domain. *J. Biol. Chem.* 274: 29960–29967, 1999.

[46] Shi, S. and Gronthos, S. Perivascular niche of postnatal mesenchymal stem cells identified in human bone marrow and dental pulp. *J. Bone Miner. Res.* 18: 696–704, 2003.

[47] Batouli, S. et al. Comparison of stem cell-mediated osteogenesis and dentinogenesis. *J. Dental. Res.* 82: 975–980, 2003.

[48] Levin, L.G. Pulpal regeneration. *Pract. Periodont. Aesthet. Dental.* 10: 621–624, 1998.

[49] About, I. et al. Pulpal inflammatory responses following non-carious class V restorations. *Oper. Dental.* 26: 336–342, 2001.

[50] About, I. et al. The effect of cavity restoration variables on odontoblast cell numbers and dental repair. *J. Dental.* 29: 109–117, 2001.

[51] Murray, P.E. et al. Restorative pulpal and repair responses. *J. Am. Dental. Assoc.* 132: 482–491, 2001.

[52] Murray, P.E. et al. Postoperative pulpal and repair responses. *J. Am. Dental. Assoc.* 131: 321–329, 2000.

[53] Rutherford, R.B. and Gu, K. Treatment of inflamed ferret dental pulps with recombinant bone morphogenetic protein-7. *Eur. J. Oral Sci.* 108: 202–206, 2000.

[54] Sloan, A.J., Rutherford, R.B., and Smith, A.J. Stimulation of the rat dentine-pulp complex by bone morphogenetic protein-7 *in vitro. Arch. Oral Biol.* 45: 173–177, 2000.

[55] Rutherford, R.B. et al. Bone morphogenetic protein-transduced human fibroblasts convert to osteoblasts and form bone *in vivo. Tissue Eng.* 8: 441–52, 2002.

[56] Iohara, K. et al. Dentin regeneration by dental pulp stem cell therapy with recombinant human bone morphogenetic protein 2. *J. Dental. Res.* 83: 590–595, 2004.

[57] Young, C.S. et al. Tissue engineering of complex tooth structures on biodegradable polymer scaffolds. *J. Dental. Res.* 81: 695–700, 2002.

[58] Duailibi, M.T. et al. Bioengineered teeth from cultured rat tooth bud cells. *J. Dental. Res.* 83: 523–528, 2004.

[59] Ohazama, A. et al. Stem-cell-based tissue engineering of murine teeth. *J. Dental. Res.* 83: 518–522, 2004.

[60] Tucker, A.S., Matthews, K.L., and Sharpe, P.T. Transformation of tooth type induced by inhibition of BMP signalling. *Science* 282: 1136–1138, 1998.

[61] Ferguson, C.A., Tucker, A.S., and Sharpe, P.T. Temporospatial cell interactions regulating mandibular and maxillary arch patterning. *Development* 127: 403–412, 2000.

[62] Thomas, B.L. et al. Role of *Dlx-1* and *Dlx-2* genes in patterning of the murine dentition. *Development* 124: 4811–4818, 1997.

[63] Grigoriou, M. et al. Expression of *Lhx6* and *Lhx7*, a novel subfamily of LIM homeodomain genes, suggests a role in mammalian head development. *Development* 125: 2063–2074, 1998.

[64] Tucker, A.S. et al. Fgf-8 determines rostral–caudal polarity in the first branchial arch. *Development* 126: 51–61, 1999.

[65] Mitsiadis, T.A. et al. Role of Islet1 in the patterning of murine dentition. *Development* 130: 4451–4460, 2003.

[66] Mucchielli, M.L. et al. *Otlx2/RIEG* expression in the odontogenic epithelium precedes tooth initiation and requires mesenchyme-derived signals for its maintenance. *Dev. Biol.* 189: 275–284, 1997.

[67] St. Amand, T.R. et al. Antagonistic signals between BMP4 and FGF8 define the expression of *Pitx1* and *Pitx2* in mouse tooth-forming anlage. *Dev. Biol.* 217: 323–332, 2000.

[68] Headon, D.J. et al. Gene defect in ectodermal dysplasia implicates a death domain adaper in development. *Nature* 414: 913–916, 2002.

[69] Sarkar, L. et al. Wnt/Shh interactions regulate ectodermal boundary formation during mammalian tooth development. *Proc. Natl Acad. Sci. USA* 97: 4520–4524, 2000.

[70] Ferguson, C.A. et al. Activin is an essential early mesenchymal signal in tooth development that is required for patterning of the murine dentition. *Genes Dev.* 12: 2636–2649, 1998.

[71] D'Souza, R.N. et al. *Cbfa1* is required for epithelial-mesenchymal interactions regulating tooth development in mice. *Development* 126: 2911–2920, 1999.

[72] Tucker, A.S. et al. Edar/Eda interactions regulate enamel knot formation in tooth morphogenesis. *Development* 127: 4691–4700, 2000.

[73] Kettunen, P. et al. Associations of FGF-3 and FGF-10 with signaling networks regulating tooth morphogenesis. *Dev. Dyn.* 219: 322–332, 2000.

[74] Kettunen, P., Karavanova, I., and Thesleff, I. Responsiveness of developing dental tissues to fibroblast growth factors: expression of splicing alternatives of FGFR1,-2,-3, and of FGFR4; and stimulation of cell proliferation by FGF-2,-4,-8, and -9. *Dev. Genet.* 22: 374–385, 1998.

[75] Åberg, T., Wozney, J., and Thesleff, I. Expression patterns of bone morphogenic proteins (bmps) in the developing mouse tooth suggest poles in morphogenesis and cell differentiation. *Dev. Dyn.* 210: 383–396, 1997.

[76] Sarkar, L. and Sharpe, P.T. Expression of wnt signaling pathway genes during tooth development. *Mech. Dev.* 85: 197–200, 1999.

[77] Snead, M.L., Luo, W., Lau, E.C., and Slavkin, H.C. Spatial and temporal-restricted pattern for amelogenin gene expression during mouse molar tooth organogenesis. *Development* 104: 77–85, 1988.

[78] Bègue-Kirn, C. et al. Dentin sialoprotein, dentin phosphoprotein, enamelysin and ameloblastin: tooth-specific molecules that are distinctively expressed during murine dental differentiation. *Eur. J. Oral Sci.* 106: 963–970, 1998.

[79] Developmental biology programme of the University of Helsinki. *Gene Expression in Tooth* [online], http://biteit.helsinki.fi, 1996.

62

Tracheal Tissue Engineering

Brian Dunham
Paul Flint
Sunil Singhal
Catherine Le Visage
Kam Leong
Johns Hopkins School of Medicine

62.1 Introduction

A seemingly simple, single-lumen structure, the trachea is the sole conduit between the supraglottic airway and the lungs. Humidified and warmed air inspired through the nose travels to the lungs through the relatively thin-walled trachea, which widens slightly at its distal end. At birth, its diameter is approximately 0.5 cm. Tracheal size grows proportionally with the height and weight of the child [1,2]. In a male human adult, the trachea is approximately 12-cm long and 1.5- to 2-cm wide. In an adult female it is approximately 11-cm long and narrower. At its distal end, the carina, it bifurcates into the two mainstem bronchi (Figure 62.1).

Mechanically, the trachea has several functions. As an air conduit one of its most important structural functions is to maintain patency; any significant obstruction of its lumen can result in rapid asphyxiation. It must also be flexible enough to accommodate cervical rotation, flexion, and extension. Furthermore, it has to withstand both negative and positive intraluminal pressures encountered in the respiratory cycle. Approximately 16 to 20 hyaline cartilage rings provide the necessary rigidity; the intervening soft tissue provides the necessary flexibility and compliance to respond to cervical motion and varying intraluminal pressure. The first and most superior ring, the cricoid cartilage, is a complete ring (Figure 62.1). The remaining cartilage rings beneath the cricoid are C-shaped and open posteriorly. The pars membrana spans the open ends of the cartilage rings and is composed of a fibroelastic ligament and longitudinally oriented smooth muscle (Figure 62.2). The ligament prevents overdistention, while contraction of the muscle reduces the size of the lumen. The latter occurs during the cough reflex; the decreased luminal size increases the velocity of the expired air, facilitating airway clearance.

The trachea is lined with a pseudostratified columnar respiratory epithelium that consists of a heterogeneous population of cells that form tight junctions; in the submucosal space are numerous mixed

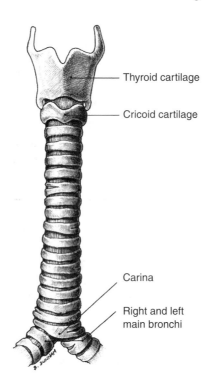

FIGURE 62.1   Anterior view of a human trachea.

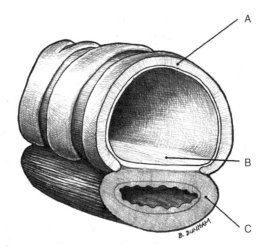

FIGURE 62.2   Cross sectional view of a human trachea segment. (A) C-shaped cartilaginous ring. (B) Pars membrana of the trachea, which is composed of a fibroelastic ligament and smooth muscle. (C) Esophagus.

sero-mucous glands, which decrease in numbers in the distal aspect of the trachea (Figures 62.3a,b). Airway epithelial cells, as well as dendritic cells found in airway epithelium, express major histocompatibility complex class I and II molecules, which endow the epithelium with the properties of an immunologic barrier [3]. The epithelium's major function was once thought to be that of a physical barrier; it is now thought to be far more complex. The airway surface epithelium does indeed possess a variety of intercellular junctional complexes that create a tight and efficient barrier against inhaled pathogens and other noxious agents [4,5]. In addition, airway epithelial cells act together to ensure mucosal defense

(a)

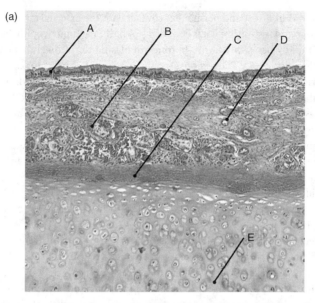

(b)

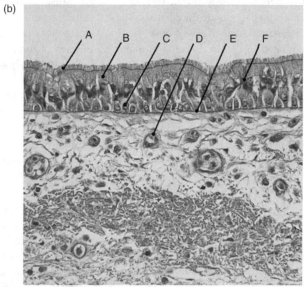

FIGURE 62.3 (a) Photomicrograph of tracheal tissue, hematoxylin and eosin stain ×200. (A) Respiratory epithelium. (B) Mixed sero-mucous glands residing in the lamina propria. (C) Perichondrium. (D) Blood vessel. The lamina propria underlying the epithelium is richly vascularized, which helps to warm the inspired air. (E) Cartilage. (b) Photomicrograph of tracheal respiratory epithelium, hematoxylin and eosin stain ×400. (A) Cilia arising from (B), the columnar ciliated epithelial cells. (C) Basal cell. (D) Blood vessel within the lamina propria. (E) Basement membrane. (F) Goblet cell.

through a variety of mechanisms such as mucociliary clearance, active secretion of ions and regulation of water balance, regulation of airway smooth muscle function, and the release of antibacterial, antioxidant, and anti-inflammatory molecules in the airway surface liquid. Airway epithelium constitutes the interface between the internal milieu and the external environment, and responds to changes in the external environment by secreting a large number of mediators that interact with cells of the immune system and underlying mesenchyme [5]. These mediators include arachidonic acid metabolites, nonprostanoid inhibitory factors, nitric oxide, endothelin, cytokines, and growth factors [3].

Since the epithelium is in direct and permanent contact with the external environment, it is frequently injured. It is capable of rapid restitution if it is denuded [6,7]. After an injury, epithelial cells dedifferentiate, flatten, and migrate rapidly beneath a fibrin–fibronectin plasma-derived gel that contains both adhesive plasma proteins and leukocytes [8]. The response to injury, however, appears to partly depend on the depth of injury. Deep injuries violating the lamina propria and reaching the perichondrial tissues are associated with excessive granulation tissue [9,10]. Bacterial and viral infections, inhaled pollutants and toxic agents, and mechanical stress can severely alter the integrity of the epithelial barrier. The response of the airway surface epithelium to an acute injury includes a succession of cellular events varying from loss of surface epithelial impermeability to partial shedding of the epithelium or even to complete denudation of the basement membrane. In response to chronic injury, the airway epithelial cells can also transdifferentiate, with a shift from serous to mucous cells, from ciliated to secretory cells, or from secretory to squamous cells. Such a remodeling illustrates the marked plasticity and capacity of the airway epithelium to regenerate [4,11]. Given its regenerative capacity, characterization of airway stem cells may eventually lead to clinical, therapeutic benefit [12].

There are at least eight morphologically distinct cells types in human respiratory epithelium. These include columnar ciliated epithelial cells, mucous goblet cells, serous cells, basal cells, Clara cells, pulmonary endocrine cells, as well as intraepithelial nerve cells, and a variety of immune cells. The latter group of cells is comprised of mast cells, intraepithelial lymphocytes, dendritic cells, and macrophages. Serous cells and Clara cells are found beyond the trachea in the more distant airway conduits. The most abundant of the tracheal epithelial cells are the ciliated columnar cells, accounting for approximately 50% of all epithelial cells. Ciliated cells, which arise from either basal or secretory cells, are no longer thought to be terminally differentiated [5,13]. In the adult human trachea, each of these ciliated columnar cells host approximately 300 cilia that beat in an organized fashion to sweep respiratory secretions upward into the larynx and oral cavity.

The second most common cell in the human trachea is the mucous goblet cell, which is characterized by acidic-mucin granules. Secretion into the airway lumen of the correct amount of mucin, a glycoprotein, and the viscoelasticity of the resulting mucus are important parameters for an efficient mucociliary clearance of mucus-entrapped foreign bodies. It is thought that the acidity, due to the sialic acid content of the glycoprotein, determines the viscoelastic profile and hence the relative ease of transport across cilia [5]. These goblet cells are thought to be capable of self-renewal and may differentiate into ciliated cells [14,15], as do the basal cells [16]. The basal cells are short, rounded cells that lie on the basal lamina without extension to the apical surface. They are the only cells in the epithelium that are firmly attached to the basement membrane and, as such, aid in the attachment of more superficial cells to the basement membrane via hemidesmosomal complexes [15,17]. The basal cell is thought to be able to function as a primary stem cell, giving rise to mucous and ciliated epithelial cells [5,18–25]. Pulmonary endocrine cells are found throughout the airway as solitary cells or in clusters. These cells secrete a variety of biogenic amines and peptides, which appear to play an important role in fetal lung development and airway function including the regulation of epithelial cell growth and regeneration.

The trachea's rich arterial blood supply is derived from fine branches of the superior and inferior thyroid arteries, of the internal thoracic arteries, and of the bronchial arteries. Returning blood from tracheal veins eventually travels into the inferior thyroid veins. The incompletion of the C-shaped rings allows the trachea to be in close apposition to the esophagus throughout its length and to share vascular supply. While it does receive its blood supply from named vessels, its vasculature is composed of a rich network of thin vessels. The profuse system of microvessels that immediately underlie the epithelium is of particular importance in the maintenance and regeneration of airway epithelium. There is thought to be a dynamic interplay between plasma-derived molecules, their receptors, airway epithelial cells, and their secretions *in vivo*, which either promotes airway defense or induces disease [26].

The smooth muscle and glands of the trachea are parasympathetically innervated by the vagus nerve, either directly or by the recurrent laryngeal nerves. Sympathetic innervation comes directly from the sympathetic trunk. Tracheal mucosa itself is richly innervated from subepithelial plexuses. The trachea is remarkably sensitive to touch and has a low threshold to elicit a reflexive cough in the presence of foreign material. The subepithelial nerves penetrate the basement membrane at focal points where they branch and spread along the basement membrane with terminal ends extending between epithelial cells and terminating in the airway lumen. The nerves have an obvious sensory role but the full breadth of their exact function is unknown; there is, however, evidence that they might be in direct apposition to pulmonary endocrine cells, with the suggestion of a bi-directional communication between these two cell types [5].

In summary, the trachea is a simple, yet elegant, structure that very effectively resists collapse from negative intraluminal pressures. It is flexible enough to accommodate distension and adapt to cervical rotation, and is lined with a metabolically active and physiologically complex respiratory epithelium that is intimately linked to the underlying mesenchyme and the immune system.

62.2   Tracheal Reconstruction: Previous Attempts

Tracheal reconstruction dates back to at least 1881 when Gluck and Zeller re-anastomosed a transected dog trachea [27]. Over 80 years later in his classic 1964 paper, Grillo described anatomic studies on human cadavers establishing the upper limits of tracheal resection that would allow a direct end-to-end anastomosis without undue anastomotic tension [28]. Subsequently, he and others refined the techniques of tracheal resection with primary anastomosis [29–37]. Today, approximately half of the human adult's and one third of the small child's trachea can safely be resected and primarily anastomosed. Even long segment tracheal stenosis can now often be handled by an operation known as a slide tracheoplasty. The need for more extensive resections is clinically rare. In the adult population, the need for replacement of greater than a half of the trachea usually arises in the setting of a low-grade neoplasm, such as adenoid cystic carcinoma of the trachea, or in the setting of unresectable diseases (such as tracheopathia osteoplastica, relapsing polychondritis, Wegener's granulomatosis, and trauma). In the neonate, it arises in the setting of tracheal agenesis, a congenital absence of tracheal tissue [38,39]. Whenever a significant length of trachea is compromised by disease, it presents a true surgical dilemma as no truly dependable and reliable replacement yet exists. Given the infrequent clinical demand, it is amazing that the literature is rich in attempts to find suitable materials with which to replace tracheal tissue. None of these have been particularly successful and none have found consistent and widely accepted clinical use. A limited review of some these attempts offers valuable insight into the physiology and pathophysiology of the trachea. They fall into several categories: implantation of foreign materials, reconstruction with autogenous tissues, reconstruction, and transplantation of autografts and allografts. The newest category is tissue engineering [38].

A wide variety of materials has been used for solid prostheses, including but not limited to stainless steel, Vitallium, glass, polyethylene, Lucite, silicone, Teflon, Ivalon, polyvinyl chloride, and polyurethane [40–54]. These materials were used as single constituents or in combination; some prostheses used cuffs draped over tracheal ends to encourage fixation of the prosthesis and prevent obstruction with granulation tissue at the anastomotic sites. The solid prostheses have been prone to migrate and dislodge, to obstruct with granulation tissue at the anastomoses, and to develop infections. In addition, they have tended to yield poor epithelialization. No solid prosthesis has ever proven reliable over time. Some may work for an unpredictable amount of time but all eventually fail. In response to the failure of solid prostheses, some groups turned to porous synthetic prostheses to allow tissue ingrowth and promote a greater prosthetic incorporation. A variety of porous prostheses have been attempted; some of these were used in conjunction with tissues such as pericardium, omentum, dermis, pleura, and fascia as well as fibrin and collagen [50,51,55–75]. The porous prostheses have also yielded unsatisfactory results. They have regularly failed to become fully epithelialized, especially in the center, which promoted central granulation, cicatrisation (scar formation), and stenosis. The porous prostheses have also shown a propensity for bacterial colonization.

There have been many attempts to replace trachea with autogenous tissues, including skin, fascia, pericardium, periosteum, buccal mucosa, aortic tissue, esophageal tissue, bronchial tissue, cartilage, bone, and bladder epithelium [38,49,57,58,70,76–92]. The implanted cartilage, despite its autogenous source, often resorbed. In addition to devascularized autogenous tissues, several authors have reported using vascularly pedicled tissue transfers. Although some yielded temporary success, none of these have become commonplace in clinical practice. Some heroic efforts have been documented in the clinical realm. There are several clinical reports of tracheal reconstruction with cutaneous troughs, as well as esophageal transfers. These are difficult procedures whose failure rates, not surprisingly, rise with their increasing complexity.

Experiments using devitalized tissues including cadaveric tracheas have also failed to produce robust results [93,94]. Cadaveric tracheal grafts have been treated in a variety of ways: irradiation, freeze-drying, and chemical treatment [58,95–102]. None has resulted in clinically reliable solutions. Devitalized tracheal tissue is inherently problematic as the cartilage is inevitably doomed to resorption, leading to tracheomalacia, a degenerative softening of the trachea. The degree of reported epithelialization is somewhat variable, but it is doubtful that any was truly and thoroughly effective. Our own laboratory has investigated the use of chemically decellularized cadaveric grafts in a rabbit model, both as anterior window grafts and circumferential grafts (unpublished data; Figures 62.4a,b). All experimental animals that underwent an anterior window replacement survived until their appointed time of sacrifice without suffering from clinically significant stenoses. The circumferential replacement was far more problematic. All grafts, if given sufficient time, gradually stenosed. Gross evaluation confirmed central malacia of the grafts, as well as centrally located mucosal stenoses. Histologic evaluation revealed a significant inflammatory response that showed a predilection for the center of the grafts; epithelial denudation also appeared to coincide with excessive granulation tissue, as is often reported in the literature.

Early experimental use of true transplants, in other words, fresh tracheal allografts in animal models has yielded uniformly poor results [57,58,78,99,103]. Even fresh autografts have been problematic. Smaller

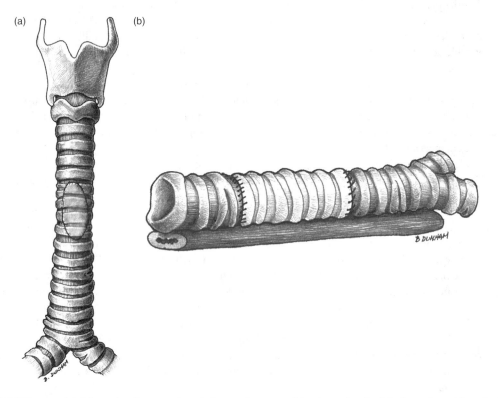

(a)   (b)

FIGURE 62.4   (a) Schematic of an anterior window replacement. (b) Schematic of a full circumferential tracheal replacment.

segments and patches tend to have a higher success rate. Fibrous degeneration of the autograft is common. Presumably, the failure partly occurs because the fine vasculature of the grafts has not reestablished rapidly enough to support the respiratory mucosa and the underlying mesenchyme before exposure to the external environment engenders a chronic inflammatory response with devolution of the mucosa. One potential solution would be the use of vascular anastomoses to allow for near immediate reconnection of a graft's vascular network. Unfortunately, although vascular anastomoses are technically feasible as recent work by Genden [104,105] has shown, they significantly increase the complexity of the surgical procedure and can increase the risk of failure in the already unforgiving milieu of the airway. Other groups have addressed this issue by incorporating thyroid tissue along with the trachea during transplantation attempts, using the thyroid's larger blood vessels to perform the anastomoses [106,107].

Without immune suppression, fresh allografts have elicited an immune rejection, resulting in ischemic necrosis of the implanted tissues. These allografts, not surprisingly, suffered from resorptive collapse of their tracheal rings and poor reepithelization leading to a short postoperative survival of the animals [57,58,103]. Some improvement in graft viability has occurred with indirect vascularization with omental flaps. This has been especially true for small grafts; longer grafts, however, still have not fared well. Allografts that have undergone cryopreservation and have been supported with an omental flap have shown improved survival, even without immunosuppression[108–110]. However, recipient chondrocytes have not repopulated the grafts' cartilage. Cryopreservation, presumably, has reduced epithelial antigenicity; this phenomenon is not yet fully understood. Bujia [111] showed evidence that the predominant locus of antigenicity is likely to reside in the epithelium and not the cartilage. Liu denuded tracheal epithelium with detergent and reported that these allografts, which were supported with an omental flap, remained viable [112,113]. Not surprisingly, given airway mucosa regenerative capacity, recipient epithelial cells have eventually repopulated the grafts' epithelium.

In an effort to induce immunotolerance, Genden and colleagues pretreated rats with a single portal-vein injection of ultraviolet-B irradiated donor splenocytes seven days prior to circumferential tracheal allograft placement. The pretreatment induced a donor-specific immune hyporesponsiveness and prevented rejection of the grafts [114]. Whether or not immune tolerance can be induced in higher animal models remains to be seen.

Tracheal obstruction is seen time and time again in tracheal reconstruction efforts. Provided that a neotrachea would be able to resist collapse, it still faces a tremendous challenge within its lumen: that of establishing a healthy mucosa, free of chronic inflammation. The luminal compromise is consistently associated with a detrimental soft tissue reaction, in which airway mucosa undergoes a significant reactive thickening with a progressive diminution of the airway lumen and a disruption of the structural integrity of the cartilaginous rings of the trachea. This reaction appears to be superficially analogous to exuberant scarring found in skin tissue. It is thought that prompt and thorough reepithelialization can prevent this complication and maintain luminal patency [115].

Our present ability to intelligently address the infrequent need for tracheal tissue replacement is hampered by our lack of understanding airway mucosal of wound healing. Significant strides have been made in the tissue engineering of cartilage; the ability to engineer a structure that is able to resist collapse and that meets the rigors of clinical application is likely to be imminent. However, a great deal remains to be understood about airway mucosal physiology and healing before true clinical utility will be possible.

Although the need for full circumferential tracheal replacement is limited, the need to address airway mucosal disease is far greater. The incidence of tracheal stenosis after an ischemic mucosal injury is far more prevalent than those etiologies requiring replacement of more than half of the trachea. Since the advent of cuffed endotracheal tubes, the incidence of tracheal stenosis has risen sharply. The presence of a foreign body within the airway, especially one that applies mucosal pressure denuding epithelium and compromising blood flow, can trigger a very poorly understood chronic mucosal inflammation, which often results in mucosal hypertrophy and luminal obstruction. The problem is compounded by the fact that the airway is constantly exposed to the bacteria-laden external environment. So, whereas the literature seems to have focused on circumferential tracheal tissue replacement, clinically there is a far greater need to address focal mucosal disease, underscoring the importance of furthering our understanding of airway mucosal physiology and pathophysiology.

62.3   Tracheal Tissue Engineering

Tracheal tissue engineering is in its infancy. The first true tissue engineering effort appeared only in 1994 [116]. As with any field in its early development, the current work is limited by a lack of detailed understanding of the physiology and pathophysiology of tracheal tissue. Current work is premised on rather crude hypotheses. Efforts in this field will undoubtedly evolve as functional replacement models begin to emerge and the critical issues become more apparent. Most efforts have centered on the construction of a cartilaginous structure that can resist collapse. Recent work has focused on finding the best cellular source and method to recreate the cartilaginous infrastructure, and attempting to introduce an epithelial lining within the lumen of a tissue-engineered construct. Some investigators have made use of mesenchymal stem cells to create cartilage as well as a respiratory epithelium. Other investigators have explored fetal surgery techniques allowing their constructs to partly mature *in utero*. There are also efforts that do not neatly fall into the category of tissue engineering but are worthy of mention.

Whereas there are many reports of attempted tracheal replacement, it was not until 1994 that the first true tissue-engineering attempt appears in the literature when Vacanti [116] and colleagues reported on the circumferential replacement of rat tracheas with tissue-engineered cartilaginous tubes. They seeded chondrocytes harvested from the shoulder of newborn calves onto sheets of nonwoven polyglycolic acid (PGA) mesh. All experimental animals died within one week of the operation. Presumably, the animals succumbed to respiratory distress. There was no discussion of postmortem histology; what happened within the lumen of the airway is not clear. It is likely that a straight cartilaginous tubular structure is inadequate for two important reasons. First, a rigid tube would place a significant mechanical demand on the anastomoses, encouraging failure at those sites. Second, it would be hard for blood vessels to penetrate directly through the cartilage to establish the robust vasculature required to meet the high metabolic demands of airway epithelium. In essence, this design requires that the vascular network arise exclusively from an intraluminal source and travel from mechanically challenged anastomoses over a considerable distance, without support from extratracheal vascular ingrowth. Nonetheless, this is a landmark paper in the evolution of tracheal engineering as it is arguably the first true translational effort to tissue engineer a trachea.

In 2002, Kojima [117] and colleagues addressed the mechanical inadequacies inherent in a straight cartilaginous tube. They isolated chondrocytes and fibroblasts from the nasal septum of 2-month-old sheep. Chondrocyte-seeded PGA mesh was placed in the grooves of a 20 by 50-mm-long helical Silastic template; the entire construct was then wrapped with a fibroblast-laden PGA mesh. In the first arm of the study, the cultured constructs were implanted into dorsal subcutaneous pockets in athymic rats and explanted after eight weeks. In this refined attempt, the rat-incubated construct yielded cartilage biochemically similar to native tissue as measured by sulfated glycosaminoglycan (GAG) content, hydroxyproline content, and cellularity. In the second arm of the study, autologous constructs were implanted underneath the sternocleidomastoid muscle of the donor sheep, allowed to mature *in vivo* for eight weeks before being harvested without preservation of a vascular pedicle and used to replace a surgically created 5-cm circumferential defect in the cervical trachea of the now four-month-old donor sheep. By contrast with the results obtained in the rat model, the sheep-incubated constructs were significantly more cellular and poorer in GAG content than native tissue. As a result the sheep-incubated constructs performed poorly once rotated into the airway, without an attached vascular supply. Postoperatively, none of the sheep survived for more than seven days. They all suffered from either stenosis or clinically significant tracheomalacia. The difference in the results obtained between the two species was tentatively attributed to an inflammatory reaction engendered by the PGA in sheep, leading to hypercellular cartilage poor in GAG content, the cartilaginous component thought to be responsible for establishing stiffness. The authors stated that their future attempts would explore less inflammatory scaffolding material and also preserve the constructs' vascular connection to the surrounding muscle. It will be interesting to see if a helical construct has the appropriate mechanical properties to allow for successful long-term integration of a tissue-engineered trachea. By its very design, a helix precludes the development of a pars membrana.

Searching for an optimal source of chondrocytes, Fuchs and colleagues [118] experimented in 2002 with the use of fetal chondrocytes to tissue engineer cartilage. Specimens of fetal ovine elastic and hyaline cartilage were harvested from ears and tracheas, respectively. Adult aural elastic cartilage served as a comparison. Isolated chondrocytes were seeded onto nonwoven biodegradable scaffolds composed of poly-L-lactic acid (PLLA)-treated PGA polymer and maintained *in vitro* for 6 to 8 weeks. The chondrocytes isolated from fetal elastic and hyaline cartilage grew significantly faster than those harvested from adult elastic cartilage. All fetal constructs showed characteristics of hyaline cartilage, both on gross and microscopic inspection, regardless of whether the cells had originated from hyaline or elastic cartilage. In the fetal constructs, the histologic pattern seen with stains for glycosaminoglycans was comparable to that seen in native hyaline cartilage. The levels of GAG and collagen type II were higher in fetal versus adult constructs. There were, however, no significant differences between GAG, collagen type II, or elastin in fetal constructs derived from hyaline or elastic cartilage. When compared to their native tissue, fetal constructs derived from elastic cartilage contained similar levels of GAG and type II collagen, but had lower levels of elastin. Fetal hyaline constructs did not differ significantly in the levels of GAG, collagen type II, or elastin when compared to their native source. Adult elastic constructs, however, were significantly lower in collagen type II and elastin than the native elastic tissue. It is interesting that chondrocytes derived from elastic cartilage eventually produced hyaline cartilage and grew faster. What governs the formation of hyaline versus elastic cartilage is unknown at this point. The authors concluded that compared with adult constructs, matrix deposition is enhanced in engineered fetal cartilage, closely mimicking native hyaline tissue.

Another study searching for an optimal source of chondrocytes was reported by Kojima and colleagues in [119] 2003 in which they compared ovine nasal and tracheal chondrocytes seeded onto PGA matrices and implanted in nude mice. Chondrocytes from the nasal septal cartilage as well as tracheal rings of 2-month old sheep were seeded onto nonwoven mesh of PGA fibers. The cell-constructs were eventually wrapped around a 7-mm diameter silicone tube and implanted subcutaneously in nude mice for 8 weeks. They evaluated the gross and histologic appearances, the GAG and the hydroxyproline contents, and the biomechanical profile of the constructs. The gross appearances from both groups were found to resemble native tracheal cartilage. The histologic evaluation revealed a mature-appearing hyaline cartilage in both cases with abundant proteoglycan production. There was no evidence of an inflammatory reaction to the implants. The GAG contents of the tracheal-derived and the nasal septum-derived constructs were 70 and 81% of the native tracheal cartilage respectively. The hydroxyproline contents were 91 and 94% for the tracheal-derived and the nasal septum-derived constructs respectively. The tensile modulus for both construct types was, however, only about 15% that of the native trachea. Nonetheless, the constructs were stiff to the touch and grossly resisted collapse. The authors suggested that other compositional features of the extracellular matrix, such as collagen crosslinking, might play an important role in the mechanical profile of tracheal tissue. This study's findings support the use of nasal septal cartilage, which is attractive since it requires a far less invasive procedure for harvest than do most other sources of cartilage.

Later in the same year, Sakata and colleagues [120] reported an attempt to line these cartilaginous tubes with a respiratory epithelium. They constructed ten tubes as previously described [116] and implanted them into the flanks of nude mice, this time for six weeks. Epithelial cells were aseptically harvested from newborn lambs' cervical tracheas and were immediately injected in the implanted cartilaginous tubes after which both ends of the cartilaginous tube were sutured shut. The epithelial cell-lined tubes were then collected at intervals of up to three weeks. Out of ten tubes, six were found to be infected and had not developed an epithelial lining as observed on hematoxylin and eosin sections. The remaining four were lined with a respiratory mucosa, including a submucosal connective tissue, which had "abundant" small blood vessels. Some of the cells had developed cilia three weeks following inoculation into the implanted cartilaginous construct. Although promising, this brief report did not provide histologic details. For example the uniformity of the epithelial lining was not commented upon, and the composition of the epithelium was not reported. The high infection rate highlights one of the challenges of engineering respiratory tissue. The airway is inherently contaminated with a significant bacterial load. Future designs might want to consider a preliminary *in vitro* incubation period of the freshly harvested epithelial cells with antibiotics to reduce the incidence of infection. It might also have been beneficial to attach silastic tubing at either end of the tubes to allow them to be flushed on a regular interval, as the epithelial lining will begin to produce mucin and the nonattached dead cells would be trapped within the lumen increasing the risk of infection. Most importantly, however, this experiment does show that it is possible to line a tissue-engineered cartilaginous lumen with a respiratory epithelium.

There is ample evidence outside the tissue engineering literature that epithelial cells can be successfully introduced into a living luminal cavity. Several investigators have made use of a heterotopic tracheal graft model developed by Terzaghi [121]. These experiments have repeatedly demonstrated that epithelium-denuded tracheal tissue that is subcutaneously implanted in nude animals can easily be repopulated with heterologous cultured rat, rabbit, and human epithelial tracheal cells [16,20,121–124]. More recently, Dupuit and colleagues used human respiratory cells to reconstitute epithelium-denuded rat tracheas, which were implanted in the flanks of nude mice. Four to five weeks postimplantation, a fully differentiated and tightly sealed pseudostratified functional epithelial barrier was documented [125]. Rainer and colleagues successfully transplanted cultured epithelial cells onto fibrotic capsules surgically created in the anterior rectus sheath of inbred Wistar Furth rats. They did so by co-culturing native rat tracheal epithelial cells with irradiated fibroblasts, then suspending them in fibrin glue, which was used as the *in vivo* delivery vehicle [126].

A subsequent study by Kojima went one step further by investigating the co-culture of epithelial cells and chondrocytes. They used ovine nasal septum chondrocytes again, but this time, added nasal septum respiratory cells suspended in a hydrogel into the lumen of the chondrocyte-seeded constructs *in vivo*. The subcutaneously implanted chondrocyte constructs were allowed to mature for six weeks. Histologic examination, four weeks post instillation of the epithelial cells, revealed that only approximately 60% of the lumen was covered with an epithelium. Although the epithelial reconstitution was not complete, this study highlighted the practicality of using a single nasal septal harvest to obtain both cell types [127].

Congenital deformities, such as long-segment stenosis and atresia, in which the tracheal lumen does not form, are relatively infrequent but bear very high mortality rates. Fuchs and colleagues [128] have begun to explore the possibility of early *in utero* intervention using harvested cells seeded onto polymer scaffolding in an ovine model. The intrauterine environment, bathed in sterile amniotic fluid, offers the advantage of avoiding the contaminated milieu of the postnatal airway. In their experiments they performed *in utero* anterior tracheal replacement using native elastic cartilage (group II) or tissue-engineered constructs seeded with heterologous fetal chondrocytes (group I).

For group I, fetal elastic or hyaline cartilage was harvested, respectively, from the ear or tracheal rings. Chondrocyte-seeded PLLA-treated nonwoven PGA mesh was maintained in a rotating oven for 6 to 8 weeks. The constructs were then trimmed into a diamond shape and used to repair a surgically created longitudinal tracheostomy spanning 4 to 5 cartilaginous rings.

In the second group, fetal auricular cartilage was used as autologous free grafts to repair the same anterior defect as created in group I. The animals were sacrificed prenatally and postnatally. The fetal and postnatal survival rates ranged from 80 to 100%. Stridor was, however, present in more than half of the surviving animals. Again, the histologic evaluation of the tissue-engineered grafts revealed hyaline cartilage formation regardless of whether the cell source was hyaline or elastic cartilage. There was mild to moderate deformation of the tracheal lumen in some of the tissue-engineered group. In the native cartilage group, however, the tracheal lumens were severely deformed. The engineered constructs displayed a time-dependent epithelialization of their lumens. Of note, there were no serous or mucinous acini that are normally found in native tissue. All the implants of group II retained their elastic cartilage characteristics, but they also developed a thinner epithelium, which lacked both ciliated cells, as well as serous and mucinous glands. It is interesting to note that the heterologous chondrocytes engrafted without obvious signs of rejection. The authors attributed that phenomenon to the immaturity of the fetal immune system and the low histocompatibility antigen expression of fetal chondrocytes. This study demonstrated the feasibility of using heterologous chondrocytes *in utero*. The authors did not comment on why group II seemed to have poorer epithelialization; it would be interesting to know if lack of rigidity and possibly central mobility of the free grafts impaired proper epithelialization and vascularization.

One important note of caution must be mentioned when evaluating anterior tracheal repair studies. The native trachea has an impressive ability to reform an epithelial mucosa when only a limited amount of tracheal tissue is removed. This phenomenon is routinely seen after tracheostomy. An epithelial membrane will quickly form after the removal of a tracheostomy tube. Studies that perform only anterior reconstruction therefore offer a limited understanding of the potential benefits or drawbacks of the graft materials used.

In 2003, Fuchs and colleagues explored the use of mesenchymal stem cells (MSCs) in tracheal tissue engineering. MSCs are attractive in tracheal tissue engineering because of their ability to form not only cartilage but also muscle with the appropriate biochemical cues. In addition, harvesting MSCs is less invasive than obtaining autologous cartilage and would obviate the need for an additional general anesthesic and its attendant risks. MSCs can be harvested from a number of sites. Umbilical cord blood has successfully been used [129,130]; adipose tissue has yielded a cell population that can undergo chondrogenesis [131]. Though there is at least one report claiming the MSCs can be collected from the peripheral circulation of an adult [132], traditionally, a bone marrow aspirate is the best means of obtaining a sufficient number of cells [133].

Fuchs and colleagues showed the feasibility of using MSCs *in* utero by comparing constructs seeded with bone marrow-derived heterologous ovine MSCs with constructs seeded with chondrocytes derived from ovine elastic cartilage. The stem cells were encouraged to differentiate into chondrocytes by exposure to carefully defined media that contained transforming growth factor as well as ascorbic acid. After 12 weeks of incubation in a rotating bioreactor, the pretreated PGA mesh-cell constructs were then implanted in heterologous fashion into a 4 to 5 ring longitudinal tracheostomy. Normal delivery of the animals was allowed. Tracheal specimens were harvested 4 days after birth. There were no significant differences found in the survival rates prenatally or postnatally. There was again a significant amount of stridor observed, this time in both groups. The engineered cartilage implants form both sources were found to engraft despite their heterologous origin; there were, however, some mononuclear infiltrates seen in some specimens. Both groups maintained their cartilaginous phenotype *in vivo* and both epithelialized their luminal surfaces. The MSC-derived cartilage had a higher GAG content *in vitro*, but after remodeling *in vivo*, both groups had comparable GAG contents.

In 2004, Kojima explored the use of augmenting an MSC-based construct with transforming growth factor β2 (TGF-β2) released from gelatin microspheres. Bone marrow-derived ovine MSCs were seeded onto a PGA nonwoven mesh and cultured for a week with exposure to both TGF-β2 and insulin growth factor 1. The cell-polymer constructs were wrapped around a silicone helical template. Constructs were then coated with glutaraldehyde-cross-linked gelatin microspheres containing TGF-β2. The entire construct was subcutaneously implanted in nude rats for six weeks. The proteoglycan content of the tissue-engineered construct was approximately 79% of that of the native tracheal cartilage. Additionally, the collagen content of the tissue-engineered product was 71% of that of the native's content. They found no statistically significant differences in glycosaminoglycan and hydroxyproline content between native and tissue-engineered tissue. In this instance, the ability to add controlled-release growth factors via microspheres is of significant value as the addition of transforming growth factor has repeatedly been shown to significantly augment chrondogenesis in MSC culture *in vitro* [134,135].

MSC are attractive not only because of their chondrogenic capacity, but also for their potential ability to support the respiratory epithelial cells. We recently described a novel *in vitro* reconstitution system for tracheal epithelium that could be useful for investigating the cellular and molecular interaction of epithelial and mesenchymal cells [136]. In this system, a porous Transwell insert was used as a basement membrane on which MSCs were cultured on the lower side whereas normal human bronchial epithelial cells were cultured on the opposite upper side (Figure 62.5). When co-cultured with MSCs, respiratory epithelial cells maintained their capacity to progressively differentiate and form a functional epithelium, leading to the differentiation of mucin-producing cells.

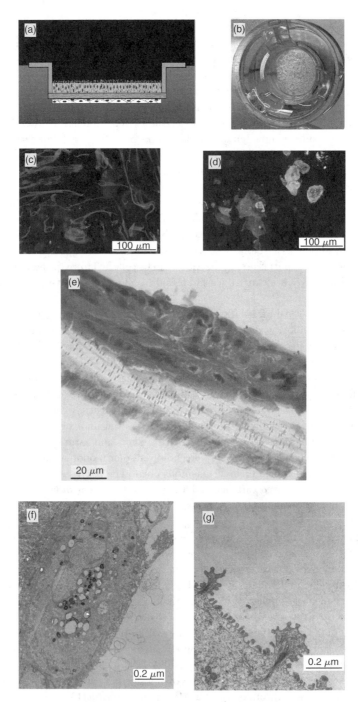

FIGURE 62.5 (a) Schematic representation of the Transwell membrane co-culture of MSCs and respiratory epithelial cells. (b) The macroscopic observation of the upper side of a Transwell membrane with a characteristic accumulation of respiratory epithelial cells. (c) Identification of MSCs during co-culture on a Transwell membrane with immuno-staining for vimentin, a mesenchymal cell marker. (d) Identification of respiratory epithelial cells during co-culture on a Transwell membrane with immunostaining for cytokeratin, an epithelial cell marker. (e) Hematoxylin and eosin paraffin section showing a monolayer of MSCs on the bottom, separated from the epithelial cells by a membrane, which is evidenced by visible pores. (f) Transmission electron microscopy (TEM) revealing the presence of granules in some epithelial cells. (g) TEM confirming the development of microvilli and actin filaments the formation of cilia.

So far most of the work has focused on the infrastructure of tracheal tissue: tracheal cartilage. There appears to be momentum gathering in this area, and it is likely that a reliable and functional infrastructure will soon be available. As of today, however, there are no standard endpoints that are commonly accepted to evaluate the overall functionality and health of the constructs. Presumptively, the ideal properties of a tissue-engineered trachea are an ability to resist negative and positive pressures, an airtight lining that promotes a healthy epithelium, torsional flexibility, good vascularization and innervation, and nonimmunogenicity and biocompatibility to ensure bioincorporation and permanence. As the work matures, endpoints are likely to routinely include thorough histological evaluation of the airway epithelium, vascular and neural networks, as well evaluation of biomechanical and biochemical function.

A major challenge in tracheal tissue engineering is the avoidance of the mucosal inflammatory response that leads to its cicatrization and an eventual reduction and obstruction of the lumen. Though recent work has begun to elucidate some of the details, the inflammatory cascade involved in this phenomenon is far from being well understood. The use of microchip arrays may help to shed some light on some of these biochemical events and guide our eventual designs. The ultimate success of a tissue-engineered trachea is likely to be dependent on future basic science efforts in airway mucosal physiology.

It is likely that the promotion of thorough vascularization and innervation will be integral to the health of the construct. So far, very little work has been done to evaluate vascularization. It is presumed, but not known, that complete coverage with a healthy respiratory epithelium at the time of airway implantation will reduce, if not eliminate, the inflammation so often seen. Considering the high metabolic nature of epithelial cells, an adequate network of blood vessels is likely to be a prerequisite. It is feasible that as our understanding of mucosal physiology matures, we might potentially avoid a two-stage operation, but, in the short term, this is unlikely to be the case. Little or no work has focused on the innervation of the tissue-engineered constructs. Though poorly understood, it is likely that neural input is integral to the healthy maintenance of airway epithelium [6]. How much time will be needed to establish robust circulation and innervation? Will growth factors be necessary? Will the development of an airway bioreactor be advantageous?

At this point, it is not known if a respiratory epithelium is an absolute must; at the very least, the surface must be airtight to prevent bacterial colonization. The presumption is that a respiratory epithelium is the ultimate lining, but could an interim lining also work until the native cells reline the lumen [137]? Respiratory epithelial restitution takes place rapidly in native tissue. Would a respiratory epithelial cell-friendly surface, such as a basement membrane, suffice? Over what length could we expect the native epithelial cells to migrate? Will tissue-engineered epithelium be functional and display coordinated movement of its cilia?

Tracheal tissue engineering is currently in the very early stages of its development. As with any new effort, there is great hope that it will produce significant advances in our ability to treat tracheal disease. Its potential, however, is inescapably restrained by our limited understanding of airway physiology and will only flourish with persistently diligent efforts in both biomaterials engineering and basic science.

References

[1] Griscom, N.T. and Wohl, M.E., Dimensions of the growing trachea related to body height. Length, anteroposterior and transverse diameters, cross-sectional area, and volume in subjects younger than 20 years of age, *Am. Rev. Respir. Dis.*, 131, 840, 1985.

[2] Chen, S.J. et al., Measurement of tracheal size in children with congenital heart disease by computed tomography, *Ann. Thorac. Surg.*, 77, 1216, 2004.

[3] Spina, D., Epithelium smooth muscle regulation and interactions, *Am. J. Respir. Crit. Care Med.*, 158, S141, 1998.

[4] Puchelle, E. and Peault, B., Human airway xenograft models of epithelial cell regeneration, *Respir. Res.*, 1, 125, 2000.

[5] Knight, D.A. and Holgate, S.T., The airway epithelium: structural and functional properties in health and disease, *Respirology*, 8, 432, 2003.

[6] Erjefalt, J.S. et al., *In vivo* restitution of airway epithelium, *Cell Tissue Res.*, 281, 305, 1995.

[7] Erjefalt, J.S. and Persson, C.G., Airway epithelial repair: breathtakingly quick and multipotentially pathogenic, *Thorax*, 52, 1010, 1997.

[8] Erjefalt, J.S. et al., Microcirculation-derived factors in airway epithelial repair *in vivo*, *Microvasc. Res.*, 48, 161, 1994.

[9] Dohar, J.E. et al., Acquired subglottic stenosis — depth and not extent of the insult is key, *Int. J. Pediatr. Otorhinolaryngol.*, 46, 159, 1998.

[10] Jung Kwon, O. et al., Tracheal stenosis depends on the extent of cartilaginous injury in experimental canine model, *Exp. Lung Res.*, 29, 329, 2003.

[11] Basbaum, C. and Jany, B., Plasticity in the airway epithelium, *Am. J. Physiol.*, 259, L38, 1990.

[12] Engelhardt, J.F. et al., Progenitor cells of the adult human airway involved in submucosal gland development, *Development*, 121, 2031, 1995.

[13] Ayers, M.M. and Jeffery, P.K., Proliferation and differentiation in mammalian airway epithelium, *Eur. Respir. J.*, 1, 58, 1988.

[14] Evans, M.J. and Plopper, C.G., The role of basal cells in adhesion of columnar epithelium to airway basement membrane, *Am. Rev. Respir. Dis.*, 138, 481, 1988.

[15] Evans, M.J. et al., The role of basal cells in attachment of columnar cells to the basal lamina of the trachea, *Am. J. Respir. Cell Mol. Biol.*, 1, 463, 1989.

[16] Liu, J.Y., Nettesheim, P., and Randell, S.H., Growth and differentiation of tracheal epithelial progenitor cells, *Am. J. Physiol.*, 266, L296, 1994.

[17] Evans, M.J. et al., Junctional adhesion mechanisms in airway basal cells, *Am. J. Respir. Cell Mol. Biol.*, 3, 341, 1990.

[18] Borthwick, D.W. et al., Evidence for stem-cell niches in the tracheal epithelium, *Am. J. Respir. Cell Mol. Biol.*, 24, 662, 2001.

[19] Nettesheim, P. et al., Pathways of differentiation of airway epithelial cells, *Environ. Health Perspect.*, 85, 317, 1990.

[20] Inayama, Y. et al., The differentiation potential of tracheal basal cells, *Lab. Invest.*, 58, 706, 1988.

[21] Inayama, Y. et al., *In vitro* and *in vivo* growth and differentiation of clones of tracheal basal cells, *Am. J. Pathol.*, 134, 539, 1989.

[22] Erjefalt, J.S., Sundler, F., and Persson, C.G., Epithelial barrier formation by airway basal cells, *Thorax*, 52, 213, 1997.

[23] Schoch, K.G. et al., A subset of mouse tracheal epithelial basal cells generates large colonies *in vitro*, *Am. J. Physiol Lung Cell Mol. Physiol.*, 286, L631, 2004.

[24] Hong, K.U. et al., Basal cells are a multipotent progenitor capable of renewing the bronchial epithelium, *Am. J. Pathol.*, 164, 577, 2004.

[25] Hong, K.U. et al., *In vivo* differentiation potential of tracheal basal cells: evidence for multipotent and unipotent subpopulations, *Am. J. Physiol. Lung Cell Mol. Physiol.*, 286, L643, 2004.

[26] Persson, C.G. et al., Plasma-derived proteins in airway defence, disease and repair of epithelial injury, *Eur. Respir. J.*, 11, 958, 1998.

[27] Gluck, T.H. and Zeller, A., Die prophylaktische resektion der trachea, *Arch. Klin. Chir.*, 26, 427, 1881.

[28] Grillo, H.C., Dignan, E.F., and Miura, T., Extensive resection and reconstruction of mediastinal trachea without prosthesis or graft: an anatomical study in man, *J. Thorac. Cardiovasc. Surg.*, 48, 741, 1964.

[29] Grillo, H.C., Circumferential resection and reconstruction of the mediastinal and cervical trachea, *Ann. Surg.*, 162, 374, 1965.

[30] Grillo, H.C., Surgical treatment of postintubation tracheal injuries, *J. Thorac. Cardiovasc. Surg.*, 78, 860, 1979.

[31] Grillo, H.C., Primary reconstruction of airway after resection of subglottic laryngeal and upper tracheal stenosis, *Ann. Thorac. Surg.*, 33, 3, 1982.

[32] Grillo, H.C., Reconstructive techniques for extensive post-intubation tracheal stenosis, *Int. Surg.*, 67, 215, 1982.

[33] Dedo, H.H. and Fishman, N.H., Laryngeal release and sleeve resection for tracheal stenosis, *Ann. Otol. Rhinol. Laryngol.*, 78, 285, 1969.

[34] Montgomery, W.W., Suprahyoid release for tracheal anastomosis, *Arch. Otolaryngol.*, 99, 255, 1974.

[35] Pearson, F.G. et al., Primary tracheal anastomosis after resection of the cricoid cartilage with preservation of recurrent laryngeal nerves, *J. Thorac. Cardiovasc. Surg.*, 70, 806, 1975.

[36] Maddaus, M.A. et al., Subglottic tracheal resection and synchronous laryngeal reconstruction, *J. Thorac. Cardiovasc. Surg.*, 104, 1443, 1992.

[37] Pearson, F.G. and Gullane, P., Subglottic resection with primary tracheal anastomosis: including synchronous laryngotracheal reconstructions, *Semin. Thorac. Cardiovasc. Surg.*, 8, 381, 1996.

[38] Grillo, H.C., Tracheal replacement: a critical review, *Ann. Thorac. Surg.*, 73, 1995, 2002.

[39] Macchiarini, P., Trachea-guided generation: deja vu all over again? *J. Thorac. Cardiovasc. Surg.*, 128, 14, 2004.

[40] Cheng, W.F., Takagi, H., and Akutsu, T., Prosthetic reconstruction of the trachea, *Surgery*, 65, 462, 1969.

[41] Borrie, J. and Redshaw, N.R., Prosthetic tracheal replacement, *J. Thorac. Cardiovasc. Surg.*, 60, 829, 1970.

[42] Demos, N.J. et al., Tracheal regeneration in long-term survivors with silicone prosthesis, *Ann. Thorac. Surg.*, 16, 293, 1973.

[43] Neville, W.E., Bolanowski, P.J., and Soltanzadeh, H., Prosthetic reconstruction of the trachea and carina, *J. Thorac. Cardiovasc. Surg.*, 72, 525, 1976.

[44] Neville, W.E., Prosthetic reconstruction of trachea, *Rev. Laryngol. Otol. Rhinol.*, 103, 153, 1982.

[45] Nelson, R.J. et al., Neovascularity of a tracheal prosthesis/tissue complex, *J. Thorac. Cardiovasc. Surg.*, 86, 800, 1983.

[46] Nelson, R.J. et al., Development of a microporous tracheal prosthesis, *Trans. Am. Soc. Artif. Intern. Organs*, 25, 8, 1979.

[47] Wykoff, T.W., A preliminary report on segmental tracheal prosthetic replacement in dogs, *Laryngoscope*, 83, 1072, 1973.

[48] Michelson, E. et al., Experiments in tracheal reconstruction, *J. Thorac. Cardiovasc. Surg.*, 41, 748, 1961.

[49] Daniel, R.A., Jr., The regeneration of defects of the trachea and bronchi. An experimental study, *J. Thorac. Surg.*, 17, 335, 1948.

[50] Shaw, R.R., Aslami, A., and Webb, W.R., Circumferential replacement of the trachea in experimental animals, *Ann. Thorac. Surg.*, 5, 30, 1968.

[51] Keshishian, J.M., Blades, B., and Beattie, E.J., Tracheal reconstruction, *J. Thorac. Surg.*, 32, 707, 1956.

[52] Spinazzola, A.J., Graziano, J.L., and Neville, W.E., Experimental reconstruction of the tracheal carina, *J. Thorac. Cardiovasc. Surg.*, 58, 1, 1969.

[53] Moncrief, W.H., Jr. and Salvatore, J.E., An improved tracheal prosthesis, *Surg. Forum*, 9, 350, 1958.

[54] Pagliero, K.M. and Shepherd, M.P., Use of stainless steel wire coil prosthesis in treatment of anastomotic dehiscence after cervical tracheal resection, *J. Thorac. Cardiovasc. Surg.*, 67, 932, 1974.

[55] Bottema, J.R. and Wildevuur, C.H., Incorporation of microporous Teflon tracheal prostheses in rabbits: evaluation of surgical aspects, *J. Surg. Res.*, 41, 16, 1986.

[56] Bottema, J.R. et al., Microporous tracheal prosthesis: incorporation and prevention of infection, *Trans. Am. Soc. Artif. Intern. Organs*, 26, 412, 1980.

[57] Bailey, B.J. and Kosoy, J., Observations in the development of tracheal prostheses and tracheal transplantation, *Laryngoscope*, 80, 1553, 1970.

[58] Greenberg, S.D., Tracheal reconstruction: an experimental study, *Arch. Otolaryngol.*, 72, 565, 1960.

[59] Poticha, S.M. and Lewis, F.J., Experimental replacement of the trachea, *J. Thorac. Cardiovasc. Surg.*, 52, 61, 1966.

[60] Beall, A.C., Jr. et al., Circumferential replacement of the trachea with marlex mesh: preliminary report, *Surg. Forum*, 11, 40, 1960.

[61] Beall, A.C., Jr. et al., Tracheal replacement with heavy Marlex mesh. Circumferential replacement of the cervical trachea, *Arch. Surg.*, 84, 390, 1962.

[62] Harrington, O.B. et al., Circumferential replacement of the trachea with Marlex mesh, *Am. Surg.*, 28, 217, 1962.

[63] Ellis, P.R. et al., The use of heavy Marlex mesh for tracheal reconstruction following resection for malignancy, *J. Thorac. Cardiovasc. Surg.*, 44, 520, 1962.

[64] Kosoy, J. et al., Proplast tracheal prosthesis: a preliminary report, *Ann. Otol. Rhinol. Laryngol.*, 86, 392, 1977.

[65] Podoshin, L. and Fradis, M., Reconstruction of the anterior wall of the cervical trachea using knitted dacron, *Ear Nose Throat J.*, 55, 42, 1976.

[66] Ike, O. et al., Experimental studies on an artificial trachea of collagen-coated poly(L-lactic acid) mesh or unwoven cloth combined with a periosteal graft, *ASAIO Trans.*, 37, 24, 1991.

[67] Mendak, S.H., Jr. et al., The evaluation of various bioabsorbable materials on the titanium fiber metal tracheal prosthesis, *Ann. Thorac. Surg.*, 38, 488, 1984.

[68] Takahama, T. et al., A new improved biodegradable tracheal prosthesis using hydroxy apatite and carbon fiber, *ASAIO Trans.*, 35, 291, 1989.

[69] Kaiser, D., Alloplastic replacement of canine trachea with Dacron, *Thorac. Cardiovasc. Surg.*, 33, 239, 1985.

[70] Suh, S.W. et al., Replacement of a tracheal defect with autogenous mucosa lined tracheal prosthesis made from polypropylene mesh, *ASAIO J.*, 47, 496, 2001.

[71] Okumura, N. et al., A new tracheal prosthesis made from collagen grafted mesh, *ASAIO J.*, 39, M475, 1993.

[72] Okumura, N. et al., Experimental reconstruction of the intrathoracic trachea using a new prosthesis made from collagen grafted mesh, *ASAIO J.*, 40, M834, 1994.

[73] Pearson, F.G. et al., The reconstruction of circumferential tracheal defects with a porous prosthesis. An experimental and clinical study using heavy Marlex mesh, *J. Thorac. Cardiovasc. Surg.*, 55, 605, 1968.

[74] Teramachi, M. et al., Porous-type tracheal prosthesis sealed with collagen sponge, *Ann. Thorac. Surg.*, 64, 965, 1997.

[75] Suh, S.W. et al., Development of new tracheal prosthesis: autogenous mucosa-lined prosthesis made from polypropylene mesh, *Int. J. Artif. Organs*, 23, 261, 2000.

[76] Glatz, F. et al., A tissue-engineering technique for vascularized laryngotracheal reconstruction, *Arch. Otolaryngol. Head Neck Surg.*, 129, 201, 2003.

[77] Rush, B.F. and Cliffton, E.E., Experimental reconstruction of the trachea with bladder mucosa, *Surgery*, 40, 1105, 1956.

[78] Barker, W.S. and Litton, W.B., Bladder osteogenesis aids tracheal reconstruction, *Arch. Otolaryngol.*, 98, 422, 1973.

[79] Ohlsen, L. and Nordin, U., Tracheal reconstruction with perichondrial grafts, *Scand. J. Plast. Reconstr. Surg.*, 10, 135, 1976.

[80] Toohill, R.J., Martinelli, D.L., and Janowak, M.C., Repair of laryngeal stenosis with nasal septal grafts, *Ann. Otol. Rhinol. Laryngol.*, 85, 600, 1976.

[81] Kato, R. et al., Tracheal reconstruction by esophageal interposition: an experimental study [see comments], *Ann. Thorac. Surg.*, 49, 951, 1990.

[82] Murakami, S. et al., An experimental study of tracheal reconstruction using a freed piece of the right bronchus, *Thorac. Cardiovasc. Surg.*, 42, 76, 1994.

[83] Carbognani, P. et al., Experimental tracheal transplantation using a cryopreserved aortic allograft, *Eur. Surg. Res.*, 31, 210, 1999.

[84] Bryant, L.R., Replacement of tracheobronchial defects with autogenous pericardium, *J. Thorac. Cardiovasc. Surg.*, 48, 733, 1958.

[85] Cohen, R.C. et al., A new model of tracheal stenosis and its repair with free periosteal grafts, *J. Thorac. Cardiovasc. Surg.*, 92, 296, 1986.

[86] Eckersberger, F., Moritz, E., and Wolner, E., Circumferential tracheal replacement with costal cartilage, *J. Thorac. Cardiovasc. Surg.*, 94, 175, 1987.

[87] Drettner, B. and Lindholm, C.E., Experimental tracheal reconstruction with composite graft from nasal septum, *Acta Otolaryngol.*, 70, 401, 1970.

[88] Martinod, E. et al., Metaplasia of aortic tissue into tracheal tissue. Surgical perspectives, *C. R. Acad. Sci. III*, 323, 455, 2000.

[89] Hubbell, R.N. et al., Irradiated costal cartilage graft in experimental laryngotracheal reconstruction, *Int. J. Pediatr. Otorhinolaryngol.*, 15, 67, 1988.

[90] Zalzal, G.H., Cotton, R.T., and McAdams, A.J., The survival of costal cartilage graft in laryngotracheal reconstruction, *Otolaryngol. Head Neck Surg.*, 94, 204, 1986.

[91] Zalzal, G.H., Cotton, R.T., and McAdams, A.J., Cartilage grafts — present status, *Head Neck Surg.*, 8, 363, 1986.

[92] Lobe, T.E. et al., The application of solvent-processed human dura in experimental tracheal reconstruction, *J. Pediatr. Surg.*, 26, 1104, 1991.

[93] Chahine, A.A., Tam, V., and Ricketts, R.R., Use of the aortic homograft in the reconstruction of complex tracheobronchial tree injuries, *J. Pediatr. Surg.*, 34, 891, 1999.

[94] Dal, T. and Demirhan, B., Reconstruction of tracheal defects with dehydrated human costal cartilage: an experimental study in rats [In Process Citation], *Otolaryngol. Head Neck Surg.*, 123, 607, 2000.

[95] Bjork, V.O. and Rodriguez, L.E., Reconstruction of the trachea and its bifurcation; an experimental study, *J. Thorac. Surg.*, 35, 596, 1958.

[96] Elliott, M.J. et al., Tracheal reconstruction in children using cadaveric homograft trachea, *Eur. J. Cardiothorac. Surg.*, 10, 707, 1996.

[97] Jacobs, J.P. et al., Pediatric tracheal homograft reconstruction: a novel approach to complex tracheal stenoses in children, *J. Thorac. Cardiovasc. Surg.*, 112, 1549, 1996.

[98] Keskin, I.G. et al., Tracheal reconstruction using alcohol-stored homologous cartilage and autologous cartilage in the rabbit model, *Int. J. Pediatr. Otorhinolaryngol.*, 56, 161, 2000.

[99] Scherer, M.A. et al., Experimental bioprosthetic reconstruction of the trachea, *Arch. Otorhinolaryngol.*, 243, 215, 1986.

[100] Jacobs, J.P. et al., Tracheal allograft reconstruction: the total North American and worldwide pediatric experiences, *Ann. Thorac. Surg.*, 68, 1043, 1999.

[101] Yokomise, H. et al., High-dose irradiation prevents rejection of canine tracheal allografts, *J. Thorac. Cardiovasc. Surg.*, 107, 1391, 1994.

[102] Yokomise, H. et al., The infeasibility of using ten-ring irradiated grafts for tracheal allotransplantation even with omentopexy, *Surg. Today*, 26, 427, 1996.

[103] Farrington, W.T., Hung, W.C., and Binns, P.M., Experimental tracheal homografting, *J. Laryngol. Otol.*, 91, 101, 1977.

[104] Genden, E.M. et al., Microvascular transplantation of tracheal allografts model in the canine, *Ann. Otol. Rhinol. Laryngol.*, 112, 307, 2003.

[105] Genden, E.M. et al., Microvascular transfer of long tracheal autograft segments in the canine model, *Laryngoscope*, 112, 439, 2002.

[106] Delaere, P.R. et al., Experimental tracheal allograft revascularization and transplantation, *J. Thorac. Cardiovasc. Surg.*, 110, 728, 1995.

[107] Khalil-Marzouk, J.F., Allograft replacement of the trachea. Experimental synchronous revascularization of composite thyrotracheal transplant, *J. Thorac. Cardiovasc. Surg.*, 105, 242, 1993.

[108] Yokomise, H. et al., Long-term cryopreservation can prevent rejection of canine tracheal allografts with preservation of graft viability, *J. Thorac. Cardiovasc. Surg.*, 111, 930, 1996.

[109] Tojo, T. et al., Tracheal replacement with cryopreserved tracheal allograft: experiment in dogs, *Ann. Thorac. Surg.*, 66, 209, 1998.

[110] Mukaida, T. et al., Experimental study of tracheal allotransplantation with cryopreserved grafts, *J. Thorac. Cardiovasc. Surg.*, 116, 262, 1998.

[111] Bujia, J. et al., Tracheal transplantation: demonstration of HLA class II subregion gene products on human trachea, *Acta Otolaryngol.*, 110, 149, 1990.

[112] Liu, Y. et al., Immunosuppressant-free allotransplantation of the trachea: the antigenicity of tracheal grafts can be reduced by removing the epithelium and mixed glands from the graft by detergent treatment, *J. Thorac. Cardiovasc. Surg.*, 120, 108, 2000.

[113] Liu, Y. et al., A new tracheal bioartificial organ: evaluation of a tracheal allograft with minimal antigenicity after treatment by detergent, *ASAIO J.*, 46, 536, 2000.

[114] Genden, E.M. et al., Portal venous ultraviolet B-irradiated donor alloantigen prevents rejection in circumferential rat tracheal allografts, *Otolaryngol. Head Neck Surg.*, 124, 481, 2001.

[115] Genden, E.M. et al., Orthotopic tracheal allografts undergo reepithelialization with recipient-derived epithelium, *Arch Otolaryngol. Head Neck Surg.*, 129, 118, 2003.

[116] Vacanti, C.A. et al., Experimental tracheal replacement using tissue-engineered cartilage, *J. Pediatr. Surg.*, 29, 201, 1994.

[117] Kojima, K. et al., Autologous tissue-engineered trachea with sheep nasal chondrocytes, *J. Thorac. Cardiovasc. Surg.*, 123, 1177, 2002.

[118] Fuchs, J.R. et al., Engineered fetal cartilage: structural and functional analysis *in vitro*, *J. Pediatr. Surg.*, 37, 1720, 2002.

[119] Kojima, K. et al., Comparison of tracheal and nasal chondrocytes for tissue engineering of the trachea, *Ann. Thorac. Surg.*, 76, 1884, 2003.

[120] Sakata, J. et al., Tracheal composites tissue engineered from chondrocytes, tracheal epithelial cells, and synthetic degradable scaffolding, *Transplant Proc.*, 26, 3309, 1994.

[121] Terzaghi, M., Nettesheim, P., and Williams, M.L., Repopulation of denuded tracheal grafts with normal, preneoplastic, and neoplastic epithelial cell populations, *Cancer Res.*, 38, 4546, 1978.

[122] Engelhardt, J.F., Allen, E.D., and Wilson, J.M., Reconstitution of tracheal grafts with a genetically modified epithelium, *Proc. Natl Acad. Sci. USA*, 88, 11192, 1991.

[123] Johnson, N.F. and Hubbs, A.F., Epithelial progenitor cells in the rat trachea, *Am. J. Respir. Cell Mol. Biol.*, 3, 579, 1990.

[124] Engelhardt, J.F., Yankaskas, J.R., and Wilson, J.M., *In vivo* retroviral gene transfer into human bronchial epithelia of xenografts, *J. Clin. Invest.*, 90, 2598, 1992.

[125] Dupuit, F. et al., Differentiated and functional human airway epithelium regeneration in tracheal xenografts, *Am. J. Physiol. Lung Cell Mol. Physiol.*, 278, L165, 2000.

[126] Rainer, C. et al., Transplantation of tracheal epithelial cells onto a prefabricated capsule pouch with fibrin glue as a delivery vehicle, *J. Thorac. Cardiovasc. Surg.*, 121, 1187, 2001.

[127] Kojima, K. et al., A composite tissue-engineered trachea using sheep nasal chondrocyte and epithelial cells, *FASEB J.*, 17, 823, 2003.

[128] Fuchs, J.R. et al., Fetal tissue engineering: in utero tracheal augmentation in an ovine model, *J. Pediatr. Surg.*, 37, 1000, 2002.

[129] Erices, A., Conget, P., and Minguell, J.J., Mesenchymal progenitor cells in human umbilical cord blood, *Br. J. Haematol.*, 109, 235, 2000.

[130] Erices, A.A. et al., Human cord blood-derived mesenchymal stem cells home and survive in the marrow of immunodeficient mice after systemic infusion, *Cell Transplant*, 12, 555, 2003.

[131] Erickson, G.R. et al., Chondrogenic potential of adipose tissue-derived stromal cells *in vitro* and *in vivo*, *Biochem. Biophys. Res. Commun.*, 290, 763, 2002.

[132] Zvaifler, N.J. et al., Mesenchymal precursor cells in the blood of normal individuals, *Arthr. Res.*, 2, 477, 2000.

[133] Wexler, S.A. et al., Adult bone marrow is a rich source of human mesenchymal "stem" cells but umbilical cord and mobilized adult blood are not, *Br. J. Haematol.*, 121, 368, 2003.

[134] Pittenger, M.F. et al., Multilineage potential of adult human mesenchymal stem cells, *Science*, 284, 143, 1999.

[135] Barry, F. et al., Chondrogenic differentiation of mesenchymal stem cells from bone marrow: differentiation-dependent gene expression of matrix components, *Exp. Cell Res.*, 268, 189, 2001.

[136] Le Visage, C., Dunham, B., Flint, P., and Leong, K.W., Co-culture of mesenchymal stem cells and respiratory epithelial cells to engineer a human composite respiratory mucosa, *Tissue Eng.*, 10, 1426–35, 2004.

[137] Kim, J. et al., Replacement of a tracheal defect with a tissue-engineered prosthesis: early results from animal experiments, *J. Thorac. Cardiovasc. Surg.*, 128, 124, 2004.

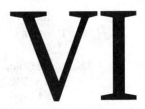

Prostheses and Artificial Organs

Pierre M. Galletti (deceased) and Robert M. Nerem
Georgia Institute of Technology

Substitutive Medicine

Over the past 50 years, humanity has progressively discovered that an engineered **device** or the transplantation of **organs**, tissues, or cells can substitute for most, and perhaps all, organs and body functions. The devices are human-made, whereas the living replacement parts can be obtained from the patient, a relative, a human cadaver, or a live animal or can be prospectively developed through genetic engineering. The concept that a disease state may be addressed not only by returning the malfunctioning organ to health using chemical agents or physical means but also by replacing the missing function with a natural or an artificial counterpart has brought about a revolution in therapeutics. Currently in the United States alone, 2 to 3 million patients a year are treated with a human-designed spare part (assist device, **prosthesis**, or **implant**), with the result that over 20 million people enjoy a longer or better quality of life thanks to artificial organs. In comparison, a shortage of donor organs limits the number of transplantation procedures to about 20,000 a year, and the total population of transplant survivors is on the order of 200,000.

The fundamental tenet of **substitutive medicine** is that beyond a certain stage of failure, it is more effective to remove and replace a malfunctioning organ than to seek in vain to cure it. This ambitious proposition is not easy to accept. It goes against the grain of holistic views of the integrity of the person. It seems at odds with the main stream of twentieth-century scientific medicine, which strives to elucidate pathophysiologic mechanisms at the cellular and molecular level and then to correct them through a specific biochemical key. The technology of organ replacement rivals that of space travel in complexity and fanfare and strikes the popular imagination by its daring, its triumphs, and its excesses. Although the artificial organ approach does not reach the fundamental objective of medicine, which is to understand and correct the disease process, it is considerably more effective than drug therapy or corrective surgery in the treatment of many conditions, for example, cardiac valve disease, heart block, malignant arrhythmia, arterial obstruction, cataract.

A priori, functional disabilities due to the destruction or wear of body parts can be addressed in two ways: the implantation of prosthetic devices or the transplantation of natural organs. For a natural **organ transplant**, we typically borrow a spare part from a living being or from an equally generous donor who before death volunteered to help those suffering from terminal organ failure. Transplanted organs benefit from refinements acquired over thousands of years of evolution. They are overdesigned, which means they will provide sufficient functional support even though the donated part may not be in perfect condition at the time of transfer to another person. They have the same shape and the same attachment needs as the body part they replace which means that surgical techniques are straightforward. The critical problem is the shortage of donors, and therefore only a small minority of patients currently benefit from this approach.

Artificial organs have different limitations. Seen on the scale of human evolution, they are still primitive devices, tested for 40 years at most. Yet they have transformed the prognosis of many heretofore fatal diseases, which are now allowed to evolve past what used to be their natural termination point. In order to design artificial organs, inventive engineers, physiologists, and surgeons think in terms of functional results, not anatomical structures. As a result, artificial organs have but a distant similarity to natural ones. They are mostly made of synthetic materials (often called **biomaterials**) which do not exist in nature. They use different mechanical, electrical, or chemical processes to achieve the same functional objectives as natural organs. They adapt but imperfectly to the changing demands of human activity. They cannot easily accommodate body growth and therefore are more beneficial to adults than to children. Most critically, artificial organs, as is the case for all machines, have a limited service expectancy because of friction, wear, or decay of construction materials in the warm, humid, and corrosive environment of the human body. Such considerations limit their use to patients whose life expectancy matches the expected service life of the replacement part or to clinical situations where repeated implantations are technically feasible. In spite of these obstacles, the astonishing reality is that millions of people are currently alive thanks to cardiac pacemakers, cardiac valves, artificial kidneys, or hydrocephalus drainage systems, all of which address life-threatening conditions. An even larger number of people enjoy the benefits of hip and knee prostheses, vascular grafts, intraocular lenses, and dental implants, which correct dysfunction, pain, inconvenience, or merely appearance. In short, the clinical demonstration of the central dogma of substitutive medicine over the span of two generations can be viewed demographically as the first step in a evolutionary jump which humans cannot yet fully appreciate.

Hybrid artificial organs, or bioartificial organs, are more recent systems which include living elements (organelles, cells, or tissues) as part of a device made of synthetic materials. They integrate the technology of natural organ transplantation and the refinements which living structures have gained through millions of years of evolution with the purposeful design approach of engineering science and the promises of newly developed synthetic materials. Table provides a current snapshot in the continuing evolution of substitutive medicine.

Depending upon medical needs and anticipated duration of use, artificial organs can be located outside of the body yet attached to it (paracorporeal prostheses or assist devices) or implanted inside the body in a appropriate location (internal artificial organs or implants). The application of artificial organs may be temporary, that is, a bridge procedure to sustain life or a specific biologic activity while waiting for either recovery of natural function (e.g., the heart-lung machine), or permanent organ replacement (e.g., left ventricular assist devices). It can be intermittent and repeated at intervals over extended periods of time when there is no biologic necessity for continuous replacement of the missing body functions (e.g., artificial kidney). It can pretend to be permanent, at least within the limits of a finite life span.

Up to 1950, organ replacement technology was relatively crude and unimaginative. Wooden legs, corrective glasses, and dental prostheses formed the bulk of artificial organs. Blood transfusion was the only accepted form of transplantation of living tissue. Suddenly, within a decade, the artificial kidney, the heart–lung machine, the cardiac pacemaker, the arterial graft, the prosthetic cardiac valve, and the artificial hip joint provided the first sophisticated examples of engineering in medicine. More recently, the membrane lung, the implantable lens, finger and tendon prostheses, total knee replacements, and soft-tissue implants for maxillo-facial, ear, or mammary reconstruction have reached the stage of broad clinical application. Ventricular assist devices and the total artificial heart have been extensively tested in animals and validated for clinical evaluation. Artificial skin is increasingly used in the treatment of ulcers and burns. Soft- and hard-tissue substitutes function effectively for several years. Sexual and sensory prostheses offer promises for the replacement of complex human functions. Interfacing of devices with the peripheral and central nervous systems appears as promising today as cardiovascular devices were 30 years ago. Perhaps the brightest future belongs to "information prostheses" which bring to the human body, signals which the organism can no longer generate by itself (e.g., pacemaker functions), signals which need to be modulated differently to correct a disease state (e.g., electronic blood pressure regulators) or signals which cannot be perceived by the nervous system through its usual channels of information gathering (e.g., artificial eye or artificial ear).

TABLE VI.1   Evolution of Organ Replacement Technology: A 1995 Perspective

Current status	Artificial organs	Transplantation
Broadly accepted clinically	Heart-lung machine	Blood transfusion
	Large-joint prostheses	Corneal transplants
	Bone fixation systems	Banked bone
	Cardiac pacemakers	Bone marrow
	Implantable defibrillators	Kidney — living related donor
	Large vascular grafts	Kidney — cadaveric donor
	Prosthetic cardiac valves	Heart
	Intra-aortic balloon pump	Liver
	Intraocular lenses	
	Middle ear ossicle chain	
	Hydrocephalus shunts	
	Dental implants	
	Skin and tissue expanders	
	Maintenance hemodialysis	
	Chronic ambulatory peritoneal dialysis	
Accepted with reservations	Breast implants	Whole pancreas
	Sexual prostheses	Single and double lung
	Small joint prostheses	Combined heart-lung
	ECMO in children	
Limited clinical application	ECMO in adults	Cardiomyoplasty
	Ventricular assist devices	Pancreatic islets
	Cochlear prostheses	Liver lobe or segment
	Artificial tendons	Small Intestine
	Artificial skin	
	Artificial limbs	
Experimental stage	Artificial pancreas	Bioartificial pancreas
	Artificial blood	Bioartificial liver
	Intravenous oxygenation	CNS implants of secreting tissue
	Artificial esophagus	Gene therapy products
	Total artificial heart	
	Nerve guidance channels	
Conceptual stage	Artificial eye	Striated muscle implants
	Neurostimulator	Smooth muscle implants
	Blood pressure regulator	Cardiac muscle implants
	Implantable lung	Functional brain implants
	Artificial trachea	Bioartificial kidney
	Artificial gut	
	Artificial fallopian tube	

Biomaterials

The materials of the first generation of artificial organs — those which are widely available at the moment — are for the most part standard commodity plastics and metals developed for industrial purposes. Engineers have long recognized the limitations of construction materials in the design and performance of machines. However, a new awareness arose when they started interacting with surgeons and biologic scientists in the emerging field of medical devices. In many cases the intrinsic and well established physical properties of synthetic materials such as mechanical strength, hardness, flexibility, or permeability to fluids and gases were not as immediately limiting as the detrimental effects deriving from the material's contact with living tissues. As a result, fewer than 20 chemical compounds among the 1.5 million candidates have been successfully incorporated into clinical devices. Yet some functional implants require material properties which exceed the limits of current polymer, ceramic, or metal alloy technology. This is an indirect tribute to the power of evolution, as well as a challenge to scientists to emulate natural materials with synthetic compounds, blends, or composites.

The progressive recognition of the dominant role of phenomena starting at the **tissue-material interface** has led to two generalizations:

1. All materials in contact with body fluids or living tissue undergo almost instantaneous and then continuing surface deposition of body components which alter their original properties.
2. All body fluids and tissues in contact with foreign material undergo a dynamic sequence of biologic reactions which evolve over weeks or months, and these reactions may remain active for as long as the contact persists and perhaps even beyond. The recognition of biologic interactions between synthetic materials and body tissues has been translated into the twin operational concepts of biomaterials and compatibility. Biomaterials is a term used to qualify materials which can be placed in intimate contact with living structures without harmful effects. **Compatibility** characterizes a set of material specifications and constraints which address the various aspects of material-tissue interactions. More specifically, **hemocompatibility** defines the ability of a biomaterial to stay in contact with blood for a clinically relevant period of time without causing alterations of the formed elements and plasma constituents of the blood or substantially altering the composition of the material itself. The term biocompatibility is often used to highlight the absence of untoward interactions with tissues other than blood (e.g., hard or soft tissues).

It is worth observing that hemocompatibility and biocompatibility are virtues demonstrated not by the presence of definable favorable properties but rather by the absence of adverse effects on blood or other tissues. Although these terms imply positive characteristics of the material, the presumption of compatibility is actually based on the accumulation of negative evidence over longer and longer periods of time, using an increasingly complex battery of tests, which must eventually be confirmed under the conditions of clinical use.

The clinical success of materials incorporated into actual devices is altogether remarkable, considering how limited our understanding is of the physical and biologic mechanisms underlying tissue-material interactions. Indeed the most substantial conclusion one can draw from a review of records of literally millions of implants is how few major accidents have been reported and how remarkably uncommon and benign have been the side effects of implanting substantial amounts of synthetic substances into the human body. Artificial organs are by no means perfect. Their performance must be appreciated within the same limits that the inexorable processes of disease and aging impose on natural organs.

Outlook for Organ Replacement

Now emerging is a second generation of implantable materials through the confluence of biomaterial science and cell biology (Figure). Cell culture technology, taking advantage of biotechnology products and progressing to tridimensional tissue engineering on performed matrices, now provides building blocks which incorporate the peptide or glycoprotein sequences responsible for cell-to-cell interactions. This combination leads to a new class of biohybrid devices which includes

1. Cellular transplants for continuing secretion of bioactive substances (e.g., transplants of insulin-producing xenograft tissue protected against immune rejection by permselective envelopes)
2. Composites of synthetic materials with living cells (often called **organoids**) to accelerate implant integration within the body (e.g. endothelial cell-lined polymer conduits designed for vascular grafts)
3. Replacement parts in which natural tissue regeneration is activated by the presence of supportive cells (e.g., Schwann cell-seeded nerve guidance channels)
4. Vehicles for gene therapy in which continued gene expression is enhanced by a synthetic polymer substrate with appropriate mechanical, chemical, or drug release properties (e.g., epicardial transplants of genetically modified skeletal or cardiac muscle grown on a distensible polymer matrix)

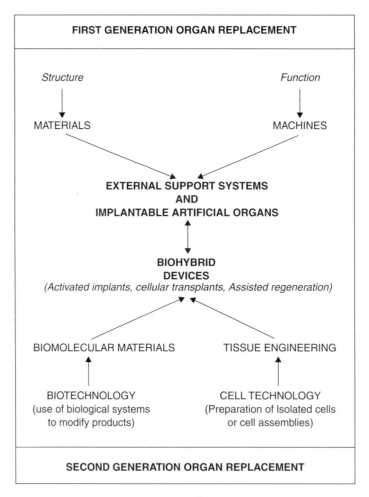

FIGURE VI.1   Schematic description of the advances in engineering, biologic, and medical technology which led to the first generation of artificial organs (read from the top) and the newer developments in body replacement parts (read from the bottom).

In many respects, the new wave of organ replacement exemplifies the synergy of the two original currents in substitutive medicine: prostheses and transplants. It expands the feasibility of cell and tissue transplantation beyond the boundaries of autografts and related donor allografts, opening the way to xenogeneic and engineered replacement parts. It also confronts the "foreign body" limitations of human-made synthetic implants by adding the molecular and cellular elements that favor permanent biointegration.

Design Considerations

Natural organ transplants, if ideally preserved, should be able to fulfill all functions of the original body part except for those mediated by the nervous system, since a transplanted organ is by definition a denervated structure. In actuality, transplants always present some degree of ischemic damage caused by interruption of the blood supply during transfer from donor to recipient. This may be reflected by a temporarily impaired function in the postoperative period or by permanent necrosis of the most delicate components of the transplant, resulting in some degree of functional limitation. In the long run, transplanted organs may also exhibit functional alterations because of cell or tissue damage associated with an underlying systemic disease. They may be damaged by the immunosuppression protocol, which at the current stage is needed for all organ replacements except for autografts, identical-twin homografts, and some types of fetal tissue transplants. The second-order limitations of transplanted organs are usually ignored, and the assumption is made that all original functions are restored in the recipient.

Artificial organs, however, can only replace those bodily functions which have been incorporated into their design because these functions were scientifically described and known to be important. Therefore, in the design of an artificial organ, the first task is to establish the specifications for the device, that is, to describe in quantitative terms the function or functions which must be fulfilled by a human-made construct and the physical constraints that apply because the device must interface with the human body. Each human organ fulfills multiple functions of unequal importance in terms of survival. Consequently, it is critical to distinguish the essential functions which must be incorporated into an effective spare part from those which can be neglected.

Defining specifications and constraints is the first step in the conceptualization of an artificial organ. Only when this is done can one think realistically about design alternatives, the limitations of available materials, and the clinical constraints which will apply, of which the key ones are connections to the body and duration of expected service.

Once all these considerations have been integrated (modeling is often useful at that stage), the next step is typically the construction of a prototype. Ideally the device should achieve everything it was expected to do, but usually it exhibits some level of performance and durability which falls short of design specifications, either because of some misjudgment in terms of required function or because of some unanticipated problem arising at the interface between the device and the body.

The following step of development may be called optimization, if the specifications were well defined from the outset, or reevaluation, if they were not. More commonly it is the reconciliation of competition and at times contradictory design criteria which leads to a second prototype.

At this point, new experiments are needed to establish the reliability and effectiveness of the device in animal models of the target disease (if such exist) or at least in animals in which the natural organ can be removed or bypassed. This is the stage of validation of the device, which is first conducted in acute experiments and must later be extended to periods of observation approximating the duration of intended use in humans. These criteria, however, cannot always be met for long-term implants, since the life expectancy of most animals is shorter than that of humans. By this point, the diverse vantage points of the theoretician, the manufacturer, the performance evaluator, and the clinical user have been articulated for some specific devices and generalized in terms of quality control for classes of devices.

The final stage of design, for many artificial organs, is individualization, that is, the ability to fit the needs of diverse individuals. Humans come in a wide range of body sizes. In some cases, the prostheses must fit very strict dimensional criteria, which implies that they must be fabricated over an extended range of sizes (e.g., cardiac valves). In other cases, there is enough reserve function in the device that one pediatric model and one adult size model may suffice (e.g., blood oxygenator for cardiac surgery).

Evaluation Process

The evaluation of an artificial organ typically is done in six phases:

1. *In vitro* bench testing
2. *Ex vivo* appraisal
3. *In vivo* studies with healthy experimental animals
4. *In vivo* studies with animal models of disease
5. Controlled clinical trials
6. General clinical use

In Vitro Bench Testing

In vitro bench testing of a completed prototype has three major purposes:

1. To observe the mode of operation of the device and assess its performance under tightly controlled circumstances

2. To define performance in quantitative terms over a wide range of environmental or input conditions
3. To assess the device's reliability and durability in a manner which can be extrapolated to the intended clinical use

For all its value, there are limitations to *in vitro* testing of devices. Devices are made to work while in contact with body fluids or body tissues. This complex environment modifies materials in ways which are not always predictable. To duplicate this effect as closely as possible a laboratory bench system can be made to match the body's environment in terms of temperature and humidity. Operating pressures and external forces can also be imitated but not perfectly reproduced (e.g., the complex pulsatile nature of cardiovascular events). Other fluid dynamic conditions such as viscosity, wall shear stress, and compliance of device-surrounding structures call for sophisticated laboratory systems and can only be approximated. The chemical environment is the most difficult to reproduce in view of the complexity of body fluids and tissue structures. Some in vitro testing systems make use of body fluids such as plasma or blood. This in turn brings in additional intricacies because these fluids are not stable outside of the body without preservatives and must be kept sterile if the experiment is to last more than a few hours.

Accelerated testing is a standard component in the evaluation of machines. It is critical for permanent implants with moving parts which are subject to the repeated action of external forces. Fatigue testing provides important information on progressive wear or catastrophic failure of device components. For example, the human heart beats about 40 million times per year. Manufacturers and regulatory agencies conduct testing of prosthetic cardiac valves over at least 400 million cycles. With a testing apparatus functioning at 1200 cycles per minute, this evaluation can be compressed by a factor of about 15, that is, to about a year.

Ex Vivo Appraisal

Because of the difficulty of keeping blood in its physiologic state in a container, the evaluation of some blood processing or blood contacting devices is performed by connecting them through the skin to an artery or vein or both if the blood must be returned to the cardiovascular system to avoid excessive hemorrhage. Such experiments retain the advantage of keeping the device under direct observation while allowing longer experiments than are feasible *in vitro*, particularly if the animal does not require general anesthesia. It is also possible in some cases to evaluate several devices in parallel or sequentially under quite realistic conditions and therefore to conduct comparative experiments under reasonably standardized conditions.

In Vivo Evaluation with Healthy Experimental Animals

There comes a stage in the development of most devices where they must be assessed in their target location in a living body. The matching of device size and shape with available experimental sites in the appropriate animal species is a necessary condition. Such experiments typically last weeks, months, or years and provide information about body-device and tissue-material interactions either through noninvasive measurement techniques or through device retrieval at the end of the observation period. Rodents, felines, and dogs raised for research purposes are usually too small for the evaluation of human-sized devices. Farm animals such as sheep, goats, pigs, and calves are commonly used. Here again the limited life expectancy of experimental animals prevents studies for periods of service as long as can be expected with permanent implants in man.

In Vivo Evaluation with Animal Models of Disease

A first approximation of the effectiveness of a device in replacing a physiologic function can be obtained after removing the target organ in a normal animal. However, when the organ failure is only the cardinal sign of a complex systemic disease, the interactions between the device and the persisting manifestations of the disease occur spontaneously in some species and in other cases can be obtained by chemical, physical, or surgical intervention. Where such models of disease exist in animals which can be fitted with a device, useful information is obtained which helps to refine the final prototypes.

Controlled Clinical Trials

Although some devices can be evaluated with little risk in normal volunteers who derive no health benefit from the experiment, our culture frowns on this approach and legal considerations discourage it. Once reliability and effectiveness have been established through animal experiments and the device appears to meet a recognized clinical need, a study protocol is typically submitted to an appropriate ethics committee or institutional review board and, upon their approval, a series of clinical trials is undertaken. The first step often concentrates on the demonstration of safety of the device with a careful watch for side effects or complications. If the device passes this first hurdle, a controlled clinical trial will be carried out with patients to evaluate effectiveness as well as safety on a scale which allows statistical comparison with a control form of treatment. This protocol may extend from a few months to several years depending upon the expected benefits of the device and the natural history of the disease.

General Clinical Use

Once a device is deemed successful by a panel of experts, it may be approved by regulatory agencies for commercial distribution. Increasingly a third stage of clinical evaluation appears necessary, namely post-market surveillance, that is, a system of clinical outcomes analysis under conditions of general availability of the device to a wide range of doctors and patients.

Postmarket surveillance is a new concept which is not yet uniformly codified. It may take the form of a data collection and analysis network, a patient registry to allow continuing follow-up and statistical analysis, a device-tracking system aimed at early identification of unforseen types of failure, or ancillary controls such as inspection of facilities and review of patient histories in institutions where devices are used. Protocols of surveillance on a large scale are difficult and costly to implement and their cost-effectiveness is therefore open to question. They are also impaired by the shortage of broadly available and minimally invasive diagnostic methods for assessing the integrity or function of a device prior to catastrophic failure. Worthwhile postmarket surveillance requires a constructive collaboration between patients, doctors, device manufacturers, government regulatory agencies, and study groups assessing health care policy issues in the public and private sectors.

Acknowledgments

The chapters that follow are derived to a substantial extent from lecture notes used in graduate courses at Brown University, the Massachusetts Institute of Technology, and the Georgia Institute of Technology. Colleagues at other institutions have also contributed chapters in their own areas of specialization. The authors are also indebted to successive generations of students of biomedical engineering who through a fresh, unencumbered look at the challenges of organ replacement have demonstrated their curiosity, their creativity, and their analytical skills.

In Memoriam

This introduction was written by Pierre Galletti, Ph.D., who passed away in 1997. It is retained here as a memorial to his significant contributions to the field of Biomedical Engineering.

Defining Terms

Artificial organs: Human-made devices designed to replace, duplicate, or augment, functionally or cosmetically, a missing, diseased, or otherwise incompetent part of the body, either temporarily or permanently, and which require a nonbiologic material interface with living tissue.

Assist device: An apparatus used to support or partially replace the function of a failing organ.

Bioartificial organ: Device combining living elements (organelles, cells, or tissues) with synthetic materials in a therapeutic system.

Bicompatibility: The ability of a material to perform with an appropriate host tissue response when incorporated for a specific application in a device, prosthesis, or implant.

Biomaterial: Any material or substance (other than a drug) or combination of materials, synthetic or natural in origin, which can be used as a whole or as a part of a system which treats, augments, or replaces any tissue, organ, or function of the body.

Compatibility: A material property which encompasses a set of specifications and constraints relative to material-tissue interactions.

Device: Defined by Congress as "an instrument, apparatus, implement, machine, contrivance, implant, in vitro reagent, or other similar or related article, including any component, part, or accessory, which is . . . intended for use in the diagnosis of disease or other conditions, or in the cure, mitigation, treatment, or prevention of disease, in man or other animals, . . . and which does not achieve any of its principal intended purposes through chemical action within or on the body of man or other animals and which is not dependent upon being metabolized for the achievement of any of its principal intended purposes."

Hemocompatibility: The ability of a biomaterial to stay in contact with blood for a clinically relevant period of time without causing alterations of the blood constituents.

Hybrid artificial organs: Synonym of bioartificial organs, stressing the combination of cell transplantation and artificial organ technology.

Implant: Any biomaterial or device which is actually embedded within the tissues of a living organism.

Organs: Differentiated structures or parts of a body adapted for the performance of a specific operation or function.

Organoid: An organlike aggregate of living cells and synthetic polymer scaffolds or envelopes, designed to provide replacement or support function.

Organ transplant: An isolated body part obtained from the patient, a living relative, a compatible cadaveric donor, or an animal and inserted in a recipient to replace a missing function.

Prosthesis: An artificial device to replace a missing part of the body.

Substitutive medicine: A form of medicine which relies on the replacement of failing organs or body parts by natural or human-made counterparts.

Tissue–material interface: The locus of contact and interactions between a biomaterial, implant, or device and the tissue or tissues immediately adjacent.

References

Cauwels, J.M. 1986. *The Body Shop: Bionic Revolutions in Medicine*, St. Louis, Mosby.

Galleti, P.M. 1991. Organ replacement: a dream come true. In R. Johnson-Hegyeli, and A.M. Marmong du Haut Champ (Eds.), *Discovering New Worlds in Medicine*, pp. 262–277, Milan, Farmitalia Carlo Erba.

Galletti, P.M. 1992. *Bioartificial organs*. Artif. Organs 16:55.

Galletti, P.M. 1993. Organ replacement by man-made devices. *J. Cardiothor. Vasc. Anesth.* 7:624.

Harker, L.A., Ratner, B.D., and Didisheim, P. 1993. Cardiovascular biomaterials and biocompatibility. A guide to the study of blood–tissue material interactions. *Cardiovasc. Pathol.* 2(suppl): IS–2245.

Helmus, M.N. 1992. *Designing Critical Medical Devices Without Failure. Spectrum, Diagnostics, Medical Equipment Supplies Opthalmics*, pp. 37-1–37-17, Decision Resources, Inc.

Richardson, P.D. 1976. Oxygenator testing and evaluation: Meeting ground of theory, manufacture and clinical concerns. In W.M. Zapol and J. Qvist (Eds.), *Artificial Lungs for Acute Respiratory Failure. Theory and Practice*, pp. 87–102, New York, Academic Press.

Further Information

The articles and books listed above provide different overviews in the filed of organ replacement. Historically most contributions to the filed of artificial organs were described or chronicled in the 40 annual volumes of the *Transactions of the American Society of Artificial Internal Organs* (1955 to present). The principal journals in the field of artificial organs are *Artificial Organs* (currently published by Blackwell Scientific Publications, Inc.), *the ASAIO Journal* (published by J.B. Lippincott Company), and the *International Journal of Artificial Organs* (published by Wichtig Editore s.r.l. Milano, Italy). Publications of the *Japanese Society for Artificial Organs* (typically in Japanese with English abstracts, Artificial Organs Today, e.g.) contain substantial information.

63

Artificial Heart and Circulatory Assist Devices

Gerson Rosenberg
Pennsylvania State University

In 1812, LeGallois [1813] postulated the use of mechanical circulatory support. In 1934, DeBakey proposed a continuous flow blood transfusion instrument using a simple roller pump [DeBakey, 1934]. In 1961, Dennis et al., performed left heart bypass by inserting cannulae into the left atrium and returning blood through the femoral artery [Dennis, 1979]. In 1961, Kolff and Moulopoulos developed the first intra-aortic balloon pump [Moulopoulos et al., 1962]. In 1963, Liota performed the first clinical implantation of a pulsatile left ventricular assist device [Liotz et al., 1963]. In 1969, Dr. Denton Cooley performed the first total artificial heart implantation in a human [Cooley et al., 1969]. Since 1969, air driven artificial hearts and ventricular assist devices have been utilized in over 200 and 600 patients, respectively. The primary use of these devices has been as a bridge to transplant. Recently, electrically powered ventricular assist devices have been utilized in humans as a bridge to transplant. These electrically powered systems utilize implanted blood pumps and energy converters with percutaneous drive cables and vent tubes.

Completely implanted heart assist systems requiring no percutaneous leads have been implanted in calves with survivals over eight months. The electric motor-driven total artificial hearts being developed by several groups in the United States are completely implanted systems employing transcutaneous energy transmission and telemetry [Rosenberg, 1991. Appendix C, The Artificial Heart, Prototypes, Policies, and Patients]. One total artificial heart design has functioned in a calf for over five months [Snyder, 1993].

There has been steady progress in the development of artificial heart and circulatory assist devices. Animal survivals have been increasing, and patient morbidity and mortality with the devices has been decreasing. It does not appear that new technologies or materials will be required for the first successful clinical application of long-term devices. There is no doubt that further advances in energy systems, materials, and electronics will provide for smaller and more reliable devices, but for the present, sound engineering design using available materials and methods appear to be adequate to provide devices satisfactory for initial clinical trials.

63.1 Engineering Design

A definition for design is given by Pahl and Beitz [1977]: "Designing is the intellectual attempt to meet certain demands in the best possible way. It is an engineering activity that impinges on nearly every sphere of human life, relies on the discoveries and laws of science, and creates the conditions for applying these laws to the manufacture of useful products." Designing is a creative activity that calls for sound grounding in mathematics, physics, chemistry, mechanics, thermodynamics, hydrodynamics, electrical engineering, production engineering, materials technology, and design theory together with practical knowledge and experience in specialist fields. Initiative, resolution, economic insight, tenacity, optimism, sociability, and teamwork are all qualities that will assist the designer. Engineering design has been broken into many steps or phases by various authors. In general, though, each of these definitions includes some common tasks. No matter what device is being designed, be it a complicated device such as a totally implantable artificial heart or a simpler device, such as a new fastener, sound engineering design principles utilizing a methodical approach will help ensure satisfactory outcome of the design process. The engineering design process can be broken down into at least four separate stages:

1. *Define the problem — clarification of the task.* At first it may appear that defining the problem or clarifying the task to be accomplished is an easy matter. In general, this is not the case. Great care should be taken in defining the problem, being very specific about the requirements and specifications of the system to be designed. Very often, a complex system can be reduced to the solution of one core problem. An excellent way to begin defining the problem or clarifying the task to be accomplished is to begin by writing a careful design specification or design requirement. This is a document that lists all the requirements for the device. Further, this design requirement may elucidate one or two specific problems which, when solved, will yield a satisfactory design.

2. *Conceptual design — plan treatment.* After the problem has been defined, the designer must plan the treatment of the problem and begin conceptual design. In this phase possible solutions to the problem at hand are examined. Various methods of determining possible solutions include brainstorming, focus groups, Delphi method. This is the phase of the design process where a thorough review of the literature and examination of similar problems is valuable. In this phase of design each of the proposed solutions to the problem should be examined in terms of a hazard analysis or failure modes and effects analysis to determine which solution appears the most feasible. Economic considerations should also be examined in this phase.

3. *Detailed design — execute the plan.* In this phase of engineering design, a detailed design is formulated. Perhaps two designs may be evaluated in the initial detailed design phase. As the detailed design or designs near completion, they must be examined with reference to the design specifications. Here, each of the proposed designs may be evaluated with regard to its ability to perform. Such aspects as system performance, reliability, manufacturability, cost, and user acceptance are all issues which must be considered before a final design is chosen.

4. *Learn and generalize.* Finally, after the design is complete, the designer should be able to learn and generalize from the design. This educational process will include manufacturing of prototypes and testing. General concepts and principles may be gleaned from the design process that can be applied to further designs.

The remainder of this chapter will deal with the application of this engineering design method to the design of artificial heart and circulatory assist devices.

63.2 Engineering Design of Artificial Heart and Circulatory Assist Devices

63.2.1 Define the Problem — Clarification of the Task

In the broadest sense, this step can best be accomplished by writing the detailed design requirement or specification for the device. In defining the problem, it is often easiest to begin with the most obvious and imperative requirements and proceed to the subtler and less demanding. A general statement of the problem for a total artificial heart or assist device is "to develop a device (perhaps totally implantable) that when implanted in the human will provide a longer and better quality of life than conventional pharmacologic or transplant therapy." The devices considered will be assumed to be permanent implantable devices, not necessarily totally implantable; they may utilize percutaneous wires or tubes. In general, it will be assumed that they will be intended for long-term use (one year or longer) but may also be utilized for short-term applications.

63.2.1.1 Fit of the System

One must first decide who the device is intended for. Will it be used in men and women, and of what size? No matter how good the device is, it must first "fit" the patient. For our example, let us assume the device will be used in men and women in the size range of 70 to 100 kg. The device must then fit in these patients and cause minimal or no pathologic conditions. When considering the fit of the implanted device, one must consider the volume and mass of the device, as well as any critical dimension such as the length, width, or height and the location of any tubes, conduits, or connectors. Careful consideration must be given to the physical attributes of the system such as whether the system should be hard, soft, rough, or smooth and the actual shape of the system in terms of sharp corners or edges that may damage tissue or organs. The design specification must give the maximum length, height, and width of the device, these dimensions being dictated by the patient's anatomy. The designer must not be limited by existing anatomy; the opportunity to surgically alter the anatomy should be considered. Nontraditional locations for devices should be considered.

The device should not project heat in such a way that surfaces in contact with tissue or blood are subjected to a temperature rise 5°C above core temperature on a chronic basis. The use of heat spreaders or fins, along with insulation, may be required. Heat transfer analysis may be helpful.

The effect of device movement and vibration should be considered in the design specification. The acceptable sound levels at various frequencies must be specified. A device should meet existing standards for electromagnetic interference and susceptibility.

The use of any percutaneous tubes will require the choice of an exit site. This site must not be in a location of constant or excessive movement or tissue breakdown will be experienced at the interface.

63.2.1.2 Pump Performance

Pump performance must be specified in terms of cardiac output range. In a 70-kg person, a normal resting cardiac output is approximately 70 ml/min/kg or 5 l/min. Choosing a maximum cardiac output of approximately 8 l/min will allow the patient the ability to perform light exercise. The cardiac output performance must be obtained at physiologic pressures, that is, the device, be it a heart assist or total artificial heart device, must be able to pump a cardiac output ranging up to 8 l/min with physiologic inlet and outlet pressures (central venous pressure ~5 mmHg mean, left atrial pressure ~7 mmHg mean, pulmonary artery pressure approximately 15 mmHg mean, aortic pressure ~100 mmHg mean).

Control of the device is critical and must be included in the design specification. For an assist pump, it may be as simple as stating that the pump will pump all the blood delivered to it by the native heart while operating under physiologic inlet and outlet pressures. Or, the design specification may include specific requirements for synchronization of the device with the natural heart. For the total artificial heart, the device must always maintain balance between the left and right pumps. It must not let left atrial pressure rise above a value that will cause pulmonary congestion (~20 mmHg). The device must respond to the patient's cardiac output requirements. The device must either passively or though an active controller vary its cardiac output upon patient demand.

63.2.1.3 Bicompatibility

Bicompatibility has already been alluded to in the design requirements by saying that the device must not cause excessive damage to the biologic system. Specifically, the device must be minimally thrombogenic and minimally hemolytic. It should have a minimal effect on the immune system. It should not promote infection, calcification, or tissue necrosis. Meeting these design requirements will require careful design of the pumping chamber and controller and careful selection of materials.

63.2.1.4 Reliability

The design specification must assign a target reliability for the device. For total artificial hearts and circulatory assist devices, the NIH has proposed a reliability of 80% with an 80% confidence for a 2-year device life. This is the value that the NIH feels is a reliability goal to be achieved before devices can begin initial clinical trials, but the final design reliability may be much more stringent, perhaps 90% reliable with 95% confidence for a 5-year life. The design specification must state which components of the system could be changed if necessary. The design specification must deal with any service that the device may require. For instance, the overall design life of the device may be 5 years, but battery replacement at 2-year intervals may be allowed. The reliability issue is very complex and involves moral, ethical, legal, and scientific issues. A clear goal must be stated and is necessary before the detailed design can begin.

63.2.1.5 Quality of Life

The design specification must address the quality of life for the patient. The designers must specify what is a satisfactory quality of life. Again, this is not an easy task. Quantitative measures of the quality of life are difficult to achieve. One person's interpretation of a satisfactory quality of life may not be the same as another's. It must always be kept in mind that the quality of life for these patients without treatment would generally be considered unsatisfactory by the general public. The prognosis for patients before receiving artificial hearts and circulatory assist devices is very poor. The quality of life must thus be considered in relation to the patient's quality of life without the device without ignoring the quality of life of individuals unaffected by cardiac disease [Rosenberg, 1991].

The design specification must state the weight of any external power supplies. The designer must consider how much weight an older patient will be able to carry. How long should this patient be able to be free-roaming and untethered? How often will the energy source require a "recharge?" What sound level will be acceptable? These are all issues that must be addressed by the designer.

All the foregoing must be considered and included in the definition of the problem and clarification of the task. Each of these issues should be clearly described in the design specification or requirement. In many instances there are no right and wrong answers to these questions.

63.2.2 Conceptual Design — Plan Treatment

In the conceptual design phase, the designer must plan the treatment of the problem and consider various designs that meet the design specification. In the design specification, it must be stated whether the blood pump is to be pulsatile or nonpulsatile. If there is no requirement in the design specification, then in the conceptual design phase, the designer may consider various nonpulsatile and pulsatile flow devices. Nonpulsatile devices include centrifugal pumps, axial flow pumps, shear flow pumps, and peristaltic pumps. Pulsatile pumps have traditionally been sac- or diaphragm-type devices. At the present time there is no definitive work describing the absolute requirement for pulsatility in the cardiovascular system; thus, both types of devices can be considered for assist and total artificial hearts.

In the conceptual design phase, the designer should consider other nontraditional solutions to the problem such as devices that employ micro-machines or magneto-hydrodynamics. Careful consideration must be given to source of energy. Sources that have been considered include electrical energy stored in batteries or derived from piezoelectric crystals, fuel cells, and thermal energy created either thermonuc-learly or through thermal storage. The performance of each of these energy sources must be considered in the conceptual design phase. Public considerations and cost for a thermonuclear source, at the present time, have essentially eliminated this as an implantable energy source. Thermal storage has been shown to be a feasible energy source, and adequate insulation has been developed and demonstrated to be reliable for short periods of time [Unger, 1989].

Steady flow devices that employ seals within the blood stream deserve very careful consideration of the seal area. These seals have been prone to failure, causing embolization. Active magnetic levitation has been proposed for component suspension and may be considered as a possible design. A device that utilities a rotating member such as a rotating electric motor that would drive an impeller or mechanical mechanism will create forces on the tissue when the patient moves due to gyroscopic or coriolis accelerations. These forces must be considered.

Pump performance, in terms of purely hydraulic considerations, can be achieved with any of the pumping systems described. Control of these devices may be more difficult. Designs that include implanted sensors such as pressure or flow sensors must deal with drift of these signals. Very often, signal-to-noise ratios are poor in devices that must operate continuously for several years. Designs that employ few or no sensors are preferable.

Systems such as sac-type blood pumps have been described as having intrinsic automatic control. That is, these devices can run in a fill limited mode, and, as more blood is returned to the pump, it will increase its stroke volume. Intrinsic control is desirable, but, unfortunately, this generally provides for only a limited control range. Nearly all devices currently being developed employ some form of automatic electronic control system. These automatic control systems are utilized on both total artificial hearts and assist devices. In some designs system parameters such as blood pump fill time, electric current, voltage, or speed are utilized to infer the state of the circulatory system. These types of systems appear to demonstrate good long-term stability and eliminate the potential for device malfunction associated with transducer drift.

Consideration of pump performance and the interaction with the biologic system is important in the conceptual design phase. Two pump designs may be capable of pumping the same in a hydrodynamic sense in terms of pressures and flows, but one pump may have much higher shear stresses than the other and thus be more hemolytic. One device may have much more mechanical vibration or movement compromising surrounding tissue.

The subject of biocompatibility for circulatory assist and artificial hearts is a very complex one. No matter what type device is designed, its interaction with the environment is paramount. Blood-contacting materials must not cause thrombosis and should have a minimal effect on formed elements in the blood. In terms of tissue biocompatibility, the device should not have sharp corners or areas where pressure necrosis can occur. Both smooth and rough exterior surfaces of devices have been investigated. It appears that devices in contact with the pleura tend to form a thinner encapsulation when they are rough surfaced. Compliance chambers form much thinner capsules when they have a rough surface. In other areas, it is not entirely clear if a rough surface is advantageous. Tissue ingrowth into a rough surface makes removal of the device difficult.

The selection of materials in the design of these devices is limited. The designer's job would be made much easier if there were several completely biocompatible materials available. If the designer only had a perfectly nonthrombogenic material that had outstanding fatigue properties, the design of these devices would be greatly simplified! Unfortunately, at the present time the designer is limited to existing materials. Traditionally, metals that have been employed in blood pumps include various stainless steels, cobalt, cobalt chromium alloys, and titanium. Each of these materials has adequate performance when in contact with tissue and blood under certain circumstances. Ceramic materials such as pyrolytic carbon, alumina, and zirconia have been used in contact with both tissue and blood with varying degrees of success. The range of polymeric materials that have been utilized for these devices is much greater. These materials include various polyurenthanes, silicone rubber, Kel-F, Teflon, Delrin, butyl rubber, Hexsyn rubber, polysulfone, polycarbonate, and others [Williams, 1981]. The designer must carefully consider all the properties of these materials when employing them. The designer must look at the strength, durability, hardness, wear resistance, modulus of elasticity, surface energy, surface finish, and biocompatibility before choosing any of these materials.

The interaction between the biologic system and these materials is complex and may be strongly influenced by fluid mechanics if in contact with blood. The designer should carefully consider surface modification of any of these materials. Surface modification can be performed, including ion implantation or grafting of various substances to the surface to promote improved compatibility. Manufacturing and fabrication processes have a profound effect on the properties of these materials and must be carefully analyzed and controlled.

The designer must give a great deal of consideration to the fluid mechanics involved. It is well known that excessive shear stresses can promote hemolysis and activation of the clotting system, as well as damage to the other formed elements in the blood. Not only the actual design of the blood pump, but the operation of the blood pump can affect phenomena such as cavitation, which can be hemolytic and destructive to system components. Thrombosis is greatly affected by blood flow. Regions of stagnation, recirculation, and low wall shear stress should be avoided. The magnitude of "low" shear stress is reported in the literature with wide range [Folie and McIntire, 1989; Hashimoto et al., 1985; Hubbell and McIntire, 1986].

Many of the analytical tools available today in terms of computational fluid dynamics and finite element analysis are just beginning to be useful in the design of these devices. Most of these systems have complex flow (unsteady, turbulent, non-Newtonian with moving boundaries) and geometries and are not easily modeled.

Once a reliability goal has been established, the designer must ensure that this goal is met. The natural heart beats approximately 40 million times a year. This means that an artificial heart or assist device with a 5-year life may undergo as may as 200,000,000 cycles. The environment in which this device is to operate is extremely hostile. Blood and extracellular fluids are quite corrosive and can promote galvanic or crevice corrosion in most metallic materials. Devices that employ polymeric materials must deal with diffusion of mass across these materials. Water, oxygen, nitrogen, carbon dioxide, and so on may all diffuse across these polymeric materials. If temperature fluctuations occur or differences exist, liquid water may form due to condensation. With carbon dioxide present, a weak acid can be formed. Many polymeric materials are degraded in the biologic environment. A careful review of the literature is imperative. The use of any "new" materials must be based upon careful testing. The designer must be aware of the difficulty in providing a sealed system. The designer may need to utilize hermetic connectors and cables which can tolerate the moist environment. All these affect the reliability of the device.

External components of the system which may include battery packs or monitoring and perhaps control functions have reliability requirements that differ from the implanted components. System components which are redundant may not require the same level of reliability as do nonredundant implanted components. Externally placed components have the advantage of being amenable to preventative maintenance or replacement. Systems that utilize transcutaneous energy transmission through inductive coupling may have advantages over systems that utilize a percutaneous wire. Although the percutaneous wire can function for long periods of time, perhaps up to 1 year, localized infection is almost always present. This infection can affect the patient's quality of life and be a source of systemic infection.

In the conceptual design phase, one must carefully weigh quality of life issues when evaluating solutions to the problem. Careful consideration needs to be given to the traditional quality of life issues such as the patient's emotional, social, and physical well-being, as well as to the details of day-to-day use of the device. What are the frequency and sound level requirements for patient prompts or alarms, and are certain kinds of alarms useful at all? For visible information for the patient, from what angles can this information be viewed, how bright does the display need to be, should it be in different languages, or should universal symbols be used? A great deal of thought must be given to all aspects of device use, from charging of the batteries to dealing with unexpected events. All these issues must be resolved in the conceptual design phase so that the detailed phase will be successful.

63.2.3 Detailed Design — Execute Plan

This is the phase of engineering design where the designer and other members of the team must begin to do what is generally considered the designer's more traditional role, that is, calculations and drawings. This phase of design may require some initial prototyping and testing before the detailed design can be complete. Akutsu and Koyangi [1993] provide several results of various groups' detailed designs for artificial hearts and circulatory assist devices.

63.2.4 Learn and Generalize

Substantial research and development of artificial hearts and circulatory assist devices has been ongoing for almost 30 years. During this period there have been literally thousands of publications related to this research, not only descriptions of device designs, but experimental results, detailed descriptions fluid dynamic phenomena, hemolysis, thrombosis, investigation of materials selection and processing, consideration of control issues, and so on. The artificial organs and biomaterials literature has numerous references to materials utilized in these devices. A thorough review of the literature is required to glean the general principles that can be applied to the design of these devices. Many of these principles or generalities apply only to specific designs. In some design circulatory assist devices, a smooth surface will function satisfactorily, whereas a rough surface may cause thrombosis or an uncontrolled growth of neointima. Yet, in other design devices, a textured or rough surface will have performance superior to that of an extremely smooth surface. Wide ranges of sheer stresses are quoted in the literature that can be hemolytic. Although considerable research has been performed examining the fluid mechanics of the artificial hearts and circulatory assist devices, there is really no current measure of what is considered a "good" blood flow within these devices. We know that the design must avoid regions of stasis, but how close to stasis one can come, or for how long, without thrombosis is unknown.

It is up to the designer to review current literature and determine what fundamental principles are applicable to his or her design. Then, when the design is complete, the designer can learn and generalize specific principles related to her or his device. Hopefully, general principles that can apply to other devices will be elucidated.

63.3 Conclusions

The design of artificial hearts and circulatory assist devices is a very complex process involving many engineering disciplines along with medicine and other life science areas. Social issues must enter into the design process. The design of such devices requires sound engineering design principles and an interdisciplinary design team dedicated to the development and ultimate clinical application of these devices.

References

Akutsu, T. and Koyanagi, H. (1993). Heart replacement. *In Artificial Heart*, Vol. 4, Tokyo, Springer-Verlag.

Cooley, D.A., Liota, D., Hallman, G.L. et al. (1969). Orthotopic cardiac prosthesis for 2-stage cardiac replacement. *Am. J. Cardiol.* 24: 723.

DeBakey, M.E. (1934). A simple continuous flow blood transfusion instrument. *New Orleans Med. Surg. J.* 87: 386.

Folie, B.J. and McIntire, L.V. (1989). Mathematical analysis of mural thrombogenesis, concentration profiles of platelet-activating agents and effects of viscous shear flow. *Biophys. J.* 56: 1121.

Hashimoto, S., Maeda, H., and Sasada, T. (1985). Effect of shear rate on clot growth at foreign surfaces. *Artif. Organs* 9: 345.

Hubbell, J.A. and McIntire, L.V. (1986). Visualization and analysis of mural thrombogenesis on collagen, polyurethane and nylon. *Biomaterials* 7: 354.

LeGallois, C.J.J. (1813). *Experience on the Principles of Life*, Philadelphia, Thomas. (Translation of CJJ Le Gallois 1812. Experiences sur les Principles de Vie. Paris, France.)

Liota, D., Hall, C.W., Walter, S.H. et al. (1963). Prolonged assisted circulation during and after cardiac and aortic surgery. Prolonged partial left ventricular bypass by means of an intra-corporeal circulation. *Am. J. Cardiol.* 12: 399.

Moulopoulos, D., Topaz, S.R., and Kolff, W.J. (1962). Extracorporeal assistance to the circulation at intra-aortic balloon pumping. *Trans. AM. Soc. Artif. Intern. Organs* 8: 86.

Pahl, G. and Beitz, W. (1977). *Engineering Design*, Berlin, Heidelberg, Springer-Verlag (First English edition published 1984 by The Design Council, London.)

Rosenberg, G. (1991). Technological opportunities and barriers in the development of mechanical circulatory support systems (Appendix C). In *Institute of Medicine, The Artificial Heart, Prototypes, Policies, and Patients*, National Academy Press.

Snyder, A.J., Rosenberg, G., Weiss, W.J. et al. (1993). *In vivo* testing of a completely implanted total artificial heart system. *ASAIO J.* 39: M415.

Unger Felix (1989). *Assisted Circulation*, Vol. 3, Berlin, Heidelberg, Springer-Verlag.

Williams, D.F. (1981). *Biocompatibility of Clinical Implant Materials*, Boca Raton, FL, CRC Press.

64

Cardiac Valve Prostheses

Gerson Rosenberg
Pennsylvania State University

The first clinical use of a cardiac valvular prosthesis took place in 1952, when Dr. Charles Hufnagel implanted the first artificial caged ball valve for aortic insufficiency. The Plexiglas cage contained a ball occluder and was inserted into the descending aorta without the need for cardiopulmonary bypass. It did not cure the underlying disease, but it did relieve regurgitation from the lower two-thirds of the body.

The first implant of a replacement valve in the anatomic position took place in 1960, with the advent of cardiopulmonary bypass. Since then, the achievements in valve design and the success of artificial heart valves as replacements have been remarkable [Roberts, 1976]. More than 50 different cardiac valves have been introduced over the past 35 years. Unfortunately, after many years of experience and success, problems associated with heart valve prostheses have not been eliminated. The most serious problems and complications [Roberts, 1976; Bodnar and Frater, 1991; Butchart, Bodnar, 1992; Giddens et al., 1993] are:

- Thrombosis and thromboembolism
- Anticoagulant-related hemorrhage

- Tissue overgrowth
- Infection
- Paravalvular leaks due to healing defects
- Valve failure due to material fatigue or chemical change

New valve designs continue to be developed. Yet to understand the future of valve replacements, it is important to understand their history.

64.1 A Brief History of Heart Valve Prostheses

This section on replacement valves highlights a relatively small number of the many various forms which have been made. However, those that have been included are either the most commonly used today or those which have made notable contributions to the advancement of replacement heart valves [Brewer, 1969; Yoganathan et al., 1992].

64.1.1 Mechanical Valves

The use of the caged-ball valve in the descending aorta became obsolete with the development in 1960 of what today is referred to as the Starr–Edwards ball-and-cage valve. Similar in concept to the original Hufnagel valve, it was designed to be inserted in place of the excised diseased natural valve. This form of intracardiac valve replacement was used in the mitral position and for aortic and multiple replacements. Since 1962, the Starr–Edwards valve has undergone many modifications to improve its performance in terms of reduced hemolysis and thromboembolic complications. However, the changes have involved materials and techniques of construction and have not altered the overall concept of the valve design in any way (Figure 64.1a).

Other manufacturers have produced variations of the ball and cage valve, notably the Smeloff–Cutter valve and the Magovern Prosthesis. In the case of the former, the ball is slightly smaller than the orifice. A subcage on the proximal side of the valve retains the ball in the closed position with its equator in the plane of the sewing ring. A small clearance around the ball ensures easy passage of the ball into the orifice. This clearance also gave rise to a mild regurgitation which was felt, but not proven, to be beneficial in preventing thrombus formation. The Magovern valve is a standard ball-and-cage format which incorporates two rows of interlocking mechanical teeth around the orifice ring. These teeth are used for inserting the valve and are activated by removing a special valve holder once the valve has been correctly located in the prepared tissue annulus. The potential hazard of dislocation from a calcified annulus due to imperfect placement was soon observed. This valve is no longer in use.

Due to the high-profile design characteristics of the ball valves, especially in the mitral position, low-profile caged disc valves were developed in the mid-1960s. Examples of the caged disc designs are the Kay–Shiley and Beall prostheses, which were introduced in 1965 and 1967, respectively (Figure 64.1b). These valves were used exclusively in the atrioventricular position. However, due to their inferior hemodynamic characteristics, caged disc valves are rarely used today.

Even after 35 years of valve development, the ball-and-cage format remains the valve of choice for some surgeons. However, it is no longer the most popular mechanical valve, having been superseded, to a large extent, by tilting-disc and bileaflet valve designs. These valve designs overcome two major drawbacks of the ball valve, namely, high profile heights and excessive occluder-induced turbulence in the flow through and distal to the valve.

The most significant developments in mechanical valve design occurred in 1969 and 1970 with the introduction of the Bjork–Shiley and Lillehei–Kaster tilting-disc valves (Figure 64.1c). Both prostheses involve the concept of a free-floating disc which in the open position tilts to an angle depending on the design of the disc-retaining struts. In the original Bjork–Shiley valve, the angle of the tilt was 60° for the aortic and 50° for the mitral model. The Lillehei–Kaster valve has a greater angle of tilt of 80° but in the closed position is preinclined to the valve orifice plane by an angle of 18°. In both cases the closed valve

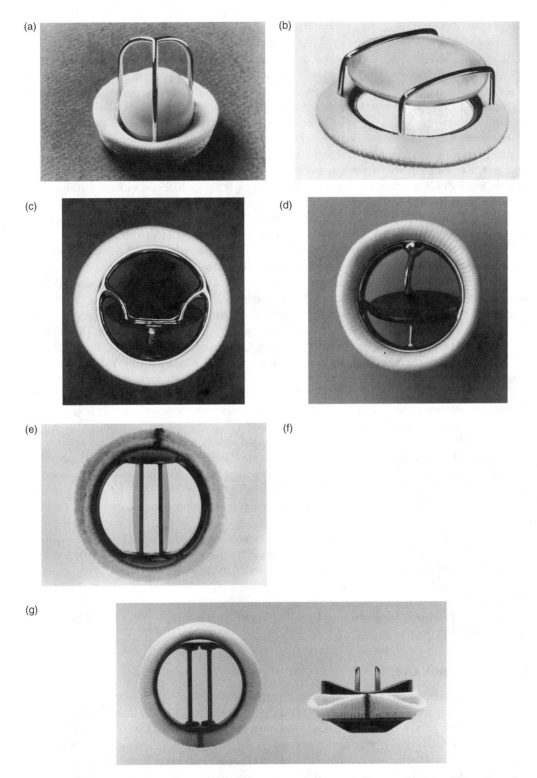

FIGURE 64.1 (a) Photograph of Starr–Edwards ball and cage valve; (b) photograph of Kay–Shiley disc valve; (c) photograph of Bjork–Shiley tilting disc valve; (d) photograph of Medtronic–Hall tilting disc valve; (e) photograph of St. Jude bileaflet valve; (f) photograph of CarboMedics bileaflet valve; (g) photograph of Parallel bileaflet valve.

configuration permits the occluder to fit into the circumference of the inflow ring with virtually no overlap, thus reducing mechanical damage to erythrocytes. A small amount of regurgitation backflow induces a "washing out" effect of "debris" and platelets and theoretically reduces the incidence of thromboemboli.

The obvious advantage of the tilting-disc valve is that in the open position it acts like an aerofoil in the blood flowing through the valve, and induced flow disturbance is substantially less than that obtained with a ball occluder. Although the original Bjork–Shiley valve employed a Delrin occluder, all present-day tilting-disc valves use pyrolitic carbon for these components. It should also be noted that the free-floating disc can rotate during normal function, thus preventing excessive contact wear from the retaining components on one particular part of the disc. Various improvements to this form of mechanical valve design have been developed but have tended to concentrate on alterations either to the disc geometry as in the Bjork–Shiley convexo-concave design or to the disc-retaining system as with the Medtronic–Hall and Omniscience valve designs (Figure 64.1d).

The Medtronic–Hall prosthesis was introduced in 1977. It is characterized by a central, disc-control strut, with a mitral opening angle of $70°$ and an aortic opening of $75°$. An aperture in the flat, pyrolitic carbon-coated disc affixes it to the central guide strut. This strut not only retains the disc but controls its opening angle and allows it to move downstream 1.5 to 2.0 mm; this movement is termed disc translation and improves flow velocity between the orifice ring and the rim of the disc. The ring and strut combination is machined from a single piece of titanium for durability. All projections into the orifice (pivot points, guide struts, and disc stop) are open-ended, streamlined, and in the region of highest velocity to prevent the retention of thrombi by valve components. The sewing ring is of knitted Teflon. The housing is rotatable within the sewing ring for optimal orientation of the valve within the tissue annulus.

Perhaps the most interesting development has been that of the bileaflet all-pyrolitic carbon valve designed by St. Jude Medical, Inc. and introduced in 1978 (Figure 64.1e). This design incorporates two semicircular hinged pyrolitic carbon occluders (leaflets) which in the open position are intended to provide minimal disturbance to flow. The leaflets pivot within grooves made in the valve orifice housing. In the fully open position the flat leaflets are designed to open to an angle of $85°$. The Duromedics valve is similar in concept to the St. Jude except that it incorporates curved leaflets.

The CarboMedics bileaflet prosthesis gained FDA approval for U.S. distribution in 1993 (Figure 64.1f). The CarboMedics valve is also made of Pyrolite, which is intended for durability and thromboresistance. The valve has a recessed pivot design and is rotatable within the sewing ring. The two leaflets are semi-circular, radiopaque, and open to an angle of $78°$. A titanium stiffening ring is used to lessen the risk of leaflet dislodgment or impingement.

The most recent bileaflet design is the Parallel valve from Medtronic, Inc. (Figure 64.1g). The significant design aspect of the Parallel valve is the ability of its leaflets to open to a position parallel to flow. This is intended to reduce the amount of turbulence that is created in the blood and therefore should improve hemodynamics and reduce thromboembolic complications. European clinical implants began in the Spring of 1994.

The most popular valve design in use today is the bileaflet. Approximately 75% of the valves implanted today are bileaflet prostheses.

64.1.2 Tissue Valves

Two major disadvantages with the use of mechanical valves is the need for life-long anticoagulation therapy and the accompanying problems of bleeding [Butchart and Bodnar, 1992]. Furthermore, the hemo-dynamic function of even the best designed valves differs significantly from that of the natural healthy heart valve. An obvious step in the development of heart valve substitutes was the use of naturally occurring heart valves. This was the basis of the approach to the use of antibiotic or cryotreated human aortic valves (homografts: from another member of the same species) removed from cadavers for implantation in place of a patient's own diseased valve.

The first of these homograft procedures was performed by Ross in 1962, and the overall results so far have been satisfactory. This is, perhaps, not surprising since the homograft replacement valve is optimum both from the point of view of structure and function. In the open position these valves provide unobstructed central orifice flow and have the ability to respond to deformations induced by the surrounding anatomical structure. As a result, such substitutes are less damaging to the blood when compared with the rigid mechanical valve. The main problem with these cadaveric allografts, as far as may be ascertained, is that they are no longer living tissue and therefore lack that unique quality of cellular regeneration typical of normal living systems. This makes them more vulnerable to long-term damage. Furthermore, they are only available in very limited quantities.

An alternative approach is to transplant the patient's own pulmonary valve into the aortic position. This operation was also the first carried out by Ross in 1967, and his study of 176 patients followed up over 13 years showed that such transplants continued to be viable in their new position with no apparent degeneration [Wain et al., 1980]. This transplantation technique is, however, limited in that is can only be applied to one site.

The next stage in development of tissue valve substitutes was the use of autologous fascia lata (a wide layer of membrane that encases the thigh muscles) either as free or frame-mounted leaflets. The former approach for aortic valve replacement was reported by Senning in 1966, and details of a frame-mounted technique were published by Ionescu and Ross in 1966 [Ionescu and Ross, 1969]. The approach combined the more natural leaflet format with a readily available living autologous tissue. Although early results seemed encouraging, Senning expressed his own doubt on the value of this approach in 1971, and by 1978 fascia lata was no longer used in either of the above, or any other, form of valve replacement. The failure of this technique was due to the inadequate strength of this tissue when subjected to long-term cyclic stressing in the heart.

In parallel with the work on fascia lata valves, alternative forms of tissue leaflet valves were being developed. In these designs, however, more emphasis was placed on optimum performance characteristics than on the use of living tissue. In all cases the configuration involved a three-leaflet format which was maintained by the use of a suitably designed mounting frame. It was realized that naturally occurring animal tissues, if used in an untreated form, would be rejected by the host. Consequently, a method of chemical treatment had to be found which prevented this antigenic response but did not degrade the mechanical strength of the tissue.

Formaldehyde has been used by histologists for many years to arrest autolysis and "fix" tissue in the state in which it is removed. It had been used to preserve biologic tissues in cardiac surgery but, unfortunately, was found to produce shrinkage and increase the stiffness of the resulting material. For these reasons, formaldehyde was not considered ideal as a method of tissue treatment.

Glutaraldehyde is another histologic fixative which has been used especially for preserving fine detail for electron microscopy. It is also used as a tanning agent by the leather industry. In addition to arresting autolysis, glutaraldehyde produces a more flexible material due to increased collagen crosslinking. Glutaraldehyde has the additional ability of reducing the antigenicity of xenograft tissue to a level at which it can be implanted into the heart without significant immunologic reaction.

In 1969, Kaiser and coworkers described a valve substitute using an explanted glutaral dehyde-treated porcine aortic valve which was mounted on to a rigid support frame. Following modification in which the rigid frame was replaced by a frame having a rigid base ring with flexible posts, this valve became commercially available as the Hancock Porcine Xenograft in 1970 (Figure 64.2a). It remains one of the two most popular valve substitutes of this type, the other being the Carpentier–Edwards Bioprosthesis introduced commercially by Edwards Laboratories in 1976. This latter valve uses a totally flexible support frame.

In 1977 production began of the Hancock Modified Orifice (M.O.) valve, a refinement of the Hancock Standard valve. The Hancock M.O. is of a composite nature — the right coronary leaflet containing the muscle shelf is replaced by a noncoronary leaflet of the correct size from another porcine valve. This high-pressure fixed valve is mounted into a Dacron-covered polypropylene stent. The Hancock II and Carpentier–Edwards supra-annular porcine bioprostheses are second-generation bioprosthetic valve designs which were introduced in the early 1980s. The porcine tissue is initially fixed at 1.5 mmHg and then at high pressure. This fixation method is designed to ensure good tissue geometry. Both valves are

(a)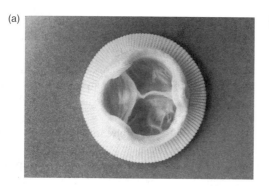

(b)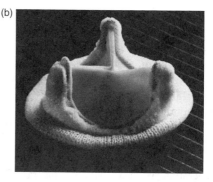

FIGURE 64.2   (a) Photograph of Hancock porcine valve; (b) photograph of Carpentier–Edwards pericardial valve.

treated with antimineralization treatments. Neither valve has been FDA approved for clinical use in the United States.

In porcine prostheses, the use of the intact biologically formed valve makes it unnecessary to manufacture individual valve cusps. Although this has the obvious advantage of reduced complexity of construction, it does require a facility for harvesting an adequate quantity of valves so that an appropriate range of valve sizes of suitable quality can be made available. This latter problem did not occur in the production of the three-leaflet calf pericardium valve developed by Ionescu and colleagues; the construction of this valve involved the molding of fresh tissue to a tricuspid configuration around a support frame. As the tissue is held in this position, it is treated with a glutaraldehyde solution. The valve, marketed in 1976 as the Ionescu–Shiley Pericardial Xenograft, was discontinued in the mid-1980s due to structural failure problems. Early clinical results obtained with tissue valves indicated their superiority to mechanical valves with respect to a lower incidence of thromboembolic complications [Bodnar and Frater, 1991]. For this reason the use of tissue valves increased significantly during the late 1970s.

The Carpentier–Edwards pericardial valve consists of three pieces of pericardium mounted completely within the Elgiloy wire stent to reduce potential abrasion between the Dacron-covered frame and the leaflets. The pericardium is retained inside the stent by a Mylar button rather than by holding sutures. Its clinical implantation began in July 1980, and it is currently approved for clinical use in the United States (Figure 64.2b).

Clinical experiences with different tissue valve designs have increasingly indicated time-dependent (5- to 7-year) structural changes such as calcification and leaflet wear, leading to valve failure and subsequent replacement [Oyer et al., 1979; Ferrans et al., 1980; Bodnar and Yacoub, 1986]. The problem of valve leaflet calcification is more prevalent in children and young adults. Therefore, tissue valves are rarely used in children and young adults at the present time. Such problems have not been eliminated by the glutaraldehyde tanning methods so far employed, and it is not easy to see how these drawbacks are to be overcome unless either living autologous tissue is used or the original structure of the collagen and elastin are chemically enhanced. On the latter point there is, as yet, much room for further work. For instance, the fixing of calf pericardium under tension during the molding of the valve cusps will inevitably produce "locked-in" stresses during fixation, thus changing the mechanical properties of the tissue.

64.2   Current Types of Prostheses

At present, over 175,000 prosthetic valves are implanted each year throughout the world. Currently, the four most commonly used basic types of prostheses are:

1. Caged ball
2. Tilting disc
3. Bileaflet
4. Bioprostheses (tissue valves)

Valve manufacturers continue to develop new designs of mechanical and tissue valves. The ideal heart valve prosthesis does not yet exist and may never be realized. However, the characteristics of the "perfect" prostheses should be noted. The ideal heart valve should:

- Be fully sterile at the time of implantation and be nontoxic
- Be surgically convenient to insert at or near the normal location of the heart
- Conform to the heart structure rather than the heart structure conforming to the valve (i.e., the size and shape of the prosthesis should not interfere with cardiac function)
- Show a minimum resistance to flow so as to prevent a significant pressure drop across the valve
- Have a minimal reverse flow necessary for valve closure, so as to keep the incompetence of the valve at a low level
- Show long resistance to mechanical and structural wear
- Be long-lasting (25 years) and maintain its normal functional performance (i.e., must not deteriorate over time)
- Cause minimal trauma to blood elements and the endothelial tissue of the cardiovascular structure surrounding the valve
- Show a low probability for thromboembolic complications without the use of anticoagulants
- Be sufficiently quiet so as not to disturb the patient
- Be radiographically visible
- Have an acceptable cost

64.3   Tissue vs. mechanical

Tissue prostheses gained widespread use during the mid-1970s. The major advantage of tissue valves compared to mechanical valves is that tissue valves have a lower incidence of thromboembolic complications [Butchart and Bodnar, 1992]. Therefore, most patients receiving tissue valves do not have to take anticoagulants long-term. The major disadvantages to tissue valves are large pressure drops compared to some mechanical valves (particularly in the smaller valve sizes), jetlike flow through the valve leaflets, material fatigue and wear of valve leaflets, and calcification of value leaflets, especially in children and young adults. Valve deterioration, however, usually takes place slowly with tissue valves, and patients can be monitored by echocardiography and other noninvasive techniques.

The clear advantage of mechanical valves is their long-term durability. Current mechanical valves are manufactured from a variety of materials, such as pyrolitic carbon and titanium. Structural failure of mechanical valves is rare, but, when it occurs, is usually catastrophic [Giddens et al., 1993]. One major disadvantage of the use of mechanical valves is the need for continuous, life-long anticoagulation therapy to minimize the risk of thrombosis and thromboembolic complications. Unfortunately, the anticoagulation therapy may lead to bleeding problems; therefore, careful control of anticoagulation medication is essential for the patient's well-being and quality of life. Another concern is the hemodynamic performance of the prosthesis. The hemodynamic function of even the best designs of mechanical valves differs significantly from that of normal heart valves.

64.4   Engineering Concerns and Hemodynamic Assessment of Prosthetic Heart Valves

In terms of considerations related to heart valve design, the basic engineering concerns are as follows:

- Hydrodynamics/hemodynamics
- Durability (structural mechanics and materials)
- Biologic response to the prosthetic implant

The ideal heart valve design from the hemodynamic point of view should [Giddens et al., 1993]

- Produce minimal pressure gradient
- Yield relatively small regurgitation
- Minimize production of turbulence
- Not induce regions of high shear stress
- Contain no stagnation or separation regions in its flow field, especially adjacent to the valve superstructure

No valve as yet, other than normal native valves, satisfies all these criteria.

64.4.1 Pressure Gradient

The heart works to maintain adequate blood flow through a prosthetic valve; a well-designed valve will not significantly impede that blood flow and will therefore have as small a pressure gradient as possible across the valve.

Because of the larger separation region inherent in flow over bluff bodies, configurations such as the caged disc and caged ball have notably large pressure gradients. Porcine bioprostheses have relatively acceptable pressure gradients for larger diameter valves because they more closely mimic natural valve geometry and motion, but the small sizes (<23 mm) generally have higher pressure gradients than their mechanical valve counterparts, as shown in Figure 64.3 [Yoganathan et al., 1984]. Tilting disc and bileaflet valve designs present a relatively streamlined configuration to the flow, and, although separation regions may exist in these designs, the pressure gradients are typically smaller than for the bluff shapes.

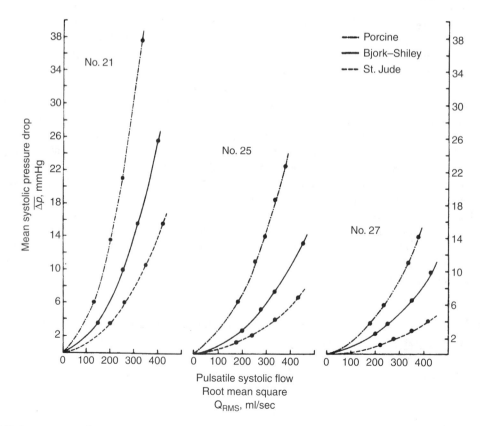

FIGURE 64.3 Examples of *in vitro* pulsatile flow pressure gradients across tilting disc (Bjork–Shiley convexo-concave), bileaflet (St. Jude Medical), and porcine aortic valves of three different sizes (27, 25, and 21 mm).

The clinical importance of pressure gradients in predicting long-term performance is not clear. The fact that these gradients are a manifestation of energy losses resulting from viscous-related phenomena makes it intuitive that minimizing pressure gradients across an artificial valve is highly desirable in order to reduce the workload of the pump (i.e., left ventricle).

64.4.2 Effective Orifice Area (EOA)

The EOA is an index of how well a valve design utilizes its primary or internal stent orifice area. In other words, it is related to the degree to which the prosthesis itself obstructs the flow of blood. A larger EOA corresponds to a smaller pressure drop and therefore a smaller energy loss. It is desirable to have as large an EOA as possible. EOA is calculated from *in vitro* pressure drop measurements for a particular valve using the following formula [Yoganathan et al., 1984].

Q_{rms} is the root mean square systolic/diastolic flow rate (cm^3/sec), D–pis the mean systolic/diastolic pressure drop (mmHg).

Table 64.1 lists EOAs obtained *in vitro*, for different size mechanical and tissue valve designs in clinical use today. These results illustrate the fact that, size for size, the newer mechanical valve designs have better pressure gradient characteristics than porcine bioprostheses in current clinical use.

64.4.3 Regurgitation

Regurgitation results from reverse flow created during valve closure and from backward leakage once closure is effected (see Figure 64.4). Regurgitation reduces the net flow through the valve. Closing regurgitation is closely related to the valve shape and closing dynamics, and the percentage of stroke volume that succumbs to this effect ranges from 2.0 to 7.5% for mechanical valves. For tissue valves it is typically less: 0.1 to 1.5%. Leakage depends upon how well the orifices are "sealed" upon closure, and it has a reported incidence of 0–10% in mechanical valves and 0.2–3% in bioprosthetic valves. The overall tendency is for regurgitation to be less for the trileaflet bioprosthetic heart valves than for mechanical valve designs.

TABLE 64.1 Effective Orifice Areas of Different Prosthetic Aortic Valve Designs

Valve sewing ring diam, mm	Medronic-hall tilting disc, cm^2	St. jude bileaflet cm^2	Carbomedics bileaflet cm^2	Hancock I porcine, cm^2	Hancock MO porcine, cm^2	Carpentier–Edwards pericardial, cm^2	Starr–Edwards 1260 ball, cm^2
19/20	1.74	1.21	1.12	1.01	1.22	1.56	1.04
21	1.74	1.81	1.66	1.31	1.43	1.88	1.23
23	2.26	2.24	2.28	1.73	1.94	2.25	1.45
25	3.07	3.23	3.14	1.93	2.16	3.25	1.59
27	3.64	4.05	3.75	2.14	—	3.70	1.75

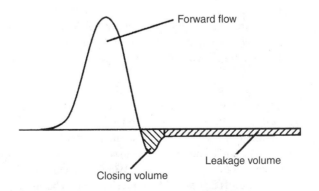

FIGURE 64.4   Flow cycle divided into forward flow, closing volume, and leakage volume.

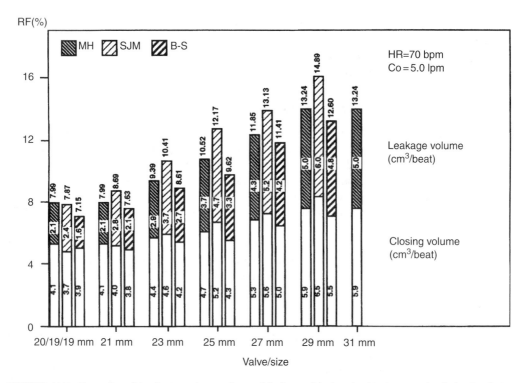

FIGURE 64.5   Examples of *in vitro* reguritant volumes (closing and leakage) with three mechanical valve designs (MH — Medtronic–Hall; SJM — St. Jude Medical; B — Bjork–Shiley mono-strut).

Figure 64.5 illustrates *in vitro* regurgitant volumes (closing and leakage) measured on three commonly used mechanical valve designs in the aortic and mitral positions.

Regurgitation has implications other than simply for flow delivery. On the negative side, back flow through a narrow slit, such as can occur in leakage regurgitation through a bileaflet valve, can create relatively high laminar shear stresses, thus increasing the tendency toward blood cell damage [Baldwin, 1990; Cape et al., 1993]. However, regurgitation can have a beneficial effect in that the back flow over surfaces may serve to wash out zones that would otherwise have stagnant flow throughout the cycle. This is particularly true for the "hinge" region in some tilting disc and bileaflet designs.

64.4.4   Flow Patterns and Turbulent Shear Stresses

Thrombosis and embolism, tissue overgrowth, hemolysis, and damage to endothelium adjacent to the valve are directly related to the velocity and turbulence fields created by various valve designs and have been addressed in detail during the past decade by investigators studying cardiovascular fluid mechanics [Chandran et al., 1983, 1984; Woo and Yoganathan, 1985, 1986; Yoganathan et al., 1986a, 1988].

It has been established that shear stresses on the order of 1500 to 4000 dynes/cm^2 can cause lethal damage to red cells [Nevaril et al., 1969]. However, in the presence of foreign surfaces, red cells can be destroyed by shear stresses on the order of 10 to 100 dynes/cm^2 [Mohandas et al., 1974]. It has also been observed that sublethal damage to red cells can occur at turbulent shear stress levels of 500 dynes/cm^2 [Sutera and Merjhardi, 1975]. Platelets appear to be more sensitive to shear and can be damaged by shear stress on the order of 100 to 500 dynes/cm^2 [Ramstack et al., 1979; Wurzinger et al., 1983]. Evidence that platelet activation, aggregation, and thrombosis is induced by fluid shear forces has been predominantly generated by viscometric studies performed under well-defined fluid mechanical conditions. In viscometers,

TABLE 64.2 Peak and Mean Turbulent Shear Stresses Measured Downstream of Different Aortic Valve Designs

Valve	Location, mm	Acceleration phase		Peak systole		Deceleration phase	
		Peak, dynes/cm^2	Mean, dynes/cm^2	Peak, dynes/cm^2	Mean, dynes/cm^2	Peak, dynes/cm^2	Mean, dynes/cm^2
Starr–Edwards (1260)	26, centerline	750	450	1800	1000	1400	700
	30, centerline	600	200	1850	1100	1300	750
Medtronic-Hall	7, major orifice	450	250	1200	450	600	300
	7, minor orifice	950	400	1000	350	850	450
	13, centerline	1200	600	1000	550	800	400
	13, major orifice	400	320	1500	370	700	300
	13, minor orifice	1250	550	1450	700	700	450
	16, centerline	300	100	2000	1000	850	450
	15, 90° rotated (Fig.)	300	170	1450	700	900	450
St. Jude	8, centerline	820	450	1150	500	600	320
	8, 6.25 mm lateral to centerline	1600	1050	2000	1000	1000	650
	13, centerline	950	470	1500	750	1400	900
	13, 6.25 mm lateral to centerline	1400	800	2000	1050	1000	700
	11, 90° rotated (Fig.)	950	550	1700	1200	1000	700
Carpentier–Edwards (2625 Porcine)	10, centerline	900	400	2750	1200	1750	1000
	15, centerline	1400	700	4500	2000	1700	900
Hancock MO (250 Porcine)	10, centerline	1000	400	2900	1100	1150	550
	15, centerline	1750	950	2450	1900	2100	1400
Carpentier–Edwards (Pericardial)	17, centerline	500	100	850	200	1000	350
	33, centerline	850	200	1130	450	900	370

the extent and reversibility of shear-induced platelet aggregation are a function of both the magnitude and duration of the applied shear stress. For example, at 150 dynes/cm^2, platelet aggregation is not observed until shear is applied for 300 sec. But, as the intensity of the applied shear stress increases, platelet activation and aggregation occur more rapidly. For example, at a shear stress of 600 dynes/cm^2, platelet aggregation occurs within 30 sec, and at 6500 dynes/cm^2, platelet activation occurs in fewer than 5 msec. As the magnitude of the applied shear increases, formed platelet aggregates tend not to separate when the shear forces are discontinued. Furthermore, platelet damage increases linearly with time of exposure to constant shear stress, indicating that shear-induced platelet damage is cumulative [Brown et al., 1977; Colantuoni et al., 1977; Anderson and Hellums, 1978].

Although the exact mechanism of turbulent stress damage to the cell is not precisely known, there is no disagreement that cell damage can be created by high turbulent stresses; minimizing these is conducive to better valve performance from the standpoints of thrombus formation, thromboembolic complications, and hemolysis and from energy loss considerations.

To illustrate the abnormal flow fields and elevated levels of turbulent shear stresses created by prosthetic valves, *in vitro* measurements conducted on 27-mm aortic valve designs in current clinical use in the United States (i.e., FDA approved) are presented below.

The figures of the *in vitro* flow field studes are presented as schematic diagrams and represent velocity and turbulence profiles obtained at peak systole, at a cardiac output of 6.0 l/min and a heart rate of 70 beats/min. All downstream distances are measured from the valve sewing ring. Table 64.2 and Table 64.3 list the maximum and cross sectionally averaged mean turbulent shear stresses measured downstream of the valves at different times during systole and diastole.

TABLE 64.3   Peak and Mean Turbulent Shear Stresses Measured Downstream of Different Mitral Valve Designs

Valve	Location, mm	Acceleration phase		Peak systole		Deceleration phase	
		Peak, dynes/cm^2	Mean, dynes/cm^2	Peak, dynes/cm^2	Mean, dynes/cm^2	Peak, dynes/cm^2	Mean, dynes/cm^2
Beall	11, centerline	500	150	1950	450	800	250
	11, 10 mm above centerline	360	150	1300	400	425	150
	17, centerline	375	125	700	225	400	175
Bjork–Shiley (cc)	8, 13 mm above centerline	320	70	235	60	240	60
	8, 10 mm below centerline	40	18	30	17	25	19
	12, centerline	100	40	330	75	150	55
	15, 90° rotated	310	85	375	100	280	60
	18, centerline	90	60	300	110	225	80
	18, 13 mm above centerline	155	80	350	240	210	140
	18, 10 mm below centerline	60	25	210	70	70	25
Medtronic-Hall	8, centerline	300	170	1800	400	650	180
	8, 12 mm above line center	850	300	1150	450	500	200
	8, 9 mm below centerline	900	230	1200	350	225	130
	14, 90° rotated	620	230	1200	320	670	230
	18, centerline	340	100	500	230	300	150
	18, 12 mm above centerline	600	230	2600	900	950	500
	18, 9 mm below centerline	280	130	670	280	360	180
St. Jude	10, centerline	170	95	250	95	175	85
	10, 10 mm above centerline	310	120	440	150	185	100
	12, 90° rotated	725	270	770	300	670	250
	19, centerline	130	80	335	130	165	90
	19, 10 mm above centerline	115	50	575	170	250	110

64.4.5   Starr–Edwards Caged-Ball Valve (Model 1260)

The flow emerging from the valve formed a circumferential jet that separated from the ball, hit the wall of the flow chamber, and then flowed along the wall. The flow had very high velocities in the annular region. The maximum velocity, measured 12 mm downstream of the valve, was 220 cm/sec at peak systole. The peak systolic velocity, measured 30 mm downstream of the valve, was 180 cm/sec, as shown in Figure 64.6. High-velocity gradients were observed at the edges of the jet. The maximum velocity gradient (1700 cm sec^{-1}/cm) was observed in the annular region adjacent to the surface of the ball during peak systole. A large-velocity defect was observed in the central part of the flow chamber as a wake developed distal to the ball. A region of low velocity reverse flow was observed at peak systole and during the deceleration phase, with a diameter of about 8 mm immediately distal to the apex of the cage. The maximum reverse velocity measured was −25 cm/sec; it occurred at peak systole 30 mm downstream of the valve (Figure 64.6). The intensity of the reverse flow during the deceleration phase was not as high as that observed at peak systole. No reverse flow was observed during the acceleration phase. However, the velocity in the central part of the flow channel was low.

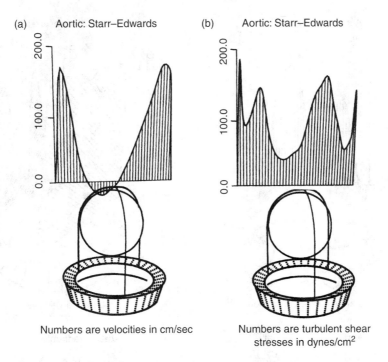

(a) Aortic: Starr–Edwards   (b) Aortic: Starr–Edwards

Numbers are velocities in cm/sec   Numbers are turbulent shear stresses in dynes/cm²

FIGURE 64.6   (a) Velocity profile 30 mm downstream on the centerline for the Starr–Edwards ball valve, at peak systole; (b) turbulent shear stress profile 30 mm downstream on the centerline for the Starr–Edwards ball valve, at peak systole.

High turbulent shear stresses were observed at the edges of the jet. The maximum turbulent shear stress measured was 1850 dynes/cm², which occurred at the location of the highest-velocity gradient (Figure 64.6). The intensity of turbulence during peak systole did not decay very rapidly downstream of the valve. Elevated turbulent shear stresses occurred during most of systole. Turbulent shear stresses as high as 3500 dynes/cm² were estimated in the annular region between the flow channel wall and the ball.

64.4.6 Medtronic–Hall Tilting Disc Valve

High-velocity jetlike flows were observed from both the major and minor orifice outflow regions. The orientation of the jets with respect to the axial direction changed as the valve opened and closed. The major orifice jet was larger than the minor orifice jet and had a slightly higher velocity. The peak velocities measured 7 mm downstream of the valve were 210 and 200 cm/sec in the major and the minor orifice regions, respectively (Figure 64.7). A region of reverse flow was observed adjacent to the wall in the minor orifice region at peak systole, which extended 2 mm from the wall with a maximum reverse velocity of −25 cm/sec. The size of this region increased during the deceleration phase to 8 mm from the wall. A small region of flow separation was observed adjacent to the wall in the major orifice region as illustrated by Figure 64.7. In the minor orifice region, a profound velocity defect was observed 7 and 11 mm distal to the minor orifice strut (Figure 64.7). Furthermore, the region adjacent to the wall immediately downstream from the minor orifice was stagnant during the acceleration and deceleration phases and had very low velocities (<15 cm/sec) during peak systole.

In the major orifice region, high turbulent shear stresses were confined to narrow regions at the edges of the major orifice jet (Figure 64.7). The peak turbulent shear stresses measured at peak systole were 1200 and 1500 dynes/cm², 7 and 13 mm downstream of the valve, respectively. During the acceleration and deceleration phases the turbulent shear stresses were relatively low. High turbulent shear stresses were more dispersed in the minor than those in the major orifice region as shown by Figure 64.7. The turbulent

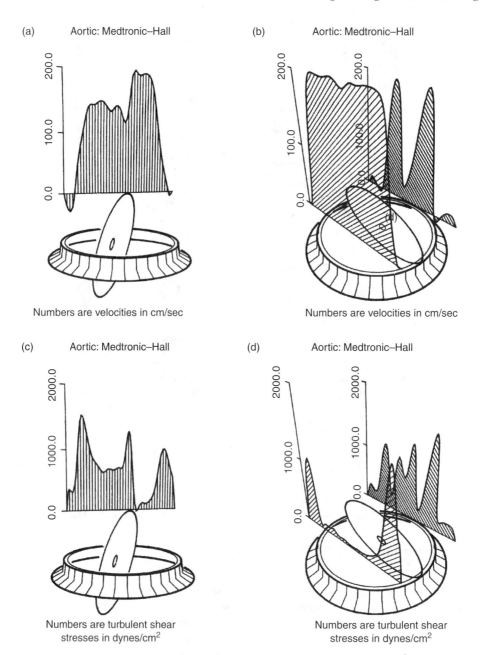

(a) Aortic: Medtronic–Hall

Numbers are velocities in cm/sec

(b) Aortic: Medtronic–Hall

Numbers are velocities in cm/sec

(c) Aortic: Medtronic–Hall

Numbers are turbulent shear
stresses in dynes/cm^2

(d) Aortic: Medtronic–Hall

Numbers are turbulent shear
stresses in dynes/cm^2

FIGURE 64.7   (a) Velocity profile 15 mm downstream on the centerline across the major and minor orifices of the Medtronic–Hall tilting disc valve (major orifice to the right), at peak systole; (b) velocity profiles 13 mm downstream in the major and minor orifices of the Medtronic–Hall tilting disc valve, at peak systole; (c) turbulent shear stress profile 15 mm downstream on the centerline across the major and minor orifices of the Medtronic–Hall tilting disc valve (major orifice to the right), at peak systole; (d) turbulent shear stress profiles 13 mm downstream in the major and minor orifices of the Medtronic–Hall tilting disc valve, at peak systole.

shear stress profiles across the major and minor orifices 15 mm downstream of the valve (Figure 64.7) showed a maximum turbulent shear stress of 1450 dynes/cm^2 at the lower edge of the minor orifice jet.

64.4.7   St. Jude Medical Bileaflet Valve

The St. Jude Medical valve has two semicircular leaflets which divide the area available for forward flow into three regions: two lateral orifices and a central orifice. The major part of the forward flow emerged from the two lateral orifices. The measurements along the centerline plane 8 mm downstream of the valve showed at peak systole a maximum velocity of 220 and 200 cm/sec for the lateral and central orifice jets, respectively. The velocity of the jets remained about the same as the flow traveled from 8 to 13 mm downstream (Figure 64.8). The velocity profiles showed two defects which corresponded to the location of the two leaflets. The velocity measurements indicated that the flow was more evenly distributed across the flow chamber during the deceleration than during the acceleration phase. Regions of flow separation were observed around the jets adjacent to the flow channel wall as the flow separated from the orifice ring. The measurements across the central orifice illustrated in Figure 64.8 show that the maximum velocity in the central orifice was 220 cm/sec. Small regions of low-velocity reverse flow were observed adjacent to the pivot/hinge mechanism of the valve (Figure 64.8). More flow emerged from the central orifice during the deceleration phase than during the acceleration phase.

High turbulent shear stresses occurred at locations of high-velocity gradients and at locations immediately distal to the valve leaflets (Figure 64.8). The flow along the centerline plane became more disturbed as the flow traveled from 8 to 13 mm downstream of the valve. The peak turbulent shear stresses measured along the centerline plane at peak systole were 1150 and 1500 dynes/cm^2 at 8 and 13 mm downstream of the valve, respectively. The profiles across the central orifice showed that the flow was very disturbed in this region. The maximum turbulent shear stress measured in the central orifice as shown in Figure 64.8 (1700 dynes/cm^2) occurred peak systole. Since these high turbulent shear stresses across the central orifice were measured 11 mm downstream, it is probable that even higher turbulent shear stresses occurred closer to the valve.

64.4.8   Carpentier–Edwards Porcine Valve (Model 2625)

The velocity profiles taken 10 mm downstream of the valve, along the centerline plane, showed that the peak velocity of the jetlike flow emerging from the valve was as high as 220 cm/sec at peak systole (Figure 64.9). The peak velocities measured during the acceleration and deceleration phases were about the same, 175 and 170 cm/sec, respectively. However, the flow was much more evenly distributed during the acceleration than during the deceleration phase. No regions of flow separation were observed throughout the systolic period in this plane of measurement. However, the annular region between the outflow surfaces of the leaflets and the flow chamber wall was relatively stagnant throughout systole. The velocity of the jet increased to about 370 cm/sec at peak systole, as the flow traveled from 10 to 15 mm downstream of the valve. This indicated that the flow tended to accelerate toward the center of the flow channel.

High turbulent shear stresses occurred at the edge of the jet (Figure 64.9). The maximum turbulent shear stress measured 10 mm downstream of the valve along the centerline plane at peak systole was 2750 dynes/cm^2. The turbulent shear stresses at the edge of the jet increased as the flow traveled from 10 to 15 mm downstream of the valve. The maximum and mean turbulent shear stress measured at peak systole increased to 4500 and 2000 dynes/cm^2, respectively (Table 64.2).

64.4.9   Hancock Modified Orifice Porcine Valve (Model 250)

In this design, a 25-mm valve was studied, since a 27-mm valve is not manufactured. The velocity measurements showed that this valve design also produced a high-velocity jetlike flow field with a maximum velocity of 330 cm/sec, which was measured along the centerline plane, 10 mm downstream. The jet, however, started to dissipate very rapidly as it flowed downstream. The maximum velocity measured 15 mm downstream of the valve was 180 cm/sec, as shown in Figure 64.10. A velocity defect was observed 15 mm

(a)   Aortic: St.Jude

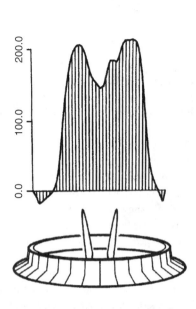

Numbers are velocities in cm/sec

(b)   Aortic: St.Jude

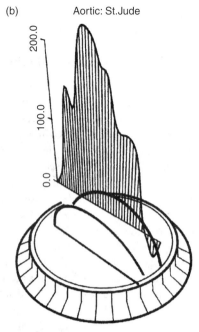

Numbers are velocities in cm/sec

(c)   Aortic: St.Jude

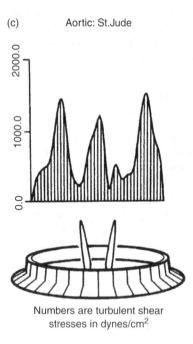

Numbers are turbulent shear
stresses in dynes/cm^2

(d)   Aortic: St.Jude

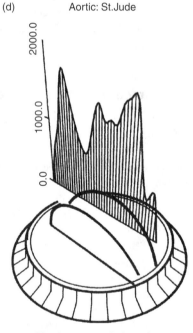

Numbers are turbulent shear
stresses in dynes/cm^2

FIGURE 64.8   (a) Velocity profile 13 mm downstream on the centerline for the St. Jude Medical bileaflet valve, at peak systole; (b) velocity profile 13 mm downstream across the central orifice for the St. Jude Medical bileaflet valve, at peak systole; (c) turbulent shear stress profile 13 mm downstream of the centerline orifice for the St. Jude Medical bileaflet valve, at peak systole; (d) turbulent shear stress profile 13 mm downstream across the central orifice for the St. Jude Medical bileaflet valve, at peak systole.

(a)   Aortic: C–E Porcine (2625)   (b)   Aortic: C–E 2625 Porcine

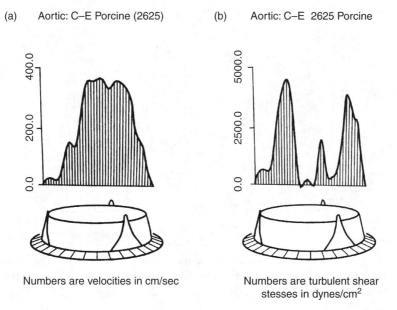

Numbers are velocities in cm/sec   Numbers are turbulent shear
                                           stesses in dynes/cm²

FIGURE 64.9   (a) Velocity profile 15 mm downstream on the centerline for the Carpentier–Edwards 2625 porcine valve, at peak systole; (b) turbulent shear stress profile 15 mm downstream on the centerline for the Carpentier–Edwards 2625 porcine valve, at peak systole.

(a)   Aortic: Hancock (MO) Porcine   (b)   Aortic: Hancock (MO) Porcine

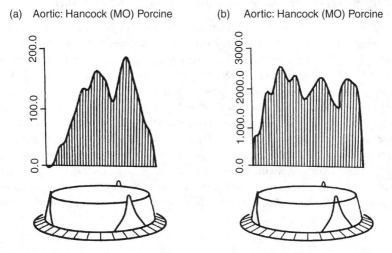

FIGURE 64.10   (a) Velocity profile 15 mm downstream on the center for the Hancock modified orifice porcine valve, at peak systole; (b) turbulent shear stress profile 15 mm downstream on the centerline for the Hancock modified orifice porcine valve, at peak systole.

downstream in the central part of the flow channel peak systole and during the deceleration phase but was not observed along the centerline plane 10 mm downstream of the valve. Once again, the annular region between the outflow surfaces of the leaflets and the flow chamber wall was relatively stagnant during systole.

Turbulent shear stress measurements showed that the high turbulent shear stresses measured 10 mm downstream of the valve were confined to a narrow region at the edge of the jet, with a peak valve of 2900 dynes/cm² (Table 64.2). This peak turbulent shear stress decreased to 2400 dynes/cm² as the flow

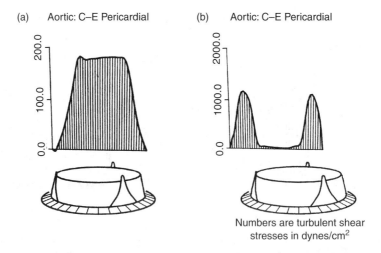

FIGURE 64.11 (a) Velocity profile 17 mm downstream on the centerline for the Carpentier–Edwards pericardial valve, at peak systole; (b) turbulent shear stress profile 17 mm downstream on the centerline for the Carpentier–Edwards pericardial valve, at peak systole.

traveled from 10 to 15 mm downstream of the valve (Figure 64.10). The region of high turbulence, however, became more diffuse as a result of energy dissipation.

64.4.10 Carpentier–Edwards Pericardial Valve (Model 2900)

The velocity profiles obtained along the centerline plane 17 mm downstream of the valve at peak systole showed a maximum velocity of 180 cm/sec. The maximum velocities measured during the acceleration and deceleration phases were 120 and 80 cm/sec, respectively. A region of flow separation which extended about 6 mm from the wall was observed at peak systole and during the deceleration phase. This region was relatively stagnant during the acceleration phase. The maximum velocity of the jet at peak systole did not change as the flow field traveled from 17 to 33 mm downstream of the valve (Figure 64.11). However, the size of the region of flow separation decreased and extended only 1 mm from the wall.

Turbulent shear stress measurements taken along the centerline plane 17 mm downstream of the valve showed that, during the deceleration phase, elevated turbulent shear stresses were spread out over a wide region (with a maximum value of 100 dynes/cm^2). At peak systole, the high turbulent shear stresses were confined to a narrow region, with a maximum value of 850 dynes/cm^2 (Figure 64.11). The intensity of turbulence at peak systole increased as the flow traveled from 17 to 33 mm downstream of the valve.

64.5 Implications for Thrombus Deposition

In the vicinity of mechanical aortic heart valves, where peak shear stresses can easily exceed 1500 dynes/cm^2 and mean shear stresses are frequently in the range of 200 to 600 dynes/cm^2 (Table 64.2), platelet activation and aggregation can readily occur. Data indicating that shear-induced platelet damage is cumulative are particularly relevant to heart valves. During an individual excursion through the replacement valve, the combination of shear magnitude and exposure time may not induce platelet aggregation. However, as a result of multiple journeys through the artificial valve, shear-induced damage may accumulate to a degree sufficient to promote thrombosis and subsequent embolization.

All the aortic and mitral valve designs (mechanical and tissue) studied created mean turbulent shear stress in excess of 200 dynes/cm^2 during the major portion of systole and diastole (Table 64.2 and Table 64.3), which could lead to damage to blood elements. In the case of mechanical prostheses, due to the presence of foreign surfaces, the chances for blood cell damage are increased. Furthermore, the regions of flow stagnation and/or flow separation that occur adjacent to the superstructures of these valve designs, could promote the deposition of damaged blood elements, leading to thrombus formation on the prosthesis.

64.6 Durability

The performance of prosthetic valves is in several ways related to structural mechanics. The design configuration affects the load distribution and dynamics of the valve components, which, in conjunction with the material properties, determine durability — notably wear and fatigue life. Valve configuration, in concert with the flow engendered by the geometry, also dictates the extent of low-wear (e.g., flow separation) and high-shear (e.g., gap leakage) regions. The hinges of bileaflet and tilting disc valves are vulnerable — their design can produce sites of stagnant flow, which may cause localized thrombosis, which may in turn restrict occluder motion. In addition, as discussed earlier, the rigid circular orifice ring is an unnatural configuration for a heart valve, since the elliptically shaped natural valve annulus changes in size and shape during the cardiac cycle.

The choice of valve materials is closely related to structural factors, since the fatigue and wear performance of a valve depends not only on its configuration and loading but on the material properties as well. In addition, the issue of biocompatibility is crucial to prosthetic valve design — and biocompatibility depends not only upon the material itself but also on its *in vivo* environment. In the design of heart valves there are engineering design trade-offs: Materials that exhibit good biocompatibility may have inferior durability and vice versa. For many patients, the implanted prosthetic valve needs to last well over a decade, and in the case of young people the need for valve durability may be even greater. Mechanical durability depends on the material properties and the loading cycle, and examples of degradation include fatigue cracks, abrasive wear, and biochemical attack on the material [Giddens et al., 1993].

64.6.1 Wear

Abrasive wear of valve parts has been and continues to be a serious issue in the design of mechanical prosthetic valves. Various parts of these valves come in contact repeatedly for hundreds of millions of cycles over the lifetime of the device. A breakthrough occurred with the introduction of pyrolitic carbon (PYC) as a valve material: It has relatively good blood compatibility characteristics and wear performance. However, although PYC wear upon PYC and upon metals is relatively low, PYC wear by metals is considerably greater [Shim and Schoen, 1974]. One example of this is a PYC disc mounted on a metallic orifice/hinge combination. The most durable wear couple is PYC–PYC, therefore PYC-coated components are very attractive. The first valve to employ a PYC–PYC couple was the St. Jude Medical valve, which has fixed pivots for the leaflets. Tests indicate that it would take 200 years to wear halfway through the PYC coating on a leaflet pivot [Gombrich et al., 1979]. By creating designs that allow wear surfaces to be distributed rather than focal (i.e., the Omnicarbon valve, which has a PYC-coated disc that is free to rotate), it is possible to reduce wear even further. Thus, materials technology continues to progress and in fact has reached the point where wear need not negatively impact the performance of prosthetic mechanical valves.

64.6.2 Fatigue

Metals are prone to fatigue failure. Their polycrystalline nature contains structural characteristics that may produce dislocations under mechanical loading. These dislocations can migrate when subjected to repeated loading cycles and can accumulate at intercrystalline boundaries, and the end result is tiny cracks. These tiny cracks are sites of stress concentration, and the fissures can worsen until fracture occurs. The Haynes 25 Stellite Bjork–Shiley valve, which used a chromium–cobalt alloy, experienced the most severe fatigue problem for a mechanical valve [Lindblom et al., 1986]. Previous investigations suggested that fatigue was not a problem for PYC; however, recent data contradict this, suggesting that cyclic fatigue-crack growth occurs in graphite/pyrolitic carbon composite material [Ritchie et al., 1990]. This work suggests a fatigue threshold that is as low as 50% of the fracture toughness, and those authors view cyclic fatigue as an essential consideration in the design and life prediction of heart valves constructed from PYC. The FDA now requires detailed characterization of PYC materials used in different valve designs (December 1993 FDA heart valve guidelines).

64.6.3 Mineralization

The major cause of both porcine aortic and pericardial bioprosthetic valve failure is calcification, which stiffens and frequently causes cuspal tears [Levy et al., 1991]. Calcific deposits occur most commonly at the commissures and basal attachments. Calcification is most extensive deep in (intrinsic to) the cusps in the spongiosa layer. Ultrastructurally, calcific deposits are associated with cuspal connective tissue cells and collagen. Degenerative cuspal calcific deposits are composed of calcium phosphates that are chemically and structurally related to physiologic bone mineral (hydroxyapatite). The flexing bladders in cardiac assist devices, flexing polymeric heart valves, and vascular grafts have also been found to be vulnerable to calcific deposits. In such cases, calcification is usually related to inflammatory cells adjacent to the blood-contacting surface, rather than to the implanted material itself.

The mechanisms of calcification, and the methods of preventing calcification are active areas of current research [Webb et al., 1991]. The most common methods of studying calcification involve valve tissue implanted either subcutaneously in 3-week old weanling rats or valves implanted as mitral replacements in young sheep or calves. Results of both types of studies show that bioprosthetic tissue calcifies in a fashion similar to clinical implants but at a greatly accelerated rate. The subcutaneous implantation mode is a well-accepted, technically convenient, economical, and quantifiable model for investigating mineralization issues. It is also very useful for determining the potential of new antimineralization treatments.

Host, implant, and biomechanical factors impact the calcification of tissue valves. Patients who are young or have renal failure are vulnerable to valve mineralization, but immunologic factors seem to be unimportant. Pretreatment of valve tissue with an aldehyde crosslinking agent has been found to cause calcification in rat subcutaneous implants; nonpreserved cusps do not mineralize. Calcification of bioprosthetic valves is greatest at the cuspal commissures and bases, where leaflet flexion is the greatest and deformations are maximal. Most data suggest that the basic mechanisms of tissue valve mineralization result from aldehyde pretreatment, which changes the tissue microstructure.

In both clinical and experimental bioprosthetic tissue, the earliest mineral deposits are observed to be localized to transplanted connective tissue cells. The collagen fibers are involved later. Mineralization of the connective tissue cells of bioprosthetic tissue is thought to result from glutaraldehyde-induced cellular "revitalization" and the resulting disruption of cellular calcium regulation. Normal animal cells have a low intracellular free calcium concentration ($\sim 10^{-7}$ M), whereas extracellular free calcium is much higher ($\sim 10^{-3}$ M), yielding a 10,000-fold gradient across the plasma membrane. In healthy cells, cellular calcium is maintained in low concentration by energy-requiring metabolic mechanisms. In addition, organellar and plasma membranes and cell nuclei, the observed sites of early nucleation of bioprosthetic tissue mineralization, contain considerable phosphorus, mainly in the form of phospholipids. In cells modified by aldehyde crosslinking, passive calcium entry occurs unimpeded, but the mechanisms for calcium removal are dysfunctional. This calcium influx reacts with the preexisting phosphorus and contributes to the mineralization [Schoen et al., 1986]. A very recent article discusses the approaches to preventing heart valve mineralization [Schoen et al., 1993].

64.7 Current Trends in Valve Design

The long-term clinical durability of bioprosthetic valves is the major impediment to their use. Before long-term durability data became available, improvement of hemodynamic performance was the focus of development. The clinical introduction of the bovine pericardial valve solved the hemodynamic problem, and such valves exhibit hemodynamics equal to or better than some mechanical prostheses.

The long-term durability of porcine and bovine bioprostheses can be improved through innovative stent designs that minimize stress concentrations and through improved processing fixation techniques that yield more pliable tissue. The most recent tissue valve design is the stentless bioprosthesis, used for aortic valve replacement. The aortic root bioprostheses are similar in concept to homografts. Absence of the stent is thought to improve hemodynamics, as there is less obstruction in the orifice. The absence of the stent is also thought to improve durability of the tissue, as there is less mechanical wear. Currently, three designs of stentless aortic valves (Medtronic's Freestyle, Baxter's Prima, and St. Jude's Toronto Non-Stented) are undergoing clinical evaluation in the United States and Europe. New antimineralization treatments are also being developed with the goal of increasing the durability of the tissue.

If the above-mentioned design challenges are met, so that bioprostheses can be produced that are durable and thromboresistant, and anticoagulant therapy is not required, there most likely will be another swing toward increased bioprosthesis use.

64.8 Conclusion

Direct comparison of the "total" performance of artificial heart valves is difficult, if not impossible. The precise definition of criteria used to benchmark valve performance varies from study to study. To study long-term performance, large numbers of patients and lengthy observation periods are required. During these periods there may be an evolution in valve materials, or design, and in the medical treatment of patients with prosthetic heart valves. The age of the patient at implant and the underlying valvular heart disease are extremely important factors in valve choice and longevity as well. A valve design suited for the aortic position may be inappropriate for the mitral position. Consequently, it is not possible to categorize a particular valve as the best. All valves currently in use, mechanical and bioprosthetic, produce relatively large turbulent stresses (that can cause lethal and or sublethal damage to red cells and platelets) and greater pressure gradients and regurgitant volumes than normal heart valves.

There are three promising directions for further advances in heart valves (and therefore three challenges for engineers designing new heart valves):

- Improved thromboresistance with new and better artificial materials
- Improved durability of new tissue valves, through the use of nonstented tissue valves, new anticalcification treatments, and better fixation treatments
- Improved hemodynamics characteristics, especially reduction or elimination of low shear stress regions near valve and vessel surfaces and of high turbulent shear stresses along the edges of jets produced by valve outflow and/or leakage of flow.

Whereas the artificial valves certainly have room for further improvement, the superior prognosis for the patient with a replacement heart valve is dramatic and convincing.

Acknowledgment

The technical writing assistance of Ms. Julie Cerlson made the writing of this chapter an enjoyable experience.

References

Anderson G.H. and Hellums J.D. 1978. Platelet lysis and aggregation in shear fields. *Blood Cells* 4: 499.

Baldwin, T. 1990. An investigation of the mean fluid velocity and Reynolds stress fields within an artificial heart ventricle. Ph.D. thesis, Penn State University, PA.

Bodnar E. and Frater R. 1991. *Replacement Cardiac Valves*, New York, Pergamon Press.

Bodnar E. and Yacoub M. 1986. *Biologic and Bioprosthetic Valves*, New York, York Medical Books.

Brewer L.A. III. 1969. *Prosthetic Heart Valves*, Springfield, Ill, Charles C Thomas.

Brown C.H. III, Lemuth R.F., Hellums J.D. et al. 1977. Response of human platelets to shear stress. *Trans. ASAIO* 21: 35.

Butchart E.G. and Bodnar E. 1992. *Thrombosis, Embolism and Bleeding*, ICR Publishers.

Cape E.G., Nanda N.C., and Yoganathan A.P. 1993. Quantification of regurgitant flow through bileaflet heart valve prostheses: theoretical and *in vitro* studies. *Ultrasound Med. Biol.* 19: 461.

Chandran K.G., Cabell G.N., Khalighi B. et al. 1983. Laser anemometry measurements of pulsatile flow past aortic valve prostheses. *J. Biomech.* 16: 865.

Chandran K.G., Cabell G.N., Khalighi B. et al. 1984. Pulsatile flow past aortic valve bioprosthesis in a model human aorta. *J. Biomech.* 17: 609.

Colantuoni G., Hellums J.D., Moake J.L. et al. 1977. The response of human platelets to shear stress at short exposure times. *Trans. ASAIO* 23: 626.

Ferrans V.J., Boyce S.W., Billingham M.E. et al. 1980. Calcific deposits in porcine bioprostheses: structure and pathogenesis. *Am. J. Cardiol.* 46: 721.

Giddens D.P., Yoganathan A.P., and Schoen F.J. 1993. Prosthetic cardiac valves. *Cardiovasc. Pathol.* 2: 167S.

Gombrich P.P., Villafana M.A., and Palmquist W.E. 1979. From concept to clinical — the St. Jude Medical bileaflet pyrolytic carbon cardiac valve. Presented at *Association for the Advancement of Medical Instrumentation, 14th Annual Meeting*, Las Vegas, Nv.

Ionescu M.F. and Ross D.N. 1969. Heart valve replacement with autologous fascia lata. *Lancet* 2: 335.

Lefrak E.A. and Starr A. 1979. *Cardiac Valve Prostheses*, New York, Appleton-Century-Crofts.

Levy R.J., Schoen F.J., Anderson H.C. et al. 1991. Cardiovascular implant calcification: a survey and update. *Biomaterials* 12: 707.

Lindblom D., Bjork V.O., and Semb K.H. 1986. Mechanical failure of the Bjork–Shiley valve. *J. Thorac. Cardiovasc. Surg.* 92: 894.

Mohandas H., Hochmuth R.M., and Spaeth E.E. 1974. Adhesion of red cells to foreign surfaces in the presence of flow. *J. Biomed. Mater. Res.* 8: 119.

Nevaril C., Hellums J., Alfrey C. Jr. et al. 1969. Physical effects in red blood cell trauma. *J. Am. Inst. Chem. Eng.* 15: 707.

Oyer P.E., Stinson E.B., Reitz B.A. et al. 1979. Long term evaluation of the porcine xenograft bioprosthesis. *J. Thorac. Cardiovasc. Surg.* 78: 343.

Ramstack J.M., Zuckerman L., and Mockros L.F. 1979. Shear induced activation of platelets. *J. Biomech.* 12: 113.

Ritchie R.O., Dauskart R.H., and Yu W. 1990. Cyclic fatigue-crack propagation, stress-corrosion, and fracture-toughness in pyrolytic carbon-coated graphite for prosthetic heart valve applications. *J. Biomed. Mater. Res.* 24: 189.

Roberts W.C. 1976. Choosing a substitute cardiac valve: type, size, surgeon. *Am. J. Cardiol.* 38: 633.

Schoen F.J., Libby P., and Diddersheim P. 1993. Future directions and therapeutic approaches. *Cardiovasc. Pathol.* 2: 2095.

Schoen F.J., Tsao J.W., and Levy R.J. 1986. Calcification of bovine pericardium used in cardiac valve bioprostheses: implications for the mechanisms of bioprosthetic tissue mineralization. *Am. J. Pathol.* 123: 134.

Shim H.S. and Schoen F.J. 1974. The wear resistance of pure and silicon alloyed isotropic carbons. *Biomater. Med. Dev. Artif. Organs* 2: 103.

Sutera S.P. and Merjhardi M.H. 1975. Deformations and fragmentation of human red cells in turbulent shear flow. *Biophys. J.* 15: 1.

Wain E.H., Greco R., Ignegen A. et al. 1980. *Int. J. Artif. Organs* 3: 169.

Webb C.L., Schoen F.J., Alfrey A.C. et al. 1991. Inhibition of mineralization of glutaraldehyde-pretreated bovine pericardium by A1C13 and other metallic salts in rat subdermal model studies. *Am. J. Pathol.* 38: 971.

Woo Y.-R. and Yoganathan A.P. 1985. *In vitro* pulsatile flow velocity and turbulent shear stress measurements in the vicinity of mechanical aortic l heart valve prostheses. *Life Support Syst.* 3: 283.

Woo Y.-R. and Yoganathan A.P. 1986. *In vitro* pulsatile flow velocity and shear stress measurements in the vicinity of mechanical mitral heart valve prostheses. *J. Biomech.* 19: 39.

Wurzinger L.J., Opitz R., Blasberg P. et al. 1983. The role of hydrodynamic factors in platelet activation and thrombotic events. In G. Schettler (Ed.), *The Effects of Shear Stress of Short Duration, Fluid Dynamics as a Localizing Factor for Atherosclerosis*, pp. 91–102, Berlin, Springer.

Yoganathan A.P., Chaux A., Gray R. et al. 1984. Bileaflet, tilting disc and porcine aortic valve substitutes: *in vitro* hydrodynamic characteristics. *JACC* 3: 313.

Yoganathan A.P., Reul H., and Black M.M. 1992. Heart valve replacements: problems and developments. In G.W. Hastings (Ed.), *Cardiovascular Biomaterials*, London, Springer-Verlag.

Yoganathan A.P., Sung H.-W., Woo Y.-R. et al. 1988. *In vitro* velocity and turbulence measurements in the vicinity of three new mechanical aortic heart valve prostheses. *J. Thorac. Cardiovasc. Surg.* 95: 929.

Yoganathan A.P., Woo Y.-R., Sung H.-W. et al. 1986a. *In vitro* haemodynamic characteristics of tissue bioprostheses in the aortic position. *J. Thorac. Cardiovasc. Surg.* 92: 198.

Yoganathan A.P., Woo Y.-R., and Sung H.-W. 1986b. Turbulent shear stress measurements in the vicinity of aortic heart valve prostheses. *J. Biomech.* 19: 433.

65

Vascular Grafts

David N. Ku
Georgia Institute of Technology

Robert C. Allen
Emory University

The use of natural or synthetic replacement parts in vascular repair and **vascular reconstruction** is extensive, with a **vascular graft** market of approximately $200 million worldwide. A multitude of biologic grafts and synthetic prostheses are available, each with distinct qualities and potential applications [Rutherford, 1989; Veith et al., 1994]. The ideal vascular graft would (1) be biocompatible, (2) be nonthrombogenic, (3) have long-term potency, (4) be durable yet compliant, (5) be infection resistant, and (6) be technically facile. There is currently no ideal conduit available, but overall, the autogenous saphenous vein is preferred for small-vessel reconstruction, and synthetic prostheses are best suited for large-vessel replacement. Large diameter (>10 mm) vascular grafts are predominantly used for aortic/iliac artery reconstruction with Dacron (80%) and PTFE (20%) being the standard construction materials. Synthetic grafts function well in these high-flow, low-resistance circuits with high long-term patencies. Small-caliber (<10 mm) vascular grafts are used for a variety of indications including lower-extremity bypass procedures, coronary artery bypass grafting (CABG), **hemodialysis access**, and extra-anatomic bypasses. Saphenous vein is the conduit of choice for lower-extremity revascularization and CABG procedures and shows superior patency rates compared to synthetic grafts. Internal mammary artery (IMA) grafts are used extensively for CABG with better long-term patency than saphenous vein grafts. Synthetic prostheses are used for hemodialysis access and **extra-anatomic bypass** grafting, especially PTFE due to its durability and resistance to external pressure. Bovine carotid heterografts are also used for hemodialysis access with fair success, but their value is questionable because of aneurysmal changes over time due to graft degeneration.

65.1 History of Vascular Grafts

Vascular surgery was first defined as a field with the initial publication of Alexis Carrel's work in 1902. Goyanes performed the first arterial graft in 1906 by using the popliteal vein *in situ* to replace an excised popliteal artery aneurysm. Lexer, in 1907, performed the first free autogenous vein graft by replacing an axillary artery defect with a segment of greater saphenous vein from the same patient. It was not until 1949, however, that Kunlin performed the first successful femoropopliteal bypass with reversed saphenous vein. The Korean War was the true advent of reconstructive surgery for arterial injuries as initiated by Shumacker and reported by Hughes and Bowers in 1952. The first report of a synthetic graft also appeared in 1952 when Voorhees described his initial work in dogs using tubes of Vinyon-N cloth to bridge arterial defects. In the late 1950s and 1960s DeBakey firmly established the clinical usefulness of Dacron grafts; Dacron arterial prostheses became commercially available in 1957. Microporous expanded polytetrafluoroethylene (ePTFE) grafts, introduced in the 1970s, were the next generation of successful synthetic grafts but bear no clear superiority to Dacron grafts.

65.2   Synthetic Grafts

Synthetic prostheses are the preferred conduit for large-vessel reconstruction and the primary alternative to saphenous vein in small-vessel repair. Thankfully, the saphenous vein is of adequate quality and length in 70 to 75% of patients requiring small-vessel grafting. the two major choices available for prosthetic reconstruction are Dacron (polyethylene terephthalate) and PTFE (polytetrafluoroethylene). The tensile strength of these grafts remains unchanged even after years of implantation, whereas Nylon (Polyamide), Ivalon, and Orlon lose significant tensile strength over a period of months.

Dacron grafts are constructed from multifilamentous yarn and fabricated by weaving or knitting [Sawyer, 1987; Rutherford, 1989]. Woven fabric is interlaced in an over-and-under pattern resulting in a nonporous graft with no stretch. Knitted fabrics have looped threads forming a continuous interconnecting chain with variable stretch and porosity. Knitted velour is a variant in which the loops of yarn extend upward at right angles to the fabric surface resulting in a velvety texture. The velour finish may be created on the internal, the external, or both surfaces to enhance preclotting and tissue incorporation. Porous knitted Dacron prostheses may be made impervious by impregnation or coating with albumin/collagen to obviate preclotting and minimize blood loss while maintaining the superior handling characteristics of knitted Dacron grafts. Dacron prostheses are often crimped to impart elasticity, maintain shape during bending, and facilitate vascular anastomosis formation. The use of external support for vascular grafts is an alternative to crimping which uses externally attached polyprophylene rings to avoid kinking with angulation and to create dimensional stability. Woven Dacron grafts possess poor handling characteristics and poor compliance and elicit a poor healing response and, therefore, are used predominantly in the repair of the thoracic aorta, ruptured abdominal aortic aneurysms, and patients with coagulation defects. Knitted Dacron prostheses are used in the remainder of cases involving the abdominal aorta, iliac, femoral, and popliteal vessels, and in extra-anatomic repair/bypass. Dacron grafts are not advocated in small-vessel reconstruction, such as the below-knee popliteal or tibial, because of poor patency rates. An active infective process or contaminated field contraindicate the use of Dacron prostheses. Vascular grafts are named after the vessel they replace or the arterial segments they connect.

Expanded Teflon (ePTFE) is a synthetic polymer of carbon and fluorine produced by mechanical stretching [Sawyer, 1987; Rutherford, 1989]. The result is a series of solid nodes of ePTFE with interconnecting small fibrils. The pore size is variable and averages 30 μm. The chief advantages of ePTFE in comparison to knitted Dacron include impermeability to blood, resistance to aneurysmal formation, and ease of declotting; ePTFE is used clinically mainly for femoropopliteal bypasses, hemodialysis angioaccess, and extra-anatomic reconstructions. The addition of an external support coil can be used to enhance graft stability against external pressure and to prevent kinking at points of angulation.

The primary area of failure in prosthetic grafting with Dacron and PTFE is the patency of small-caliber grafts, which remains poor. The inherent thrombogenicity of these prosthetic grafts in conjunction with **neointimal hyperplasia**, which is limited to the anastomotic area, are the prime factors. The seeding of prosthetic grafts with endothelial cells and subsequent proliferation of these cells into a confluent monolayer along the graft has been suggested as an attractive solution to this problem for a number of years. The technology and techniques devoted to develop this solution to small-caliber graft patency have

TABLE 65.1   Patency Data for Representative Vascular Grafts

Graft	Conduit	5-year patency, %
Aortiobifemoral	Dacron	90
	ePTFE	90
Femorofemoral	Dacron	80
	ePTFE	80
Femoropopliteal	Saphenous vein	70
	ePTFE	50
	ePTFE	40
Dialysis access	ePTFE	60 (3 years)
	Bovine heterograft	25 (3 years)

been impressive, but the results have been variable and certainly not the panacea envisioned by early investigators. The clinical utility of endothelial cell seeding onto prosthetic grafts remains to be defined.

65.3   Regional Patency

Patency data for any vascular graft depend on multiple factors including the conduit and vessel size. Large-diameter vessels have a high rate of patency, and therefore, synthetic grafts are the conduit of choice and display high short- and long-term patencies. Saphenous vein is the primary graft for small-caliber vessel reconstruction with good patency rates, and prosthetic grafts demonstrate acceptable short-term patencies but poor long-term results. Extra-anatomic bypasses utilize synthetic conduits with external support to reduce kinking. Dacron vs. PTFE graft trials have shown no significant difference in patency rates [Rutherford, 1989]. Hemodialysis access grafts are constructed primarily of PTFE with a minority of bovine carotid heterografts still present. PTFE is preferred due to resistance to infection, decreased pseudoaneurysm formation, and improved patency rates. Patency data for representative vascular grafts is summarized in Table 65.1 by anatomical location and conduit [Imparato et al., 1972; Rutherford, 1989; Veith et al., 1994].

Vascular grafts have a finite life span which is usually reported in the form of a life-table of graft patency. The patency rate falls to about 50% in 4 years after implantation for the most common PTFE femoral-popliteal grafts. Graft failures are typically caused by (1) thrombosis in the early postoperative period of 1 month, (2) tissue ingrowth or neointimal hyperplasia at the anastomoses after several years, and (3) graft infections. Thrombosis in the early postoperative period is usually caused by a technical error at time of implantation and is readily fixed. The longer-term growth of tissue at the anastomoses is more insidious. Late failure of these grafts as a result of neointimal hyperplasia is a major problem confronting the vascular surgeon. Increasing the longevity of these grafts would greatly benefit the patient and have an important economic impact, nationally.

65.4   Thrombosis

When an artificial vascular graft is first exposed to blood, a clot will typically form at the surface. The clot is formed initially of platelet aggregates, and then the coagulation cascade is activated to lay down fibrin and thrombin. The tissue which forms this inner lining of the graft is often called **pseudointimal hyperplasia**. Pseudointimal hyperplasia is devoid of cellular ingrowth and is composed mainly of fibrin, platelet debris, and trapped red blood cells [Greisler, 1991]. The blood clots immediately on contract and will occlude the vessel if the blood is stagnant or very sluggish. Platelet activity is generally most intense during the first 24 h and subsidies to a very low level after 1 week.

Various artificial surfaces are more or less thrombogenic. Many approaches have been developed in an attempt to make the grafts less thrombogenic [Greisler, 1991]. Typically, the surface characteristics have been modified to prevent adherence or activation of platelets. The surfaces have been modified by seeding with endothelial cells and other exotic treatments such as photopolymerization, plasma-gas coatings, and antisense genetics. Although many of these theories have promise, few have been shown to yield long-term improvements over the existing materials of Dacron and PTFE.

65.5   Neointimal Hyperplasia

Tissue ingrowth onto the artificial surface of a PTFE graft occurs at the anastomoses and is called neointimal hyperplasia. Initially, platelets and thrombin/fibrin cover the entire graft surface within the first 24 h. After this initial phase, smooth-muscle cells migrate from the native artery into the graft, variously referred to as **pannus** ingrowth, neointimal hyperplasia, and fibromuscular hyperplasia. The pannus advances from the edge of the graft at a rate of approximately 0.1 mm per week but does not cover the entire surface in humans. Typically, the maximum extent of ingrowth in humans is 1 to 2 cm. In the first few hours, a thrombotic stage of platelet, fibrin, and red blood cell accumulation occurs (stage I). Days 3 to 4 consist of cellular recruitment in which the thrombus is coated with an endothelial layer (stage II). Cell proliferation of actin-positive cells which resorb and replace the residual thrombus are the major events in stage III, at approximately 7 to 9 days. This description leads to a conclusion that thrombosis and cell proliferation are the two controlling events affecting graft patency. However, this process is one of normal healing which creates no significant **stenosis** in most cases. Recent findings indicate that a fourth stage should be added in which the tissue growths in volume primarily by synthesis and deposition of large amounts of extracellular substance over the following months, as shown in Figure 65.1. This stage IV leads to a hemodynamically significant stenosis.

The ingrowth has been characterized by Glagov as having two different forms: intimal fibromuscular hypertrophy (IFMH) and intimal hyperplasia (IH) [Glagov et al., 1991]. The first form of IFMH is basically a normal healing process which consistently takes place on all grafts and does not become highly stenotic. Initial healing is well organized with smooth-muscle cells organized in lamellae and little

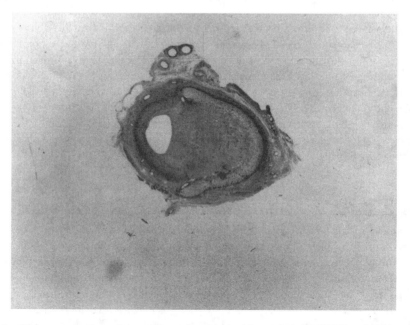

FIGURE 65.1   High-power sections of the anastomotic neointimal hyperplasia in a PTFE graft. This endothelium-lined layer is formed of highly disorganized spindle-shaped cells surrounded by a large amount of extracellular matrix material.

extracellular proteins or mucopolysaccharide material. A second form of abnormal healing creates stenotic and occlusive thickening, called intimal hyperplasia (IH). Intimal hyperplasia is characterized by a chaotic appearance of randomly oriented cells embedded in a field of extracellular matrix material. The histologic appearance is one of hyperplasia or tumor-like behavior. Little is known on the exact stimulant which causes healing to proceed by IFMH or IH, although Glagov speculates that hemodynamic shear stress may play a role. The events in graft neointimal hyperplasia appear to be similar to that of restenotic hyperplasia.

Although the underlying etiology of neointimal hyperplasia has not been fully elucidated, a large number of theories have been proposed to explain this process. The theories generally fall into several broad categories: platelet deposition with local release of PDGF, other growth factor stimulation of SMC proliferation (e.g., TGF-, FGF), monocyte recruitment, complement activation, leukocyte deposition, chronic inflammation, and mechanical stimuli such as stress and shear abnormalities [Greisler, 1991].

Many studies have focused on preventing graft intimal thickening by attacking either thrombosis or cell proliferation. Cell culture studies clearly demonstrate that certain pharmacologic agents can profoundly affect the platelet adhesiveness and cell proliferation. However, the effectiveness of these agents *in vivo* is variable, depending on which animal species is used. A large number of human restenosis trials using a wide variety of antithrombotic agents, steroids, lipid-lowering therapies, and ACE inhibitors have largely been negative. Arteriovenous fistula graft studies in baboons suggest that modifying graft surfaces and infusing antithrombotic agents have little effect on the rate of obstruction of the prostheses.

Compliance mismatch, medial tension, and hemodynamic shear stress are additional putative agents which have been hypothesized to be important in arterial adaptation and neointimal hyperplasia. Arteries tend to adapt in size to maintain a specific wall shear stress under conditions of increased blood flow. Wall shear stress appears to play a major role in the pathogenesis of atherosclerosis and in arterially transplanted autogenous veins, and elevations in shear stress inhibits SMC proliferation and neointimal thickening in porous PTFE grafts in baboons.

We have recently characterized the quantitative relationship between the amount of shear stress and the associated neointimal thickness, shown graphically in Figure 65.2.

This relationship can be written as the mathematical relationship

$$\text{Intimal thickness} = A \times \frac{1}{\text{wall shear rate}} + C \tag{65.1}$$

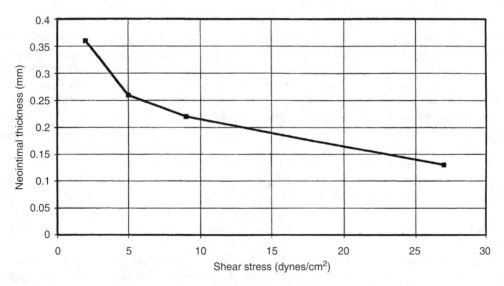

FIGURE 65.2 Graph of neointimal thickness vs. mean shear stress for PTFE tapered grafts in a canine model of intimal hyperplasia.

where C is a constant which would depend on the implantation age of the graft. This relationship appears to be dominant over proximal or distal positioning or absolute flow rate. This inverse, nonlinear relationship between neointimal thickening and wall shear stress shown in Figure 65.2 is strikingly similar to that seen for early atherosclerotic intimal thickening in arteries [e.g., Ku and Zhu, 1993]. Thus, neointimal hyperplasia appears to respond to low shear stress in the same consistent, stereotypic way as do other vascular cells *in vivo*. Since wall shear is primarily determined by the graft diameter, selection of an optimal-size graft for typical flow rates may increase the long-term patency of prosthetic grafts [Binns et al., 1989]. These results apply to *in vivo* PTFE grafts composed of the pore-size and material configuration used most commonly in clinical vascular surgery today.

Surprisingly, the pseudointima of thrombus material consistently shows the same thickening as the anastomotic neointima, even though there are no nucleated cells in the pseudointima [Binns et al., 1989]. The advancing front exhibits an unusual shape in which the endothelial cells grow over the existing thrombus at the lumen, but the smooth-muscle cells stay at the graft surface underneath the thrombus. Thus, the two cell types do not touch each other at the advancing edge of the pannus. The distances between the two types of cells suggest that direct cellular communication is not present at the advancing edge.

Although there is clearly a large body of knowledge on intimal hyperplasisa, the more general question of what biologic material is actually causing occlusions is not clear. The *in vitro* cell culture studies are elegant in their ability to probe the molecular regulators of synthesis and proliferation. However, the response of cells grown as monolayers on plastic may be different from tissue growing in the complex milieu *in vivo*. Small animal studies are useful for initial testing of a wide variety of potential therapeutic agents. Unfortunately, many agents which are successful in rats and rabbits turn out to be unsuccessful in large animals or humans. Large animals such as dogs, pigs, and baboons appear to develop lesions similar to humans and respond to therapies in a similar manner. The major drawback, however, is that the lesions typically take approximately 1 year to develop into advanced stenoses which mimic the clinical human problem. An accurate large-animal model of high-grade neointimal hyperplastic lesions is needed in order to generate a comprehensive characterization of lesion development *in vivo*.

The cellular mechanism by which shear stress influences the development of neointimal hyperplasia is not well understood. The pannus ingrowth is likely to be composed predominantly of smooth-muscle cells. However, the fluid–wall shear stress interface is primarily experienced by endothelial cell. One mechanism for neointimal thickening may be that the endothelial cells sense the local wall shear and regulate the amount of underlying smooth muscle cell growth. Clearly, endothelial cells can change their physiologic behavior and morphologic appearance in response to wall shear stress [Nerem, 1992]. Shear-sensitive endothelial cells mechanoreceptors have been postulated as regulators of the adaptation process seen in arteries in response to increased shear stress. Such receptors, however, have not been identified. An "endothelial-derived relaxation factor" and an "endothelial-derived constriction factor" appear to play an important role in the acute response of the arterial wall to alterations in shear stress. A separate humoral factor acting on the media in response to alterations in shear stress has been suggested. The fact that most of these mediators are endothelium-derived or endothelium-dependent may explain the localization of neointimal hyperplasia in PTFE grafts to the juxta-anastomotic region. In contrast to native vessels, the commonly used human prosthetic grafts are rarely, if ever, fully lined with endothelium except for a short distance adjacent to the anastomosis.

The morphology of endothelial cells grown in low shear or static conditions are random in orientation without a preferred direction. As the intimal thickening progresses, one would expect the deeper layers to be more insulated from the shear effects of hemodynamics and to experience a more static environment. PTFE grafts are essentially nondistensible under physiologic pressure conditions. Thus, the perigraft cells would be expected to experience the least amount of stress from pressure pulses and circumferential stretch as well.

Recently, there has been greater recognition of the importance of extracellular matrix (ECM) in vascular lesions [Bell, 1992]. In general, we have observed that the deepest layers of cells in the perigraft region exhibited the most disorganization and extracellular matrix material. The appearance of the intimal hyperplasia in this region strongly suggests that growth of neointima in this region from the production of extracellular matrix is the dominant mechanism by which intimal hyperplasia becomes occlusive. ECM is dominant in advanced lesions, often to the virtual exclusion of cellular elements. The ECM is also directly responsible for a variety of tissue signals which can augment or reduce cellular proliferation and protein production. The ECM can act directly or act as a repository for other growth factors. Several investigators are attempting to recreate the detailed architecture of ECM in order to develop future biologic substrates for arteries.

Low compliance of PTFE grafts are associated with higher rates of intimal hyperplasia. Rodbard [1970] has hypothesized that the normal adaptive response of cells to static conditions is the production of large amounts of ECM. It is possible that the lack of stretch in the PTFE graft removes any mechanical stimulus to the smooth-muscle cells in this layer and transforms the cells into a synthetic mode with production of large amounts of ECM. The highly synthetic mode of these cells and the hypocellularity in this region would suggest that the major culprit of late graft occlusion is synthesis instead of proliferation. Studies of the response of endothelial cells to very low levels of wall shear stress and the response of underlying smooth muscle cells to endothelial cell products should provide important information on the cellular and molecular mechanisms producing the transformation of thin, organized healing into occlusive growth.

65.6 Graft Infections

Vascular graft infections are catastrophic and challenging problems that threaten life and limb. The incidence of synthetic graft infection is ∼2% and has remained stable despite advances in aseptic surgical technique, vascular graft production, and immunology. Prosthetic grafts are involved in infections four times as often as autogenous vein. The infection rates for PTFE and Dacron prostheses are about the same. The mechanism of infectious complications may involve direct inoculation during surgery or hematogenous seeding, but most occur due to contamination at the time of surgery. Contact of the prosthesis with the skin of the patient is felt to be a key event. The highest incidence anatomically occurs in the inguinal areas due to perineal proximity, lymphatic disruption, and poor wound healing. Antibiotic prophylaxis, both systemically and locally, decreases the incidence of graft infection. The bonding of antibiotics to the prosthesis has been attempted in various forms to prevent prosthetic graft infection but to date is not clinically available. *Staphylococcus epidermidis* is the most common organism involved in graft infections, which *Staphylococcus aureus* also a prevalent organism. Early graft infections commonly are superficial infections (inguinal) with virulent organisms such as *S. aureus* or *Pseudomonas aeruginosa*. Late graft infections usually involve contamination of an abdominal graft with less virulent species such as *S. epidermidis*. The reported mortality rates vary with the anatomic location of the graft and the aggressiveness of the infecting organism. These may range from 5 to 10% for femoropopliteal grafts to 50 to 75% for aortobifemoral grafts. The associated amputation rate varies from 25 to 75%.

Vascular grafts are important tools in the clinical treatment of end-stage arteriosclerosis. Large-diameter grafts made of artificial material have high success and longevity. For small-diameter grafts, autogenous venous grafts are superior in longevity and patency than artificial grafts. The main problems for artificial vascular grafts are early thrombosis, late neointimal hyperplasia, and iatrogenic infection. Some active areas of research include the prevention of flowing blood thrombosis on surfaces, control of the pathogenic process causing neointimal hyperplasia occlusions, and facilitation of the immunogenic response to bacterial infection of a graft.

Defining Terms

Extra-anatomic bypass: Vascular graft used to bypass a blocked artery where the graft is placed in a different location than the original artery. One example is an axillo-femoral graft which brings blood from the arm to the leg though a tube placed under the skin along the side of the person.

Hemodialysis access: Arterial-venous connection surgically placed to provide a large amount of blood flow for hemodialysis. These are often loops of ePTFE placed in the arm.

Neointimal hyperplasia: Fibroblast and smooth-muscle cell growth covering a vascular graft on the inside surface.

Pannus: Neointimal hyperplasia tissue ingrowth at the anastomoses.

Pseudointimal hyperplasia: Fibrin/thrombin deposition on the inside surface of an arterial vascular graft. This accumulation of material is acellular.

Stenosis: Tissue ingrowth into vessel causing a narrow lumen and reduction of blood flow.

Vascular graft: Tube replacement of an artery or vein segment.

Vascular reconstruction: Reconstruction of an artery or vein after trauma, surgery, or blockage of blood flow from disease.

References

Bell, E. 1992. *Tissue Engineering, Current Perspectives*, Boston, Birkhauser.

Binns, R.L., Du, D.N., Stewart, M.T. et al. 1989. Optimal graft diameter: effect of wall shear stress on vascular healing. *J. Vasc. Surg.* 10: 326.

Glagov, S., Giddens, D.P., Bassiouny, H. et al. 1991. Hemodynamic effects and tissue reactions at grafts to vein anastomosis for vascular access. In B.G. Sommer and M.L. Henry (Eds), *Vascular Access for Hemodynamics — II*, pp. 3–20, Precept Press.

Greisler, H.P. 1991. *New Biologic and Synthetic Vascular Prosthesis*, Austin, TX, RG Landes.

Imparato, A.M., Bracco, A., Kim, G.E. et al. 1972. Intimal and neointimal fibrous proliferation causing failure of arterial reconstructions. *Surgery* 72: 1007.

Ku, D.N. and Zhu, C. 1993. The mechanical environment of the artery. In B. Sumpio (Ed.), *Hemodynamic Forces and Vascular Cell Biology*, pp. 1–23, Austin, TX, RG Landes.

Nerem, R.M. 1992. Vascular fluid mechanics, the arterial wall, and atherosclerosis. *J. Biomech. Eng.* 114: 274.

Rodbard, S. 1970. Negative feedback mechanisms in the architecture and function of the connective and cardiovascular tissues. *Perspect. Biol. Med.* 13: 507.

Rutherford, R.B. 1989. *Vascular Surgery*, pp. 404–486, Philadelphia, PA, Saunders.

Sawyer, P.N. 1987. *Modern Vascular Grafts*, New York, McGraw-Hill.

Veith, F.J., Hobson, R.W., Williams, R.A. et al. 1994. *Vascular Surgery*, pp. 523–535, New York, McGraw-Hill.

Further Information

Ku, D.N., Salam, T.A., and Chen, C. 1994. The development of intimal hyperplasia in response to hemodynamic shear stress. Second World Congress of Biomechanics, 31b, Amsterdam.

66

Artificial Lungs and Blood–Gas Exchange Devices

Pierre M. Galletti
Clark K. Colton
Massachusetts Institute of
Technology

The natural lung is the organ in which blood exchanges oxygen and carbon dioxide with the body environment. In turn, blood brings oxygen to all body tissues, so as to oxidize the nutrients needed to sustain life. The end products of the chemical reactions that take place in tissues (globally referred to as **metabolism**) include carbon dioxide, water, and heat, which must all be eliminated. In mammals, oxygen is obtained from the air we breathe through diffusion at the level of the pulmonary alveoli and then carried to the tissues by the hemoglobin in the red blood cells. The carbon dioxide produced by living cells is picked up by the circulating blood and brought to the pulmonary capillaries from where it diffuses into the alveoli and is conveyed out by ventilation through the airways. These processes can be slowed down to a fraction of resting levels by hypothermia or accelerated up to 20-fold when the demand for fuel increases, as for instance with hypothermia, fever, and muscular exercise.

Only a fraction of the oxygen in the air is actually transferred from the pulmonary alveoli to the pulmonary capillary blood, only a fraction of the oxygen carried by arterial blood is actually extracted by the tissues, and only a fraction of the oxygen present in tissues is actually replenished in a single blood pass. Similarly, only a fraction of the CO_2 present in tissues is conveyed to the circulating blood, only a fraction of the mixed venous blood CO_2 content is actually discharged in the alveoli, and only a fraction of the CO_2 in the aveolar gas is eliminated into each breath. Delicately poised physiologic mechanisms, further balanced by chemical buffer systems, maintain the gas exchange system in equilibrium.

The challenge of replacing the function of the natural lungs by an exchange device allowing continuous blood flow and continuous blood **arterialization** was first outlined by physiologists at the end of the 19th century but could not be met reliably until the 1950s. The large transfer areas needed for blood-gas exchange in an **artificial lung** were initially obtained by continuous foaming and defoaming in a circulating blood pool or by spreading a thin film of blood in an oxygen atmosphere. Because the direct blood–gas interface was found to be damaging to blood as well as difficult to stabilize over extended periods, membrane-mediated processes were introduced and are now almost universally preferred.

66.1   Gas Exchange Systems

Artificial lungs are often called **blood oxygenators** because oxygen transfer has traditionally been seen as the most important function being replaced and, in most situations, has proved more limiting than CO_2 transfer. The change in blood color between inlet and outlet also encourages the term oxygenator, considering that changes in blood CO_2 content are not visible to the eye and are more difficult to measure than oxygen transfer.

As is the case for most artificial organs, artificial lungs may be called upon to replace entirely the pulmonary gas exchange function (when the natural organ is totally disabled or, while still sound, must be taken out of commission for a limited time to allow a surgical intervention) or to assist the deficient gas transfer capacity of the natural organ, either temporarily, with the hope that the healing process will eventually repair the diseased organ, or permanently, when irreversible lung damage leaves the patient permanently disabled.

Since most artificial lungs cannot be placed in the anatomical location of the natural lung, venous blood must be diverted from its normal path through the central veins, right heart, and pulmonary vascular bed and rerouted, via **catheters** and tubes, through an extracorporeal circuit which includes the artificial lung before being returned, by means of a pump, to the arterial system.

The procedure in which the pulmonary circulation is temporarily interrupted for surgical purposes and gas exchange is provided by an artificial lung is often referred to as **extracorporeal circulation** (ECC) because, for convenience sake in the operating room, the gas exchange device as well as the pumps which circulate the blood are located outside the body.

The vision of coupling extracorporeal blood pumping with extracorporeal gas exchange at a level of performance sufficient to permit unhurried surgical interventions in adult patients originated with Gibbon [1939] whose initial laboratory models relied on rotating cylinders to spread blood in a continuously renewed thin film, in the tradition of 19th-century physiologists. Gibbon's clinical model [1954], built with technical support from IBM, was a stationary **film oxygenator**, a bulky device in which venous blood was evenly smeared over a stack of vertical wire screen meshes in an oxygen atmosphere, flowing gently downward to accumulate in a reservoir from where blood could be returned to a systemic artery. The main problems with that design, besides its cumbersome dimensions, were to avoid blood streaming and to maintain a constant blood–gas exchange area. Other investigators tried to increase the flexibility of the system by replacing the stationary film support with rotating screens or rotating discs partly immersed in a pool of blood. This allowed some control of gas transfer performance by changing the rational speed, but minimizing the blood content of the device dictated a tight fit between the discs and the horizontal glass cylinder surrounding them. Foaming and **hemolysis** were encountered at high disc spinning velocity, and these designs were eventually abandoned.

The very first strategy of physiologists for exchanging oxygen and carbon dioxide in venous blood had been to bubble pure oxygen through a stationary blood pool. To turn this batch process into a continuous operation for totally body **perfusion**, blood was collected through cannulae from the central veins by a syphon or a pump, driven upward in a vertical chimney, mixed with a stream of oxygen gas bubbles, and finally passed through filters and defoaming sponges so as to collect bubble-free arterialized blood, which could then be used to perfuse the arterial tree. The efficiency of **bubble oxygenators** is extremely high because the smaller the bubbles, the larger the blood–oxygen exchange area developed by a steady current of gas. In the limiting case, it is even possible to saturate venous blood by introducing no more oxygen into the blood than is consumed by the tissues. This process, however, doe not remove any carbon dioxide. Since the partial pressure of CO_2 in the excess gas vented from the bubble oxygenator cannot exceed the CO_2 partial pressure in arterialized blood (and in actuality is much lower), it follows the carbon dioxide transfer rate of bubble oxygenators is a direct function of the volume inflow rate of oxygen, which must exceed oxygen uptake severalfold to transfer both O_2 and CO_2. Thus, the operating conditions for a bubble oxygenator are dictated to a major extent by the requirements for adequate CO_2 removal.

Three major advances propelled bubble oxygenators ahead of film oxygenators in the pioneer decades of cardiac surgery. The first was the identification of silicone-based defoaming compounds which could be smeared on top of the bubble chimney and proved much more effective in coalescing the blood foam than previously used chemicals. The second was the quantitative process analysis by Clark [1950] and Gollan [1956] which showed that, since small bubbles favor oxygen transfer and large bubbles are need for CO_2 removal, an optimum size could be found in between, or alternatively a mix of small and large bubbles should be used. The third and practically decisive advance was made simultaneously by Rygg and Kyvsgaard [1956] and DeWall [1957], who replaced the assembly of glass, steel, and ceramic parts of early bubble oxygenators with inexpensive plastic components and thereby paved the way for the industrial manufacturing of disposable bubble oxygenators. As a result, reusable stationary film and disc oxygenators, which require careful cleaning and sterilization, slowly disappeared, and disposable bubble oxygenators dominated the field of extracorporeal gas exchange from 1960 to the early 1980s. The oxygenator and pumps designed during the pioneer phase of extracorporeal circulation are described in a book by Galletti and Brecher [1962].

In the 1970s, the bubble oxygenator was integrated with a heat exchanger (usually a stainless steel coil) and placed within a clean plastic container that also served as a venous reservoir with a capacity of several liters of blood. The level of blood–air interface allowed direct observation of changes of blood volume in the extracorporeal circuit. This simple design feature gave the equipment operator (who eventually became known as the **perfusionist**) plenty of time in which to react to a sudden blood loss and make compensating changes in operation.

Yet a number of problems occurred with bubble oxygenators because of their large blood-gas interface. If the blood foam did not coalesce completely, a gaseous microemboli could be carried into the arterialized bloodstream. Plasma proteins were denatured at the gas interface, leading to blood trauma associated with platelet activation and aggregation, complement activation, and hemolysis. These problems could be ameliorated by placement of a gas-permeable **membrane** between the blood and gas phases. The idea of using membranes permeable to respiratory gases in order to separate the blood phase from the gas phase in an artificial lung, and consequently avoid the risk of foaming or the formulation of thick blood rivulets inherent in bubble or film oxygenators, was stimulated after World War II by the growing availability of commercially produced thin plastic films for the packaging industry. The two major challenges for membrane oxygenators were, and indeed remain, that no synthetic membrane could be fabricated as thin as the pulmonary alveolar wall, and manifolding and blood distribution system could match the fluid dynamic efficiency of the pulmonary circulation, where a single feed vessel — the pulmonary artery — branches over a short distance and with minimal resistance to flow into millions of tiny gas exchange capillaries the size of an erythrocyte. Membrane oxygenators have progressively captured the largest share of the market for clinical gas exchange devices not only because their operation is less traumatic for blood but also because the blood content of the gas exchange unit is fixed, thereby limiting volume fluctuations to calibrated reservoirs and minimizing the risk of major shifts in intracorporeal blood volume during **total body perfusion**.

The interposition of a membrane between flowing gas and flowing blood reduces the gas transfer efficiency of the system as a consequence of the additional mass transfer resistances associated with the membrane itself and the geometry of the blood layer. The permeability of various polymeric materials to oxygen and carbon dioxide is summarized in Table 66.1. The very first plastic films used, such as thin

TABLE 66.1 O_2 and CO_2 permeability of Various Materials

Chemical composition	Common name	O_2 permeability $\frac{cm^3 (STP).mil}{min.m^2.atm}$	$\frac{CO_2 \text{ permeability}}{O_2 \text{ permeability}}$
Air		5×10^7	0.8
Polydimethylsiloxane	Silicone rubber	1100	5
Water		150	18
Polystyrene		55	5
Polyisoprene	Natural rubber	50	6
Polybutadiene		40	7
Regenerated cellulose	Cellophane	25	18
Polyethylene		12	5
Polytetrafluoroethylene	Teflon	8	3
Polyamide	Nylon	0.1	4
Polyvinylidene chloride	Saran	0.01	6

Permeability is the product of the diffusion coefficient D and the Bunsen solubility coefficient α. The gas flux J ($cm^3(STP)/min\,m^2$) across a membrane of thickness h with a partial pressure difference Δr is given by $J = P\Delta r/h$.

sheets of polyethylene and polytetrafluoroethylene (PTFE), showed such a low diffusional permeability that 5–10 m^2 were needed to meet even the minimal oxygen needs of an anesthetized hypothermic adult [Clowes et al., 1956]. The advent of silicone elastomer films (either as solid sheets or cast over a textile support mesh) in the 1960s established the technical feasibility of membrane oxygenators [Bramson et al., 1965; Galletti et al., 1966; Peirce, 1967]. Silicone rubber is about 140 times more permeable to oxygen and 230 times more permeable to CO_2 than is PTFE for equivalent thickness. Even though silicone rubber and related elastomers cannot be cast as thin as PTFE, their permeability is so high that they became the standard material for early membrane oxygenator prototypes.

Extensive research was carried out in the 1960s and 1970s to develop improved membrane oxygenator designs with more efficient oxygen transport across the blood **boundary layer**. These designs are discussed later in this chapter. The clinical motivation was to provide continuous full or partial replacement of pulmonary gas exchanges for periods of weeks to patients with advanced respiratory failure, with the hope that in the interval the natural lung would recover. Since extensive blood trauma limited the use of blood oxygenators beyond 12–24 h, membrane oxygenators became the key to this application. In the mid-1970s, an NIH-sponsored clinical study [Zapol, 1975] demonstrated that with the protocols used lung function was not regained after 1–3 weeks of extracorporeal circulatory with a membrane oxygenator. The major intended application of membrane oxygenators having vanished, and the high cost of silicone rubber making these devices much more expensive than bubble oxygenators, research and development almost came to a halt, leaving bubble oxygenators in control of the remaining field of use, namely cardiopulmonary **bypass**.

Two technical advances have over the following two decades reversed this trend (1) the discovery that hydrophobic microporous membranes, through which gas can freely diffuse, have a high enough surface tension to prevent plasma filtration at the moderate pressures prevailing in the blood phase of an artificial lung; (2) the large-scale fabrication of defect-free **hollow fibers** of microporous polypropylene, which can be assembled in bundles, potted and manifolded at each extremity to form an artificial capillary bed of parallel blood pathways immersed in a cylindrical hard shell through which oxygen circulates.

Microporous hollow fiber membrane oxygenators now dominate the market. The most common embodiment of the hollow fiber membrane oxygenator features gas flow through the lumen of the fibers and blood flow in the interstices between fibers. This arrangement not only utilizes the larger outer surface area of the capillary tubes as gas transfer interface, instead of the luminal surface, it also promotes blood mixing in a manner which enhances oxygen transport, as will become apparent later.

66.2 Cardiopulmonary Bypass

Cardiopulmonary bypass (CPB), also called heart-lung bypass, allows the temporary replacement of the gas exchange function of the lungs and the blood-pumping function of the heart. As a result blood no longer flows through the heart and lungs, which then presents the surgeon with a bloodless operative field.

The terms **pump-oxygenator** and **heart–lung machine** graphically describe the equipment used. Cardiopulmonary bypass is the procedure. Open-heart surgery strictly speaking refers to interventions inside the heart cavities, which once provided the most frequent demand for cardiopulmonary bypass technology. By extension, the term is also applies to surgical procedures which take place primarily on the external aspects of the heart, such as creating new routes for blood to reach the distal coronary arteries from the aorta, for example, **coronary artery bypass grafting (CABG)** or, popularly, bypass surgery. In these operations the cardiac cavities are temporarily vented (i.e., open to atmospheric pressure) to avoid the build-up of pressure which could damage the cardiac muscle.

As usually employed for cardiac surgery, the heart–lung machine is part of a total, venoarterial cardiopulmonary bypass circuit, meaning that all the venous blood returning to the right heart cavities is collected in the extracorporeal circuit and circulated through the gas exchange device, from where it is pumped back into the arterial tree, thereby "bypassing" the heart cavities and the pulmonary circulation. On the blood side, this procedure usually involves **hemodilution**, some degree of hypothermia, nonpulsatile arterial perfusion at a flow rate near the resting cardiac output, and continuous recirculation of blood in an extracorporeal circuit in series with the systemic circulation of the patient. On the gas side, oxygen or an oxygen-enriched gas mixture (with or without a low concentration of CO_2) flows from a moderately pressurized source in a continuous, nonrecycling manner and is vented to the room atmosphere.

CPB hinges on twin postulates: that blood circulation can be sustained by mechanical pumps while the heart is arrested and that venous blood can be artificially arterialized in an extracorporeal gas exchange device while blood flow is excluded from the lungs. Each of these claims was established separately through animal experimentation over the course of over 100 years (see Galletti and Brecher [1962]). Then surgeons and engineers combined the advances made by physiologists and pharmacologists and turned them, in the 1950s, into the basic tool of cardiac surgery. A recent update on the evolution of artificial membrane lungs for CPB surgery has been provided by Galletti [1993]. It is estimated that each year about 650,000 disposable membrane lungs are used in the operating room worldwide, with each gas exchange unit selling for a price in the range of $250 to 400, that is, a market close to $2 billion.

Typical operating conditions for total cardiopulmonary bypass in an adult are summarized in Figure 66.1 and Table 66.2. Most notable are the large differences in driving forces for O_2 and CO_2. An approximate comparison can be made using the inlet conditions. Thus, under normothermia and with pure oxygen fed to the gas phase, initial driving force is approximately $45 - 0 = 45$ mmHg for CO_2 and $760 - 47 = 713$ mmHg for O_2 yielding a ratio of CO_2 to O_2 driving forces of about 0.06. The ratio of CO_2 to O_2 permeability for silicone rubber is roughly 5 (Table 66.2), and the corresponding flux ration is 0.35, less than half of the metabolically determined **respiratory quotient**. Under these conditions, CO_2 is the limiting gas, and the device should be sized on the basis of CO_2 transport rather than O_2 transport requirements. This is why silicone rubber membranes have been replaced by microporous polypropylene membrane, where the solubility of CO_2 in the membrane material, and consequently its permeability, is no longer the limiting factor. Indeed, with some modern membrane oxygenators, gas flow through the device may have to be controlled to avoid an excessive loss of CO_2.

66.3 Artificial Lung vs. Natural Lung

In the natural lungs, the factors underlying exchange across the alveolo-capillary barrier and transport by the blood can be grouped into four classes:

1. The ventilation of the lungs (the volume flow rate of gas) and the composition of the gas mixture to which mixed venous (pulmonary artery) blood will be exposed

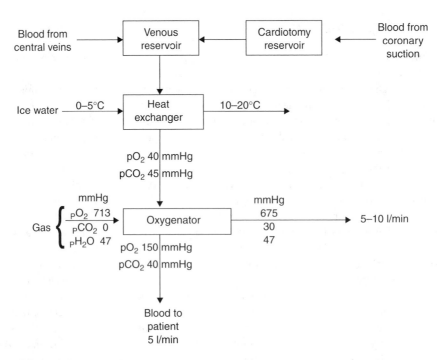

FIGURE 66.1 Scheme of standard operating conditions during cardiopulmonary bypass.

TABLE 66.2 Typical Operating Parameters for Cardiopulmonary Bypass in an Adult

Oxygen transfer requirement		250 ml/min
CO_2 elimination requirement		200 ml/min
Respiratory gas exchange ratio (respiratory quotient)		0.8
Blood flow rate		5 l/min
Gas flow rate		5–10 l/min
Gas partial pressures (in mmHg)		
Blood in	$pO_2 = 40$	$pCO_2 = 45$
Blood out	$pO_2 = 100–300$	$pCO_2 = 30–40$
Gas in (humidified)	$pO_2 = 250–713$	$pCO_2 = 0–20$
Gas out	$pO_2 = 150–675$	$pCO_2 = 10–30$

2. The permeability of the materials which separate the gas phase from the blood phase in the pulmonary alveoli
3. The pattern of pressure and flow through the airways and through the pulmonary vascular bed and the distribution of inspired air and circulating blood among the various zones of the exchange system
4. The gas carrying capacity of the blood as regards oxygen and carbon dioxide (and secondarily nitrogen and anesthetic gases)

In an artificial lung, replacing the gas transfer function of the natural organ implies that blood circulation can be sustained by mechanical pumps for extended periods of time to achieve a continuous, rather than a batch process, and that venous blood can be arterialized in that device by exposure to a gas mixture of appropriate composition. The external gas supply to an artificial lung does not pose particular problems, since pressurized gas mixtures are readily available. Similarly the components of blood which provide its gas-carrying capacity are well identified and can be adapted to the task at hand. In clinical

TABLE 66.3 Comparison of Nature and Artificial Membrane Lung

Natural lung	Hollow fiber oxygenator
Performance	
Must meet demand at rest and during exercise, fever, etc.	Must meet demand at rest and under anesthesia
Constant temperature process around 37°C	Can be coupled with heat exchanger to lower body temperature
O_2 and CO_2 transfer are matched to achieve the respiratory quotient imposed by foodstuff metabolism (around 0.8)	O_2 and CO_2 transfer are largely independent of each other and must be controlled by the operator
Continuous over a lifetime	Usually limited to few hours
Exchange surface area	
Wide transfer area ($\sim$70 m^2)	Limited transfer area (1–3 m^2)
Highly permeable alveolar–capillary membrane	Diffusion barriers in synthetic membrane and blood **oxygenation boundary layer**
Short diffusion distances (1–2 μm)	Relatively thick membranes (50–100 μm)
Hydrophilic membrane	Hydrophobic polymers
No hemocompatibility problems	Hemocompatibility problems
Self-cleaning membrane	Protein build-up on membrane
Gas side	
To-and-fro ventilation	Steady cross flow gas supply
Operates with air	Operates with oxygen-rich mixture
Membrane structure sensitive to high oxygen partial pressure	Membrane insensitive to high oxygen partial pressure
Pressure below that in blood phase to avoid capillary collapse	Pressure below that on blood side to avoid bubble formation
Operates under water vapor saturation conditions	Can be clogged by water vapor condensation
Ventilation linked to perfusion by built-in control mechanisms	Ventilation dissociated from perfusion, with risks of hyper- or hypoventilation
Can be used for gaseous anesthesia	Can be used for gaseous anesthesia
Blood side	
Short capillaries (0.5–1 mm)	Long blood path (10–15 cm)
Narrow diameter (3–7 μm)	Thick blood film (150–250 μm)
Short exposure time (0.7 sec)	Long exposure time (5–15 sec)
Low resistance to blood flow	Moderate to high resistance to blood flow
Sophisticated branching	Crude manifolding of entry and exit ports
Minimal priming volume	Moderate to large priming volume
Capillary recruitment capability	Fixed geometry of blood path
No recirculation	Possibility of recirculation
Limited venous admixture	Risk of uneven perfusion of parallel beds
No on-site blood mixing	Possibility of blood stirring and mixing
Operates with normal hemoglobin concentration	Hemodilution is common
Does not require anticoagulation	Requires anticoagulation

practice, it is important to minimize the amount of donor blood needed to fill the extracorporeal circuit, or **priming volume**. Therefore a heart–lung machine is generally filled with an electrolyte or plasma expander solution (with or without donor blood), resulting in hemodilution upon mixing of the contents of the extracorporeal and intracorporeal blood circuits. The critical aspects for the operation of an artificial lung are blood distribution to the exchanger, diffusion resistances in the blood mass transfer boundary layer, and stability of the gas exchange process.

Artificial lungs are expected to perform within acceptable limits of safety and effectiveness. The most common clinical situation in which an artificial lung is needed is typically of short duration, with resting or basal metabolism in anesthetized patients. Table 66.3 compares the structures and operating conditions of the natural lung and standard hollow fiber artificial membrane lungs with internal blood flow.

An artificial lung designed to replace the gas exchange function of the natural organ during cardiac surgery must meet specifications which are far less demanding than the range of capability of the mammalian lung would suggest. Nonetheless, these specifications must embrace a range of performance to cover all metabolic situations which a patient undergoing cardiopulmonary bypass might present. These conditions range in terms of metabolic rate from the slightly depressed resting metabolism characteristic of an anesthetized patient, lightly clad in a cool operating room, to moderate (25 to 28°C) and occasionally deep (below 20°C) hypothermia. Hypothermia and high blood flow are occasionally encountered in patients with septic shock. In terms of body mass, patients range from 2 to 5-lb newborn with congenital cardiac malformations to the 250-lb obese, diabetic elderly patient suffering from coronary artery disease and scheduled for aortocoronary bypass surgery.

Whereas it is appropriate to match in advance the size and therefore the transfer capability of the gas exchange unit in the heart-lung machine to the size of the patient (largely out of concern for the volume of fluid needed to fill or "prime" the extracorporeal circuit), each gas exchange unit, once in use, must be capable of covering the patient's requirement under any circumstances. This is the responsibility of the perfusionist, who controls the system in the light of what is happening to the patient in the operative field. In fact, the perfusionist substitutes his or her own judgment for the natural feedback mechanisms which normally control ventilation and circulation to the natural lungs. The following analysis indicates how there requirements can be met in the light of the gas transport properties of blood and the characteristics of diffusional and convective transport in membrane lung devices.

66.4 Oxygen Transport

The starting point for analysis of O_2 transport is the conservation of mass relation, which is derived from a material balance in a differential element within the flowing blood. By way of example, the relation commonly employed for oxygen transport of blood flowing in a tube is

$$V \left(\frac{\partial [O_2]}{\partial x} + \frac{\partial [HbO_2]}{\partial x} \right) = DO_2 \frac{1}{r} \frac{\partial}{\partial r} \left(r \frac{\partial [O_2]}{\partial x} \right) \tag{66.1}$$

where x is the axial coordinate, r is the radial coordinate, V is the velocity in the axial direction, DO_2 is the effective diffusion coefficient of O_2 in flowing blood, $[O_2]$ is the concentration of physically dissolved O_2, and $[HbO_2]$ is the concentration of O_2 bound to hemoglobin. The terms on the left side of Equation 66.1 represent convection in the axial direction of O_2 in its two forms, dissolved in aqueous solution and bound to hemoglobin. The right-side term represents the diffusion of dissolved O_2 in the radial direction.

By making the usual assumption that the concentration of dissolved O_2 is linearly proportional to the O_2 partial pressure p, $[O_2] = \alpha p$, where α is the Bunsen solubility coefficient, and by using the definition of oxyhemoglobin saturation: $[HbO_2] = C_T$ where C_T is the oxygen-carrying capacity of hemoglobin (per unit volume of blood) and S is its fractional saturation, Equation 66.1 can be rewritten in a modified form

$$V \frac{\partial p}{\partial x} \left(1 + \frac{C_T}{a} \frac{\partial S}{\partial P} \right) = DO_2 \frac{1}{r} \frac{\partial}{\partial r} \left(r \frac{\partial p}{\partial x} \right) \tag{66.2}$$

which shows that the convective contribution is proportional to the slope of the saturation curve. Equation 66.2 must be solved subject to the appropriate initial and boundary conditions, which for a tube are

$$x = 0, \quad p = p_i \tag{66.3}$$

$$r = 0, \quad \frac{\partial p}{\partial r} = 0 \tag{66.4}$$

$$r = R, \quad \alpha DO_2 \frac{\partial p}{\partial r} = P_m(p_o - p) \tag{66.5}$$

where p_i and p_o are the oxygen partial pressures in the inlet blood and in the gas, respectively, and P_m is the membrane permeability for O_2 diffusion, defined so as to include the membrane thickness. These conditions represent, in order, a uniform inlet concentration, symmetry about the tube axis, and the requirement that the O_2 diffuison flux at the blood-membrane interface be equal to the O_2 diffusion flux through the membrane.

Implicit in the derivation of Equation 66.2 are two important assumptions. The first is that, on a macroscopic scale, blood can be treated as a homogenous continuum, even though as a suspension of red blood cells in plasma, blood is microscopically heterogeneous. This simplification is acceptable as long as the volume element in which oxygen transport occurs is large compared to the size of a single red cell but small compared to the size of the overall diffusion path. This seems reasonable when applied to transport in membrane lungs, where the blood diffusion path thickness is usually equivalent to 20 to 30 red cell diameters or more.

The second important assumption is that the rate of reaction between O_2 and hemoglobin is sufficiently fast, when compared to the rate of diffusion of O_2 within the red cell, that the reaction can be considered at equilibrium, with the concentration of hemoglobin-bound O_2 in the red blood cells directly related to the concentration of dissolved O_2 in plasma via the oxyhemoglobin dissociation curve (ODC). Implicit in the use of this relationship is the assumption that the O_2 diffusion resistance of the red cell membrane is insignificant.

The human ODC for normal physiologic conditions is shifted to the right by increased temperature or decreased pH because of decreased hemoglobin affinity for O_2. The ODC is shifted to the right by an increase in the concentration of various organic phosphates, especially 2,3-diphosphoglycerate (DPG).

Under typical venous physiologic conditions (37°C, boundary O_2 partial pressures of 40 and 95 mmHg), the reaction between hemoglobin and oxygen reaches equilibrium during the time of contact between the blood and the gas phase. The ratio of the effective permeability of blood to that of plasma in a model system is 0.87 at the hematocrit of 45%; without any facilitation within the red cell, the ratio would be 0.75. Using the most reliable data for the O_2 solubility and diffusion coefficient in plasma leads to an estimate of 1.7×10^{-5} cm^2/sec for the effective diffusion coefficient of O_2 in normal whole blood.

We can now return to the analysis of convective transport of oxygen in a membrane lung, specifically the solution of Equation 66.2 or its equivalent for other geometrics, on the assumption of equilibrium for the hemoglobin oxygenation reaction in such devices. The various theoretical analyses that have been carried out differ primarily in the means by which the saturation curve is handled. The most common approach is to retain its intrinsic nonlinearity and to approximate it by a suitable analytical expression. The resulting nonlinear partial differential equation does not permit analytical solution, and it is therefore necessary to resort to numerical solution with a finite difference scheme on a digital computer. This approach yields numerical values for p and S as a function of x and r. To relate theoretical prediction with experimental measurement, one must calculate the velocity-weighted bulk average values of p and S [Colton, 1976]. The average O_2 partial pressure, p, and oxyhemoglobin saturation, S, that would be measured if the blood issuing from the tube were physically mixed are then calculated from

$$\frac{1}{\int_0^R Vr\,dr}\left[\alpha\int_0^R Vpr\,dr + C_T\int_0^R VSr\,dr\right] = \alpha\bar{p} + C_T\bar{S} \tag{66.6}$$

Numerical solutions provide accurate predictions. However, they apply only to specific operating conditions and cannot be generalized for design purposes. Two methods have been used to simplify the ODC and provide approximate yet useful analytical solutions.

The first is known as the **advancing front theory** [Thews, 1957; Marx et al., 1960]. The oxyhemoglobin saturation curve is approximated as a step function between the saturation values corresponding to the O_2 partial pressure and that of the gas phase or the blood-membrane interface. The blood is treated as two regions of uniform oxyhemoglobin saturation separated by a front that moves rapidly inward. Outside the front, blood is saturated at a value corresponding to the blood–gas or blood-membrane interface, and the rest of the blood is relatively unsaturated. Oxygen diffuses through the saturated blood to the interface, where it reacts with unsaturated hemoglobin. The advancing front approximation reasonably represents the calculated saturation profiles and has proved useful in developing analytical design expressions for membrane lungs in terms of saturation changes effected. However, it can be in error by a very wide margin for the prediction of O_2 partial pressure changes. A modification of advancing front theory, involving approximation of the partial pressure changes. A modification of advancing front theory, involving approximation of the ODC by several straight line segments, retains the ability to provide an analytical solution and gives better accuracy than the conventional step function approximation of the ODC.

The second type of simplification is to approximate the ODC by a straight line drawn between the inlet and boundary O_2 partial pressures, which make $\partial S/dp$, the slope of the saturation curve constant and renders Equation 66.2 linear. Use can then be made of existing solutions for analogous convective heat and mass transfer problems without chemical reaction.

For typical operating conditions in the clinic, the initial and boundary O_2 partial pressures lie on the upper portion of the ODC, and the advancing front solution provides an overestimation of the rate of O_2 transport, whereas the constant slope solution provides an underestimate. Conversely, on the lower portion of the ODC at very low O_2 partial pressures, the advancing front estimate of O_2 transport rate is too low and constant slope too high. The constant slope approximation is most accurate over the steep portion of the saturation cure, where it is nearly linear. Since the O_2 transport rate per unit membrane surface area is much more sensitive to blood inlet O_2 partial pressure than would be expected solely from the change in the overall driving force, comparative testing of membrane lungs must be carried out with identical inlet blood O_2 partial pressure and oxyhemoglobin saturation.

Theoretical prediction of membrane lung performance is useful for design purposes and for providing a guide to the effect of permissive design variables. However, theoretical prediction cannot substitute for experimental data under closely controlled conditions where control of pH, temperature, and CO_2 partial pressure in fresh blood allow the definition of the appropriate ODC.

66.5 CO_2 Transport

The CO_2 dissociation curve for normal human blood is far more linear in its normal operating range than the ODC. The fractional volume of CO_2 that is removed in the process of arterialization of venous blood is also considerably less than the corresponding fractional loss of oxygen (about 10% of blood CO_2 content, vs. 25% for oxygen). As is the case for oxygen, the total CO_2 concentration is far larger than that of gas physically dissolved in the aqueous component of blood. Plasma accounts for about two-thirds of all the CO_2 carried in blood, whereas typically about 98% of O_2 is carried in the red cells.

The main vehicles for CO_2 transport in blood are bicarbonate, the primary carrier in both plasma and red cells, and carbamino hemoglobin, where CO_2 is combined with the amino groups of hemoglobin (Figure 66.2a). Arrows on Figure 66.2b indicate the direction and relative rate of each reaction whereby CO_2 is removed in a membrane lung. Carbonate and hydrogen ions form bicarbonate, which decomposes to CO_2 or combines with another hydrogen ion to form carbonic acid; the latter is dehydrated to liberate CO_2. Since the reactions that form CO_2 in plasma are very slow, biocarbonate is the predominant species. Biocarbonate can diffuse into the red cell, albeit slowly, in exchange for chloride, leading to the same chain of reactions. In the red cell, however, dehydration of carbonic acids is catalyzed by the enzyme carbonic anhydrase. This reaction liberates CO_2, which, in turn, diffuses out of the red cell into the plasma and then across the blood–membrane interface. Decomposition of carbamino hemoglobin is a significant additional source of CO_2. Carbamate compounds that arise from combination of CO_2 with plasma proteins have a much smaller effect because of the relatively unfavorable equilibria for their formation. Finally, various ionic species, such as organic and inorganic phosphates, amino acids, and proteins, behave as weak acids at pH 7.4. The buffering power of hemoglobin is particularly strong and has a marked effect in influencing the shape of the CO_2 dissociation curve.

(a)

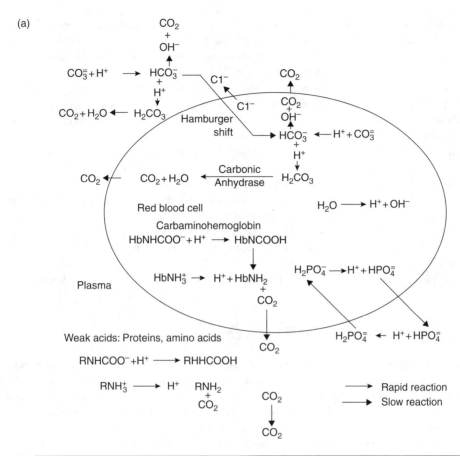

(b)

CO$_2$ transport form		Mixed venous blood		Arterial blood		Veno-arterial difference	
		mM/l	%	mM/l	%	mM/l	%
Bicarbonate	Plasma	14.41	61.8	13.42	62.4	.99	55.0
	RBC	5.92	25.4	5.88	27.3	.04	2.2
Dissolved CO$_2$	Plasma	.76	3.3	.66	3.1	.10	5.6
	RBC	.51	2.2	.44	2.0	.07	3.9
Carbamino CO$_2$	Plasma	-	-	-	-	-	-
	RBC	1.70	7.3	1.10	5.1	.60	33.3
Total in whole blood		23.30	100	21.50	100	1.80	100

FIGURE 66.2   (a) Schematic representation of CO$_2$ transfer from the red blood cell to plasma and into alveolar gas, emphasizing the various buffer systems involved. (b) Blood CO$_2$ content. CO$_2$ transport forms in mixed venous and arterial blood, and as components of the veno-arterial CO$_2$ difference. Observe that the red blood cells (RBC) bicarbonate content, although it represents a large fraction of CO$_2$ transport, does not contribute significantly to the arteriovenous difference in CO$_2$ content. Conversely hemoglobin-bound CO$_2$, though less abundant than bicarbonate in red blood cells, constitutes a larger fraction of the veno-arterial difference.

Under clinical conditions of O_2 and CO_2 countertransport, two reciprocal phenomena occur which affect CO_2 and O_2 exchange. A decrease of CO_2 partial pressure causes a shift to the left of the oxyhemoglobin dissociation curve, leading to an increased affinity of hemoglobin when CO_2 is removed (Bohr effect). Meanwhile, because oxyhemoglobin is a stronger acid than hemoglobin, uptake of O_2 decreases the affinity of hemoglobin for CO_2, thereby releasing additional CO_2 from carbamino hemoglobin (Haldane effect). At the same time, increased acidity favors the conversion of more biocarbonate into carbonic acid, which then dissociates, releasing CO_2. The simultaneous occurrence of these two effects enhances transport rates of both gases.

If the entire reaction scheme in Figure 66.2 is assumed to be at equilibrium, the CO_2 dissociation curve can be used to relate the total blood concentration of CO_2 (in all forms) to the CO_2 partial pressure. The CO_2 dissociation curve can be linearized in the same manner as the constant slope approximation for O_2 transport described above. A relation similar to Equation 66.2 results, except that p refers to the CO_2 partial pressure, and the term $(C_T/a)\,(\partial S/\partial p)$ is replaced by the derivative of the total CO_2 concentration with respect to the concentration of dissolved CO_2. The equation is now linear, and the same simplifications hold as for the O_2 problem with a constant slope approximation. The membrane-limited case becomes particularly simple, and the membrane lung can be treated as simple mass or heat exchanger with a constant transport coefficient. This approach has been successfully used to correlate experimental data.

66.6   Coupling of O_2 and CO_2 Exchange

In the conceptual representation of Figure 66.3 [Colton, 1976], the ratio of the CO_2 transport rates is plotted against an index of the blood-side mass transfer efficiency divided by the membrane permeability on a logarithmic scale. With a constant slope approximation for both O_2 and CO_2 transport, a unique curve is obtained for a specific membrane lung design if the abscissa is taken to be the ratio of the blood-side log-mean average CO_2 mass transfer coefficient divided by the CO_2 membrane permeability, and the curve is parameterized by unique values of three dimensionless quantities (1) the ratio of the membrane permeabilities for O_2 and CO_2, (2) the ratio of the average blood-side transfer coefficients for O_2 and CO_2, and (3) the ratio of the log-mean average O_2 and CO_2 partial pressure driving force. The asymptotic limits plotted are very approximate characteristic values of a capillary or flat plate (sandwich) gas exchange

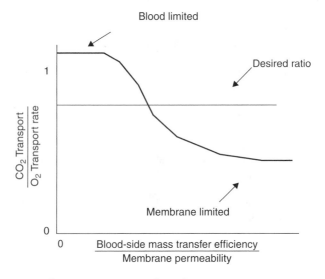

FIGURE 66.3   Relative CO_2 and O_2 transport in a membrane lung.

device in which the limiting factor is either the blood mass transfer boundary layer or the membrane itself.

When transport of both O_2 and CO_2 is blood phase-limited — that is a relatively low blood-side mass transfer coefficient or high membrane permeability — the CO_2 transport rate is higher than the O_2 rate, and it is necessary to add CO_2 to the inlet gas or to decrease gas flow rate to prevent excessive CO_2 removal. At the other extreme, if gas transport in membrane limited, the ratio of CO_2 to O_2 transport is always lower than the physiological value (0.8), because no existing gas-permeable membrane has a sufficiently high CO_2/O_2 permeability ratio to overcome the unfavorable driving force ratio of the O_2 and CO_2 partial pressures (14 : 1) under the actual operating conditions of a membrane lung. Under either limiting condition, it is necessary to design the membrane lung on the basis of the gas that limits transport, O_2, for blood-limited conditions and CO_2 for membrane-limited conditions.

A priori, it seems undesirable to operate under blood-limited conditions because full advantage is not taken of the membrane permeability. Therefore, an increase in the blood-side mass transfer efficiency is valuable, but only to the point where the ratio of CO_2 to O_2 transport rates is equal to the respiratory quotient. Beyond that point, further improvements in design will not reduce the size of the device required unless membrane permeability to CO_2 is increased, thereby moving the operating point on the curve to the left and justifying the use of a more efficient exchange device. For example, conventional solid silicone rubber membranes cannot take advantage of high-efficiency designs because gas transport is membrane limited and has to be designed on the basis of CO_2 transport rate. To make effective use of the most effective devices, it is necessary to employ microporous membranes or ultrathin membranes on microporous substrates where the CO_2 permeability is no longer a limiting factor.

66.7 Shear-Induced Transport Augmentation and Devices for Improved Gas Transport

There is evidence that flow-dependent properties of blood can substantially influence the transport of O_2 and CO_2. The presence of velocity gradient in a stream can enhance mass transfer through blood either by shear-induced collision diffusion wherein interactions between red blood cells produce net lateral displacements and associated motions in the surrounding phase or by rotation of individual cells, which gives rise to local mechanical stirring of the adjacent fluid. Both mechanisms can lead to transport augmentation of species present in the dispersed or continuous phases. Only the first mechanism can cause dispersive migration of the particles themselves, and available evidence suggests that it is the dominant factor [Cha and Bessinger, 1994]. The shear-induced diffusion coefficient of particles in suspension increases linearly with the shear rate and can be orders-of-magnitude larger than the Brownian motion diffusivity. The effect of lateral cell movement in oxygen transport in capillary tubes depends on both the shear rate and the slope of the ODC, with a maximum at the steepest portion of the curve, that is, below the operating range of a clinical oxygenator. The extent to which such phenomena occur in blood under the clinical operating conditions of membrane lungs in cardiopulmonary bypass has not been investigated, but the effect on oxygen transport is thought to be significant.

The earliest oxygenator configurations featuring rubber membranes made the blood flow in simple enclosed geometries, such as a flat plate or hollow fiber, that were inherently inefficient from a mass transfer standpoint. It was soon recognized that the gas transport rate was limited almost entirely by transport within the blood oxygenation boundary layer. There followed extensive efforts in the 1960s and early 1970s to investigate new approaches for improving gas transfer in membrane oxygenators, as summarized in Table 66.4. These approaches relied on one or more mechanisms (1) increasing shear rate or producing turbulence; (2) keeping the oxygenation boundary layer very thin by using an appropriate contacting geometry or pulsatile blood flow; and (3) making use of **secondary flow**, which incorporates significant velocity components normal to the membrane surface. All these approaches are demonstrably effective under laboratory conditions, but few have achieved successful commercialization because of the

TABLE 66.4   Approaches for Improving Mass Transport in Membrane Oxygenators

Passive designs	Active designs
Obstacles in blood path	Oscillating toroidal chamber
Membrane undulations from external supports	Enclosed rotating disc
Membrane texturing or embossing	Pulsed flow vortex shedding
Helical flow systems	Couette flow
External blood flow over hollow fibers	Annulus, inner cylinder rotating axial flow, tangential flow

constraints imposed by the geometry of available membrane materials (flat sheets and capillary tubes) and the clinical demand for simple, reliable, and inexpensive devices.

In Table 66.4, passive designs for inducing secondary flows are those for which no energy source is needed except that required for steady blood flow. A common technique has been to place obstacles, for example screens, in the blood path to induce secondary fluid movements and/or flow separation on a small scale and thereby increase blood mixing in flat plate devices. A similar result has been obtained by creating undulations in a flat membrane with grooved or multiple point supports or by using textured membranes to direct blood flow through the exchanger.

Active signs are those in which there is energy input to achieve high shear rates or create secondary flows. Highly efficient oxygenator prototypes have been described, and at least two, the enclosed rotating disc and a pulsed-flow vortex shedding device, have been commercialized, but neither has achieved widespread clinical acceptance, in part because of the complexity or cumbersomeness of their operating mechanisms in an operating room setting.

Another widely investigated approach has been to use flow geometries that naturally induce secondary flow, for example helical coils, where, superimposed on the primary flow, is a swirling motion in each half of the tube. The secondary flow trajectory which results from centrifugal effects takes particles from the periphery and carries them into the core, back to the periphery, back to the core in a continuously repeated fashion. Such secondary motion, by continuously sweeping oxygenated blood away from the membrane and replacing it with venous blood from the central core of the channel, can be extremely effective in increasing gas transport rates to the point where the dominant resistance to diffusion lies in the membrane. However, the practical difficulty of constructing such complex devices which are also disposable has thus far prevented industrial development.

When the potential market for continuous extracorporeal membrane oxygenation collapsed, so did the intensive research and development effort in developing new devices. However, three developments, two technical and one marketing-related, over the next decade eventually led to dominance of membrane oxygenators for cardiopulmonary bypass.

The first major technical advance was the fabrication of hydrophobic microporous capillary hollow fiber membranes at prices considerably lower than for silicon rubber membranes. The driving force for the initial development of these materials was their potential in another technology, membrane plasmapheresis for the separation of plasma from the cellular components of blood. Hollow fibers for the application had nominal pore sizes, around 0.5 mm, which were too large for membrane oxygenation because plasma could seep through the fiber wall under pressure leading to a catastrophic decrease in membrane permeability (Table 66.1). In the early 1980s, microporous polypropylene hollow fibers with a nominal pore size around 0.1 mm became available and proved satisfactory for membrane oxygenation. In addition to reduced trauma and competitive pricing with bubble oxygenators, membrane lungs could be employed with a reduced, fixed blood-priming volume, thereby minimizing transfusion and hemodilution problems. Surprisingly, this advantage was initially viewed as a drawback by perfusionists who were used to having a large venous blood reservoir with a visible gas-blood interface.

The key marketing development of the mid-1980s was to make a membrane oxygenator by attaching it, along with a heat exchanger, to a clear plastic venous reservoir with a visible gas-blood interface. The astute move was breakthrough which put membrane oxygenators into the operating room. Their clear advantage

TABLE 66.5 Comparison of Membrane Oxygenator Performance (Blood Flow Rate = Gas Flow Rate = 5 l/min; AAMI Conditions)

Model	Membrane form	Blood path configuration	O_2, flux cm^3(STP)/min-m^3	CO_2/O_2 flux ratio
Silicone Rubber				
Sci Med SM35	Sheet	Spiral coil embedded failure	90	0.6
Microporous polypropylene				
Cobe CMI	Sheet	Flat plate	130	1.4
Shiley M-2000	Sheet	Blood screens	120	1.0
Bentley Bos CM-40	Hollow fiber	Internal flow	70	0.7
Terumo Capiox II 43	Hollow fiber	Internal flow	60	0.9
Bard William Harvey 4000	Hollow fiber	External cross flow	140	0.9
Johnson and Johnson Maxima	Hollow fiber	External cross flow	150	0.9
Sarns	Hollow fiber	External cross flow	150	1.0
Bentely Univox	Hollow fiber	External cross flow	160	1.0

in minimizing blood trauma and postoperative complications was so overwhelming that within a year membrane oxygenators captured the dominant market share. Shortly thereafter, bubble oxygenators were virtually eliminated from the U.S. marketplace.

The most recent technical development has been the inversion of the usual internal flow arrangement so that, now, gas flows through the lumen of the hollow fibers while blood is pumped over the external surface of the capillary membrane. This arrangement is most effective when the blood flow is at right angles to the hollow fiber. In that configuration the flowing blood successively encounters different fibers, and a new oxygenation boundary layer forms on each fiber. Because the boundary layer is thinnest where it begins (in this case, at the front of each fiber), and the mass transfer rate is correspondingly highest, the transport of oxygen averaged over the periphery of each fiber is much higher than with the conventional internal (luminal) flow of blood. Thus the transport of oxygen averaged over the periphery of each fiber is much higher than with the conventional internal (luminal) flow of blood. The performance of various membrane oxygenators is compared in Table 66.5. The data clearly demonstrate the superior performance attainable with microporous hollow fibers operated with external crossflow of blood.

The state of the art is now fairly advanced for membrane blood oxygenators, but there is still room for improvement. Further increases in flux would further reduce cost and minimize priming volume and blood consumption. Now that membrane oxygenators are fully entrenched, it is more likely that the reduced priming volume and improved control of a closed system can be realized. Lastly, the residual gas-blood interface that still exists at the microporous membrane surface could be eliminated by coating with a very thin skin in a n asymmetric or composite structure.

Defining Terms

Advancing front theory: A type of exchanger theory addressing the limitation of oxygen transport in a blood film through a fully saturated boundary layer leading to a front where the hemoglobin in flowing blood reacts with the dissolved oxygen.

Arterialization: A gas exchange process whereby oxygen and carbon dioxide concentrations in venous blood are changed to levels characteristic of arterial blood.

Artificial lung: A device which allows for continuous exchange for oxygen and carbon dioxide between circulating blood and a controlled gas atmosphere.

Blood oxygenator: Synonymous with artificial lung, with the accent placed on oxygen transport, which is the most critical aspect of natural lung replacement, since the body oxygen reserves are very limited. Depending upon the physical process used for blood–gas transfer, artificial lungs are classified as bubble oxygenators, stationary or rotating film oxygenators, and membrane oxygenators.

Boundary layer: The film of blood adjacent to a permeable membrane, which, by reason of local fluid dynamics, is not renewed at the same rate as blood in the core of the flow path, thereby creating an additional diffusion barrier between the blood and the gas phase.

Bubble oxygenator: Blood–gas transfer device in which a large exchange surface is obtained by the dispersion of oxygen bubbles in a venous blood stream, followed by coalescence of the foam and venting of excess gas (cocurrent blood and gas flow) or by spreading of venous blood over a continuously renewed column of foam generated by bubbling oxygen at the bottom of a reservoir (countercurrent blood and gas flow).

Bypass: Derivation or rerouting of blood around an organ or body part, to diminish its blood supply, to abolish local circulation for the duration of a surgical intervention, or to increase blood flow permanently beyond an obstruction. The qualifier used with the word bypass designates the organ so isolated (e.g., left ventricular bypass, coronary artery bypass).

Cardiopulmonary bypass (CPB): A procedure whereby blood is prevented from circulating through the heart cavities and the lungs. Cardiopulmonary bypass (also known as **heart–lung bypass**) can be partial if no obstacle is placed on venous return to the right heart cavities and consequently some of the blood continues to flow through the pulmonary circulation. In that case the arterial system is fed in part by left ventricular output and in part by the arterialized blood perfusion from the hear–lung machine. The balance between the internal and extracorporeal blood circuits depends on the setting of the pumps and the relative resistance to flow in the two venous drainage pathways. During total cardiopulmonary bypass, the cardiac muscle must receive arterial blood from the extracorporeal circuit (intermittently or continuously) to prevent hypoxic myocardial damage. Since coronary venous blood drains into the cardiac cavities, this blood must be drained to the outside to prevent an intracavitary pressure increase which could be damaging to the heart.

Catheter: A long hollow cylinder designed to be introduced in a body canal to infuse or withdraw materials into or out of the body.

Coronary artery bypass graft (CABG): The construction of new blood conduits between the aorta (or other major arteries) and segments of coronary arteries beyond lesions which partially or totally obstruct the lumen of those vessels, for the purpose of providing an increased blood supply to regions of the myocardium made ischemic by those lesions.

Extracorporeal circulation: Artificial maintenance of blood circulation by means of pumps located outside of the body, with blood fed through catheters advanced in an appropriate blood vessel and returning the blood to another blood vessel.

Film oxygenator: Blood–gas transfer device in which a large exchange surface is obtained by spreading venous blood in a thin film over a stationary or moving physical support in an oxygen-rich atmosphere.

Heart–lung bypass: Synonymous with cardiopulmonary bypass.

Heart–lung machine: A mechanical system capable of pumping venous blood around the heart and the lungs and arterializing it in an appropriate gas exchange unit.

Hemodilution: Temporary reduction in blood erythrocyte concentration (and consequently hemoglobin content, hematocrit, oxygen-carrying capacity, and viscosity) resulting from mixing with the erythrocyte-free or erythrocyte-poor content of the liquid used to prime an extracorporeal circuit.

Hemolysis: The destruction of red blood cells with liberation of hemoglobin in surrounding plasma, caused by mechanical damage of the erythrocyte membrane, osmotic imbalance between intracorpuscular and extracorpuscular ion concentration, or uncontrolled freezing-thawing cycles.

Hollow fiber: A capillary tube of polymeric material produced by spinning a melted or dissolved polymer through an annular orifice.

Membrane: A solid or liquid phase which acts as a barrier to prevent coalescence of neighboring compartments while allowing restricted or regulated passage of one or more molecular species.

Membrane lung or Membrane oxygenator: Blood–gas transfer device in which the blood compartment is shielded from the gas phase by a porous or solid, hydrophobic polymer membrane permeable to gases but not to liquids (in particular, blood plasma).

Metabolism: The sum of the chemical reactions occurring within a living body including build up (anabolism) and break down (catabolism) of chemical substances.

Open heart surgery: Interventions taking place inside the cardiac cavities, such as for the replacement or reconstruction of cardiac valves, or the closure of abnormal communications between cardiac chambers, and which for reasons of convenience and safety, require the interruption of blood flow through the heart. By extension this stem is often used for cardiac interventions under total cardiopulmonary bypass, which address structures on the outside surface of the heart (such as coronary arteries) when drainage of the cardiac cavities through a vent is needed to avoid accumulation of coronary venous blood.

Oxygenation boundary layer: Stationary or slowly moving blood layer adjacent to a gas-permeable membrane, which progressively develops along the blood path and, once enriched with oxygen diffusion through the membrane, effectively becomes a barrier to oxygen transport perpendicular to the direction of flow.

Perfusion: A technique for keeping an organ or body part alive, though severed from its normal blood circulation, by introducing blood under pressure into the appropriate feeder artery.

Perfusionist: The operator of the heart–lung machine during cardiac surgery or respiratory assist procedures.

Priming volume: The volume of liquid (blood, plasma, synthetic plasma expanders, or electrolyte solutions) needed to fill all components of an extracoporeal circuit (oxygenator, heat exchanger, blood pumps, filter, tubing, and catheters) so as to avoid exsanguination once the intracorporeal and extracorporeal circulation systems are joined.

Pump-oxygenator: Equipment used to circulate blood through an extracorporeal circuit by means of mechanical blood pumps and to arterialize mixed venous blood by means of a gas exchange device. In most embodiments, the pump-oxygenator also serves to control blood temperature by means of a heat exchanger, typically incorporated in the gas exchange device. Synonymous with heart–lung machine.

Respiratory quotient: The ratio of carbon dioxide produced by tissues or eliminated by the lungs to oxygen consumed by tissues or taken in through the lungs.

Secondary flow: Any type of fluid motion, steady or periodic, in which the fluid is moving in a direction different from that of the primary flow. Secondary flow systems may be continuous in distribution, occupying the entire flow path, or comprise local elements that produce periodic remixing of the fluid.

Total body perfusion: Maintenance of blood circulation through the arterial and venous system by means of a positive displacement pump introducing blood into an artery under pressure and collecting it from a vein for continuous recirculation.

References

Bartlett R.h., Drinker P.A., and Galletti P.M. (eds). 1971. *Mechanical Devices for Cardiopulmonary Assistance*, Basel, Karger.

Bramson M.L., Osborn J.J., Main F.B. et al. 1995. A new disposable membrane oxygenator with integral heat exchange. *J. Thorac Cardiovasc. Surg.* 50: 391.

Cha W. and Beissinger R.L. in press. Augmented mass transport of macromolecules in sheared suspension to surfaces: part B (Borine serum interface). *J. Colloid Interface Sci.*

Clark L.C. Jr., Gollan F., and Gupta V. 1950. The oxygenation of blood by gas dispersion. *Science* 111: 85.

Clowes G.H.A. Jr, Hopkins A.L., and Neville W.E. 1956. An artificial lung dependent upon diffusion of oxygen and carbon dioxide through plastic membranes. *J. Thorac Surg.* 32: 630.

Colton C.K. 1976. Fundamentals of gas transport in blood. In W.M. Zapol and J. Qvist (eds), *Artificial Lungs for Acute Respiratory Failure. Theory and Practice*, pp 3–41, New York, Academic Press.

Colton C.K. and Drake R.F. 1971. Effect of boundary conditions on oxygen transport to flowing blood in a tube. *Chem. Eng. Prog. Symp.* 67(114): 88.

Curtis R.M. and Eberhart R.C. 1974. Normalization of oxygen transfer data in membrane oxygenators. *Trans. Am. Soc. Artif. Intern Organs* 20: 210.

Dawids S. and Engell H.C. (eds). 1976. *Physiological and Clinical Aspects of Oxygenator Design*, Amsterdam, Elsevier.

DeWall R.A., Lillelei C.W., Vareo R.L. et al. 1957. The helix reservoir pump-oxygenator. *Surg. Gyn. Obstet.* 104: 699.

Dorson W.J. Jr and Voorhees M.E. 1974. Limiting models for the transfer of CO_2 and CO_2 in membrane oxygenators. *Trans. Am. Soc. Artif. Intern. Organs* 20: 219.

Dorson W.J. Jr and Voorhees M.E. 1976. Analysis of oxygen and carbon dioxide transfer in membrane lungs. In W.M. Zapol and J. Qvist (eds), *Artificial Lungs for Acute Respiratory Failure. Theory and Practice*, pp 43–68.

Galletti P.M. 1993. Cardiopulmonary bypass: a historical perspective. *Artif. Organs* 17: 675.

Galletti P.M. and Brecher G.A. 1962. *Heart-Lung Bypass, Principles and Techniques of Extracorporeal Circulation*, New York, Grune & Stratton.

Galletti P.M., Richardson P.D., Snider M.T. et al. 1972. A standardized method for defining the overall gas transfer performance of artificial lungs. *Trans. Am. Soc. Artif. Intern. Organs* 18: 359.

Galletti P.M., and Snider M.T., Silbert-Aidan D. 1966. Gas permeability of plastic membrane for artificial lungs. *Med. Res. Eng.* 20.

Gibbon J.H. Jr. 1939. An oxygenator with a large surface-volume ratio. *J. Lab. Clin. Med.* 24: 1192.

Gibbon J.H. Jr. 1954. Application of a mechanical heart and lung apparatus to cardiac surgery. *Minnesota Med.* 37: 71.

Gollan F. 1956. Oxygenation of circulating blood by dispersion, coalescence and surface tension separation. *J. Appl. Physiol.* 8: 571.

Hagl S., Klovekorn W.P., Mayr N. et al. (eds). 1984. *Thirty Years of Extracorporeal Circulation*, Munich, Deutches Herzzentrum.

Harris G.W., Tompkins F.C., and de Filippi R.P. 1970. Development of capillary membrane blood oxygenators. In D Hershey (ed), *Blood Oxygenation*, pp. 333–354, New York, Plenum.

Marx T.I., Snyder W.E., St John A.D. et al. 1960. Diffusion of oxygen into a film of whole blood. *J. Appl. Physiol.* 15: 1123.

Mockros L.F., Gaylor J.D.S. 1975. Artificial lung design: tubular membrane units. *Med. Biol. Eng.* 13: 171.

Peirce E.C. II. 1967. The membrane lung, its excuse, present status, and promise. *J. Mt. Sinai. Hosp.* 34: 437.

Richardson P.D. 1971. Effects of secondary flows in augmenting gas transfer in blood. Analytical considerations. In RH Bartlett, P.A. Drinker, and P.M. Galletti (eds), *Mechanical Devices for Cardiopulmonary Assistance*, pp. 2–16, Basel, Karger.

Richardson P.D. 1976. Oxygenator testing and evaluation: Meeting ground of theory, manufacture and clinical concerns. In W.M. Zapol and J. Qvist, (eds), *Artificial Lungs for Acute Respiratory Failure. Theory and Practice*, pp. 87–102, New York, Academic Press.

Richardson P.D. and Galletti P.M. 1976. Correlation of effects of blood flow rate, viscosity, and design features on artificial lung performance. In S.G. Davids and H.C. Engell (eds), *Physiological and Clinical Aspects of Oxygenator Design*, pp. 29–44, Amsterdam, Elsevier.

Rygg I.H. and Kyvsgaard E. 1956. A disposable polyethylene oxygenator system applied in a heart–lung machine. *Acta Chir. Second* 112: 433.

Snider M.T., Richardson P.D., Friedman L.I. et al. 1974. Carbon dioxide transfer rate in artificial lungs. *J Appl Physiol* 36: 233.

Spaan J.A.E., and Oomens J.M.M. 1976. Scaling rules for flat plate and hollow fiber membrane oxygenators. In S.G. Dawids and H.C. Engell (eds), *Physiological and Clinical Aspects of Oxygenator Design*, pp 13–28, Amsterdam, Elsevier.

Thews G. 1957. Verfahren zur Berechnung des O_2-Diffusionskoeffizienten aus Messungen der Sauer-stoffdiffusion in Hemoglobin und Myoglobin Loesungen. *Pfluegers Arch* 2: 138.

Villarroel F., Lanhyam C.E., Bischoff K. et al. 1970. A mathematical model for the prediction of oxygen, carbon dioxide, and pH profiles with augmented diffusion in capillary blood oxygenators. In D Hershey (ed.), *Blood Oxygenation*, pp. 321–333, New York, Plenum.

Zapol W.M. 1975. Membrane lung perfusion for acute respiratory failure. *Surg. Clin. N. Am.* 55: 603.

Zapol W.M., Qvist J. (ed.) 1967. *Artificial Lungs for Acute Respiratory Failure. Theory and Practice,* New York, Academic Press.

Further Information

Over the years, a number of books and monographs have reviewed the scientific and technical literature on gas exchange devices and their application. These include J.G. Allen, ed., *Extracorporeal Circulation*, Thomas, Springfield, 1958; P.M. Galletti and G.A. Brecher, Heart-Lung Bypass, Principles and Techniques of Extracorporeal Circulation, Grune and Stratton , New York, 1962; D. Hershey, ed., *Blood Oxygenation*, Plenum, New York, 1970; R.H. Bartlett, P.A. Drinker and P.M. Galletti, eds., *Mechanical Devices for Cardiopulmonary Assistance*, Karger, Basel, 1971; W.M. Zapol and J. Qvist, eds., *Artificial Lungs for Acute Respiratory Failure. Theory and Practice.* Academic Press, New York, 1976; G.G. Dawids and H.G. Engell, *Physiological and Clinical Aspects of Oxygenator Design*, Elsevier, Amsterdam, 1967; S. Hagl, W.P. Klövekorn, N. Mayr, and F. Sebening, *Thirty Years of Extracorporeal Circulation*, Deutsches Herzzentrum, Munich, 1984; P.A. Casthely and D. Bregman, *Cardiopulmonary Bypass: Physiology, Related Complications and Pharmacology*, Futura, Mount Kisco, NY, 1991.

Topical advances in artificial lungs are typically published in the *Transactions of the American Society for Artificial Internal Organs* or in journals such as the *ASAIO Journal*, the International Journal of Artificial Organs, the Japanese of Artificial Organs, and the *Journal of Thoracic and Cardiovascular Surgery*, as well as the *Proceedings of the American Institute for Chemical Engineering* and, occasionally, Chemically Engineering Symposium Series.

67

Artificial Kidney

C. Mavroidis
Northeastern University

67.1 Structure of Function of the Kidney

The key separation functions of the kidney are:

1. To eliminate the water-soluble nitrogenous end-products of protein metabolism
2. To maintain electrolyte balance in body fluids and get rid of the excess electrolytes
3. To contribute to obligatory water loss and discharge excess water in the urine
4. To maintain acid-base balance in body fluids and tissues

To fulfill these functions, the kidney processes blood — or more accurately, plasma water — which in turn exchanges water and solutes with the extravascular water compartments: extracellular, intracellular, and transcellular. The solute concentrations in body fluids vary from site to site, yet all compartments are maintained remarkably constant in volume and composition despite internal and external stresses. The global outcome of normal renal function is a net removal of water, electrolyte, and soluble waste products from the blood stream. The kidney provides the major regulatory mechanisms for the control of volume, osmolality, and electrolyte and nonelectrolyte composition as well as pH of the body fluids and tissues.

Renal function is provided by paired, fist-sized organs, the kidneys, located behind the peritoneum against the posterior abdominal wall on both sides of the aorta. Each kidney is made up of over a million parallel mass transfer units which receive their common blood supply from the renal arteries, return the processed blood to the systemic circulation through the renal veins, and collect the waste fluids and solutes through the calyx of each kidney into the ureter and from there into the urinary bladder. These functional units are called nephrons and can be viewed as a sequential arrangement of mass transfer devices (glomerulus, proximal tubule, and distal tubule) for two fluid streams: blood and urine.

Kidney function is served by two major mechanisms: **ultrafiltration**, which results in the separation of large amounts of extracellular fluid through plasma filtration in the glomeruli, and a combination of passive and active tubular transport of electrolytes and other solutes, together with the water in which they are dissolved, in the complex system provided in the rest of the nephron.

67.1.1   Glomerular Filtration

The volume of blood flowing into the natural kidneys far exceeds the amount needed to meet their requirements for oxygen and nutrients: the primary role of the kidneys is chemical processing. As blood flows through the glomerular capillaries, about one-fifth of the plasma water is forced through permeable membranes to enter the proximal portion of the renal tubule and form the primary urine, which henceforth becomes the second fluid phase of the renal mass exchanger. The concentrated blood remaining in the vascular system is collected in the efferent arterioles and goes on to perfuse the tubules via the peritubular capillaries of the "vasa recta" system, where it recovers some of the lost water and eventually coalesces with the other blood drainage channels to form the renal vein. The plasma water removed from the blood in the glomerulus is termed the glomerular filtrate, and the process of removal is called glomerular filtration. Glomerular filtrate normally contains no blood cells and very little protein. Glomerular filtration is a passive process driven by the differences in hydrostatic and oncotic pressures across the glomerular **membrane**. Solutes which are sufficiently small and not bound to large molecules pass quite freely through the glomerular membrane. All major ions, glucose, amino acids, urea, and creatinine appear in the glomerular filtrate at nearly the same concentrations as prevail in plasma.

The normal **glomerular filtration rate** (GFR) averages 120 ml/min. This value masks wide physiological fluctuations (e.g., up to 30% decrease during the night, and a marked increase in the postprandial period). Although the kidneys produce about 170 l of glomerular filtrate per day, only 1 to 2 l of urine is formed. A minimum volume of about 400 ml/day is needed to excrete the metabolic wastes produced under normal conditions (often called obligatory water loss).

67.1.2   Tubular Function

In the tubule, both solute and water transport take place. Some materials are transported from the lumen across the tubular epithelium into the interstitial fluid surrounding the tubule and thence into the blood of the peritubular capillaries. This process is called reabsorption and results in the return of initially filtered solutes to the blood stream. Other substances are transported from the peritubular blood to the interstitial fluid across the tubular epithelium and into the lumen. This process is called secretion and leads to elimination of those substances to a greater extent than would be possible solely through glomerular filtration. The return of filtered molecules from the kidney tubule to the blood is accompanied by the passive reabsorption of water through osmotic mechanisms.

The proximal tubule reabsorbs about two-thirds of the water and salt in the original glomerular filtrate. The epithelial cells extrude Na+ (and with it Cl–) from the glomerular filtrate into the interstitial fluid. Water follows passively and in proportionate amounts because of the osmotic pressure gradient (the proximal tubular membrane is freely permeable to water). In the loop of Henle, the glomerular filtrate, now reduced to onethird of its original volume, and still isoosmotic with blood, is processed to remove another 20% of its water content. The active element is the ascending limb of the loop of Henle, where cells pump out Na+, K+, and Cl− from the filtrate and move the Na+ and Cl− to the interstitial fluid. Because the ascending limb is not permeable to water, tubular fluid becomes increasingly more dilute along the ascending loop. The blood vessels around the loop do not carry back all the extruded salt to the general circulation, and therefore the Na+ concentration builds up down the descending limb of the loop of Henle, reaching a concentration four to five times higher than isoosmolar. As a result, the Na+ concentration in tubular fluid increases as its volume is decreased by passive transport into interstitial fluid and from there into the blood.

Countercurrent multiplication refers to the fact that the more Na+ the ascending limb extrudes the higher the concentration in the interstitial fluid, the more water removed from the descending limb by osmosis, and the higher the Na+ concentration presented to the ascending limb around the bend of the loop. Overall, the countercurrent multiplier traps salt in the medullary part of the nephron because it recirculates its locally. Countercurrent exchange refers to the interaction of the descending and ascending branches of the circulatory loops (vasa recta) with the loop of Henle which flows in the opposite direction. Substances which pass from the tubule into the blood accumulate in high concentrations in the medullary tissue fluid. Na+ and urea diffuse into the blood as it descends along the loop but then diffuse out of the ascending vessels and back into the descending vessels where the concentration is lower. Solutes are therefore recirculated and trapped (short-circuited) in the medulla, but water diffuses out of the descending vessel and into the ascending vessel to be transported out.

The distal tubule of the kidney, located in the cortex, is the site of fine adjustments of renal excretion. Here again the primary motor is the Na+/K+ pump in the baso-lateral membrane, which creates a Na+ concentration gradient. The walls of the collecting duct, which traverses through a progressively hypertonic renal medulla tissue, are permeable to water but not to Na+ and Cl−. As a result, water is drawn out and transported by capillaries to the general circulation. The osmotic gradient created by the countercurrent multiplier system provides the force for water reabsorption from the collecting duct. However, the **permeability** of the cell membrane in the collecting duct is modulated by the concentration of antidiuretic hormone (ADH). A decrease in ADH impairs the reabsorption of water and leads to the elimination of a larger volume of more dilute urine.

The terms reabsorption and secretion denote direction of transport rather than a difference in physiologic mechanism. In fact, a number of factors may impact on the net transport of any one particular solute. For example, endogenous creatinine (an end product of protein metabolism) is removed from plasma water through glomerular filtration in direct proportion to its concentration in plasma. Since it is neither synthesized nor destroyed anywhere in the kidney, and it is neither reabsorbed nor secreted in the tubule, its eventual elimination in the urine directly reflects glomerular filtration. Therefore, creatinine **clearance** can be used to measure glomerular filtration rate. However, glucose, which initially passes in the glomerular filtrate at the same concentration as in plasma, is completely reabsorbed from the tubular urine into peritubular capillaries as long as its plasma concentration does not exceed a threshold value somewhat above the level prevailing in normal subjects. As a result, there should be no glucose in the urine. When the threshold is exceeded, the amount of glucose excreted in the urine increases proportionately, producing glycosuria.

Several weak organic acids such as uric acid and oxalic acid, and some related but not naturally occurring substances such as p-aminohippuric acid (PAH), barbiturates, penicillates, and some x-ray contrast media, have the special property of being secreted in the proximal tubule. For example, PAH concentration in glomerular filtrate is the same as in plasma water. So avid is the tubular transport system for PAH that tubular cells remove essentially all the PAH from the blood perfusing them. Therefore, the removal of PAH is almost complete, and the rate of appearance of PAH in the urine mirrors the rate of presentation of PAH to the renal glomeruli, that is to say, renal plasma flow. Therefore, PAH clearance can be used, in association with the hematocrit, to estimate the rate of renal blood flow.

Urea appears in the glomerular filtrate at the same concentration as in plasma. However, one-third of urea diffuses back into the blood in the proximal tubule. In the distal nephron, urea (as an electrically neutral molecule without specific transport system) follows the fate of water (solvent drag). If large amounts of water are reabsorbed in the distal tubule and the collecting duct, then an additional third of the urea can be reabsorbed. However, if water diuresis is large, then correspondingly more urea is excreted.

67.2   Kidney Disease

The origin of kidney disease may be infectious, genetic, traumatic, vascular, immunologic, metabolic, or degenerative [Brenner and Rector, 1986]. The response of the kidneys to a pathologic agent may be rapid or slow, reversible or permanent, local or extensive. Under most circumstances, an abnormal body fluid composition is more likely to arise from the unavailability or excess of a raw material than from some intrinsic disturbance of renal function. This is why many clinical problems are corrected by fluid or electrolyte therapy and secondarily by dietary measures and pharmacologic agents which act on the kidney itself. Only as a treatment of last resort, where kidney disease progresses to renal failure, do clinicians use extracorporeal body fluid processing techniques that come under the generic concept of **dialysis**. These invasive procedures are intended to reestablish the body's fluid and electrolyte homeostasis and to eliminate toxic waste products. Processing can address the blood (e.g., **hemodialysis**) or a proxy fluid introduced in body cavities (e.g., **peritoneal dialysis**).

Even in healthy subjects, the GFR falls steadily from age 40 onward. Beyond age 80, it is only half of its adult value of 120 ml/min. However this physiologic deterioration is not extensive enough to cause symptoms. Since nature has provided kidneys with an abundance of overcapacity, patients do not become identifiably sick until close to 90% of original function has been lost. When kidneys keep deteriorating and functional loss exceeds 95%, survival is no longer possible without some form of replacement therapy.

Supplementation (as distinct from replacement) of renal function by artificial means is occasionally used in case of poisoning. Toxic substances are often excreted into the urine of glomerular filtration and active tubular secretion, but the body load at times exceeds the kidneys' clearing capacity. There are no methods known to accelerate the active transport of poisons into urine. Similarly, enhancement of passive glomerular filtration is not a practical means to facilitate elimination of toxic chemicals. Processing of blood in an extracorporeal circuit may be life-saving when the amount of poison in the blood is large compared to the total body burden and binding of the compound to plasma proteins is not extensive. In such cases (e.g., methanol, ethylene glycol, or salicylates poisoning) extracorporeal processing of blood for removing the toxic element from the body is indicated. If the poison is distributed in the entire extracellular space or tightly bound to plasma proteins, dialytic removal is unlikely to affect the clinical outcome because it can only eliminate a small fraction of the toxic solute.

Unfortunately in some situations either the glomerular or the tubular function of the kidneys, or both, fails and cannot be salvaged by drug and diet therapy. Failure can be temporary, self-limiting and potentially reversible, in which case only temporary substitution for renal function will be needed. Failure can also be the expression of progressive, intractable structural damage, in which case permanent replacement of renal function will eventually be needed for survival. However, the urgency of external intervention in end-stage renal disease (**ESRD**) is never as acute as is the case for the replacement of cardiac or respiratory function: The signs of renal dysfunction (water retention, electrolyte shifts, accumulation of metabolic end products normally eliminated by the kidneys) develop over days, weeks, or even months and are not immediately life threatening. Even in the end stage, renal failure can be addressed by intermittent rather than continuous treatment.

67.3   Renal Failure

There are two types of renal failure: acute (days or weeks) and chronic (months or years). Acute renal failure is typically associated with ischemia (reduction in blood flow), acute glomerulonephritis, tubular necrosis, or poisoning with "nephrotoxins" (e.g., heavy metals, some aminoglycosides, and excessive loads of free hemoglobin). Chronic renal failure is usually caused by chronic glomerulonephritis (of infectious or immune origin), pyelonephritis (ascending infection of the urinary tract), hypertension (leading to nephrosclerosis), or vascular disease (most commonly secondary to diabetes).

Renal insufficiency elicits the clinical picture of **uremia**. Although the word uremia means that there is too much urea in the blood, urea level in itself is not the cause of the problem. Uremia, often expressed in the United States as **blood urea nitrogen** concentration or BUN (which is actually half the urea concentration), serves as an indicator of the severity of renal disease. Urea is a metabolic end product in the catabolism of proteins that is hardly toxic even in high concentration. However, it mirrors the impaired renal elimination and the resulting accumulation in body fluids of other toxic substances, some of which have been identified (e.g., phenols, guanidine, diverse polypeptides); others remain unknown and are therefore referred to as **uremic toxins** or, for reasons to be discussed later, **middle molecules**. The attenuation of uremic symptoms by protein restriction in the diet and by various dialytic procedures underscores the combined roles of retention, removal, and metabolism in the constellation of signs of uremia. Toxicity may result from the synergism of an entire spectrum of accumulated molecules [Vanholder and Ringoir, 1992]. It may also reflect the imbalance that results from a specific removal through mechanisms which eliminate physiologic compounds together with potential toxins.

Not until the GFR (as estimated by its proxy, creatinine clearance) falls much below a third of normal do the first signs of renal insufficiency become manifest. At that point the plasma or extracellular concentration of substances eliminated exclusively through the glomeruli, such as creatinine or urea, increase measurably, and the possibility of progressive renal failure must be considered. In such cases, over a period of months to years, the kidneys lose their ability to excrete waste materials, to achieve osmoregulation, and to maintain water and electrolyte balance. The signs of ESRD become recognizable as creatinine clearance approaches 15 ml/min, eventually leading to uremic coma as water and solute retention depress the cognitive functions of the central nervous system. Empirically, it appears that the lowest level of creatinine clearance that is compatible with life is on the order of 8 ml/min, or 11.5 l/day, or 80 l/per week. (These numbers have a bearing on the definition of adequate dialysis in ERSD patients, because they represent the time-averaged clearance which must be achieved by much more effective but intermittent blood processing.) Human life cannot be sustained for more than 7 to 10 days in the total absence of kidney function. Clinical experience also shows that even a minimum of **residual renal clearance** (KR) below the level necessary for survival can be an important factor of well-being in dialyzed patients, perhaps because the natural kidney, however sick, remains capable of eliminating middle molecular weight substances, whereas the **artificial kidney** is mostly effective in eliminating water and small molecules.

The incidence of ESRD (incidence is defined as the number of new patients entering treatment during a given year) has increased dramatically in the past 25 years in the United States and elsewhere. Whereas in the 1960s it was estimated at 700 to 1000 new cases a year in the United States (nearly three quarters of them between the ages of 25 and 54), the number of new patients reached 16,000 per year at the end of the 1970s (still with the majority of cases under age 54) and 40,000 at the end of the 1980s, with the largest contingent between 65 and 74 years old. Serious kidney disease now strikes between in 1 in 5,000 and 1 in 10,000 people per year in our progressively aging population. The fastest rate of growth is in the age group over 75, and the incidence of ESRD shows no signs of abating.

The prevalence of ESRD (prevalence is defined as the total number of patients present in the population at a specific time) has grown apace: In the United States, about 1,000 people were kept alive by dialysis in 1969; 58,253 in 1979; 163,017 in 1989; close to 200,000 now. This is the result of a combination of factors which include longer survival of patients on hemodialysis and absolute growth of an elderly population suffering from an increasing incidence of diseases leading to ESRD such as diabetes. Worldwide, over 500,000 people are being kept alive by various modalities of "artificial kidney" treatment: about a third in the United States, a third in Europe, and a third in Japan and Pacific Rim countries. Another 500,000 or so have benefitted from dialytic treatment in the past but have since died or received transplants [Lysaght and Baurmeister, 1993]. Close to 85% of current patients are treated by maintenance hemodialysis, and 15% are on peritoneal dialysis. These numbers do not include about 100,000 people with a functional renal transplant, most of whom required hemodialysis support while waiting for a donor organ, and who may need it again, if only for a limited period, in case of graft rejection.

The mortality of ESRD patients in the United States has inched upward from 12 to 16% per year in the 1970s and 1980s and has risen abruptly in recent years to levels in the order of 20 to 25%. This has led to extensive controversy as to the origin of this deterioration, which has not been observed to the same extent in other regions with a similarly large population of ESRD patients, such as Western Europe and Japan, and may reflect for the United States insufficient dialysis as well as the burden of an increasingly older population.

67.4   Treatment of Renal Failure

Profound uremia, whether caused by an acute episode of renal failure or by the chronic progressive deterioration of renal function, used to be a fatal condition until the middle of the twentieth century. The concept of clearing the blood of toxic substances while removing excess water by a membrane exchange process was first suggested by the experiments of Abel, Rowntree, and Turner at the Johns Hopkins Medical School. Back in 1913, these investigators demonstrated the feasibility of blood dialysis to balance plasma solute concentrations with those imposed by an appropriately formulated washing solution. However, their observation was not followed by clinical application, perhaps because experiments were limited by the difficulty of fabricating suitable exchange membranes, and blood anticoagulation was then extremely precarious. Collodion, a nitrocellulose film precipitated from an alcohol, ether, or acetone solution was the sole synthetic permeable membrane material available until the advent of cellophane in the 1930s. The unreliability of anticoagulants before the discovery of heparin also made continuous blood processing a hazardous process even in laboratory animals.

In 1944, Kolff in the Netherlands developed an artificial kidney of sufficient yet marginal capacity to treat acute renal failure in man. This device consisted of a long segment of cellophane sausage tubing coiled around a drum rotating in the thermostabilized bath filled with a hypertonic, buffered electrolyte solution, called the **dialysate**. Blood was allowed to flow from a vein into the coiled cellophane tube. Water and solute exchange occurred through the membrane with a warm dialysate pool, which had to be renewed every few hours because of the risk of bacterial growth. The cleared blood was returned to the circulatory system by means of a pump. After World War II, a somewhat similar system was developed independently by Alwall in Sweden. Because of the technical difficulty of providing repeated access to the patient's circulation, and the overall cumbersomeness of the extracorporeal clearing process, hemodialysis was limited to patients suffering from acute, and hopefully reversible, renal failure, with the hope that their kidneys would eventually recover. To simplify the equipment, Inouye and Engelberg [1953] devised a coiled cellophane tube arrangement that was stationary and disposable, and shortly thereafter Kolff and Watschinger (by then at the Cleveland Clinic) reported a variant of this design, the Twin Coil, that became the standard for clinical practice for a number of years.

Repeated treatment, as needed for chronic renal failure, was not possible until late 1959, when Scribner and Quinton introduced techniques for chronic access to the blood stream which, combined with improvements in the design and use of hemodialysis equipment, allowed the advent of chronic intermittent hemodialysis for long-term maintenance of ESRD patients. This was also the time when Kiil first reported results with a flat plate dialyzer design in which blood was made to flow between two sheets of cellophane supported by solid mats with grooves for the circulation of dialysate. This design — which had been pioneered by Skeggs and Leonard, McNeill, and Bluemle and Leonard — not only needed less blood volume to operate then the coiled tube devices, it also had the advantage of requiring a relatively low head of pressure to circulate the blood and the dialysate. This meant that the two fluids could circulate without high pressure differences across the membrane. Therefore, in contrast to coil dialyzers, where a long blood path necessitated a high blood pressure at the entrance of the exchanger, flat plate dialyzers could transfer metabolites through the membrane by diffusion alone, without coupling it with the obligatory water flux deriving from high transmembrane pressure. When ultrafiltration was needed, it could be achieved by circulating the dialysate at subatmospheric pressures.

Device development was also encouraged by the growing number of home dialysis patients. By 1965, the first home dialysate preparation and control units were produced industrially. Home dialysis programs based on the twin coil or flat plate dialyzers were soon underway. At that time the cost of home treatment was substantially lower than hospital care, and in the United States, Social Security was not yet underwriting the cost of treatment of ESRD.

In 1965 also, Bluemle and coworkers analyzed means to pack the maximum membrane area in the minimum volume, so as to reduce the bulkiness of the exchange device and diminish the blood loss associated with large dialyzers and long tubing. They concluded that a tightly packed bundle of parallel capillaries would best fit this design goal. Indeed by 1967, Lipps and colleagues reported the initial clinical experience with hollow fiber dialyzers, which have since become the mainstay of hemodialysis technology.

In parallel developments. Henderson and coworkers [1967] proposed an alternative solution to the problem of limited mass transfer achievable by diffusion alone with hemodialysis equipment. They projected that a purely convective transport (ultrafiltration) through membranes more permeable to water than the original cellulose would increase the effective clearance of metabolites larger than urea. The lost extracellular volume was to be replaced by infusing large volumes of fresh saline into the blood at the inlet or the outlet of the dialyzer to replace the lost water and electrolytes. The process was called **hemodiafiltration** or, sometimes, diafiltration. (The procedure in which solutes and water are removed by convective transport alone, using large pore membranes and without substantial replacement of the fluid, is now known as **hemofiltration** and is used primarily in patients presenting with massive fluid retention.)

As is intuitively apparent, the effectiveness of hemodialysis with a given devices is related to the duration of the procedure. In the pioneer years, dubbed "the age of innocence" by Colton [1987], patients were treated for as many as 30 h a week. Economics and patient convenience promoted the development of more efficient transfer devices. Nowadays, intermittent maintenance dialysis can be offered with 10 h (or even less) of treatment dividend in 3 sessions per week. Conversely, nephrologists have developed (mostly for use in the intensive care unit) the procedure known as continuous arterio-venous hemodialysis (with its variant continuous arterio-venous hemofiltration) in which blood pressure from an artery (aided or not by a pump) drives blood through the exchange device and back into a vein. Continuous operation compensates for the relatively low blood flow and achieves stable solute concentrations, as opposed to the seesaw pattern that prevails with periodic treatment.

The concept of using a biologic membrane and its blood capillary network to exchange water and solutes with a washing solution underlies the procedure known as peritoneal dialysis, which relies on the transfer capacity of the membranelike tissue lining the abdominal cavity and the organs it contains. In 1976, Popovich and Moncrief described **continuous ambulatory peritoneal dialysis** (CAPD), a procedure in which lavage of the peritoneal cavity is conducted as a continuous form of mass transfer through introduction, equilibration, and drainage of dialyzate on a repetitive basis 4 to 6 times a day. In CAPD, a sterile solution containing electrolytes and dextrose is fed by gravity into the peritoneal cavity through a permanently installed transcutaneous **catheter**. After equilibriation with capillary blood over several hours, this dialyzate is drained by gravity into the original container and the process is repeated with a fresh solution. During the dwell periods, toxins and other solutes are exchanged by diffusional processes. Water transfer is induced by the osmotic pressure difference due to the high dextrose concentration in the treatment fluid. This procedure is analyzed in detail in Chapter 70.

Plasmapheresis, that is, the extraction of plasma from blood by separative procedures (see Chapter 71), has been used in the treatment of renal disease [Samtleben and Gurland, 1989]. However, the cost of providing fresh plasma to replace the discarded material renders plasmapheresis impractical for frequent, repeated procedures, and plasmapheresis is used mainly for other clinical indications.

Most hemodialysis is performed in free-standing treatment centers, although it may also be provided in a hospital or performed by the patient at home. The hemodialysis circuit consists of two fluid pathways. The blood circuitry is entirely disposable, though many centers reuse some or all circuit components in order to reduce costs. It comprises a 16-gauge needle for access to the circulation (usually through an **arteriovenous fistula** created in the patient's forearm), lengths of plasticized polyvinyl chloride tubing (including a special segment adapted to fit into a peristaltic blood pump), the hemodialyzer itself, a bubble trap and an open mesh screen filter, various ports for sampling or pressure measurements at the blood outlet, and a return cannula. Components of the blood side circuit are supplied in sterile and nonpyrogenic conditions. The dialysate side is essentially a machine capable of (1) proportioning out glucose and electrolyte concentrates with water to provide a dialysate of appropriate composition; (2) sucking dialysate past a restrictor valve and through the hemodialyzer at subatmospheric pressure; and (3) monitoring temperature, pressures, and flow rates. During treatment the patient's blood is anticoagulated with heparin. Typical blood flow rates are 200 to 350 ml/min; dialysate flow rates are usually set at 500 ml/min. Simple techniques have been developed to prime the blood side with sterile saline prior to use and to return to the patient nearly all the blood contained in the extracorporeal circuit after treatment. Whereas most mass transport occurs by diffusion, circuits are operated with a pressure on the blood side, which may be 100 to 500 mmHg higher than on the dialysate side. This provides an opportunity to remove 2 to 4 l of fluid along with solutes. Higher rates of fluid removal are technically possible but physiologically unacceptable. Hemodialyzers must be designed with high enough hydraulic permeabilities to provide adequate fluid removal at low transmembrane pressure but not so high that excessive water removal will occur in the upper pressure range.

Although other geometries are still employed, the current preferred format is a "hollow fiber" hemodialyzer about 25 cm in length and 5 cm in diameter, resembling the design of a shell and tube heat exchanger. Blood enters at the inlet manifold, is distributed to a parallel bundle of capillary tubes (potted together with polyurethane), and exits at a collection manifold. Dialysate flows countercurrent in an external chamber. The shell is typically made of an acrylate or polycarbonate resin. Devices typically contain 6,000–10,000 capillaries, each with an inner diameter of 200–250 μm and a dry wall thickness as low as 10 μm. The total membrane surface area in commercial dialyzers varies from 0.5 to 1.5 m^2, and units can be mass-produced at a relatively low cost (selling price around $10–15, not including tubing and other disposable accessories). Several reference texts (see For Further Information) provide concise and comprehensive coverage of all aspects of hemodialysis.

67.5   Renal Transplantation

The uremic syndrome resembles complex forms of systemic poisoning and is characterized by multiple symptoms and side effects. Survival requires that the toxins be removed, and the resulting quality of life depends on the quantity of toxins which are actually eliminated. Ideally, one would like to clean blood and body fluids to the same extent as is achieved by normal renal function. This is only possible at the present time with an organ transplant.

The feasibility of renal transplantation as a therapeutic modality for ESRD was first demonstrated in 1954 by Murray and coworkers in Boston, and Hamburger and coworkers in Paris, in homozygous twins. Soon the discovery of the first immunosuppressive drugs led to the extension of transplantation practice to kidneys of live, related donors. Kidney donation is thought to be innocuous since removal of one kidney does not lead to renal failure. The remaining kidney is capable of hypertrophy, meaning that the glomeruli produce more filtrate, and the tubules become capable of increased reabsorption and secretion. A recent Canadian study indicates that the risk of ESRD is not higher among living kidney donors than in the general population, meaning that a single kidney has enough functional capacity for a lifetime. Nonetheless, cadaver donors now constitute the main organ source for the close to 10,000 renal transplants performed in the United States every year. Even though under ideal circumstances each cadaver donor allows two kidney transplants, the scarcity of donors is the major limitation to this form of treatment of ESRD. Most patients aspire to renal transplant because of the better quality of life it provides and the freedom from the time constraints of repeated procedures. However, the incidence of ESRD is such that only one patient in five can be kept alive by transplantation. Dialysis treatment remains a clinical necessity while waiting for a transplant, as a safety net in case of organ rejection, and for the many patients for whom transplantation is either contraindicated or simply not available.

67.6 Mass Transfer in Dialysis

In artificial kidneys, the removal of water and solutes from the blood stream is achieved by:

1. Solute diffusion in response to concentration gradients
2. Water ultrafiltration and solute convection in response to hydrostatic and osmotic pressure gradients
3. Water migration in response to osmotic gradients

In most cases, these processes occur simultaneously and in the same exchange device, rather than sequentially as they do in the natural kidney with the cascade of glomerular filtration, tubular reabsorption, and final adjustments in the collecting tubule.

Mechanistically, the removal of water and solutes from blood is achieved by passive transport across thin, leaky, synthetic polymer sheets or tubes similar to those used in the chemical process call dialysis. Functionally, an artificial kidney (also called hemodialyzer, or dialyzer or filter for short) is a device in which water and solutes are transported from one moving fluid stream to another. One fluid stream is blood; the other is dialysate: a human-made solution of electrolytes, buffers, and nutrients. The solute concentration as well as the hydrostatic and osmotic pressures of the dialysate are adjusted to achieve transport in the desired direction (e.g., to remove urea and potassium ions while adding glucose or bicarbonate to the bloodstream).

Efficiency of mass transfer is governed by two and only two independent parameters. One, which derives from mass conservation requirements, is the ratio of the flow rates of blood and dialysate. The other is the rate constant for solute transport between the two fluid streams. This rate constant depends upon the overall surface area of membrane available for exchange, its leakiness or permeability, and such design characteristics as fluid channel geometry, local flow velocities, and **boundary layer** control, all of which affect the thickness of stationary fluid films, or diffusion barriers, on either side of the membrane.

67.7 Clearance

The overall mass transfer efficiency of a hemodialyzer is defined by the fractional depletion of a given solute in the blood as it passes through the unit. Complete removal of a solute from blood during a single pass defines the dialyzer clearance for that solute as equal to dialyzer blood flow. In other terms, dialyzer blood flow asymptotically limits the clearance of any substance in any device, however efficient.

Under conditions of steady-state dialysis, the mass conservation requirement is expressed as

$$N = Q_B(C_{Bi} - C_{Bo}) = Q_D(C_{Do} - C_{Di}) \tag{67.1}$$

where N is the overall solute transfer rate between blood and dialysate, Q_B and Q_D are blood flow and dialysate flow rates, respectively, and C_{Bi}, C_{Bo}, C_{Di}, and C_{Do}, are the solution concentrations C in blood, B, or dialysate, D, at the inlet, i, or the outlet, o of the machine.

Equation 67.1 about mass conservation leads to the first and oldest criterion for dialyzer effectiveness, namely clearance K, modeled after the concept of renal clearance. Dialyzer clearance is defined as the mass transfer rate N divided by the concentration gradient prevailing at the inlet of the artificial kidney.

$$K = \frac{N}{C_{Bi} - C_{Di}} \tag{67.2}$$

Since mass transfer rate also means the amount of solute removed from the blood per unit of time, which in turn is equal to the amount of solute accepted in the dialysate per unit of time, there are two expressions for dialysance

$$K_B = \frac{Q_B(C_{Bi} - C_{Bo})}{C_{Bi} - C_{Di}} \tag{67.3}$$

$$K_D = \frac{Q_D(C_{Do} - C_{Di})}{C_{Bi} - C_{Di}} \tag{67.4}$$

which afford two methods for measuring it. Any discrepancy must remain within the error of measurements, which under the conditions of clinical hemodialysis easily approaches $\pm10\%$. As in the natural kidney, the clearance of any solute is defined by the flow rate of blood which is completely freed of that solute while passing through the exchange device. The dimensions of clearance are those of flow (a virtual flow, one may say), which can vary only between zero and blood flow (or dialysate flow, whichever is smaller), much in the way the renal clearance of a substance can only vary between zero and effective renal plasma flow.

Since dialyzer clearance is a function of blood flow, a natural way to express the efficiency of a particular exchange device consists of "normalizing" clearance with respect to blood flow as a dimensionless ratio

$$\frac{K}{Q_B} = \frac{C_{Bi} - C_{Bo}}{C_{Bi} - C_{Di}} \tag{67.5}$$

or

$$\frac{K}{Q_B} = \frac{C_{Do} - C_{Di}}{C_{Bi} - C_{Di}} \quad \text{(extraction fraction)} \tag{67.6}$$

K/Q_B can vary only between zero and one and represents the highest attainable solute depletion in the blood which is actually achieved in a particular device for a particular solute under a particular set of circumstances.

Another generalization of the dialysance concept may be useful in the case where the direction of blood flow relative to the direction of dialysate flow is either parallel, random, or undetermined, as occurs with the majority of clinical hemodialyzers. Under such circumstances, the best performance which can be achieved is expressed by the equality of solute concentration in outgoing blood and outgoing dialysate ($C_{Bo} = C_{Do} = C_e$ or equilibrium concentration). This limit defines, after algebraic rearrangement of Equation 67.3 and Equation 67.4, the maximal achievable clearance at any combination of blood and dialysate flow rates without reference to solute concentrations.

$$K_{max} = \frac{Q_B \times Q_D}{Q_B + Q_D} \tag{67.7}$$

Since blood and dialysate flows can usually be measured with a reasonable degree of accuracy, the concept of K_{max} provides a practical point of reference against which the effectiveness of an actual dialyzer can be estimated.

67.8 Filtration

So far we implicitly assumed that differences in concentration across the membrane provide the sole driving force for solute transfer. In clinical hemodialysis, however, the blood phase is usually subject to a higher hydrostatic pressure than the dialysate phase. As a result, water is removed from the plasma by ultrafiltration, dragging with it some of the solutes into the dialysate. Ultrafiltration capability is a necessary consequence of the transmural pressure required to keep the blood path open with flat sheet or wide tubular membranes. It is also clinically useful to remove the water accumulated in the patient's body in the interval of dialysis. Ultrafiltration can be enhanced by increasing the resistance to blood flow at the dialyzer outlet, and thereby raising blood compartment pressure, by subjecting the dialysate to a negative pressure or by utilizing membranes more permeable to water than the common cellophanes.

Whenever water is removed from the plasma by ultrafiltration, solutes are simultaneously removed in a concentration equal to or lower than that present in the plasma. For small, rapidly diffusible molecules such as urea, glucose, and the common electrolytes, the rate of solute removal almost keeps pace with that of water, and ultrafiltrate concentration is the same as that in plasma. With compounds characterized by a larger molecular size, the rate of solute removal lags behind that of water. Indeed with some of the largest molecules of biological interest, ultrafiltration leads to an actual increase in plasma concentration during passage through the artificial kidney.

Defining ultrafiltration as the difference between blood flow entering the dialyzer and blood flow leaving the dialyzer

$$F = Q_{Bi} - Q_{Bo}$$

one can rewrite the mass conservation requirement as

$$Q_{Bi} C_{Bi} \text{(amount of solute in the incoming blood)}$$

$$= Q_{Bo} C_{Bo} \text{(amount of solute in the outgoing blood)}$$

$$+ K_B (C_{Bi} - C_{Di}) \text{(amount cleared in the dialyzer)}$$

The clearance equations can then be rewritten as

$$K_B = \frac{Q_{Bi}(C_{Bi} - (Q_{Bo}/Q_{Bi})C_{Bo})}{C_{Bi} - C_{Di}} \tag{67.8}$$

$$K_D = \frac{Q_{Di}((Q_{Do}/Q_{Di})C_{Do} - C_{Di})}{C_{Bi} - C_{Di}} \tag{67.9}$$

The clearance is now defined as the amount of solute removed from the blood phase per unit of time, regardless of the nature of the driving force, divided by the concentration difference between incoming blood and incoming dialysate.

When $C_{Di} = 0$

$$K_B = Q_{Bi} - Q_{Bo} \left(\frac{Q_{Bo}}{Q_{Bi}} \right) \tag{67.10}$$

$$K_D = \frac{Q_{Do} C_{Do}}{C_{Bi}} \tag{67.11}$$

When $C_{Di} = 0$ and $C_{Bo} = C_{Bi}$

$$K_B = F \tag{67.12}$$

The practical value of these equations is somewhat limited, since their application requires a high degree of accuracy in the measurement of flows and solute concentrations. The special case where there is no solute in the incoming dialysate ($C_{Di} = 0$) is important for *in vitro* testing of artificial kidneys.

67.9 Permeability

The definition of clearance is purely operational. Based upon considerations of conservation of mass, it is focused primarily on the blood stream from which a solute must be removed, thus, in final analysis, on the patient herself or himself. Clearance describes the artificial kidney as part of the circulatory system and of the fluid compartments which must be cleared of a given solute. To relate the performance of a hemodialyzer to its design characteristics, clearance is of limited value.

To introduce into the picture the surface area of membrane and the continuously variable (but predictable) concentration difference between blood and dialysate within the artificial kidney, one must define the rate constant of solute transfer, or permeability P_Σ.

$$P_\Sigma = \frac{N}{A \times \Delta C} \tag{67.13}$$

where N is the overall solute transport rate between blood dialysate, A is the membrane area, and ΔC is the average solute concentration difference between the two moving fluids.

Permeability is defined by Equation 67.13 as the amount of solute transferred per unit area and per unit of time, under the influence of a unit of concentration driving force. The proper average concentration, ΔC — drivingforceis the logarithmic mean of the concentration differences prevailing at the inlet and at the outlet

$$\overline{\Delta C} = \frac{\Delta C_i - \Delta C_o}{\ln(\Delta C_i / \Delta C_o)} \tag{67.14}$$

The boundary conditions on the concentration driving force (Δ_{Ci} and Δ_{Co}) are uniquely determined by the geometry of the dialyzer. The three most common cases to consider are (1) cocurrent flow of blood and dialysate; (2) laminar blood flow, with completely mixed dialysate flow; and (3) countercurrent blood and dialysate flow. The boundary conditions on concentration driving force as follows:

Cocurrent flow is

$$C_{Bi} - C_{Di} \quad \text{and} \quad C_{Bo} - C_{Do}$$

Mixed dialysate flow is

$$C_{Bi} - C_{Do} \quad \text{and} \quad C_{DBo} - C_{Do}$$

Countercurrent flow is

$$C_{Bi} - C_{Do} \quad \text{and} \quad C_{Bo} - C_{Di}$$

Thus permeability can be expressed as in the following equations. Cocurrent flow is

$$P_\Sigma = \frac{N(\ln(C_{Bi} - C_{Di})/(C_{Bo} - C_{Do}))}{A(C_{Bi} - C_{Di}) - (C_{Bo} - C_{Do})} \tag{67.15}$$

Mixed dialysate flow is

$$P_\Sigma = \frac{N(\ln(C_{Bi} - C_{Do})/(C_{Bo} - C_{Do}))}{A(C_{Bi} - C_{Do}) - (C_{Bo} - C_{Do})} \tag{67.16}$$

Countercurrent flow is

$$P_\Sigma = \frac{N(\ln(C_{Bi} - C_{Do})/(C_{Bo} - C_{Di}))}{A(C_{Bi} - C_{Do}) - (C_{Bo} - C_{Di})} \tag{67.17}$$

By simultaneous solution of Equation 67.3, Equation 67.4, and Equation 67.12, and use of the formal definition of the logarithmic mean concentration driving force 67.14, the clearance ratio (K/Q_B) can be expressed as a function of two dimensionless parameters (Z and R), neither of which involves solute concentration terms [Leonard and Bluemle, 1959; Michaels, 1966]. Cocurrent flow is

$$\frac{K}{Q_B} = \frac{1}{1+Z}[1 - \exp(-R(1 + Z))] \tag{67.18}$$

Mixed dialysate flow is

$$\frac{K}{Q_B} = \frac{1 - \exp(-R)}{1 + Z[1 - \exp(-R)]} \tag{67.19}$$

Countercurrent flow is

$$\frac{K}{Q_B} = \frac{1 - \exp[R(1-Z)]}{Z - \exp[R(1-Z)]} \tag{67.20}$$

where $Z = Q_B/Q_D$ and $R = P_\Sigma A/Q_B$.

Michaels has expressed graphically Equation 67.8 to Equation 67.20 as plots of clearance ratio (K/Q_B) vs. flow ratio (Q_B/Q_D) with various solute transport ratios (P_Σ, A/Q_B) as parameters. These plots give an appreciation of the relative importance of the variables affecting dialyzer efficiency and permit one to recognize readily the factors which limit mass transfer under a particular set of conditions.

For the computation of actual permeability coefficients, from pooled data obtained at varying solute concentrations, Equation 67.15 to Equation 67.17 can be rearranged, using definitions of N, C_{Bo}, and C_{Do} from Equation 67.2 to Equation 67.4. Cocurrent flow is

$$P_\Sigma = \frac{Q_B Q_{Di}}{A(Q_B + Q_D)} \ln \frac{1}{1 - K/Q_B - K/Q_D} \tag{67.21}$$

Mixed dialysate flow is

$$P_\Sigma = \frac{Q_B}{A} \ln \frac{1 - K/Q_D}{1 - K/Q_B - K/Q_D} \tag{67.22}$$

Countercurrent flow is

$$P_\Sigma = \frac{Q_B Q_D}{A(Q_D - Q_B)} \ln \frac{1 - K/Q_D}{1 - K/Q_B} \tag{67.23}$$

As remarked by Leonard and Bluemle [1959], when, and only when, Q_D is much greater than Q_B, Equation 67.18 to Equation 67.23 reduce to Renkin's [1956] formula

$$P_\Sigma = \frac{Q_B}{A} \ln \frac{1}{1 - K/Q_B} \tag{67.24}$$

or

$$\frac{K}{Q_B} - 1 - \exp\left(\frac{p_\Sigma A}{Q_B}\right) \tag{67.25}$$

Historically, Equation 67.25 played an important role in pointing out to designers that the clearance ratio (K/Q_B) can be improved equally well by an increase in exchange area (A) or in permeability (P). However, caution is required in applying the equation to some of the efficient modern dialyzers. First, the assumption that dialysate flow is "infinitely" large with respect to blood flow is seldom verified. Furthermore, the functions relating permeability to dialysance, Equation 67.21 to Equation 67.24, or to the individual solute concentrations and flows, Equation 67.15 to Equation 67.17, have an exponential form. When the overall permeability approaches that of the membrane alone, when the outgoing solute concentrations approach the equilibrium conditions, or when clearance approaches blood flow, one deals with the steep part of that exponential function. Any slight error in the experimental measurements will lead to a disproportionately larger error in calculated permeability.

67.10 Overall Transport

In a dialyzer, separation occurs because small molecules diffuse more rapidly than larger ones and because the degree to which membranes restrict solute transport usually increases with permeant size (**permselectivity**). Fick's equation states that solute will move from a region of greater concentration to a region of lower concentration in a rate proportional to the difference in concentration on opposite sides of the membrane

$$\phi = -D\frac{\partial c}{\partial x} \tag{67.26}$$

where f is the unit solute flux in g/cm^2 sec; D the diffusion coefficient cm^2/sec; c the concentration in g/cm^3; and x the distance in cm. The minus sign accounts for the convention that flux is considered positive in the direction of decreasing concentration. Diffusion coefficient decreases roughly in proportion to the square root of molecular weight.

Ignoring boundary layer effects for the moment, and assuming that diffusion within the membrane is analogous to that in free solution, Equation 67.26 can be integrated across a homogeneous membrane of thickness d to yield

$$\phi = \frac{SD_{\mathrm{m}}\Delta c}{d} \tag{67.27}$$

where S represents the dimensionless solute partition coefficient, that is, the ratio of solute concentration in external solution to that at the membrane surface, and D_{m} represents solute diffusion within the membrane and is assumed to be independent of solute concentration in the membrane. If two or more solutes are dialysing at the same time, the degree of separation or enrichment will be proportional to the ratio of their permeabilities. The closer the permeability of a membrane is to that of an equivalent thickness of free solution, the more rapid will be the resultant dialytic transport. Equation 67.27 is often further simplified to this expression for flux per unit of membrane area

$$\phi = P_{\Sigma}\overline{\Delta C} \tag{67.28}$$

where thickness is incorporated into an overall membrane mass transfer coefficient with units of cm/sec, and $\overline{\Delta C}$ is the logarithmic mean concentration.

Chemical engineers provided a firm foundation for describing the overall performance of hemodialyzers recognizing the importance of understanding and describing mass transfer in each of the three phases of a hemodialyzer (blood, membrane, dialysate), the individual mass transfer resistances of which sum to the overall mass transfer resistance of the device [Colton, 1987]. Solutions adjacent to the membranes are rarely well mixed, and the resistance to transport resides not just in the membrane but also in the fluid regions termed boundary layers, on both the dialysate and blood side. Moreover, some dialyzers are designed to direct flow parallel to the surface of the membrane rather than expose it to a well-mixed bath. Boundary layer effects typically account for 25 to 75% of the overall resistance to solute transfer [Lysaght and Baurmeister, 1993]. In many exchanger designs, boundary layer effects can be minimized by rapid convective flow targeted to the surface of the membrane where fluid pathways are thin, flow near the membrane is laminar, and boundary layer resistance decreases with increasing wall shear rates. When geometry permits higher Reynolds numbers, flow becomes turbulent, and fluid resistance varies with net tangential velocity. Geometric obstacles (e.g., properly spaced obstacles) or fluid mechanical modulation (e.g., superimposed pulsation) are often-used tactics to minimize boundary layer effects, but all result in higher energy utilization. Quantitatively, the membrane resistance becomes part of an overall mass transfer parameter P_{Σ} which for conceptual purposes can be broken down into three independent and reciprocally additive components for the triple laminate: blood boundary layer (subscript B), membrane (subscript M), and dialysate boundary layer (subscript D), such that

$$\frac{1}{P_{\Sigma}} = \frac{1}{P_{\mathrm{B}}} + \frac{1}{P_{\mathrm{M}}} + \frac{1}{P_{\mathrm{D}}} \tag{67.29}$$

or reciprocally

$$R_{\Sigma} = R_{\mathrm{B}} + R_{\mathrm{M}} + R_{\mathrm{D}} \tag{67.30}$$

where P_{Σ} is the device-averaged mass transfer coefficient (or permeability) in cm/sec and R_{Σ} is the device-averaged resistance in sec/cm. DB can be estimated for many relevant conditions of geometry and flow using mass transport analysis based upon wall Sherwood numbers [Colton et al., 1971]. PM is best obtained by measurements employing special test fixtures in which boundary layer resistances are negligible or known [Klein et al., 1977]. PD is more problematic and is usually obtained by extrapolations based upon Wilson plots [Leonard and Bluemle, 1960]. Boundary layer theory, as well as technique for correlation, estimation, and prediction of the constituent mass transfer coefficients, is reviewed in detail by Colton and coworkers [1971] and Klein and coworkers [1977]. Overall solute transport is obtained from local flux by mass balance and integration; for the most common case of countercurrent flow

$$\Phi = (C_{Bi} - C_{Di}) \frac{Q_B}{A} \frac{\exp[(p_\Sigma A/Q_B)(1 - Q_B/Q_D)] - 1}{\exp[(P_\Sigma A/Q_B)(1 - Q_B/Q_D)] - Q_B/Q_D} \tag{67.31}$$

where C_{Bi} and C_{Di} represent inlet concentrations in the blood and dialysate streams in g/cm^3, A represents membrane surface area in cm^2, Q_B and Q_D are blood and dialysate flow rates in cm^3/min, and F and P_Σ are as defined in Equation 67.28 and Equation 67.29. Derivations of this relationship and similar expressions for cocurrent or crossflow geometries can be found in reviews by Colton and Lowrie [1981] and Gotch and colleagues [1972].

As pointed out by Lysaght and Baurmeister [1993], hemodialysis is a highly constrained process. Molecular diffusion is slow, and the driving forces are set by the body itself, decreasing in the course of purification and not amenable to extrinsic augmentation. The permeant toxic species are not to be recovered, and their concentrations are necessarily more dilute in the dialysate than in the incoming blood. The flow and gentle nature of dialysis has a special appeal for biologic applications, particularly when partial purification of the feed stream, rather than recovery of a product, is intended.

67.11 Membranes

Hemodialysis membranes vary in chemical composition, transport properties, and, as we will see later, biocompatibility. Hemodialysis membranes are fabricated from these classes of materials: regenerated cellulose, modified cellulose, and synthetics [Lysaght and Baurmeister, 1993]. Regenerated cellulose is most commonly prepared by the cuproamonium process and are macroscopically homogenous. These extremely hydrophilic structures sorb water, bind it tightly, and form a true hydrogel. Solute diffusion occurs through highly water-swollen amorphous regions in which the cellulose polymer chains are in constant random motion and would actually dissolve if they were not tied down by the presence of crystalline regions. Their principles advantage is low unit cost, complemented by the strength of the highly crystalline cellulose, which allows polymer films to be made very thin. These membranes provided effective small-solute transport in relatively small exchange devices. The drawbacks of regenerated cellulose are their limited capacity to transport middle molecules and the presence of labile nucleophilic groups which trigger complement activation and transient leukopenia during the first hour of exposure to blood. The advantages appear to outweigh the disadvantages, since over 70% of all hemodialyzers are still prepared from cellulosics, the most common of which is supplied by Akso Faser AG under the trade name Cuprophan.

A variety of other hydrophilic polymers account for 20% of total hemodialyzer production, including derivatized cellulose, such as cellulose acetate, diacetate, triacetate, and synthetic materials such as polycarbonate (PC), ethylenevinylalcohol (EVAL), and polyacrylonitrile-sodium methallyl sulfonate copolymer (PAN-SO3), which can all be fabricated into homogeneous films.

At the opposite end of the spectrum are membranes prepared from synthetic engineered thermoplastics, such as polysulfones, polyamides, and polyacylonitrile-polyvinylchloride copolymers. These hydrophobic materials, which account for about 10% of the hemodialyzer market, form asymmetric and anisotropic membranes with solid structures and open void spaces (unlike the highly mobile polymeric structure of regenerated cellulose). These membranes are characterized by a skin on one surface, typically a fraction of a micron thick, which contains very fine pores and constitutes the discriminating barrier determining the hydraulic permeability and solute retention properties of the membrane. The bulk of the membrane is composed of a spongy region, with interstices that cover a wide size range and with a structure ranging from open to closed cell foam. The primary purpose of the spongy region is to provide mechanical strength; the diffusive permeability of the membrane is usually determined by the properties of this matrix. As the convective and diffusive transport properties of these membranes are, to a large extent, associated independently with the properties of the skin and spongy matrix, respectively, it is possible to vary independently the convective and diffusive transport properties with these asymmetric structures. There is often a second skin on the other surface, usually much more open than the primary barrier. These materials are usually less activating to the complement cascade than are cellulosic membranes. The materials are also less restrictive to the transport of middle and large molecules. Drawbacks are increased cost and such high hydraulic permeability as to require special control mechanisms to avoid excess fluid loss and to raise concerns over the biologic quality of dialysate fluid because of the possibility of back filtration carrying pyrogenic substances to the blood stream.

The discovery of asymmetry membrane structures launched the modern era of membrane technology by motivating research on new membrane separation processes. Asymmetric membranes proved useful in ultrafiltration, and a variety of hydrophobic materials have been used including polysulfone (PS), polyacrylonitrile (PAN), its copolymer with polyvinylchloride (PVC), polyamide (PA), and polymethyl methacrylate (PMMA). PMMA does not form an obvious skin surface and should perhaps be placed in a class of its own.

67.12   Hemofiltration

Although low rates of ultrafiltration have been used routinely for water removal since the beginning of hemodialysis, the availability of membranes with very high hydraulic permeabilities led to radically new approaches to renal substitutive therapy. Such membranes allowed uniformly high clearance rates of solutes up to moderate molecular weights (several thousands) by the use of predominantly convective transport, thereby mimicking the separation capabilities of the natural kidney glomeruli. Progress in the development of this pressure-driven technique, which has come to be known as hemofiltration, has been reviewed by Henderson [1982], Lysaght [1986], and Ofsthum et al. [1986].

In ultrafiltration, the solute flux J_s (the rate of solute transport per unit membrane surface area) is equal to the product of the ultrafiltrate flux J_F (the ultrafiltrate flow rate per unit membrane surface area) and the solute concentration in the filtrate, c_F. In turn c_F is related to the retentate concentration C_R in the bulk solution above the membrane by the observed rejection coefficient R:

$$J_s = J_F c_F = J_F(1 - R)c_R \qquad (67.32)$$

Thus, knowledge of the ultrafiltrate flux and observed rejection coefficient permits prediction of the rate of solute removal.

With increasing transmembrane pressure difference, the ultrafiltrate flux increases and then levels off to a pressure-independent value. This behavior arises from the phenomenon of concentration polarization [Colton, 1987]. Macromolecules (e.g., proteins) that are too large to pass through the membrane build up in concentration in a region near the membrane surface. At steady state, the rate at which these rejected macromolecules are convected by the flow of fluid towards the membrane surface must be balanced by the rate of convective diffusion away from the surface. Estimation of the ultrafiltrate flux reduces largely to the problem of estimating the rate of back transport of macromolecules away from the membrane surface

$$J_F = k \ln \frac{c_{pw}}{c_{pb}} \qquad (67.33)$$

where k is the mass transfer coefficient for back transport of the rejected species, and c_{pw} and c_{pb} are the plasma concentrations of rejected species at the membrane surface and in the bulk plasma, respectively. Attainment of an asymptotic, pressure-independent flux is consistent with the concentration at the wall c_{pw} reaching a constant value. As with diffusive membrane permeability, solute rejection coefficients must be measured experimentally, since the available theoretical models and details of membrane structure are inadequate for prediction.

In hemofiltration the magnitude of the maximum clearance is determined by the blood and ultrafiltrate flow rates and whether the substitution fluid is added before or after filtration. Solutes with molecular weights up to several thousand are cleared at essentially the same rate in hemofiltration, whereas there is a monotonic decrease with increasing molecular weight in hemodialysis. If a comparison is made with devices of equal membrane surface area, it is generally found that hemodialysis provides superior clearance for low-molecular-weight solutes such as urea. The superiority of hemofiltration becomes apparent at molecular weights of several hundred.

Hemodialysis and hemofiltration represent two extremes with membranes having relatively low and relatively high hydraulic permeabilities, respectively. As a variety of new membranes became available with hydraulic permeabilities greater than that of regenerated cellulose, various groups began to examine new treatment modalities in which hemodialysis was combined with controlled rates of ultrafiltration which were higher than those employed in conventional hemodialysis but smaller than those used in hemofiltration [Funck-Brenato et al., 1972; Ota et al., 1975; Lowrie et al., 1978]. The advantage of such an approach is that it retains the high clearance capabilities of hemodialysis for low-molecular-weight solutes while adding enhanced clearance rates for the high-molecular-weight solutes characteristic of hemofiltration. A variety of systems is now commercially available and in clinical use, mainly in Europe and Japan. The proliferation of mixed-mode therapies has led to a panopoly of acronyms: hemodialysis (HD), hemofiltration (HF), high-flux dialysis (HFD), hemodiafiltration (HDF), biofiltration (BF), continuous arteriovenous hemofiltration (CAVH), **continuous arteriovenous hemodialysis** (CAVHD), slow continuous ultrafiltration (SCUF), simultaneous dialysis and ultrafiltration (SDUF), and so on.

Rigorous description of simultaneous diffusion and convection in artificial kidneys has not yet been carried out. Available analyses span a wide range of complexity and involve, to varying degrees, simplifying assumptions. Their predictions have not been systematically compared with experimental data. In view of the growing interest in various "high-flux" membranes and their application for enhanced solute removal rates and/or shortened treatment times, further refinement may be helpful.

67.13   Pharmacokinetics

Whereas the above analysis is founded on understanding the solute-removal capabilities of hemodialyzers, clinical application must also consider the limitations imposed by the transport of solute between body fluid compartments. The earliest physiologic models were produced by chemical engineers [Bell et al., 1965; Dedrick and Bischoff, 1968] using techniques which had been developed to describe the flow of material in complex chemical processes and were applied to the distribution of drugs and metabolites in biologic systems. This approach has progressively found its way into the management of uremia by hemodialysis [e.g., Farrell, 1983; Gotch and Sargent, 1983; Lowrie et al., 1976; Sargent et al., 1978].

Pharmacokinetics summarizes the relationships between solute generation, solute removal, and concentration in the patient's blood stream. It is most readily applied to urea as a surrogate for other uremic toxins in the quantitation of therapy and in attempts to define its adequacy. In the simplest case, the patient is assumed to have no residual renal function and to produce no urea during the relatively short periods of dialysis. Urea is generated in the body from the breakdown of dietary protein, which empirically has been found to approximate

$$G = 0.11I - 0.12 \qquad (67.34)$$

where G is the urea generation rate and I the protein intake (both in mg/min). If reliable measurements of I are not available, one assumes an intake of 1 g of protein per kilogram of body weight per day.

Urea accumulates in a single pool equivalent to the patient's total body water and is removed uniformly from that pool during hemodialysis. Mass balance yields the following differential equation:

$$\frac{\mathrm{d}(cV)}{\mathrm{d}t} = G - Kc \tag{67.35}$$

where c is the blood urea concentration (equal to total body water urea concentration) in mg/ml; V is the urea distribution volume in the patient in ml; G is the urea generation rate in mg/min; t is the time from onset of hemodialysis in minutes; and K is the urea clearance in ml/min. V can be measured by tritiated water dilution studies but is usually 58% of body weight. Generation is calculated from actual measurement or estimate of the patient's protein intake (each gram of protein consumed produces about 250 mg of urea). Therefore, a 70-kg patient, consuming a typical 1.0 g of protein per kilogram of body weight per day, would produce 28 g of urea distributed over a fluid volume of 40.6 l. In the absence of any clearance, urea concentration would increase by 70 mg/100 ml every 24 h. The reduction of urea concentration during hemodialysis is readily obtained from Equation 67.32 by neglecting intradialytic generation and changes in volume:

$$c^t = c^i \exp\left(\frac{Kt}{V}\right) \tag{67.36}$$

where c^i and c^t represent the urea concentrations in the blood at the beginning and during the course of treatment. A 3-1/2-h treatment of a 70-kg patient ($V = 40.6$ l) with a urea clearance of 200 ml/min would lead to a 64% reduction in urea concentration or a value of 0.36 for the c^t/c^i ratio. (This parameter almost always falls between 0.30 and 0.45.)

The increase in urea concentration between hemodialysis treatments is obtained from Equation 67.33, again assuming a constant V:

$$c^t = c^f + \frac{G}{V}t \tag{67.37}$$

where c^f is the urea concentration in the patient's blood at the end of the hemodialysis and c^t the concentration at time t during the intradialytic interval. Urea concentration typically increases by about 50 to 100 mg/100 ml/24 h. Even a small residual renal clearance will prove numerically significant. Therefore in oliguric patients who still exhibit a minimum of kidney function, one should use the slightly more complex equations given by Sargent and Gotch [1989] or Farrell [1988].

The exponential decay constant in Equation 67.33, Kt/v, expresses the net normalized quantity of hemodialysis therapy received by a uremic patient. It is calculated simply by multiplying the urea clearance of the dialyzer (in ml/min) by the duration of hemodialysis (in min) and dividing by the distribution volume (in ml) which in the absence of a better estimate is taken as 0.58 times body weight. Gotch and Sargent [1983] first recognized that this parameter provides an index of the adequacy of hemodialysis. Based upon a retrospective analysis of various therapy formats, they suggested a value of 1.0 or greater as representing an adequate amount of hemodialysis for most patients. Although not immune to criticism, this approach has found widespread clinical acceptance and represents the current prescriptive norm in hemodialysis therapy.

TABLE 67.1 Uremic Syndrome under Dialysis

Adverse effects of uremia can be attributed to:

1. Retention of solutes normally degraded or excreted by the kidneys
2. Overhydration associated with inadequate balance between fluid intake and water removal
3. Absence of factors normally synthesized by the kidneys
4. Pathophysiologic response to the decline in renal function on the part of other organ systems
5. Pathologic response of the organism to repeated exposure to damaging procedures and foreign materials

TABLE 67.2   Uremic Solutes with Potential Toxicity

Urea	Middle molecule
Guanidines	Ammonia
Methylguanidine	Alkaloids
Guanidine	Trace metals (e.g., bromine)
β-Guanidinipropionic acid	Uric acid
Guanidinosuccinic acid	Cyclic AMP
Gamma-guanidinobutyric acid	Amino acids
Taurocyanine	Myoinositol
Creatinine	Mannitol
Creatine	Oxalate
Arginic acid	Glucuronate
Homoarginine	Glycols
N-a-acetylarginine	Lysozyme
Phenols	Hormones
O-cresol	Parathormone
P-cresol	Natriuretic factor
Benzylalcohol	Glucagon
Phenol	Growth hormone
Tyrosine	Gastrin
Phenolic acids	Prolactin
P-hydroxyphenylacetic acid	Catecholamines
β-(m Hydroxyphenyl)-	Xanthine
hydracrylic acid	Hypoxanthine
Hippurates	Furanpropionic acid
p-(OH)hippuric acid	Amines
o-(OH)hippuric acid	Putrescine
Hippuric acid	Spermine
Benzoates	Spermidine
Polypeptides	Dimethylamine
$β_2$-Microglobulin	Polyamines
Indoles	Endorphins
Indol-3-acetic acid	Pseudouridine
Indoxyl sulfate	Potassium
5-Hydroxyindol acetic acid	Phosphorus
Indo-3-acrylic acid	Calcium
5-Hydroxytryptophol	Sodium
N-acetyltryptophan	Water
Tryptophan	Cyanides

67.14   Adequacy of Dialysis

As outlined in Table 67.1, the uremic syndrome under dialysis is more complex than observed in ESRD before the institution of treatment. The pathology observed not only is related to insufficient removal of toxic solutes but also comprises some unavoidable adverse effects of extracorporeal blood processing, including the interactions of blood with foreign materials [Colton et al., 1994]. The attenuation of uremic syndrome symptoms by protein restriction in the patient's diet and by various dialytic procedures underscores the combined roles of retention, removal, and metabolism in the constellation of signs of the disease. Toxicity may result from the synergism of the entire spectrum of accumulated molecules, which is surprisingly large (see Table 67.2 and Vanholder and Ringoir [1992]). The uremic syndrome resembles complex forms of systemic poisoning and is characterized by multiple symptoms and side effects. Survival requires that the toxins be removed, and survival quality depends on the quantity of toxins that are actually eliminated. Ideally, one would like to clean blood and body fluids to the same extent as is achieved by normal renal function. This is possible with an organ transplant that works without interruption but is only asymptotically approached with intermittent dialysis.

TABLE 67.3   Factors Influencing Solute Concentration in Dialyzed Patients

Solute-related factors	Patient-related factors
Compartmental distribution	Body weight
Intracellular concentration	Distribution volume
Resistance of cell membrane	Intake and generation of solutes metabolic precursors
Protein binding	Residual renal function
Electrostatic charge	Quality of vascular access
Steric configuration	Absorption from the intestine
Molecular weight	Hematocrit
Dialysis-related factors	Blood viscosity
Dialysis duration	Absorption of solutes on the membrane, on other parts of the circuit
Interdialytic intervals	Ultrafiltration rate
Blood flow	Intradialytic changes in efficiacy
Mean blood flow	Changes with indirect effect on solute-related factors
Blood flow pattern	Blood pH
Concentration gradients	Heparinization
Dialysate flow	Free fatty acid concentration
Dialyzer surface	
Dialyzer volume	
Dialyzer membrane resistance	
Dialyzer pore size	

There is a compelling need for objective definition of the adequacy of ESRD treatment: How much removal in how much time is necessary for each individual? The answer is indirect and approximate. Some define adequacy of dialysis by clinical assessment of patient well-being. More sophisticated procedures, such as electromyography, electroencephalography, and neuropsychologic tests, may refine the clinician's perception of inadequate dialysis. Yet inadequate therapy can remain unrecognized when therapeutic decisions are based exclusively on clinical parameters. The inverse is also true, and follow-up of dialysis adequacy should never be restricted to static markers of toxicity or dynamic biochemical parameters such as clearance, kinetic modeling, and the like.

Most patients undergoing dialysis do not work or function as healthy people do, and often their physical activity and employment status does not go beyond the level of taking care of themselves. In many centers, the best patients in a hemodialysis program are selectively removed for transplantation. Hospitalization rate is an approximate index of dialysis inadequacy. About 25% of all hospitalizations are due to vascular access problems. Comparison among centers may be difficult, however, because of differences in local conditions for hospital admission. Vanholder and Ringoir [1992] have attempted to relate the adequacy of dialysis to the relevant solute concentrations in blood and distinguish among solute-related factors, patient-related factors, and dialysis-related factors (Table 67.3). Their analysis constitutes a useful point of departure for adjusting the quantity of dialysis to the specific needs of an individual patient, which is a complex problem, since it requires not only an appreciation of what the removal process can do, but also of the generation rate of metabolic end products (related to nutrition, physical activity, fever, etc.) and the dietary load of water and electrolytes. Dialysis patients are partially rehabilitated, but their condition rarely compares to that of recipients of a successful renal transplant.

67.15   Outlook

The treatment of chronic renal failure by artificial kidney dialysis represents one of the most common, and certainly the most expensive, component of substitutive medicine. From an industrial viewpoint, 500,000 patients each "consuming" perhaps 100 hemodialysis filters per year (allowing for some reuse from the 150 units per year that would be needed for 3 times per week treatment) means a production of 50 million filters. With each unit selling for an approximate price of $15, the world market is on the order of $750 million. From a public health viewpoint, if one is to take the U.S. figure of

$30,000 for the world average annual cost of a single dialysis patient, the aggregate economic impact of the medical application of hemodialysis approaches $15 billion a year (of which <10% is spent on the purchase of technology; health care personnel costs are the most expensive component of the treatment).

Yet "maintenance dialysis on the whole is non-physiological and can be justified only because of the finiteness of its alternative" [Burton, 1976]. Dialytic removal remains nonspecific, with toxic as well as useful compounds eliminated indiscriminately. A better definition of disturbed metabolic pathways will be necessary to formulate treatment hypotheses and design adapted equipment. Sensors for on-line monitoring of appropriate markers may also help to evaluate the modeling of clearance processes. The confusing interference of interactions between the patient and the foreign materials in the dialysis circuit may be reduced as more compatible materials become available. A better clinical condition of the ESRD patient remains the ultimate goal of dialysis therapy because at the moment it seems unlikely that either preventative measures or organ transplantation will reduce the number of patients whose lives depend on the artificial kidney.

Defining Terms

Arteriovenous fistula: A permanent communication between an artery and an adjacent vein, created surgically, leading to the formation of a dilated vein segment which can be punctured transcutaneously with large bore needles so as to allow connecting the circulatory system with an extracorporeal blood processing unit.

Artificial kidney: A blood purification device based on the removal of toxic substances through semipermeable membranes washed out by an acceptor solution which can safely be discarded.

Blood urea nitrogen (BUN): The concentration of urea in blood, expressed as the nitrogen content of the urea (BUN is actually 0.47 times, or approximately half, the urea concentration).

Boundary layer: The region of fluid adjacent to a permeable membrane, across which virtually all (99%) of the concentration change within the fluid occurs.

Catheter: A tube used to infuse a fluid in or out of the vascular system or a body cavity.

Clearance: A measure of the rate of mass removal expressed as the volume of blood which per unit of time is totally cleared of a substance through processing in a natural or artificial kidney. Clearance has the dimensions of a flow rate and can be defined only in relation to a specific solute. Clearance can also be viewed as the minimal volume flow rate of blood which would have to be presented to a processing device to provide the amount actually recovered in the urine or the dialysate if extraction of that material from blood were complete. Clearance is measured as the mass transfer rate of a substance divided by the blood concentration of that substance.

Continuous ambulatory peritoneal dialysis: A modality of peritoneal dialysis in which uninterrupted — although not evenly effective — treatment is provided by 4 to 6 daily cycles of filling and emptying the peritoneal cavity with a prepared dialysate solution. Solute removal relies on diffusive equalization with molecular species present in capillary blood. Water removal relies on the use of hyperosmotic dialysate.

Continuous arteriovenous hemodialysis: A dialytic procedure in which blood, propelled either by arterial pressure or by a pump, flows continuously at a low flow rate through a dialyzer, from where it returns to a vein, providing for uninterrupted solute and fluid removal and nearly constant equilibration of body fluids with the dialysate solution.

Dialysate: A buffered electrolyte solution, usually containing glucose at or above physiologic concentration, circulated through the water compartment of a hemodialyzer to control diffusional transport of small molecules across the membranes and achieve the blood concentrations desired.

Dialysis: A membrane separation process in which one or more dissolved molecular species diffuse across a selective barrier in response to a difference in concentration.

Dwell time: The duration of exposure of a solution used to draw waste products and excessive water out of the blood during peritoneal dialysis.

ESRD: End-stage renal disease.

Glomerular filtration rate: The volume of plasma water, or primary urine, filtered in the glomerulus per unit of time. Measured, for instance, by creatinine clearance, it expresses the level of remaining renal function in end-stage renal disease.

Hemodiafiltration: Removal of water and solutes by a combination of diffusive and convective transport (paired filtration-dialysis) across a dialysis membrane to achieve effective transport of small and middle molecules. To compensate for the water loss, a large volume of saline or balanced electrolyte solution must be infused in the blood circuit to prevent hemoconcentration.

Hemodialysis: A modality of extracorporeal blood purification in which blood is continuously circulated in contact with a permeable membrane, while a large volume of balanced electrolyte solution circulates on the other side of the membrane. Diffusion of dissolved substances from one stream to the other removes molecules that are in excess in the blood and replaces those for which there is a deficiency. Increased removal can be achieved by increasing the duration of the procedure, the overall membrane area, or the membrane permeability.

Hemofiltration: Removal of water and solutes by convective transport, controlled by a large hydrostatic pressure difference between blood and a liquid compartment across a large-pore, high-water-flux membrane.

Membrane: A thin film of natural or synthetic polymer which allows the passage of dissolved molecules and solvents in response to a concentration or pressure difference (diffusion or filtration) across the polymer.

Middle molecules: Molecules of intermediate molecular weight (roughly of 1000 to 30,000 Da) which are presumed to be responsible for the toxic manifestations of end-stage renal disease and therefore should be eliminated by substitutive therapy.

Peritoneal dialysis: A process in which metabolic waste products, toxic substances, and excess body water are removed through a membranelike tissue that lines the internal abdominal wall and the organs in the abdominal cavity.

Permeability: The ability of a membrane to allow the passage of certain molecules while maintaining a physical separation between two adjacent phases.

Permselectivity: The property of a membrane whereby a differential rate of molecular transport between two phases is achieved based on characteristics such as molecular weight, molecular size, degree of hydration, affinity for membrane material, and electric charge. The most common feature leading to permselectivity is membrane pore size.

Residual renal clearance: The small level of renal function (measured as creatinine clearance by the diseased kidneys) remaining in some patients in end-stage renal disease, particularly in the early years of dialytic treatment.

Ultrafiltration: The process whereby plasma water flows through a membrane in response to a hydrostatic pressure gradient, dragging with it solute molecules at concentrations equal or lower to that prevailing in plasma.

Uremia: A condition in which the urea concentration in blood is chronically elevated, reflecting an inability to remove from the body the end products of protein metabolism.

Uremic toxins: Partly unidentified and presumably toxic substances appearing in the blood of patients in end-stage renal failure, which can be eliminated to a variable extent by chemical processing of body fluids.

References

Abel J.J., Rowntree L.G., and Turner B.B. 1913. On the removal of diffusible substances from the circulating blood by means of dialysis. *Trans. Assoc. Am. Phys.* 28: 50.

Babb A.L., Maurer C.J., Fry D.L. et al. 1968. The determination of membrane permeabilities and solute diffusivities with application to hemodialysis. *Chem. Eng. Prog. Symp. Ser* 63: 59.

Brunner H. and Mann H. 1985. What remains of the "middle molecule" hypothesis today? *Contr. Nephrol.* 44: 14.

Burton B.J. 1976. Overview of end stage renal disease. *J. Dial.* 1: 1.

Chenoweth D.E. 1984. Complement activation during hemodialysis: clinical observations, proposed mechanisms and theoretical implications. *Artif. Organs.* 8: 281.

Colton C.K. 1987a. Analysis of membrane processes for blood purification. *Blood Purif.* 2: 202.

Colton C.K. 1987b. Technical foundations of renal prostheses. In H.G. Gurland (ed.), *Uremia Therapy*, pp. 187–217, Berlin, Heidelberg; Springer Verlag.

Colton C.K., Smith K.A., Merril E.W. et al. 1971. Permeability studies with cellulosic membranes. *J. Biomed. Mat. Res.* 5: 459.

Colton C.K., Ward R.A., and Shaldon S. 1994. Scientific basis for assessment of biocompatibility in extracorporeal blood treatment. *J. Nephol. Dial. Transplant.* 9 (Suppl 2): 11.

Dedrick R.A. and Bischoff K.B. 1968. Pharmacokinetics in applications of the artificial kidney. *Chem. Eng. Prog. Ser.* 64: 32.

Gotch F.A., Autian J., Colton C.K. et al. 1972. The Evaluation of Hemodialyzers, Washington, DC, Department of Health, Education and Welfare Publ. No. NIH-72-103.

Gotch F.A., Sargent J.A., Keen M.L. et al. 1974. Individualized, quantified dialysis therapy of uremia. *Proc. Clin. Dial. Trans. Forum* 4: 27.

Jaffrin M.Y., Butruille Y., Granger A., et al. 1978. Factors governing hemofiltration (HF) in a parallel plate exchanger with highly permeable membranes. *Trans. Am. Soc. Artif. Intern. Organs.* 24: 448.

Jaffrin M.Y., Gupta B.B., and Malbraneq J.M. 1981. A one-dimensional model of simultaneous hemodialysis and ultrafiltration with highly permeable membranes. *J. Biomech. Eng.* 103: 261.

Kedem O. and Katchalsky A. 1958. Thermodynamic analysis of the permeability of biological membranes to nonelectrolytes. *Biochim. Biophys. Acta* 27: 229.

Kiil F. 1960. Development of a parallel flow artificial kidney in plastics. *Acta. Chir. Scand.* (Suppl) 253: 143.

Klein E., Holland F.F., Donnaud A. et al. 1977. Diffusive and hydraulic permeabilities of commercially available cellulosic hemodialysis films and hollow fibers. *J. Membr. Sci.* 2: 349–364.

Leonard E.F. and Bluemle L.W. 1960. The permeability concept as applied to dialysis. *Trans. Am. Soc. Artif. Intern. Organs* 6: 33.

Lysaght M.J., Colton C.K., Ford C.A. et al. 1978. Mass transfer in clinical blood ultrafiltration devices — a review. In T.H. Frost (ed.), *Technical Aspects of Renal Dialysis*, pp. 81–95, London, Pittman Medical.

Michaels A.S. 1966. Operating parameters and performance criteria for hemodialyzers and other membrane separation devices. *Trans. Am. Soc. Artif. Intern. Organs* 12: 387.

Quinton W., Dillard D., and Scribner B.H. 1960. Cannulation of blood vessels for prolonged hemodialysis. *Trans. Am. Soc. Artif. Intern. Organs* 6: 104.

Renkin E.M. 1956. The relationship between dialysance, membrane area, permeability, and blood flow in the artificial kidney. *Trans. Am. Soc. Artif. Intern. Organs* 2: 102.

Sargent J.A., Gotch F.A., Borah M. et al. 1978. Urea kinetics: a guide to nutritional management of renal failure. *Am. J. Clin. Nutr.* 31: 1692.

Solomon B.A., Castino F., Lysaght M.J. et al. 1978. Continuous flow membrane filtration of plasma from whole blood. *Trans. Am. Soc. Artif. Intern. Organs* 24: 21.

Vanholder R., Hsu C., and Ringoir S. 1993. Biochemical definition of the uremic syndrome and possible therapeutic implications. *Artif. Organs* 17: 234.

Vanholder R. and Ringoir S. 1992. Adequacy of dialysis, a critical analysis. *Kidney Int.* 42: 540.

Vanholder R.C., De Smet R.V., and Ringoir S.M. 1992. Validity of urea and other "uremic markers" for dialysis quantification. *Clin. Chem.* 38: 1429.

Wilson E.E. 1915. A basis for rational design of heat transfer apparatus. *Trans. Am. Soc. Mech. Eng.* 37: 47.

Further Information

An extensive review of renal pathophysiology is to be found in B.M. Brenner and F.C. Rector, Eds., *The Kidney*, 3rd ed., Saunders Publishing Co., Philadelphia PA, 1986. Two volumes addressing the clinical aspects of dialysis are A.R. Nissanson, R. Fine, and D. Gentile, *Clinical Dialysis*, Appleton Lange Century Crofts, Norwalk, 1984; and H.J. Gurland, Ed., *Uremia Therapy*, Springer-Verlag, Berlin, 1987. The principles of designs and functions of dialysis therapy are outlined in P.C. Farrel, *Dialysis Kinetics, ASAIO Primers in Artificial Organs*, vol. 4, J.B. Lippincott, Philadelphia, PA, 1988; and J.F. Maher, *Replacement of Renal Function of Dialysis*, 3rd ed., Klumer, Boston, 1989. Recent reviews of specific aspects in the operation of artificial kidneys are C.K. Colton, "Analysis of Membrane Processes for Blood Purification," *Blood Purification* 5: 202–51, 1987; C.K. Colton and E.G. Lowrie, "Hemodialysis Physical Principles and Technical Considerations," in B.M. Brenner and F.C. Rector, Jr., Eds., *The Kidney*, 2nd ed., vol 2, Saunders, Philadelphia, PA; and C.K. Colton, R.A. Ward, and S. Shaldon, "Scientific Basis for Assessment of Biocompatibility in Extracorporeal Blood Treatment," *Nephrology Dialysis, Transplantation*, 9(Suppl. 2): 11, 1994.

Ongoing contributions to the field of artificial kidney therapy are often found in biomaterials journals (e.g., the *Journal of Biomaterials Research*) and in artificial organ publications (e.g., the *Transactions of the American Society for Artificial Organs*, the *ASAIO Journal*, the *International Journal of Artificial Organs*, and *Artificial Organs*). Clinical contributions can be found in Kidney International, Nephron, and Blood Purification.

68

Peritoneal Dialysis Equipment

Michael J. Lysaght
Brown University

John Moran
Vasca Inc.

Irreversible end-stage kidney disease occurs with an annual frequency of about 1 in 5,000 to 10,000 in general population, and this rate is increasing. Until the 1960s, such disease was universally fatal. In the last four decades various interventions have been developed and implemented for preserving life after loss of all or most of a patient's own kidney function. **Continuous ambulatory peritoneal dialysis (CAPD)**, the newest and most rapidly growing of renal replacement therapies, is one such process in which metabolic waste products, electrolytes, and water are removed through the **peritoneum**, an intricate *membrane* like tissue that lines the abdominal cavity and covers the liver, intestine, and other internal organs. This review begins with a brief summary of the development of CAPD and its role in the treatment of contemporary renal failure. The therapy format and its capacity for solute removal are then described in detail. Bioengineering studies of peritoneal transport, in which the peritoneum is described in terms analogous to the mass transfer properties of a planar membrane separating well-mixed pools of blood and dialysate, are then reviewed. The transport properties of the equivalent peritoneal membrane are summarized and compared to those of **hemodialysis** membranes. Mode's to describe and predict fluid and solute removal rates are examined. Finally, current developments and emerging trends are summarized.

The early history of peritoneal dialysis, as reviewed by Boen [1985], is contemporaneous with that of hemodialysis (HD). Small-animal experiments were reported in the 1920s and 1930s in the United States and Germany. Earliest clinical trials in acute reversible cases of kidney failure began in the late 1930s in the form of a continuous "lavage" in which dialysate was continuously infused and withdrawn from dual trochar access sites. Acute treatments were continued through the 1940s, and about 100 case reports appeared in the literature by 1950; sequential inflow, dwell, and withdrawal was increasingly favored over continuous flow. Chronic therapy was introduced in the early 1960s, followed shortly by indwelling peritoneal catheters. From 1960 onward, peritoneal dialysis clearly lagged behind HD, as the latter became more streamlined, efficient, and cost-effective. Although endorsed by a small group of enthusiasts and

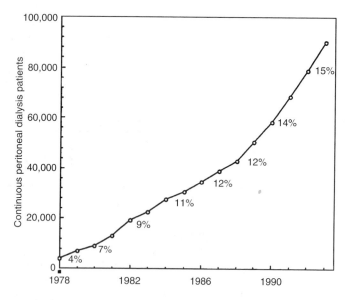

FIGURE 68.1   The growth of peritoneal dialysis. Line and points refer to the total estimated worldwide peritoneal dialysis population; the numbers adjacent to the points are PD patients as a percent of total dialysis population. At the end of 1993, 14,000 of the 90,000 peritoneal dialysis patients utilized some version of APD; the remainder were treated with CAPD. Data compiled taken from various patient registries and industrial sources.

proponents, peritoneal dialysis had evolved into a specialized or niche therapy. This changed dramatically in 1976 when Popovich, a biomedical engineer, and Moncrief, a clinical nephrologist, announced the development of a new form of peritoneal dialysis in which ambulatory patients were continuously treated by two liters of dialysis dwelling in the **peritoneal cavity** and exchanged four times daily [Popovich et al., 1976]. Two years later Baxter began to offer CAPD fluid in flexible plastic containers, along with necessary ancillary equipment and supplies. The rapid subsequent growth of the process is tabulated in Figure 68.1. At this writing, approximately 90,000 patients are treated by CAPD (vs. 490,000 by HD and 130,000 with kidney transplants). A more recent development is the introduction of **automated peritoneal dialysis (APD)**, in which all fluid exchanges are performed by a simple pump console, usually while the patient sleeps. About one peritoneal dialysis patient in six now receives some form of APD; this approach is discussed more fully in a later section on emerging developments.

   Both CAPD and HD have advantages and disadvantages, and neither therapy is likely to prove better for all the patients all the time. The principal attraction of CAPD is that it frees the patient from the pervasive life-style invasions associated with thrice weekly in-center HD. CAPD is particularly popular with patients living in rural areas distant from a hemodialysis treatment center. The continuous nature of CAPD eliminates fluctuations in the concentrations of uremic metabolites and avoids the sawtooth pattern of hemodialysis peak toxin concentrations. Fluid and dietary constraints are less restrictive for patients on CAPD than those on HD. A major complication of CAPD is peritonitis. The rate of peritonitis was initially around 2 episodes per patient year; this has fallen to fewer than 0.5 episodes per patient year due to advances in administration set design and use. The morbidity of peritonitis has also decreased with increased experience in its treatment. In most cases, detected early and treated promptly, peritonitis can be managed without requiring hospitalization. Peritonitis caused by certain organisms including *Staphylococcus aureus*, Pseudomonas, and fungi remains a clinical problem. Other drawbacks of CAPD include the daily transperitoneal administration of 100 to 150 g of glucose providing ~600 calories, and the tedium of the exchanges. APD and new solution formulations are being developed to address both issues. Little doubt now exists that risk-adjusted survival and morbidity for patients treated by CAPD is equivalent to that for patients treated with HD. On balance, the therapy seems well suited to many patients, and it continues to grow more rapidly than alternative treatment modalities.

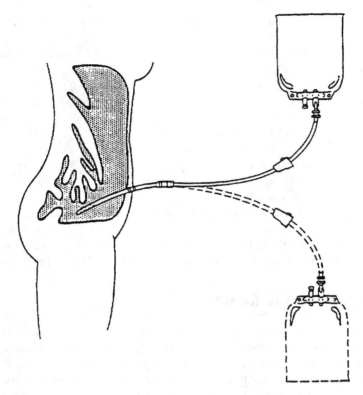

FIGURE 68.2 Illustration of the three steps involved in a single CAPD exchange fluid infusion, dwell, and drain. Some administration sets require the bag to stay connected during dwell (it is rolled and fits in a girdle around the waist); others allow it to be disconnected. Drain and infusion take about 10 min each; three daytime dwells are 4–6 h each; the overnight dwell lasts 8–10 h.

68.1 Therapy Format

The process of CAPD is technically simple. Approximately 2 l of a sterile, nonpyrogenic, and hypertonic solution of glucose and electrolyte are instilled via gravity flow into the peritoneal cavity through an indwelling catheter 4 times per day. A single exchange is illustrated in Figure 68.2. Intraperitoneal fluid partially equilibrates with solutes in the plasma, and plasma water is ultrafiltered due to osmotic gradients. After 4–5 h, except at night where the exchange is lengthened to 9–11 h to accommodate sleep, the peritoneal fluid is drained and the process repeated. Patients perform the exchanges themselves in 20–30 min, at home or in the work environment after a training cycle which lasts only 1–2 weeks. In APD, 10–15 l are automatically exchanged overnight; 2 l remain in the peritoneal cavity during the day for a "long dwell" exchange.

As will be discussed in more detail below, the drained fluid contains solute at concentrations around 90–100% of plasma for urea, 65–70% for creatinine, and 15–25% for inulin and β_2 microglobulin. Net fluid removal ranges up to 1000 ml per exchange. CAPD generally removes the same quantity of toxins and fluid as HD (a little thought will show that this is a requirement of steady state, provided that generation is unaltered between the two treatment formats); however, CAPD requires a higher plasma concentration as the driving force for this removal. Steady-state concentrations during CAPD are typically close to the peak, that is, pretreatment, concentrations of small solutes during HD but much lower than the corresponding peaks for larger species.

Access to the peritoneum is usually via a double-cuff Tenchkhoff catheter, essentially a 50–100 cm length of silicone tubing with side holes at the internal end, a Dacron mesh flange at the skin line, and connector fittings at the end of the exposed end. Several variations have evolved, but little hard evidence supports the selection of one design format over another [Dratwa et al., 1986]. Most are implanted in a routine surgical procedure requiring about 1 h and are allowed to heal for 1–2 weeks prior to routine clinical use. Sterile and nonpyrogenic fluid is supplied in 2-l containers fabricated from dioctyl phthalate plasticized polyvinyl chloride. The formulation is essentially potassium-free lactated Ringers to which has been added from 15 to 42.5 g/l of glucose (dextrose monohydrate). The solution is buffered to a pH of 5.1–5.5, since the glucose would caramelize during autoclaving at higher pH levels. Several different exchange protocols are in use. In the original design, the patient simply rolls up the empty bag after instillation and then drains into the same bag following exchange. The bag filled with drain fluid is disconnected and a fresh bag is reconnected. Patients are trained to use aseptic technique to perform the connect and disconnect. Many ingenious aids were developed to assist in minimizing breaches of sterility including enclosed ultraviolet-sterilized chambers and heat splicers. More recent approaches, known as the "O" set and "Y" set or more generically as "flush before fill" disconnect, invoke more complex tubing sets to allow the administration set to be flushed (often with antiseptic) prior to installation of dialysate and generally permit the patient to disconnect the empty bag during the dwell phase. Initial reports of the success of the protocols in reducing peritonitis were regarded with skepticism, but definite improvement over earlier systems has now been documented in a well-designed and carefully controlled clinical trials [Churchill et al., 1989].

68.2   Fluid and Solute Removal

The rate at which solutes are removed during peritoneal dialysis depends primarily upon the rate of equilibration between blood and instilled peritoneal fluid. This is usually quantified as the ratio of dialysate to plasma concentration as a function of dwell time, often in graphs called simply "D over P" (dialysate over plasma) curves. A typical plot of dialysate-to-plasma ratio for solutes of various molecular weight is given in Figure 68.3. Smaller species equilibrate more rapidly than do larger ones, because **diffusion** coefficient varies in inverse proportion to the square root of a solute's molecular weight. Dialysate equilibrium rates vary considerably from patient to patient; error bars on the plot represent standard error of the mean for duplicate determinations with five patients.

The rate of mass removal during dialysis, ϕ, is simply the volume of fluid, V_D, removed from the peritoneal cavity at the end of a dwell period lasting time t, multiplied by the concentration C_D of the solute in the removed fluid

$$\phi = V_D C_D \tag{68.1}$$

The whole blood **clearance**, Cl, is the rate of mass removal divided by the solute concentration in blood C_B

$$Cl = \frac{\phi}{t C_B} = \frac{V_D C_D}{t C_B} \tag{68.2}$$

In Equation 68.1 and Equation 68.2, time conventionally is reported in minutes, volume in milliliters, and concentration in any consistent units. Equation 68.1 and Equation 68.2 are based on mass balances; they are thus general and unaffected by the complexity of underlying phenomena such as bidirectional selective connective transport and lymphatic uptake. Equation 68.2 requires that solute concentration in the denominator be reported as whole blood concentration, rather than as plasma concentration, which is often reported clinically. With many small solutes (urea, creatinine, and uric acid), only small error is introduced by considering blood and plasma concentration as interchangeable. With larger solutes, especially those excluded from the red blood cell, care must be taken to correct for differences in plasma and blood concentrations.

Since urea is nearly completely equilibrated during CAPD, that is, $c_D/c_B =\sim 1.0$, urea clearance is commonly equated with total drainage volume. Four 2-l exchanges and 2 l of ultrafiltration would thus result in a continuous urea clearance of 10 l/day or $\sim$7 ml/min. The situation is more complex with APD, which involves several (4 to 6) short exchanges at partial equilibrium and one very long exchange. In any case, no meaningful direct or a priori comparison of clearance with hemodialysis is possible because one therapy is intermittent and the other continuous.

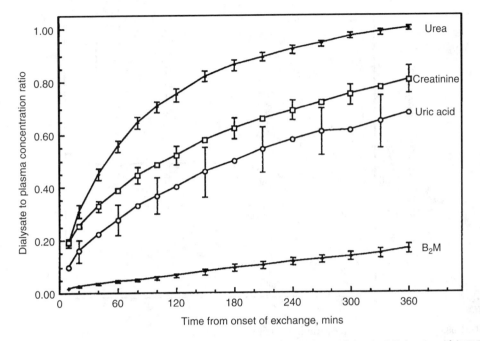

FIGURE 68.3 Ratio of plasma to dialysate concentration for urea (60 Da), creatinine (113 Da), uric acid (158 Da), and β_2 microglobulin ($\sim$12,000 Da). Data were obtained by withdrawing and analyzing a sample of dialysate at each time point and comparing it to plasma concentration. Each point is the average of two determinations on five patients. Error bars are standard error of the mean [Lysaght, 1989].

The volume of fluid in the peritoneal cavity increases during an exchange but at a decreasing rate. The driving force for fluid transfer from the blood to the peritoneal cavity is the osmotic pressure of the glucose in the infused dialysate. Typical CAPD solutions contain $\sim$1.5, $\sim$2.5, or $\sim$4.25 by weight of glucose monohydrate, leading to an initial maximum osmotic force (across an ideally semipermeable membrane) of approximately 1000–5000 mmHg. In the first few minutes of an exchange, the rate of ultrafiltration may be as high as 10–30 ml/min. The driving force rapidly dissipates as glucose diffuses from the peritoneal cavity into the bloodstream. After the first hour, rates of 1.0–2.0 ml/min are common. Throughout the exchange, the peritoneal lymphatics are draining fluid from the peritoneal cavity at a rate of 0.5–2.0 ml/min. Fluid balance is thus the difference between removal by a time-dependent rate of ultrafiltration and return via a more constant lymphatic drainage. Net fluid removal is very easily determined in the clinical setting simply by comparing the weight of fluid drained to that instilled. Instantaneous rates of ultrafiltration may be estimated in study protocols by a series of tedious mass balances around high-molecular-weight radiolabled markers added to the dialysate fluid. The results of a typical study are plotted in Figure 68.4 and Figure 68.5 showing both the instantaneous rate of ultrafiltration and the net intraperitoneal volume as a function of time. On average, these patients removed 500 ml of fluid in a single 6-h exchange or roughly 2 l/day, which permits far more liberal fluid intake than is possible with patients on HD. But here again patient variation is high. Commercial CAPD fluid is available in a variety of solute concentrations; physicians base their prescription for a particular patient on his or her fluid intake and residual urine volume.

68.3 The Peritoneal Membrane: Physiology and Transport Properties

In contrast to synthetic membranes employed during HD, the peritoneum is not a simple selective barrier between two phases. As implied by its Latin root (peritonere = to stretch tightly around), the primary

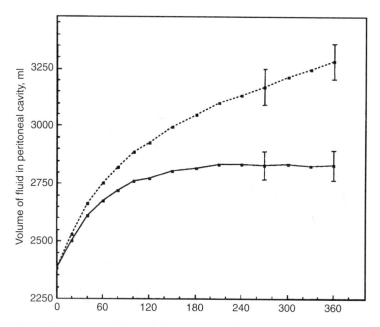

FIGURE 68.4 Volume of fluid in the peritoneal cavity vs. time during an exchange with ~2.5% glucose dialysis fluid. Solid line is actual volume. Dotted line represents estimate of the volume in the absence of lymphatic flow. Results represent an average of duplicate determinations on five patients. Volume was estimated by dilution of radiolabeled tracers (too large to diffuse across the peritoneal membrane) added to dialysate prior to installation; lymphatic flow was calculated from a mass balance on net recovered marker. Each point is the average of two determinations on five patients. Error bars are standard error of the mean [Lysaght, 1989].

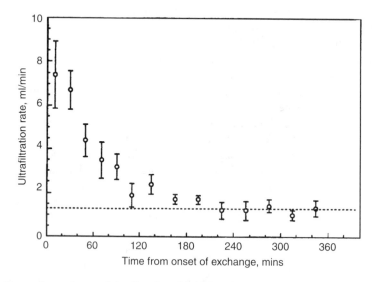

FIGURE 68.5 Comparisons of rates of ultrafiltration of fluid into the peritoneal cavity (open circles) and lymphatic drainage of fluid from the peritoneal cavity back to the patient (dotted line). Same study and methods as in Figure 68.4.

physiologic function of the peritoneum is to line the walls of the abdominal cavity and encapsulate its internal organs (stomach, liver, spleen, pancreas, and parts of the intestine). Most CAPD literature, including this review, uses the terms peritoneum and peritoneal membrane interchangeably and conveniently extends both expressions to include underlying and connective tissue. Overall adult peritoneal surface is approximately 1.75 ± 0.5 m^2, which generally is considered equal on an individual basis to skin surface area.

The peritoneum is not physically homogenous. The visceral portion (~80%) covering the internal organs differs somewhat from the parietal portion overlaying the abdominal walls, which in turn is different from the folded or pleated mesentery connecting the two.

The physiology of the peritoneum, its normal ultastructure, and variations induced by CAPD have been increasingly elucidated over the past decade. Morphologically, the peritoneum is a smooth, tough, somewhat translucent sheath. Its thickness ranges from under 200 to over 1000 μm. The topmost layer, which presents to the dialysate during CAPD, is formed from a single layer of mesothelial cells, densely covered by microvilli (hairlike projections), although the latter tend to disappear gradually during the first few weeks of CAPD. Immediately underneath is the interstitium, a thick sheath of dense mucopolysaccharide hydrogel interlaced with collagenous fibers, microfibrillar structures, fibroblasts, adipocytes, and granular material. Most important for CAPD, the interstitium is perfused with a network of capillaries through which blood flows from the mesenteric arteries and the vasculature of the abdominal wall to the portal and systemic venous circulations. Blood-flow rate has been estimated to be in the range of 30 to 60 ml/min, but this is not well established. The interstitial layer is a hydrogel; its water content, and thus its transport properties, will vary in response to the osmolarity of the peritoneal dialysate.

Peritoneal mass transfer characteristics are most commonly obtained by back-calculating basic membrane properties from results in standard or modified peritoneal dialysis. Three membrane parameters will be described: Lp, the hydraulic permeability; R, the rejection coefficient; and K_0A, the **mass transfer coefficient** (=area A × diffusive permeability K_0). The formal definitions of these parameters are given in Equation 68.3 through Equation 68.5, with R and K_0A defined for the limiting conditions of pure convection and pure diffusion.

$$Lp = \frac{\text{Filtration rate}}{\text{Area} \cdot \text{pressure driving force}} = \frac{J_F}{A(\Delta P - \Sigma\sigma_i\Pi_i)} \tag{68.3}$$

$$R = 1 - \frac{\text{Concentration in bulk filtrate}}{\text{Concentration in bulk retentate}} = \left[\frac{C_B - C_D}{C_B}\right]_{\Phi d=0} \tag{68.4}$$

$$K_0A = \frac{\text{Solute transport}}{\text{Concentration driven force}} = \left[\frac{\phi_d}{C_B - C_D}\right]_{J_F R=0} \tag{68.5}$$

where J_F is the filtration rate, A the area, σ the Staverman reflection coefficient, π the osmotic pressure, and other terms are as defined previously.

At the onset of a CAPD exchange using 4.25% dextrose, the ultrafiltration rate is 10 to 30 ml/min. Relative to a perfectly semipermeable membrane, the glucose osmotic pressure of the solution is 4400 mmHg. Overall membrane hydraulic permeability is the quotient of these terms and is thus of the order of 0.2 ml/h-mmHg, in the units commonly employed for HD membranes. This estimate needs to be corrected for the osmotic back-pressure, which is primarily due to urea in the blood (conc. ~1.3 g/l) as well as the fact that the membrane is only partially semipermeable. The best results are not obtained from a single point measurement but either from curve fitting to the ultrafiltration profile during the entire course of dialysis or from data taken at different osmotic gradients. A review [Lysaght and Farrell, 1989] of reports from several different investigators suggests an average value of ~2 ml/h-mmHg or, roughly, 2 gal/ft^2/day (GSFD) at 100 PSI. This is higher than desalination membranes, just slightly lower than conventional regenerated cellulose hemodialysis membranes, and much lower than anisotropic ultrafiltration membranes.

Rejection coefficients, R, numerically equal to unity minus sieving coefficient are obtained either from kinetic modeling as described below or experimentally by infusing a hypertonic solution into the peritoneum with a permeant concentration equal to that in the plasma. After a suitable period of ultrafiltration, the ration of solute to water flux is calculated from the dilution of the recovered solution. Both methods are approximate and results from different investigators may vary substantially. Reported values are observed average rejection coefficients. These are often described as the Staverman reflection coefficient, σ, which is somewhat overreaching, since filtration velocity is not recorded and differences between bulk and wall concentrations are not known. Representative values, from a review of the literature [Lysaght and

TABLE 68.1   Equivalent Transport Coefficients for the Peritoneal
Membrane

Permeant species, MW	Rejection coefficient, dimensionless	K_0A cm^3/min
Urea, 60	0.26 ± 0.08	21 ± 4
Creatinine, 113	0.35 ± 0.07	10 ± 2
Uric acid, 158	0.37	10
B-12, 1,355		5
Inulin, 5,200	0.5 ± 0.2 4 ± 1.5	
$\beta_2$microglobulin, 12,000		0.8 ± 0.4
Albumin, 69,000	0.99	

Note: SD not given if $n < 3$. Equivalent ultrafiltration coefficient is ~2.0 ml/min-m^2-mmHg. Data taken from a review by Lysaght and Farrell [1989].

Farrell, 1989], are summarized in Table 68.1. Thus the membrane appears quite tight, possibly rejecting about 10 to 20% of urea and other small molecules, about 50% of intermediate-molecular-weight species, and over 99% of plasma proteins.

The diffusive permeability of the membrane is obtained by back calculation from measurements of blood and dialysate concentration vs. time during an exchange, as will be further elaborated below. Values are given as the product of membrane permeability and estimated peritoneal area (K_0A), and the results of various investigators have been reasonably consistent. Critical values from a review of the literature are summarized in Table 68.1. A K_0A value of about 20 ml/min for urea is around one order of magnitude less than comparable values for contemporary hollow-fiber hemodialyzers. If the area of the peritoneum is taken as 1.75 m^2, then urea transfers through the peritoneum analogously to urea diffusing through a stagnant film of water roughly a centimeter thick. Alternatively, given a peritoneal thickness range of 200 to 2000 μm, the diffusion of urea inside the membrane is about 20% of what would be found in a film of stagnant water of the same thickness.

It should once more be noted that the physiologic peritoneum is a complex and heterogeneous barrier, and its transport properties would be expected to vary over different regions of its terrain. For example, studies in animal models have suggested that transport during peritoneal dialysis is little affected when large segments of the visceral membrane are surgically excised. It is also repeated for emphasis that the terms Lp, R, and K_0A do not describe this membrane itself but rather a hypothetical barrier that is functionally and operationally equivalent and thus capable of producing the same mass transfer characteristics in response to the same driving forces.

68.4 Transport Modeling

Several investigators have developed mathematic models to describe, correlate, and predict relationships among the time-course of solute removal, fluid transfer, treatment variables, and physiologic proper-ties [Lysaght and Farrell, 1989; Vonesh et al., 1991; Waniewski et al., 1991].Virtually all kinetic studies start with the model illustrated in Figure 68.6. The patient is considered to be a well-mixed compart-ment with a distribution volume V_B set equal to some fraction of total body weight. (For example, urea distributes over total body water, which is ~0.58 times body weight.) Dialysate occupies a second, much smaller compartment, $V_D = 2$ to 3 l, which is also considered well-mixed but which changes in size during the course of exchange. These two compartments are separated by a planar membrane capable of supporting bidirectional transport and characterized by the terms Lp, R, and K_0A previously defined by Equation 68.3 to Equation 68.5. Fluid drains from the peritoneum to the blood at a rate of Q_L. From this point forward, the complexity and appropriate utility of the models depend upon the investigators' choices of simplifying assumptions. The simplest model, proposed by Henderson and Nolph [1969], considers ultrafiltration rate and lymphatic flow to be negligible and treats all parameters except dialysate concentration as constant with time. The basic differential equation describing this

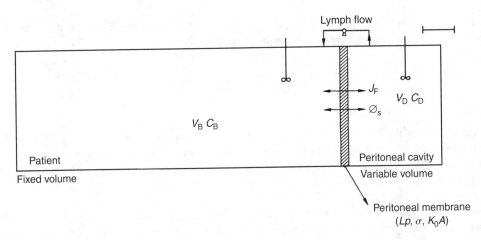

FIGURE 68.6 Single pool model for peritoneal dialysis. Solute diffuses across a planar selective membrane from a large well-mixed plasma space at constant volume and concentration to a smaller well-mixed space in which concentration and volume both increase with time. Fluid and solute are selectively ultrafiltered across the peritoneal membrane from plasma to dialysate; they are also nonselectively transported by the lymphatics from the dialysate to the body compartment.

model is

$$\frac{d(V_D C_D)}{dt} = V_D \frac{dC_D}{dt} = K_0 A (C_B - C_D) \tag{68.6}$$

Equation 68.6 may be readily solved, either to obtain $K_0 A$ from a knowledge of concentration vs. time data 68.7, or to predict dialysate concentration from a knowledge of mass transfer coefficient, blood concentration, and initial dialysate concentration 68.8 where:

$$K_0 A = \frac{V_D}{t} \ln \left(\frac{C_B - C_D^0}{C_B - C_D^t} \right) \tag{68.7}$$

$$C_D^t = C_B - (C_B - C_D^0)^{-K_0 At/V_D} \tag{68.8}$$

In these equations, the superscript t represents the value at time t, and the superscript 0 designates the value at $t = 0$. This model provides a very easy way of measuring $K_0 A$ if it is applied during the isovolemic interval that often occurs ~30 to 90 min after the beginning of an exchange.

Several years later, investigators at the University of New South Wales [Garred et al., 1983] proposed a slightly more complex model that included ultrafiltration, subject to the assumptions that (1) blood concentration was constant, (2) the membrane was nonselective ($R = O$), and (3) lymphatic involvement could be ignored. The appropriate differential equation is now:

$$\frac{d(V_D C_D)}{dt} = K_0 A (C_B - C_D) + C_B \frac{dV_D}{dt} \tag{68.9}$$

This equation can be solved in two ways. Over either relatively short time intervals or small differences in dialysate volume, an average volume V_D is obtained as the mean of initial and final volumes. In that case $K_0 A$ is given by

$$C_D^t = \bar{C}_B - \frac{V_D^0}{V_D^t} (\bar{C}_B - C_D^0) e^{-K_0 At/V_D} \tag{68.10}$$

where variables overlined with a solid diachrin are treated as constant during the integration of Equation 68.9. The similarity of Equation 68.9 and Equation 68.10 to Equation 68.7 and Equation 68.8

should be noted. Where a series of data points for blood and dialysate concentrations are available at various times during the treatment, Equation 68.10 may be rewritten as

$$C_D^t = \bar{C}_B - \frac{V_D^0}{V_D^t}(\bar{C}_B - C_D^0)e^{-K_0At/V_D} \qquad (68.11)$$

Data in the form of this equation may be readily regressed to obtain K_0A from a knowledge of V_D, C_B, and C_D at various times in an exchange. The values for peritoneal volume V_D may be obtained experimentally from tracer dilution studies, calculated from an algorithm, in which case it varies with time, or simply averaged between initial and final values, in which case it is assumed constant. Equation 68.11 and Equation 68.12 are recommended for routine modeling of patient kinetics.

Several investigators, reviewed by Lysaght and Farrell [1989], have produced far more elaborate models which incorporate lymphatic drainage, deviations from ideal semipermeability of the peritoneal membrane, time-dependent ultrafiltration rates, and coupling between bidirectional diffusive and connective transport. Although potent in the hands of their developers, none of the numerical models has been widely adopted, and the current trend is toward simpler approaches. In comparative studies [Lysaght, 1989; Waniewski et al., 1991], only small differences were found between the numeric values of transport parameters calculated from simple analytic models (Equation 68.6 to Equation 68.12) and those we obtained by far more complex numerical methods. In peritoneal dialysis, solute is being exchanged through an inefficient membrane between a large body compartment through an inefficient membrane and a second compartment only 5% as large, and treatment times have been chosen so that the smaller compartment will reach saturation. These physical circumstances, and the very forgiving nature of exponential asymptotes, perhaps explain why simple analytic solutions perform nearly as well as their more complex numeric counterparts.

68.5 Emerging Developments

Modified therapy formats and new formulations for exchange solutions constantly are being proposed and evaluated. APD is the most successful of the new formats; at the end of 1993, about one in six peritoneal dialysis patients received some variant of automated overnight treatment. APD is carried out by a small console (Figure 68.7) which automatically instills and drains dialysate at 1.5–3-h intervals while the patient sleeps, typically over 8–10 h each night. The peritoneum is left full during the day. Since the short exchanges do not permit complete equilibration even for urea, the process is somewhat wasteful of dialysate. However, reference to Figure 68.3 will readily demonstrate that small-solute removal is most efficient in the early portion of an exchange; for example, two 2-h exchanges will provide 75% more urea clearance than one 4-h exchange. As currently prescribed, APD requires 84–105 l per week of dialysate (vs. 56 for CAPD) and increases total small-solute clearance per 24 h by up to 50% over that achieved by CAPD. The number of patients on APD is increasing by half every year, a phenomenon driven by two main factors. The first relates to quality of life; APD is far-and-away the least invasive of the maintenance dialysis protocols. The patient performs one connection at night and one disconnection in the morning and is thereby freed from the tedium and inconvenience of daily exchanges or the need to spend a significant portion of 3 days per week at an HD treatment facility. In addition, small-solute clearance is higher than in other continuous peritoneal therapies, which helps address increasing concern about the adequacy of the standard four 2-l CAPD exchanges per day, especially with large muscular patients and those with no residual renal function. A group of patients who may benefit from APD are those who have rapid transport of glucose across the peritoneal membrane; because of the consequent loss of the osmotic gradient, they have difficulty achieving adequate ultrafiltration. The short dwell times of ADP circumvent this problem. The counterbalancing disadvantage of APD is increased expense associated with the larger fluid consumption and the fluid cyclers.

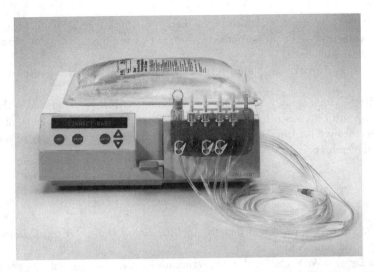

FIGURE 68.7 Contemporary equipment module for APD (Home Choice, Renal division, Baxter Healthcare) which automatically controls and monitors the delivery of 10 to 15 l of dialysate from 5-l bags via a multipronged disposable administration set. The console incorporates a diaphragm pump used to emulate gravity, and a derivative of the ideal gas law measures fluid volume, eliminating the need for scales. Setup and operation are designed to be straightforward and convenient.

Virtually all solution development comprises attempts to replace glucose with an alternative osmotic agent, preferably one which diffuses more slowly and thus provides a more stable osmotic gradient and one which obviates the obligatory load of about 600 calories of sugar. However glucose is cheap and safe, and it will be difficult to find a satisfactory alternative. A competing osmotic agent must be safe to administer in amounts of tens of grams per day over years to patients who have little or no ability to clear accumulated material via the kidney — but an osmotic agent which is readily metabolizable provides no caloric "advantage" over glucose. A glucose polymer, termed polyglucose, has been recently introduced in England [Mistry and Gokal, 1993]. This disperse oligodextrin has a weight-averaged MW of 18,700 Da and number-averaged molecular weight of 7,300 Da. At a concentration of 7.5% (i.e., 30 g per 2-l exchange), it provides more stable ultrafiltration during long dwell exchanges; however, administration is limited to one exchange per day because of the accumulation of maltose and higher MW polysaccharides; an alternative approach, recently introduced in Europe and in clinical trials in the United States, is a solution in which glucose is replaced with 1.1% amino acids, enriched for essential amino acids [Jones et al., 1992]. This solution also improves nitrogen balance, a significant feature, since dialysate patients are frequently malnourished. Concern about excessive nitrogen intake, however, limits its use to one or two exchanges per day, and the amino acid solution is necessarily more expensive than glucose.

Defining Terms

Automated peritoneal dialysis (APD): A recent variant of CAPD in which fluid exchanges are performed by simple pumps, usually at night while the patient sleeps.

Clearance: The rate of mass removal divided by solute concentration in the body. Clearance represents the virtual volume of blood or plasma cleared of a particular solute per unit time.

Continuous ambulatory peritoneal dialysis (CAPD): A continuous process for the treatment of chronic renal failure in which metabolic waste products and excess body water are removed through the peritoneum with four exchanges of up to 3 l every 24 h.

Diffusion: The molecular movement of matter from a region of greater concentration to lesser concentration at a rate proportional to the difference in concentration.

Hemodialysis (HD):   Intermittent extracorporeal therapy for chronic renal failure. See Chapter 67.

Mass transfer coefficient: The proportionality constant between the rate of solute transport per unit area and the driving force.

Membrane: A thin barrier capable of providing directional selective transport between two phases.

Peritoneal cavity: A topologically closed space in the abdomen which is surrounded by the peritoneum.

Peritoneum: An intricate, vascularized, membranelike tissue that lines the internal abdominal walls and covers the liver, intestine, and other internal organs. Used interchangeably with the expression peritoneal membrane.

References

Boen S.T. 1985. History of peritoneal dialysis. In K.D. Nolph (Ed.), *Peritoneal Dialysis*, pp. 1–22, The Hague, Martinus Nijhoff.

Churchill D.N., Taylor D.W., Vas S.I. et al. 1989. Peritonitis in continuous ambulatory peritoneal dialysis (CAPD): a multi-centre randomized clinical trial comparing the Y connector disinfectant system to standard systems. *Perit. Dial. Int.* 19: 159.

Dratwa M., Collart F., and Smet L. 1986. CAPD peritonitis and different connecting devices: a statistical comparison. In J.F. Maher and J.F. Winchester (Eds.), *Frontiers in Peritoneal Dialysis*, pp. 190–197, New York, Field Rich.

Garred L.J., Canaud B., and Farrell P.C. 1983. A simple kinetic model for assessing peritoneal mass transfer in chronic ambulatory peritoneal dialysis. *ASAIO J.* 6: 131.

Henderson L.W. and Nolph K.D. 1969. Altered permeability of the peritoneal membrane after using hypertonic peritoneal dialysis fluid. *J. Clin. Invest.* 48: 992.

Jones M.R., Martis L., Algrim C.E. et al. 1992. Amino acid solutions for CAPD: rationale and clinical experience. *Miner. Electrolyte. Metab.* 18: 309.

Lysaght M.J. 1989. *The Kinetics of Continuous Peritoneal Dialysis*. PhD thesis, Center for Biomedical Engineering, University of New South Wales.

Lysaght M.J. and Farrell P.C. 1989. Membrane phenomena and mass transfer kinetics in peritoneal dialysis. *J. Membr. Sci.* 44: 5.

Mistry C.D. and Gokal R. 1993. Single daily overnight (12-h dwell) use of 7.5% glucose polymer (MW 18,700; Mn 7,300) + 0.35% glucose solution: a 3-month study. *Nephrol. Dial. Transplant.* 8: 443.

Popovich R.P., Moncrief J.W., Decherd J.F. et al. 1976. The definition of a novel portable/wearable equilibrium peritoneal technique. *Abst. AM Soc. Artif. Intern. Organs* 5: 64.

Vonesh E.F., Lysaght M.J., Moran J. et al. 1991. Kinetic modeling as a prescription aid in peritoneal dialysis. *Blood Purif.* 9: 246.

Waniewski J., Werynski A., Heimburger O. et al. 1991. A comparative analysis of mass transport models in peritoneal dialysis. *ASAIO Trans.* 37: 65.

Further Information

The literature on continuous peritoneal dialysis is abundant. Among several reference texts the most venerable and popular is *Peritoneal Dialysis*, edited by K. Nolph and published by Kluwer; this is regularly updated. Also recommended is *Continuous Ambulatory Peritoneal Dialysis*, edited by R. Gokal and published by Churchill Livingston. The journal *Peritoneal Dialysis International* (published by MultiMed; Toronto) is published quarterly and is devoted exclusively to CAPD. The continuing education department of the University of Missouri–Columbia organizes a large annual conference on peritoneal dialysis with plenary lecture and submitted papers. The International Society of Peritoneal Dialysis holds its conference biannually and usually publishes proceedings. Peritoneal dialysis is also discussed in the meeting and journals of the other major artificial organ societies (American Society of Artificial Internal Organs; European Dialysis and Transplant Association; Japanese Society of Artificial Organs) and the American and International Societies of Nephrology. Blood Purification (published by Karger; Basel) attracts many outstanding papers dealing with engineering and transport issues in peritoneal dialysis. For the insatiable, Medline now contains over 10,000 citations to CAPD and peritoneal dialysis.

69

Therapeutic Apheresis and Blood Fractionation

Andrew L. Zydney
University of Delaware

Apheresis is the process in which a specific component of blood (either plasma, a plasma component, white cells, platelets, or red cells) is separated and removed with the remainder of the blood returned to the patient (often in combination with some type of replacement fluid). **Donor apheresis** is used for the collection of specific blood cells or plasma components from blood donors, resulting in a much more effective use of limited blood-based resources. Donor apheresis developed during World War II as a means for increasing the supply of critically needed plasma, and clinical trials in 1944 demonstrated that it was possible to safely collect donations of a unit of plasma ($\sim$300 ml) on a weekly basis if the cellular components of blood were returned to the donor. **Therapeutic apheresis** is used for the treatment of a variety of diseases and disorders characterized by the presence of abnormal proteins or blood cells in the circulation which are believed to be involved in the progression of that particular condition. Therapeutic apheresis thus has its roots in the ancient practice of bloodletting, which was used extensively well into the 19th century to remove "bad humors" from the patient's body, thereby restoring the proper balance between the "blood, yellow bile, black bile, and phlegm."

The term **plasmapheresis** was first used by Abel, Rowntree, and Turner in 1914 in their discussion of a treatment for toxemia involving the repeated removal of a large quantity of plasma, with the cellular components of blood returned to the patient along with a replacement fluid [Kambic and Nosé, 1993]. The first successful therapeutic applications of plasmapheresis were reported in the late 1950s in the management of macroglobulinemia (a disorder characterized by a large increase in blood viscosity due to the accumulation of high-molecular-weight globulins in the blood) and in the treatment of multiple myeloma (a malignant tumor of the bone marrow characterized by the production of excessive amounts of immunoglobulins).

By 1990, there were well over 50 diseases treated by therapeutic apheresis [Sawada et al., 1990] with varying degrees of success. Plasmapheresis is used in the treatment of (1) protein-related diseases involving excessive levels of specific proteins (e.g., macroglobulins in Waldenstrom's syndrome and lipoproteins in familial hypercholesterolemia) or excessive amounts of protein-bound substances (e.g., toxins in hepatic failure and thyroid hormone in thyrotoxicosis), (2) antibody-related or **autoimmune diseases** (e.g., glomerulonephritis and myasthenia gravis), and (3) immune-complex-related diseases (e.g., rheumatoid arthritis and systemic lupus erythematosus).

Cytapheresis involves the selective removal of one (or more) of the cellular components of blood, and it has been used in the treatment of certain leukemias (for the removal of leukocytes) and in the treatment of polycythemia. Table 69.1 provides a more complete listing of some of the diseases and blood components that are removed during therapeutic apheresis. This list is not intended to be exhaustive, and there is still considerable debate over the actual clinical benefit of apheresis for a number of these diseases.

The required separation of blood into its basic components (red cells, white cells, platelets, and plasma) can be accomplished using centrifugation or membrane filtration; the more specific removal of one (or more) components from the separated plasma generally involves a second membrane filtration or use of an appropriate sorbent. The discussion that follows focuses primarily on the technical aspects of the different separation processes currently in use. Additional information on the clinical aspects of therapeutic apheresis is available in the references listed at the end of this chapter.

69.1 Plasmapheresis

The therapeutic application of plasmapheresis can take one of two forms: **plasma exchange** or **plasma perfusion**. In plasma exchange therapy, a relatively large volume of plasma, containing the toxic or immunogenic species, is separated from the cellular components of blood and replaced with an equivalent volume of a replacement fluid (either fresh frozen plasma obtained from donated blood or an appropriate plasma substitute). In plasma perfusion, the separated plasma is treated by an adsorptive column or second membrane filtration to remove a specific component (or components) from the plasma. This treated plasma is then returned to the patient along with the blood cells, thereby eliminating the need for exogenous replacement fluids. The different techniques that can be used for plasma perfusion are discussed subsequently.

The reduction in the concentration (C_i) of any plasma component during the course of a plasmapheresis treatment can be described using a single compartment pharmacokinetic model as

$$V_p \frac{dC_i}{dt} = -\alpha_i Q_p C_i + G_i \tag{69.1}$$

where V_p is the volume of the patient's plasma (which is assumed to remain constant over the course of therapy through the use of a replacement fluid or through the return of the bulk of the plasma after a plasma perfusion), Q_p is the volumetric rate of plasma collection, G_i is the rate of component generation, and α is a measure of the effectiveness of the removal process. In membrane plasmapheresis, α, is equal to the observed membrane sieving coefficient, which is defined as the ratio of the solute concentration in the filtrate collected through the membrane to that in the plasma entering the device; α_i is thus equal to 1 for a small protein that can pass unhindered through the membrane but can be less than 1 for large proteins and immune complexes. In plasma perfusion systems, α_i is equal to the fraction of the particular component removed from the collected plasma by the secondary (selective) processing step. The generation rate is typically negligible over the relatively short periods (fewer than 3 h) involved in the actual plasmapheresis; thus the component concentration at the end of a single treatment is given as

$$\frac{C_i}{C_{i0}} = \exp\left(-\frac{\alpha_i Q_p t}{V_p}\right) = \exp\left(-\frac{\alpha_i V_{exc}}{V_p}\right) \tag{69.2}$$

TABLE 69.1 Disease States Treated by Therapeutic Apheresis

Disease	Components removed
Hematologic	
Hemophilia	AntiFactor VIII Ab
Idiopathic thrombocytopenia purpura	Antiplatelet Ab, **immune complexes**
Thrombotic thrombocytopenia purpura	Antiplatelet Ab, immune complexes
AIDS, HIV	Antilymphocyte Ab, immune complexes
Autoimmune hemolytic Anemia	Anti-red cell Ab, red cells
Rh incompatibility	Anti-Rh Ab
Cryoglobulinemia	Cryoglobulins
Hyperviscosity syndrome	Macroglobulins, immunglobulin M
Waldenstrom's syndrome	Immunoglobulin M
Paraproteinemia	Paraproteins
Sickle cell anemia	Red blood cells
Thrombocythemia	Platelets
Collagen/rheumatologic	
Systemic lupus erythematosus	Anti-DNA Ab, immune complexes
Progressive systemic sclerosis	Antinonhistone nuclear Ab
CREST syndrome	Anticentromere Ab
Sjorgen syndrome	Antimitochondrial Ab
Rheumatoid arthritis	Rheumatoid factor, cryoglobulins, immunoglobulins
Periarteritis nodosa	Cryoglobulins, immune complexes
Raynaud's disease	Cryoglobulins, macroglobulins
Scleroderma	Immune complexes
Mixed connective tissue diseases	Immunoglobulins
Neurologic	
Myasthenia gravis	Antiacetylcholine receptor Ab, cryoglobulins
Multiple sclerosis	Antimyelin Ab
Guillain-Barre syndrome	Antimyelin Ab
Polyneuropathy	Cryoglobulins, macroglobulins
Polyradiculoneuropathy	Antibodies
Lambert-Eaton syndrome	Antibodies
Hepatic	
Chronic active hepatitis	Antimitochondrial Ab
Hepatic failure	Protein-bound toxins
Primary biliary cirrhosis	Protein-bound toxins, antimitochondrial Ab
Renal	
Goodpasture's syndrome	Antiglomerular basement membrane Ab
Glomerulonephritis	Immune complexes
Lupus nephritis	Immune complexes
Transplant rejection	Immune complexes, anti-HLA Ab
Malignant diseases	
Cancer	Tumor-specific Ab, immune complexes
Multiple myeloma	Immunoglobulins
Leukemia	Leukocytes
Miscellaneous	
Addison's disease	Antiadrenal Ab
Autoimmune thyroiditis	Antimicrosomal Ab
Chronic ulcerative colitis	Anticolonic epithelial cell Ab
Diabetes mellitus	Antiinsulin receptor Ab
Hashimoto's disease	Antithyroglobulin Ab
Insulin autoimmune syndrome	Antiinsulin Ab
Pemphigus	Antiepidermal cell membrane Ab
Ulcerative colitis	Anticolonic lipopolysaccharide Ab
Asthma	Immunoglobulin E
Hypercholesterolemia	Cholesterol, lipoproteins
Hyperlipidemia	Low- and very low-density lipoproteins
Thyrotoxicosis	Thyroid hormone

where $V_{exc} = Q_p t$ is the actual volume of plasma removed (or exchanged) during the process. Plasma exchange thus reduces the concentration of a given component by 63% after an exchange of one plasma volume (for $\alpha_i = 1$) and by 86% after two plasma volumes. This simple single compartment model has been verified for a large number of plasma components, although immunoglobulin G actually appears to have about 50% extravascular distribution with the reequilibration between these compartments occurring within 24 to 28 h following the plasmapheresis.

There is still considerable variability in the frequency and intensity of the plasmapheresis used in different therapeutic applications, and this is due in large part to uncertainties regarding the metabolism, pharmacokinetics, and pathogenicity of the different components that are removed during therapeutic apheresis. The typical plasma exchange therapy currently involves the removal of 2–3 l of plasma (approximately one plasma volume) at a frequency of two to four times per week, with the therapy continued for several weeks. There have also been a number of studies of the long-term treatment of several diseases via plasmapheresis, with the therapy performed on a periodic basis (ranging from once per week to once every few months) over as much as 5 years (e.g., for the removal of cholesterol and lipoproteins in the treatment of severe cases of hypercholesterolemia).

69.1.1 Centrifugal Devices

Initially, all plasmapheresis was performed using batch centrifuges. This involved the manual removal of approximately one unit (500 ml) of blood at a time, with the blood separated in a centrifuge so that the target components could be removed. The remaining blood was then returned to the patient before drawing another unit and repeating the entire process. This was enormously time-consuming and labor-intensive, requiring as much as 5 h for the collection of only a single liter of plasma. Batch centrifugation is still the dominant method for off-line blood fractionation in most blood-banking applications, but almost all therapeutic plasmapheresis is performed using online (continuous) devices.

The first continuous flow centrifuge was developed in the late 1960s by IBM in conjunction with the National Cancer Institute, and this basic design was subsequently commercialized by the American Instrument Co. (now a division of Travenol) as the Aminco Celltrifuge [Nosé et al., 1983]. A schematic diagram showing the general configuration of this, and most other continuous flow centrifuges is shown in Figure 69.1. The blood is input at the bottom of the rotating device and passes through a chamber in which the actual separation into plasma, white cells/platelets, and red cells occurs. Three separate exit ports are located at different radial positions to remove the separated components continuously from the top of the chamber using individual roller pumps. The position of the buffy coat layer (which consists of the white cells and platelets) is controlled by adjusting the centrifugal speed and the relative plasma and red cell flow rates to obtain the desired separation. Probably the most difficult engineering problem in the development of the continuous flow centrifuge was the design of the rotating seals through which the whole blood and separated components must pass without damage. The seal design in the original NCI/IBM device used saline lubrication to prevent intrusion of the cells between the contacting surfaces.

In order to obtain effective cell separation in the continuous flow centrifuge, the residence time in the separation chamber must be sufficiently large to allow the red cells to migrate to the outer region of the device. The degree of separation can thus be characterized by the packing factor

$$P = \frac{G V_{sed} t}{h} \tag{69.3}$$

where G is the g-force associated with the centrifugation, V_{sed} is the sedimentation velocity at 1 g, t is the residence time in the separation chamber, and h is the width of the separation chamber (i.e., the distance over which the sedimentation occurs). The packing factor thus provides a measure of the radial migration compared to the width of the centrifuge chamber, with adequate cell separation obtained when $P > 1$.

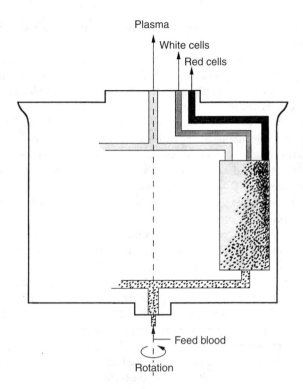

FIGURE 69.1 Schematic diagram of a generic continuous flow centrifuge for fractionation of blood into red cells, white cells/platelets, and plasma.

The residence time in the separation chamber is inversely related to the blood flow rate (Q_B) as

$$t = \frac{AL}{Q_B} \qquad (69.4)$$

where L and A are the length and cross-sectional area of the chamber, respectively.

Rotational speeds in most continuous flow centrifuges are maintained around 1500 rpm (about 100 g) to obtain a relatively clean separation between the red cells and buffy coat, to avoid the formation of a very highly packed (and therefore highly viscous) region of cells at the outer edge of the chamber, and to minimize excessive heating around the rotating seals [Rock, 1983]. The width of the separation chamber must be large enough to permit effective removal of the different blood components from the top of the device, while minimizing the overall extracorporeal blood volume. For example, a packing factor of ten requires a residence time of about 20 sec for a device operated at 100 g with a 0.1-cm-wide separation chamber. The blood flow rate for this device would need to be maintained below about 120 ml/min for a chamber volume of 40 ml. Most of the currently available devices operate at $Q_B \approx 50$ ml/min and can thus collect a liter of plasma in about 30 to 40 min.

More recent models for the continuous flow centrifuge have modified the actual geometry of the separation chamber to enhance the cell separation and reduce the overall cost of the device [Sawada et al., 1990]. Examples include tapering the centrifuge bowl to improve flow patterns and optimizing the geometry of the collection region to obtain purer products. The IBM 2997 (commercialized by Cobe Laboratories) uses a disposable semirigid plastic rectangular channel for the separation chamber, which eliminates some of the difficulties involved in both sterilizing and setting up the device. Fenwal Laboratories developed the CS-3000 Cell Separator (subsequently sold by Baxter Healthcare), which uses a continuous J-shaped mulitchannel tubing connected directly to the rotating element. This eliminates the need for a rotating seal, thereby minimizing the possibility of leaks. The tubing in this device actually rotates around the centrifuge bowl during operation, using a "jump rope" principle to prevent twisting of the flow lines during centrifugation.

In addition to the continuous flow centrifuge, Haemonetics has developed a series of intermittent flow centrifuges [Rock, 1983]. Blood flows into the bottom of a separation chamber similar to that shown in Figure 69.1, but the red cells simply accumulate in this chamber while the plasma is drawn to the center of the rotating bowl and removed through an outlet port at the top of the device. When the process is complete, the pump action reverses, and the red cells are forced out of the bowl and reinfused into the patient (along with any replacement fluid). The entire process is then automatically repeated to obtain the desired level of plasma (or white cell) removal. This device was originally developed for the collection of leukocytes and platelets, but it is now used extensively for large-scale plasmapheresis as well. Maximum blood flow rates are typically about 70 to 80 ml/min, and the bowl rotates at about 5000 rpm. The device as a whole is more easily transported than most of the continuous flow centrifuges, but it requires almost 50% more time for the collection of an equivalent plasma volume due to the intermittent nature of the process. In addition, the total extracorporeal volume is quite high (about 500 ml compared to only 250 ml for most of the newer continuous flow devices) due to the larger chamber required for the red cell accumulation [Sawada et al., 1990].

All these centrifugal devices have the ability to carry out effective plasma exchange, although the rate of plasma collection tends to be somewhat slower than that for the membrane devices discussed in the next section. These devices can also be used for the collection of specific cell fractions, providing a degree of flexibility that is absent in the membrane systems. The primary disadvantage of the centrifugal units is the presence of a significant number of platelets in the collected plasma (typically about 105 platelets per microliter). Not only can this lead to considerable platelet depletion during repeated applications of plasma exchange, it can also interfere with many of the secondary processing steps employed in plasma perfusion.

69.1.2 Membrane Plasmapheresis

The general concept of blood filtration using porous membranes is quite old, and membranes with pores suitably sized to retain the cellular components of blood and pass the plasma proteins have been available since the late 1940s. Early attempts at this type of blood filtration were largely unsuccessful due to severe problems with membrane plugging (often referred to as fouling) and red cell lysis. Blatt and coworkers at Amicon recognized that these problems could be overcome using a cross-flow configuration [Solomon et al., 1978] in which the blood flow was parallel to the membrane and thus perpendicular to the plasma (filtrate) flow as shown schematically in Figure 69.2. This geometry minimizes the accumulation of retained cells at the membrane surface, leading to much higher filtration rates and much less cell damage than could be obtained in conventional dead-end filtration devices [Solomon et al., 1978]. This led to the development of a large number of membrane devices using either flat sheet or hollow-fiber membranes made from a variety of polymers including polypropylene (Travenol Laboratories, Gambro, Fresenius), cellulose diacetate (Asahi Medical), polyvinyl alcohol (Kuraray), polymethylmethacrylate (Toray), and polyvinyl chloride (Cobe Laboratories).

These membrane devices all produce essentially cell-free plasma with minimal protein retention using membranes with pore sizes of 0.2 to 0.6 μm. In addition, these devices must be operated under conditions that cause minimal red cell lysis, while maintaining a sufficiently high plasma filtrate flux to reduce the cost of the microporous membranes. Typical experimental data for a parallel plate membrane device are shown in Figure 69.3 [Zydney and Colton, 1987]. The results are plotted as a function of the mean transmembrane pressure drop (ΔP_{TM}) at several values of the wall shear rate (γ_w), where γ_w is directly proportional to the inlet blood flow rate (Q_B). The filtrate flux initially increases with increasing ΔP_{TM} reaching a maximum pressure independent value which increases with increasing shear rate. The flux under all conditions is substantially smaller than that obtained when filtering pure (cell-free) saline under identical conditions (dashed line in Figure 69.3). No measurable hemolysis was observed at low ΔP_{TM} even when the flux was in the pressure-independent regime. Hemolysis does become significant at higher

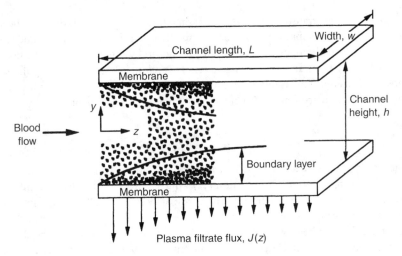

FIGURE 69.2 Schematic diagram of a parallel plate device for cross-flow membrane plasmapheresis.

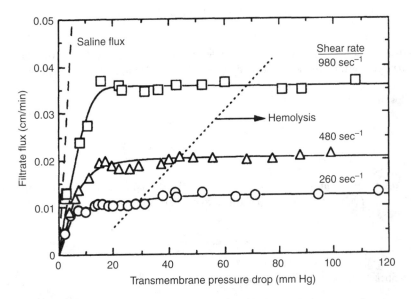

FIGURE 69.3 Experimental data for the filtrate flux as a function of the applied transmembrane pressure drop in a parallel plate membrane plasmaphersis device. Red cell hemolysis, defined as a filtrate hemoglobin concentration exceeding 20 mg/dl, occurs to the right of the dashed line. Data have been adapted from Zydney and Colton [1987].

pressures, with the extent of hemolysis decreasing with increasing γ_w and with decreasing membrane pore size [Solomon et al., 1978]. The dashed diagonal line indicates the pressure at which the filtrate hemoglobin concentration exceeds 20 mg/dl.

The pressure-independent flux at high ΔP_{TM} generally has been attributed to the formation of a concentration polarization boundary layer consisting of a high concentration of the formed elements in blood, mainly the red blood cells, which are retained by the microporous membrane (Figure 69.2). This dynamic layer of cells provides an additional hydraulic resistance to flow, causing the flux to be substantially smaller than that obtained during filtration of a cell-free solution. At steady-state, this boundary layer is in dynamic equilibrium, with the rate of convection of formed elements toward the membrane balanced by the rate of mass transport back into the bulk suspension. There has been some debate in the literature over the actual mechanism of cell transport in these devices, and the different models that have been developed for the plasma flux during membrane plasmapheresis are discussed elsewhere [Zydney and Colton, 1986].

Zydney and Colton [1982] proposed that cell transport occurs by a shear-induced diffusion mechanism in which cell–cell interactions and collisions give rise to random cell motion during the shear flow of a concentrated suspension. This random motion can be characterized by a shear-included diffusion coefficient, which was evaluated from independent experimental measurements as

$$D = a^2 \gamma f(c) \tag{69.5}$$

where γ is the local shear rate (velocity gradient), a is the cell radius ($\sim 4.2 \ \mu$m for the red blood cells), and C is the local red cell concentration. The function $f(c)$, which reflects the detailed concentration dependence of the shear-induced diffusion coefficient, is approximately equal to 0.03 for red cell suspensions over a broad range of cell concentrations.

The local filtrate flux can be evaluated using a stagnant film analysis in which the steady-state mass balance is integrated over the thickness of the concentration boundary layer yielding [Zydney and Colton, 1986]

$$J(z) = k_{\mathrm{m}} \ln \frac{C_{\mathrm{w}}}{C_{\mathrm{b}}} \tag{69.6}$$

where z is the axial distance measured from the device inlet, and C_{w} and C_{b} are the concentrations of formed elements at the membrane surface and in the bulk suspension, respectively. The bulk mass transfer coefficient (k_{m}) can be evaluated using the Leveque approximation for laminar flow in either a parallel plate or hollow fiber device

$$k_{\mathrm{m}} = 0.516 \left(\frac{D^2 \gamma_{\mathrm{w}}}{z} \right)^{1/3} = 0.047 \left(\frac{a^4}{z} \right)^{1/3} \gamma_{\mathrm{w}} \tag{69.7}$$

where the second expression has been developed using the shear-induced diffusion coefficient given by Equation 69.5 with $f(C) = 0.03$. The wall shear rate is directly proportional to the blood flow rate with

$$\gamma_{\mathrm{w}} = \frac{4 Q_{\mathrm{B}}}{N \pi R^3} \tag{69.8}$$

for a hollow-fiber device with N fibers of inner radius R and

$$\gamma_{\mathrm{w}} = \frac{6 Q_{\mathrm{B}}}{w h^2} \tag{69.9}$$

for a parallel plate device with channel height h and total membrane width w.

At high pressures, C_{w} approaches its maximum value which is determined by the maximum packing density of the cells (about 95% under conditions typical of clinical plasmapheresis). The plasma flux under these conditions becomes independent of the transmembrane pressure drop, with this pressure-independent flux varying linearly with the wall shear rate and decreasing with increasing bulk cell concentration as described by Equation 69.6 and Equation 69.7. A much more detailed numerical model for the flux [Zydney and Colton, 1987], which accounts for the concentration and shear rate dependence of both the blood viscosity and shear-induced cell diffusion coefficient as well as the compressibility of the blood cell layer that accumulates at the membrane, has confirmed the general behavior predicted by Equation 69.6 and Equation 69.7.

The volumetric filtrate (plasma) flow rate (Q_{p}) in a hollow-fiber membrane filter can be evaluated by integrating Equation 69.6 to Equation 69.8 along the length of the device accounting for the decrease in the blood flow rate (and thus γ_w) due to the plasma removal [Zydney and Colton, 1986]. The resulting expression for the fractional plasma yield is

$$\frac{Q_P}{Q_B} = 1 - \exp\left[-0.62\left(\frac{a^2 L}{R^3}\right)\ln\frac{C_w}{C_b}\right]$$ (69.10)

An analogous expression can be evaluated for a parallel plate device with the channel height h replacing R and the coefficient 0.62 becoming 0.84. Even though the development leading to Equation 69.10 neglects the detailed variations in the bulk cell concentration and velocity profiles along the fiber length, the final expression has been shown to be in good agreement with experimental data for the plasma flow rate in actual clinical devices [Zydney and Colton, 1986]. Equation 69.10 predicts that the volumetric plasma flow rate is independent of the number of hollow fibers (or the membrane width for a parallel plate membrane device), a result which is consistent with a number of independent experimental investigations.

According to Equation 69.10, the plasma flow rate increases significantly with decreasing fiber radius. There are, however, a number of constraints on the smallest fiber radius that can actually be employed in these hollow-fiber membrane devices. For example, blood clotting and fiber blockage can become unacceptable in very narrow bore fibers. The blood flow in such narrow fibers also causes a very high bulk shear stress, which potentially can lead to unacceptable levels of blood cell damage (particularly for white cells and platelets). Finally, the hollow-fiber device must be operated under conditions which avoid hemolysis.

Zydney and Colton [1982] developed a model for red cell lysis during membrane plasmapheresis in which the red cells are assumed to rupture following their deformation into the porous structure of the membranes. A given red cell is assumed to lyse if it remains in a pore for a sufficient time for the strain induced in the red cell membrane to exceed the critical strain for cell lysis. Since the red cell can be dislodged from the pore by collisions with other cells moving in the vicinity of the membrane or by the fluid shear stress, the residence time in the pore will be inversely related to the wall shear rate.

The tension (σ) in the red cell membrane caused by the deformation in the pore is evaluated using Laplace's law [Zydney and Colton, 1987]

$$\sigma = \frac{\Delta P_{TM} R_P}{2}$$ (69.11)

where R_p is the pore radius. Hemolysis is assumed to occur at a critical value of the strain in the red cell membrane (S); thus the time required for lysis is given implicitly by

$$S = \sigma g(t) = \sigma\{0.0010 + 0.0012[1 - \exp(-8t)] + 4.5 \times 10^{-6}t\}$$ (69.12)

The function $g(t)$ represents the temporal dependence of the lytic phenomenon and has been evaluated from independent experimental measurements [Zydney and Colton, 1982]. Cell lysis occurs when $S \geq 0.03$ in Equation 69.12 where σ is given in dyne/cm and t is in sec. This simple model has been shown to be in good agreement with experimental data for red cell lysis during cross-flow membrane plasmapheresis [Zydney and Colton, 1987].

This physical model for red cell lysis implies that hemolysis can be avoided by operating at sufficiently high shear rates to reduce the residence time in the membrane pores. However, operation at high shear rates also causes the inlet transmembrane pressure drop to increase due to the large axial pressure drop associated with the blood flow along the length of the device [Zydney and Colton, 1982]:

$$\Delta P_{TM}(0) = \Delta P_{TM}(L) + 2\mu\gamma_w\frac{L}{R}$$ (69.13)

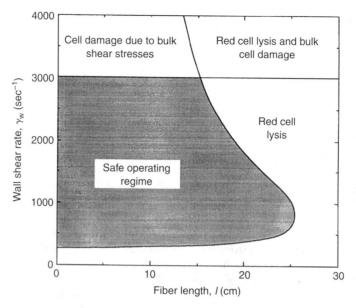

FIGURE 69.4 Schematic representation of the safe operating regime for a clinical membrane plasmapheresis device.

where $\Delta P_{TM}(0)$ and $\Delta P_{TM}(L)$ are the inlet and exit transmembrane pressure drops, respectively, and μ is the average blood viscosity. $\Delta P_{TM}(L)$ is typically maintained at a small positive value (about 20 mmHg) to ensure that there is a positive transmembrane pressure drop along the entire length of the device. Since the increase in $\Delta P_{TM}(0)$ with increasing γ_w has a greater effect on hemolysis than the reduction in the residence time for the red cells in the membrane pores, there is also an upper bound on the shear rate for the safe operation of any given clinical device.

The predicted safe operating regime for a clinical membrane plasmapheresis device can be determined using Equation 69.11, with the maximum transmembrane pressure drop occurring at the device inlet, Equation 69.13. The results are shown schematically in Figure 69.4. Hemolysis occurs at very low shear rates due to the long residence time in the membrane pores, whereas lysis at high shear rates is due to the large value of the inlet transmembrane pressure drop associated with the axial flow. Note that there is a critical fiber length (at fixed values of the fiber radius and $\Delta P_{TM}(L)$) above which there is no longer any safe operating condition.

To avoid some of the constraints associated with the design of both parallel plate and hollow-fiber membrane devices. Hemasciences developed a rotating membrane filter for use in both donor and therapeutic plasmapheresis. A nylon membrane is placed on an inner cylinder and rotated at about 3600 rpm inside a concentric outer cylindrical chamber using a magnetic coupling device. The rotating membrane causes a very high shear rate (on the order of 10,000 sec^{-1}) in the narrow gap between the cylinders. However, these high shear rates do not result in a large axial pressure drop, as found in the parallel plate and hollow-fiber devices, due to the decoupling of the axial blood flow and the shear rate in this system (the shear is now due almost entirely to the membrane rotation). The fluid flow in this rotating cylinder system also leads to the development of fluid instabilities known as Taylor vortices, and these vortices dramatically increase the rate of cell mass transport away from the membrane and back into the bulk suspension. This leads to a dramatic increase in the plasma filtrate flux and a dramatic reduction in the required membrane area. The Autopheresis-C (the rotating filter currently sold by Baxter Healthcare) uses only 70 cm^2 of membrane, which is more than an order of magnitude less than that required in competitive hollow-fiber and parallel plate devices. The mathematical analysis of the plasma filtrate flux and the corresponding design equations for the rotating cylinder plasma filter are provided by Zeman and Zydney [1996].

69.2 Plasma Perfusion

In repeated applications of plasma exchange, it is necessary to use replacement fluids that contain proteins to avoid the risks associated with protein depletion. One approach to minimizing the cost of these protein-containing replacement fluids (either albumin solutions, fresh frozen plasma, or plasma protein fraction) is to use a saline or dextran solution during the initial stages of the process and to then switch to a protein-containing replacement fluid toward the end of the treatment. Alternatively, a number of techniques have been developed to selectively remove specific toxic or immunogenic components from the plasma, with this treated plasma returned to the patient along with the cellular components of blood. This effectively eliminates the need for any expensive protein-containing replacement fluids.

Plasma perfusion (also known as online plasma treatment) is typically performed using either membrane or sorbent-based systems. Membrane filtration separates proteins on the basis of size and is thus used to selectively remove the larger molecular weight proteins from albumin and the small plasma solutes (salts, sugars, amino acids, and so on). A variety of membranes have been employed for this type of plasma fractionation including cellulose acetate (Terumo), cellulose diacetate (Asahi Medical and Teijin), ethylene vinyl alcohol (Kuraray), and polymethylmetharcrylate (Toray). These membranes are generally hydrophilic to minimize the extent of irreversible protein adsorption, with pore sizes ranging from 100 to 600 Å depending on the specific objectives of the membrane fractionation.

The selectivity that can be obtained with this type of plasma filtration can be examined using available theoretical expressions for the actual sieving coefficient (S_a) for a spherical solute in a uniform cylindrical pore:

$$S_a = (1 - \lambda)^2[2 - (1 - \lambda)^2]\exp(-0.711 \neq \lambda^2) \tag{69.14}$$

where λ is the ratio of the solute to pore radius. Equation 69.14 is actually an approximate expression which has been shown to be in good agreement with more rigorous theoretical analyses. This expression for the actual sieving coefficient, where S_a is defined as the ratio of the protein concentration in the filtrate to that at the upstream surface of the membrane, is valid at high values of the plasma filtrate flux, since it implicitly assumes that the diffusive contribution to protein transport is negligible. To avoid excessive albumin loss, it is desirable to have $S_a > 0.8$, which can be achieved using a membrane with an effective pore size greater than about 160 Å (albumin has a molecular weight of 69,000 and a Stokes–Einstein radius of 36 Å). This membrane would be able to retain about 80% of the immunglobulin M (which has a molecular weight of about 900,000 and a Stokes–Einstein radius of 98 Å), but it would retain less than 40% of the immunglobulin G (with MW = 155,000 and a radius of 55 Å).

The protein retention obtained during an actual plasma filtration is substantially more complex than indicated by the above discussion. The polymeric membranes used in these devices actually have a broad distribution of irregularly shaped (noncylindrical) pores. Likewise, the proteins can have very different (nonspherical) conformations, and their transport characteristics also can be affected by electrostatic, hydrophobic, and van der Waals interactions between the proteins and the polymeric membrane, in addition to the steric interactions that are accounted for in the development leading to Equation 69.14. Protein–protein interactions can also significantly alter the observed protein retention. Finally, the partially retained proteins will tend to accumulate at the upstream surface of the membrane during filtration (analogous to the concentration polarization effects described previously in the context of blood cell filtration).

This type of secondary plasma filtration, which is generally referred to in the literature as **cascade filtration**, is primarily effective at removing large immune complexes (molecular weight of $\sim$700,000) and immunglobulin M (MW of 900,000) from smaller proteins such as albumin. Several studies have, however, found a higher degree of albumin–immunoglobulin G separation than would be expected based on purely steric considerations (Equation 69.14). This enhanced selectivity is probably due to some type of long-range (e.g., electrostatic) interaction between the proteins and the membrane.

A number of different techniques have been developed to enhance the selectivity of these plasma filtration devices. For example, Malchesky and coworkers at the Cleveland Clinic [Malchesky et al., 1980] developed the process of cryofiltration in which the temperature of the plasma is lowered to about 10°C prior to filtration. A number of diseases are known to be associated with the presence of large amounts of cryo- (cold-) precipitable substances in the plasma, including a number of autoimmune diseases such as systemic lupus erythematosus and rheumatoid arthritis. Lowering the plasma temperature causes the aggregation and/or gelation of these cryoproteins, making it much easier for these components to be removed by the membrane filtration. About 10 g of cryogel can be removed in a single cryofiltration, along with significant amounts of the larger-molecular-weight immune complexes and IgM. The actual extent of protein removal during cyrofiltration depends on the specific composition of the plasma and thus on the nature as well as the severity of the particular disease state [Sawada et al., 1990]. There is thus considerable uncertainty over the actual components that are removed during cryofiltration under different clinical and/or experimental conditions. The cryogel layer that accumulates on the surface of the membrane also affects the retention of other plasma proteins, which potentially could lead to unacceptable losses even of small proteins such as albumin.

It is also possible to alter the selectivity of the secondary membrane filtration by heating the plasma up to or even above physiologic temperatures. This type of thermofiltration has been shown to increase the retention of low- (LDL) and very low (VLDL) density lipoproteins, and this technique has been used for the online removal of these plasma proteins in the treatment of hypercholesterolemia. LDL removal can also be enhanced by addition of a heparin/acetate buffer to the plasma, which causes precipitation of LDL and fibrinogen with the heparin [Sawada et al., 1990]. These protein precipitates can then be removed relatively easily from the plasma by membrane filtration. The excess heparin is subsequently removed from the solution by adsorption, with the acetate and excess fluid removed using bicarbonate dialysis.

An attractive alternative to secondary membrane filtration for the selective removal of plasma components is the use of sorbent columns such as (1) activated charcoal or anion exchange resins for the removal of exogenous toxins, bile acids, and bilirubin; (2) dextran sulfate cellulose for the selective removal of cholesterol, LDL, and VLDL; (3) immobilized protein A for the removal of immunoglobulins (particularly IgG) and immune complexes; and (4) specific immobilized ligands like DNA (for the removal of anti-DNA Ab), tryptophan (for the removal of antiacetylcholine receptor antibodies), and insulin (for the removal of anti-insulin antibodies). These sorbents provide a much more selective separation than is possible with any of the membrane processes; thus they have the potential to significantly reduce the side effects associated with the depletion of needed plasma components. The sorbent columns generally are used in combination with membrane plasmaphersis, since the platelets that are present in the plasma collected from available centrifugal devices can clog the columns and interfere with the subsequent protein separation.

The development of effective sorbent technology for online plasma treatment has been hindered by the uncertainties regarding the actual nature of the plasma components that must be removed for the clinical efficacy of therapeutic apheresis in the treatment of different disease states. In addition, the use of biologic materials in these sorbent systems (e.g., protein A or immobilized DNA) presents particular challenges, since these materials may be strongly immunogenic if they desorb from the column and enter the circulation.

69.3 Cytapheresis

Cytapheresis is used to selectively remove one (or more) of the cellular components of blood, with the other components (including the plasma) returned to the patient. For example, leukocyte (white cell) removal has been used in the treatment of leukemia, autoimmune diseases with a suspected cellular immune mechanism (e.g., rheumatoid arthritis and myasthenia gravis), and renal allograft rejection. Erythrocyte (red cell) removal has been used to treat sickle cell anemia, severe autoimmune hemolytic anemia, and severe parasitemia. Plateletapheresis has been used to treat patients with thrombocythemia.

Most cytapheresis is performed using either continuous or intermittent flow centrifuges, with appropriate software and/or hardware modifications used to enhance the collection of the specific cell fraction. It is also possible to remove leukocytes from whole blood by depth filtration, which takes advantage of the strong adherence of leukocytes to a variety of polymeric materials (e.g., acrylic, cellulose acetate, polyester, or nylon fibers). Leukocyte adhesion to these fibers is strongly related to the configuration and the diameter of the fibers, with the most effective cell removal obtained with ultrafine fibers less than 3 μm in diameter. Available leukocyte filters (Sepacel, Cellsora, and Cytofrac from Asahi Medical Co.) have packing densities of about 0.1 to 0.15 g fiber/cm^3 and operate at blood flow rates of 20 to 50 ml/min, making it possible to process about 2 l of blood in 1.5 h.

Leukocyte filtration is used most extensively in blood-banking applications to remove leukocytes from the blood prior to transfusion, thereby reducing the likelihood of antigenic reactions induced by donor leukocytes and minimizing the possible transmission of white-cell associated viral diseases such as cytomegalovirus. The absorbed leukocytes can also be eluted from these filters by appropriate choice of buffer solution pH, making it possible to use this technique for the collection of leukocytes from donated blood for use in the subsequent treatment of leukopenic recipients. Depth filtration has also been considered for online leukocyte removal from the extracorporeal circuit of patients undergoing cardiopulmonary bypass as a means to reduce the likelihood of postoperative myocardial or pulmonary reperfusion injury which can be caused by activated leukocytes.

A new therapeutic technique that involves online cytapheresis is the use of extracorporeal photochemotherapy, which is also known in the literature as **photopheresis**. Photopheresis can be used to treat a variety of disorders caused by aberrant T-lymphocytes [Edelson, 1989], and it has become an established therapy for the treatment of advanced cutaneous T-cell lymphoma in the United States and several European countries. In this case, the therapy involves the use of photoactivated 8-methoxypsoralen, which blocks DNA replication causing the eventual destruction of the immunoactive T-cells. The psoralen compound is taken orally prior to the phototherapy. Blood is drawn from a vein and separated by centrifugation. The white cells and plasma are collected, diluted with a saline solution, and then pumped through a thin plastic chamber in which the cells are irradiated with a high-intensity UV light that activates the psoralen. The treated white cells are then recombined with the red cells and returned to the patient. Since the photoactivated psoralen has a half-life of only several microseconds, all its activity is lost prior to reinfusion of the cells, thereby minimizing possible side effects on other organs. The removal of the red cells (which have a very high adsorptivity to UV light) makes it possible to use a much lower energy UV light, thereby minimizing the possible damage to normal white cells and platelets.

Photopheresis has also been used in the treatment of scleroderma, systemic lupus erythematosus, and pemphigus vulgaris. The exact mechanism for the suppression effect induced by the photo-therapy in these diseases is uncertain, although the T-cell destruction seems to be highly specific for the immunoactive T-cells [Edelson, 1989]. The response is much more involved than simple direct photoinactivation of the white cells; instead, the photo-treated cells appear to undergo a delayed form of cell death which elicits an immunologic response possibly involving the production of anti-idiotypic antibodies or the generation of clone-specific suppressor T-cells. This allows for an effective "vaccination" against a particular T-cell activity without the need for isolating or even identifying the particular cells that are responsible for that activity [Edelson, 1989].

Phototherapy has also been used for virus inactivation, particularly in blood-banking applications prior to transfusion. This can be done using high-intensity UV light alone or in combination with specific photoactive chemicals to enhance the virus inactivation. For example, hematoporphyrin derivatives have been shown to selectively destroy hepatitis and herpes viruses in contaminated blood. This technique shows a high degree of specificity toward this type of enveloped virus, which is apparently due to the affinity of the photoactive molecules for the lipids and glycolipids that form an integral part of the viral envelope.

Another interesting therapeutic application involving cytapheresis is the *ex vivo* activation of immunologically active white cells (lymphokine-activated killer cells, tumor-infiltrating lymphocytes, or activated killer macrophages) for the treatment of cancer. The detailed protocols for this therapy are still being developed, and there is considerable disagreement regarding its actual clinical efficacy. A pool of activated cells is generated *in vivo* by several days of treatment with interleukin-2. These cells are then collected from the blood by centrifugal cytapheresis and further purified using density gradient centrifugation. The activated cells are cultured for several days in a growth media containing additional interleukin-2. These *ex vivo* activated cells are then returned to the patient, where they have been shown to lyse existing tumor cells and cause regression of several different metastatic cancers.

69.4 Summary

Apheresis is unique in terms of the range of diseases and metabolic disorders which have been successfully treated by this therapeutic modality. This broad range of application is possible because apheresis directly alters the body's immunologic system though the removal or alteration of specific immunologically active cells and proteins.

Although there are a number of adverse reactions that can develop during apheresis (e.g., fluid imbalance, pyrogenic reactions, depletion of important coagulation factors, and thrombocytopenia), the therapy is generally well tolerated even by patients with severely compromised immune systems. This has, in at least some instances, led to the somewhat indiscriminate use of therapeutic apheresis for the treatment of diseases in which there was little physiologic rationale for the application of this therapy. This was particularly true in the 1980s, where dramatic advances in the available technology for both membrane and centrifugal blood fractionation allowed for the relatively easy use of apheresis in the clinical milieu. In some ways, apheresis in the 1980s was a medical treatment that was still looking for a disease. Although apheresis is still evolving as a therapeutic modality it is now a fairly well-established procedure for the treatment of a significant number of diseases (most of which are relatively rare) in which the removal of specific plasma proteins or cellular components can have a beneficial effect on the progression of that particular disease. Furthermore, continued advances in the equipment and procedures used for blood fractionation and component removal have, as discussed in this chapter, provided a safe and effective technology for the delivery of this therapy.

The recent advances in sorbent-based systems for the removal of specific immunologically active proteins and in the development of treatment for the activation or inactivation of specific cellular components of the immune system has provided exciting new opportunities for the alteration and even control of the body's immunologic response. This includes (1) the direct removal of specific antibodies or immune complexes (using membrane plasmapheresis with appropriate immunosorbent columns), (2) the inactivation or removal of specific lymphocytes (using centrifugal cytapheresis in combination with appropriate extracorporeal phototherapy or chemotherapy), and/or (3) the activation of a disease-specific immunologic response (using cytapheresis and *ex vivo* cell culture with appropriate lymphokines and cell stimuli). New advances in our understanding of the immune system and in our ability to selectively manipulate and control the immunologic response should thus have a major impact on therapeutic apheresis and the future development of this important medical technology.

Defining Terms

Autoimmune diseases: A group of diseases in which pathological antibodies are produced that attack the body's own tissue. Examples include glomerulonephritis (characterized by inflammation of the capillary loops in the glomeruli of the kidney) and myasthenia gravis (characterized by an inflammation of the nerve/muscle junctions).

Cascade filtration: The combination of plasmapheresis with a second online membrane filtration of the collected plasma to selectively remove specific toxic or immunogenic components from blood based primarily on their size.

Cytapheresis: A type of therapeutic apheresis involving the specific removal of red blood cells, white cells (also referred to as leukapheresis), or platelets (also referred to as plateletapheresis).

Donor apheresis: The collection of a specific component of blood (either plasma or one of the cellular fractions), with the return of the remaining blood components to the donor. Donor apheresis is used to significantly increase the amount of plasma (or a particular cell type) that can be donated for subsequent use in blood banking and/or plasma fractionation.

Immune complexes: Antigen-antibody complexes that can be deposited in tissue. In rheumatoid arthritis this deposition occurs primarily in the joints, leading to severe inflammation and tissue damage.

Photopheresis: The extracorporeal treatment of diseases characterized by aberrant T-cell populations using visible or ultraviolet light therapy, possibly in combination with specific photoactive chemicals.

Plasma exchange: The therapeutic process in which a large volume of plasma (typically 3 l) is removed and replaced by an equivalent volume of a replacement fluid (typically fresh frozen plasma, a plasma substitute, or an albumin-containing saline solution).

Plasma perfusion: The therapeutic process in which a patient's plasma is first isolated from the cellular elements in the blood and then subsequently treated to remove specific plasma components. This secondary treatment usually involves a sorbent column designed to selectively remove a specific plasma component or a membrane filtration designed to remove a broad class of plasma proteins.

Plasmapheresis: The process in which plasma is separated from the cellular components of blood using either centrifugal or membrane-based devices. Plasmapheresis can be employed in donor applications for the collection of source plasma for subsequent processing into serum fractions or in therapeutic applications for the treatment of a variety of disorders involving the presence of abnormal circulating components in the plasma.

Therapeutic apheresis: A process involving the separation and removal of a specific component of the blood (either plasma, a plasma component, or one of the cellular fractions) for the treatment of a metabolic disorder or disease state.

References

Edelson R.L. 1989. Photopheresis: a new therapeutic concept. *Yale. J. Biol. Med.* 62: 565.

Kambic H.E. and Nosé Y. 1993. Plasmapheresis: historical perspective, therapeutic applications, and new frontiers. *Artif. Organs* 17: 850.

Malchesky P.S., Asanuma Y., Zawicki I. et al. 1980. On-line separation of macromolecules by membrane filtration with cryogelation. *Artif. Organs* 400: 205.

Nosé Y., Kambic H.E., and Matsubara S. 1983. Introduction to therapeutic apheresis. In Y. Nosé, P.S. Malchesky, J.W. Smith et al. (Eds.), *Plasmapheresis: Therapeutic Applications and New Techniques*, pp. 1–22, New York, Raven Press.

Rock G. 1983. Centrifugal apheresis techniques. In Y. Nosé, P.S. Malchesky, J.W. Smith et al. (Eds.), *Plasmapheresis: Therapeutic Applications and New Techniques*, pp. 75–80, New York, Raven Press.

Sawada K., Malchesky P., and Nosé Y. 1990. Available removal systems: state of the art. In U.E. Nydegger (Ed.), *Therapeutic Hemapheresis in the 1990s*, pp. 51–113, New York, Karger.

Solomon B.A., Castino F., Lysaght M.J. et al. 1978. Continuous flow membrane filtration of plasma from whole blood. *Trans. Am. Soc. Artif. Intern. Organs* 24: 21.

Zeman L.J. and Zydney A.L. 1986. *Microfiltration and Ultrafiltration: Principles and Applications*, pp. 471–489, New York, Marcel Dekker.

Zydney A.L. and Colton C.K. 1982. Continuous flow membrane plasmaphersis: theoretical models for flux and hemolysis prediction. *Trans. Am. Soc. Artif. Intern. Organs* 28: 408.

Zydney A.L. and Colton C.K. 1986. A concentration polarization model for filtrate flux in cross-flow microfiltration of particulate suspensions. *Chem. Eng. Commun.* 47: 1.

Zydney A.L. and Colton C.K. 1987. Fundamental studies and design analyses of cross-flow membrane plasmapheresis. In J.D. Andrade, J.J. Brophy, and D.E. Detmer (Eds.), *Artif. Organs*, pp. 343–358, VCH Publishers.

Further Information

Several of the books listed above provide very effective overviews of both the technical and clinical aspects of therapeutic apheresis. In addition, the Office of Technology Assessment has published Health Technology Case Study 23: *The Safety, Efficacy, and Cost Effectiveness of Therapeutic Apheresis,* which has an excellent discussion of the early clinical development of apheresis. Several journals also provide more detailed discussions of current work in apheresis, including *Artificial Organs* and the *Journal of Clinical Apheresis.* The abstracts and proceedings from the meetings of the *International Congress of the World Apheresis Association* and the *Japanese Society for Apheresis* also provide useful sources for current research on both the technology and clinical applications of therapeutic apheresis.

70

Liver Support Systems

Pierre M. Galletti
Hugo O. Jauregui
Rhode Island Hospital

70.1 Morphology of the Liver

The liver is a complex organ that operates both in series and in parallel with the gastrointestinal tract. After entering the portal system, the products of digestion come in contact with the liver **parenchymal** cells, or hepatocytes, which remove most of the carbohydrates, amino acids, and fats from the feeder circulation, therefore preventing excessive increases throughout the body after a meal. In the liver, these products are then stored, modified, and slowly released to the better advantage of the whole organism.

The liver can be considered a complex large-scale biochemical reactor, since it occupies a central position in the **metabolism**, that is, the sum of the physical and chemical processes by which living matter is produced, maintained, and destroyed, and whereby energy is made available for the functioning of liver cells as well as tissues from all other organs.

The adult human liver (weighing 1500 g) receives its extensive blood supply (on the order of 1 l/min or 20% of cardiac output) from two sources: the portal vein (over two-thirds) and the hepatic artery (about one-third). Blood from the liver drains through the hepatic veins into the inferior vena cava. Macroscopically, the liver is divided into four or five lobes with individual blood supply and bile drainage channels. Some of these lobes can be surgically separated, although not without difficulty.

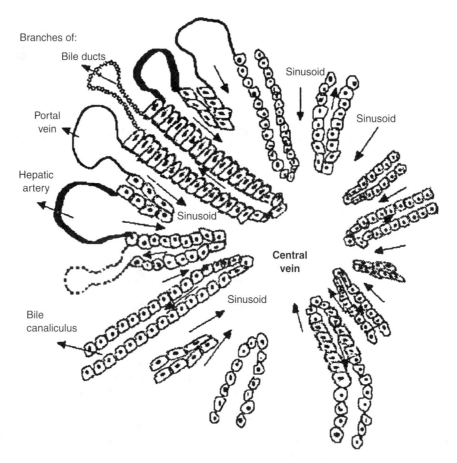

FIGURE 70.1   The liver lobule.

Microscopically, human hepatocytes (250–500 × 109 in. each liver) are arranged in plates (Figure 70.1) that are radially distributed around the central (drainage) vein [Jones and Spring-Mills, 1977] and form somewhat hexagonal structures, or liver lobules, which are much more clearly demarcated in porcine livers. Present in the periphery of these lobules are the so-called **portal triads**, in the ratio of three triads for each central vein. In each portal triad, there are tributaries of the portal vein, branches of the hepatic artery, and collector ducts for the bile (Figure 70.1). Blood enters the liver lobule at the periphery from terminal branches of the portal vein and the hepatic arteries and is distributed into capillaries which separate the hepatocyte plates. These capillaries, called sinusoids, characteristically have walls lined by layers of endothelial cells that are not continuous but are perforated by small holes (fenestrae). Other cells are present in the sinusoid wall, for example, phagocytic Kuppfer cells, fat-storing Ito cells, and probably a few yet undefined **mesenchymal cells**. It is important to emphasize that blood-borne products (with the exception of blood cells) have free access to the perisinusoidal space, called the space of Disse, which can be visualized by electron microscopy as a gap separating the sinusoidal wall from the hepatocyte plasma membrane (Figure 70.2). In this space, modern immunomicroscopic studies have identified three types of collagens: Type IV (the most abundant), Type I, and Type III. Fibronectin and glycosaminoglycans are also found there, but laminin is only present in the early stages of liver development not in adult mammalian livers [Martinez-Hernandez, 1984].

The hepatocytes themselves are large (each side about 25 μm), multifaceted, polarized cells with an apical surface which constitutes the wall of the bile canaliculus (the channel for bile excretion) and basolateral surfaces which lie in close proximity to the blood supply. Hepatocytes constitute 80 to 90% of the liver cell mass. Kuppfer cells (about 2%) belong to the reticulo-endothelial system, a widespread class

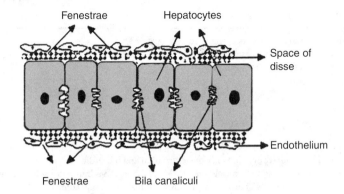

FIGURE 70.2 Hepatocyte relationships with the space of Disse and the sinusoid wall.

of cells which specialize in the removal of particulate bodies, old blood cells, and infectious agents from the blood stream.

The cytoplasm of hepatocytes contains an abundance of smooth and rough endoplasmic reticulum, ribosomes, lysosomes, and mitochondria. These organelles are involved in complex biochemical processes: fat and lipid metabolism, synthesis of lipoproteins and cholesterol, protein metabolism, and synthesis of complex proteins, for example, serum albumin, transferrin, and clotting factors from amino acid building blocks. The major aspects of detoxification take place in the cisternae of the smooth endoplasmic reticulum, which are the site of complex oxidoreductase enzymes known collectively as the cytochrome P-450 system. In terms of excretion, hepatocytes produce bile, which contains bile salts and **conjugated** products. Hepatocytes also store large pools of essential nutrients such as folic acid, retinol, and cobalamin.

70.2 Liver Functions

The liver fulfills multiple and finely tuned functions that are critical for the **homeostasis** of the human body. Although individual pathways for synthesis and breakdown of carbohydrates, lipids, amino acids, proteins, and nucleic acids can be identified in other mammalian cells, only the liver performs all these biochemical transformations simultaneously and is able to combine them to accomplish its vital biologic task. The liver is also the principal site of biotransformation, activation or inactivation of drugs and synthetic chemicals. Therefore, this organ displays a unique biologic complexity. When it fails, functional replacement presents one of he most difficult challenges in substitutive medicine.

Under normal physiologic requirements, the liver modifies the composition and concentration of the incoming nutrients for its own usage and for the benefit of other tissues. Among the major liver functions, the detoxification of foreign toxic substances (**xenobiotics**), the regulation of essential nutrients, and the secretion of transport proteins and critical plasma components of the blood coagulation system are probably the main elements to evaluate in a successful organ replacement [Jauregui, 1991]. The liver also synthesizes several other critical proteins, excretes bile, and stores excess products for later usage, functions that can temporarily be dispensed with but must eventually be provided.

The principal functions of the liver are listed in Table 70.1. The challenge of liver support in case of organ failure is apparent from the complexity of functions served by liver cells and from our still imperfect ability to rank these functions in terms of urgency of replacement.

70.3 Hepatic Failure

More than any other organ, the liver has the property of regeneration after tissue damage. Removal or destruction of a large mass of hepatic parenchyma stimulates controlled growth to replace the missing tissue. This can be induced experimentally, for example, two-thirds of a rat liver can be excised with no

TABLE 70.1 Liver Functions

Carbohydrate metabolism: glyconeogenesis and glycogenolysis
Fat and lipid metabolism: synthesis of lipoproteins and cholesterol
Synthesis of plasma proteins, for example:
    Albumin
    Globulins
    Fibrinogen
    Coagulation factors
    Transferrin
    α-fetoprotein
Conjugation of bile acids; conversion of heme to bilirubin and biliverdin
Detoxification: Transformation of metabolites, toxins, and hormones into water-soluble compounds
    (e.g., cytochrome P-450 P-450 oxidation, glucuronyl transferase conjugation)
Biotransformation and detoxification of drugs
Metabolism and storage of vitamins
Storage of essential nutrients
Regeneration

ill effects and will be replaced within 6 to 8 days. The same phenomenon can be observed in humans and is a factor in the attempted healing process characteristic of the condition called liver **cirrhosis**. Recent attempts at liver transplantation using a liver lobe from a living donor rely on the same expectation of recovery of lost liver mass. Liver regeneration is illustrated by the myth of Prometheus, a giant who survived in spite of continuous partial hepatectomy through the good auspices of a vulture (a surgical procedure inflicted on him as punishment for having stolen the secret fire from the gods and passing it on to humanity).

Hepatic failure may be acute or chronic according to the time span it takes for the condition to develop. Mechanisms and toxic by-products perpetuating these two conditions are not necessarily the same. Acute fulminant hepatic failure (FHF) is the result of massive necrosis of hepatocytes induced over a period of days or weeks by toxic substances or viral infection. It is characterized by jaundice and mental confusion which progresses rapidly to stupor or coma. The latter condition, hepatic encephalopathy (HE), is currently thought to be associated with diminished hepatic **catabolism**. Metabolites have been identified which impair synaptic contacts and inhibit neuromuscular and mental functions (Table 70.2). Although brain impairment is the rule in this condition, there is no anatomic damage to any of the brain structures, and therefore, the whole process is potentially reversible. The mortality rate of FHF is high (70 to 90%), and death is quite rapid (a week or two). Liver transplantation is currently the only effective form of treatment for FHF. Transplantation procedures carried out in life-threatening circumstances are much more risky than interventions in relatively better compensated patients. The earlier the transplantation procedure takes place, the greater is the chance for patient survival. However, 10 to 30% of FHF patients will regenerate their liver under proper medical management without any surgical intervention. Hence, liver transplantation presents the dilemma of choosing between an early intervention, which might be unnecessary in some cases, or proceeding to a late procedure with a statistically higher mortality [Jauregui et al., 1994].

Chronic hepatic failure, the more common and progressive form of the disease, is often associated with morphologic liver changes known as cirrhosis in which fibrotic tissue gradually replaces liver tissue as the result of long-standing toxic exposure (e.g., alcoholism) or secondary to viral hepatitis. More than 30,000 people died of liver failure in the United States in 1990.

In chronic hepatic failure, damaged hepatocytes are unable to detoxify toxic nitrogenous products that are absorbed by intestinal capillaries and carried to the liver by the portal system. Ammonia probably plays the major role in the deterioration of the patient's mental status, leading eventually to "hepatic coma." An imbalance of conventional amino acids (some abnormally high, some low) may also be involved in the pathogenesis of the central nervous system manifestation of hepatic failure, the most dramatic of which is cerebral edema. Impaired blood coagulation (due to decreased serum albumin and clotting factors),

TABLE 70.2 Metabolic Products with Potential Effects in Acute Liver Failure

Substance	Mode of action
Ammonia	Neurotoxic interaction with other neurotransmitters
	Contributes to brain edema
Benziodiazepine like substances	Neural inhibition
GABA	Neural inhibition
Mercaptans	Inhibition of Na–K ATPase
Octopamine	Acts as a false neurotransmitter

hemorrhage in the gastro-intestinal system (increased resistance to blood flow through the liver leads to portal hypertension, ascites formation, and bleeding from esophageal varices), and hepatic encephalopathy with glial cell damage in the brain are the standard landmarks of chronic hepatic failure. In fact, HE in chronic liver failure is often precipitated by episodes of bleeding and infection, and progression to deep coma is an ominous sign of impending death.

Intensive management of chronic liver failure includes fluid and hemodynamic support, correction of electrolyte and acid–base abnormalities, respiratory assistance, and treatment of cerebral edema if present. Aggressive therapy can diminish the depth of the coma and improve the clinical signs, but the outcome remains grim. Eventually, 60 to 90% of the patients require transplantation. About 2500 liver transplants are performed every year in the United States, with a survival rate ranging from 68 to 92%. The most serious limitation to liver transplantation (besides associated interrelated diseases) remains donor scarcity. Even if segmented transplants and transplants from living related donors become acceptable practices, it is unlikely that the supply of organs will ever meet the demand. Further, the problem of keeping a patient alive with terminal hepatic failure, either chronic or acute, while waiting for an adequately matched transplant is much more difficult than the parallel problem in end-stage renal disease, where dialysis is a standardized and effective support modality.

An appreciation of the modalities of presentation of the two types of hepatic coma encountered in liver failure is needed for a definition of the requirements for the proper use of liver assist devices. In the case of FHF, the hepatologist wants an extracorporeal device that will circulate a large volume of blood through a detoxifying system [Jauregui and Muller, 1992] allowing either the regeneration of the patient's damaged liver (and the avoidance of a costly and risky liver transplantation procedure) or the metabolic support needed for keeping the patient alive while identifying a cadaveric donor organ. In the first option, the extracorporeal liver assist device functions as an organ substitute for the time it takes the liver to regenerate and recover its function; in the second, it serves as temporary bridge to transplantation.

In the case of chronic liver failure today, spontaneous recovery appears impossible. The damaged liver needs to be replaced by a donor organ, although not with the urgency of FHF. The extracorporeal liver assist device (LAD) is used as a bridge while waiting for the availability of a transplant. It follows that the two different types of liver failure may require different bioengineering designs.

70.4 Liver Support Systems

The concept of artificial liver support is predicated on the therapeutic benefit of removing toxic substances accumulating in the circulation of liver failure patients. These metabolites reflect the lack of detoxification by damaged hepatocytes, the lack of clearance of bacterial products from the gut by impaired Kupffer cells, and possibly the release of necrotic products from damaged cells which inhibit liver regeneration. Systemic endotoxemia as well as massive liver injury give rise to an inflammatory reaction with activation of monocytes and macrophages and release of cytokines which may be causally involved in the pathogenesis of multiorgan failure commonly encountered in liver failure.

Technologies for temporary liver support focus on the detoxifying function, since this appears to be the most urgent problem in liver failure. The procedures and devices which have been considered for this purpose include the following.

70.4.1 Hemodialysis

Hemodialysis with conventional cellulosic membranes (cut-off point around 2000 Da) or more permeable polysulfone or polyacrylonitrile [de Groot et al., 1984] (cut-off 1500 to 5000 Da) helps to restore electrolyte and acid–base balance and may decrease the blood ammonia levels but cannot remove large molecules and plasma protein-bound toxins. Improvement of the patient's clinical condition (e.g., amelioration of consciousness and cerebral edema) is temporary. The treatment appears to have no lasting value and no demonstrated effect on patient survival. In addition, hemodialysis may produce a respiratory distress syndrome caused by a complement-mediated poly-morphonuclear cell aggregation in the pulmonary circulatory bed. Because some of the clinical benefit seems related to the removal of toxic molecules, more aggressive approaches focused on detoxification have been attempted.

70.4.2 Hemofiltration

Hemofiltration with high cut-off point membranes (around 50,000 Da with some polyacrylonitrile–polyvinyl chloride copolymers, modified celluloses, or polysulfones) clears natural or abnormal compounds within limits imposed by convective transport across the exchange membrane. These procedures again have a temporary favorable effect on hepatic encephalopathy (perhaps because of the correction of toxic levels of certain amino acids) with reversal of coma, but they do not clearly improve survival rates.

70.4.3 Hemoperfusion

Hemoperfusion, that is, extracorporeal circulation of blood over nonspecific sorbents (e.g., activated charcoal) [Chang, 1975] or more complex biochemical reactors which allow the chemical processing of specific biologic products, such as ammonia, have not yet met clinical success in spite of encouraging experimental results, except in the case of hepatic necrosis induced by poisonous mushrooms such as Amanita phalloides. Anion exchange resins and affinity columns similar to those used in separative chromatography may help in removing protein-bound substances (e.g., bilirubin) which would not pass through dialysis or hemofiltration membranes, but nonspecific sorbents may also deplete the plasma of biologically important substances. Further, these techniques are complicated by problems of hemocompatibility, related in part to the entrainment of dust ("fines") associated with the sorbent material itself and in part to platelet activation in patients with an already compromised coagulation status. To minimize this problem direct blood or plasma contact with the sorbent material can be avoided by polymer coating of the sorbent particles using either albumin, cellulose nitrate, or similar thin films, but hemocompatibility remains a concern. Here again, there is anecdotal evidence of clinical improvement of hepatic failure with hemoperfusion, with some reports claiming a higher survival rate in hepatic encephalopathy, but these reports have not been supported by well-controlled studies. As is the case for hemodialysis and hemofiltration, the possible beneficial effect of hemoperfusion should be evaluated in the context of the clinical variability in the course of FHF.

70.4.4 Lipophilic Membrane Systems

Because lipophilic toxins dominate in fulminant hepatic failure, it is conceibable to eliminate such compounds with a hydrophobic (e.g., polysulfone) membrane featuring large voids filled with a nontoxic oil [Brunner and Tegtimeier, 1984]. After diffusion, the toxins can be made water-soluble through reaction with a NaOH-based acceptor solution, thereby preventing their return to the blood stream. A standard, high-flux dialyzer in series with the lipophilic membrane device allows the removal of hydrophilic solutes. Such a system has proved effective in removing toxins such as phenol and p-cresol as well as fatty acids without inducing detrimental side effects of its own.

70.4.5 Immobilized Enzyme Reactors

To address the problem of specificity in detoxification, enzymes such as urease, tyrosinase, L-asparaginase, glutaminase, and UDP-glucuronyl transferase have been attached to hollow fibers or circulated in the closed dialysate compartment of an artificial kidney or still incorporated into microcapsules or "artificial cells" exposed to blood. There is considerable in vitro evidence for the effectiveness of this approach, and some indication of therapeutic value from *in vivo* animal experiments [Brunner et al., 1979]. However, no clinical report has documented the superiority of enzyme reactors over the various modalitites of dialysis. Again there are clinical observations of clearing of the mental state of patients in hepatic coma, but no statistically demonstrated effect on survival. It is unclear whether the lack of success is due to the inability of specific enzymes to remove all offending toxins or is evidence of the need for more than detoxification for effective treatment.

70.4.6 Parabiotic Dialysis

Also referred to as cross-dialysis, parabolic dialysis is a variant of hemodialysis in which the dialysate compartment of a solute exchange device is perfused continuously with blood from a living donor. Because of membrane separation of the two blood streams, the procedure can be carried out even if the two subjects belong to different blood groups or different animal species. However, the risk of the procedure to a human donor (control of blood volume, transfer of toxic substances, mixing of blood streams in case of dialyzer leak) and the difficulty of introducing a live animal donor into the hospital environment have relegated this approach to the class of therapeutic curiosities.

70.4.7 Exchange Transfusion

Exchange transfusion, that is, the quasi-total replacement of the blood volume of a patient in liver failure by alternating transfusion and bleeding, is occasionally used in severe hyperbilirubinemia of the newborn, which used to carry an ominous prognosis because of its association with cerebral edema. The rationale is that exchange transfusion will reduce the level of toxins and replenish the deficient factors in the blood stream while the underlying condition is corrected by natural processes or drugs [Trey et al., 1966]. With the advent of blood component therapy, specific plasma components can also be administered to treat identified deficiencies. Mortality rates of patients treated with exchange blood transfusions have been reported as greater than those observed with conventional therapies.

70.4.8 Plasmapheresis

Plasmapheresis, that is, the combination of withdrawal of blood, centrifugation, or membrane processing to separate and discard the patient's plasma, and return of autologous cells diluted with donor plasma, was practiced initially as a batch process. Techniques now exist for a continuous exchange process, in which plasma and cells are separated by physical means outside of the body (membrane separation or centrifugation), and the patient's plasma replaced by banked plasma (up to 5000 ml per day) [Lepore et al., 1972]. There is evidence from controlled clinical trials for the effectiveness of this form of therapy, but the mortality rate remains high in patients with hepatic failure, whether from insufficient treatment or the risks of the procedure. It appears, however, that plasma exchange can be beneficial in the preoperative period prior to liver transplantation so as to correct severe coagulopathy. Plasmapheresis is used in conjunction with the placement of a hepatocyte-seeded extracorporeal hollow-fiber device to treat acute and chronic liver failure [Rozga et al., 1993].

70.4.9 Combined Therapy

Endotoxins and cytokines can be removed by hemoperfusion over activated charcoal and absorbent resins, but it may be more effective to process plasma than whole blood. This has led to the concept of combining plasmapheresis with continuous plasma treatment for removal of substances such as tumor necrosis factor (TNF), interleukin-6 (IL-6), and bile acids by a resin column, and then ultrafiltration or dialysis for fluid removal, since patients with liver failure often develop secondary renal failure.

70.5   Global Replacement of Liver Function

Because of the complexity and interplay of the various functions of the liver, more success can be expected from global approaches, which allow many or all hepatic functions to be resumed. These include the following.

70.5.1   Cross-Criculation

Cross-circulation of the patient in hepatic coma with a compatible, healthy donor is one approach. This procedure is more than a prolonged exchange transfusion since it allows the donor's liver to substitute for the patient's failing organ and to process chemicals from the patient's blood stream as long as the procedure lasts [Burnell, 1973]. It had been attempted in isolated cases, but reports of effectiveness are entirely anecdotal and the procedure has not been accepted clinically because of ambiguous results and the perceived risk for the donor.

70.5.2   Hemoperfusion over Liver Tissue Slices

The incorporation of active hepatocytes in a hemoperfusion circuit was suggested by the laboratory practice of biochemists who, since Warburg, have investigated metabolic pathways in tissue slices. For liver replacement, this technology has been pioneered primarily in Japan as a substitute for organ transplantation, which is culturally frowned upon in that country in spite of a major incidence of severe liver disease. The procedure may improve biochemical markets of liver failure but has no demonstrated clinical value [Koshino et al., 1975].

70.5.3   *Ex Vivo* Perfusion

Ex vivo perfusion uses an isolated animal liver (pig or baboon) connected to the patient's cardiovascular system [Saunders et al., 1968]. This is a cleaner and more acceptable form of treatment than cross-circulation of hemoperfusion over tissue pieces. Nevertheless, it is limited by the need for thorough washing of the animal's blood from the excised liver, the requirement for a virus-free donor organ source, the limited survival capacity of the excised, perfused organ, which must be replaced at intervals of approximately 24 h, and the cost of the procedure. Success has recently been reported in isolated clinical trials [Chari, 1994].

70.5.4   Heterotopic Hepatocyte Transplantation

This procedure may someday offer an alternative to whole organ transplantation, especially in cases of chronic liver failure, if a sufficient number of cells can be grafted. Freshly isolated hepatocytes have damaged cell surfaces and must be cultured to regain their integrity and display the surface receptors needed for attachment or binding of xenobiotics or endogenous toxic products [McMillan et al., 1988]. At the clinical level, this procedure could rely in part on banking frozen hepatocytes from livers which are not usable for whole organ transplants but constitute a reliable source of cells [Bumgardener et al., 1988]. The procedure does not require removal of the recipients's liver and provides the following advantages: (1) minimal surgery, (2) repeatability as needed, and (3) interim strategy to whole organ transplant. There is no agreement as to the best anatomic site for hepatocyte transplantation, the type of matrix needed for cell attachment and differentiation, and the number of cells needed. It has been reported that hepatocyte culture supernatants were as effective as transplanted hepatocytes in treating rats with chemically induced liver failure [LaPlante-O'Neill et al., 1982]. The tridemensional reconstruction of high-density, functional liver tissue will be the greatest challenge in view of the cell mass required. Structural organization and differentiated functions may be achieved by using an asialoglycoprotein model polymer as the synthetic substrate for a primary culture of hepatocytes to develop functional modules for implantation in humans [Akaike et al., 1989].

70.5.5 Whole Organ *In Situ* Transplantation

This is currently the procedure of choice, most particularly in children. Although progress in clinical and surgical skills certainly accounts in large part for the growing success rate of this procedure over the past 20 years, it is worth noting that the introduction of extracorporeal ciruclation techniques in the surgical protocol to support the donor organ while waiting for completion of the anastomosis has paralleled the steepest increase in success rate of liver transplantation in the past few years. Whereas most liver transplants rely on the availability of cadaver organs, the recent advent of segmented transplants allows consideration of living related donors and possibly the sharing of a donor organ among two or more recipients.

70.6 Hybrid Replacement Procedures

The complexity of hepatic functions, coupled with shortage of human donor organs, has encouraged the development of procedures and devices which rely on xenogeneic living elements attached to synthetic structures and separated from the most host by a permselective membrane to replace temporarily, and perhaps someday permanently, the failing organ.

The incorporation of liver microsomes in microcapsules, hydrogels, or polymer sheets, with or without additonal enzymes or pharmacologic agents, goes one step beyond the immobilized enzyme reactor inasmuch as it calls on cell components endowed with a variety of enzymatic properties to process blood or other body fluids. The feasibility of this technique has been demonstrated *in vitro* [Denti et al., 1976] but has not been investigated extensively in animal experiments.

Cellular hybrid devices — the incorporation of functional cells in a device immersed in body fluids or connected to the vascular system (extracorporeally or somewhere inside the body of the recipient) — are a promising application of the concept of bioartificial organs. However, the problems faced by the "hepatocyte bioreactor" are formidable:

1. The mass of functional cells required is much larger than in the case of secretory or endocrine organs, since a normal liver weighs about 1.5 kg and since as much as 10 to 30% of that mass (i.e., several billion cells) may be required for life-sustaining replacement of function. Taking into account the need for supporting structures, the sheer size of the device will be an obstacle to implantation.
2. The liver features a double feeder circulation (portal and hepatic) and a complex secretory–excretory system which utilizes both blood and bile to dispose of its waste products. How to duplicate such a complex manifolding in an artificial organ and whether it is worth the resulting complexity are questions not yet resolved.
3. With membrane separation of recipient and donor cells, the size of some natural macromolecules to be exchanged (e.g., low-density lipoproteins) precludes the use of standard diffusion membranes. Allowing relatively free solute exchange between the compartments in a device without endangering the immune sequestration of the donor tissue remains a challenge for membrane technology. However, the low immunogenicity of hepatocytes (which lack type I HLA antigens) allows the consideration of relatively open membranes for the construction of extracorporeal reactors.

At the moment, most of the extracorporeal liver assist devices (**ELAD**) utilize xenogeneic mammalian hepatocytes seeded on solid, isotropic hollow fibers. Membrane selectivity limits the rate of diffusion of liposoluble toxins which are bound to plasma proteins for transport. Hence manipulation of membrane transport properties and concentrations of acceptor protiens can affect the clearance of polar materials.

Also, most devices focus on replacing the detoxification function of the natural liver and avoid the more complex "cascade" dialysis circuitry which could either (1) allow the macromolecules synthesized by hepatocytes to return to the blood stream (or another body fluid compartment) though a high cut-off point membrane or (2) provide an excretory path to clear toxic products manufactured by the hepatoctyes, on the model of the bile excretory system. Nonetheless, such circuitry might be valuable to prolong the life of the seeded cells, since the combination of bile salts and bile acids has a damaging detergent effect on the lipid components of the hepatocyte membrane.

The development of bioreactors including cells capable of performing liver functions, and therefore capable of providing temporary liver support, finds applications in the treatment of acute, reversible liver failure or as a bridge for liver transplantation. Designs for a **bioartificial liver** can be classified according to (1) the type of cells selected to replace the hepatic functions or (2) the geometry and chemical nature of the polymer structure used organize the hepatocytes.

70.6.1 Source of Functional Cells

Two main methods of hepatocyte isolation (mechanical and enzymatic) can be used, separately or in combination. Mechanical methods (tissue dissociation) have largely failed in terms of long-term cell viability, although this is not always recognized by investigators developing liver assist systems. Collagenase perfusion [Seglen, 1976] is today the method of choice, yet there is evidence that hepatocytes lose some of their oligosaccharide–lectin binding capacity in the process and do not recover their glycocalyx until after a day or two in culture. Collagenase is thought to loosen cell junctions and secondarily to digest the connective tissue around the hepatocytes. Chemical methods using citrate, EDTA, and similar substances weaken cell junctions by depleting calicum ions without altering the cell membranes and presumably result in better preservation of natural enzymatic functions. Although the yield of chemical methods is lower than that of enzymatic dissociation methods, it may be of interest once a reliable technology for separating viable from nonviable cells on a large scale is perfected.

A priori, an effective bioartificial liver would require either all the multifunctional characteristics of normal hepatocytes *in vivo* or only the specific functional activity that happens to be missing in the patient. Unfortunately, in most cases, clinical signs do not allow us to distinguish between these two extremes, justifying a preference for highly diffrentiated cells.

Differentiation and proliferation are usually at opposite ends of a biologic continuum in most cell types (Figure 70.3) [Jauregui, 1991]. Hence, there is a difficulty of obtaining large numbers of multifunctional hepatocytes. Several options are available:

1. The simplest approach is to use adult mammalian liver cells isolated in sufficient number from large animals. Porcine hepatocytes are preferred for clinical applications because of the availability of virus-free donors. Large-scale isolation of porcine hepatocytes is becoming a routine procedure, and Demetriou has been able to treat several patients with such a system. The expectation is that hepatocytes in suspension or attached to synthetic microcarriers will remain metabolically active even though separated from neighboring cells and normal supportive structures. This approach, which appeared almost beyond practicality a few years ago, seems now less formidable because of expanded knowledge of the molecular factors which favor both hepatocyte attachment to polymeric substrates and functional differentiation. The potential contribution of Kupffer cells to a bioartificial liver has not yet been extensively investigated.

2. The use of liver tumor cells — preferably nonmalignant hepatoma — has been pioneered by Wolfe and Munkelt [1975] because such cells can proliferate indefinitely and therefore require a minimal seeding dose. They are also less anchor-dependent than normal cells. The drawbacks are the loss of specialized hepatic functions often encountered in tumor cell lines, and the theroretical risk of escape of tumor cells in the recipient.

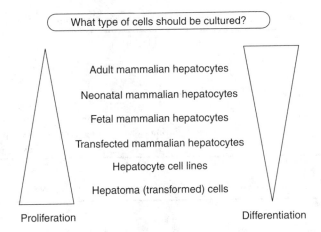

FIGURE 70.3 Cellular choices based on proliferation and differentiation.

3. A modified, functionally differentiated, human hepatoblastoma cell line capale of growing to high densities, yet strongly contact-inhibited by containment with membranes, has been patented and used in animals and man by Sussman et al. [1992]. Evidence for metabolic effectiveness has been reported, and clinical trials are now in progress. The uncertainty associated with the use of a human tumor cell line remains a source of concern.

4. Potentially replicating hepatocytes, such as those obtained from embryonic liver, neonatal animals, or recently hepatectomized adults, have been proposed as a means to obtain a stem cell population with enhanced proliferation capacity. Neonatal hepatocyte-based bioartificial devices have been built on that principle [Hager et al., 1983] and have shown to produce albumin, to metabolize urea, to deaminate cytidine, and to detoxify drugs such as a diazepam. The reliance on "juvenile" cells has become less important with the identification of molecular mechanisms for growth control mitogens such as EGF, TGFa, hepatopoieten B, HSS (hepatic stimulatory substance) and HGF (hepatoctye growth factor), co-mitogenic factors such as norepinephrine and growth inhibitors such as TGFb, and interleukin-1b.

5. Transfected or transgeic hepatocytes may provide the ultimate solution to the cell supply problem. However, they are usually selected for the monoclonal expression of a single function and therefore may not be suitable except when a single cause of hepatic failure has been identified. Alternatively, a combination of different transfected hepatocytes may be considered.

Table 70.3 illustrates the choices made by three different groups of investigators for clinical liver assist devices.

70.6.2 Supporting Structures

Microencapsulation in a nutrient liquid or a polymer gel surrounded by a conformal membrane provides a suspension of metabolically active units which can either be placed in a container for extracorporeal hemoperfusion, introduced into the peritoneal cavity for implantation, or even infused into the portal vein for settling in the patient's liver. The blood or tissue reaction to multiple implants and the long-term in vivo stability of hydrogels based on polyelectrolytes remain unresolved problems.

A flat sheet of membrane or a spongy matrix coated with attachment factors can be used to anchor a suspension of functional cells. The limitation of this approach is the need for vascularization of the implant, since the cells are metabolically active and therefore are quite avid of oxygen and nutrients.

Microcarrier-attached hepatocytes are attractive because the technology of suspension cultures is amenable to the proliferation of a large number of cells. The bulk of the carrier beads probably limits this approach to the extracorporeal circuits similar to those used for hemoperfusion [Rozga et al., 1993].

TABLE 70.3 Present Choice of the Cellular Component for Extracorporeal Liver Assist Devices

Sussman and Kelly [1993]	Neuzil et al. [1993]	Jauregui and Muller [1992]
Hepatoblastoma-derived cell line	Porcine hepatocytes separated via portal vein perfusion	Porcine hepatocytes separated via hepatic vein perfusion
Cells divide indefinitely	Hepatocyte division has not been tested (5 to 8)	Limited number of hepatocyte doublings
Cells are cultured in the device	Hepatocytes are seeded on microcarriers and introduced in the device immediately before clinical use	Hepatocytes may be seeded or cultured in the device through a proprietary technology

TABLE 70.4 Consideration in the Choice of the Cellular Component of Extracorporeal Liver Assist Devices

Advantages	Disadvantages
Hepatoblastoma cell lines are easy to culture and are free of other cell contaminants	Hepatoblastoma cell lines are tumorigenic
Tumor cell lines are not anchorage dependent	Tumor cell lines may not respond to physiologic regulation
Porcine or primary hepatocytes respond to physiologic stimulation	Porcine hepatocytes have limited proliferation ability
Porcine hepatocytes express P450 (detoxification activity)	Porcine hepatocytes show limited life span

Hollow-fiber ELADs are constructed by filling the interstices within a bundle of parallel hollow fibers with liver cells, using the lumen of the tubes to provide metabolic support and an excretion channel, typically by circulating blood from an extracorporeal circuit. Alternatively, a hybrid organ can be built by filling the lumen of the hollow fibers with functional cells and implanting the bundle in the body cavity to allow exchanges with the surrounding fluid. One could combine such a device with an oxygenation system, for example, by filling the peritoneal cavity with a high-oxygen-capacity fluid such as a fluorocarbon and a gas exchange system for that fluid analogous to the intravenous oxygenator (IVOX).

70.7 Outlook

Medical trials with extracorporeal hollow-fiber systems are already in progress, although there are some unanswered questions in the proper design of a hepatocyte-seeded ELAD. A review of Table 70.4 will indicate that there is no consensus for implementing cellular choices in the construction of such systems.

Some researchers believe that the culture of hepatocytes on a synthetic matrix prior to chemical application is a complicated proposition that impairs the practical application of this technology. An alternative could be the isolation, freezing, and shipping of porcine hepatocytes to the medical centers treating patients with acute and chronic liver failure (usually transplantation centers). This approach may offer a direct and economically sound solution. Unfortunately, many FHF patients require emergency liver support and are managed in secondary care medical institutions which have neither a transplantation program nor a tissue culture facility for the seeding of hollow-fiber devices. Part of the argument for the porcine hepatocyte isolation, shipment, seeding, and immediate use in a bioartificial liver system relies on the earlier concept that primary mammalian hepatocytes do not grow *in vitro* or are very difficult to maintain in hollow-fiber devices. In fact, rodent hepatocytes have shown excellent detoxification activities when cultured on perfused hollow fiber cultures. Rabbit hepatocytes also survive in hollow-fiber bioreactors which have proved successful in treating one of the most representative animal modes of human FHF.

The technology for manufacturing ELADs may also need further attention. For instance, the efficiency of hollow fibers in maintaining hybridoma cultures and producing specific proteins is known to be inferior to that of cellular bioreactors based on microcarrier technology. The surface of hollow fibers has been optimized for blood compatibility but not for hepatocyte attachment, and therefore new materials or structures may have to be developed.

At the conceptual level, primary hepatocytes may need to be cultured either in combination with other cells that will provide parabiotic support or on substrates that imitate the composition of the extracellular matrix found *in situ* in the space of Disse. Our own experience [Naik et al., 1990] and that of others [Singhvi et al., 1994] raise some questions about the role of substrates in maintaining long-term hepatocyte viability *in vitro*. In fact, most of them operate in a rather indiscriminate fashion by providing an anchor for hepatocytes. Collagen, types I, III, IV, and fibonectin contribute to cytoplasmic spreading which in the long term does not favor maintenance of the pheontypic expression of hepatocytes. Polymer compositions expressing surface sugar residues responsible for hepatocyte attachment through the asailoglycoprotein receptor (a plasma membrane complex present mainly in the bile canalicular area which internalizes plasma asiaglycoprotein) appear able to maintain hepatocytes in culture with extended functional activities [Akaike et al., 1989]. Other investigators have shown the value of extracellular glycoproteins and glycosaminoglycans rich in laminin (e.g., Matrigel) [Caron and Bissell, 1989]. Hepatocytes immobilized on these substraes do not spread but maintain their tridimensional morphology, as well as their functional activity. Such observations suggest that long-term expression of hepaotcyte-specific functions depend on maintaining the in situ cell shape and their spacial interrelations [Koide et al., 1990]. Future ELAD designs should provide not only ideal polymer substrates for cell attachment but also a special configuration that will maintain the tridimensional structure of hepatic tissue.

Experience with artificial organs shows that the development of these devices tends to underestimate the effort and the technical advances needed to pass from a "proof of principle" prototype for animal evaluation to fabrictaion of a clinically acceptable system for human use. Full-scale design, cell procurement, cell survival, and device storage are all major bottlenecks on the way to a clinical product. One of the gray areas remains in the molecular weight cut-off of the hollow fiber wall. Which substances are responsible for the development of FHF and must therefore be cleared? Are they protein-bound, middle-molecular-, or low-molecular-size compounds? In the absence of clear answers to these questions, the designer of separation membranes is in an ambigous position; some investigators use low molecular cut-off membranes to guarantee immunoseparation of the xenograft, whereas others prefer high-molecular cut-off to enhance functionality. The use of microporous membranes in human subjects has not led, as of yet, to any hypersensitivity reactions in spite of potential passage of immunglobulins.

A reliable way to restore consciousness in animal models of FHF is to cross-circulate the blood with a normal animal. To the extent that ELADs may function in patients as in these animal models, they may prove successful only in relieving the symptoms of the disorder without increasing the survival rate. For instance, when 147 patients with advanced stages of HE were treated with charcoal hemoperfusion over a 10-year period, all showed symptomatic improvement, but the survival rate of 32% was the same as in five control groups. Therefore, enthusiasm generated by preliminary human trials with hollow-fiber devices should be tempered with a cautious approach. Without reliable control studies, we will remain in the position defined by Benhamou et al. [1972], "The best future one can wish for a sufferer from severe acute hepatic failure is to undergo a new treatment and have his case published — Be published or perish!"

Defining Terms

Bioartificial liver: A liver assist or liver replacement device incorporating living cells in physical or chemical processes normally performed by liver tissue.

Catabolism: The aspect of metabolism in which substances in living tissues are transformed into waste products or solutes of simpler chemical composition. (The opposite process is called anabolism.)

Cirrhosis: A degenerative process in the liver marked by excess formation of connective tissue destruction of functional cells, and, often, contraction of the organ.

Conjugated: The joining of two compounds to produce another compound, such as the combination of a toxic product with some substance in the body to form a detoxified product, which is then eliminated.

ELAD: Extracorporeal liver assist device.

Homeostasis: A tendency of stability in the normal body states (internal environment) of the organism. This is achieved by a system of control mechanisms activated by negative feedback, for example, a high level of carbon dioxide in extracellular fluid triggers increased pulmonary ventilation, which in turn causes a decrease in carbon dioxide concentration.

Mesenchymal cells: The meshwork of embryonic connective tissue in the mesoderm from which are formed the connective tissues of the body and the blood vessels and lymphatic vessels.

Metabolism: The sum of all the physical and chemical processes by which living organized substance is produced and maintained (anabolism) and the transformation by which energy is made available for the uses of the organism (catabolism).

Parenchymal: The essential elements of an organ.

Phagoctyic: Pertaining to or produced by any cells that ingest microrganisms of other cells and foreign particles.

Portal triad: These are microscopic areas of collagen type I-III fibroblasts as well as other connective tissue elements. These triads have a branch of the portal vein, a branch of the hepatic artery, and intermediate caliber bile ducts.

Xenobiotic: A chemical foreign to the biologic system.

References

Akaike T., Kobayashi A., Kobayashi K., et al. 1989. Separation of parenchymal liver cells using a lactose-substituted styrene polymer substratum. *J. Bioact. Compat. Polym.* 4: 51.

Benhamou J.P., Rueff B., and Sicot C. 1972. Severe hepatic failure: a critical study of current therapy. In F. Orlandi, A.M. Jezequel (Eds.), *Liver and Drugs*, New York, Academic Press.

Brunner G., Holloway C.J., and Lösgen H. 1979. The application of immobilized enzymes in an artificial liver support system. *Artif. Organs* 3: 27.

Brunner G., and Tegtimeier F. 1984. Enzymatic detoxification using lipophilic hollow fiber membranes. *Artif. Organs* 8: 161.

Bumgardner G.L., Fasola C., and Sutherland D.E.R. 1988. Prospects for hepatocyte transplantation. *Hepatology* 8: 1158.

Burnell J.M., Runge C., Saunders F.C. et al. 1973. Acute hepatic failure treated by cross circulation. *Arch. Intern. Med.* 132: 493.

Caron J.M. and Bissel D.M. 1989. Extracellular matrix induces albumin gene expression in cultured rat hepatocytes. *Hepatology* 10: 636.

Chang T.M.S. 1975. Experience with the treatment of acute liver failure patients by hemoperfusion over biocompatible microencapsulated (coated) charcoal. In R. Williams, I.M. Murray-Lyon (Eds.), Artificial Liver Support, Tunbridge Wells, England, Pitman Medical.

Chari R.S., Collins B.H., Magee J.C. et al. 1994. Brief report: treatment of hepatic failure with ex vivo pig-liver perfusion followed by liver transplantation. *N. Engl. J. Med.* 331: 134.

De Groot G.H., Schalm S.W., Schicht I. et al. 1984. Large-pore hemodialytic procedures in pigs with ischemic hepatic necrosis; a randomized study. *Hepatogastroenterology* 31: 254.

Denti E., Freston J.W., Marchisi M. et al. 1976. Toward a bioartificial drug metabolizing system: gel immobilized liver cell microsomes. *Trans. Am. Soc. Artif. Intern. Organs* 22: 693.

Hager J.C., Carman R., Porter L.E. et al. 1983. Neonatal hepatocyte culture on artificial capillaries: a model for drug metabolism and the artificial liver. *ASAIO J.* 6: 26–35.

Jauregui H.O. 1991. Treatment of hepatic insufficiency based on cellular therapies. *Int. J. Artif. Organs* 14: 407.

Jauregui H.O. and Muller T.E. 1992. Long-term cultures of adult mammalian hepatocytes in hollow fibers as the cellular component of extracorporeal (hybrid) liver assist devices. *Artif. Organs* 16: 209.

Jauregui H.O., Naik S., Santangini H. et al. 1994. Primary cultures of rat hepatocytes in hollow fiber chambers. *In Vitro Cell Dev. Biol.* 30A: 23.

Jones A.l. and Spring-Mills E. 1977. The liver and gallbladder. In Weiss, R.O. Greep (Eds.), Histology, 4th ed., New York, McGraw-Hill.

Koide N.H., Sakaguchi K., Koide Y. et al. 1990. Formation of multicellular spheroids composed of adult rat hepatocytes in dishes with positively charged surfaces and under other nonadherent environments. *Exp. Cell Res.* 186: 227.

Koshino I., Castino F., Yoshida K. et al. 1975. A biological extracorporeal metabolic device for hepatic support. *Trans. Am. Soc. Artif. Intern. Organs* 21: 492.

LaPlante-O'Neill P., Baumgarner D., Lewis W.I. et al. 1982. Cell-free supernatant from hepatocyte cultures improves survival of rats with chemically induced acute liver failure. *J. Surg Res.* 32: 347.

Lepore M.J., Stutman L.J., Bonnano C.A. et al. 1972. Plasmapheresis with plasma exchange in hepatic coma. II. Fulminant viral hepatitis as a systemic disease. *Arch. Intern. Med.* 129: 900.

Martinez-Hernandez A. 1984. The hepatic extracellular matrix. I. Electron immunohistochemical studies in normal rat liver. *Lab. Invest.* 51: 57.

McMillan P.N., Hevey K.A., Hixson D.C. et al. 1988. Hepatocyte cell surface polarity as demonstrated by lectin binding to isolate and cultured hepatocytes. *J. Histochem. Cytochem.* 36: 1561.

Naik S., Santangini H., and Jauregui H.O. 1990. Culture of adults rabbit hepatoctyes in perfused hollow membranes. *In Vitro Cell Dev. Biol.* 26: 107.

Neuzil D.F., Rozga J., Moscioni A.D., Ro M.S., hakim R., Arnaout W.S., and Demetriou A.A. 1993. Use of a novel bioartificial liver in a patient with acute liver insufficiency. *Surgery* 113: 340.

Rozga J., Williams F., Ro M.-S., et al. 1993. Development of a bioartificial liver: properties and function of a hollow-fiber module inoculated with liver cells. *Hepatology* 17: 258.

Saunders S.J., Bosman S.C.W., Terblanche J. et al. 1968. Acute hepatic coma treated by cross ciruclation with a baboon and by repeated exchange transfusions. *Lancet* 2: 585.

Seglen P.O. 1976. Preparation of isolated rat liver cells. *Meth. Cell Biol.* 13: 29.

Singhvi R., Kumar A., Lopez G.P. et al. 1994. Engineering cell shape and function. *Science* 264: 696.

Sussman N.L., Chong M.G., Koussayer T. et al. 1992. Reversal of fulminant hepatic failure using an extracorporeal liver assist device. *Hepatology* 16: 60.

Sussman N.L., and Kelly J.H. 193. Extracorporeal liver assist in the treatment of fulminant hepatic failure. *Blood Purif.* 11: 170.

Trey C., Burns D.G., and Saunders S.J. 1966. Treatment of hepatic coma by exchange blood transfusion. *N. Eng. J. Med.* 274: 473.

Wolf C.F.W. and Munkelt B.E. 1975. Bilirubin conjugation by an artificial liver composed of cultured cells and synthetic capillaries. *Trans. Am. Soc. Artif. Intern. Organs* 21: 16.

Further Information

Two books of particular interest in hepatic encephalopathy are *Hepatic Encephalopathy: Pathophysiology and Treatment* edited by Roger F. Butterworth and Gilles Pomier Layrargues, published by The Humana Press [1989], and *Hepatology: A Textbook of Liver Disease* edited by David Zakim and Thomas D. Boyer, published by W.B. Saunders Company [1990].

Articles pertaining to extracorporeal liver assist devices appear periodically in the following journals: *ASAIO Journal*, the official journal for the American Society for Artificial Internal Organs (for subscription information, write to J.B. Lippincott, P.O. Box 1600, Hagerstown, MD 21741-9932); *Artificial Organs*, official journal of the International Society for Artificial Organs (for subscription information, write to Blackwell Scientific Publications, Inc., 328 Main Street, Cambridge, MA 02142); and *Cell Transplantation*, official journal of the Cell Transplantation Society (for subscription information, write to Elsevier Science, P.O. Box 64245, Baltimore, MD, 21264-4245).

71

Artificial Pancreas

Pierre M. Galletti
Clark K. Colton
Massachusetts Institute of Technology

Michel Jaffrin
Université de Technologie de Compiègne

Genard Reach
Hôpital Hostel-Dieu Paris

71.1 Structure and Function of the Pancreas

The pancreas is a slender, soft, lobulated gland (ca. 75 g in the adult human), located transversally in the upper abdomen in the space framed by the three portions of the duodenum and the spleen. Most of the pancreas is an exocrine gland which secretes proteolytic and lipolytic enzymes, conveying more than 1 l per day of digestive juices to the gastrointestinal tract. This liquid originates in cell clusters called acini and is collected by a system of microscopic ducts, which coalesce in a channel (the canal of Wirsung) which courses horizontally through the length of the organ and opens into the duodenum next to, or together with, the main hepatic duct (choledocous). Interspersed throughout the exocrine tissue are about 1 million separate, highly vascularized and individually innervated cell clusters known as islets of Langerhans, which together constitute the endocrine pancreas (1 to 2% of the total pancreatic mass). Blood is supplied to the islets by the pancreatic artery and drained into the portal vein. Therefore the entire output of pancreatic hormones is first delivered to the liver.

Human islets average 150 μm in diameter, each cluster including several endocrine cell types. Alpha cells (about 15% of the islet mass) are typically located at the periphery of the cluster. They are the source of glucagon, a fuel-mobilizing (catabolic) hormone which induces the liver to release into the circulation energy-rich solutes such as glucose and aceto-acetic and β-hydroxybutyric acids. Beta cells, which occupy the central portion of the islet, comprise about 80% of its mass. They secrete insulin, a fuel-storing (anabolic) hormone that promotes sequestration of carbohydrate, protein, and fat in storage depots in the liver, muscle, and adipose tissue. Delta cells, interposed between alpha and beta cells, produce somatostatin, one role of which seems to be to slow down the secretion of insulin and digestive juices, thereby prolonging the absorption of food. The PP cells secrete a "pancreatic polypeptide" of yet unknown significance. Other cells have the potential to produce gastrin, a hormone that stimulates the production of gastric juice.

71.2   Endocrine Pancreas and Insulin Secretion

The term **artificial pancreas** is used exclusively for systems aimed at replacing the endocrine function of that organ. Although the total loss of exocrine function (following removal of the gland for polycystic disease, tumor, or trauma) can be quite debilitating, no device has yet been designed to replace the digestive component of the pancreas. Since insulin deficiency is the life-threatening consequence of the loss of endocrine function, the artificial pancreas focuses almost exclusively on insulin supply systems, even though some of the approaches used, such as islet transplantation, of necessity include an undefined element of delivery of other hormones.

Insulin is the most critical hormone produced by the pancreas because, in contradistinction to glucagon, it acts alone in producing its effects, and survival is not possible in its absence. **Endogenous** insulin secretion is greatest immediately after eating and is lowest in the interval between meals. Coordination of insulin secretion with fluctuating demands for energy production results from beta-cell stimulation by metabolites, other hormones, and neural signals. The beta cells monitor circulating solutes (in humans, primarily blood glucose) and release insulin in proportion to needs, with the result that in normal individuals, blood glucose levels fluctuate within quite narrow limits. The response time of pancreatic islets to an increase in blood glucose is remarkably fast: 10 to 20 sec for the initial burst of insulin release (primarily from intracellular stores), which is then followed, in a diphasic manner, by a gradual increase in secretion of newly synthesized hormone up to the level appropriate to the intensity and duration of the stimulus. Under fasting condition the pancreas secretes about 40 μg (1 unit) of insulin per hour to achieve a concentration of insulin of 2 to 4 μg/ml (50 to 100 μU/ml) in portal blood and of 0.5 μg/ml (12 μU/ml) in the peripheral circulation.

71.3   Diabetes

Insulin deficiency leads to a disease called diabetes mellitus, which is the most common endocrine disease in advanced societies, affecting as many as 3 to 5% of the population in the United States, with an even higher incidence in specific ethnic groups.

Diabetes is a chronic systemic disease resulting from a disruption of fuel metabolism either because the body does not produce enough insulin or because the available insulin is not effective. In either case, the result is an accumulation of glucose in the blood or **hyperglycemia**, and, once the renal tubular threshold for glucose is exceeded, a spillover of glucose into the urine or "glycosuria." Hyperglycemia is thought to be the main determinant of microvascular alterations which affect several organs (renal glomerulus, retina, myocardium). It is considered as an important factor in large-blood-vessel pathology (aorta and peripheral arteries, such as carotid and lower limb vessels) often observed in diabetes. Neuropathies of the autonomic, peripheral, and central nervous systems are also common in diabetics, although the pathogenic mechanism is not known.

When blood glucose levels are abnormally high, an increasing fraction of hemoglobin in the red blood cells tends to conjugate with glucose forming a compound identifiable by chromatography and called HbAIC. This reaction serves as a tool in diabetes management and control. The fraction of hemoglobin that is normally glycosylated (relative to total Hb) is between 6 and 9%. If elevated, HbAIC reflects the time-averaged level of hyperglycemia over the lifetime of the red blood cells (3 to 4 months). It can be interpreted as an index of the severity of diabetes or the quality of control by dietary measures and insulin therapy.

There are two main forms of diabetes: Type I, juvenile onset diabetes (typically diagnosed before age 30), or insulin-dependent diabetes; and type II, maturity onset diabetes (typically observed after age 40), or noninsulin-dependent diabetes.

Type I appears abruptly (in a matter of days or weeks) in children and young people, although there is evidence that the islet destruction pattern may start much earlier but remain undiagnosed until close to 90% of the islets have been rendered ineffective. Type I represents only 10% of all cases of diabetes, yet it still affects close to 1 million patients in the United States alone. Endogenous insulin is almost totally absent, and an **exogenous** supply is therefore required immediately to avoid life-threatening metabolic accidents (**ketoacidosis**) as well as the more insidious degenerative processes which affect the cardiovascular system, the kidneys, the peripheral nervous system and the retina. For some unknown reason, 15% of juvenile diabetics never develop complications. Because the cellular and molecular mechanisms of hyperglycemic damage appear experimentally to be reversible by tight control of glucose levels, and the progress of vascular complications is said to be proportional to the square of the blood glucose concentration, early and rigorous control of insulin administration is believed to be essential to minimize the long-term consequences of the disease.

In contrast, type II diabetes, which affects close to 90% of all patients, develops slowly and can often be controlled by diet alone or by a combination of weight loss and oral hypoglycemic drugs. Endogenous insulin is often present in normal and sometimes exaggerated amounts, reflecting an inability of cells to make use of available insulin rather than a true hormonal deficiency. Only 20 to 30% of type II diabetics benefit from insulin therapy. Keto-acidosis is rare, and the major problems are those associated with vascular wall lesions and arterial obstruction. Adult onset diabetics develop the same vascular, renal, ocular, and neural complications as type I diabetics, suggesting that even if the origin of the disease is not identical, its later evolution is fundamentally the same as in juvenile diabetics (Table 71.1).

Diabetes is the leading cause of blindness in the United States. It is also responsible for the largest fraction of the population of patients with end-stage renal disease who are being keep alive by maintenance dialysis. It is one of the most frequent causes of myocardial infraction and stroke, and the most common factor in arterial occlusion and gangrene of the lower extremities leading to limb amputation. With the diabetic population increasing by about 5% per year, diabetes has become one of the major contributors to health expenditures in advanced societies.

It is currently thought that destruction of the pancreatic islets in juvenile diabetes is the result of an autoimmune process, occurring in genetically predisposed individuals, perhaps in relation to an

Table 71.1 Pathogenesis of Diabetes

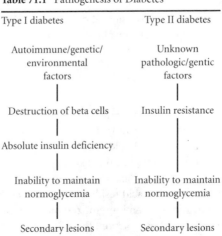

intercurrent infectious disease. This has led to clinical attempts to salvage the remaining intact islets at the earliest recognizable stage of the disease using standard immunosuppressive drugs such as cyclosporin A. The effectiveness of this approach has not been demonstrated.

Diabetologists have also recognized that, at the onset of juvenile diabetes, hyperglycemia exerts a deleterious effect on the function of the still surviving islets, and that in the short term, intensive exogenous insulin therapy may actually lead to an apparent cure of the disease. However, this phenomenon, occasionally referred to as the honeymoon period of insulin treatment is transitory. After a period of weeks to months, diabetes reappears, and an exogenous source of insulin administration becomes necessary for survival. The need for insulin to protect borderline functioning islets against hyperglycemic damage has also been recognized in the early stage of islet transplantation.

71.4   Insulin

Insulin is the mainstay for the treatment of diabetes type I and, to a lesser extent, type II. Since it is the key substance produced by beta cells, it is important to define its chemical nature and its mode of action.

Insulin is a 51 amino acid peptide with a molecular weight of about 5800 Da, made up of two chains (A and B) connected by disulfide bridges. Insulin is formed in the beta cell as a cleavage product of a larger peptide, proinsulin, and is stored there as crystals in tiny intracellular vesicles until released into the blood. The other cleavage product, the "connecting" or C-peptide, though biologically inactive, passes into the blood stream together with insulin, and therefore its concentration reflects, in a patient receiving exogenous insulin, the amount of insulin secreted by the pancreas itself, if any.

Active extracts of islet tissue, obtained from animals following ligation of the pancreation duct to avoid **autolysis**, were first prepared by Banting and Best in 1922. Insulin was crystallized by Abel in 1926. In 1960, Sanger established the sequence of amino acids that make up the molecule shortly thereafter the hormone was synthesized.

The extract composition of insulin varies slightly among animal species. The presence of disulfide bonds between the A and the B chain is critical. Loss of the C-terminal alanine of the B chain by carboxypeptidase hydrolysis results in no loss of biologic activity. The octapeptide residue that remains after splitting off the last eight amino acids of the B chain has a biologic activity amounting to about 15% of the original insulin molecule. About one-half of the insulin disappears in its passage through the liver. Only a small fraction normally goes to peripheral tissues. Plasma half-life is on the order of 40 min, most of the degradation occurring in the liver and kidneys. No biologically active insulin is eliminated in the urine.

Since insulin is a polypeptide, it cannot be taken orally because it would be digested and inactivated in the gastrointestinal tract. In an emergency, insulin can be administered intravenously, but standard treatment relies on subcutaneous administration. This port of entry differs from physiologic secretion of insulin in two major ways: The adsorption is slow and does not mimic the rapid rise and decline of secretion in response to food ingestion, and the insulin diffuses into the systemic veins rather than into the portal circulation.

71.5   Insulin Therapy

Preparations of insulin are classified according to their species of origin and their duration of action. Human insulin (synthesized by recombinant DNA techniques) and porcine insulin (which is obtained by chemical extraction from slaughterhouse-retrieved organs and differs from human insulin by only one amino-acid at the carboxyl-terminus of the B chain) are in principle preferable to bovine insulin (which differs from the human form by three amino acid residues). In practice, all three are equipotent, and all three can, in a minority of patients, stimulate an immune response and cause hypersensitivity reactions. Because of insulin's relatively short duration of action, formulations delaying the absorption of subcutaneously injected hormone and hence prolonging its effectiveness have greatly facilitated the treatment of diabetes. The mode of administration of insulin influences its plasma concentration and bioavailability. The usual treatment schemes rely on the use of one or more types of insulin (Table 71.2).

Pharmacologists classify the available insulin formulations according to their latency and duration of action as fast acting, intermediate-acting, and slow acting using a terminology of regular, semilente, lente, and ultralente (Table 71.3). Crystalline insulin is prepared by precipitating the polypeptide in the presence of zinc in a suitable buffer solution. Insulin complexed with a strongly basic protein, protamine, and stabilized with zinc is relatively insoluble at physiological pH and is therefore released only slowly from the site of injection. However, one must keep in mind that onset and duration of action may be quite variable from one patient to another.

Whereas insulin was hailed as a life-saving drug in the years following its discovery (which it was, as evidenced by the much reduced incidence of hyperglycemic coma and the much longer life expectancy of juvenile diabetics, as compared to the period before 1930), it has not turned out to be quite the universal panacea it was expected to be. Some of the problems that have surfaced relate to the limitations associated with the mode of administration of the drug. Other problems are thought to derive from our inability to mimic the finely tuned feedback system which normally maintains the blood glucose levels within very narrow limits (Table 71.4).

TABLE 71.2 Types of Insulin

Fast acting	Multiple injections (basal and preprandial)
Intermediate	Two injections (morning and evening)
Slow acting	One injection (to prevent hyperglycemia at night)

TABLE 71.3 Properties of Insulin Preparations

Type	Appearance	Added protein	Zinc content mg/100 U	Time of action (h)		
				Onset	Peak	Duration
Rapid						
Crystalline (regular)	Clear	None	0.01–0.04	0.3–0.7	2–4	5–8
Insulin–zinc suspension (semilente)	Cloudy	None	0.2–0.25	0.5–1.0	2–8	12–16
Intermediate						
NPH (Isophane insulin suspension)	Cloudy	Protamine	0.016–0.04	1–2	6–12	18–24
Lente (insulin zinc suspension)	Cloudy	None	0.2–0.25	1–2	6–12	18–24
Slow						
Ultalente (extended insulin zinc suspension)	Cloudy	None	0.2–0.25	4–6	16–18	20–36
PZI (Protamine zinc insulin suspension)	Cloudy	Protamine	0.2–0.25	4–6	14–20	24–36

Source: Modified from Table 71.1 in *The Pharmacological Basis of Therapeutics*, 3rd ed., Goodman and Gillman.

TABLE 71.4 Problems with Insulin Treatment

Problem	Answers
Poor compliance with multiple injections	Better syringes and needles
	Subcutaneous ports
	Intravenous ports
	Insulin pens
Inadequate pharmacokinetics of insulin preparations	Enhance immediate effect
	Prolong duration of effect
Hyperinsulinemia	Release insulin in portal circulation
Lack of feedback control	Servo-controlled administration
	Natural control by transplant
	Bioartificial pancreas

TABLE 71.5 Potential
Approaches to Diabetes Treatment

Prevent destruction of beta cells
Prevent beta cell exhaustion
Increase insulin output
Amplify glucose signal
Overcome insulin resistance
Replace beta cells by:
    Insulin administration
    Electromechanical delivery system
    Whole organ transplantation
    Islet transplantation
    Biohybrid device

71.6 Therapeutic Options in Diabetes

Experimental studies of blood glucose regulation and empirical observations in diabetic patients have revealed three major characteristics of blood glucose regulation by the pancreas:

1. The natural system operates as a closed-loop regulatory mechanism within narrow limits
2. Portal administration is more effective than systemic administration because insulin reaches the liver first
3. Pulsatile administration of insulin is more effective than continuous administration

There are several stages in the evolution of diabetes where a medical intervention might be helpful (Table 71.5). Many interventions have been attempted with various degrees of success. Since diabetes expresses a disturbance of biologic feedback mechanism between blood glucose levels and insulin secretion, there might be possibilities to influence the biologic regulation process through its natural sensing or amplifying mechanisms. However, no practical solution has yet emerged from this approach. As a result the accent has been placed primarily on pharmacologic forms of treatment (diverse insulin formulations and routes of administration), engineered delivery systems (extracorporeal or implanted pumps), and substitution by natural insulin production sources (organ, islet, or individual beta cell transplantation, with or without genetic manipulation and with or without membrane immunoprotection). An overview of the recently investigated approaches is given in Table 71.6.

71.7 Insulin Administration Systems

71.7.1 Syringes and Pens

Insulin traditionally has been administered subcutaneously by means of a syringe and needle, from a vial containing insulin at a concentration of 40 units per ml.

When insulin was first proposed to treat diabetic patients in 1922, glass syringes were used. The burden linked to repeated sterilization disappeared when disposable syringes became available in the early 1970s. Yet patients still had to perform the boring and, for some, difficult task of refilling the syringe from a vial. From a pragmatic viewpoint the development of pens in which insulin is stored in a cartridge represented a major advance in diabetes management. In France, for instance, a recent survey indicates that more than half of the patients use a pen for daily therapy. A needle is screwed on the cartridge and should ideally be replaced before each injection. Cartridges containing either 1.5 or 3 ml of 100 U/ml regular or intermediate insulin are available. Unfortunately, long-acting insulin cannot be used in pens because it crystallizes at high concentrations. Attempts are being made toward developing soluble, slow-actin analogs of insulin to overcome this problem.

TABLE 71.6 Biologic and Engineered Insulin Delivery Systems Insulin Administration Systems

Insulin Administration Systems	
Standard Insulin	Routes of administration (subcutaneous, intravenous, intraperitoneal, nasal spray)
	Injection systems (syringes, pens)
Insulin release systems	Passive release from depot forms
	Bioresponsive insulin depot
	Implanted, permeable reservoirs
	Programmed release systems
Insulin delivery pumps	
Open loop	Osmotic pumps
	Piston and syringe pumps
	Peristaltic (roller) pumps
	Bellow frame pumps
	Pressurized reservoir pumps
Closed loop	Glucose sensors
	Electromechanical, servo-controlled delivery systems
Insulin Synthesis Systems	
Pancreas transplantation	Simultaneous with kidney transplant
	After kidney transplant
	Before kidney transplant
Islet transplantation	Autologous tissue
	Allogeneic tissue
	Xenogeneic tissue
Encapsulated islets or beta cell transplants	Microencapsulated cells
	Macroencapsulated cells
Genetically engineered cell transplants	Unprotected gene therapy
	Protected gene therapy

A common insulin regimen consists of injecting regular insulin before each meal with a pen and long-acting insulin at bedtime with a syringe. Typically half of the daily dosage is provided in the form of regular insulin. Since patients often need 50 units of insulin per day, a pen cartridge of 150 units of regular insulin must be replaced every 6 days or so. The setting of the appropriate dose is easy. However, most pens cannot deliver more than 36 units of insulin at a time, which in some patients may place a limit on their use. In those countries where insulin comes in vials of 40 U/ml for use with syringes, patients must be aware that insulin from cartridges is 2.5 times more concentrated than standard vial insulin. The major advantage of insulin pens is that they do not require refilling and therefore can be used discretely. Pens are particularly well accepted by teenagers.

71.7.2 Reservoirs, Depots, and Sprays

Attempts have been made to develop distensible, implantable reservoirs or bags made of silicone elastomers, fitted with a small delivery catheter, and refillable transcutaneously. In the preferred embodiment, insulin drains at a constant rate into the peritoneal cavity. Assuming uptake by the capillary beds in the serosal membranes which line the gastrointestinal tract, insulin reaches first the portal valve and hence the liver which enhances its effectiveness. This is an attractive concept but not without serious handicaps. The implanted reservoir may elicit an untoward tissue reaction or become a site of infection. The delivery catheter may be plugged by insulin crystals if a high insulin concentration is used, or the catheter may be obstructed by biologic deposits at the tip. The system only provides a baseline insulin delivery and needs to be supplemented by preprandial injections. Its overall capacity constitutes a potential risk should the reservoir accidentally rupture and flood the organism with an overdose of insulin.

Insulin depots, in the form of bioerodible polymer structures in which insulin — amorphous or in crystalline form — is entrapped and slowly released as hydrolytic decay of the carrier of the polymer progressively liberates it, present some of the same problems as reservoirs. In addition, the initial burst which often precedes zero-order release can prove unpredictable and dangerous. No reliable long-term delivery system has yet been developed on that principle.

New routes of introduction of insulin are being investigated, in particular, transmucosal adsorption. Nasal sprays of specially formulated insulin may become a practical modality of insulin therapy if means are found to control reliably the dose administered.

71.7.3 Insulin Pumps

Externally carried portable pumps, based on the motorized syringe or miniature roller pump designs, were evaluated in the 1970s with the anticipation that they could be both preprogrammed for baseline delivery and overridden for bolus injections at the time of meals without the need for repeated needle punctures. In actual practice, this system did not find wide acceptance on the part of patients, because it was just too cumbersome and socially unacceptable.

The first implantable insulin pump was evaluated clinically in 1980. Unlike heparin delivery or cancer chemotherapy, insulin administration requires programmable pumps with adjustable flow rates. Implantable pumps provide better comfort for the patient than portable pumps, since the former are relatively unobtrusive and involve no danger of infection at the skin catheter junction. They also permit intraperitoneal insulin delivery, which is more efficient than subcutaneous administration. However, these pumps operate without feedback control, since implantable glucose sensors are not yet available, and the patient must program the pump according to his/her needs.

The vapor pressure driven Infusaid pump relies on a remarkably astute mechanism for an implantable device. A rigid box is separated in two compartments by a metal bellow with a flat diaphragm and an accordion-pleated seal (bellow frame). One compartment is accessible from the outside through a subcutaneously buried filling port and contains a concentrated insulin solution. The other compartment (the bellows itself) is filled with a liquid freon which vaporizes at 37°C with a constant pressure of 0.6 bar. With no other source of energy but body heat (which is continuously replenished by metabolism and blood circulation), the freon slowly evaporates, and the pressure developed displaces the diaphragm and forces insulin at a constant flow rate through a narrow delivery catheter. The freon energy is restored each time the insulin reservoir is refilled, since the pressure needed to move the bellow liquefies the freon vapor within a smaller compartment.

The housing is a disc-shaped titanium box. The insulin reservoir contains 15 to 25 ml of insulin stabilized with polygenol at a concentration of either 100 or 400 U/ml, providing an autonomy of 1 to 3 months. The self-sealing septum on the filling port can be punctured through the skin up to 500 times. The pump is implanted under general or local anesthesia between skin and muscle in the lateral abdominal area. The tip of the catheter can be located subcutaneously or intraperitoneally.

The original device provided a constant flow of insulin which still needed to be supplemented by the patient at meal time. The most recent model (Infusaid 1000) weighs 272 g, contains 22 ml of insulin, and has a diameter of 9 cm and a height of 2.2 cm. It is designed for 100 U/ml insulin and is equipped with a side port which allows flushing of the catheter when needed. To dissipate the pressure generated by freon evaporation before it reaches the catheter, the insulin must cross a 0.22 μm bacteriologic filter and pass through a steel capillary 3 cm long and 50 μm in diameter. Basal flow rate can be adjusted from 0.001 to 0.5 ml/h, and a bolus can be superposed by releasing a precise amount of insulin stored in a pressurized accumulator through the opening of a valve leading to the catheter. These control features require an additional source of energy in the form of lithium thionile batteries with a service life of about 3 years. Control is achieved with a handheld electronic module or programs connected to the pump by telemetry.

The current Minimed pump (INIP 2001) has a dry weight of 162 g and a diameter of 8.1 cm and contains 14 ml of insulin at a concentration of 400 U/ml, allowing up to 3 months' autonomy between refills. This pump relies on a reservoir from which insulin can be delivered in a pulsatile form by a piston mechanism under the control of solenoid-driven valves. The basal rate can be adjusted 0.13–30 U/h (0.0003–0.07 ml/h), and boluses from 1 to 32 U over intervals 1–60 min can be programmed. The reservoir is permanently under negative pressure to facilitate filling.

The Siemens Infusor (1D3 model) replaced an earlier type based on a peristaltic miniature roller pump (discontinued in 1987). It is somewhat similar in design and dimensions to the minimed pumps, but it has now been withdrawn from the market.

The Medtronic Synchromed pump, which was originally designed for drug therapy and relied on a roller pump controlled by an external programmer, was evaluated for insulin therapy but is seldom used for that purpose because it lacks the required flexibility.

Between 1989 and 1992, 292 insulin pumps were implanted in 259 patients in France, where most of the clinical experience has been collected (205 Minimed, 47 Infusaid, and 7 Siemens). The treatment had to be permanently discontinued in 14 patients (10 because of poor tissue tolerance, 3 due to catheter obstruction, and 1 due to pump failure). The pump was replaced in 33 patients, with 28 cases of component failure; battery, microelectronic control, flow rate decline due to insulin precipitation in Infusaid pumps, insulin reflux in Minimed pumps, and perceived risk of leak from septum. The overall frequency of technical problems was 0.10 per patient-year. There were 46 surgical interventions without pump replacement because of catheter obstructions, and 24 related to poor tissue tolerance at the site of implantation. Glucose regulation was satisfactory in all cases, and the mean blood glucose concentration dropped appreciably after 6 and 18 months of treatment. A major gain with the intraperitoneal delivery was the reduction in the incidence of severe **hypoglycemia** associated with improved metabolic control. For the sake of comparison, other methods used for intensive insulin therapy showed a threefold increase in the frequency of serious hypoglycemic episodes.

71.7.4 Servo-Controlled Insulin Delivery Systems

Sensor-actuator couples which allow insulin delivery in the amount needed to maintain a nearly constant blood glucose level are sometimes designated as the **artificial beta cell** because of the analogy between the components of the electromechanical system and the biologic mechanisms involved in sensing, controlling, and delivering insulin from the pancreas (Table 71.7).

From a technology viewpoint, the key aspects are the glucose sensor, the control systems applicable to a biologic situation where both hyperglycemia and hypoglycemia must be prevented, and the practicality of the overall system.

71.7.4.1 Glucose Sensors

A glucose sensor provides a continuous reading of glucose concentration. The device consists of a detection part, which determines for the specificity of the glucose measurement, and a transducing element, which transforms the chemical or physical signals associated with glucose recognition into an electric signal. The most advanced technology is based on enzymatic and amperometric detection of glucose. Glucose is recognized by a specific enzyme, usually glucose oxidase, layered on the anode of an electrode, generating hydrogen peroxide which is then oxidized and detected by the current generated in the presence of

TABLE 71.7 Component Mechanisms of Insulin Delivery Systems

	Natural beta cell	Artificial beta cell
Sensor of glucose level	Intracellular glycolysis	Polarographic or optoelectronic sensor
Energy source	Mitochondria	Implantable battery
Logic	Nucleus	Minicomputer chip
Insulin reserve	Insulin granules	Insulin solution reservoir
Delivery system	Cell membrane	Insulin pump
Set point	Normally 80–120 mg%	Adaptable
Fail-safe	Glucagon and hunger	Glucose infusion

a fixed potential between the anode and the cathode. Alternatively, a chemical mediator may serve as a shuttle between the enzyme and the electrode to avoid the need for a potential difference at which other substances, such as ascorbate or acetaminophen, may be oxidized and generate an interfering current. Other approaches such as the direct electrocatalytic oxidation of glucose on the surface of the electrode or the detection of glucose by a combination with a lectin have not reached the stage of clinical evaluation.

Ideally a blood glucose sensor would be permanently installed in the bloodstream. Because of the difficulty of building a hemocompatible device and the inconvenience of a permanent blood access, several investigators have turned to the subcutaneous site for glucose sensing. Indeed, glucose concentration in the interstitial fluid is very close to that of blood and reflects quite directly changes associated with meals or physical activity as observed in diabetic patients. Two types of subcutaneous glucose sensors have been developed. Those with electrodes at the tip of a needle may be shielded from their environment by the inflammatory reaction in tissues contacting the electrode membrane and occasionally cause pain or discomfort. Nonetheless, reliable measurements have been obtained for up to 10 days, whereupon the sensor needed to be changed. Sensing can also be based on microdialysis through an implanted, permeable hollow fiber, providing fluid which is then circulated to a glucose electrode. This system has not yet been miniaturized and industrialized.

In either case, the concept is to develop an external monitor such as a wrist watch, which could receive its analyte from the implanted catheter or sensor and trigger a warning when glucose concentration is abnormally high or low. Such a monitor could eventually be incorporated in a closed-loop insulin delivery system, but this objective is not yet realizable.

Noninvasive technology has been suggested to monitor blood glucose, for example, by near-infrared spectroscopy or optical rotation applied to transparent fluid media of the eye. No reliable technology has yet emerged.

71.7.4.2   The Artificial Beta Cell

The standard equipment for feedback-controlled insulin administration is the artificial beta cell, also referred to in the literature as the **extracorporeal artificial pancreas**. It consists of a system for continuous blood sampling, a blood glucose sensor, and minicomputer which, through preestablished algorithms, drives an insulin infusion pump according to the needs of the patient. Accessories provide a minute-by-minute recording of blood glucose levels, insulin delivery, and glucose delivery.

In the first clinically oriented artificial beta cell (Miles Laboratories' Bioslator), the glucose sensor was located in a flow-through chamber where blood from a patient's vein was sucked continuously, at the rate of 2 ml/h, through a double-lumen catheter. The double lumen allowed the infusion of a minute dose of heparin at the tip of the catheter to prevent thrombosis in the glucose analyzer circuit. Glucose diffused through a semipermeable membrane covering the electrode and was oxidized by the enzyme. The hydrogen peroxide generated by this reaction crossed a second membrane, the role of which was to screen off substances such as urate and ascorbate. The resulting electric current was fed to a computer which controlled the flow rate of the insulin pump when the readings were in the hyperglycemic range and administered a glucose solution in case of hypoglycemia.

Three forms of oversight of blood glucose levels and insulin needs can be achieved with the artificial beta cell:

Blood glucose monitoring is the technique employed to investigate the time course of blood glucose levels in a particular physiologic situation without any feedback control from the artificial beta cell, that is, without insulin administration to correct the fluctuations of blood glucose levels.

Blood glucose control is the standard feedback mode of application of the artificial beta cell, which entails an arbitrary choice of the level of blood glucose desired and provides a recording of the rate of administration and the cumulative dose of intravenous insulin needed to achieve a constant blood glucose level.

Blood glucose clamp involves intravenous insulin administration at a constant rate to obtain a stable, high blood insulin level. The desired value of blood glucose level is arbitrarily selected (typically in the normal range), and the feedback-control capability of the artificial beta cell is used to measure the amount of exogenous glucose needed to "clamp" blood glucose at the desired level in the presence of a slight excess of insulin. With this technique, a decrease in the rate of glucose administration signals a decrease in insulin biologic activity.

The artificial beta cell is primarily a clinical research tool, applicable also for therapy in high-risk conditions such as pregnancy in poor controlled diabetic mothers or cardiac surgery in brittle diabetics [Galletti et al., 1985], where hypothermia and a massive outpouring of adrenergic agents alter the response to insulin [Kuntschen et al., 1986]. The primary drawbacks of current servo-controlled insulin delivery systems are the instability of the glucose sensor (in terms of both risk of thrombosis and the need for intermittent recalibration), the complexity of the system (up to four pumps can be needed for continuous blood sampling, heparinization, insulin administration, and glucose administration), and the risks involved. The dose of intravenous insulin required for rapid correction of hyperglycemia may cause an overshoot, which in turn calls for rapid administration of glucose. Such fluctuations may also influence potassium uptake by cells and in extreme conditions lead to changes in potassium levels which must be recognized and corrected [Kuntschen et al., 1983]. Finally, the general cumbersomeness of the extracorporeal system, to which the patient must be tethered by sampling and infusion lines, limits its applicability. Modeling of blood glucose control by insulin has allowed the development of algorithms that are remarkably efficient in providing metabolic feedback in most clinical situations. The physiologic limits of closed-loop systems have been lucidly analyzed by Sorensen and coworkers [1982] and Kraegen [1983].

71.8 Insulin Production Systems

The exacting requirement placed on insulin dosage and timing of administration in diabetic patients, as well as the many years of safe and reliable treatments expected from the insulin delivery technology, have pointed to the advantages of implantable systems in which insulin would be synthesized as needed and made available to the organism on demand.

As already outlined in Table 71.6 four avenues have been considered and undergone chemical evaluation: whole organ transplantation, human islet and xenogeneic islet transplantation, immunoisolation of normal or tumoral insulin-secreting tissue, and transplantation of cells genetically engineered to replace the functions of the beta cells.

71.8.1 Pancreas Transplantation

Human allograft transplantation, first attempted over 20 years ago, has been slow in reaching clinical acceptance because of the difficulty of identifying healthy cadaver organs (the pancreas is also a digestive gland which undergoes autolysis soon after death) and the need to deal with the gland exocrine secretion, which serves no useful purpose in diabetes but nonetheless must be disposed of. After many ingenious attempts to plug the secretory channels with room-temperature vulcanizing biopolymers, a preferred surgical technique has been developed whereby the pancreas is implanted in the iliac fossa, its arterial supply and venous drainage vessels anastomosed to the iliac artery and vein, and the Wirsung canal implanted in the urinary bladder. Surprisingly, the bladder mucosa is not substantially damaged by pancreatic enzymes, and the exocrine secretion dries up after a while.

The success rate of pancreatic tranplantation is now approaching that of heart and liver transplantation. Since it is mostly offered to immunosuppressed uremic diabetic patients who previously received or concurrently receive a kidney transplant, preventative therapy against organ rejection does not constitute an additional risk. The main limitation remains the supply of donor organs, which in the United States will probably not exceed 2000 per year, that is to say, very far from meeting the incidence of new cases of juvenile diabetes [Robertson and Sutherland, 1992]. Therefore, human organ transplantation is not a solution to the public health problems of diabetes and ensuing complications.

71.8.2 Human Islet Transplantation

Interest in the transplantation of islets of Langerhans, isolated from exocrine, vascular, and connective tissue by enzymatic digestion and cell separation techniques, has received a boost following the clinical demonstration that it can lead to insulin independence in type I diabetic patients [Scharp et al., 1990]. However, this "proof of principle" has not been followed by widespread application. Not only is the overall supply of cadaveric organs grossly insufficient in relating to the need (by as much as two orders of magnitude), but the islet separation techniques are complex and incompletely standardized. Therefore, it is difficult to justify at this point cutting into the limited supply of human pancreata for whole organ transplantation, the more so that whole organ replacement has become increasingly successful. Autologous islet transplantation can be successfully performed in relatively uncommon cases of pancreatic and polycystic disease, where the risk of spilling pancreatic juice in the peritoneal cavity necessitates the removal of the entire organ. Allogeneic islet transplantation under the cover of pharmacologic immunosuppression is useful inasmuch as it provides a benchmark against which to evaluate islet transplantation from animal sources and the benefits of membrane **immunoisolation**.

71.8.3 Xenogeneic Islet Transplantation

The term **bioartificial pancreas** refers to any insulin-production-glycemia-regulation system combining living pancreatic beta cells or equivalents with a synthetic polymer membrane of gel to protect the transplant against immune rejection. A wide variety of device designs, cell sources and processing techniques, implant location, and biomaterial formulation and characterization have been investigated (Table 71.8). Common to all is the belief that if transplantation of insulin-producing tissue is to serve the largest number of insulin-dependent diabetic patients possible, xenogeneic tissue sources will have to be identified. In that context, protection by a semipermeable membrane may be the most effective way to dispense with drug immunosuppression therapy [Lysaght et al., 1994]. However, a number of issues

TABLE 71.8 Membrane-Encapsulated Cell Transplants

Technology	Microencapsulation	
	Macroencapsulation	
	Coextrusion	
Location	Vascular release	Intravascular
		Perivascular
	Portal release	Intraperitoneal
		Intrahepatic
		Intrasplenic
	Systemic release	Subcutaneous
		Intramuscular
Cell source	Human islets or beta cells ⎫ fetal or adult	
	Animal islets or beta cells ⎭	
	Functionally active tumor tissue	
	Immortalized cell lines	
	Genetically engineered cell lines	
Cell processing	Isolation and purification	
	Culture and banking	
	Cryopreservation	
	Implant manufacturing	
Membrane characterization	Envelope mechanical stability	
	Envelope chemical stability	
	Diffusion and filtration kinetics	
	Immunoprotection	
	Bioacceptance	

must be addressed and resolved before the bioartificial pancreas becomes a clinically acceptable treatment modality [Colton, 1994].

71.8.3.1 Tissue Procurement

In the evolution of type I diabetes, the oral glucose tolerance test does not become abnormal until about 70% of the islets are destroyed. Therefore, roughly 250,000 human islets, or about 3,500 islets per kilogram of body weight, should suffice to normalize blood glucose levels. In reality, clinical observations of transplanted patients indicate a need for a considerably larger number (3,500 to 6,000 islets/kg, and perhaps more). This suggests that many processed islets are either nonviable or not functional because they have been damaged during the isolation procedure or by the hyperglycemic environment of the transplanted patient [Eizirik et al., 1992].

To procure such large numbers of islets an animal source must be identified. Porcine islets are favored because of the size of the animal, the availability of virus-free herds, and the low antigenicity of porcine insulin. Pig islet separation procedures are not yet fully standardized, and there are still considerable variations in terms of yield, viability, and insulin secretory function. Quality control and sterility control present serious challenges to industrialization.

Alternative tissue sources are therefore being investigated. **Insulinomas** provided the first long-term demonstration of the concept of encapsulated endocrine tissue transplant [Altman et al., 1984]. Genetically engineered cell lines which can sense glucose concentration and regulate it within the physiologic range have been reported, but so far none has matched the secretory ability of normal pancreatic tissue or isolated islets. This approach remains nonetheless attractive for large-scale device production, even though no timetable can be formulated for successful development.

71.8.3.2 Device Design

Immunoisolation of allogeneic or xenogeneic islets can be achieved by two main classes of technology: microencapsulation and macroencapsulation. Microencapsulation refers to the formation of a spherical gel around each islet, cell cluster, or tissue fragment. Calcium alginate, usually surrounded with a polyanion such as poly-L-lysine to prevent biodegradation, and at times overcoated with an alginate layer to improve the biocompatibility, has been the most common approach, although other polymers may be substituted. Suspension of microcapsules are typically introduced in the peritoneal cavity to deliver insulin to the portal circulation.

Technical advances have permitted the fabrication of increasingly smaller microcapsules (order of 150 to 200 μm) which do not clump, degrade, or elicit too violent a tissue reaction. Control of diabetes has been achieved in mice, rats, dogs, and, on pilot basis, in humans [Soon-Siong et al., 1994]. An obstacle to human application has been the difficulty, if not the impossibility, of retrieving the very large number of miniature implants, many of which adhere to tissue. There is also a concern for the antigenic burden that may arise upon polymer degradation and liberation of islet tissue, whether living or necrotic.

Macroencapsulation refers to the reliance on larger, prefabricated envelopes in which a slurry of islets or cell clusters is slowly introduced and sealed prior to implantation. The device configuration can be tubular or planar. The implantation site can be perivascular, intravascular, intraperitoneal, subcutaneous, or intravascular.

71.8.3.3 Intravascular Devices

In the most successful intravascular device (which might be more accurately designated as perivascular), a semipermeable membrane is formed into a wide-bore tube connected between artery and vein or between the severed ends of an artery as if it were a vascular graft. The islets are contained in a gel matrix within a compartment surrounding the tube through which blood circulates. In other embodiments, the islets are contained in semipermeable parallel hollow fibers or coiled capillaries attached to the external wall of a macroporous vascular prosthesis. In all cases, a rising glucose concentration in the blood stream leads to glucose diffusion into the islet compartment, which stimulates insulin production, raises its concentration in the gel matrix, and promotes diffusion into the blood stream.

In an earlier type of perivascular device, blood is forced to circulate through the lumina of a tight bundle of hollow fibers, and the islet suspension is placed in the extracapillary space between fibers and circumscribed by a rigid shell, as was the case in the design which established the effectiveness of immunoprotected islets [Chick et al., 1977]. A truly intravascular device design has been proposed in which the islets are contained within the lumina of a bundle of hollow fibers which are plugged at both ends and placed surgically in the blood stream of a large vein or artery, in a mode reminiscent of the intravenous oxygenator (IVOX). Hemocompatibility has been the major challenge with that approach.

There have also been attempts to develop extracorporeal devices with a semipermeable tubular membrane connected transcutaneously, through flexible catheters, to an artery or vein. The islets are seeded in the narrow "extravascular" space separating the membrane from the device external wall and can therefore be inspected and, in case of need, replaced. This concept has evolved progressively to wider-bore (3 to 6 mm ID), spirally coiled tubes in a disc-shaped plastic housing. Such devices have remained patent for several months in dogs in the absence of anticoagulation and have shown the ability to correct hyperglycemia in spontaneous or experimentally induced diabetes.

In order to accelerate glucose and insulin transport across synthetic membranes and shorten the reactive time lag of immuno-protective islets, Reach et al. [1984] have proposed to take advantage of a Starling-type ultrafiltration cycle made possible, in blood-perfused devices, by the arteriovenous pressure difference between device inlet and outlet. An outward-directed ultrafiltration flux in the first half of the blood conduit is balanced by a reverse readsorption flux in the second half, since the islet compartment is fluid-filled, rigid, and incompressible. An acceleration of the response time to fluctuations in blood glucose levels has been demonstrated both by modeling and experimentally. This system may also enhance the transport of oxygen and nutrients and improve the metabolic support of transplanted tissue.

The primary obstacle to clinical acceptance of the intravascular bioartificial pancreas is the risk of thrombosis (including obstruction and embolism) of a device expected to function for several years. The smaller the diameter of the blood channel, and the greater the surface of polymeric material exposed to blood, the more likely are thrombotic complications. These devices also share with vascular grafts the risk of a small but definite incidence of infection of the implant and the potential sacrifice of a major blood vessel. Therefore, their clinical application is likely to remain quite limited.

71.8.3.4 Intratissular Devices

Tubular membranes with diameters on the order of 0.5 to 2 mm have also been evaluated as islet containers for subcutaneous, intramuscular, or intracavitary implantation: the islets are contained inside the membrane envelope at a low-volume fraction in a gel matrix. A problem is that small-diameter tubes require too much length to be practical. Large-diameter tubes are mechanically fragile and often display a core of necrotic tissue because diffusion distances are too long for adequate oxygen and nutrient transport to the islets. Both systems are subject to often unpredictable foreign body reactions and the development of scar tissue which further impairs metabolic support of the transplanted tissue. However materials that elicit a minimal tissue reaction have been identified [Galletti, 1992], and further device design and evaluation is proceeding at a brisk pace [Scharp et al., 1994].

Some microporous materials display the property of inducing neovascularization at the tissue–material interface and in some cases within the voids of a macroporous polymer. This phenomenon is thought to enhance mass transport for nutrient and secretory products by bringing capillaries in closer proximity to immuno-seperated cells. Pore size, geometry, and interconnections are critical factors in vascularization [Colton, 1994]. Some encapsulated cell types also stimulate vacularization beyond the level observed with empty devices. Chambers made by laminating a 5-μm porosity expanded polytetrafluoroethylene (Gore PTFE) on a 9.45-μm Biopore (Millipore) membrane have shown the most favorable results [Brauker et al., 1992]. The laminated, vascualrized membrane structure has been fabricated in a sandwichlike structure that can be accessed through a port to inject an islet suspension once the empty device has been fully integrated in the soft tissues of the host. This **organoid** can nonetheless be separated from adjacent tissues, exteriorized, and retrieved.

TABLE 71.9   Polymer Technology for Cell Transplantation

Component	Function	Polymer
Scaffold	Synthetic or semisynthetic extracellular matrix	Collagen
		Gelatin
		Alginate
		Agarose
	Physical separation of cells or cell aggregates	Chitosan
		Hyaluronan
Envelope		
Microencapsulation	Stabilization of cell suspension and immunoseperation	Alginate
		Poly-L-lysine
Macroencapsulation	Physical immunoseperation	Polyacrylonitrile
		Polyvinyl copolymers
		Polysulfones
		Modified celluloses
	Transport-promoting tissue–material interface	PTFE-Biopore laminate

71.8.3.5 Polymers for Immunoisolation

The polymeric materials used in bioartificial endocrine devices serve two major purpose (1) as a scaffold and an extracellular matrix, they favor the attachment and differentiation of functional cells or cell clusters, and keep them separate from one another, which in some cases has proven critical; (2) as permselective envelopes they provide immunoisolation of the transplant from the host, while inducing a surrounding tissue reaction which will maximize the diffusional exchange of solutes between the transplant and its environment. A number of materials can be used for these purposes (Table 71.9).

The matrix materials typically are gels made of natural or synthetic polyelectrolytes, with quite specific requirements in terms of viscosity, porosity, and electric charge. In some cases specific attachment or growth factors may be added.

For immunoisolation, the most commonly used envelopes are prepared from polyacrylonitrile–polyvinyl chloride copolymers. These membranes display the anistropic structure typical of most ultrafiltration membranes, in which a thin retentive skin is supported on a spongy matrix [Colton, 1994]. The shape and dimensions of the interconnecting voids and the microarchitecture of the inner and outer surfaces of the membrane are often critical characteristics for specific cell types and implant locations.

71.8.3.6 Protection from Immune Rejection

The central concept of immunoisolation is the placement of a semipermeable barrier between the host and transplanted tissue. It has been tacitly assumed that membranes with a nominal 50,000 to 100,000-Da cutoff would provide adequate protection, because they would prevent the passage of cells from the host immune system and impair the diffusion of proteins involved in the humoral component of immune rejection.

This belief has been largely supported by empirical observations of membrane-encapsulated graft survival, with occasional failures rationalized as membrane defects.

However, the cut-off point of synthetic semipermeable membranes is not as sharp as one may believe, and there is often a small number of pores which theoretically at least allow the transport of much larger molecules than suggested by the nominal cut-off definition. Therefore, complex issues of rate of transport, threshold concentration of critical proteins, adsorption and denaturation in contact with polymeric materials, and interactions between proteins involved in immune reactions in an environment where their relative concentrations may be far from normal may all impact in immunoprotection. The possibility of antigen release from living or necrotic cells in the sequestered environment must also be considered. The cellular and luminal mechanisms of immunoseperation by semipermeable membranes and the duration of the protection they afford against both immune rejection of the graft and sensitizations of the host call for considerably more study.

71.9 Outlook

Replacement of the endocrine functions of the pancreas presents a special challenge in substitutive medicine. The major disease under consideration, diabetes, is quite common, but a reasonably effective therapy already exists with standard insulin administration. The disease is not immediately life-threatening, and therefore optimization of treatment is predicated on the potential for reducing the long-term complications of diabetes. Therefore, complete clinical validation will require decreases of observations, not merely short-term demonstration of effectiveness in controlling blood glucose levels.

Standard insulin treatment is also relatively inexpensive. Competitive therapeutic technologies will therefore be subject to a demanding cost–benefit analysis before they are widely recognized. Finally, the patient self-image will be a major factor in the acceptance of new diagnostic or treatment modalities. Already some demonstrably useful devices, such as subcutaneous glucose sensors, portable insulin pumps, and the extracorporeal artificial beta cell, have failed in the marketplace for reasons of excessive complexity, incompatibility with all activities of daily life, physicians' skepticism, or cost. Newer technologies involving the implantation of animal tissue or genetically engineered cells will bring about a new set of concerns, whether justified or imaginary. There is perhaps no application of the artificial organ concept where human factors are so closely intertwined with the potential of science and technology as is already the case with the artificial pancreas.

Defining Terms

Anabolism: The aspect of metabolism in which relatively simple building blocks are transformed into more complex substances for the purpose of storage or enhanced physiologic action.

Artificial beta cell: A system for the control of blood glucose levels based on servo-controlled administration of exogenous insulin based on continuous glucose level monitoring.

Artificial pancreas: A device or system designed to replace the natural organ. By convention, this term designates substitutes for the endocrine function of the pancreas and specifically glucose homeostasis though the secretion of insulin.

Autolysis: Destruction of the components of a tissue, following cell death, mediated by enzymes normally present in that tissue.

Bioartificial pancreas: A device or implant containing insulin-producing, glycemia-regulating cells in combination with polymeric structures for mechanical support and immune protection.

Catabolism: The aspect of metabolism in which substances in living tissues are transformed into waste products or solutes of simpler chemical composition.

Endogenous: Originating in body tissues.

Exogenous: Introduced in the body from external sources.

Extracorporeal artificial pancreas: An apparatus including a glucose sensor, a minicomputer with appropriate algorithms, an insulin infusion pump, and a glucose infusion pump, the output of which are controlled so as to maintain a constant blood glucose level. (Synonymous with artificial beta cell.)

Hyperglycemia: Abnormally high blood glucose level (in humans, above 140 mg/100 ml).

Hypoglycemia: Abnormally low blood glucose level (in humans, below 50 mg/100 ml).

Immunoisolation: Separation of transplanted tissue from its host by a membrane or film which prevents immune rejection of the transplant by forming a barrier against the passage of immunologically active solutes and cells.

Insulinoma: A generally benign tumor of the pancreas, originating in the beta cells and functionally characterized by a secretion of insulin and the occurrence of hypoglycemic coma. Insulinoma cells are thought to have lost the feedback function and blood-glucose-regulating capacity of normal cells, or to regulate blood glucose around an abnormally low set point.

Ketoacidosis: A form of metabolic acidosis encountered in diabetes mellitus, in which fat is used as a fuel instead of glucose (because of lack of insulin), leading to high concentration of metabolites such as aceto-acetic acid, β-hydroxybutyric acid, and occasionally acetone in the blood and intestinal fluids.

Organoid: A device — typically an implant — in which cell attachment and growth in the scaffold provided by a synthetic polymer sponge or mesh leads to a structure resembling that of a natural organ including, in many cases, revascularization.

References

Altman J.J., Houlbert D., Callard P. et al. 1986. Long-term plasma glucose normalization in experimental diabetic rats using microencapsulated implants of benign human insulinomas. *Diabetes* 35: 625.

Altman J.J., Houlbert D., Chollier A. et al. 1984. Encapsulated human islet transplantation in diabetic rats. *Trans. Am. Soc. Artif. Intern. Organs* 30: 382.

Brauker J.H., Martinson L.A., Young S. et al. 1992. Neovascularization at a membrane–tissue interface is dependent on microarchitecture. *Abstracts, Fourth World Biomaterials Congress*, Berlin FRG, p. 685.

Chick W.L., Like A.A., Lauris V. et al. 1975. Artificial pancreas using living beta cells: effects on glucose homeostasis in diabetic rats. *Science* 197: 780.

Chick W.L., Perla J.J., Lauris V. et al. 1977. Artificial pancreas using living beta cells: effects on glucose homeostasis in diabetic rats. *Science* 197: 780.

Colton C.K. 1992. The engineering of xenogeneic islet transplantation by immunoisolation. *Diab. Nutr. Metab.* 5: 145.

Colton C.K. 1994. Engineering issues in islet immunoisolation. In R. Lanza and W. Chick (Eds.), *Pancreatic Islet Transplantation, Vol. III: Immunoisolation of Pancreatic Islets*, RG Landes.

Colton C.K. and Avgoustiniatos E.S. 1991. Bioengineering in development of the hybrid artificial pancreas. *J. Biomech. Eng.* 113: 152.

Dionne K.E., Colton C.K., and Yarmush M.L. 1993. Effect of hypoxia on insulin secretion by isolated rat and canine islets of Langerhans. *Diabetes* 42: 12.

Eizirik D.L., Korbutt G.S., and Hellerstrom C. 1992. Prolonged exposure of human pancreatic islets to high glucose concentrations *in vitro* impairs the β-cell function. *J. Clin. Invest.* 90: 1263.

Galletti P.M. 1992. Bioartificial organs. *Artif. Organs* 16: 55.

Galletti P.M. and Altman J.J. 1984. Extracorporeal treatment of diabetes in man. *Trans. Am. Soc. Artif. Intern. Organs* 30: 675.

Galletti P.M., Kuntschen F.R., and Hahn C. 1985. Experimental and clinical studies with servo-controlled glucose and insulin administration during cardiopulmonary bypass. *Mt. Sinai. J. Med.* 52: 500.

Jaffrin M.Y., Reach G., and Notelet D. 1988. Analysis of ultrafiltration and mass transfer in a bioartificial pancreas. *ASME J. Biomech. Eng.* 110: 1.

Kraegen E.W. 1983. Closed loop systems: physiological and practical considerations. In P. Brunetti, K.G.M.M. Albeti, A.M. Albisser et al. (Eds.), *Artificial Systems for Insulin Delivery*, New York, Raven Press.

Kuntschen F.R., Galletti P.M., and Hahn C. 1986. Glucose–insulin interactions during cardiopulmonary bypass. Hypothermia versus normothermia. *J. Thorac. Cardiovas. Surg.* 91: 45.

Kuntschen F.R., Taillens C., Hahn C. et al. 1983. Technical aspects of Biostator operation during coronary artery bypass surgery under moderate hypothermia. In *Artificial Systems for Insulin Delivery*, pp. 555–559, New York, Raven Press.

Lanza R.P., Butler D.H., Borland K.M. et al. 1991. Xenotransplantation of canine, bovine, and porcine islets in diabetic rats without immunosuppression. *PNAS* 88: 11100.

Lanza R.P., Sullivan S.J., and Chick W.L. 1992. Islet transplantation with immunoisolation. *Diabetes* 41: 1503.

Lysaght M.J., Frydel B., Winn S. et al. 1994. Recent progress in immunoisolated cell therapy. *J. Cell Biochem.* 56: 1.

Mikos A.G., Papadaki M.G., Kouvroukogiou S. et al. 1994. Mini-review: Islet transplantation to create a bioartificial pancreas. *Biotechnol. Bioeng.* 43: 673.

Pfeiffer E.F., Thum C.I., and Clemens A.H. 1974. The artificial beta cell. A continuous control of blood sugar by external regulation of insulin infusion (glucose controlled insulin infusion system). *Horm. Metab. Res.* 6: 339.

Reach G., Jaffrin M.Y., and Desjeux J.-F. 1984. A U-shaped bioartificial pancreas with rapid glucose-insulin kinetics. *In vitro* evaluation and kinetic modeling. *Diabetes* 33: 752.

Ricordi C. (Ed.). 1992. *Pancreatic Islet Transplantation*, Austin, TX, RG Landes.

Robertson R.P. and Sutherland D.E. 1992. Pancreas transplantation as therapy for diabetes mellitus. *Annu. Rev. Med.* 43: 395.

Scharp D.W., Lacy P.E., Santiago J.V. et al. 1990. Insulin independence after islet transplantation into a Type I diabetes patient. *Diabetes* 39: 515.

Scharp D.W., Swanson C.J., Olack B.J. et al. 1994. Protection of encapsulated human islets implanted without immunosuppression in patients with Type I and II diabetes and in nondiabetic controls. *Diabetes* (accepted for publication in September 1994 issue).

Soon-Siong P., Heintz R.E., Meredith N. et al. 1994. Insulin independence in a type 1 diabetic patient after encapsulated islet transplantation. *Lancet* 343: 950.

Sorensen J.T., Colton C.K., Hillman R.S. et al. 1982. Use of physiologic pharmacokinetic model of glucose homeostasis for assessment of performance requirements for improved requirements for improved insulin therapies. *Diab. Care* 5: 148.

Sullivan S.J., Maki T., Boreland K.M. et al. 1991. Biohybrid artificial pancreas: Long-term implantation studies in diabetic, pancreatectomized dogs. *Science* 252: 718.

Further Information

A useful earlier review of insulin delivery systems is to be found in *Artificial Systems for Insulin Delivery*, edited by P. Brunetti, K.G.M.M. Alberti, A.M. Albisser, K.D. Hepp, and M. Massi Benedetti, Serono Symposia Publications from Raven Press, New York, 1983. An upcoming review, focused primarily on islet transplantation will be found in *Pancreatic Islet Transplantation, Vol. III: Immunoisolation of Pancreatic Islets*, edited by R.P. Lanza and W.L. Chick, R.G. Landes Company, Austin, Texas, 1994. A volume entitled *Implantation Biology: The Host Response and Biomedical Devices*, edited by R.S. Greco, from CRC Press, 1994, provides a background in the multiple aspects of tissue response to biomaterials and implants.

Individual contributions to the science and technology of pancreas replacement are likely to be found in the following journals: *Artificial Organs, the Journal of Cell Transplantation*, and *Transplantation*. Reports on clinically promising devices are often published in *Diabetes* and *Lancet*.

72

Nerve Guidance Channels

Robert F. Valentini
Brown University

In adult mammals, including humans, the peripheral nervous system (PNS) is capable of regeneration following injury. The PNS consists of neural structures located outside the central nervous system (CNS), which is comprised of the brain and spinal cord. Unfortunately, CNS injuries rarely show a return of function, although recent studies suggest a limited capacity for recovery under optimal conditions. Neural regeneration is complicated by the fact that neurons, unlike other cell types, are not capable of proliferating. In successful regeneration, sprouting axons from the proximal nerve stump traverse the injury site, enter the distal nerve stump, and make new connections with target organs. Current surgical techniques allow surgeons to realign nerve ends precisely when the lesion does not require excision of a large nerve segment. Nerve realignment increases the probability that extending axons will encounter an appropriate distal neural pathway, yet the incidence of recovery in the PNS is highly variable, and the return of function is never complete. Surgical advances in the area of nerve repair seem to have reached an impasse, and biologic rather than technical factors now limit the quality of regeneration and functional recovery. The use of synthetic nerve guidance channels facilitates the study of nerve regeneration in experimental studies and shows promise in improving the repair of injured human nerves. Advances in the synthesis of biocompatible polymers have provided scientists with a variety of new biomaterials which may serve as nerve guidance channels, although the material of choice for clinical application has not yet been identified.

The purpose of this chapter is to review the biologic aspects of PNS regeneration (CNS regeneration will be discussed in a subsequent chapter) and the influence of nerve guidance channels on the regeneration process. The biologic mechanisms and the guidance channel characteristics regulating regeneration will

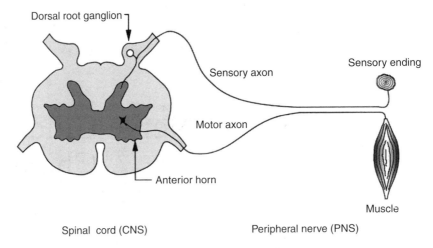

FIGURE 72.1 Spinal cord in cross-section. Relationship between motor and sensory cell bodies and their axons. Motor neurons (black) are located in the anterior horn of the gray matter within the spinal cord. Sensory neurons (white) are located in dorsal root ganglia just outside the spinal cord. Axons exit via dorsal (sensory) and ventral (motor) spinal roots and converge to form peripheral nerves, which connect to target structures (sensory endings and muscles). Note that the distance between axons and their corresponding cell bodies can be quite long.

be emphasized, since the rational design of guidance systems hinges on the integration of engineering (polymer chemistry, materials science, and so on) and biologic (cellular and molecular events) principles.

72.1 Peripheral Nervous System

Peripheral nerve trunks are responsible for the innervation of the skin and skeletal muscles and contain electrically conductive fibers termed axons, whose cell bodies reside in or near the spinal cord (Figure 72.1). Nerve cells are unique in that their cellular processes may extend for up to one meter or longer (e.g., for axons innervating the skin of the foot). Three types of neuronal fibers can be found in peripheral nerves (1) motor fibers, whose axons originate in the anterior horn of the spinal cord and terminate in the neuromuscular ending of skeletal muscle; (2) sensory fibers, which are the peripheral projections of dorsal root ganglion neurons and terminate at the periphery either freely or in a variety of specialized receptors; and (3) sympathetic fibers, which are the postganglionic processes of neurons innervating blood vessels or glandular structures of the skin. These three fiber types usually travel within the same nerve trunk, and a single nerve can contain thousands of axons. All axons are wrapped by support cells named Schwann cells. Larger axons are surrounded by a multilamellar sheath of myelin, a phospholipid-containing substance which serves as an insulator and enhances nerve conduction. An individual Schwann cell may ensheath several unmyelinated axons but only one myelinated axon, within its cytoplasm. Schwann cells are delineated by a fine basal lamina and are in turn surrounded by a complex structure made of collagen fibrils interspersed with fibroblasts and small capillaries, forming a tissue termed the endoneurium. A layer of flattened cells with associated basement membrane and collagen constitute the perineurium, which envelops all endoneurial constituents. The presence of tight junctions between the perineurial cells creates a diffusion barrier for the endoeurium and thus functions as blood–nerve barrier. The perineurium and its endoneurial contents constitute a fascicle, which is the basic structural unit of a peripheral nerve. Most peripheral nerves contain several fascicles, each containing numerous myelinated and unmyelinated axons. Since the fascicular tracts branch frequently and follow a tortuous pathway, the cross-sectional fascicular pattern changes significantly along a nerve trunk. Outside the perineurium is the epineurium, a protective, structural connective tissue sheath made of several layers of flattened fibroblastic cells interspersed with collagen, blood vessels, and adipocytes (fat cells). Peripheral nerves are well vascularized, and their blood supply is derived either from capillaries located within the epineurium and endoneurium (i.e., vasa nervosum) or from peripheral vessels which penetrate into the nerve from surrounding arteries and veins.

72.2   PNS Response to Injury

Nerves subjected to mechanical, thermal, chemical, or ischemic insults exhibit a typical combination of degenerative and regenerative responses. The most severe from of injury results from complete transaction of the nerve, which interrupts communication between the nerve cell body and its target, disrupts the interrelations between neurons and their support cells, destroys the local blood–nerve barrier, and triggers a variety of cellular and humoral events. Injuries close to the nerve cell body are more detrimental than injuries occurring more peripherally.

The cell bodies and axons of motor and sensory nerves react in a characteristic fashion to transection injury. The central cell body (which is located within or just outside the spinal cord) and its nucleus swell. Neurotransmitter (e.g., the chemicals which control neuronal signaling) production is diminished drastically, and carbohydrate metabolism is shifted to the pentose-phosphate cycle. These changes indicate a metabolic shift toward production of the substrates necessary for reconstituting the cell membrane and other structural components. For example, the synthesis of the protein tubulin, which is the monomeric elements of the microtubule, the structure responsible for axoplasmic transport, is increased dramatically. Following injury, tubulin and other substrates produced in the cell soma are transported, via slow and fast axoplasmic transport, to the distal nerve fiber.

Immediately after injury, the tip of the proximal stump (i.e., the nerve segment closest to the spinal cord) swells to two or three times its original diameter, and the severed axons retract. After several days, the proximal axons begin to sprout vigorously and growth cones emerge. Growth cones are axoplasmic extrusions of the cut axons which flatten and spread when they encounter a solid, adhesive surface. They elicit numerous extensions (fillipodia) which extend outward in all directions until the first sprout reaches an appropriate target (i.e., Schwann cell basal lamina). The lead sprout is usually the only one to survive, and the others quickly die back.

In the distal nerve stump, the process of Wallerian degeneration begins within 1 to 2 h after transection. The isolated axons and their myelin sheaths are degraded and phagocytized by Schwann cells and macrophages, leading to a complete dissociation of neurotubules and neurofilaments. This degradation process is accompanied by a proliferation of Schwann cells which retain the structure of the endoneurial tube by organizing themselves into ordered columns termed bands of Bunger. While the Schwann cells multiply, the other components of the distal nerve stump atrophy or are degraded, resulting in a reduction in the diameter of the overall structure. Severe retrograde degeneration can lead to cell atrophy and, eventually, cell death. Peripheral nerve transection also leads to marked atrophy of the corresponding target muscle fibers.

72.3   PNS Regeneration

In successful regeneration, axons sprouting from the proximal stump bridge the injury gap and encounter an appropriate Schwann cell column (band of Bunger). In humans, axons elongate at an average rate of 1 mm day. The bridging axons are immediately engulfed in Schwann cell cytoplasm, and some of them become myelinated. Induction of myelogenesis by the Schwann cell is thought to depend on axonal contact. Some of the axons reaching the distal stump traverse the length of the nerve to form functional synapses, but changes in the pattern of muscular and sensory reinnervation invariably occur. The misrouting of growing fibers occurs primarily at the site of injury, since once they reach the distal stump their paths do not deviate further. The original Schwann cell basal lamina in the distal stump persists and may aid in the migration of axons and proliferating Schwann cells. Axons which fail to reach an appropriate end organ or fail to make a functional synapse eventually undergo Wallerian degeneration. Abnormal regeneration may lead to the formation of a neuroma, a dense, irregular tangle of axons which can cause painful sensations. Some nerve injuries result from clean transections of the nerve which leave the fascicular pattern intact. More often, a segment of nerve is destroyed (e.g., during high-energy trauma or avulsion injuries in which tissue is torn), thus creating a nerve deficit. The resulting nerve gap is the separation between the proximal and distal stumps of a damaged nerve that is due to elastic retraction of the nerve stumps and tissue loss. The longer the nerve gap, the less likely regeneration will occur.

72.4 Surgical Repair of Transected Peripheral Nerves

In the absence of surgical reconnection, recovery of function following a transection or gap injury to a nerve is negligible, since (1) the cell bodies die due to severe retrograde effects, (2) the separation between nerve ends precludes sprouting axons from finding the distal stump, (3) connective tissue ingrowth at the injury site acts as physical barrier to neurite elongation, and (4) the proximal and distal fascicular patterns differ so much that extending axons cannot find an appropriate distal pathway.

Efforts to repair damaged peripheral nerves by surgical techniques date back many years although histologic evidence of regeneration was not reported by Ramon y Cajal until the first part of this century. Early attempts to reconnect severed peripheral nerves utilized a crude assortment of materials, and anatomic repair rarely led to an appreciable return of function. In the 1950s, the concept of end-to-end repair was refined by surgeons who directly reattached individual nerve fascicles or groups of fascicles. Further refinements occurred during the 1960s with the introduction of the surgical microscope and the availability of finer suture materials and instrumentation. Microsurgical nerve repair led to a significant improvement in the return of motor and sensory function in patients to the point that success rates of up to 70% can currently be achieved. In microsurgical nerve repair the ends of severed nerves are apposed and realigned by placing several strands of very fine suture material through the epineurial connective tissue without entering the underlying nerve fascicles. Nerve-grafting procedures are performed when nerve retraction or tissue loss prevents direct end-to-end repair. Nerve grafts are also employed when nerve stump reapproximation would create tension along the suture line, a situation which is known to hinder the regeneration process. In grafting surgery, an autologous nerve graft from the patient, such as the sural nerve (whose removal results in little functional deficit), is interposed between the ends of the damaged nerve.

72.5 Repair with Nerve Guidance Channels

In repair procedures using nerve guidance channels, the mobilized ends of a severed nerve are introduced in the lumen of a tube and anchored in place with sutures (Figure 72.2). Tubulation repair provides (1) a direct, unbroken path between nerve stumps; (2) prevention of scar tissue invasion into the regenerating environment; (3) directional guidance for elongation neurites and migrating cells; (4) proximal-distal stump communication without suture-line tension in cases of extensive nerve deficit; (5) minimal number of epineurial stay sutures, which are known to stimulate connective tissue proliferation; and (6) preservation, within the guidance channel lumen, of endogenous trophic or growth factors released by the traumatized nerve ends. Guidance channels are also useful from an experimental perspective (1) the gap distance between the nerve stumps can be precisely controlled; (2) the fluid and tissue entering the channel can be evaluated; (3) the properties of the channel can be varied; and (4) the channel can be filled with various drugs, gels, and the like. Nerves with various dimensions from several mammalian species, including mice, rats, rabbits, hamsters, and nonhuman primates have been tested. The regenerated tissue in the guidance channel is evaluated morphologically to quantify the outcome of regeneration. Parameters analyzed include the cross-sectional area of the regenerated nerve cable, the number of myelinated and unmyelinated axons, and the relative percentages of cellular constituents (i.e., epineurium, endoneurium, blood vessels, and so on). Electrophysiologic and functional evaluation can also be performed in studies conducted for long periods (e.g., several weeks or more).

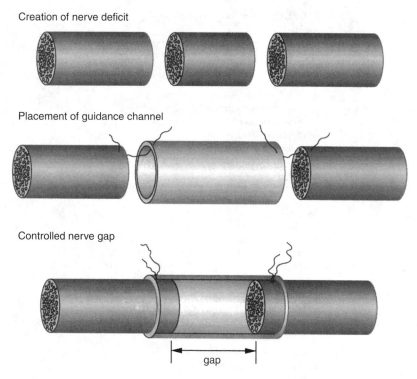

Creation of nerve deficit

Placement of guidance channel

Controlled nerve gap

gap

FIGURE 72.2 Tube to repair nerve. Surgical placement of nerve guidance channel.

The frequent occurrence of nerve injuries during the world wars of this century stimulated surgeons to seek simpler, more effective means of repairing damaged nerves. A variety of biologic and synthetic materials shaped into cylinders were investigated (Table 72.1). Bone, collagen membranes, arteries, and veins (either fresh or freeze-dried to reduce antigenicity) were used from the late 1800s through the 1950s to repair nerves. These materials did not enhance the rate of nerve regeneration when compared to regular suturing techniques, so clinical applications were infrequent. Magnesium, rubber, and gelatin tubes were evaluated during World War I, and cylinders of parchment paper and tantalum were used during World War II. The poor results achieved with these materials can be attributed to poor biocompatibility, since the channels elicited an intense tissue response which limited the ability of growing axons to reach the distal nerve stump. Following World War II, polymeric materials with more stable mechanical and chemical properties became available. Millipore (cellulose acetate) and Silastic (silicone elastomer) tubing received the greatest attention. Millipore, a filter material with a maximum pore size of 0.45 μm, showed early favorable results. In human trials, however, Millipore induced calcification and eventually fragmented several months after implantation so that its use was discontinued. Silastic tubing, a biologically inert polymer with rubberlike properties, was first tested in the 1960s. Thin-walled Silastic channels were reported to support regeneration over large gaps in several mammalian species. Thick-walled tubing was associated with nerve necrosis and neuroma production. The material showed no long-term degradation nor did it elicit a sustained inflammatory reaction. As a result, thin-walled Silastic tubing has been used, on a very limited basis, in the clinical repair of severed nerves.

72.6 Recent Studies with Nerve Guidance Channels

The availability of a variety of new biomaterials has led to a resurgence of tubulation studies designed to elucidate the mechanisms of nerve regeneration. The spatial-temporal progress of nerve regeneration

TABLE 72.1   Materials Used for Nerve Guidance
Channels

Synthetic materials
Nonresorbable
   Nonporous
      Ethylene-Vinyl Acetate Copolymer (EVA)
      Polytetrafluoroethylene (PTFE)
      Polyethylene (PE)
      Silicone elastomers (SE)
      Polyvinyl chloride (PVC)
      Polyvinylidene fluoride (PVDF)
   Microporous
      Gortex, expanded polytetrafluoroethylene (ePTFE)
      Millipore (cellulose filter)
   Semipermeable
      Polyacrylonitrile (PAN)
      Polyacrylonitrile/Polyvinyl chloride (PAN/PVC)
      Polysulfone (PS)
Bioresorbable
   Polyglycolide (PGA)
   Polylactide (PLLA)
   PGA/PLLA blends

Biologic materials
Artery
Collagen
Hyaluronic acid derivatives
Mesothelial tubes
Vein

Metals
Stainless steel
Tantalum

across a 10-mm rat sciatic nerve gap repaired with a silicone elastomer tube has been analyzed in detail (Figure 72.3). During the first hours following repair, the tube fills with a clear, protein-containing fluid exuded by the cut blood vessels in the nerve ends. The fluid contains the clot-forming protein, fibrin, as well as factors known to support nerve survival and outgrowth. By the end of the first week, the lumen is filled with a longitudinally oriented fibrin matrix which coalesces and undergoes syneresis to form a continuous bridge between the nerve ends. The fibrin matrix is soon invaded by cellular elements migrating from the proximal and distal nerve stumps, including fibroblasts (which first organize along the periphery of the fibrin matrix), Schwann cells, macrophages, and endothelial cells (which form capillaries). At 2 weeks, axons advancing from the proximal stump are engulfed in the cytoplasm of Schwann cells. After 4 weeks some axons have reached the distal nerve stump, and many have become myelinated. The number of axons reaching the distal stump is related to the distance the regenerating nerve has to traverse and the length of original nerve resected. Silicone guidance channels do not support regeneration if the nerve gap is greater than 10 mm and if the distal nerve stump is left out of the guidance channel. The morphology and structure of the regenerated nerve is far from normal. The size and number of axons and the thickness of myelin sheaths are less than normal. Electroymyographic evaluation of nerves regenerated through silicone tubes reveals that axons can make functional synapses with distal targets, although nerve conduction velocities and signal amplitudes are slower than normal, even after many months. Attempts to improve the success rate and quality of nerve regeneration have led to the use of other tubular biomaterials as guidance channels (Table 72.1). biodurable materials such as acrylic copolymers, polyethylene, and porous stainless steel and bioresorbable materials including polyglycolides, polylactides, and other polyesters have investigated. There is some concern that biodurable materials may cause long-term complications via compression injury to nerves or soft tissues. Biodegradable materials

Filling of tube by blood derived fluid and proteins (day 1)

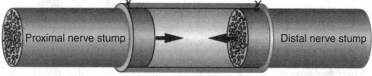

Formation and coalescence of fibrin cable (days 2–6)

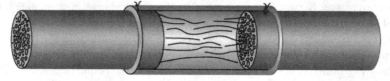

Invasion of cable by schwann cells, fibroblasts, and endothelial cells (days 7–14)

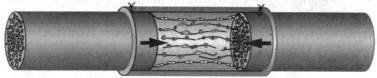

Axonal elongation and myelination (days 15–28)

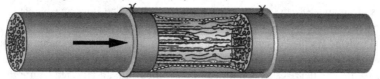

FIGURE 72.3 Regeneration process. Nerve regeneration through a guidance channel.

offer the advantage of disappearing once regeneration is complete, but success thus far has been limited by swelling, increased scar tissue induction, and difficulty in controlling degradation rates. In all cases, these materials have displayed variable degrees of success in bridging transected nerves, and the newly formed nerves are morphologically quite different from normal peripheral nerves. The general spatial-temporal progress of nerve regeneration, however, resembles that described for the silicone channel model.

72.7 Enhancing Regeneration by Optimizing Nerve

72.7.1 Guidance Channel Properties

Manipulating the physical, chemical, and electrical properties of guidance channels allows control over the regenerating environment and optimization of the regeneration process. The following features of synthetic nerve guidance channels have been studied (1) transmual permeability, (2) surface texture or microgeometry, (3) electric charges, (4) release of soluble factors, (5) inclusion of insoluble factors, and (6) seeding with neuronal support cells.

72.7.1.1 Transmural Permeability

The synthetic nerve guidance channel controls the regeneration process by influencing the cellular and metabolic aspects of the regenerating environment. Since transected nerves lose the integrity of their blood-nerve barrier (which controls oxygen and carbon dioxide tensions, pH, and the concentrations of nutrients and essential proteins), the guidance channel's transmural mass transfer characteristics modulate solute exchange between the regenerating tissue and the surrounding fluids. Nerves regenerated through permselective tubes display more normal morphologic characteristics than nerves regenerated in impermeable silicone elastomer (SE) and polyethylene (PE) or freely permeable expanded polytetrafluoroethylene (ePTFE) tubes. Nerves found in semipermeable tubes feature more myelinated axons and less connective tissue. Nerve cables regenerated in semipermeable or impermeable tubes are both round-shaped and free from attachment to the inner wall of the guidance channel. Nerves regenerated in highly porous, open structures do not form a distinct cable but contain connective tissue and dispersed neural elements. The range of permselectivity is very important, and optimal regeneration is observed with a molecular weight (MW) cut-off of 50,000 to 100,000 Da (D). Permselective PAN/PVC channels with an MW cut-off of 50,000 D support regeneration even in the absence of a distal nerve stump.

These observations suggest that controlled solute exchange between the internal regenerative and external wound-healing environments is essential in controlling regeneration. The availability of oxygen and other nutrients may minimize connective tissue formation in permeable PAN/PVC and PS tubes. Decreased oxygen levels and waste buildup may increase connective tissue formation in SE and PE tubes. Regeneration may also be modulated by excitatory and inhibitory factors released by the wound-healing environment. Semipermeable channels may sequester locally generated growth factors while preventing the inward flux of molecules inhibitory to regeneration.

72.7.1.2 Surface Texture or Microgeometry

The microgeometry of the luminal surface of the guidance channel plays an important role in regulating tissue outgrowth. Expanded microfibrilar polytetrafluorethylene (ePTFE) tubes exhibiting different internodal distances (1, 5, and 10 μm) were compared to smooth-walled impermeable PTFE tubes. Larger internodal distances result in greater surface irregularity and increased transmural porosity. Rough-walled tubes contained isolated fascicles of nerves disperses within a loose connective tissue stroma. The greater the surface roughness, the greater the spread of fascicles. In contrast, smooth-walled, impermeable PTFE tubes contained a discrete nerve cable delineated by an epineurium and located within the center of the guidance channel. Similar results were observed with semipermeable PAN/PVC tubes with the same chemistry and MW cut-off but with either smooth or rough surfaces. Nerves regenerated in tubes containing alternating sections of smooth and rough inner walls showed similar morphologies with an immediate change from single-cable to numerous fascicle morphology at the interface of the smooth and rough segments.

These studies suggest that the microgeometry of the guidance channel lumen also modulates the nerve regeneration process. Wall structure changes may alter the protein and cellular constituents of the regenerating tissue bridge. For example, the orientation of the fibrin matrix is altered in the presence of a rough inner wall. Instead of forming a single, longitudinally oriented bridge connecting the nerve ends, the fibrin molecules remain dispersed throughout the lumen. As a result, cells migrating in from the nerve stumps loosely fill the entire lumen rather than form a dense central structure.

72.7.1.3 Electric Charge Characteristics

Applied electric fields and direct dc stimulation are known to influence nerve regeneration *in vitro* and *in vivo*. Certain dielectric polymers may be used to study the effect of electric activity on nerve regeneration *in vivo* and *in vitro*. These materials are advantageous in that they provide electric charges without the need for an external power supply, can be localized anatomically, are biocompatible, and can be formed into a variety of shapes including tubes and sheets.

Electrets are a broad class of dielectric polymers which can be fabricated to display surface charges because of their unique molecular structure. True electrets, such as polytetrafluorethylene (PTFE), can be modified to exhibit a static surface charge due to the presence of stable, monopolar charges located in the bulk of the polymer. The sign of the charge depends on the poling conditions. Positive, negative, or combined charge patterns can be achieved. The magnitude of surface charge density is related to the number and stability of the monopolar charges. Charge stability is related to the temperature at which poling occurs. Crystalline piezoelectric materials such as polyvinylidene fluoride (PVDF) display transient surface charges related to dynamic spatial reorientation of molecular dipoles located in the polymer bulk. The amplitude of charge generation depends on the degree of physical deformation (i.e., dipole displacement) of the polymer structure. The sign of the charge is dependent on the direction of deformation, and the materials show no net charge at rest.

Negatively and positively poled PVDF and PTFE tubes have been implanted as nerve guidance channels. Poled PVDF and PTFE channels contain significantly more myelinated axons than unpoled, but otherwise identical, channels. In general, positively poled channels contained larger neural cables with more myelinated axons than negatively poled tubes. It is not clear how static or transient charge generation affects the regeneration process. The enhancement of regeneration may be due to electrical influences on protein synthesis, membrane receptor mobility, growth core mobility, cell migration, and other factors.

72.7.1.4 Release of Soluble Factors

The release of soluble agents, including growth factors and other bioactive substances from synthetic guidance channels, may improve the degree and specificity of neural outgrowth. Using single or multiple injections of growth factors has disadvantages including early burst release, poor control over local drug levels, and degradation in biologic environments. Guidance channels can be prefilled with drugs or growth factors, but the aforementioned limitations persist. Advantages of using a local, controlled delivery system are that the rate and amount of factor release can be controlled and that the delivery can be maintained for long periods (several weeks). Channels composed of an ethylene–vinyl acetate (EVA) copolymer have been fabricated and designed to release incorporated macromolecules in a predictable manner. The amount of drug loaded, its molecular weight, and geometry of the drug-releasing structure affect the drug release kinetics. It is also possible to restrict drug release to the luminal side of the guidance channel by coating its outer wall with a film of pure polymer.

Growth or neurontrophic factors that ensure the survival and general growth of neurons are produced by support cells (e.g., Schwann cells) or by target organs (e.g., muscle fibers). Some factors support neuronal survival, other support nerve outgrowth, and some do both. Numerous growth factors have been identified, purified, and synthesized through recombinant technologies (Table 72.2). *In vivo*, growth factors are found in solution in the serum or extracellular fluid or bound to extracellular matrix (ECM) molecules. Nerve guidance channels fabricated from EVA and designed to slowly release basic fibroblast growth factor (bFGF) or nerve growth factor (NGF) support regeneration over a 15-mm gap in a rat model. Control EVA tubes supported regeneration over a maximum gap of only 10 mm with no regeneration in 15-mm gaps. The concurrent release of growth factors which preferentially control the survival and outgrowth of motor and sensory neurons may further enhance regeneration, since the majority of peripheral nerves contain both populations. For example, NGF and b-FGF control sensory neuronal survival and outgrowth, whereas brain-derived growth factor (BDGF) and ciliary neurontrophic factor (CNTF) control motor neuronal survival and outgrowth. Growth factors released by guidance channels may also allow regeneration over large nerve deficits, and important consideration in nerve injuries with severe tissue loss. The local release of other pharmacologic agents (e.g., anti-inflammatory drugs) may also be useful in enhancing nerve growth.

72.7.1.5 Inclusion of Insoluble Factors

Several neural molecules found on cell membranes and in the extracellular matrix are potent modulators of neural attachment and outgrowth (Table 72.3). Proteins responsible for eliciting and stimulating axon elongation are termed neurite promoting factors. The glycoprotein laminin, an ECM component present in the balsa lamina of Schwann cells, has been reported to promote nerve elongation *in vitro* and *in vivo*. Other ECM products, including the glycoprotein fibronectin and the proteoglycan heparan sulphate, also

TABLE 72.2   Growth Factors Involved in Peripheral Nerve Regeneration

Growth Factor	Possible function
NGF — nerve growth factor	Neuronal survival, axon-Schwann cell interaction
BDNF — brain-derived neurotrophic factor	Neuronal survival
CNTF — ciliary neuronotrophic factor	Neuronal survival
NT-3 — neuronotrophin 3	Neuronal survival
NT-4 — neuronotrophin 4	Neuronal survival
IGF-1 — insulinlike growth factor-1	Axonal growth, Schwann cell migration
IGF-2 — Insulinlike growth factor-2	Motoneurite sprouting, muscle reinnervation
PDGF — platelet-derived growth factor	Cell proliferation, neuronal survival
aFGF — acidic fibroblast growth factor	Neurite regeneration, cell proliferation
bFGF — basic fibroblast growth factor	Neurite regeneration, neovascularization

TABLE 72.3   Neuronal Attachment and Neurite-Promoting Factors

Factor	Minimal peptide sequence
Collagen	RGD
Fibronectin	RGD
Laminim	RGD, SIKVAV, YIGSR
Neural cell adhesion molecule (N-CAM)	Unknown
N-caherin	Unknown

have been reported to promote nerve extension *in vitro*. Some subtypes of the ubiquitous protein collagen also support neural attachment. Filling guidance channels with gels of laminin and collagen has been shown to improve and accelerate nerve repair. The addition of longitudinally oriented fibrin gels to SE tubes has also been shown to accelerate regeneration. Collagen, laminin, and glycosaminoglycans (another ECM component) introduced in the guidance channel lumen support some degree of regeneration over a 15 to 20 mm gap in adult rats. The concentration of ECM gel is important, as thicker gels impede regeneration in semipermeable tubes.

The activity of these large, insoluble ECM molecules (up to 106 D MW) can be mimicked by short sequences only 3 to 10 amino acids long (e.g., RGD, YIGSR) (Table 72.3). The availability of small, soluble, bioactive agents allows more precise control over the chemistry, conformation, and binding of neuron-specific substances. Additionally, their stability and linear structure facilitate their use instead of labile (and more expensive) proteins which require three-dimensional structure for activity. Two- and three-dimensional substrates containing peptide mimics have been shown to promote neural attachment and regeneration *in vitro* and *in vivo*.

72.7.1.6   Seeding Neuronal Support Cells

Adding neural support cells to the lumen of guidance channels is another strategy being used to improve regeneration or to make regeneration possible over otherwise irreparable gaps. For example, Schwann cells cultured in the lumen of semipermeable guidance channels have been shown to improve nerve repair in adult rodents. Cells harvested from inbred rats were first cultured in PAN/PVC tubes using various ECM gels as stabilizers. The Schwann cells and gel formed a cable at the center of the tube after several days in culture. Once implanted, the cells were in direct contact with the nerve stumps. A dose-dependent relationship between the density of seeded cells and the extent of regeneration was noted. Another approach toward nerve repair involves the use of Schwann cells, fibroblasts, and the like which are genetically engineered to secrete growth factors. The use of support cells which release neuronotrophic and neurite-promoting molecules may enable regeneration over large gaps. There is increasing evidence that PNS elements, especially Schwann cells, are capable of supporting CNS regeneration as well. For example,

Schwann-cell-seeded semipermeable channels support regeneration at the level of the dorsal and ventral spinal cord roots and the optic nerve, which are CNS structures.

72.8 Summary

The permeability, textural, and electrical properties of nerve guidance channels can be optimized to impact favorably on regeneration. The release of growth factors, addition of growth substrates, and inclusion of neural support cells and genetically engineered cells also enhance regeneration through guidance channels. Current limitations in PNS repair, especially the problem of repairing long gaps, and in CNS repair, where brain and spinal cord trauma rarely result in appreciable functional return, may benefit from advances in engineering and biology. The ideal guidance system has not been identified but will most likely be a composite device that contains novel synthetic or bioderived materials and that incorporates genetically engineered cells and new products from biotechnology.

References

Aebischer, P., Salessiotis, A.N., and Winn, S.R. (1989). Basic fibroblast growth factor released from synthetic guidance channels facilitates peripheral nerve regeneration across nerve gaps. *J. Neurosci. Res.* 23: 282.

Dyck, P.J. and Thomas, P.K. (1993). *Peripheral Neuropathy*, 3rd ed., Vol. 1, Philadelphia, London, W.B. Saunders.

Guenard, V., Kleitman, N., and Morrissey, T.K. et al. (1992). Syngeneic Schwann cells derived from adult nerves seeded in semi permeable guidance channels enhance peripheral nerve regeneration. *J. Neurosci.* 12: 3310–3320.

LeBeau, J.M., Ellisman, M.H., and Powell, H.C. (1988). Ultrastructural and morphometric analysis of long-term peripheral nerve regeneration through silicone tubes. *J. Neurocytol.* 17: 161.

Longo, F.M., Hayman, E.G., Davis, G.E. et al. (1984). Neurite-promoting factors and extracellular matrix components accumulating *in vivo* within nerve regeneration chambers. *Exp. Neurol.* 81: 756.

Lundborg, G. (1987). Nerve regeneration and repair: a review. *Acta. Orthop. Scand.* 58: 145.

Lundborg, G., Dahlin, L.B., Danielsen, N. et al. (1982). Nerve regeneration in silicone chambers: influence of gap length and of distal stump components. *Exp. Neurol.* 76: 361.

Lundborg, G., Longo, F.M., and Varon, S. (1982). Nerve regeneration model and trophic factors *in vivo*. *Brain Res.* 232: 157.

Raivich, G. and Kreutzberg, G.W. (1993). Peripheral nerve regeneration: role of growth factors and their receptors. *Int. J. Dev. Neurosci.* 11: 311.

Sunderland, S. (1991). *Nerve Injuries and Their Repair*, Edinburgh, London, Churchill Livingstone.

Valentini, R.F. and Aebischer, P. (1991). The role of materials in designing nerve guidance channels and chronic neural interfaces. In P. Dario, G. Sandini, and P. Aebischer (Eds.), *Robots and Biological Systems: Towards a New Bionics?* pp. 625–636, Berlin, Germany, Springer-Verlag.

Valentini, R.F., Aebischer, P., Winn, S.R. et al. (1987). Collagen- and laminin-containing gels impede peripheral nerve regeneration through semi-permeable nerve guidance channels. *Exp. Neurol.* 98: 350.

Valentini, R.F., Sabatini, A.M., Dario, P. et al. (1989). Polymer electret guidance channels enhance peripheral nerve regeneration in mice. *Brain Res.* 480: 300.

Weiss, P. (1944). The technology of nerve regeneration: a review. Sutureless tubulation and related methods of nerve repair. *J. Neurosurg.* 1: 400.

Williams, L.R., Longo, F.M., Powell, H.C. et al. (1983). Spatial-temporal progress of peripheral nerve regeneration within a silicone chamber: parameters for a bioassay. *J. Comp. Neurol.* 218: 460.

73

Tracheal, Laryngeal, and Esophageal Replacement Devices

Tatsuo Nakamura
Yasuhiko Shimizu
Kyoto University

As the ability to reconstruct parts of the body has increased, so has the potential for complications associated with the replacement devices used to do so. Some of the most significant complications associated with replacement devices, such as vascular prostheses, cardiac valves, and artificial joints, are caused by infections at the implantation site. It is well known that the presence of a foreign material impairs host defenses and that prolonged infections cannot be cured unless the foreign material is removed from the site of infection. As the trachea, larynx, and esophagus are located at sites facing the "external environment," these prostheses are exposed to a high risk of infections and severe complications. The development of an artificial trachea, esophagus, and larynx is way behind that of artificial vascular grafts even though they are all tubular organs. In this chapter, we review conventional prostheses and their problems and limitations and discuss the current state of developments in this field.

73.1 Tracheal Replacement Devices

End-to-end anastomosis has been one of the standard operations for tracheal reconstruction. However, in patients in whom a large length of trachea has to be resected, this procedure is often difficult (the resectable limit is now considered to be approximately 6 cm). In such patients, alternative methods are required to reconstruct the airway. Such reconstructive methods can be classified into the following three categories (1) reconstruction with autologous tissue, (2) reconstruction with nonautologous trachea (i.e., transplantation), and (3) reconstruction with artificial material. The only one of these operative techniques which achieves good clinical results in the long term is the first (reconstruction with autologous tissue), particularly cervical tracheal reconstruction using an autologous skip flap conduit.

73.1.1 Designs of Artificial Tracheae

The artificial tracheae developed previously were designed according to one of two concepts. One is that the implanted prosthesis alone replaces the resected area of trachea, and the inner surface of the reconstructed trachea is not endothelialized. The other is that the implanted prosthesis is incorporated by the host tissue and its inner surface is endothelialized. These two types of prosthesis are called nonporous and mesh types, respectively, which reflect the materials from which they are made.

73.1.2 Nonporous Tube — Type Artificial Tracheae

The study of nonporous tube-type trachea has a long history, and many materials have been tried repeatedly for artificial tracheae. However, the results have been unsatisfactory, and now only one prosthesis of this type remains on the market, the Neville artificial trachea, which comprises a silicone tube with two suture rings attached to each of its ends (Figure 73.1). Neville used this trachea in 62 patients, from 1970 to 1988, some of whom survived for a long time [1]. However, late complications, such as migration of the artificial trachea and granular tissue formation at the anastomosis, were inevitable in many cases and occurred within several months and even as late as 2 years after implantation. Therefore, the Neville prosthesis is not used for patients with benign tracheal disease, because clinically, even if a large portion of the trachea up to the bifurcation has to be resected, the airway can be reconstructed easily by tracheotomy using a skin flap with sternal resection. For the alleviation of tracheal stenosis, **silicone T-tubes** (Figure 73.2) are widely indicated. The major advantage of such nonporous tubular prostheses is that airway patency can be

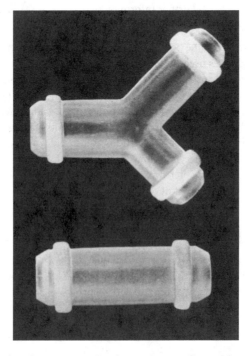

FIGURE 73.1   Neville artificial trachea constructed with a nonporous silicone tube with Dacron suture rings.

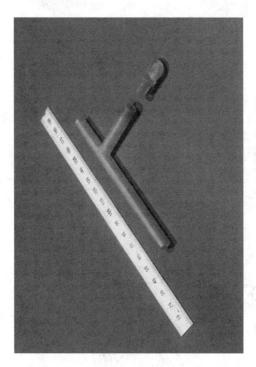

FIGURE 73.2 Silicone T-Tube.

ensured. Therefore, for patients for whom end-to-end anastomosis is impossible, nonporous prostheses may be used at last resort to avoid threatened suffocation (asphyxiation).

Tracheal replacement using the Neville artificial trachea requires the following operative procedure:

1. Right-sided posterolateral skin incision and 4th or 5th intercoastal thoracotomy. Up to the stage of tracheal resection, the operative procedure is similar to that for standard tracheal resection. However, because the tension at anastomosis is not as high as that with an end-to-end anastomosis, neither **hilar** nor **laryngeal release** is often necessary.
2. Reconstruction with an artificial trachea. After resection of the tracheal lesion, the oral intubation tube is drawn back, and the trachea is reintubated via the operative field (Figure 73.3). In patients who require resection that reaches to near the bifurcation, the second intubation tube should be placed in the left main bronchus. An artificial trachea with a diameter similar to that of the tracheal end is used. Any small differences in their diameters can be compensated for by suturing. Anastomosis is carried out using 4 to 0 absorbable sutures, 2 mm apart, with interrupted suturing. The tracheal sutures are attached to the tracheal cartilage. On completion of the anastomosis on one side, the oral intubation tube is readvanced, and the other side is anastomosed under oral ventilation. After anastomosis, an air leakage test at pressure of 30 cm H_2O is carried out. In order to avoid rupture of the great vessels near the implanted artificial trachea, they should not be allowed to touch each other. In cases at risk of this occurring, wrapping of the artificial trachea with the grater omentum is also recommended.
3. Postoperative care. Frequent postoperative boncofiberscopic checks should be performed to ensure sputum does not come into contact with the anastomosis sites. The recurrent laryngeal nerves on both sides are often injured during the operation, so the movement of the vocal cord should be checked at extubation.

   The major reason for the poor results with the Neville tracheal prosthesis during long-term follow-up was considered to be the structure of the prosthesis, that is, the nonelasticity of the tube and suture rings. A variety of improvements to this prosthesis have been tried, especially at the areas

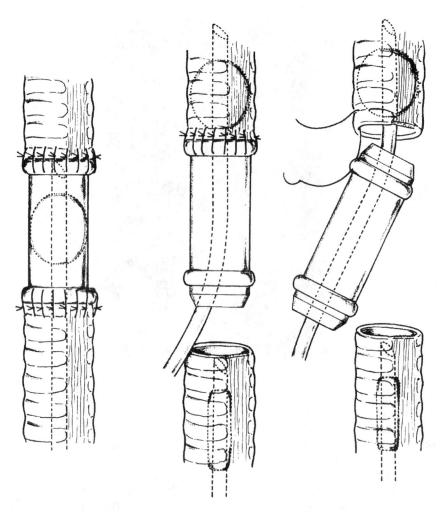

FIGURE 73.3 Operation proceeding of tracheal reconstruction using an artificial trachea.

of interface with the host tissue by suture reinforcement with mesh skirts, increasing the flexibility of the tube, and application of **hydroxyapatite** to the suture rings. However, the problems at the anastomosis have not been conquered yet.

In attempt to overcome the problems described above, a new mesh-type artificial trachea has been designed that is intended to be incorporated into the host tissue so that eventually there is no foreign-body–external-environment interface.

73.1.3 Mesh-Type Artificial Tracheae

Porous artificial tracheae are called mesh-type because the prosthetic trunk is made of mesh. In the 1950s, several trials of tracheal reconstruction using metallic meshes made of tantalum and stainless steel were conducted. In the 1960s, **heavy Marlex mesh** was used clinically for tracheal reconstruction, and good short-term results were reported. However, long-term observations showed that this mesh caused rupture of the adjacent graft vessels, which was fatal, so it fell gradually out of use for tracheal reconstruction. When used clinically, because the heavy mesh was rough and not air-tight, other tissues, such as autografted pericardium, fascia, or dura mater, were applied to seal it until the surrounding tissue grew into it and made it air-tight. The pore size of materials conventionally used for artificial vessels, such as **expanded PTFE** (**polytetrafluoroethylene**, pore size of 15 to 30 μm), is so small that the host tissue cannot penetrate the

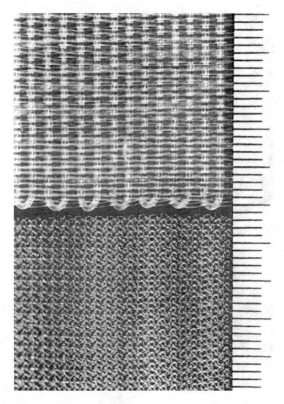

FIGURE 73.4 Marlex Mesh, fine (left) and heavy (right) (division of the scale; mm).

mesh, which is rejected eventually. The optimal pore size for tracheal replacement mesh is 200 to 300 μm. **Fine Marlex** mesh is made of polypropylene with a pore size 200 to 300 μm (Figure 73.4). It is now widely used clinically for abdominal wall reconstruction and reinforcement after inguinal herniation. **Collagen**-grafted fine Marlex mesh is air-tight, and clinically, good tissue regeneration is achieved when it is used to patch-graft of the trachea. The grafted collagen has excellent biocompatibility and promotes connective tissue infiltration into the mesh. However, the fine mesh alone is too soft to keep the tube open, so a tracheal prosthesis was made of collagen-grafted fine Marlex mesh reinforced with a continuous polypropylene spiral (Figure 73.5). In dogs, complete surgical resection of a 4-cm length of trachea, which was replaced with a 5-cm long segment of this type of artificial trachea, was performed, and the prostheses were incorporated completely by the host trachea and confluent formation of respiratory epithelium on each prosthetic lumen was observed (Figure 73.6) [2]. These results indicate that this artificial trachea is highly biocompatible and promising for clinical application.

73.2 Laryngeal Replacement Devices

Total laryngectomy is one of the standard operations for laryngeal carcinomas. As radiation therapy and surgery have progressed, the prognosis associated with laryngeal carcinoma has improved. The curability of total laryngeal carcinoma is now almost 70%, and therefore many patients survive for a long time after surgery. Individuals who have undergone laryngectomy are called laryngectomees or laryngetomized patients, and for them, laryngeal reconstruction is of the utmost importance. However, because the larynx is situated just beneath the oral cavity, where the danger of infection is high, successful reconstruction with foreign materials is very difficult. As yet, no total replacement device for the larynx has been developed, and laryngeal transplantation, although apparently feasible, is still at the animal experimental stage.

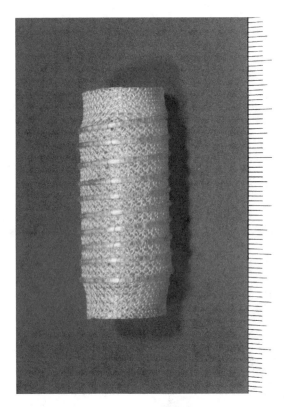

FIGURE 73.5 New artificial trachea made from collagen-conjugated fine Marlex mesh.

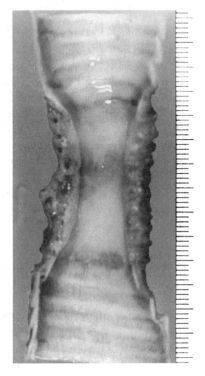

FIGURE 73.6 Macroscopic inner view of the reconstructed trachea 6 months after operation. Inner surface is covered with smooth and lustrous soft regenerated tissue.

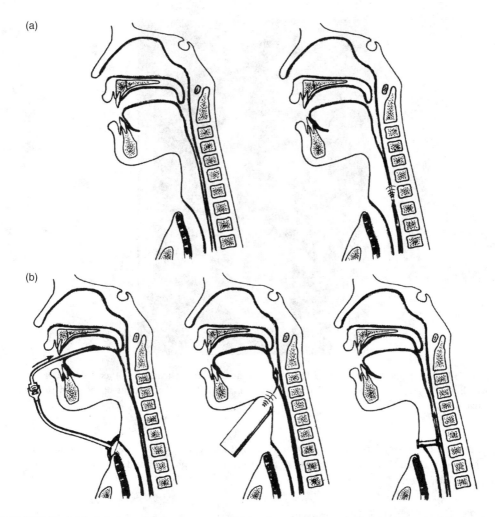

FIGURE 73.7 (a) Sagital views of the laryngectomee (left) and esophageal speech (right). Air flow from the esophagus makes the sound. (b) Pneumatic larynx (reed type) (left); electric artificial larynx (transcervical type), (center); voice prosthesis (T-E shut) of Blom & Singer method, right.

The larynx has three major functions (1) phonation, (2) respiration, and (3) protection of the lower airway during swallowing. Of these, phonation is considered to be the most important. The conventional so-called artificial larynx can only substitute phonation. A variety of methods have been developed to recover phonation after total larygectomy, which is called vocal rehabilitation. Methods for vocal rehabilitation are classified as (1) esophageal speech, (2) artificial larynx, and (3) surgical laryngoplasty. Two-thirds of laryngectomees learn esophageal speech as their means of communication. For the rest, an artificial larynx and surgical laryngoplasty are indicated. The typical devices are the pneumatic and electrical larynx which are driven by the expiratory force and electric energy, respectively. Tracheo-esophageal (T-E) fistula with voice prosthesis is the most popular method in surgical laryngoplasty. Figure 73.7 illustrates the mechanical structures of typical artificial larynxes.

73.2.1 Pneumatic Larynxes

The first pneumatic mechanical device was developed by Tapia in 1883. Several variations of pneumatic larynxes are now used. In Figure 73.8, the pneumatic device uses expired air from the tracheo stoma to vibrate a rubber band or reed to produce a low frequency sound, which is transmitted to the mouth via a

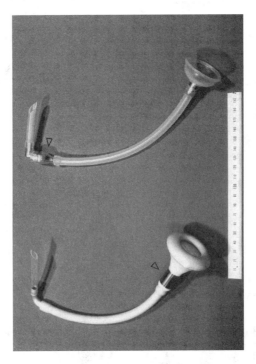

FIGURE 73.8 Pneumatic larynxes: Myna (left) (Nagashima Medical Instrument Tokyo, Japan) and Okumura Artificial larynx (Okumura, Osaka, Japan) (right). Arrow marks indicate the portions of reed and rubber band, respectively.

tube. Pneumatic transoral larynxes produce excellent natural speech, which is better than that with other artificial larynxes, but their disadvantages are that they are conspicuous and that regular cleaning and mopping of saliva leakage is necessary.

73.2.2 Electric Artificial Larynxes

The transcervical electrolarynx is an electric, handheld vibrator that is placed on the neck to produce sound (Figure 73.9). The frequency used is 100 to 200 Hz. The vibrations of the electrolarynx are conducted to the neck tissue and create a low-frequency sound in the hypopharynx. This is the most popular artificial larynx. The transoral artificial laryngeal device is a handheld electric device that produces a low-pitched sound which is transmitted to the back of the mouth by a connecting tube placed in the patient's mouth. As microelectronic science progresses, great hopes of applying microelectric techniques to the artificial larynx are now entertained, and some devices have been designed, although implantable laryngeal prostheses have not achieved widespread use.

73.2.3 Voice Prostheses

As well as the artificial larynxes described above, tracheo-esophageal (T-E) fistula prostheses are now widely used for vocal rehabilitation, and excellent speech and voice results have been achieved. In 1980, Singer and Blom developed and introduced the first simple method, which is called Blom and Singer's voice prosthesis. The principle of the T-E fistula technique is to shunt expired pulmonary air through a voice prosthesis device into the esophagus to excite the mucosal tissue to vibrate. A fistula is made by puncturing the posterior wall of the trachea 5 mm below the upper margin of the tracheal stoma, and when a patient speaks, he/she manually occludes the stoma to control the expiratory flow through the fistula to the oral cavity. The voice prosthesis has a one-way value to prevent saliva leakage (Figure 73.10).

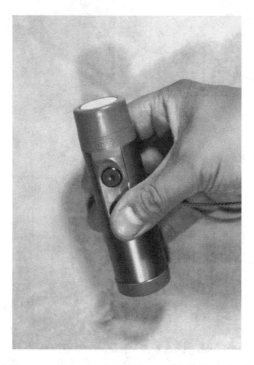

FIGURE 73.9 Electric artificial larynx (transcervical type): Servox (Dr Kuhn & Co. GmBH, Köln, Germany).

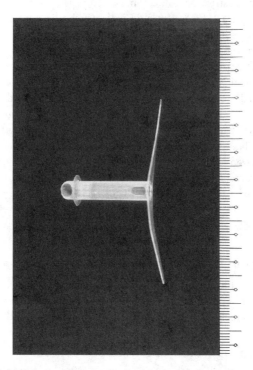

FIGURE 73.10 Voice prosthesis (Bivona, Indiana, USA). This valved tube is inserted into a surgically placed T-E fistula for voice restoration following laryngectomy.

(a)   (b)

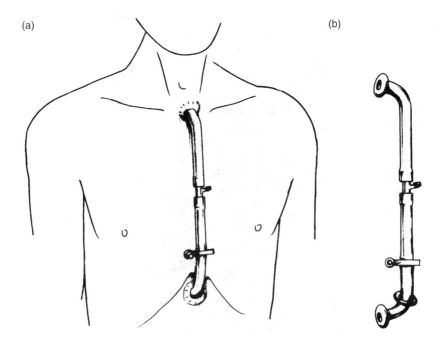

FIGURE 73.11   Extracorporeal artificial esophagus (Tokyo University type).

73.3   Artificial Esophagi (Esophageal Prostheses)

In patients with esophageal cancer, the esophagus is resected and reconstructed using a piece of pediculated alimentary tract, such as the gastric conduit, colon, or ileum. However, in some cases, it is impossible to use autologous alimentary tract, for example, in patients who have undergone gastrectomy. In such cases, an artificial esophagus is indicated. However, with the exception of extracorporeal-type esophagi and intraesophageal stent tubes, the esophageal replacement devices developed have remained far from useful in clinical reconstructive practice. The main reason is anastomosis dehiscence, which often leads to fatal infections, as well as prosthetic dislodgment, migration, and narrowing at a late stage.

The conventional artificial esophagi now used in the clinic can be broadly classified into two types: extracorporeal and intraesophageal stents. Extracorporeal artificial esophagi are used as bypasses from cervical esophageal to gastric fistulae (Figure 73.11). They are used during the first stage of two-stage esophageal reconstruction. They are made of latex rubber or silicone, but since the development of **IVH** method, their use is now extremely rare.

Intraesophageal stent types of artificial esophagus are made from a rubber or plastic tube, which is inserted in the stenotic part of the esophagus (Figure 73.12). They are used only for unresectable esophageal carcinoma, that is, they are not indicated for resectable cases. Therefore, conventional artificial esophagi are only palliative devices for use as stop-gap measures.

73.3.1   Development of New Artificial Esophagi

In contrast to the palliative artificial esophagi, the ideal artificial esophagus would replace the resected part of the esophagus by itself. The artificial esophagi of this type are classified according to the materials from which they are made, namely natural substances, artificial materials, and their composites (hybrids).

73.3.2   Artificial Esophagi Made of Natural Substances

The first report of an artificial esophagus made of a natural substance was the skin conduit developed by Bircher in 1907. Subsequently, esophageal reconstruction using a variety of natural substances — muscle

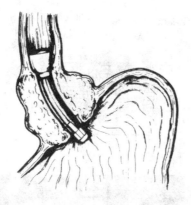

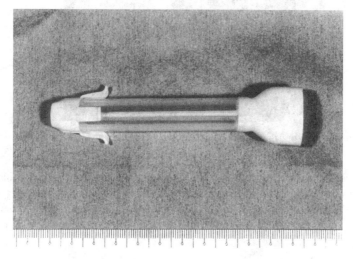

FIGURE 73.12   Intraesophageal type of artificial esophagus. (Sumitomo Bakelite Co., Ltd., Tokyo, Japan.)

fasciae, isolated jejunum, autologous aorta, aortic homograft, autologous esophagus, connective tissue conduit, trachea, and freeze-dried dura mater homograft — has been reported. However, non of these has overcome the problems of stenosis, which necessitates continuous bougieing, and other complications at the anastomosis sites.

73.3.3 Artificial Esophagi Made of Artificial Materials

The first trial of an esophagus made of an artificial material was carried out by Neuhof, who, in 1922, used a rubber tube to reconstruct the cervical esophagus. Subsequently, several artificial materials have been tried repeatedly, such as polyethylene, Dacron, stainless steel mesh, tantalum mesh, dimethylopolysiloxane, polyvinylformal sponge, Teflon, nylon, silicone rubber, collagen-silicone, Dacron-silastic, acrylresin, and expanded PTFE tubes, but all the trials ended in failure. These materials were foreign bodies, after all, and the host tissues continuously rejected them, which caused anastomotic dehiscence followed by infections. Even rare cases, whose artificial esophagi escaped early rejection, did not avoid the late complications, such as prosthetic migration and esophageal stenosis.

73.3.4 Hybrid Artificial Esophagi

Cultured cells are now widely used for hybrid artificial organs, especially for metabolic organs, such as the liver and pancreas. A hybrid artificial esophagus comprising a latissimus dorsi muscle tube, the inner

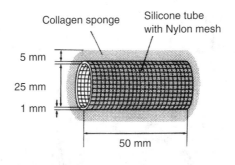

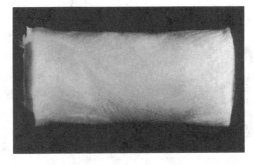

FIGURE 73.13   An artificial esophagus made of collagen sponge which is intended to be replaced with host tissue.

surface of which is epithelialized by human cultured esophageal epithelial cells, is being studied by the Keio University group [3]. Human esophageal epithelial cells cultured on collagen gel for 10 days were transplanted onto the surfaces of the lattisimus dorsi muscles of athymic mice, and new epithelial cells were observed, which indicates it may be possible to develop an artificial esophagus incorporating cultured epithelial cells.

73.3.5   New Concepts in Artificial Esophageal Design

The previous studies on artificial esophagi are a history of how to prevent the host tissue from recognizing the artificial esophagus as a foreign body, and all the trials, without exception, resulted in failure. Currently, an artificial esophagus made according to a completely new design concept is undergoing trials. The outer collagen sponge layer of the prosthesis is intended to be replaced with host tissue over a period of time, and its inner tube acts as a palliative (temporary) stent until the outer layer has been replaced by host tissue. This type of artificial esophagus comprises an inner silicone tube and an outer tube of collagen sponge (Figure 73.13), which is nonantigenic and has excellent biocompatibility, as well as promoting tissue regeneration in the form of an **extracellular matrix**. In dogs implanted with a 5-cm length of this artificial esophagus, esophageal regeneration was accomplished in 3 weeks, and all the early complications at the anastomosis were overcome. However, in dogs from which the inner stents were removed as soon as mucosal regeneration was accomplished, stenosis developed rapidly, and the regenerated esophagus began to constrict. Such stenosis and constriction could not be overcome, even when autologous buccal mucosal cells were seeded onto the collagen sponge. Accordingly, on the basis of the hypothesis that stenosis and constriction depend on the maturity of the regenerated submucosal tissue, stent removal was postponed for at least 1 week after mucosal epithelialization of the artificial esophagus was complete. Late stenotic complications did not occur, and regeneration of muscle tissue and esophageal glands was observed (Figure 73.14) [4]. The regenerated esophagus showed adequate physiologic function and pathologically satisfactory results. The limit to the length of the esophagus that can be resected successfully was reported to be 9 cm, and the longest successful artificial esophagus developed hitherto was 5 cm. In order to achieve more widespread use, artificial esophagi which can be used for longer reconstructions are needed. Although

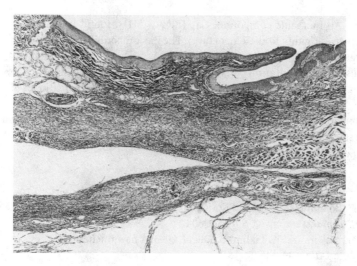

FIGURE 73.14 Pathologic finding of a regenerated esophageal tissue in a dog using the artificial esophagus (Figure 73.13). Continuous epithelial layer and the muscle and esophageal gland were regenerated at the interposed area.

still at the stage of animal experiments, the long-term observations indicate that typical difficulties, such as anastomotic leakage, ablation, and dislocation of the prosthesis, have been overcome, which suggests this type of prosthesis will have a promising future in clinical practice.

Defining Terms

Collagen: A main supportive protein of connective tissue, bone, skin, and cartilage. One-third of protein of vertebrate animal consists of collagen.

End-to-end anastomosis: An operative union after resecting the lesion, each end to be joined in a plane vertical to the ultimate flow through the structures.

Expanded PTFE (polytetrafluorethylene): PTFE is polymer made from tetrafluoroethylene (CF2 = CF2), with the structure of −CF2−CF2−. It provides excellent stability chemically and thermally. Teflon is the trade mark of PTFE of Du Pont Co. Expanded PTFE has a microporous structure which has elasticity and antithrombogenisity in the body and is medically applied for vascular grafts or surgical seats.

Extracellular matrix (ECM): The substances which are produced by connective tissue cells. The two major components of the extracellular matrix are collagen and proteoglycans. There are a number of other macromolecules which provide important functions such as tissue growth, regeneration or aging.

Heavy Marlex mesh and fine Marlex mesh: Surgical mesh is used for reconstruction of the defect that results from massive resection. Most popular surgical meshes are Marlex meshes. Heavy mesh is made of high-density polyethylene and has been used for reconstruction of chest wall. Fine mesh is made of polypropylene and is now widely used for abdominal wall reconstruction or reinforcement of inguinal herniation operation.

Hilar release and laryngeal release: The pulmonis hilus is the depression of the mediastinal surface of the lung where the blood vessels and the bronchus enter. The hilus is fixed by the pulmonary ligament to downward. In order to reduce the tension at the tracheal anastomoses, the pulmonary ligament is released surgically. This method is called hilar release. At the resection and reconstruct of upper trachea, the larynx can be also released from its upper muscular attachment. This method is called laryngeal release and up to 5 cm of tracheal mobilization may be achieved.

Hydroxyapatite: An inorganic compound, $Ca_{10}(PO_4)_6(OH)_2$, found in the matrix of bone and the teeth which gives rigidity to these structures. The biocompatibility of hydroxyapatite has attracted special interest.

IVH (intravenous hyperalimentation): An alimentation method for patients who cannot eat. A catheter is placed in the great vessel, through which high concentration alimentation is given continuously.

Silicone T-tube: A self-retaining tube in the shape of a T which is made of silicone. Tracheal T-tube is used popularly for tracheal stenotic disease and serves both as a tracheal stent and tracheotomy tube. One side branchi of T-tube projects from the tracheotomy orifice.

References

[1] Neville, W.E., Bolanowski, P.J.P., and Kotia, G.G. 1990. Clinical experience with the silicone tracheal prosthesis. *J. Thorac. Cardiovasc. Surg.* 99: 604.

[2] Okumura, N., Nakamura, T., Takimoto, Y. et al. 1993. A new tracheal prosthesis made form collagen grafted mesh. *ASAIO J.* 39: M475.

[3] Sato, M., Ando, N., Ozawa, S. et al. 1993. A hybrid artificial esophagus using cultured human esophageal cells. *ASAIO J.* 39: M554.

[4] Takimoto, Y., Okumura, N., Nakamura, T. et al. 1993. Long-term follow up of the experimental replacement of the esophagus with a collagen-silicone composite tube. *ASAIO J.* 39: M736.

Further Information

Proceedings of the American Society of Artificial Internal Organs Conference are published annually by the American Society of Artificial Internal Organs (ASAIO). These proceedings include the latest developments in the field of reconstructive devices each year. The monthly journal *Journal of Thoracic and Cardiovascular Surgery* reports advances in tracheal and esophageal prosthetic instruments. An additional reference is H.F. Mahieu, "Voice and speech rehabilitation following larygectomy, Groningen," the Netherlands, Rijksuniversiteit Groningen, 1988.

74

Artificial Blood

Marcos Intaglietta
University of California

Robert M. Winslow
SANGRAT Inc.

Blood is a key component of surgery and treatment of injury, and its availability is critical for survival in the presence of severe blood losses. Its present use under conditions of optimal medical care delivery is one unit (0.5 l) per 20 person-year. On a world-wide basis, however, its availability and use is limited to one unit per 100 person-year according to statistics from the World Health Organization. The gap between current optimal need and actual availability is further aggravated by the fact that the blood supply in many locations is not safe. Even in conditions of optimal testing and safeguards, blood per se has a number of inherent risks [Dodd, 1992], ranging from about 3% (3 adverse outcomes per 100 units transfused) for minor reactions, to a probability of 0.001% of undergoing a fatal hemolytic reaction. Superimposed on these risks is the possibility of transmission of infectious diseases such as hepatitis B (0.002%) and hepatitis non-A non-B (0.03%). The current risk of becoming infected with the human immunodeficiency virus (HIV) is about 1 chance in 400,000 under optimal screening conditions. These are risks related to the transfusion of one unit of blood, and become magnified in surgical interventions requiring multiple transfusions.

The HIV epidemic caused many fatalities due to blood transfusion before stringent testing was introduced in 1984. The danger of contamination of the blood supply led the U.S. military to develop blood substitutes starting in 1985 with the objective of finding a product for battlefield conditions that was free of contamination, could be used immediately, and did not need special storage. The end of the Cold War, changes in the nature of military engagements, the slow progress in the development of a blood substitute, and the fact that blood testing caused the blood supply to be again safe and abundant in both the United States and Europe lowered the interest of the U.S. military in artificial blood, and the development passed almost exclusively into the hands of private industry.

While about a dozen products have been tested in humans, at present only three are in clinical trials for blood replacement. These products have side effects whose relevance is difficult to assess in the absence of massive clinical trials. A side effect common to hemoglobin-based products is hypertension, which was proposed to be of additional therapeutic value in the treatment of hypotensive conditions associated with severe blood losses and hemorrhagic shock. However, extensive clinical trials led by Baxter Healthcare, with their product HemAssist™ showed that their product caused twice the mortality found with the use of conventional therapies for volume resuscitation. This unfortunate outcome was fully predicted by results in academic research showing that hypertension per se causes a severe impairment of microvascular function.

The key transport parameters that determine the exchange of oxygen in the microcirculation were, until recently, incompletely understood. Most experimental studies underlying the development of artificial blood emphasized systemic, whole organ methods in order to assess efficacy and biocompatibility, without quantitative analysis of transport phenomena inherent to blood function, or data from the microcirculation. Advances in instrumentation and *in vivo* methods (Figure 74.1) during the past few years have provided new understanding of how oxygen is distributed to the tissues by the microscopic blood vessels, and this information has proven to be crucial in identifying the transport characteristics needed for artificial blood to work effectively, and to counteract some of its inherent problems.

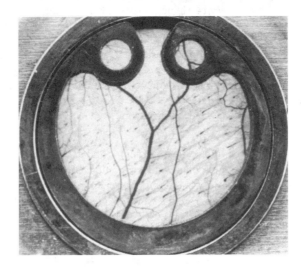

FIGURE 74.1 Experimental hamster skinfold model for the analysis of the microvasculature in the awake animal, without anesthesia and after the effects of surgery have subsided. This technology allows to quantify blood flow, blood and tissue pO_2, leukocyte activation, blood vessel permeability to macromolecules, and blood vessel tone throughout the arterioles, capillaries, and venules. The tissue under study consists of skeletal muscle and subcutaneous connective tissue. Arterial and venous catheters are used to monitor systemic data.

74.1 Oxygen Carrying Plasma Expanders and the Distribution of Transport Properties in the Circulation

To the present it has not been possible to obtain an artificial fluid with the same properties as blood, primarily due to its cellular nature. Consequently, artificial blood or blood substitutes are plasma expanding fluids that carry more oxygen than that dissolved in water or plasma. Their physical properties are significantly different from those of natural blood, and therefore it is necessary to determine the positive or negative effects on circulatory function and tissue oxygenation that may arise from these differences.

Under normal conditions, the transport properties of blood, such as hydraulic pressure, partial pressure of oxygen, oxygen content and viscosity, are distributed (Figure 74.2). The distribution of transport properties of blood is matched to anatomical features of the macro- and microcirculation and set within narrow limits throughout the life of the organism. Hydraulic blood pressure, which changes continuously in the circulation due to viscous losses, is an example of this situation. Each branching order of the vasculature is adapted to recognize a narrow range of hydraulic blood pressures and react if pressure changes and the normal set point is not met. The distribution of blood pressure influences the cellular composition of blood vessels, and is regulated by the so-called myogenic response [Johnson, 1996], which causes vessels to constrict, thus increasing viscous losses, if pressure increases and vice versa.

The same type of matching is present for the distribution of oxygen tension and blood oxygen content in the vasculature. The shape of the oxygen dissociation curve for hemoglobin and the distribution of

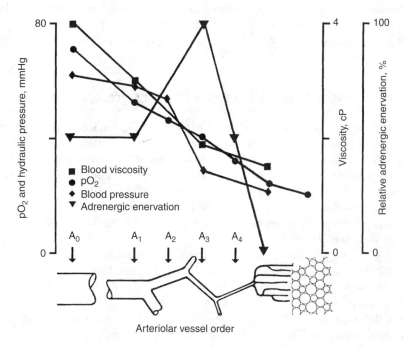

FIGURE 74.2 Distributed nature of transport properties in the hamster skinfold microcirculation. Arterial blood vessels are classified according to their hierarchical position starting with the A_0 small arteries (100 μm and greater diameter), and ending with A_4 terminal arterioles. Blood pressure, blood viscosity, and blood pO_2 fall continuously from the systemic value. Furthermore, the characteristics of the oxygen saturation of hemoglobin curve correspond to specific microvascular locations. This distribution is maintained through the life of an organism and is autoregulated by central and peripheral controls, including adrenergic nerve endings which have the highest density in the A_3 arterioles. Introduction of a molecular plasma expander fundamentally changes the distribution of viscosity, blood pressure, **shear stress**, and the availability of oxygen to the vessel wall. Autoregulatory processes sense these changes and cause the microcirculation to react. Data on viscosity is derived from Lipowsky, 1987, data on blood pressure is from the hamster cheek pouch from [Joyner et al., 1972], other data is from our studies.

enervation of arterioles is such that the knee of the oxygen dissociation curve for hemoglobin is located in arterioles that present the highest density of adrenergic enervation [Saltzman et al., 1992].

Blood viscosity and blood flow velocity in the circulation are also distributed in such a fashion that together with the anatomical features of the local blood vessels, shear stress is caused to be virtually uniform throughout the circulation. This is also the consequence of the continuous variation of hematocrit from the systemic value in the larger blood vessels, to about half this value in the capillaries, due to the Faraheus–Lindquist effect (a property due to the cellular composition of blood) and the very strong dependance of blood viscosity on hematocrit. In larger arterioles, blood viscosity is about 3.5 to 4.0 centipoise (cP), while in the smaller arterioles viscosity falls to about that of plasma (1.1 to 1.2 cP). This has large effects on shear stress and shear stress dependant release of endothelial dependant relaxing factors (EDRF, NO, and prostaglandins), since the circulation is designed to maintain shear stress constant. In other words, shear stress is also present in a prescribed way in the microcirculation when the system is perfused by normal blood.

A molecular oxygen carrying plasma expander is not subjected to the Fahraeus–Lindquist effect (which determines the progressive decrease of hematocrit in the microcirculation), causing the whole microcirculation to be exposed to a uniform viscosity (see the mathematical model) and significantly changing shear stress distribution.

The significance of the mechanical traction at the interface between flowing blood and tissue is that shear stress modulates the production of vasoactive materials such as nitric oxide (NO) and prostacyclin [Frangos et al., 1985; Kuchan et al., 1994] and therefore is an active control of blood flow and the oxygen supply. Furthermore, NO is also a major regulator of mitochondrial metabolism [Shen et al., 1995], acting as a brake for tissue oxygen consumption. These considerations show that the transport properties of blood are intertwined with the physical and biological regulation of oxygen delivery and the level of tissue oxygen consumption.

74.2 The Distribution of Oxygen in the Circulation

Oxygenation of tissue as a whole has been extrapolated from the so-called Krogh model, which is focused on how gases are exchanged between blood flowing in a cylindrical conduit, the single capillary, and a surrounding tissue cylinder. It is generally assumed that most of the oxygen is exchanged at this level, implying the existence of large blood/tissue oxygen gradients in a substantial portion of tissue capillaries. However, capillary/tissue O_2 gradients are maximal in the lung (50 mmHg/μm) and minimal in the tissues (0.5 mmHg/μm). Most tissue capillaries appear to be in near oxygen concentration equilibrium with the tissue; thus, large oxygen gradients are not present, suggesting that capillaries may not be the primary mechanism for tissue oxygenation.

The technology of phosphorescence quenching for measuring oxygen partial pressure optically in the microvessels and the surrounding tissue [Torres and Intaglietta, 1994; Wilson, 1993], when used in conjunction with the awake hamster skinfold model, allows for *in vivo* analysis of the assumptions in the Krogh model. Current findings indicate that in the hamster skinfold connective tissue and skeletal muscle at rest, most of the oxygen is delivered by the arterioles and that little oxygen is contributed by the capillaries. In this tissue average capillary pO_2 is about 25 mmHg and venular pO_2 is higher. This indicates that at least half of the oxygen in blood exits the blood vessels prior to arrival in the tissue. In summary, these results and previous findings from other laboratories [Intaglietta et al., 1996] show that:

1. Capillary blood pO_2 is only slightly higher (about 5 mmHg) than tissue pO_2.
2. Arterio/venous capillary pO_2 differences are very small because tissue pO_2 is essentially uniform, and capillaries are close to pO_2 equilibrium with the tissue.
3. The only tissue domain where pO_2 exhibits large gradients is the immediate vicinity of the microvessels (vessels with diameter 80 μm and smaller), a tissue compartment whose main constituent is the microvascular wall.
4. A major portion of blood oxygen exits the circulation via the arterioles.

74.3   Oxygen Gradients in the Arteriolar Wall

The phosphorescence optical technology allows us to make an accurate mass balance between the decrease of oxygen content in the arterioles and the diffusion flux of oxygen out of the microvessels determined by the oxygen gradients in the surrounding tissue. These measurements made simultaneously inside and outside of the vessels show that oxygen exiting from arterioles is driven by steep oxygen gradients at the arteriolar wall, which is consistent with the hypothesis that the arteriolar wall is a high metabolism tissue and therefore a large oxygen sink [Tsai et al., 1998]. These steep gradients are present in arterioles, but not in capillaries and venules. The large oxygen consumption is due to biological activity in the endothelium and smooth muscle [Kjellstrom et al., 1987]. These findings lead to the following conceptualization for the design of artificial blood:

1. Endothelium and smooth muscle serve as a metabolic barrier to the passage of oxygen from blood to tissue, which in part protects the tissue from the high oxygen content (pO_2) of blood.
2. One of the goals of basal tissue perfusion is to supply oxygen to the endothelium and smooth muscle.
3. Oxygenation of working tissue (exercising skeletal muscle) results from three events:
   - Lowering of the vessel wall metabolic barrier
   - Increased perfusion with oxygenated blood
   - Deployment of a biochemical process that protects the tissue from high pO_2 levels
4. Under basal conditions, tissue capillaries only partially serve to supply oxygen to the tissue. They may be a structure to expose the endothelium to blood in order to fulfill the large oxygen demand of these cells and provide for the extraction of CO_2.
5. The physical and biological properties of blood affect the oxygen consumption of the vessel walls.

74.4   Mathematical Modeling of Blood/Molecular Oxygen Carrying Plasma Expander

The previous discussion shows that tissue oxygenation is the result of the interplay of quantifiable physical events, and therefore it may be subjected to analytical modeling to identify key parameters and set the stage for rational design. The critical issue is to understand the changes due to the presence of molecular oxygen carriers. These changes are (a) change in availability of oxygen to the vessel wall due to the molecular nature of the carrier; (b) distortion of the pattern of intraluminal oxygen distribution in the microcirculation; (c) lowered viscosity and decreased generation of EDRF due to lowered shear stress; (d) increased colloid osmotic pressure; and (e) increased vessel wall pO_2 gradient. The mathematical model is based on oxygen mass balance in subsequent vessel segments, starting with a major arterial vessel and terminating in the capillaries, with the objective of calculating the oxygen tension of blood in the capillaries, which should correspond to tissue pO_2.

The result of this analysis is the following equation, which expresses how the total loss of oxygen from the arterial and arteriolar network K_n is related to anatomical and transport features of the blood vessels and blood [Intaglietta, 1997]. Total oxygen exit is the summation of losses from n individual vascular segments i. This equation gives the functional relationship between transport parameters that determine capillary blood pO_2 for given changes in the physical properties of blood:

$$K_n = \sum k_i = \frac{128\mu}{F(Htc, C)m_t} \sqrt{\frac{g_0 \alpha D}{2}} \sum_1^n \frac{L_i^2}{n_i d_i^3 \Delta P_i} \qquad (74.1)$$

where μ is blood viscosity, $F(Htc, C)$ is the concentration of hemoglobin (red blood cells + molecular), m_t is the maximum amount of oxygen that can be dissolved in blood under normal conditions, D is the diffusion constant for oxygen in tissue, a is the solubility of oxygen in tissue, g_0 is the oxygen consumption by the vessel wall, L_i is the length of each vessel segment, d_i is the diameter of each segment, and n_i is the slope of the oxygen dissociation curve for hemoglobin.

The summation shows two distinct groups of terms. One group is common to all vessel segments and includes blood viscosity, hematocrit or blood **oxygen carrying capacity**, and vessel wall metabolism. The second group is a summation where each term is specific to each vascular segment. This expression shows that, in principle, better capillary oxygenation results from lowering viscosity. However, increased capillary oxygenation is a signal that triggers auto regulatory mechanisms which strive to maintain capillary oxygen constant through vasoconstriction. Thus, lowering blood viscosity should be expected to lead to vasoconstriction.

The factor g_0 represents vessel wall metabolism which is directly affected by the composition of blood and flow velocity. Furthermore g_0 has a basal value representative of the baseline activity necessary for the living processes of the tissue in the microvessel wall and alteration of this activity, such as by an inflammatory process or increased tone, leads to an increase in tissue metabolism and therefore lowering of tissue oxygenation (since the increase in K_n lowers capillary pO_2).

74.5   Blood Substitutes and Hemodilution

In general, it is possible to survive very low hematocrits, corresponding to losses of the red blood cell mass of the order of 70%; however, our ability to compensate for comparatively smaller losses of blood volume is limited. A 30% deficit in blood volume can lead to irreversible shock if not rapidly corrected.

Maintenance of normovolemia is the objective of most forms of blood substitution or replacement, leading to the dilution of the original blood constituents. This **hemodilution** produces systemic and microvascular phenomena that underlie all forms of blood replacement and provides a physiological reference for comparison for blood substitutes. The fluids available to accomplish volume restitution can be broadly classified as crystalloid solutions, colloidal solutions, and oxygen carrying solutions. All of these materials significantly change the transport properties of blood, and therefore it is important to determine how these changes affect tissue oxygenation, a phenomenon that takes place in the microvasculature. Therefore, hemodilution must be analyzed in terms of systemic effects and how these, coupled with the altered composition of blood, influence the transport properties of the microcirculation.

74.6   Hematocrit and Blood Viscosity

Blood viscosity is primarily determined by the hematocrit in the larger vessels while it is a weaker function of the systemic hematocrit in the microcirculation. At a given shear rate, blood viscosity is approximately proportional to the hematocrit squared according to the relationship:

$$\mu = a_s + b_s H^2 \tag{74.2}$$

while microvascular blood viscosity can be empirically described by a relation of the form:

$$\mu = a_m + b_m H \tag{74.3}$$

where μ is the blood viscosity in centipoise and a_i and the b_i are parameters that are shear rate and vessel size dependent [Dintenfass, 1979; Quemada, 1978]. In the microcirculation, blood viscosity is relatively insensitive to shear rate. These relationships show that when hematocrit is reduced, systemic viscous pressure losses decrease much more rapidly than those in the microvasculature, while in the microcirculation the A–V pressure drop is not very much affected. The net result is that if arterial pressure remains constant, hemodilution produces a significant pressure redistribution in the circulation [Mirhashemi et al., 1987].

Hemodilution increases central venous pressure, which improves cardiac performance and increases cardiac output [Richardson and Guyton, 1959]. This effect causes increased blood flow velocity and therefore the maintenance of oxygen delivery capacity, since a lesser number of red blood cells arrive at a greater frequency. As a consequence of hemodilution, both systemic and capillary oxygen carrying capacities improve up to hematocrit 33% and are at the normal value at arterial hematocrits of the order of 27%. The maximum improvement in oxygen carrying capacity is about 10%.

This behavior of the heart and the circulation as determined by the viscosity of the circulating blood has been subjected to exhaustive experimental and clinical verification. The consequence of the adaptability of the circulation to changes in blood viscosity is that, in general, oxygen delivery capacity is not compromised up to red blood cell losses of about 50%. This fact determines the **transfusion trigger**, currently set at about 7 g Hb/dl. It should be noted that up to the transfusion trigger blood losses can be corrected with the use of a molecular plasma expander. Furthermore, if artificial blood is based on a molecular oxygen carrying material, its introduction in the circulation once the transfusion trigger is passed should be analyzed also as a phenomenon of extreme hemodilution. Conversely, introduction of an oxygen carrying plasma expander prior to reaching the transfusion trigger should show no improvement on oxygenation, since this point is the limit for compensatory adjustments in the circulation.

74.7 Regulation of Capillary Perfusion During Extreme Hemodilution in Hamster Skinfold Microcirculation by High Viscosity Plasma Expander

Although capillaries do not appear to be the determinant structure for the supply of oxygen, our studies [Kerger et al., 1996] have shown that maintenance of functional capillary density (FCD, defined as the number of capillaries that possess red blood cell transit in a mass of tissue) in shock is a critical parameter in determining the outcome in terms of survival vs. nonsurvival, independent of tissue pO_2, suggesting that extraction of products of metabolism may be a more critical function of capillaries than oxygenation (Figure 74.3).

When hemodilution is carried to extreme conditions, defined as the replacement of more than 80% of the red blood cell mass, blood viscosity falls to near plasma levels. A concomitant effect is the reduction of FCD to near pathological levels. The decrease in FCD observed in blood substitutions with plasma expanders is in part due to the lowered viscosity of the resulting blood in circulation. This has been demonstrated with conventional plasma expanders such as dextran 70 kDa, where reductions of systemic hematocrit were to 75% of control and final plasma viscosities of 1.38 cP lowered FCD to 53% of control, while hemodilution with a combination of dextrans of different molecular weights yielding a final **plasma viscosity** of 2.19 cP maintained FCD to near normal levels. In these experiments, vessel wall shear stress was not changed after low viscosity hemodilution while it increased by a factor of 1.3 in arterioles and 2.0 in venules relative to baseline with high viscosity [Tsai et al., 1998] exchanges. Therefore increased shear stress dependant release of endothelium derived relaxing factors are a possible mechanism that reverses the constrictor effects and decreased FCD due to low blood viscosity.

74.8 Crystalloid and Colloidal Solutions as Volume Expanders

Crystalloids are among the most widely used fluids for volume replacement. Ringer's lactate, for example, is administered in volumes that are as much as three times the blood loss, since the dilution of plasma proteins lowers the plasma **oncotic** pressure causing an imbalance of the fluid exchange favoring microvascular fluid extravasation and edema. The advantage of crystalloid solutions is that large volumes can be given over a short period of time with low danger of increasing pulmonary wedge pressure. Excess volumes are rapidly cleared from the circulation by diuresis, which in many instances is a beneficial side effect in the treatment of trauma. Blood volume replacement with Ringer's lactate lowers blood viscosity.

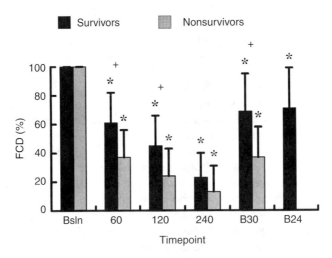

FIGURE 74.3 Changes of FCD in the hamster skinfold model during shock and resuscitation. FCD is the number of capillaries with red blood cell transit in a microscopic field of view. Hamsters were subjected to 4 h hemorrhagic shock to 40 mmHg and resuscitated with their own blood. FCD was the principal microvascular parameter that was the predictor of outcome, while microvascular and tissue pO_2 was the same for survivors and nonsurvivors. This result indicates that resuscitation solutions should ensure the restoration of FCD as well as reestablish tissue oxygenation [Kerger et al., 1996]. Bsln: Baseline. Timepoint: Time after induction of hemorrhage. B30: 30 min after resuscitation. B24: 24 h after resuscitation. *: Significantly different from control, $p > .05$. +: Significantly different between survivors and nonsurvivors, $p > .05$.

The rapid clearance of crystalloid solutions from the intravascular compartment is at the expense of the expansion of the tissue compartment and edema. Peripheral edema has been speculated to impair oxygen delivery, wound healing, and the resistance to infection. Microvascular flow may be impaired by capillary compression from edema. However, given the wide clinical experience with the use of crystalloids, it appears that these are not major effects. A more important effect is the development of pulmonary edema, or adult respiratory distress syndrome (ARDS); however, the relationship between the use of large volumes of salt solutions and ARDS is not firm.

Larger colloidal molecular weight materials such as albumin have the advantage of longer retention time, they do not extravasate and therefore do not cause edema. Albumin is used as a plasma expander for emergency volume restitution, but due to cost considerations the synthetic colloids dextran and hydroxyethyl starch are used more frequently. These materials are free of viral contaminations, but may cause anaphylactic reactions and have a tendency to alter platelet function thus interfering with hemostasis. It is not well established whether these materials increase bleeding per se or the effect is due to improved perfusion.

The beneficial effect of this form of volume replacement resides in the high oncotic pressure which they generate, maintaining intravascular volume in the amount of about 20 ml of fluid per gram of circulating colloid. In this context, dextran 70 kDa and hydroxyethyl starch have the highest retention capacity, 22 and 17 ml/g, respectively, while albumin is 15 ml/g. Furthermore, this form of volume replacement lowers blood viscosity with all the associated positive transport effects described for hemodilution [Messmer et al., 1972].

74.9 Artificial Oxygen Carriers

The amount of oxygen carried in simple aqueous solutions is inconsequential in the overall oxygen requirements of the tissue, and therefore when intrinsic oxygen carrying capacity has to be restored, it is necessary to include an oxygen carrier. This can be presently accomplished through the use of modified hemoglobins which bind oxygen chemically and reversibly, and fluorocarbons which have a high capacity for dissolving oxygen. These compounds present important differences which will ultimately determine in what form of blood substitution and replacement they will be used.

Hemoglobin separated from the red cell membrane, that is, **stroma-free hemoglobin**, carries oxygen with a high affinity. These materials have intrinsically high oxygen carrying capacity; however, they are based on a biologically active molecule, which in most instances requires specialized storage procedures. By contrast, fluorocarbons carry a limited amount of oxygen under normal atmospheric conditions, but are biologically inert, can be stored at room temperature, and are excreted as gas through the lungs.

74.10   Fluorocarbons

Fluorocarbons (perfluorochemicals, PFCs) are compounds that have a very high solubility of oxygen and their oxygen transport capacity is directly proportional to their concentration and pO_2. They are formulated in stable water soluble emulsions that are metabolically inert. These PFC emulsions consist in droplets of fluorochemicals in the range of 0.1 to 0.2 μm diameter coated by a thin film of egg yolk phospholipids. These products are heat sterilized and can be stored under ambient conditions ready for use. The technology for large scale manufacture is well established and the necessary materials for production are well characterized and commercially available. Their half life in the circulation is in the range of 6 to 9 h.

Pure PFCs have oxygen solubilities of the order of 50 ml O_2/100 ml at 37°C and 760 mmHg oxygen pressure. The solubility varies linearly as a function of gas pressure. These materials carry about 30% more oxygen than blood when diluted to 60% (the recommended clinical form of administration) and with 100% inspired oxygen. They have been given clinically at a maximal dosage of 2 g PFC/kg (vs. 15 g hemoglobin/kg for normal blood in humans) [Lamy et al., 1998]. At this dosage, in an isovolemic exchange they increase intrinsic oxygen carrying capacity of blood by about 20%, provided that 100% oxygen is inspired. Since normal tissues and the microcirculation operate in the range of 20 to 50 mmHg, the effect of this fundamentally altered blood pO_2 and oxygen content on the normal distribution of oxygen tension in the circulation is not known. However, since tissues regulate their blood oxygen supply and pO_2, it is unlikely that microvascular blood pO_2 would be much greater than 50 mmHg without eliciting autoregulatory adjustments; therefore, in the absence of hypertensive effects it may be assumed that microvascular blood pO_2 in the presence of PFCs does not exceed 50 mmHg and therefore in terms of tissue oxygen delivery the contribution is small relative to hemoglobin since at pO_2 50 mmHg they carry about 2 ml O_2/dl, while hemoglobin carries 15 ml O_2/dl.

The viscosity of PFCs is only slightly higher than water; therefore, when used in the amounts described they behave as low viscosity plasma expanders, and therefore should exhibit some of the beneficial effects to be derived from moderate hemodilution.

74.11   Hemoglobin for Oxygen Carrying Plasma Expanders

The hemoglobin molecule in solution presents unique characteristics as an oxygen carrying plasma expander, since it has a molecular weight similar to that of albumin and therefore comparable intravascular retention. Its ability to chemically bind oxygen determines that large amounts of oxygen can be associated chemically at relatively low pO_2, and its molecular weight is such that it does not extravasate. Consequently, it should provide an extended period of colloid osmotic effects that prevent the passage of water into the interstitium and therefore edema. However, when hemoglobin is diluted from the concentration present in red blood cells, the tetrameric molecule tends to spontaneously dissociate into smaller molecular weight dimers and monomers which rapidly extravasates from the vascular compartment. Until recently it was assumed that when hemoglobin is free in the circulation it has an oxygen affinity that is too high for tissue oxygenation. As a consequence, strategies for the modification of hemoglobin by chemical means at present are aimed at prolonging intravascular retention and reducing oxygen affinity [Winslow, 1997].

Hemoglobin can be prevented from dissociating by chemically crosslinking the tetramers such as the widely used agent glutaraldehyde. Direct crosslinking with this agent produces a spectrum of different high molecular weight hemoglobin derivatives since glutaraldehyde is nonspecific and reacts with any amino group. A more homogenous product can be obtained by reacting human hemoglobin first with the 2,3-DPG analog PLP, which reduces oxygen affinity and then polymerizing the compound with glutaraldehyde. This product is called PLP-polyHB and has near normal oxygen carrying capacity and a plasma half-time retention (in rats) of about 20 h.

Diaspirins are another group of crosslinking agents. The reaction of native hemoglobin with *bis*(3,5-dibromosalicy)fumarate (DBBF) leads to the linking of the two a chains of the hemoglobin molecule, producing a compound called aaHb which has an oxygen affinity (P50) of 30 mm Hg and an intravascular retention time of the order of 12 h in rats. Phosphorylated compounds added to purified hemoglobin also change the P50 value of the resulting compound and have been studied extensively. There is an increasing variety of hemoglobin compounds that is being developed; however, at this time aaHb is the most widely studied compound since it was produced in quantity by the U.S. Army Letterman Institute, San Francisco, and a similar compound was developed and used in extensive clinical trials by Baxter Healthcare Inc.

Hemoglobin can be produced as a recombinant protein leading to the construction of either the naturally occurring molecule or variants that have different crosslinking and oxygen affinity. It is presently possible to produce both alpha and beta chains of human hemoglobin in bacteria, yeast, and transgenic animals. While it is in principle possible to produce large amounts of a specific product by these means, there remain problems of purification, elimination of other bacterial products, and endotoxins that may be expressed in parallel.

Human hemoglobin genes have been induced into transgenic mammals, leading to the potential production of large amounts of human hemoglobin. However, the production is not 100% pure and some of the original animal material is also present, causing an important purification problem. This problem may be compounded by potential immunogenicity of animal hemoglobin and the potential transmission of animal diseases to humans.

A unique form of hemoglobin modification is the process of pegylation, consisting of attaching polyethylene glycol polymeric strands to the surface of the hemoglobin molecule. The resulting product termed PEG–hemoglobin interacts with the surrounding water, producing an aqueous barrier that surrounds the molecule. This phenomenon causes several beneficial effects, namely (1) renders the molecule invisible to the immune system; (2) draws water into the circulation increasing blood volume; (3) increases molecular size of the molecule, thus further limiting its capacity to extravasate; (4) decreases the diffusive oxygen delivery from HbO_2 by increasing path length; and (5) increases plasma viscosity. This type of molecule is presently manufactured by Sangart, Inc., La Jolla, and Apex Bioscience Inc., North Carolina, who uses human hemoglobin and Enzon Inc., New Jersey, who uses bovine hemoglobin.

74.12   Hemoglobin-Based Artificial Blood

Many hemoglobin-based artificial blood substitutes are being developed which may be classified relative to the technology used and whether the hemoglobin is either of human, animal, or bacterial origin. It is now established that hemoglobin containing red blood cell substitutes deliver oxygen to the tissue and maintain tissue function. However, problems of toxicity and efficacy are not yet resolved, and are shared by many of the hemoglobin solutions presently available. Renal toxicity is one of the primary problems because hemoglobin toxicity to the kidney is a classic model for kidney failure. The mechanism of toxicity includes tubular obstruction, renal arterial vasospasm, and direct toxicity to tubular cells. It is not clear whether hemoglobin must be filtered by the kidney to be toxic, and the tolerance of the kidney to different types of hemoglobins and concentrations is not established [Paller, 1988].

There are many reports of anaphylaxis/anaphylactoid reactions to hemoglobin infusion. This may result from heme release from hemoglobin, the presence of endotoxins bound to hemoglobin or preexisting in the circulation, or from oxygen-derived free radicals released after exposure to hemoglobin. Vasoconstriction of coronary, cerebral, and renal vessels has also been attributed to the presence of free hemoglobin in the circulation, a phenomenon that may be due to the intrinsic capacity of hemoglobin to scavenge nitric oxide or metabolic autoregulation.

Toxicity of hemoglobin may be due to special characteristics of the manufacturing procedure, the given molecule, or problems due to purification. It may also be inherent to the presence of large quantities of a molecular species for which the circulation has a very limited tolerance when present in solution. This problem may be circumvented by separating hemoglobin from the circulation by encapsulating this material in a synthetic membrane, in the same way that the red cell membrane encapsulates hemoglobin.

Encapsulation of hemoglobin has been accomplished by introducing the molecule into a **liposome**. To the present this technology presents several problems, namely (1) poor efficiency of hemoglobin incorporation into the liposome; (2) physical instability of liposomes in storage; and (3) chemical instability of the lipid–hemoglobin interface leading to lipid peroxidation and hemoglobin denaturation. These factors translate in decreased oxygen carrying capacity, increased viscosity of the circulating blood/liposome mixture, and reticuloendothelial blockade. This situation notwithstanding, lipid encapsulation may ultimately provide the artificial blood of choice once a quality hemoglobin becomes consistently available and liposome production can be scaled up to quantities commensurate with demand.

74.13 Results in the Microcirculation with Blood Substitution with aa-Hemoglobin

The effectiveness of aa-Hb (cell-free o-raffinose cross-linked) as a blood carrying plasma expander was tested in the microcirculation by implementing isovolemic hemodilution up to an exchange of 75% of the original cell mass. Exchanges with dextran 70 kDa molecular weight were used as control. Experiments were carried out in the microcirculation of the hamster window preparation, which was evaluated in terms of hemodynamic parameters and oxygen distribution at three successive levels of exchange. The oxygen delivery capacity of the microcirculation was determined in terms of the rate of arrival of hemoglobin (in red blood cells + molecular) to the capillaries. It was found that using molecular solutions of about 10 g/dl concentration, the oxygen delivery capacity of the microcirculation was identical to that of dextran 70 for substitutions up to 60% of the red blood cell mass. This was a consequence of the lack of increased cardiac output with the Hb solutions, which should be expected when viscosity is lowered, as is the case with colloidal solutions (starch and dextran).

This hemoglobin caused hypertension, and at the highest level of exchange exhibited abnormally low tissue pO_2, which fell from a normal value of 22.4 mmHg to about 5 mmHg. This lowered tissue pO_2 was accompanied by a significant decrease in functional capillary density, and increased vessel wall gradients. Consequently, this hemoglobin does not appear to function as a tissue oxygenator in the microcirculation, although the total amount of hemoglobin and its capacity to transport oxygen is similar to that of natural blood. The principal reasons for this outcome are hypertension elicited by lowered blood viscosity with consequent decrease of production of NO, increased scavenging of NO, and increased availability of oxygen to the vessel wall, which promotes autoregulatory responses aimed at limiting over oxygenation of the vessel wall. The linkage between blood supply and oxygen demand is due to the existence of chemical vasodilator signals transmitted from the tissue cells to the resistance vessels, which relax (increase their diameter) causing blood flow to increase when tissue oxygen tension falls below critical levels. Conversely, increasing blood oxygen tension over normal levels elicits vasoconstriction.

The most critical side effect in terms of microvascular function is the finding that molecular hemoglobin solutions significantly lower functional capillary density.

74.14 Hemoglobin and Nitric Oxide (NO) Binding

The principal adverse effect of hemoglobin in solution is to produce vasoconstriction. This is based on two fundamental observations (1) Hb has a very high affinity to bind NO at heme sites, and (2) Hb has been shown to produce constriction of isolated aortic rings. However, there is no direct proof that these mechanisms exists because NO has a very short half-life in the circulation (1.8 msec) [Liu et al., 1998], making its detection difficult. Further complicating the story is the observation that NO can also bind to hemoglobin at its sulfhydryl residues [Stamler et al., 1997], and that this mechanism might be oxygen-linked. It should also be noted that NO binding as a cause for vasoconstriction has been primarily deduced from studies that have shown constriction of isolated aortic rings when exposed to hemoglobin solutions. However, *in vivo* the situation is more complicated, particularly because most of the important diameter reductions occur in specific microvessels. Alternative explanations are that this effect can be produced directly on the blood side of the endothelium, where the presence of molecular hemoglobin in the red cell free plasma layer could significantly distort the diffusion field from the endothelial cell, diverting NO from smooth muscle into blood. Another effect could arise if the protein leaves the vascular space and enters the interstitium, there to interfere with the diffusion of NO from endothelium to its target, vascular smooth muscle. Thus, Rohlfs et al. [1997] found that hemoglobins with differing effects on mean arterial blood pressure all had similar reaction kinetics with NO. These findings are consistent with the autoregulation hypothesis, and suggest that there is more to the story than NO scavenging.

A different explanation is that altered blood properties in extreme hemodilution affect the production of NO and prostacyclin (and other cytokines) in endothelial cells, which is dependent on the maintenance of some level of shear stress. Such shear stress, in a flowing system such as blood, is dependent on a number of factors, including the viscosity of the solution. Thus, it would be expected that hemoglobin solutions with low viscosity, such as aa-Hb, would decrease NO synthesis and induce vasospasm. In fact, vasoconstriction is probably a natural reaction of the organism to reduced blood viscosity.

The difficulties associated with the measurement of NO directly in biological systems has led to the formulation of theoretical models. This type of analysis shows that NO distribution between blood and smooth muscle is the consequence of its high diffusivity, the fact that its half-life is limited by its reaction with oxygen and hemoglobin, its diffusion into red cells, and the geometry of vessels in the microcirculation. A tentative conclusion, in part supported by direct studies in the microcirculation, indicates that effects should be maximal in arterioles of the order of 30 to 100 μm in diameter.

Thus far, the NO physiology has not been completely translated into the design of blood substitutes [Winslow, 1998]. The group at Somatogen have designed a series of hemoglobin mutants with a range of NO affinity and shown that there is a correlation between NO binding and the blood pressure response in rats [Doherty et al., 1998]. However, Rohlfs et al. [1998] have shown that a different series of chemically modified hemoglobins with different vasoactivities have essentially the same NO reactivity.

74.15   Rational Design of an Oxygen Carrying Molecular Plasma Expander

The products presently in clinical trials reflect the physiological know-how of the 1970s, when their effects could not be analyzed at the level of microscopic blood vessels, blood flow regulation by NO was unknown, the theory of microvascular autoregulation had just been formulated, and the endothelium was viewed as a passive cellular lining which prevented the extravasation of plasma proteins. At that time, systemic experimental findings and the clinical experience with low viscosity plasma expanders used in hemodilution established that lowering blood viscosity was a safe and efficacious method for restoring blood volume, particularly if oncotic pressure was maintained within the physiological range through the use of colloids. These well-established tenets were incorporated into the design of artificial blood, or blood substitute, which was conceived as a fluid of low viscosity (i.e., lower than blood and closer to plasma in order to obtain the beneficial effects of hemodilution), moderate oncotic pressure (i.e., of the order of 25 mmHg), a right-shifted oxygen dissociation curve, and a concentration of hemoglobin, or equivalent oxygen carrying capacity, of 10 g Hb/dl.

This scenario was firmly established because there were no practical methods for assessing tissue pO_2 clinically, other than direct measurement of venous blood pO_2, while in experimental conditions tissue pO_2 could only be determined by extremely laborious and difficult to implement microelectrode methods.

Thus, the distribution of oxygen in the tissue, even at the experimental level, was not known and related fundamental mechanisms directly involved with survival at the level of the microcirculation were equally unknown or misunderstood.

High resolution methods for measuring tissue pO_2 became available at the beginning of the 1990s, and when these were applied to the analysis of the effects of hemoglobin-based blood substitutes, they reversed several of the established principles. It was found that oxygen is delivered by the arterioles and not the capillaries, and that this rate of delivery was modulated by the consumption of oxygen in the arteriolar wall. Vasoconstrictor effects were found to increase the oxygen consumption of the arterioles to the detriment of tissue oxygenation. This was particularly true for hemoglobin solutions formulated with small molecules, such as the aa-crosslinked hemoglobin, which also presented another of the presumed required properties, namely low viscosity.

To the present, the vasoconstrictor effect has been attributed to NO scavenging by hemoglobin; however, other mechanisms may be involved and superimposed on the scavenging effect. The molecular nature of the presently developed hemoglobin solutions determines that the oxygen source in blood is very close to the endothelium, since the barrier determined by the plasma layer is no longer present. This configuration increases the oxygen availability to the microvascular wall, potentially eliciting autoregulatory vasoconstriction aimed at regulating oxygen delivery. It is now apparent that right-shifted materials further increase oxygen availability, thus enhancing the vasoconstrictor stimulus.

Concerning NO scavenging, it may well be that this shall remain an intrinsic property of the hemoglobin molecule dictated by the physical similarity of NO and O_2. In this context, two solutions to the problem may be implemented directly at the level of the oxygen carrier: One consists of producing an elevated (relative to normal) plasma viscosity, in such a fashion that shear stress dependant NO production remains constant or is elevated. Second, physically separating the hemoglobin molecule from the endothelial barrier as may be obtained with a pegylated material may retard hemoglobin–NO interaction.

There is increasing evidence that low viscosity is of no benefit once the transfusion trigger is passed, particularly if combined with vasoconstrictor effects that impede the increase of cardiac output. In fact, conditions of extreme hemodilution, as those that obtain purely on the basis of viscosity considerations when the red blood cell mass is reduced, can only survive when plasma viscosity is increased, so that blood viscosity is near normal, which has the effect of maintaining functional capillary density at basal levels. This beneficial effect is further augmented by added production of shear stress dependant NO, which induces vasodilation and adequate blood flow. The physiological consequences of introducing molecular solutions of hemoglobin in the circulation can be seen in full perspective when the products are ranked according to size (Figure 74.4), where it becomes apparent that side effects such as hypertension and retention time are a direct result of molecular dimensions, which in turn determine viscosity and diffusivity.

In these conditions, tissue oxygenation is enhanced by the use of a left-shifted hemoglobin which effectively "hides" oxygen from the arterioles and facilitates its unloading in the regions of the microcirculation where oxygen consumption by the vessel wall is smaller.

Finally, a critical issue is how much hemoglobin is necessary to obtain the desired effects. Experimental evidence presently indicates that when the "counter-intuitive" formulation of product is implemented, the actual amount of hemoglobin needed may be as low as 3 g Hb/dl [Winslow et al., 1998]. This consideration impacts on the cost of the product and the potential for production, since most hemoglobin modifications have at most a 50% yield. This is critical for products based on human blood, where the principal source is outdated material, which would impose an inherent limitation on the total production capacity if the product is formulated with 7 to 10 g Hb/dl concentration.

74.16 Conclusions

Lethality consequent to blood losses results from hypovolemia and not anemia, and a number of plasma expanders exist that restitute volume and ensure survival even though they carry oxygen only to the extent of its plasma solubility. This is a consequence of the "derived" increase of oxygen carrying capacity resulting

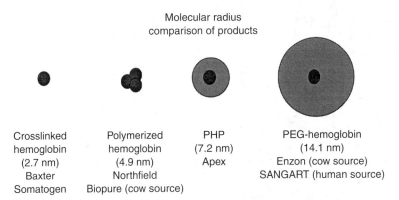

FIGURE 74.4 The physiological reaction to the presence of even small amounts of circulating hemoglobin can be predicted by grouping the products according to molecular dimension. Systemic blood pressure rise is maximal for the smallest molecules and virtually absent for the largest molecules. The effect on blood viscosity correlates with both the rise of blood pressure and the maintenance of functional capillary density, where small molecules, which lower blood viscosity, also significantly lower FCD, while the larger molecules, causing blood viscosity to remain similar to that of whole blood, have no effect on FCD. Intravascular retention time is also directly proportional to molecular size, varying from about 12 h for the smaller molecules to more than 48 h for PEG-hemoglobin. Products are identified according to their manufacturer, namely: Baxter Healthcare, Round Lake, IL; Somatogen, Inc., Boulder, CO; Northfield Laboratories Inc., Chicago, IL; Hemosol Ltd., Toronto, Canada; Biopure Pharmaceuticals Corp., Boston, MA; Apex Bioscience Inc., Research Triangle Park, NC; Enzon Inc., Piscataway, NJ; SANGART Inc., La Jolla, CA. [Data from Vandegriff et al., 1997.]

from lowered viscosity and increased cardiac output. This approach serves as hemoglobin concentration reaches the transfusion trigger, beyond which restoration of oxygen carrying capacity is needed.

The use of oxygen carrying plasma expanders made with molecular solutions of hemoglobin, when the red blood cell mass is reduced below the transfusion trigger, causes extreme hemodilution associated with a significant reduction of blood viscosity and NO production, and reflex vasoconstriction, leading to decreased functional capillary density. This combination of events is difficult to survive because decreased NO availability increases the intrinsic oxygen consumption of the tissue. An oxygen carrying volume replacement with a capacity commensurate to blood is presently the perceived sine qua necessity for extreme blood losses. However, new findings indicate that this may not necessarily be the case.

Recent developments in the understanding of the physiology of extreme hemodilution, and the physical events associated with the substitution of red blood cells with molecular hemoglobin solutions have determined a shift in paradigm, indicating that a viable "artificial blood" will be obtained from a counterintuitive formulation of the product. In this formulation, viscosity is near normal for blood, the dissociation curve is left-shifted, oncotic pressure is high, and the concentration of hemoglobin is in the range of 3 to 5 g Hb/dl [Winslow and Intaglietta, 1998].

Defining Terms

Hemodilution: The replacement of natural blood with a compatible fluid that reduces the concentration of red blood cells

Stroma-free hemoglobin: Hemoglobin derived from red blood cells where all materials related to cell membrane and other components within the red blood cells have been removed.

Liposome: Microscopic phospholipid vesicle used to encapsulate materials for slow release. The use of liposomes to encapsulate hemoglobin is a departure from the conventional use of liposomes, exploiting encapsulation, and requires their modification to ensure sustained entrapment.

Oncotic: Refers to colligative properties due to the presence of macromolecules, for instance oncotic pressure, which is differentiated from osmotic pressure, which is that due to the presence of all molecular species in solution.

Oxygen carrying capacity: The total amount of oxygen that may be transported by blood or the fluid in the circulation. Differentiated from oxygen delivery capacity which involves considerations of flow rate.

Plasma viscosity: Viscosity of blood devoid of cellular elements, a parameter that is critically impacted by the introduction of molecular hemoglobin solutions.

Shear stress: Force per unit area parallel to the vessel wall or traction, experienced by the endothelium due to blood flow and blood viscosity.

Transfusion trigger: Concentration of blood hemoglobin beyond which blood is required to restore circulatory function.

Acknowledgment

This work was supported in part by USPHS Grant HLBI 48018.

References

Dintenfass, L. *Blood Microrheology: Viscosity Factors in Blood Flow, Ischemia and Thrombosis*. Appleton-Century-Crofts, New York, 1971.

Doherty, D.H., Doyle, M.P., Curry, S.R., Vali, R.J., Fattor, T.J., Olson, J.S., and Lemon, D.D. Rate of reaction with nitric oxide determines the hypertensive effect of cell-free hemoglobin. *Nat. Biotechnol.* 16: 672, 1998.

Frangos, J.A., Eskin, S.G., McIntire, L.V., and Ives, C.L. Flow effects on prostacyclin production in cultured human endothelial cells. *Science* 227: 1477, 1985.

Intaglietta, M., Johnson, P.C., and Winslow, R.M. Microvascular and tissue oxygen distribution. *Cardiovasc. Res.* 32: 632, 1996.

Intaglietta, M. Whitaker lecture 1996: microcirculation, biomedical engineering and artificial blood. *Ann. Biomed. Eng.* 25: 593, 1997.

Johnson, P.C. Brief review: autoregulation of blood flow. *Circ. Res.* 59: 483, 1996.

Joyner, W.L., Davis, M.J., and Gilmore, J.P. Intravascular pressure distribution and dimensional analysis of microvessels in the hamsters with renovascular hypertension. *Microvasc. Res.* 22: 1, 1974.

Kerger, H., Saltzman, D.J., Menger, M.D., Messmer, K., and Intaglietta, M. Systemic and subcutaneous microvascular pO_2 dissociation during 4-h hemorrhagic shock in conscious hamsters. *Am. J. Physiol.* 270: H827, 1996.

Kjellstrom, B.T., Ortenwall, P., and Risberg, R. Comparison of oxidative metabolism *in vitro* in endothelial cells from different species and vessels. *J. Cell. Physiol.* 132: 578, 1987.

Kuchan, M.J., Jo, H., and Frangos, J.A. Role of G proteins in shear stress-mediated nitric oxide production by endothelial cells. *Am. J. Physiol.* 267: C753, 1994.

Lamy, M., Mathy-Hartert, M., and Deby-Dupont, G. Perfluorocarbons as oxygen carriers. In *Update in Intensive Care Medicine*, Vol. 33, J.-L. Vincent, Ed., Springer-Verlag, Berlin, 1998, p. 332.

Lipowsky, H.H. Mechanics of blood flow in the microcirculation. In *Handbook of Bioengineering*, R. Skalak and S. Chien, Eds., McGraw-Hill, New York, 1987, Chap. 8.

Liu, X., Miller, M.J., Joshi, M.S., Sadowska-Krowicka, H., Clark, D.A., and Lancaster, J.R.J. Diffusion-limited reaction of free nitric oxide with erythrocytes. *J. Biol. Chem.* 273: 18709, 1998.

Messmer, K., Sunder-Plasman, L., Klövekorn, W.P., and Holper, K. Circulatory significance of hemodilution: rheological changes and limitations. *Adv. Microcirc.*, 4: 1, 1972.

Mirhashemi, S., Messmer, K., and Intaglietta, M. Tissue perfusion during normovolemic hemodilution investigated by a hydraulic model of the cardiovascular system. *Int. J. Microcirc.: Clin. Exp.* 6: 123, 1987.

Paller, M.S. Hemoglobin and myoglobin-induced acute renal failure: Role of iron nephrotoxicity. *Am. J. Physiol.* 255: F539, 1988.

Quemada, D. Rheology of concentrated dispersed systems: III. General features of the proposed non-Newtonian model: comparison with experimental data. *Rheol. Acta* 17: 643, 1978.

Richardson, T.Q. and Guyton, A.C. Effects of polycythemia and anemia on cardiac output and other circulatory factors. *Am. J. Physiol.* 197: 1167, 1959.

Rohlfs, R., Vandegriff, K., and Winslow, R. The reaction of nitric oxide with cell-free hemoglobin based oxygen carriers: physiological implications. In *Industrial Opportunities and Medical Challenges*, R.M. Winslow, K.D. Vandegriff, and M. Intaglietta, Eds., Birkhäuser, Boston, 1997, p. 298.

Rohlfs, R.J., Bruner, E., Chiu, A., Gonzales, A., Gonzales, M.L., Magde, D., Magde, M.DJ., Vandegriff, K.D., and Winslow, R.M. Arterial blood pressure responses to cell-free hemoglobin solutions and the reaction with nitric oxide. *J. Biol. Chem.* 273: 12128, 1998.

Saltzman, D., DeLano, F.A., and Schmid-Schönbein, G.W. The microvasculature in skeletal muscle. VI. Adrenergic innervation of arterioles in normotensive and spontaneously hypertensive rats. *Microvasc. Res.* 44: 263, 1992.

Shen, W., Hintze, T.H., and Wolin, M.S. Nitric oxide: an important signaling mechanism between vascular endothelium and parenchymal cells in the regulation of oxygen consumption. *Circulation* 92: 3505, 1995.

Stamler, J.S., Jia, L., Eu, J.P., McMahon, T.J., Demchenko, I.T., Bonaventura, J., Gernert, K., and Piantadosi, C.A. Blood flow regulation by S-nitrosohemoglobin in the physiological oxygen gradient. *Science* 276: 2034, 1997.

Torres Filho, I.P. and Intaglietta, M. Micro vessel pO_2 measurements by phosphorescence decay method. *Am. J. Physiol.* 265: H1434, 1994.

Tsai, A.G., Friesenecker, B., Mazzoni, M.C., Kerger, H., Buerk, D.G., Johnson, P.C., and Intaglietta, M. Microvascular and tissue oxygen gradients in the rat mesentery. *Proc. Natl Acad. Sci. USA* 95: 6590, 1998.

Tsai, A.G., Friesenecker, B., McCarthy, M., Sakai, H., and Intaglietta, M. Plasma viscosity regulates capillary perfusion during extreme hemodilution in hamster skin fold mode. *Am. J. Physiol.*, 275: H2170, 1998.

Vandegriff, K.D., Rohlfs, R.J., and Winslow, R.M. Colloid osmotic effects of hemoglobin-based oxygen carriers. In *Advances in Blood Substitutes. Industrial Opportunities and Medical Challenges*, R.M. Winslow, K.D. Vandegriff, and M. Intaglietta, Eds., Birkhäuser, Boston, MA, 1997.

Wilson, D.F. Measuring oxygen using oxygen dependent quenching of phosphorescence: a status report. *Adv. Exp. Med. Biol.* 333: 225, 1993.

Winslow, R.M. Blood substitutes. *Sci. Med.* 4: 54, 1997.

Winslow, R.M. Artificial blood: ancient dream, modern enigma. *Nature Biotechnology.* 16: 621, 1998.

Winslow, R.M. and Intaglietta, M. U.S. Patent 5,814,601. Methods and compositions for optimization of oxygen transport by cell free systems, 1998.

Further Information

Winslow, R.M., Vandegriff, K.D., and Intaglietta, M. Eds., Birkhäuser, Boston, 1995.

Winslow, R.M., Vandegriff, K.D., and Intaglietta, M., Eds., *Blood Substitutes. New Challenges* Birkhäuser, Boston, 1996.

Winslow, R.M., Vandegriff, K.D., and Intaglietta, M., Eds. *Advances in Blood Substitutes. Industrial Opportunities and Medical Challenges* Birkhäuser, Boston, 1997.

75

Artificial Skin and Dermal Equivalents

Ioaniss V. Yannas
*Massachusetts Institute
of Technology*

75.1 The Vital Functions of Skin

Skin is a vital organ, in the sense that loss of a substantial fraction of its mass immediately threatens the life of the individual. Such loss can result suddenly, either from fire or from a mechanical accident. Loss of skin can also occur in a chronic manner, as in skin ulcers. Irrespective of the time scale over which skin loss is incurred, the resulting deficit is considered life threatening primarily for two reasons: Skin is a barrier to loss of water and electrolytes from the body, and it is a barrier to infection from airborne organisms. A substantial deficit in the integrity of skin leaves the individual unprotected either from shock, the result of excessive loss of water and electrolytes, or from sepsis, the result of a massive systemic infection. It has been reported that burns alone account for 2,150,000 procedures every year in the United States. Of these, 150,000 refer to individuals who are hospitalized, and as many as 10,000 die.

Four types of tissue can be distinguished clearly in normal skin. The **epidermis**, outside, is a 0.1-mm-thick sheet, comprising about ten layers of keratinocytes at levels of maturation which increase from the inside out. The **dermis**, inside, is a 2- to 5-mm-thick layer of vascularized and innervated connective tissue with very few cells, mostly quiescent fibroblasts. The dermis is a massive tissue, accounting for

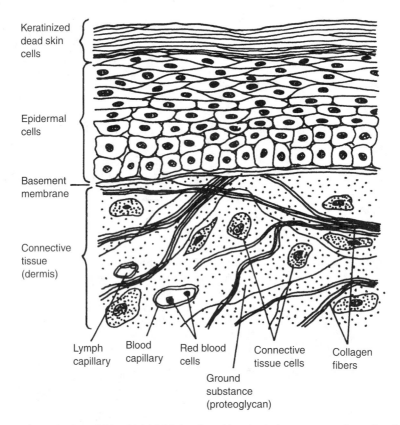

Keratinized dead skin cells

Epidermal cells

Basement membrane

Connective tissue (dermis)

Lymph capillary | Blood capillary | Red blood cells | Connective tissue cells | Collagen fibers

Ground substance (proteoglycan)

FIGURE 75.1   Schematic view of skin which highlights the epidermis, the basement membrane interleaved between the epidermis and the dermis, and the dermis underneath. Only a small fraction of the thickness of the dermis is shown. (Redrawn with permission from J. Darnell, J. Lodish, and D. Baltimore, *Molecular Cell Biology*, Scientific American Books, New York, Chapter 5, Fig. 552, 1986.)

15 to 20% of total body weight. Interleaved between the epidermis and the dermis is the **basement membrane**, an approximately 20-nm-thick multilayered membrane (Figure 75.1). A fourth layer, the **subcutis**, underneath the dermis and 0.4- to 4-mm in thickness, comprises primarily fat tissue. In addition to these basic structural elements, skin contains several appendages (**adnexa**), including hair follicles, sweat glands, and sebaceous glands. The latter are mostly embedded in the dermis, although they are ensheathed in layers of epidermal tissue.

The functions of skin are quite diverse, although it can be argued that the single function of skin is to provide a viable interface with the individual's environment. In addition to the specific vital functions mentioned above (protection from water and electrolyte loss, and from infection), skin also protects from heat and cold, mechanical friction, chemicals, and from UV radiation. Skin is responsible for a substantial part of the thermoregulatory and communication needs of the body, including the transduction of signals from the environment such as touch, pressure, and temperature. Further, skin transmits important emotional signals to the environment, such as paleness or blushing of the face and the emission of scents (pheromones). Far from being a passive membrane that keeps the internal organs in shape, skin is a complex organ.

75.2   Current Treatment of Massive Skin Loss

The treatment of skin loss has traditionally focused on the design of a temporary wound closure. Attempts to cover wounds and servere burns have been reported from historical sources at least as far back as 1500 BC, and a very large number of temporary wound dressings have been designed. These include membranes or sheets fabricated from natural and synthetic polymers, skin grafts from human cadavers (homografts, or **allografts**), and skin grafts from animals (heterografts, or **xenografts**). Although a satisfactory temporary dressing helps to stem the tide, it does not provide a permanent cover. Polymeric membranes which lack specific biologic activity, such as synthetic polymeric hydrogels, have to be removed after several days due to incidence of infection and lack of formation of physiologic structures. Patients with cadaver allografts and xenografts are frequently immunosuppressed to avoid rejection; however, this is a stop-gap operation which is eventually terminated by removal of the graft after several days. In all cases where temporary dressings have been used, the routine result has been an open wound. Temporary dressings are useful in delaying the time at which a permanent graft, such as an **autograft**, is necessary and are therefore invaluable aids in the management of the massively injured patient.

The use of an autograft has clearly shown the advantages of a permanent wound cover. This treatment addresses not only the urgent needs but also the long-term needs of the patient with massive skin loss. The result of treatment of a third-degree burn with a **split-thickness autograft** is an almost fully functional skin which has become incorporated into the patient's body and will remain functional over a lifetime. Autografts usually lack hair follicles and certain adnexa as well. However, the major price paid is the removal of the split thickness graft from an intact area of the patient's body: The remaining dermis eventually becomes epithelialized but not without synthesis of **scar** over the entire area of trauma (**donor site**). To alleviate the problem associated with the limited availability of autograft, surgeons have resorted to meshing, a procedure in which the **sheet autograft** is passed through an apparatus which cuts slits into the sheet autograft, allowing the expansion of the graft by several times and thereby extending greatly the area of use. An inevitable long-term result of use of these **meshed autografts** is scar synthesis in areas coinciding with the open slits of the meshed graft and a resulting pattern of scar which greatly reduces the value of the resulting new organ (Figure 75.2). An important aspect of the use of the autograft is the requirement for early excision of dead tissue and the provision, thereby, of a viable wound bed to "**take**" the autograft.

The term "**artificial skin**" has been used to describe a cell-free membrane comprising a highly porous graft copolymer of type I collagen and chondroitin 6-sulfate which degrades at a specific rate in the wound and regenerates the dermis in dermis-free wounds in animal models and patients (see below: **dermis regeneration template**, DRT). "**Skin equivalent**" (SE) refers to a collagen lattice which has been

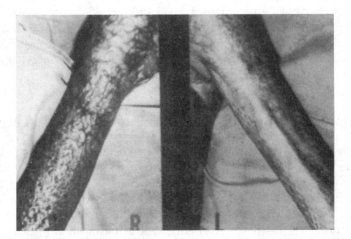

FIGURE 75.2   Comparision between treatment with the meshed autograft (R) and treatment with the artificial skin (L). Autograft is usually meshed before grafting; scar forms in areas coinciding with the open slits of the autograft. The artificial skin treatment consists of grafting the excised wound bed with a skin regeneration template, followed by grafting on about day 14 with a very thin epidermal autograft. (Photo courtesy of J.F. Burke.)

prepared by contraction of a collagen gel by heterologous fibroblasts ("**dermal equivalent**" or DE) and has subsequently been overlayed with a keratinocyte culture to induce formation of a mature, cornified epidermis in vitro prior to grafting of skin wounds. **Cultured epithelial autografts** (CEA) consist of a mature, cornified epidermis which has been produced by culturing keratinocytes in vitro, prior to grafting on skin wounds. The major goal of these treatments has been to replace definitively the use of the autograft in the treatment of patients with massive skin loss.

75.3 Two Conceptual Stages in the Treatment of Massive

75.3.1 Skin Loss by Use of the Artificial Skin

Loss of the epidermis alone can result from a relatively mild burn, such as an early exposure to the sun. Controlled loss of epidermis in a laboratory experiment with an animal can result from the repeated use of adhesive tape to peel off the keratinocyte layers. In either case, the long-term outcome is an apparently faithful regeneration of the epidermis by migration of epithelial cells from the wound edge, and from roots of hair follicles, over the underlying basement membrane and dermis. It has been shown that the epidermis can regenerate spontaneously provided there is a dermal substrate over which epithelial migration and eventual anchoring to the underlying connective tissue can occur.

Loss of the dermis has quite a different outcome. Once lost, the dermis does not regenerate spontaneously. Instead, the wound closes by contraction of the wound edges toward the center of the skin deficit, and by synthesis of scar. Scar is a distinctly different type of connective tissue than is dermis. The depth of skin loss is, therefore, a critical parameter in the design of a treatment for a patient who has a skin deficit. In the treatment of burns, physicians distinguish among a first-degree burn (loss of epidermis alone), a second-degree burn (loss of epidermis and a fraction of the thickness of the dermis), and a third-degree burn (loss of the epidermis and the entire dermis down to muscle tissue). A similar classification, based on depth of loss, is frequently applied to mechanical wounds, such as abrasion. The area of skin which has been destroyed needs also to be specified in order to assess the clinical status of the patient.

A massively injured patient, such as a patient with about 30% body surface area or more destroyed from fire through the full thickness of skin, presents an urgent problem to the clinician, since the open wound is an ongoing threat to survival. A large number of temporary wound coverings have been used to help the patient survive through this period while waiting for availability of autografts which provide permanent cover. If autograft is unavailable over a prolonged period while the patient has survived the severe trauma, contraction and scar synthesis occur over extensive areas. In the long run, the patient therefore has to cope with deep, disfiguring scars or with crippling contractures. Thus, even though the patient has been able to survive the massive trauma and has walked out of the clinic, the permanent loss of skin which has been sustained prevents, in many cases, resumption of an active, normal life.

75.4 Design Principles for a Permanent Skin Replacement

The analysis of the plight of the patient who has suffered extensive skin loss, presented above, leads logically to a wound cover which treats the problem in two stages. Stage 1 is the early phase of the clinical experience, one in which protection against severe fluid loss and against massive infection are defined as the major design objectives. Stage 2 is the ensuing phase, one in which the patient needs protection principally against disfiguring scars and crippling contractures. Even though the conceptual part of the design is separated in two stages for purposes of clarity, the actual treatment is to be delivered continuously, as will be become clear below. The sequential utilization of features inherent in stages 1 and 2 in a single device can be ensured by designing the graft as a bilayer membrane (Figure 75.3). In this approach, the top layer incorporates the features of a stage 1 device, while the bottom layer delivers the performance expected from a stage 2 device. The top layer is subject to disposal after a period of about 10 to 15 days,

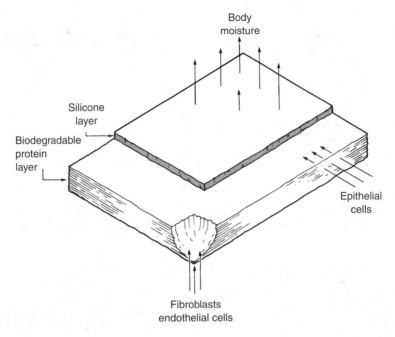

FIGURE 75.3 Schematic of the bilayer membrane which has become known as the artificial skin. The top layer is a silicone film which controls moisture flux through the wound bed to nearly physiologic levels, controls infection of the wound bed by airborne bacteria, and is strong enough to be sutured on the wound bed. The bottom layer is the skin regeneration template, which consists of a graft copolymer of type I collagen and chondroitin 6-sulfate, with critically controlled porosity and degradation rate. About 14 days after grafting, the silicone layer is removed and replaced with a thin epidermal autograft. The bottom layer induces synthesis of a nearly physiologic dermis and eventually is removed completely by biodegradation. (From Yannas IV, Burke J.F., Orgill D.P., et al. 1982. *Science* 215: 74.)

during which time the bottom layer has already induced substantial synthesis of new dermis. Following removal of the top layer, the epidermal cover is provided either by covering with a thin epidermal graft or by modifying the device (cell seeding) so that an epidermis forms spontaneously by about 2 weeks after grafting.

75.4.1 Stage 1 Design Parameters

The overriding design requirement at this stage is based on the observation that air pockets ("dead space") at the graft-wound bed interface readily become sites of bacterial proliferation. Such sites can be prevented from forming if the graft surface wets, in the physicochemical sense, the surface of the wound bed on contact and thereby displaces the air from the graft-tissue interface (Figure 75.4). It follows that the physicochemical properties of the graft must be designed to ensure that this leading requirement is met, not only when the graft is placed on the wound bed but for several days thereafter, until the function of the graft has moved clearly into its stage 2, in which case the graft-wound bed interface has been synthesized *de novo* and the threat of dead space has been thereby eliminated indefinitely.

First, the flexural rigidity of the graft, that is, the product of Young's modulus and moment of inertia of a model elastic beam, must be sufficiently low to provide for a flexible graft which drapes intimately over a geometrically nonuniform wound bed surface and thus ensures that the two surfaces will be closely apposed. In practice, these requirements can be met simply by adjusting both the stiffness in tension and the thickness of the graft to appropriately low values. Second, the graft will wet the wound bed if the surface energy of the graft-wound bed interface is lower than that of the air-wound bed surface, so that

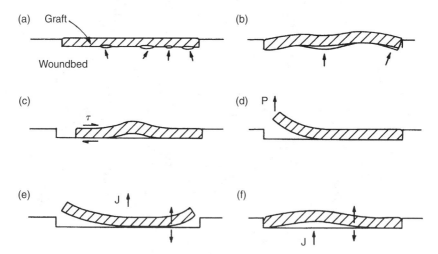

FIGURE 75.4 Certain physicochemical and mechanical requirements in the design of an effective closure for a wound bed with full-thickness skin loss. (a) The graft (cross-hatched) does not displace air pockets (arrows) efficiently from the graft-wound bed interface. (b) Flexural rigidity of the graft is excessive. The graft does not deform sufficiently, under its own weight and the action of surface forces, to make good contact with depressions on the surface of the wound bed; as a result, air pockets form (arrows). (c) Shear stresses t (arrows) cause buckling of the graft, rupture of the graft-wound bed bond and formation of an air pocket. (d) Peeling force P lifts the graft away from the wound bed. (e) Excessively high moisture flux rate J through the graft causes dehydration and development of shrinkage stresses at the edges (arrows), which cause lift-off away from the wound bed. (f) Very low moisture flux J causes fluid accumulation (edema) at the graft-wound bed interface and peeling off (arrows). (From Yannas I.V. and Burke J.F. 1980. *J. Biomed. Mater. Res.* 14: 65.)

the graft can adequately displace air pockets from the air-wound bed surface. Although the measurement of a credible value of the surface energy is not a simple matter when the graft is based on certain natural polymers in the form of a hydrated gel, the requirement of adequate adhesion can be met empirically by chemical modification of the surface or by proper use of structural features such as porosity.

Third, the moisture flux through the graft must be maintained within bounds which are set by the following considerations. The upper bound to the moisture flux must be kept below the level where excessive dehydration of the graft occurs, thereby leading to alteration of the surface energy of the graft-wound bed interface and loss of the adhesive bond between graft and wound bed. Further, when the moisture flux exceeds the desired level, the graft is desiccated, and shrinkage stesses develop which pull the graft away from the wound bed. An estimate of the maximum normal stress sm can be obtained by modeling the desiccating graft in one dimension as a shrinking elastic beam bonded to a rigid surface

$$\sigma_m = 0.45\alpha(V_2 - V_1)E \tag{75.1}$$

In Equation 75.1, a is the coefficient of expansion of a graft which swells in water, V_1 and V_2 are initial and final values of the volume fraction of moisture in the graft, and E is Young's modulus of the graft averaged over the range V_1 to V_2, the latter range being presumed to be narrow. If, by contrast, the moisture flux through the graft is lower than the desired low bound, water accumulates between the graft and the wound bed, and edema results with accompanying loss of the adhesive bond between the two surfaces.

75.4.2 Stage 2 Design Parameters

The leading design objectives in this stage are two: synthesis of new, physiologic skin and the eventual disposal of the graft.

The lifetime of the graft, expressed as the time constant of biodegradation t_b, was modeled in relation to the time constant for normal healing of a skin incision t_h. The latter is about 25 days. In preliminary studies with animals, it was observed that when matrices were synthesized to degrade at a very rapid rate, amounting to $t_b \ll t_h$, the initially insoluble matrix was reduced early to a liquidlike state, which was incompatible with an effective wound closure. At the other extreme, matrices were synthesized which degraded with exceptional difficulty within 3 to 4 weeks, compatible with $t_b \gg t_h$. In these preliminary studies it was observed that a highly intractable matrix, corresponding to the latter condition, led to formation of a dense fibrotic tissue underneath the graft which eventually led to loss of the bond between graft and wound bed. Accordingly, it was hypothesized that a rule of **isomorphous matrix replacement**, equivalent to assuming a graft degradation rate of order of magnitude similar to the synthesis rate for new tissue, and represented by the relation

$$\frac{t_b}{t_h} = 1 \qquad (75.2)$$

would be optimal. Control of t_b is possible by adjustment of the crosslink density of the matrix. Equation 75.2 is the defining equation for a biodegradable scaffold which is coupled with, and therefore interacts with, the inflammatory process in a wound.

Migration of cells into the matrix is necessary for synthesis of new tissue. Such migration can proceed very slowly, defeating Equation 75.2, when fibroblasts and other cells recruited below the wound surface are required to wait until degradation of a potentially solid-like matrix has progressed sufficiently. An easier pathway to migrating cells can be provided by modifying a solid-like matrix into one which has an abundance of pore channels, where the average pore is at least as large as one cell diameter (about 10 μm) for ready access. Although this rationale is supported by experiment, results with animal studies have shown that not only is there a lower limit to the average pore diameter, but there is also an upper limit (see below).

Migration of cells into the porous graft can proceed only if nutrients are available to these cells. Two general mechanisms are available for transport of nutrients to the migrating cells, namely, diffusion from the wound bed and transport along capillaries which may have sprouted within the matrix (angiogenesis). Since capillaries would not be expected to form for at least a few days, it is necessary to consider whether a purely diffusional mode of transport of nutrients from the wound bed surface into the graft could immediately supply the metabolic needs of the invading cells adequately. The cell has been modled as a reactor which consumes a critical nutrient with a rate r, in units of mol/cm^3/sec; the nutrient is transported from the wound bed to the cell by diffusion over a distance l, the nutrient concentration at or near the surface of the wound bed is c_0, in units of mole/cm^3, and the diffusivity of the nutrient is D, in cm^2/sec. The appropriate conditions were expressed in terms of a dimensionless number S, the **cell lifeline number**, which expresses the relative importance of reaction rate for consumption of the nutrient by the cell to rate of transport of the nutrient by diffusion alone:

$$S = \frac{rl^2}{Dc_0} \qquad (75.3)$$

Equation 75.3 suggests that when $S = 1$, the critical value of the path length, l_c, corresponds to the maximum distance along which cells can migrate inside the graft without requiring angiogenesis (vascularization) for nutrient transport. The value of l_c defines the maximum thickness of graft that can be populated with cells within a few hours after grafting, before angiogenesis has had time to occur.

These conceptual objectives have been partially met by designing the graft as an analog of **extracellular matrix** (ECM) which possesses morphogenetic activity since it leads to partial regeneration of dermis. The discovery of the specific ECM analog that possesses this activity has been based on the empirical observation that, whereas the vast majority of ECM analogs apparently do not inhibit wound contraction almost at all, one of the analogs does. The activity of this analog, for which the term regeneration template has been coined, is conveniently detected as a significant delay in the onset of wound contraction. When seeded with (uncultured) autologous keratinocytes, an active regeneration template is capable of inducing simultaneous synthesis both of a dermis and an epidermis in the guinea pig and in the swine (Yorkshire pig). The regeneration is almost complete; however, hair follicles and other skin adnexa are not formed. The resulting integument performs the two vital functions of skin, that is, control of infection and moisture loss, while also providing physiologic mechanical protection to the internal organs and, additionally, providing a cosmetic effect almost identical to that of intact skin.

The morphogenetic specificity of the dermis regeneration template depends sensitively on retention of certain structural characteristics. The overall structure is that of an insoluble, three-dimensional covalently crosslinked network. The primary structure can be described as that of a graft-copolymer of type I collagen and a glycosaminoglycan (GAG) in the approximate ratio 98/2. The GAG can be either chondroitin 6-sulfate or dermatan sulfate; other GAGs appear capable of contributing approximately equal increments to morphogenetic specificity. The collagen fibers lack banding almost completely although the integrity of the triple helical structure is retained through the network. The resistance of the network to collagenase degradation is such that approximately two-thirds of the mass of the network becomes solubilized in vivo within about 2 weeks. The structure of the network is highly porous. The pore volume fraction exceeds 95% while the average pore diameter is maintained in the range 20 to 125 μm. The regeneration template loses its activity rapidly when these structural features are flawed deliberately in control studies.

The dermis regeneration template, a porous matrix unseeded with cells, induces synthesis of a new dermis and solves this old surgical problem. Simultaneous synthesis of a new, confluent epidermis occurs by migration of epithelial cell sheets from the wound edges, over the newly synthesized dermal bed. With wounds of relatively small characteristic dimension, for example, 1 cm, epithelial cells migrating at speeds of about 0.5 mm/day from each wound edge can provide a confluent epidermis within 10 days. In such cases, the unseeded template fulfills all the design specifications set above. However, the wounds incurred by a massively burned patient are typically of characteristic dimension of several centimeters, often more than 20 to 30 cm. These wounds are large enough to preclude formation of a new epidermis by cell migration alone within a clinically acceptable timeframe, say 2 weeks. Wounds of that magnitude can be treated by seeding the porous collagen-GAG template, before grafting, with at lest 5×10^4 keratinocytes per square centimeter wound area. These uncultured, autologous cells are extracted by applying a cell separation procedure, based on controlled trypsinization, to a small epidermal biopsy.

Details of the synthesis of the dermis regeneration template, as well as of other templates which regenerate peripheral nerves and the knee meniscus, are presented elsewhere in this handbook. The dermis regeneration template described in this section was first reported as a **synthetic skin** and as an artificial skin.

75.5 Clinical Studies of a Permanent Skin Replacement (Artificial Skin)

75.5.1 Clinical Studies

The skin regeneration template has been tested clinically on two occasions. In the first, conducted in the period 1979 to 1980, one clinical center was involved, and ten severely burned patients were studied. In the second, conducted during 1986 to 1987, 11 clinical centers were involved, and 106 severely burned patients were treated in a prospective, randomized manner. In each case the results have been published in some detail. The second study led to a surgical report, a histologic report, and an immunologic report. There is now adequate information available to discuss the advantages and disadvantages of this prototype artificial skin in the treatment of the severely burned patient.

The artificial skin used in clinical studies so far consists of the bilayer device illustrated in Figure 75.3. The outer layer is a silicone film, about 100 μm in thickness, which fulfills the requirements of stage 1 of the design (see above), and the inner layer is the skin regeneration template. In these clinical studies this device has not been seeded with keratinocytes. Closure of the relatively large wounds by formation of an epidermis has been achieved instead by use of a 100-μm-thin layer of the patient's epidermis (autoepidermal graft). The latter has been excised from an intact area of the patient's skin; the donor site can, however, be harvested repeatedly, since the excised epidermis regenerates spontaneously in a few days over the relatively intact dermal bed. Briefly, the entire procedure consists of preparation of the wound bed prior to grafting by excision of thermally injured tissue (**eschar**), followed by immediate grafting of the unseeded template on the freshly excised wound and ending, 3 weeks later, by replacing the outer, silicone layer of the device with a thin epidermal graft. The results of studies with a guinea pig model and a swine model have shown that seeding of the dermis regeneration template with fresh, uncultured autologous keratinocytes prior to grafting leads to simultaneous synthesis of an epidermis as well as a dermis in about 2 weeks. However, definitive clinical studies of the keratinocyte-seeded template have yet to be performed.

The discussion below focuses on the advantages and disadvantages of the (unseeded) artificial skin, as these emerge from clinical observations during the treatment as well as from a limited number of follow-up observations extending over several years after the treatment. The controls used in the clinical studies included meshed autograft, allograft, and xenografts. Comparative analysis of the clinical data will focus on each of the two stages of treatment for the massively burned patient, that is, the early (acute) stage and the long term stage, the conceptual basis for which has been discussed above.

75.5.2 Clinical Parameters Used in the Evaluation

The clinical parameters during the early stage of treatment (about 3 weeks) include the take of the graft, expressed as a percentage of graft area which formed an adhesive bond of sufficient strength with the wound bed and became vascularized. In the case of the artificial skin treatment, two different measures of take are reported, namely, that of the bilayer membrane on the freshly excised wound bed and the take of the epidermal graft applied on the neodermal bed about 3 weeks later. Another parameter is the thickness of dermis that has been excised from the donor site in order to obtain the autograft that is used to close the wound definitively. An additional parameter which characterizes the cost of the donor site to the patient is the time to heal the donor site. The surgeon's overall qualitative evaluation of the treatment (relative to controls) during the early stage is also reported.

The long-term evaluation has extended at least 1 year in approximately one-quarter of the patients. The first long-term parameter is based on the patients' reports of the relative incidence of nonphysiologic sensations, including itching, dryness, scaliness, lack of elasticity (lack of deformability), sweating, sensation, and erythema. The second parameter is based on the physicians' report of the relative presence of hypertrophic scarring in the grafted area. A third parameter is the patient's evaluation of the physiologic feel and appearance of the donor sites. Finally, there is an overall evaluation and preference of the patients for a given grafted site as well as the physicians' evaluation of the same grafted site.

75.5.3 Short-Term Clinical Evaluation of Artificial Skin

The median percentage take of the artificial skin was 80%, compared with the median take of 95% for all controls. Use of the Wilcoxin Rank Sum Test for the bimodally distributed data led to the conclusion that the take of the artificial skin was lower than that of all controls with a p value of $<.0001$. The reported difference reflected primarily the significantly lower take of the artificial skin relative to the meshed autograft. There was no significant difference in take when the artificial skin was compared with allograft (Wilcoxin Rank Sum $p > .10$). The take of the epidermal autograft was 86%.

Mean donor site thickness was 0.325 ± 0.045 mm for control sites and only 0.15 ± 0.0625 mm for epidermal grafts which were harvested for placement over the newly synthesized dermis; the difference was found to be significant by t test with a *p* value of <.001. The thinner donor sites used in the artificial skin procedures healed, as expected, significantly faster, requiring 10.6 ± 5.8 d compared to 14.3 ± 6.9 d for control sites, with a *p* value of <.001 by *t* test. It is worth noting that donor sites used in the artificial skin procedure were frequently reharvested sites from previous autografting; reharvested donor sites healed more slowly than primary sites.

The subjective evaluation of the operating surgeons at the conclusion of the acute stage of treatment was a response to the question, "Was artificial dermis (artificial skin) advantageous in the management of this particular patient?" Sixty-three percent of the comments were affirmative, whereas in 36% of the responses, the acute (early) results were believed to be no better than by use of routine methods. The physicians who responded positively to the use of artificial skin commented on the ability to use thin donor sites that healed quickly, relative to the thicker donor sites which were harvested in preparation for an autograft. Positive comments also cited the handling characteristics of the artificial skin relative to the allograft as well as the ability to close the wound without fear of rejection while awaiting healing of the donor site. Negative comments included a less-than-adequate drainage of serum and blood through the unperforated silicone sheet, the seemingly poor resistance of the artificial skin to infection, and the need for a second operation.

75.5.4 Long-Term Clinical Evaluation of Artificial Skin

One year after treatment, the allografted and xenografted sites had been long ago covered definitively with autograft; therefore, the experimental sites included, in the long term, either autografts (referred to occasionally as controls below) or the test sites, comprising the new integument induced as a result of treatment with the artificial skin (partially regenerated dermis closed with an epidermal graft).

The patients reported that itching was significantly less (Wilcoxin Rank Sum test $p < .02$) in the artificial skin site than in control sites. Dryness, scaliness, elasticity (deformability), sweating, sensation, and erythema were similar at both control and artificial skin sites. Hypertrophic scarring was reported to be less in artificial skin in 42% of sites and was reported to be equivalent on test and control sites 57% of the time. No patient reported that the artificial skin sites had more hypertrophic scar than the autografted sites. Even though donor sites that were used during treatment with the artificial skin were harvested repeatedly (recropping), 72% of patients reported that these artificial skin donor sites felt "more normal," 17% felt that there was no difference, and 11% felt that the control donor site was "more normal."

The results of the histologic study on this patient population showed that, in sites where the artificial skin was used, an intact dermis was synthesized as well as definitive closure of a complete epidermal layer with a minimum of scarring had occurred. The results of the immunologic study led to the conclusion that, in patients who had been treated with the artificial skin, there was increased antibody activity to bovine skin collagen, bovine skin collagen with chondroitin sulfate, and human collagen; however, it was concluded that these increased levels of antibodies were not immunologically significant.

The overall evaluation by the patients showed that 26% preferred the new integument generated by use of the artificial skin whereas 64% found that the sites were equivalent and 10% showed preference for the autografted site. Physician's overall evaluation showed that 39% preferred the artificial skin site, 45% found the sites to be equivalent, and 16% preferred the autografted site.

75.5.5 Clinical Results

The take of the artificial skin was comparable to all other grafts and was inferior only to the meshed autograft. The latter showed superior take in part because meshing reduces drastically the flexural rigidity of the graft (see above) leading thereby to greater conformity with the wound bed (see Figure 75.4). The interstices in the meshed autograft also provided an outlet for drainage of serum and blood from the wound, thereby allowing removal of these fluids. By contrast, the continuity of the silicone sheet in the artificial skin accounted for the increased flexural rigidity of the graft and prevented drainage of wound fluids with a resulting increased incidence of fluid accumulation underneath the graft. Fluid accumulation was probably the cause of the reduced take of the artificial skin, since immediate formation of a physiochemical bond between the graft and the wound bed was thereby prevented (see Figure 75.4). The development of infection underneath the artificial skin, noted by physicians in certain cases, can also be explained as originating in the layer of wound fluid which presumptively collected underneath the artificial skin. This analysis suggests that meshing of the silicone layer of the artificial skin, without affecting the continuity of the collagen-GAG layer, could lead to improved take and probably to reduced incidence of infection.

The healing time for donor sites associated with use of the artificial skin was shorter by about 4 days than for donor sites that were used to harvest autograft. An even shorter healing time for donor sites for artificial skin can be realized by reducing the thickness of the epidermal graft which is required to close the dermal bed. The average epidermal graft thickness reported in this study, 0.15 mm, was significantly higher than thicknesses in the range 0.05 to 0.07 mm, corresponding to an epidermal graft with adequate continuity but negligible amount of attached dermis. Increasing familiarity of surgeons with the procedure for harvesting these thin epidermal grafts is expected to lead to harvesting of thinner grafts in future studies. The importance of harvesting a thin graft cannot be overestimated, since the healing time of the donor site decreases rapidly with decreasing thickness of harvested graft. It has been reported that the mean healing time for donor sites for the artificial skin reported in this study, about 11 days, is reduced to 4 days provided that a pure epidermal graft, free of dermis, can be harvested.

Not only does the time to heal increase, but the incidence of hypertrophic scarring at a donor site also increases with the thickness of the harvested graft. This observation explains the higher incidence of hypertrophic scarring in donor sites associated with harvesting of autografts, since the latter were thicker by about 0.175 mm than the epidermal grafts used with the artificial skin. An additional advantage associated with use of a thin epidermal graft is the opportunity to reharvest (recropping) within a few days; this reflects the ability of epithelial tissues to regenerate spontaneously provided there is an underlying dermal bed. When frequent recropping of donor graft is possible, the surface area of a patient that can be grafted within a clinically acceptable period increases rapidly. In the clinical study described here, a patient with deep burns over as much as 85% body surface area was covered with artificial skin grafts for 75 days while the few donor sites remaining were being harvested several times each.

In the long term rarely did a patient or a physician in this clinical study prefer the new skin provided by the autograft to that provided by the artificial skin treatment. This result is clearly related to the use of meshed autografts, a standard procedure in the treatment of massively burned patients. Meshing increases the wound area which can by autografted by between 1.5 and 6 times, thereby alleviating a serious resource problem. However, meshing destroys the dermis as well as the epidermis; although the epidermis regenerates spontaneously and fills in the defects, the dermis does not. The long-term result is a skin site with the meshed pattern permanently embossed on it. The artificial skin is a device that, in principle, is available in unlimited quantity; accordingly, it does not suffer from this problem (Figure 75.2). The result is a smooth skin surface which was clearly preferred on average by patients and physicians alike.

It has been established that the artificial skin regenerates the dermis and, therefore, its use leads to complete inhibition of scar formation in full-thickness skin wounds. The regeneration is partial because skin adenexa (hair follicles, sweat glands) are not recovered. The results of studies of the mechanism by which the artificial skin regenerates the dermis in full-thickness skin wounds in animal models have been described elsewhere.

75.5.6 Summary

The artificial skin leads to a new skin which appears closer to the patient's intact skin than does the meshed autograft. Take of the artificial skin is as good as all comparative materials except for the unmeshed autograft, which is superior in this respect. Donor sites associated with the artificial skin treatment heal faster, can be recropped much more frequently, and eventually heal to produce sites that look closer to the patient's intact skin than do donor sites harvested for the purpose of autografting. In comparison to the allograft, the artificial skin is easier to use, has the same take, does not get rejected, and is free of the risk of viral infection associated with use of allograft.

75.6   Alternative Approaches: Cultured Epithelial Autografts (CEA) and Skin Equivalents (SE)

The use of cultured epithelial autografts has been studied clinically. In this approach autologous epidermal cells are removed by biopsy and are then cultured *in vitro* for about 3 weeks until a mature keratinizing epidermis has formed; the epidermis is then grafted onto the patient. The epithelial cells spread and cover the dermal substrate, eventually covering the entire wound. Early reports on two pediatric patients were very encouraging, describing the life-saving coverage of one-half of body surface with cultured epithelial autografts and the technique was eventually used in a very large number of clinical centers in several countries. Later studies showed that the "take" of CEA was very good on partial thickness wounds but was questionable in full thickness wounds. In particular, blisters formed within 2 weeks in areas grafted by CEA, a problem which has recurred persistently in clinical studies. The mechanical fragility of the resulting integument resulting from use of CEA has been traced to lack of three structural features which are required for formation of a physiological dermal–epidermal junction at the grafted site, namely, the 7-S domain of type IV collagen, anchoring fibrils, and rete ridges. Early studies of the connective tissue underlying the CEA grafts have shown lack of a convincing dermal architecture as well as lack of elastin fibers.

In another development, a skin equivalent has been prepared by populating a collagen lattice with heterologous fibroblasts, observing the contraction of the lattice by the cells and finally seeding the surface of the lattice with a suspension of epidermal cells from an autologous source or from cell banks. The latter attach, proliferate, and differentiate to form a multilayered epidermis in 7 to 10 days of exposure to the atmosphere and the resulting skin equivalent is then grafted on wounds. Clinical studies of the SE have been limited. In an early study (1988), the SE was used to cover partially full-thickness burn wounds covering over 15% of body surface area on eight patients. In every patient grafted with SE, an extensive lysis of the SE grafts was observed at the first dressing (48 h). In one patient only, a significant percentage of "take" (40%) was observed 14 days after grafting. It was concluded that the SE was not completely appropriate to serve routinely as a substitute for the autograft. In a later study (1995), the wounds treated were acute, mostly the result of excision of skin cancers. Twelve patients had clinical "takes" at the time of grafting and there was no evidence of rejection or toxicity following grafting with the SE. The wounds grafted with SE contracted by 10 to 15%, an extent larger than that observed following grafting with full-thickness skin. Biopsies of the grafted sites showed formation of scar tissue. The authors hypothesized that the SE was eventually replaced by host tissue. Recent studies of the SE have focused on patients with venous ulcers; these studies are in progress.

An attempt has been made to correct the erratic cover provided by split-thickness autografts; the latter are normally applied in a meshed form (meshed autograft) and, consequently, fail to cover the entire wound bed with a dermal layer. The attempted improvement consisted in grafting underneath the meshed autograft a **living dermal tissue replacement**, consisting of a synthetic polymeric mesh (polyglactin-910) which had been cultured in vitro over a period of 2 to 3 weeks with fibroblasts isolated from neonatal foreskin. Seventeen patients with full-thickness burn wounds were included in a preliminary clinical trial. Epithelialization of the interstices of the meshed autograft led to complete wound closure in 14 days in sites where the dermal living replacement had been grafted underneath the meshed autograft (experimental sites) and in those where it was omitted (control sites). Take of the meshed autograft was slightly reduced when the living dermal tissue replacement was underneath. Basement membrane structures developed both in control and experimental sites. Elastic fibers (elastin) were not observed in neodermal tissue either in control or experimental sites at periods up to one year after grafting. A subsequent clinical study explored the use of this device for the temporary closure of excised burn wounds. This 66-patient multicenter trial showed that the biosynthetic skin replacement was equivalent or superior to cadaver skin graft (frozen human cadaver allograft) with respect to its ability to prepare wounds for eventual closing with autograft.

Allograft is a human cadaver skin, which is frequently stored in frozen state in a skin bank. It is a temporary cover. If left on the wound longer than about 2 weeks, allograft is rejected by the severely burned patient, even though the latter is in an immunocompromised condition. When rejection is allowed to occur, the wound bed is temporarily ungraftable and is subject to infection. In a modification of this basic use of the allograft, the latter has been used as a dermal equivalent prior to grafting with cultured epithelia. Since the allograft is rejected if allowed to remain on the wound long enough for the epithelia to spread across the wound bed, the allograft has been treated in a variety of media in an effort to eliminate its immunogenicity.

Defining Terms

Adnexa: Accessory parts or appendages of an organ. Adnexa of skin include hair follicles and sweat glands.

Allograft: Human cadaver skin, usually maintained frozen in a skin bank and used to provide a temporary cover for deep wounds. About 2 weeks after grafting, the allograft is removed and replaced with autograft which has become available by that time. Previously referred to as homograft.

Artificial skin: A bilayer membrane consisting of an upper layer of silicone and a lower layer of dermis regeneration template. The template is a cell-free, highly porous analog of extracellular matrix.

Autograft: The patient's own skin, harvested from an intact area in the form of a membrane and used to graft an area of severe skin loss.

Basement membrane: An approximately 20-nm-thick multilayered membrane interleaved between the epidermis and the dermis.

Cell lifeline number: A dimensionless number which compares the relative magnitudes of chemical reaction and diffusion. This number, defined as S in Equation 75.3 above, can be used to compute the maximum path length, lc , over which a cell can migrate in a scaffold while depending on diffusion alone for transport of critical nutrients that it consumes. When the critical length is exceeded, the cell requires transport of nutrients by angiogenesis in order to survive.

Cultured epithelial autografts: A mature, keratinizing epidermis synthesized in vitro by culturing epithelial cells removed from the patient by biopsy. A relatively small skin biopsy (1 cm^2) can be treated to yield an area larger by about 10,000 in 2–3 weeks and is then grafted on patients with burns.

Dermal equivalent: A term which has been loosely used to describe a device that replaces, usually temporarily, the functions of the dermis following injury.

Dermis: A 2 to 5 mm-thick layer of connective tissue populated with quiescent fibroblasts which lies underneath the epidermis. It is separated from the former by a very thin basement membrane. The dermis of adult mammals does not regenerate spontaneously following injury.

Dermis regeneration template: A graft copolymer of type I collagen and chondroitin 6-sulfate, average pore diameter 20 to 125 μm, degrading *in vivo* to an extent of about 50% in 2 weeks, which induces partial regeneration of the dermis in wounds from which the dermis has been fully excised. When seeded with keratinocytes prior to grafting, this analog of extracellular matrix has induced simultaneous synthesis both of a dermis and an epidermis.

Donor site: The skin site from which an autograft has been removed with a dermatome.

Epidermis: The cellular outer layer of skin, about 0.1-mm thick, which protects against moisture loss and against infection. An epidermal graft, for example, cultured epithelium or a thin graft removed surgically, requires a dermal substrate for adherence onto the wound bed. The epidermis regenerates spontaneously following injury, provided there is a dermal substrate underneath.

Eschar: Dead tissue, typically the result of a thermal injury, which covers the underlying, potentially viable tissue.

Extracellular matrix: A largely insoluble, nondiffusible macromolecular network, consisting mostly of glycoproteins and proteoglycans.

Isomorphous matrix replacement: A term used to describe the synthesis of new, physiologic tissue within a skin regeneration template at a rate which is of the same order as the degradation of the template. This relation, Equation 75.2 above, is the defining equation for a biodegradable scaffold which biologically interacts with the inflammatory process of the wound bed.

Living dermal replacement: A synthetic biodegradable polymeric mesh, previously cultured with fibroblasts, which is placed underneath a conventional meshed autograft.

Meshed autograft: A sheet autograft which has been meshed and then expanded by a factor of 1.5 to 6 to produce grafts with a characteristic pattern.

Regeneration template: A biodegradable scaffold which, when attached to a missing organ, induces its regeneration.

Scar: The result of a repair process in skin and other organs. Scar is morphologically different from skin, in addition to being mechanically less extensible and weaker than skin. The skin regeneration template induces synthesis of nearly physiologic skin rather than scar.

Sheet autograft: A layer of the patient's skin, comprising the epidermis and about one-third of the dermal thickness, which has not been meshed prior to grafting areas of severe skin loss.

Skin: A vital organ which indispensably protects the organism from infection and dehydration while also providing other functions essential to physiologic life, such as assisting in thermoregulation and providing a tactile sensor for the organism.

Skin equivalent: A collagen gel which has been contracted by fibroblasts cultured therein. Following culturing with keratinocyte, until a cornified epidermis is formed over the contracted collagen lattice, it is grafted on skin wounds.

Split-thickness autograft: An autograft which is about one-half or one-third as thick as the full thickness of skin.

Subcutis: A layer of fat tissue underneath the dermis.

Synthetic skin: A term used to describe the artificial skin in the early literature.

Take: The adhesion of a graft on the woundbed. Without adequate take, there is no physicochemical or biologic interaction between graft and wound bed.

Xenograft: Skin graft obtained from a different species: for example, pig skin grafted on human. Synthetic polymeric membranes are often referred to as xenografts. Previously referred to as heterograft.

References

Boykin J.V., Jr. and Molnar J.A. 1992. Burn scar and skin equivalents. In I.K. Cohen, R.F. Diegelmann and W.J. Lindblad (Eds.) *Wound Healing*, pp. 523–540, Philadelphia, W.B. Saunders.

Burke J.F., Yannas I.V., Quinby W.C., Jr., Bondoc C.C., and Jung W.K. 1981. Successful use of a physiologically acceptable artificial skin in the treatment of extensive burn injury. *Ann. Surg.* 194: 413–428.

Compton C.C. 1992. Current concepts in pediatric burn care: the biology of cultured epithelial autografts: An eight-year study in pediatric burn patients. *Eur. J. Pediatr. Surg.* 2: 216–222.

Compton C.C., Gill J.M., Bradford D.A., Regauer S., Gallico G.G., and O'Connor N.E. 1989. Skin regenerated from cultured epithelial autografts on full-thickness burn wounds from 6 days to 5 years after grafting. *Lab. Invest.* 60: 600–612.

Eaglstein W.H., Iriondo M., and Laszlo K. 1995. A composite skin substitute (Graftskin) for surgical wounds. *Dermatol. Surg.* 21: 839–843.

Gallico G.G., O'Connor N.E., Compton C.C., Kehinde O., and Green H. 1984. Permanent coverage of large burn wounds with autologous cultured human epithelium, *N. Engl. J. Med.* 311: 448–451.

Hansbrough J.F., Dore C., and Hansbrough W.B. (1992b). Clinical trials of a living dermal tissue replacement placed beneath meshed, split-thickness skin grafts on excised burn wounds, *J. Burn Care Rehab.* 13: 519–529.

Heimbach D., Luterman A., Burke J., Cram A., Herndon D., Hunt J., Jordan M., McManus W., Solem L., Warden G., and Zawacki B. 1988. Artificial dermis for major burns. *Ann. Surg.* 208: 313–320.

Michaeli D. and McPherson M. 1990. Immunologic study of artificial skin used in the treatment of thermal injuries, *J. Burn Care Rehab.* 11: 21–26.

Purdue G.F., Hunt J.L., Still J.M. Jr, Law E.J., Herndon D.N., Goldfarb I.W., Schiller W.R., Hansbrough J.F., Hickerson W.L., Himel H.N., Kealey P., Twomey J., Missavage A.E., Solem L.D., Davis M., Totoritis M., and Gentzkow G.D. 1997. A multicenter clinical trial of a biosynthetic skin replacement, Dermagraft-TC, compared with cryopreserved human cadaver skin for temporary coverage of excised burn wounds. *J Burn Care Rehab.* 18: 52–57.

Sabolinski M.L., Alvarez O., Auletta M., Mulder G., and Parenteau N.L. 1996. Cultured skin as a 'smart material' for healing wounds: experience in venous ulcers. *Biomaterials* 17: 311–320.

Stern R., McPherson M., and Longaker M.T. 1990. Histologic study of artificial skin used in the treatment of full-thickness thermal injury, *J. Burn Care Rehab.* 11: 7–13.

Tompkins R.G. and Burke J.F. 1992. Artificial Skin. *Surg. Rounds* 881–890.

Waserman D., Sclotterer M., Toulon A., Cazalet C., Marien M., Cherruau B., and Jaffray P. 1988. Preliminary clinical studies of a biological skin equivalent in burned patients. *Burns* 14: 326–330.

Yannas I.V. and Burke J.F. 1980. Design of an artificial skin I. Basic design principles, *J. Biomed. Mater. Res.* 14: 65–81.

Yannas I.V., Burke J.F., Warpehoski M., Stasikelis P., Skrabut E.M., Orgill D., and Giard D.J. 1981. Prompt, long-term functional replacement of skin. *Trans. Am. Soc. Artif. Internal Organs* 27: 19–22.

Further Information

Bell E., Erlich H.P., Buttle D.J., and Nakatsuji T. 1981. Living skin formed *in vitro* and accepted as skin-equivalent tissue of full thickness. *Science* 211: 1052–1054.

Bell E., Ivarsson B., and Merrill C. 1979. Production of a tissue-like structure by contraction of collagen lattices by human fibroblasts of different proliferative potential in vitro. *Proc. Natl Acad. Sci. USA* 76: 1274–1278.

Boyce S.T. and Hansbrough J.F. 1988. Biologic attachment, growth, and differentiation of cultured human keratinocytes on a graftable collagen and chondroitin 6-sulfate substrate. *Surgery* 103: 421–431.

Eldad A., Burt A., and Clarke J.A. 1987. Cultured epithelium as a skin substitute, *Burns* 13: 173–180.

Green H., Kehinde O., and Thomas J. 1979. Growth of cultured human epidermal cells into multiple epithelia suitable for grafting. *Proc. Natl Acad. Sci. USA* 76: 5665–5668.

Langer R. and Vacanti J.P. 1993. Tissue engineering. *Science* 260: 920–926.

O'Connor N.E., Mulliken J.B., Banks-Schlegel S., Kehinde O., and Green H. 1981. Grafting of burns with cultured epithelium prepared from autologous epidermal cells. *Lancet* 1: 75–78.

Woodley D.T., Peterson H.D., Herzog S.R., Stricklin G.P., Bergeson R.E., Briggaman R.A., Cronce D.J., and O'Keefe E.J. 1988. Burn wounds resurfaced by cultured epidermal autografts show abnormal reconstitution of anchoring fibtils. *JAMA* 259: 2566–2571.

Woodley D.T., Briggaman R.A., Herzog S.R., Meyers A.A., Peterson H.D., and O'Keefe E.J. 1990. Characterization of "neo-dermis" formation beneath cultured human epidermal autografts transplanted on muscle fascia. *J. Invest. Dermatol.* 95: 20–26.

Yannas I.V., Lee E., Orgill D.P., Skrabut E.M., and Murphy G.F. 1989. Synthesis and characterization of a model extracellular matrix that induces partial regeneration of adult mammalian skin. *Proc. Natl Acad. Sci. USA* 86: 933–937.

Yannas I.V., Burke J.F., Gordon P.L., and Huang C. 1977. Multilayer membrane useful as synthetic skin, US Patent no. 4,060,081, Nov. 29.

Yannas I.V. 1982. Wound tissue can utilize a polymeric template to synthesize a functional extension of the skin. *Science* 215: 174–176.

VII

Ethics

David E. Reisner

76

Beneficence, Nonmaleficence, and Medical Technology

Joseph D. Bronzino
Trinity College/Biomedical Engineering Alliance and Consortium (BEACON)

Two moral norms have remained relatively *constant across* the various moral codes and oaths that have been formulated for health-care deliverers since the beginnings of Western medicine in classical Greek civilization, namely beneficence — the provision of benefits — and nonmaleficence — the avoidance of doing harm. These norms are traced back to a body of writings from classical antiquity known as the *Hippocratic Corpus*. Although these writings are associated with the name of Hippocrates, the acknowledged founder of Western medicine, medical historians remain uncertain whether any, including the *Hippocratic Oath*, were actually his work. Although portions of the Corpus are believed to have been authored during the 6th century BC, other portions are believed to have been written as late as the beginning of the Christian Era. Medical historians agree, though, that many of the specific moral directives of the *Corpus* represent neither the actual practices nor the moral ideals of the majority of physicians of ancient Greece and Rome.

Nonetheless, the general injunction, "As to disease, make a habit of two things — to help or, at least, to do no harm," was accepted as a fundamental medical ethical norm by at least some ancient physicians. With the decline of Hellenistic civilization and the rise of Christianity, beneficence and nonmaleficence became increasingly accepted as the fundamental principles of morally sound medical practice. Although beneficence and nomaleficence were regarded merely as concomitant to the craft of medicine in classical Greece and Rome, the emphasis upon compassion and the brotherhood of humankind, central to Christianity, *increasingly made* these norms the only acceptable motives for medical practice. Even today the provision of benefits and the avoidance of doing harm are stressed just as much in virtually all contemporary Western codes of conduct for health professionals as they were in the oaths and codes that guided the health-care providers of the centuries past.

Traditionally, the ethics of medical care have given greater prominence to nomaleficence than to beneficence. This priority was grounded in the fact that, historically, medicine's capacity to do harm far exceeded its capacity to protect and restore health. Providers of health care possessed many treatments that posed clear and genuine risks to patients but that offered little prospect of benefit. Truly effective therapies were all too rare. In this context, it is surely rational to give substantially higher priority to avoiding harm than to providing benefits.

The advent of modern science changed matters dramatically. Knowledge acquired in laboratories, tested in clinics, and verified by statistical methods has increasingly dictated the practices of medicine. This *ongoing alliance* between medicine and science became a critical source of the plethora of technologies that now pervades medical care. The impressive increases in therapeutic, preventive, and rehabilitative capabilities that these technologies have provided have pushed beneficence to the forefront of medical morality. Some have.even gone so far as to hold that the old medical ethic of "Above all, do no harm" should be superseded by the new ethic that "The patient deserves the best." However, the rapid advances in medical technology capabilities have also produced great uncertainty as to what is most beneficial or least harmful for the patient. In other words, along with increases in ability to be beneficent, medicine's technology has generated much debate about what actually counts as beneficent or nonmaleficent treatment. To illustrate this point, let us turn to several specific moral issues posed by the use of medical technology [Bronzino, 1992, 1999].

76.1 Defining Death: A Moral Dilemma Posed by Medical Technology

Supportive and resuscitative devices, such as the respirator, found in the typical modern intensive care unit provide a useful starting point for illustrating how technology has rendered medical morality more complex and problematic. Devices of this kind allow clinicians to sustain respiration and circulation in patients who have suffered massive brain damage and total permanent loss of brain *function*. These technologies force us to ask: precisely when does a human life end? When is a human being indeed dead? This is not the straightforward factual matter it may appear to be. All of the relevant facts may show that the patient's brain has suffered injury grave enough to destroy its functioning forever. The facts may show that such an individual's circulation and respiration would permanently cease without artificial support. Yet these facts do not determine whether treating such an individual as a corpse is morally appropriate. To know this, it is necessary to know or perhaps to decide on those features of living persons that are essential to their status as "living persons." It is necessary to know or decide which human qualities, if irreparably lost, make an individual identical to a corpse in all morally relevant respects. Once those qualities have been specified, deciding whether total and irreparable loss of brain function constitutes death becomes a straightforward factual matter. Then, it would simply have to be determined if such loss itself deprives the individual of those qualities. If it does, the individual is morally identical to a corpse. If not, then the individual must be regarded and treated as a living person.

The traditional criterion of death has been irreparable cessation of heartbeat, respiration, and blood pressure. This criterion would have been quickly met by anyone suffering massive trauma to the brain prior to the development of modem supportive technology. Such technology allows indefinite artificial maintenance of circulation and respiration and, thus, forestalls what once was an inevitable consequence of severe brain injury. The existence and use of such technology therefore challenges the traditional criterion of death and forces us to consider whether continued respiration and circulation are in themselves sufficient to distinguish a living individual from a corpse. Indeed, total and irreparable loss of brain function, referred to as "brainstem death," "whole brain death," and, simply, "brain death," has been widely accepted as the legal standard for death. By this standard, an individual in a state of brain death is legally indistinguishable from a corpse and may be legally treated as one even though respiratory and circulatory functions may be sustained through the intervention of technology. Many take this legal standard to be the morally appropriate one, noting that once destruction of the brainstem has occurred, the brain *cannot function* at all, and the body's regulatory mechanisms will fail unless artificially sustained. Thus mechanical sustenance of an individual in a state of brain death is merely postponement of the inevitable and sustains nothing of the personality, character, or consciousness of the individual. It is merely the mechanical intervention that differentiates such an individual from a corpse and a mechanically ventilated corpse is a corpse nonetheless.

Even with a consensus that brainstem death is death and thus that an individual in such a state is indeed a corpse, hard cases remain. Consider the case of an individual in a persistent vegetative state — the condition known as "neocortical death." Although severe brain injury has been suffered, enough brain function remains to make mechanical *sustenance* of respiration and circulation unnecessary. In a persistent vegetative state, an individual exhibits no purposeful response to external stimuli and no evidence of self-awareness. The eyes may open periodically and the individual may exhibit sleep–wake cycles. Some patients even yawn, make chewing motions, or swallow spontaneously. Unlike the complete unresponsiveness of individuals in a state of brainstem death, a variety of simple and complex responses can be elicited from an individual in a persistent vegetative state. Nonetheless, the chances that such an individual will regain consciousness virtually do not exist. Artificial feeding, kidney dialysis, and the like make it possible to sustain an individual in a state of neocortical death for decades. This sort of condition and the issues it raises were exemplified by the famous case of Karen Ann Quinlan. James Rachels [1986] provided the following description of the situation created by Quinlan's condition:

> In April 1975, this young woman ceased breathing for at least two 15-minute periods, for reasons that were never made clear. As a result, she suffered severe brain damage, and, in the words of the attending physicians, was reduced to a "chronic vegetative state" in which she "no longer had any cognitive function." Accepting the doctors' judgment that there was no hope of recovery, her parents sought permission from the courts to disconnect the respirator that was keeping her alive in the intensive care unit of a New Jersey hospital.
>
> The trial court, and then the Supreme Court of New Jersey, agreed that Karen's respirator could be removed. So it was disconnected. However, the nurse in charge of her care in the Catholic hospital opposed this decision and, anticipating it, had begun to wean her from the respirator so that by the time it was disconnected she could remain alive without it. So Karen did not die. Karen remained alive for ten additional years. In June 1985, she finally died of acute pneumonia. Antibiotics, which would have fought the pneumonia, were not given.

If brainstem death is death, is neocortical death also death? Again, the issue is not a straightforward factual matter. For, it too, is a matter of specifying which features of living individuals distinguish them from corpses and so make treatment of them as corpses morally impermissible. Irreparable cessation of respiration and circulation, the classical indications of death, would entail ensuring that an individual in a persistent vegetative state is not a corpse and so, morally speaking, not to be treated as one. The brainstem death criterion for death would also entail that a person in a state of neocortical death is not yet a corpse. On this criterion, what is crucial is that brain damage is severe enough to cause failure of the body's regulatory mechanisms.

Is an individual in a state of neocortical death any less in possession of the characteristics that distinguish the living from cadavers than one whose respiration and circulation are mechanically maintained? Of course, it is a matter of what the relevant characteristics are, and it is a matter that society must decide. It is not one that can be settled by greater medical information or more powerful medical devices. Until society decides, it will not be clear what would count as beneficent or nonmaleficent treatment of an individual in a state of neocortical death.

76.2 Euthanasia

A long-standing issue in medical ethics, which has been made more pressing by medical technology, is euthanasia, the deliberate termination of an individual's life for the individual's own good. Is such an act ever a permissible use of medical resources? Consider an individual in a persistent vegetative state. On the assumption that such a state is not death, withdrawing life support would be a deliberate termination of a human life. Here a critical issue is whether the quality of a human life can be so low or so great a liability to the individual that deliberately taking action to hasten death or at least not to postpone death is morally defensible. Can the quality of a human life be so low that the value of extending its quantity is totally negated? If so, then Western medicine's traditional commitment to providing benefits and avoiding harm would seem to make cessation of life support a moral requirement in such a case.

Consider the following hypothetical version of the kind of case that actually confronts contemporary patients, their families, health-care workers, and society as a whole. Suppose a middle-aged man suffers a brain hemorrhage and loses consciousness as a result of a ruptured aneurysm. Suppose that he never regains consciousness and is hospitalized in a state of neocortical death, a chronic vegetative state. He is maintained by a surgically implanted gastronomy tube that drips liquid nourishment from a plastic bag directly into his stomach. The care of this individual takes seven and one-half hours of nursing time daily and includes (1) shaving, (2) oral hygiene, (3) grooming, (4) attending to his bowels and bladder, and so forth.

Suppose further that his wife undertakes legal action to force his care givers to end all medical treatment, including nutrition and hydration, so that complete bodily death of her husband will occur, She presents a preponderance of evidence to the court to show that her husband would have wanted this result in these circumstances.

The central moral issue raised by this sort of case is whether the quality of the individual's life is sufficiently compromised by neocortical death to make intentioned termination of that life morally permissible. While alive, he made it clear to both family and friends that he would prefer to be allowed to die rather than be mechanically maintained in a condition of irretrievable loss of consciousness. Deciding whether the judgment in such a case should be allowed requires deciding which capacities and qualities make life worth living, which qualities are sufficient to endow it with value worth sustaining, and whether their absence justifies deliberate termination of a life, at least when this would be the wish of the individual in question. Without this decision, the traditional norms of medical ethics, beneficence and nonmaleficence, provide no guidance. Without this decision, it cannot be determined whether termination of life support is a benefit or harmful to the patient.

An even more difficult type of case was provided by the case of Elizabeth Bouvia. Bouvia, who had been a lifelong quadriplegic sufferer of cerebral palsy, was often in pain, completely dependent upon others, and was bedbound all the time. Bouvia, after deciding that she did not wish to continue such a life, entered Riverside General Hospital in California. She desired to be kept comfortable while starving to death. Although she remained adamant during her hospitalization, with the legal sanction of the courts, Bouvia's requests were denied by hospital officials.

Many who might believe that neocortical death renders the quality of life sufficiently low to justify termination of life support, especially when this is in agreement with the individual's desires, would not arrive at this conclusion in a case like Bouvia's. Whereas neocortical death completely destroys consciousness and makes purposive interaction with the individual's environment impossible, Bouvia was fully aware and mentally alert. She had previously been married and had even acquired a college education. Televised interviews with her portrayed a very intelligent person who had great skill in presenting persuasive arguments to support her wish not to have her life continued by artificial means of nutrition. Nonetheless, she judged her life to be of such low quality that she should be allowed to choose to deliberately starve to death. Before the existence of life support technology, maintenance of her life against her will might not have been possible at all and at least would have been far more difficult.

Should Elizabeth Bouvia's judgment have been accepted? Her case is more difficult than the care of a patient in a chronic vegetative state because, unlike such an *individual, she* was able to engage in meaningful interaction with her environment. Regarding an individual who cannot speak or otherwise meaningfully interact with others as nothing more than living matter, as a "human vegetable," is not especially difficult. Perceiving Bouvia this way is not easy. Her awareness, intelligence, mental acuity, and ability to interact with others mean that although her life is one of discomfort, indignity, and complete dependence, she is not a mere "human vegetable."

Despite the differences between Bouvia's situation and that of someone in a state of neocortical death, the same issue is posed. Can the quality of an individual's life be so low that deliberate termination is morally justifiable? How that question is answered is a matter of what level of quality of life, if any, is taken to be sufficiently low to justify deliberately acting to end it. If there is such a level, the conclusion that it is not always beneficent or even nonmaleficent to use life-support technology must be accepted.

Another important issue here is respect for individual autonomy. For the cases of Bouvia and the hypothetical instance of neocortical death discussed above, both concern voluntary euthanasia, that is, euthanasia voluntarily requested by the patient. A long-standing commitment, vigorously defended by various schools of thought in Western moral philosophy, is the notion that competent adults should be free to conduct their lives as they please as long as they do not impose undeserved harm on others. Does this commitment include a right to die? Some clearly believe that it does. If at all one owns anything, surely one owns one's life. In the two cases discussed above, neither individual sought to impose undeserved harm on anyone else, nor would satisfaction of their wish to die do so. What justification can there then be for not allowing their desires to be fulfilled?

One plausible answer is based upon the very respect of individual autonomy at issue here. A necessary condition, in some views, of respect for autonomy is the willingness to take whatever measures are necessary to protect it, including measures that restrict autonomy. An autonomy-respecting reason offered against laws that prevent even competent adults from voluntarily entering life-long slavery is that such an exercise of autonomy is self-defeating and has the consequence of undermining autonomy altogether: same token, an individual who acts to end his own life thereby exercises his autonomy in a manner that places it in jeopardy of permanent loss. Many would regard this as justification for using the coercive force of the law to prevent suicide. This line of thought does not fit the case of an individual in a persistent vegetative state because his/her autonomy has been destroyed by the circumstances that rendered such a person neocortically dead. It does fit Bouvia's case though. Her actions indicate that she is fully competent and her efforts to use medical care to prevent the otherwise inevitable pain of starvation is itself an exercise of her autonomy. Yet, if allowed to succeed, those very efforts would destroy her autonomy as they destroy her. Along this line of reasoning, her case is a perfect instance of limitation of autonomy being justified by respect for autonomy and of one where, even against the wishes of a competent patient, the life-saving power of medical technology should be used.

76.2.1 Active vs. Passive Euthanasia

Discussions of the morality of euthanasia often distinguish active from passive euthanasia in light of the distinction made between killing a person and letting a person die, a distinction that rests upon the difference between an act of commission and an act of omission. When failure to take steps that could effectively forestall death results in an individual's demise, the resultant death is an act of omission and a case of letting a person die. When a death is the result of doing something to hasten the end of a person's life (giving a lethal injection, for example), that death is caused by an act of commission and is a case of killing a person. When a person is allowed to die, death is a result of an act of omission, and the motive is the person's own good, the omission is an instance of passive euthanasia. When a person is killed, death is the result of an act of commission, and the motive is the person's own good, the commission is an instance of active euthanasia.

Does the difference between passive and active euthanasia, which reduces to a difference in how death comes about, make any moral difference? It does in the view of the American Medical Association. In a statement adopted on December 4, 1973, the House of Delegates of the American Medical Association (AMA) asserted the following [Rachels, 1978]:

> The intentional termination of the life of one human being by another — mercy killing — is contrary to that for which the medical profession stands and is contrary to the policy of the American Medical Association (AMA).

The cessation of extraordinary means to prolong the life of the body where there is irrefutable evidence that biological death is imminent is the decision of the patient and immediate family. The advice of the physician would be freely available to the patient and immediate family.

In response to this position, Rachels [1978, 1986] answered with the following:

The AMA policy statement isolates the crucial issue very well, the crucial issue is "intentional termination of the life of one human being by another." But after identifying this issue and forbidding "mercy killing," the statement goes on to deny that the cessation of treatment is the intentional termination of a life. This is where the mistake comes in, for what is the cessation of treatment in those circumstances (where the intention is to release the patient from continued suffering), if it is not "the intentional termination of the life of one human being by another?"

As Rachels correctly argued, when steps that could keep an individual alive are omitted for the person's own good, this omission is as much the intentional termination of life as taking active measures to cause death. Not placing a patient on a respirator due to a desire not to prolong suffering is an act intended to end life as much as the administration of a lethal injection. In many instances, the main difference between the two cases is that the latter would release the individual from his pain and suffering more quickly than the former. Dying can take time and involve considerable pain even if nothing is done to prolong life. Active killing can be done in a manner that causes death painlessly and instantly. This difference certainly does not render killing, in this context, morally worse than letting a person die, Insofar as the motivation is merciful (as it must be if the case is to be a genuine instance of euthanasia) because the individual is released more quickly from a life that is disvalued than otherwise, the difference between killing and letting one die may provide support for active euthanasia. According to Rachels, the common rejoinder to this argument is the following:

The important difference between active and passive euthanasia is that in passive euthanasia the doctor does not do anything to bring about the patient's death. The doctor does nothing and the patient dies of whatever ills already afflict him. In active euthanasia, however, the doctor does something to bring about the patient's death: he kills the person. The doctor who gives the patient with cancer a lethal injection has himself caused his patient's death; whereas if he merely ceases treatment, the cancer is the cause of death.

According to this rejoinder, in active euthanasia someone must do something to bring about the patient's death, and in passive euthanasia the patient's death is caused by illness rather than by anyone's conduct. Surely this is mistaken. Suppose a physician deliberately decides not to treat a patient who has a routinely curable ailment and the patient dies. Suppose further that the physician were to attempt to exonerate himself by saying, "I did nothing. The patient's death was the result of illness. I was not the cause of death." Under current legal and moral norms, such a response would have no credibility. As Rachels noted, "it would be no defense at all for him to insist that he didn't do anything. He would have done something very serious indeed, for he let his patient die."

The physician would be blameworthy for the patient's death as surely as if he had actively killed him. If causing death is justifiable under a given set of circumstances, whether it is done by allowing death to occur or by actively causing death is morally irrelevant. If causing someone to die is not justifiable under a given set of circumstances, whether it is done by allowing death to occur or by actively causing death is also morally irrelevant. Accordingly, if voluntary passive euthanasia is morally justifiable in the light of the duty of beneficence, so is voluntary active euthanasia. Indeed, given that the benefit to be achieved is more quickly realized by means of active euthanasia, it may be preferable to passive euthanasia in some cases.

76.2.2 Involuntary and Nonvoluntary Euthanasia

An act of euthanasia is involuntary if it hastens the individual's death for his own good but against his wishes. To take such a course would be to destroy a life that is valued by its possessor. Therefore, it is no different in any morally relevant way from unjustifiable homicide. There are only two legitimate reasons for hastening an innocent person's death against his will: self-defense and saving the lives of a larger number of other innocent persons. Involuntary euthanasia does not fit either of these justifications. By definition, it is done for the good of the person who is euthanized and for self-defense or saving innocent others. No act that qualifies as involuntary euthanasia can be morally justifiable. Hastening a person's death for his own good is an instance of nonvoluntary euthanasia when the individual is incapable of agreeing or disagreeing. Suppose it is clear that a particular person is sufficiently self-conscious to be regarded a person but cannot make his wishes known. Suppose also that he is suffering from the kind of ailment that, in the eyes of many persons, makes one's life unendurable. Would hastening his death be permissible? It would be if there was substantial evidence that he has given prior consent. This person may have told friends and relatives that under certain circumstances efforts to prolong his life should not be undertaken or continued. He might have recorded his wishes in the form of a Living Will (below) or on audio- or videotape. Where this kind of substantial evidence of prior consent exists, the decision to hasten death would be morally justified. A case of this scenario would be virtually a case of voluntary euthanasia.

To My Family, My Physician, My Clergyman, and My Lawyer:

If the time comes when I can no longer take part in decisions about my own future, let this statement stand as testament of my wishes: If there is no reasonable expectation of my recovery from physical or mental disability. I, _____, request that I be allowed to die and not be kept alive by artificial means or heroic measures. Death is as much a reality as birth, growth, maturity, and old age — it is the one certainty. I do not fear death as much as I fear the indiginity of deterioration, dependence, and hopeless pain. I ask that drugs be mercifully administered to me for the terminal suffering even if they hasten the moment of death.

This request is made after careful consideration. Although this document is not legally binding, you who care for me will, I hope, feel morally bound to follow its mandate. I recognize that it places a heavy burden of responsibility upon you, and it is with the intention of sharing that responsibility and of mitigating any feelings of guild that this statement is made.

Signed:_____
Date: _____

Witnessed by:
_____
_____

But what about an instance in which such evidence is not available? Suppose the person at issue has never had the capacity for competent consent or dissent from decisions concerning his life. It simply cannot be known what value the individual would place on his life in his present condition of illness. What should be done is a matter of what is taken to be the greater evil — mistakenly ending the life of an innocent person for whom that life has value or mistakenly forcing him to endure a life that he radically disvalues.

Living Will statutes have been passed in at least 35 states and the District of Columbia. For a Living Will to be a legally binding document, the person signing it must be of sound mind at the time the will is made and shown not to have altered his opinion in the interim period between the signing and his illness. The witnesses must not be able to benefit from the individual's death.

76.2.3 Should Voluntary Euthanasia be Legalized?

Recent events have raised the question: "Should voluntary euthanasia be legalized?" Some argue that even if voluntary euthanasia is morally justifiable, nonetheless, it should be prohibited by social policy.

According to this position, the problem with voluntary euthanasia is its impact on society as a whole. In other words, the overall disutility of allowing voluntary euthanasia outweighs the good it could do for its beneficiaries. The central moral concern is that legalized euthanasia would eventually erode respect for human life and ultimately become a policy under which "socially undesirable" persons would have their deaths hastened (by acts of omission or commission). The experience of Nazi Germany is often cited in support of this fear. What began there as a policy of euthanasia soon became one of eliminating individuals deemed racially inferior or otherwise undesirable. The worry, of course, is that what happened there can happen here as well. If social policy encompasses efforts to hasten the deaths of people, respect for human life in general is eroded and all sorts of abuses become socially acceptable, or so the argument goes.

No one can provide an absolute guarantee that the experience of Nazi Germany would not be repeated, but there is reason to believe that its likelihood is negligible. The medical moral duty of beneficence justifies only voluntary euthanasia. It justifies hastening an individual's death only for the individual's benefit and only with the individual's consent. To kill or refuse to save people judged socially undesirable is not to engage in euthanasia at all and violates the medical moral duty of nomaleficence. As long as only voluntary euthanasia is legalized, and it is clear that involuntary euthanasia is not and should never be, no degeneration of the policy need occur. Furthermore, such degeneration is not likely to occur if the beneficent nature of voluntary euthanasia is clearly distinguished from the maleficent nature of involuntary euthanasia and any policy of exterminating the socially undesirable. Euthanasia decisions must be scrutinized carefully and regulated strictly to ensure that only voluntary cases occur, and severe penalties must be established to deter abuse.

References

Bronzino, J.D. Beneficence, nonmaleficence and technological progress. *The Biomedical Engineering Handbook*. CRC Press, Boca Raton, FL, 1995; 2000, chap. 190.

Bronzino, J.D. Medical and ethical issues in clinical engineering practice. *Management of Medical Technology*. Butterworth, 1992, chap. 10.

Bronzino, J.D. Moral and ethical issues associated with medical technology. *Introduction to Biomedical Engineering*. Academic Press, 1999, chap. 20.

Rachels, J. Active and passive euthanasia, In: *Moral Problems*, 3rd ed., Rachels, J. (Ed.), Harper and Row, New York, 1978.

Rachels, J. *Ethics at the End of Life: Euthanasia and Morality*, Oxford University Press, Oxford, 1986.

Further Information

Dubler, N.N. and Nimmons D. *Ethics on Call*. Harmony Books, New York, 1992.

Jonsen, A.R. *The New Medicine and the Old Ethics*. Harvard University Press, Cambridge, MA, 1990.

Seebauer, E.G. and Barry R.L. *Fundamentals of Ethics for Scientists and Engineers*. Oxford University Press, Oxford, 2001.

77

Ethical Issues Related to Clinical Research

Joseph D. Bronzino
Trinity College/Biomedical
Engineering Alliance and
Consortium (BEACON)

The Medical Device Amendment of 1976, and its updated 1990 version, requires approval from the Food and Drug Administration (FDA) before new devices are marketed and imposes requirements for the clinical investigation of new medical devices on human subjects. Although the statute makes interstate commerce of an unapproved new medical device generally unlawful, it provides an exception to allow interstate distribution of unapproved devices in order to conduct clinical research on human subjects. This investigational device exemption (IDE) can be obtained by submitting to the FDA "a protocol for the proposed clinical testing of the device, reports of prior investigations of the device, certification that the study has been approved by a local institutional review board, and an assurance that informed consent 'will be obtained from each human subject"[Bronzino et al., 1990a,b; 1992; 1995; 1999; 2000].

With respect to clinical research on humans, the FDA distinguishes devices into two categories: devices that pose significant risk and those that involve insignificant risk. Examples of the former included orthopedic implants, artificial hearts, and infusion pumps. Examples of the latter include various dental devices and daily-wear contact lenses. Clinical research involving a significant risk device cannot begin until an institutional review board (IRB) has approved both the protocol and the informed consent form and the FDA itself has given permission. This requirement to submit an IDE application to the FDA is waived in the case of clinical research where the risk posed is insignificant. In this case, the FDA requires only that approval from an IRB be obtained certifying that the device in question poses only insignificant risk. In deciding whether to approve a proposed clinical investigation of a new device, the IRB and the FDA must determine the following:

1. Risks to subjects are minimized
2. Risks to subjects are reasonable in relation to the anticipated benefit and knowledge to be gained

3. Subject selection is equitable
4. Informed consent materials and procedures are adequate
5. Provisions for monitoring the study and protecting patient information are acceptable

The FDA allows unapproved medical devices to be used without an IDE in three types of situations: emergency use, treatment use, and feasibility studies. However, in each instance there are specific ethical issues.

77.1 Ethical Issues in Feasibility Studies

Manufacturers seeking more flexibility in conducting investigations in the early developmental stages of a device have submitted a petition to the FDA, requesting that certain limited investigations of significant risk devices be subject to abbreviated IDE requirements. In a feasibility study, or "limited investigation," human research on a new device would take place at a single institution and involve no more than ten human subjects. The sponsor of a limited investigation would be required to submit to the FDA a "Notice of Limited Investigation," which would include a description of the device, a summary of the purpose of the investigation, the protocol, a sample of the informed consent form, and a certification of approval by the responsible IRB. In certain circumstances, the FDA could require additional information, or require the submission of a full IDE application, or suspend the investigation [Bronzino et al., 1990a,b].

Investigations of this kind would be limited to certain circumstances (1) investigations of new uses of existing devices, (2) investigations involving temporary or permanent implants during the early developmental stages, and (3) investigations involving modification of an existing device.

To comprehend adequately the ethical issues posed by clinical use of unapproved medical devices outside the context of an IDE, it is necessary to utilize the distinctions between practice, nonvalidated practice, and research elaborated in the previous pages. How do those definitions apply to feasibility studies?

Clearly, the goal of this sort of study, that is, generalizable knowledge, makes it an issue of research rather than practice. Manufacturers seek to determine the performance of a device with respect to a particular patient population in an effort to gain information about its efficacy and safety. Such information would be important in determining whether further studies (animal or human) need to be conducted, whether the device needs modification before further use, and the like. The main difference between use of an unapproved device in a feasibility study and use under the terms of an IDE is that the former would be subject to significantly less intensive FDA review than the latter. This, in turn, means that the responsibility for ensuring that use of the device is ethically sound would fall primarily to the IRB of the institution conducting the study.

The ethical concerns posed here are best comprehended with a clear understanding of what justifies research. Ultimately, no matter how much basic research and animal experimentation has been conducted on a given device, the risks and benefits it poses for humans cannot be adequately determined until it is actually used on humans.

The benefits of research on humans lie primarily in the knowledge that is yielded and the generalizable information that is provided. This information is crucial to medical science's ability to generate new modes and instrumentalities of medical treatment that are both efficacious and safe. Accordingly, for necessary but insufficient condition for experimentation to be ethically sound, it must be scientifically sound [Capron, 1978, 1986].

Although scientific soundness is a necessary condition of ethically acceptable research on humans, it is not of and by itself sufficient. Indeed, it is widely recognized that the primary ethical concern posed by such investigation is the use of one person by another to gather knowledge or other benefits where these benefits may only partly or not at all accrue to the first person. In other words, the human subjects of such research are at risk of being mere research resources, as having value only for the ends of the research. Research upon human beings runs the risk of failing to respect them as people. The notion that human beings are not mere things but entities whose value is inherent rather than wholly instrumental is one of the most widely held norms of contemporary Western society. That is, human beings are not valuable wholly or solely for the uses to which they can be put. They are valuable simply by being the kinds of entities they are. To treat them as such is to respect them as people.

Respecting individuals as people is generally agreed to entail two requirements in the context of biomedical experimentation. First, since what is most generally taken to make human beings people is their autonomy — their ability to make rational choices for themselves — treating individuals as people means respecting that autonomy. This requirement is met by ensuring that no competent person is subjected to any clinical intervention without first giving voluntary and informed consent. Second, respect for people means that the physician will not subject a human to unnecessary risks and will minimize the risks to patients in required procedures.

Much of the ethical importance of the scrutiny that the FDA imposes upon use of unapproved medical devices in the context of an IDE derives from these two conditions of ethically sound research. The central ethical concern posed by use of medical devices in a feasibility study is that the decreased degree of FDA scrutiny will increase the likelihood that either or both of these conditions will not be met. This possibility may be especially great because many manufacturers of medical devices are, after all, commercial enterprises, companies that are motivated to generate profit and thus to get their devices to market as soon as possible with as little delay and cost as possible. These self-interested motives are likely, at times, to conflict with the requirements of ethically sound research and thus to induce manufacturers to fail (often unwittingly) to meet these requirements. Note that profit is not the only motive that might induce manufacturers to contravene the requirements of ethically sound research on humans. A manufacturer may sincerely believe that his product offers great benefit to many people or to a population of especially needy people and so from this utterly altruistic motive may be prompted to take shortcuts that compromise the quality of the research. Whether the consequences being sought by the research are desired for reasons of self-interest, altruism, or both, the ethical issue is the same. Research subjects may be placed at risk of being treated as mere objects rather than as people.

What about the circumstances under which feasibility studies would take place? Are these not sufficiently different from the "normal" circumstances of research to warrant reduced FDA scrutiny? As noted above, manufacturers seek to be allowed to engage in feasibility studies in order to investigate new uses of existing devices, to investigate temporary or permanent implants during the early developmental stages, and to investigate modifications to an existing device. As also noted above, a feasibility study would take place at only one institution and would involve no more than ten human subjects. Given these circumstances, is the sort of research that is likely to occur in a feasibility study less likely to be scientifically unsound or to fail to respect people in the way that normal research upon humans does in "normal" circumstances?

Such research would be done on a very small subject pool, and the harm of any ethical lapses would likely affect fewer people than if such lapses occurred under more usual research circumstances. Yet, even if the harm done is limited to a failure to respect the ten or fewer subjects in a single feasibility study, the harm would still be ethically wrong. To wrong ten or fewer people is not as bad as to wrong in the same way more than ten people but it is to engage in wrongdoing nonetheless. In either case, individuals are reduced to the status of mere research resources and their dignity as people is not properly respected.

Are ethical lapses more likely to occur in feasibility studies than in studies that take place within the requirements of an IDE? Although nothing in the preceding discussion provides a definitive answer to this question, it is a question to which the FDA should give high priority in deciding whether to allow this type of exception to IDE use of unapproved medical devices. The answer to this question might be quite different when the device at issue is a temporary or permanent implant than when it is an already approved device being put to new uses or modified in some way. Whatever the contemplated use under the feasibility studies mechanism, the FDA would be ethically advised not to allow this kind of exception to IDE use of an unapproved device without a reasonably high level of certainty that research subjects would not be placed in greater jeopardy than in "normal" research circumstances.

77.2   Ethical Issues in Emergency Use

What about the mechanism for avoiding the rigors of an IDE for emergency use?

> The FDA has authorized emergency use where an unapproved device offers the only alternative for saving the life of a dying patient, but an IDE has not yet been approved for the device or its use, or an IDE has been approved but the physician who wishes to use the device is not an investigator under the IDE [Bronzino et al., 1990a,b].

Because the purpose of emergency use of an unapproved device is to attempt to save a dying patient's life under circumstances where no other alternative is at hand, this sort of use constitutes practice rather than research. Its aim is primarily to benefit the patient rather than provision of new and generalizable information. Because this sort of use occurs prior to the completion of clinical investigation of the device, it constitutes a nonvalidated practice. What does this mean?

First, it means that while the aim of the use is to save the life of the patient, the nature and likelihood of the potential benefits and risks engendered by use of the device are far more speculative than in the sort of clinical intervention that constitutes validated practice. In validated practice, thorough investigation, including preclinical studies, animal studies, and studies on human subjects of a device has established its efficacy and safety. The clinician thus has a well-founded basis upon which to judge the benefits and risks such an intervention poses for his patients.

It is precisely this basis that is lacking in the case of a nonvalidated practice. Does this mean that emergency use of an unapproved device should be regarded as immoral? This conclusion would follow only if there were no basis upon which to make an assessment of the risks and benefits of the use of the device. The FDA requires that a physician who engages in emergency use of an unapproved device must "have substantial reason to believe that benefits will exist. This means that there should be a body of preclinical and animal tests allowing a prediction of the benefit to a human patient."

Thus, although the benefits and risks posed by use of the device are highly speculative, they are not entirely speculative. Although the only way to validate a new technology is to engage in research on humans at some point, not all nonvalidated technologies are equal. Some will be largely uninvestigated, and assessment of their risks and benefits will be wholly or almost wholly speculative. Others will at least have the support of preclinical and animal tests. Although this is not a sufficient support for incorporating the use of a device into regular clinical practice, it may however represent sufficient support to justify use in the desperate circumstances at issue in emergency situations. Desperate circumstances can justify desperate actions, but desperate actions are not the same as reckless actions, hence the ethical soundness of the FDA's requirement that emergency use be supported by solid is due to from preclinical and animal tests of the unapproved device.

A second requirement that the FDA imposes on emergency use of unapproved devices is the expectation that physicians "exercise reasonable foresight with respect to potential emergencies and make appropriate arrangements under the IDE procedures. Thus, a physician should not 'create' an emergency in order to circumvent IRB review and avoid requesting the sponsor's authorization of the unapproved use of a device."

From a Kantian point of view, which is concerned with protecting the dignity of people, it is a particularly important requirement to create an emergency in order to avoid FDA regulations which prevent the patient being treated as a mere resource whose value is reducible to a service of the clinician's goals. Hence, the FDA is quite correct to insist that emergencies are circumstances that reasonable foresight would not anticipate.

Also especially important here is the nature of the patient's consent. Individuals facing death are especially vulnerable to exploitation and deserve greater measures for their protection than might otherwise be necessary. One such measure would be to ensure that the patient, or his legitimate proxy, knows the highly speculative nature of the intervention being offered. That is, to ensure that it is clearly understood that the clinician's estimation of the intervention's risks and benefits is far less solidly grounded than in the case of validated practices. The patient's consent must be based upon an awareness that the particular device has not undergone complete and rigorous testing on humans and that estimations of its potential are based wholly upon preclinical and animal studies. Above all, the patient must not be led to believe that there is complete understanding of the risks and benefits of the intervention. Another important point here is to ensure that the patient is aware that the options he is facing are not simply life or death but may include life of a severely impaired quality, and therefore that even if his life is saved, it may be a life of significant impairment. Although desperate circumstance may legitimize desperate actions, the decision to take such actions must rest upon the informed and voluntary consent of the patient, in particular when he/she is an especially vulnerable patient.

It is important here for a clinician involved in emergency use of an unapproved device to recognize that these activities constitute a form of nonvalidated practice and not research. Hence, the primary obligation is to the well-being of the patient. The patient enters into the relationship with the clinician with the same trust that accompanies any normal clinical situation. To treat this sort of intervention as if it were an instance of research and hence justified by its benefits to science and society would be to abuse this trust.

77.3   Ethical Issues in Treatment Use

The FDA has adopted regulations authorizing the use of investigational new drugs in certain circumstances — where a patient has not responded to approved therapies. This "treatment use" of unapproved new drugs is not limited to life-threatening emergency situations, but rather is also available to treat "serious" diseases or conditions.

The FDA has not approved treatment use of unapproved medical devices, but it is possible that a manufacturer could obtain such approval by establishing a specific protocol for this kind of use within the context of an IDE.

The criteria for treatment use of unapproved medical devices would be similar to criteria for treatment use of investigational drugs: (1) the device is intended to treat a serious or life-threatening disease or condition, (2) there is no comparable or satisfactory alternative product available to treat that condition, (3) the device is under an IDE, or has received an IDE exemption, or all clinical trials have been completed and the device is awaiting approval, and (4) the sponsor is actively pursuing marketing approval of the investigational device. The treatment use protocol would be submitted as part of the IDE, and would describe the intended use of the device, the rationale for use of the device, the available alternatives and why the investigational product is preferred, the criteria for patient selection, the measures to monitor the use of the device and to minimize risk, and technical information that is relevant to the safety and effectiveness of the device for the intended treatment purpose.

Were the FDA to approve treatment use of unapproved medical devices, what ethical issues would be posed? First, because such use is premised on the failure of validated interventions to improve the patient's condition adequately, it is a form of practice rather than research. Second, since the device involved in an instance of treatment use is unapproved, such use would constitute nonvalidated practice. As such, like emergency use, it should be subject to the FDA's requirement that prior preclinical tests and animal studies have been conducted that provide substantial reason to believe that it will result in the benefit of the patient. As with emergency use, although this does not prevent assessment of the intervention's benefits and risks from being highly speculative, it does prevent assessment from being totally speculative. Here too, although desperate circumstances can justify desperate action, they do not justify reckless action. Unlike emergency use, the circumstances of treatment use involve serious impairment of health rather than the threat of premature death. Hence, an issue that must be considered is how serious such impairment must be to justify resorting to an intervention whose risks and benefits have not been solidly established.

In cases of emergency use, the FDA requires that physicians not use this exception to an IDE to avoid requirements that would otherwise be in place. This particular requirement would be obviated in instances of treatment use by the requirement that a protocol for such use be previously addressed within an IDE.

As with emergency use of unapproved devices, the patients involved in treatment use would be particularly vulnerable. Although they are not dying, they are facing serious medical conditions and are thereby likely to be less able to avoid exploitation than patients under less desperate circumstances. Consequently, it is especially important that patients be informed of the speculative nature of the intervention and of the possibility that treatment may result in little or no benefit to them.

77.4   The Safe Medical Devices Act

On November 28, 1991, the Safe Medical Devices Act of 1990 (Public Law 101-629) went into effect. This regulation requires a wide range of health-care institutions, including hospitals, ambulatory-surgical facilities, nursing homes, and outpatient treatment facilities, to report information that "reasonably suggests" the likelihood that the death, serious injury, or serious illness of a patient at that facility has been caused or contributed to by a medical device. When a death is device-related, a report must be made directly to the FDA *and* to the manufacturer of the device. When a serious illness or injury is device-related, a report must be made to the manufacturer *or* to the FDA in cases where the manufacturer is not known. In addition, summaries of previously submitted reports must be submitted to the FDA on a semiannual basis. Prior to this regulation, such reporting was voluntary. This new regulation was designed to enhance the FDA's ability to quickly learn about problems related to medical devices. It also supplements the medical device reporting (MDR) regulations promulgated in 1984. MDR regulations require that reports of device-related deaths and serious injuries be submitted to the FDA by manufacturers and importers. The new law extends this requirement to users of medical devices along with manufacturers and importers. This act represents a significant step forward in protecting patients exposed to medical devices.

References

Bronzino, J.D., Flannery, E.J. and Wade, M.L. "Legal and ethical issues in the regulation and development of engineering achievements in medical technology,"*IEEE Engineering in Medicine and Biology*, Part I, 1990a.

Bronzino, J.D. Flannery, E.J. and Wade, M.L. "Legal and ethical issues in the regulation and development of engineering achievements in medical technology," *IEEE Engineering in Medicine and Biology*, Part II, 1990b.

Bronzino, J.D. Chapter 10 "Medical and ethical issues in clinical engineering practice." *Management of Medical Technology*. Butterworth. 1992.

Bronzino, J.D. Chapter 20 "Moral and ethical issues associated with medical technology" *Introduction to Biomedical Engineering*. Academic Press. 1999.

Bronzino, JD. Chapter 192. "Regulation of medical device innovation." *The Biomedical Engineering Handbook*. CRC Press, Boca Raton, FL, 1995; 2000.

Capron, A. "Human experimentation: basic issues." *The Encyclopedia of bioethics*, vol. II. The Free Press, Glencoe, II. 1978.

Capron, A. "Human experimentation." (J.P. Childress, et al., Eds.) University Publications of America, 1986.

Further Information

Dubler, N.N. and Nimmons, D. *Ethics on Call*. Harmony Books, New York, 1992.

Jonsen, A.R. *The New Medicine and the Old Ethics*. Harvard University Press, Cambridge, MA, 1990.

Index